Dr. miriam stoppard's

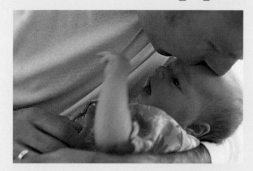

Family Health Guide

Dr. miriam stoppard's

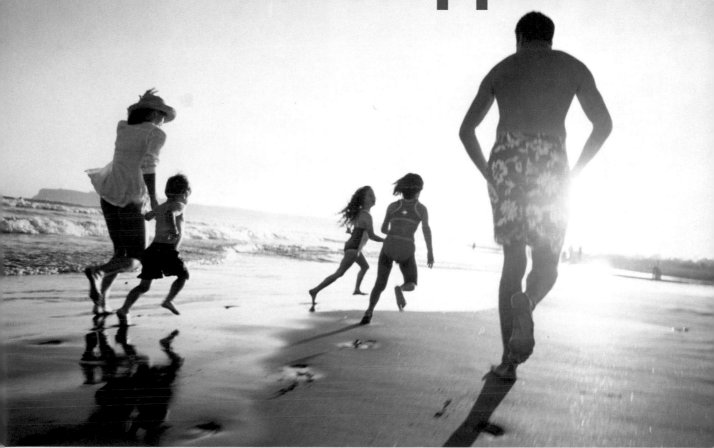

Family Health Guide

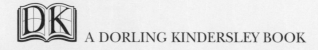

A DORLING KINDERSLEY BOOK

For Eden, Violet, Brodie and Zac

LONDON, NEW YORK, MUNICH, MELBOURNE, DELHI

Senior Managing Art Editor: Lynne Brown
Senior Editor: Julia North
Senior Art Editor: Rosamund Saunders
Art Editor – Life Stages section: Kathryn Gammon
DTP Designer: Karen Constanti
Editors: Jinny Johnson, Kathy Fahey
Picture Research: Samantha Nunn
Picture Library: Charlotte Oster, Scott Stickland
Production: Heather Hughes

Special Photography: Trish Gant
Photographic Coordination: Sally Smallwood
Illustrations: Richard Tibbitts

This book is not intended to be a substitute for medical diagnosis and you are advised to consult your doctor for specific information concerning your health.

All photography in this book uses models.

First published in Great Britain in 2002

This edition published 2006
By Dorling Kindersley Limited
A Penguin company
80 Strand
London
WC2R 0RL

ISBN 13: 978-1-40532-012-5
ISBN 10: 1-40532-012-5

Reproduced by GRB
Jacket reproduced by Colourscan
Printed and bound in China by Hung Hing

See our complete catalogue at
www.dk.com

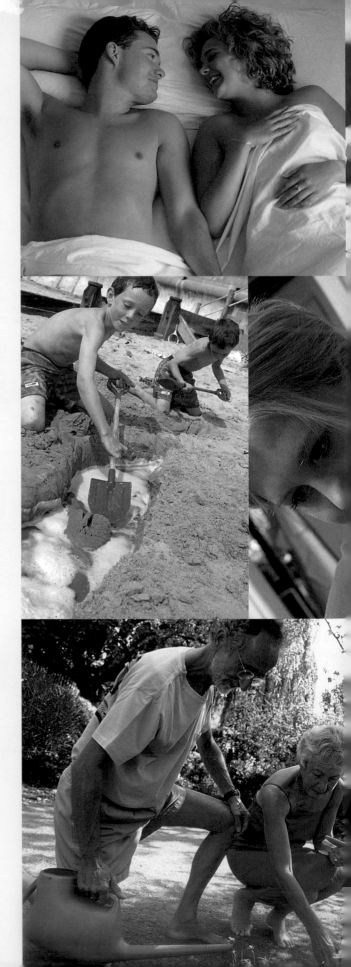

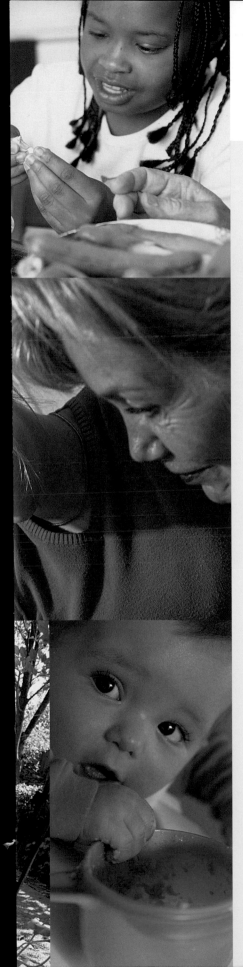

Contents

How to use this book

The Family Health Guide is about how you can stay well as much as it is about what to do if you are ill. It has been planned so that you can find topics that interest you quickly and easily, with boxed text to highlight areas of special interest, such as tests and treatments, information on what you can do to help yourself and important points to note. The book is also easy to browse with related topics listed in section openers, overview articles at the beginning of each section and cross-references between articles.

Section Opener

Throughout the book, the main topics that are covered in each section are listed in section openers, making it easy to find a subject that interests you and enabling you to see at a glance other topics that are related to it.

Sections include
• Golden Rules
• Life Stages
• Symptom Guides
• Directory
• Reference
• Useful Addresses
• Index

SECTION OPENER

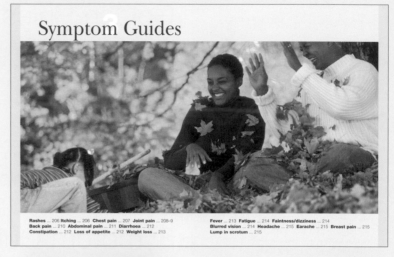

Symptom Guides

Rashes ... 206 Itching ... 206 Chest pain ... 207 Joint pain ... 208-9   Fever ... 213 Fatigue ... 214 Faintness/dizziness ... 214
Back pain ... 210 Abdominal pain ... 211 Diarrhoea ... 212   Blurred vision ... 214 Headache ... 215 Earache ... 215 Breast pain ... 215
Constipation ... 212 Loss of appetite ... 212 Weight loss ... 213   Lump in scrotum ... 215

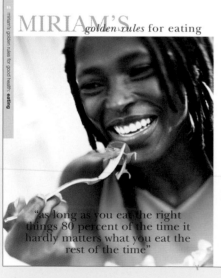

MIRIAM'S *golden rules* for eating

"as long as you eat the right things 80 percent of the time it hardly matters what you eat the rest of the time"

◄ **Golden Rules** Guidelines to a healthy lifstyle are easy to understand and easy to follow.

"drink plenty of fluids"

"eat whole fruit as well as drinking fruit juices"

▲ **Explanation** Supporting information explains the whys and hows of the rules.

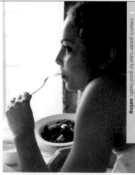

Golden Rules

The Golden Rules section of the book gives Dr Stoppard's concise, essential guidelines for maintaining a lifetime of good health. Each rule is supported by facts that explain why it is important and precise instructions on what you need to do to stay on track.

Topics include:
• Eating • Exercise • Safe drinking limits • Giving up smoking • Safe sex • Restful sleep • Avoiding stress

Life Stages

The Life Stages section offers advice and information on issues affecting health and wellbeing at each stage of life.

Stages covered
- 0–1 years • 1–4 years • 4–11 years
- 11–18 years • 18–40 years • 40–60 years • 60+ years

MINI CONTENTS

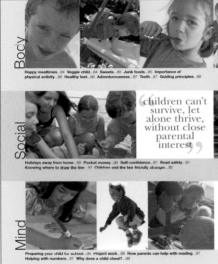

Body

Happy mealtimes...84 Veggie child...84 Sweets...85 Junk foods...85 Importance of physical activity...86 Healthy feet...86 Adventurousness...87 Teeth...87 Guiding principles...88

> *children can't survive, let alone thrive, without close parental interest*

Social

Holidays away from home...90 Pocket money...90 Self-confidence...91 Road safety...91
Knowing where to draw the line...92 Children and the less friendly stranger...92

Being considerate...93 Changing patterns of friendship...93 Bullying...94 Problem behaviour...94
A healthy attitude to nudity...95 Masturbation is normal...95

> *tell your children the facts of life as soon as they begin to ask*

Mind

Preparing your child for school...96 Project work...96 How parents can help with reading...97
Helping with numbers...97 Why does a child cheat?...98

Why does a child lie?...98 Hyperactivity...99 Why does a child steal?...99 Sex play is normal...100
Answering questions about sex...101 Television?...101

CHAPTER OPENER

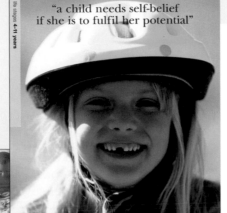

> "a child needs self-belief if she is to fulfil her potential"

life stages: 4 to 11 years

Between the ages of 4 and 11 your energetic, loving, mischievous pre-schooler is going to grow and develop into a reflective, kind, industrious, cooperative adolescent with whom you can have a serious conversation, on whom you can rely and whose company everyone enjoys. That's a tough assignment for any 4-year-old and there are many complex skills to acquire along the way, not the least of which are self-control and self-discipline.

Most important, milestones can only be achieved if parents show loving care to their children. Children can't survive let alone thrive without close parental interest. They can get by of course and most do, even if parental care isn't forthcoming.

Achieving self-belief

But there are some milestones that are exceedingly difficult for a child to master alone and they can go astray without feedback and guidance. Let me give you just one example of a milestone that involves an important step in personal development – achieving self-belief.

Call it self-confidence, call it self-assurance, but without it a child will not only fail to fulfil her potential, she could get into all kinds of trouble because she won't know how to control her emotions or how to re-channel her frustrations and anger to gainful purpose.

You may think, well, she'll grow into a shy child, unsure of herself. That would be bad enough, but you're wrong, it's worse than that.
- She grows into a child who becomes a loner without friends, which is heartbreaking for any parent to see.
- She may seek attention and affection to bolster her waning ego with all kinds of inappropriate behaviour, sometimes being labelled as **hyperactive**.
- And then, if no one helps her to build belief in herself, she resorts to lying, stealing, bullying, even to drinking and taking drugs to feel good about herself.

You can see that without achieving **self-belief**, there are problems ahead. So important is this

milestone, and several other crucial milestones, that I call them **islands of development**. If a child doesn't reach the haven of these islands, there can be disastrous fallout later.

Think of your child as bobbing along on a river of development trying to negotiate the equivalent of white water, the flow sometimes fast as she goes through a spurt of skill acquisition, or slower and more placid as she consolidates her achievements.

These islands make the river navigable. They're places where your child can rest up, so to speak, take stock and move on to the next milestone – with lots of encouragement and praise from you of course.

The islands are also an insurance policy. If you can help your child to reach one she'll tackle the next stretch of white water with determination, courage and good sense. And, having enjoyed the security of reaching one of these islands, your child can safely be given responsibilities of increasing gravitas both for herself and others.

In the pages that follow, I offer guidelines where appropriate, advice where I feel there may be a need and strategies for dealing with difficult situations.

The right age to...

- A child is ready to learn to tie her own shoelaces at about 4 years old.
- A child may be able to cope with sleeping like a grown-up bed at about 5 years old.
- A 6-year-old is probably ready to receive pocket money and decide how to spend it.
- At 7 a child can learn to cross the street alone.
- A child of 8 can sleep over at a friend's house.
- A 9-year-old is ready to learn about puberty.
- A child of 10 may enjoy the responsibility of looking after a pet.
- An 11-year-old can be left at home alone for short periods.

▲ **Life Stages** Dr Stoppard outlines and gives her views on the most significant health-related issues that arise at each stage of life.

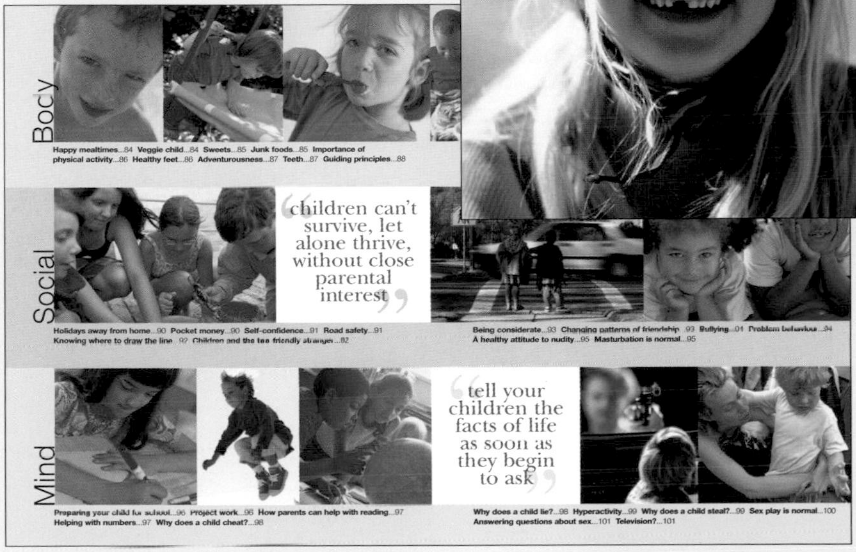

◀ **Contents** Picture timelines help you to pick out the subjects that interest you most.

BODY

SOCIAL

MIND

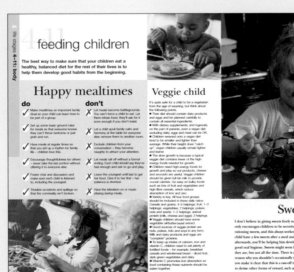

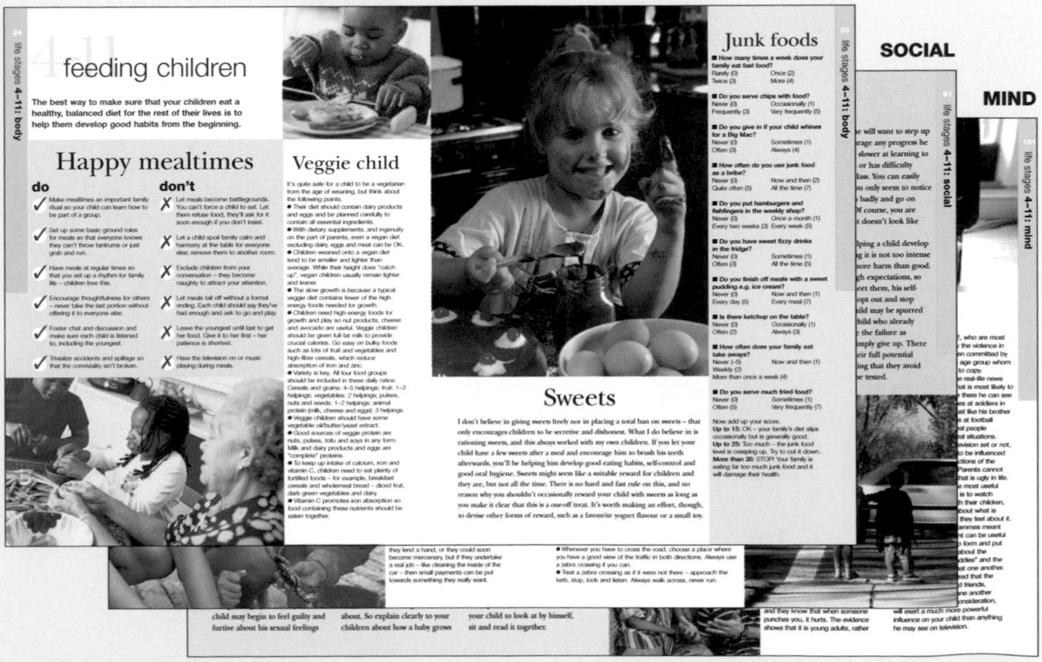

4–11 feeding children

The best way to make sure that your children eat a healthy, balanced diet for the rest of their lives is to help them develop good habits from the beginning.

Happy mealtimes

do	don't
✓ Make mealtimes an important family ritual so your child can learn how to be part of a group.	✗ Let meals become battlegrounds. You can't force a child to eat. Let them refuse food, they'll ask for it soon enough if you don't insist.
✓ Set up some basic ground rules for meals so that everyone knows they can't throw tantrums or just grab and run.	✗ Let a child spoil family calm and harmony at the table for everyone else; remove them to another room.
✓ Have meals at regular times so that you set up a rhythm for family life – children love this.	✗ Exclude children from your conversation – they become naughty to attract your attention.
✓ Encourage thoughtfulness for others – never take the last portion without offering it to everyone else.	✗ Let meals tail off without a formal ending. Each child should say they've had enough and ask to go and play.
✓ Foster chat and discussion and make sure each child is listened to, including the youngest.	✗ Leave the youngest until last to get her food. Give it to her first – her patience is shortest.
✓ Treat accidents and spillage so that the conviviality isn't broken.	✗ Have the television on or music playing during meals.

Veggie child

It's quite safe for a child to be a vegetarian from the age of weaning, but think about the following points.
- Their diet should contain dairy products and eggs and be planned carefully to contain all essential ingredients.
- With dietary supplements, and ingenuity on the part of parents, even a vegan diet excluding dairy, eggs and meat can be OK.
- Children weaned onto a vegan diet tend to be smaller and lighter than average. While their height does "catch up", vegan children usually remain lighter and leaner.
- The slow growth is because a typical veggie diet contains lower of the high-energy foods needed for growth.
- Children need high-energy foods for growth and play so nut products, cheese and avocado are useful. Veggie children should be given full fat milk to provide crucial calories. Go easy on bulky foods such as lots of fruit and vegetables and high-fibre cereals, which reduce absorption of iron and zinc.
- Variety is key. All four food groups should be included in these daily ratios. Cereals and grains: 4–5 helpings; fruit: 1–3 helpings; vegetables: 2 helpings; pulses, nuts and seeds: 1–2 helpings; animal protein (milk, cheese and eggs): 3 helpings. Veggie children should have some vegetable oil/butter/yeast extract.
- Good sources of veggie protein are nuts, pulses, tofu and soya in any form. Milk and dairy products and eggs are "complete" proteins.
- To keep up intake of calcium, iron and vitamin C, children need to eat plenty of fortified foods – for example, breakfast cereals and wholemeal bread – diced fruit, dark green vegetables and dairy.
- Vitamin C promotes iron absorption so food containing these nutrients should be eaten together.

Sweets

I don't believe in giving sweets freely nor in placing a total ban on them – that only encourages children to be secretive and dishonest. What I do believe in is rationing sweets, and this always worked with my own children. If you let your child have a few sweets after a meal and encourage him to brush his teeth afterwards, you'll be helping him develop good eating habits, self-control and good oral hygiene. Sweets might seem like a suitable reward for children and they are, but not all the time. There is no hard and fast rule on this, and no reason why you shouldn't occasionally reward your child with sweets as long as you make it clear that this is a one-off treat. It's worth making an effort, though, to devise other forms of reward, such as a favourite yogurt flavour or a small toy.

Junk foods

- How many times a week does your child eat fast food?
  Rarely (1)   Once (2)
  Twice (3)   More (4)
- Do you serve chips with food?
  Never (0)   Occasionally (1)
  Frequently (3)   Very frequently (5)
- Do you give in if your child whines for a Big Mac?
  Never (0)   Sometimes (1)
  Often (3)   Always (4)
- How often do you use junk food as a bribe?
  Never (0)   And all the time (7)
  Quite often (5)
- Do you put hamburgers and fishfingers in the weekly shop?
  Never (0)   Once a month (1)
  Every two weeks (3) Every week (5)
- Do you have sweet fizzy drinks in fridge?
  Never (0)   Sometimes (1)
  Often (3)   All the time (5)
- Do you finish off meals with a sweet pudding e.g. ice cream?
  Never (0)   Now and then (1)
  Every day (5)   Every meal (7)
- Is there ketchup on the table?
  Never (0)   Occasionally (1)
  Often (2)   Always (3)
- How often does your family eat take aways?
  Never (-5)   Now and then (5)
  Weekly (2)
  More than once a week (4)
- Do you serve much fried food?
  Never (2)   Sometimes (7)
  Often (3)   Very frequently (7)

Now add up your score.
Up to 15: OK – your family's diet aligns occasionally but in generally good.
Up to 25: Too much – the junk food level is creeping up. Try to cut it down.
More than 35: STOP! Your family is eating far too much junk food and it will damage their health.

Social

He will want to step up your age progress he is slower at learning to or has difficulty than. You can easily only seem to notice badly and go on of course, you are doesn't look like.

ping a child develop it is not too intense more harm than good. gh expectations, so ...en them, this self-...opt out and stop ...ild may be spurred ...child who already ...the failure as ...simply give up. There ...eir full potential ...ng that they avoid ...e tested.

Mind

...who are most ...the evidence in ...situations. ...there he can see ...at football ...people ...evision set or not, ...be influenced ...that is ugly in life. ...e most useful ...e to watch ...about the children, ...about what is ...can be useful ...lem and put ...about the ...ckles" and the ...st one another. ...that the ...e another ...consideration, ...a much more powerful ...influence on your child than anything ...he may see on television.

▶ **Category** For each life stage Dr Stoppard discusses health implications related to mind, body and social development. Life stages are colour-coded so that you can find the one that interests you at a glance.

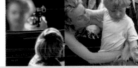

Symptom Guides

These guides help you make sense of the most common symptoms you and your family are likely to experience and direct you to the right information.

Charts include:
• Fatigue • Faintness • Fever
• Headache • Weight loss • Blurred vision • Earache • Chest pain
• Back pain • Joint pain • Abdominal pain • Loss of appetite • Diarrhoea
• Constipation • Rash • Itching
• Breast pain • Lump in scrotum

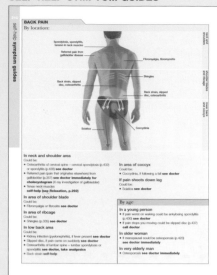

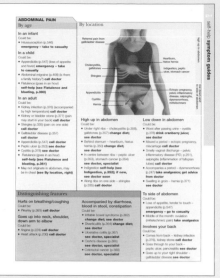

SELF-HELP SYMPTOM GUIDES

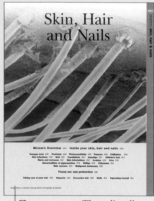

Chapter openers These list all conditions covered.

Directory

With a strong emphasis on prevention and cure, the Directory covers over 280 of the most common medical conditions. These are grouped by body system and are explained in friendly, non-specialist language.

Chapters include:
• Heart, Blood & Circulation • Sexuality & Fertility • Threats to Mental

Wellbeing • Allergies & the Immune System • Infections • Digestion • Kidneys & Bladder • Chest & Air Passages • Brain & Nervous System • Bones, Joints & Muscles • Skin, Hair & Nails • Eyes & Vision • Ears, Nose & Throat • Teeth & Gums • Hormones

Plus:
A special section on children's conditions

▶ **Essay & Anatomy**
These pages give Dr Stoppard's personal view of each medical area, with a guide to the basic anatomy of the body system dealt with in the chapter.

▶ **Directory**
Each entry gives an explanation of the condition, how and why it occurs, how a doctor might treat it and what you can do to help yourself.

▶ **Focus On**
Focus On pages give Dr Stoppard's personal view of a topic of special concern, helping you to understand it in greater depth.

ESSAY

ANATOMY

DIRECTORY

FOCUS ON

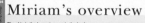

Special section on children's conditions

▶ **Children's conditions**
This section gives advice on what to do when your child is ill and includes over 50 common medical conditions and developmental problems that occur in childhood.

▶ **Development**
Key aspects of behaviour and development that may cause concern include dyslexia and dyspraxia, developmental delay and attention deficit hyperactivity disorder.

CHILDREN'S CONDITIONS

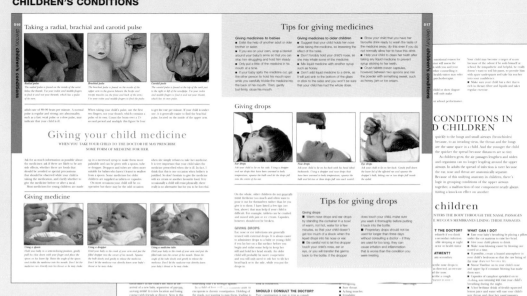

Reference

This section includes First Aid for common emergencies, how to keep healthy when travelling abroad and a list of useful addresses and websites relating to topics covered in the book.

Features

• First Aid • Travel health • Useful addresses, telephone numbers and websites • Index • Acknowledgments

▶ **Step-by-step** The First Aid section gives step-by-step instructions to help you deal with minor and more serious medical emergencies.

FIRST AID

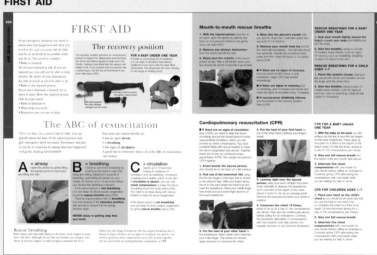

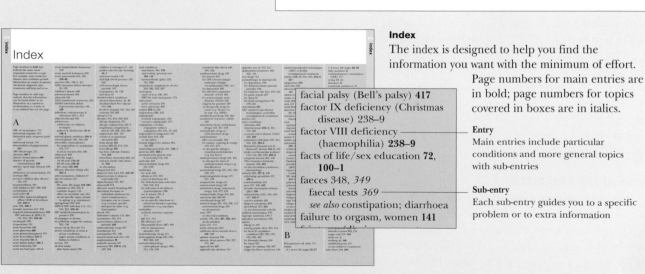

Index

The index is designed to help you find the information you want with the minimum of effort.

Page numbers for main entries are in bold; page numbers for topics covered in boxes are in italics.

Entry
Main entries include particular conditions and more general topics with sub-entries

Sub-entry
Each sub-entry guides you to a specific problem or to extra information

MIRIAM'S introduction

Why another health book you may ask. There are many answers, the first being that my aim is to inform parents and through them promote healthy families. So while you'll find many topics and issues that affect you yourself, there are many others that are important to you because they affect your children and your parents.

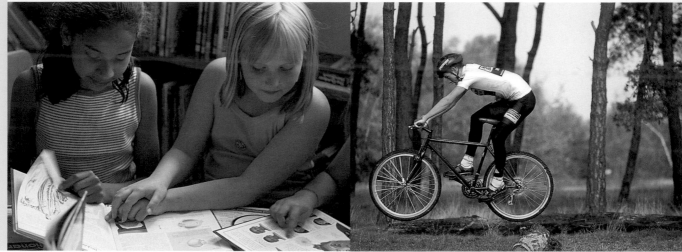

When I wrote this book I had you in mind: the mum or dad who has growing children at one end of the scale and ageing parents at the other. You are the person who has the most need of good, accurate, usable information that will clarify, reassure and inform you about the health and wellbeing of all your family on a day-to-day basis.

Towards this end I've included a section in the book called Life Stages, which takes a look at the major issues that arise from birth to death. It's aimed at giving you warning of the sorts of questions you may face as you go through each decade. It offers you the opportunity to look back, say from your 40s or 50s, at your children as they grow through their teenage years and beyond, and on to what your parents may be experiencing now and what you yourself will in the future.

LOOK AFTER YOURSELF

As the most pivotal person in your family you have a responsibility to yourself and to them to stay fit and healthy. When I was disinclined to look after my own health, my mother would remind me that the family would fall apart if I became ill. "Who will look

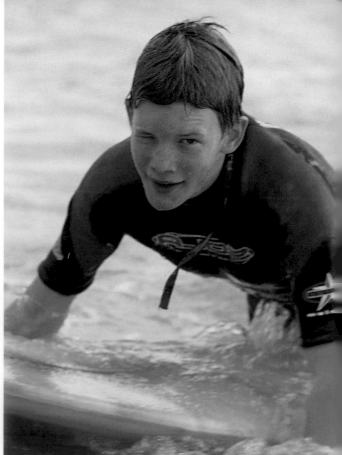

"your lifestyle can easily give you ten more years of life"

"improve the health and wellbeing of the whole family"

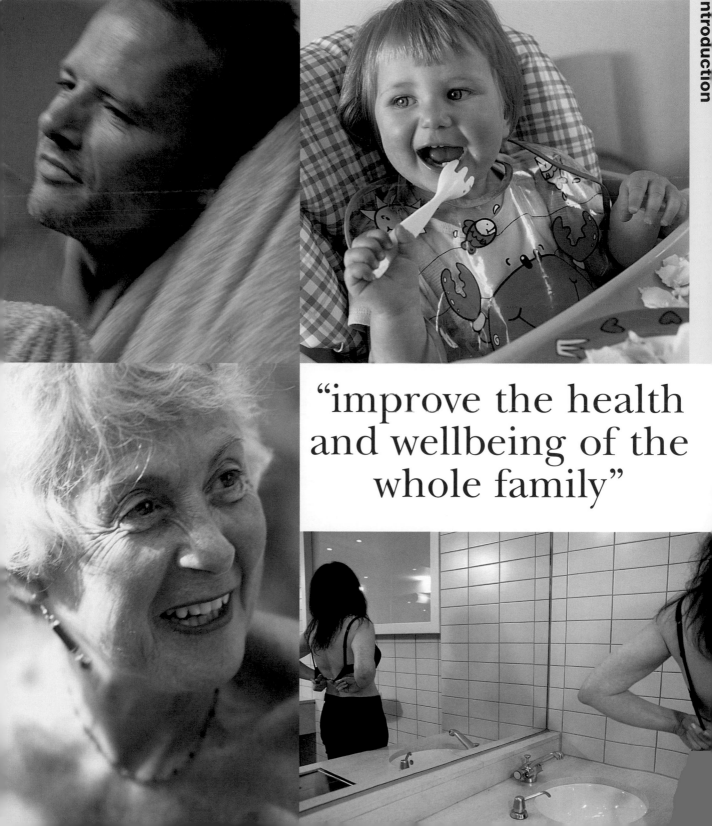

"those tough workouts in the gym aren't life expanding at all"

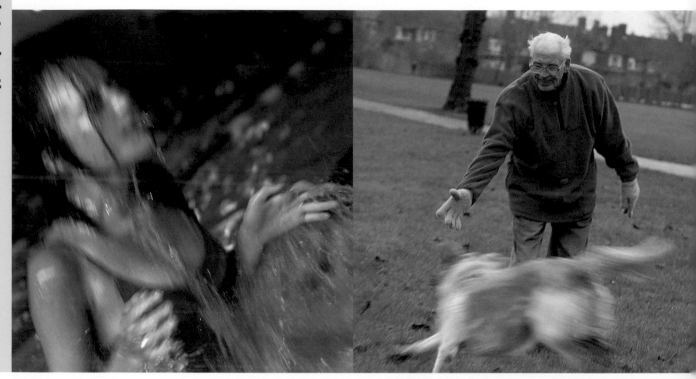

after your four little boys?" she'd ask, and that was usually a good enough corrective to make me pay attention to what I was eating and to take exercise.

"healthy eating needn't be a chore"

SMALL CHANGES – HUGE DIFFERENCES

These days healthy eating needn't be a chore. Quite the opposite in fact. There are a few very simple tips (what I've called Golden Rules) about eating which, if followed even approximately, will improve the health and wellbeing of the whole family. Small changes in eating make huge differences, especially as a list of what can truly be called power foods has emerged in the last few years and no person should go without them. No one would claim that simply by

eating a plentiful supply of these power foods that we can live longer. Food alone won't do that, but evidence is emerging that your lifestyle can easily give you ten more years of life – or take ten away.

CLUES TO A LONG LIFE

Long-term studies on the Okinawan people, the longest-living race on the planet, give us plenty of clues about how to increase our lifespan and defy the biological markers of age. The Okinawans, who live on an island off the coast of Japan, are, decade for decade, biologically younger than we are in the West. Many of the beneficial aspects of Okinawan life are the direct opposite of what we pursue here.

They don't smoke, for instance, and they drink very little. They don't eat just five portions of fruit and vegetables as we're exhorted to do, but anything from 9 to 19. They are the opposite of sedentary – our most life-shortening habit is sitting down – and they potter all day long, walking, gardening, dancing and engaging in gentle martial arts.

In fact we now know that those tough workouts in the gym aren't life expanding at all. Keeping moving, even gently, is. If I had to recommend just one life change to instantly improve your health and life expectancy it would be to take more exercise in the way the Okinawans do. Nothing onerous, three or four sessions a week of gentle cycling or brisk walking will do. The pay-offs are quite surprising.

First, you won't be fat. Second, you won't be in danger of developing type II diabetes and you'll lower your chances of a heart attack or stroke. Osteoporosis and fractures will probably pass you by. If, in addition, you follow my Golden Rules for your lifestyle, you could find you've avoided many cancers.

KEEP INFORMED

Despite our best efforts we are prey to illness and you'll find most of the common ones in the ready-reference disease directory. I hope you'll dip in and out of it to make sure you're well enough informed to know a potentially serious symptom when it arises, what to do in a household emergency, and how to be an equal negotiator with your doctors and carers.

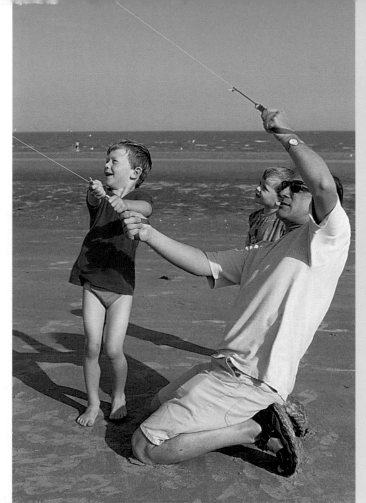

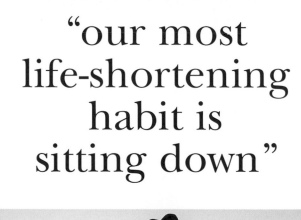

"our most life-shortening habit is sitting down"

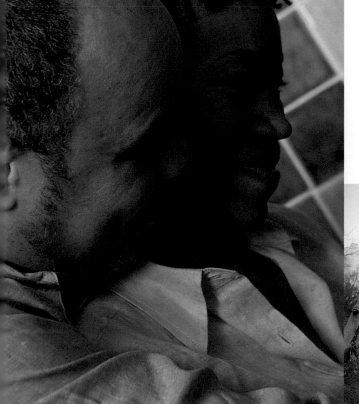

Golden Rules

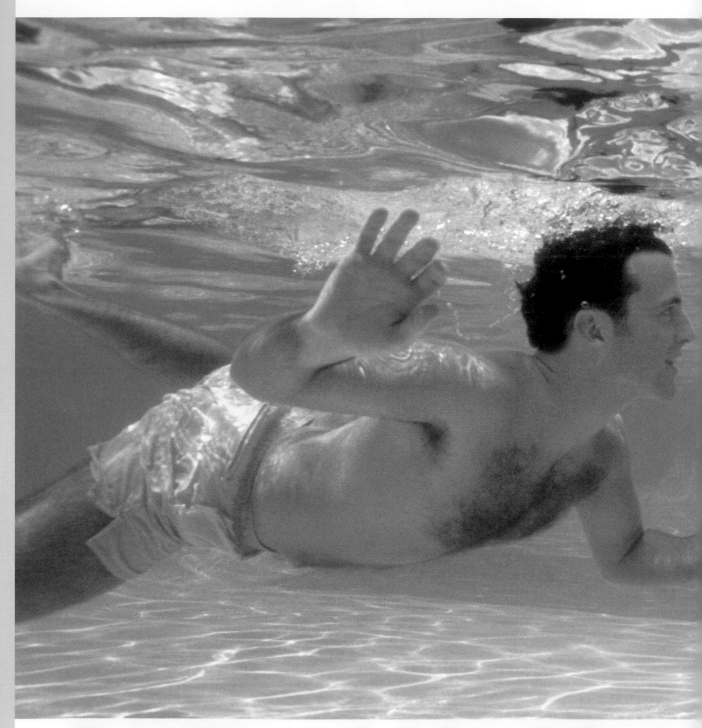

for Good Health

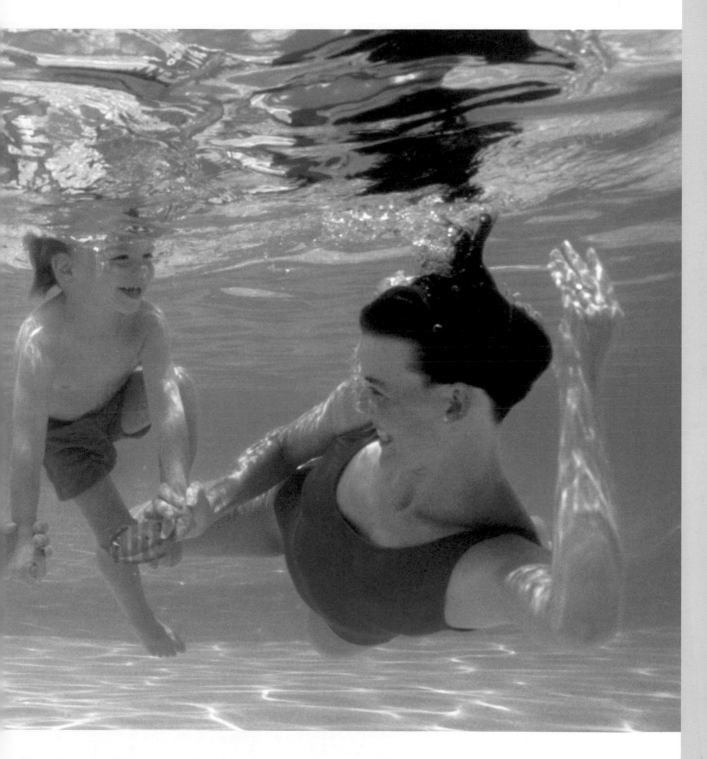

MIRIAM'S *golden rules* for eating

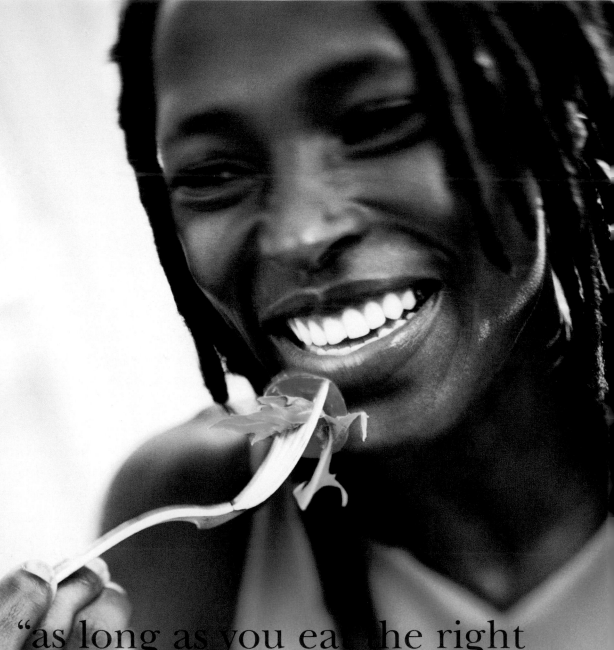

"as long as you eat the right things 80 percent of the time it hardly matters what you eat the rest of the time"

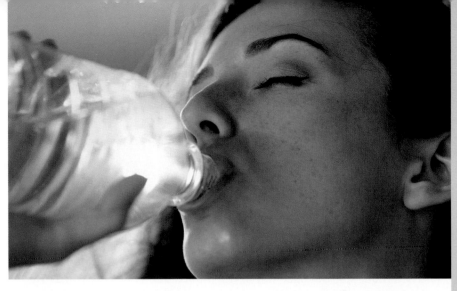

"drink plenty of fluids"

✻ Our bodies don't need balanced meals every time we eat, but **eating a variety of different foods each day promotes good health**. Don't get too worried about picky children who go through food fads – their diet usually balances out over a week.

✻ As long as you **eat the right things 80 percent of the time** it hardly matters what you eat the rest of the time.

✻ **Eat an orange fruit or vegetable every day** for the carotenoids, which help to protect against cancer.

• **Drink at least 6–8 large glasses of fluid a day** – any liquid will do. Vary water with fruit juice and low-fat milk. A few cups of tea can count too.

✻ No healthy person who **eats a balanced diet** needs vitamin supplements.

✻ For children of two and up, start to moderate fatty foods. Use semi-skimmed milk, **cut the fat off meat**, don't fry – grill.

✻ Always eat some breakfast. Research shows that **breakfast eaters tend to be slimmer** and have healthier diets. Don't eat a heavy meal too late in the evening – it will stop you sleeping.

✻ **Small changes in eating habits reap great rewards**, so there's no need to go overboard and make dietary changes you can't stick to. **Make one or two small adjustments a week** – change from white to wholemeal bread, full cream to semi-skimmed milk, butter to an olive-oil spread.

✻ We really do all need at least **five helpings of fruit and vegetables a day** – fresh, frozen, canned, dried or juiced. There's no alternative.

✻ **Eat oily fish at least once a week**. It is very good for you because it helps to maintain a healthy heart. Have a little olive oil on your salad too.

✻ Drink tea for the flavonoids, which **seem to help reduce the risk of heart disease** and stroke and may even slow ageing.

✻ Around **half of our calories should come from unrefined carbohydrates** – that is, wholewheat bread, oats in any form, rice in any form, pasta, wholegrain cereals, potatoes (in jackets especially good), peas, beans and fruit.

✻ Treat protein like a condiment – a little goes a long way. **Eat some lean red meat a few times a week.** Remember that red meat is an excellent source of protein, easily absorbed iron and zinc, and B vitamins.

✻ Start reading labels for food values, especially fat and sugar. **Sugar adds variety, but is a non-essential food** – don't give your children sugar-coated cereals as this may encourage a sweet tooth for life.

✻ Stop adding salt to food and keep your blood pressure at a healthy level. **The healthy limit for salt is 6g (⅕oz) per day** (equivalent to 2.4g (⅒oz) sodium – salt is usually listed as "sodium" on food labels). But your doctor may advise you to reduce it even further.

✻ Read labels for salt content, too, and **never give foods with a high salt content to babies** and young children; their kidneys can't handle it.

"eating a healthy diet helps you control your weight"

How to eat healthily

Changing from an unhealthy to a healthy diet is not difficult; it simply involves making some different choices and emphasizing certain foods. It does require a little effort and determination, but once you start following the golden rules, you'll really enjoy it, feel marvellous and be encouraged to continue.

Most of the foods you should eat are easily available and, contrary to what you might have thought, you can eat more of some of them. You will soon find that a healthy diet can be delicious and satisfying. It doesn't involve starvation pangs, which would

only lead to excessive snacking and over-eating later. In fact, you'll find that your desire to snack will gradually decrease and that eating a healthy diet helps you to control your weight without effort.

There are very few foods we need to eat every day. I'd narrow them down to:

✽ at least two fruits, more if possible; one should be orange in colour
✽ at least two veg, more if possible
✽ a large bowl of green leaves.

Otherwise, eat a variety of foods each day from the other three main food groups: meat, fish or pulses; breads,

potatoes and cereals; and milk and dairy foods. Most of us eat enough meat and dairy products but need to increase the amount of fruit and vegetables as well as cereals and grains.

Fruit and vegetables

Fresh fruits and vegetables provide lots of vitamins, minerals and fibre. Eat more of them and a greater variety – aim for at least five portions each day.

Eat more salads of all kinds: try beans, corn, potato, celery, apple, carrot, bean sprouts, beetroot, rice, cress and chickpeas as delicious alternatives to the familiar lettuce, cucumber and tomato.

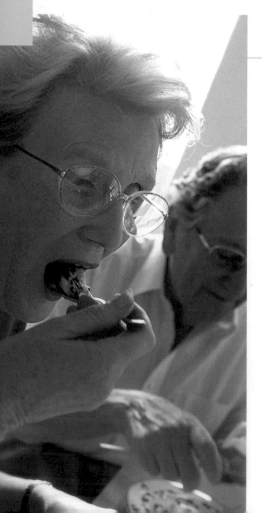

Superfoods

avocados • Contain vitamins B1, B6 and E, potassium, magnesium and healthy fatty acids that help regulate cholesterol levels. Make a great first food for babies. Beware, though, they are high in calories.

broccoli • Contains vitamins C, A and E, calcium and folic acid.

tomatoes • Good source of vitamin C and flavonoids. Contain the antioxidant lycopene, which helps protect against prostate cancer and heart disease.

sweetcorn • Contains fibre, potassium and lutein, which may help protect against cataracts and macular degeneration (deterioration in vision).

grapefruit • One half contains half your daily requirement of vitamin C. Eat the pith – the soluble fibre lowers cholesterol and contains folic acid and bioflavonoids to keep cancer at bay.

red onions • Contain folic acid, B6 and potassium as well as flavonoids to help reduce risk of heart disease. May help raise HDL ("good" cholesterol).

beetroot • Fresh, not pickled, beetroot contains folic acid.

strawberries • Rich in vitamin C and ellagic acid, a compound with anti-cancer effects.

blackcurrants • Very rich in vitamin C, vitamin K and body-protecting flavonoids.

carrots • Contain carotenoids, which protect against cancer, as do all orange foods. Eat at least one every day.

prunes • Contain iron, fibre, potassium, vitamin A.

cranberries • Juice stops bacteria clinging to the lining of the bladder. Ace for women who are cystitis-prone.

Use fresh fruits as your snack food and try a greater variety – have you tasted mango, papaya, passion fruit, ugli fruit or kiwi fruit? Eat whole fruits as well as drinking fruit juices, and avoid squashes and cordials, many of which contain only fruit flavours.

Choose a variety of yellow and orange vegetables, beans and pulses, and green leafy vegetables each week. Don't add salt to your vegetables, and steam or reduce the boiling time for green vegetables.

Eat fresh, unprocessed nuts as snacks and put them in salads. Nuts contain essential fatty acids not found in many other foods, and therefore are a vital part of your diet. They are also high in calories so don't eat too many, and limit the roasted, dry-roasted and salted ones.

Potatoes, cereals and grains

As well as potatoes, this group includes wheat, oats, barley, rye and rice and the foods made of them, such as bread, pasta, biscuits and breakfast cereals. Wholegrain products are the most nutritious and contain a lot of dietary fibre. Increase the amount of wholegrain foods you eat.

∗ Choose wholemeal pasta and brown or basmati rice.
∗ Eat at least four slices of wholemeal bread a day.
∗ Buy unsweetened breakfast cereals.
∗ Use wholemeal flour for making pastry (or use half white and half wholemeal).
∗ Eat fewer cakes and biscuits, even when they are made with wholemeal flour, because of their high fat and sugar content. Choose scones, currant buns, fruit and nut cakes and malt loaves, which are lower in sugar and fat than cream-filled and iced cakes.

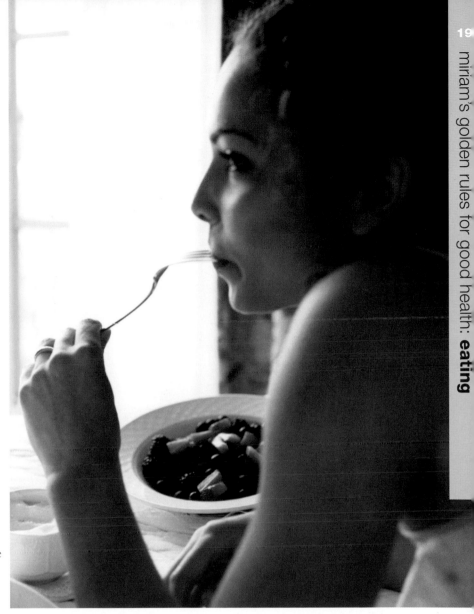

"eat whole fruit as well as drinking fruit juices"

∗ Eat more potatoes. Try them thinly sliced and steamed, or boiled or baked in their skins, and eat them with low-fat yogurt and herbs rather than butter. Mashed potatoes are tasty made with skimmed milk or low-fat yogurt, parsley and pepper.

The only other comment I'd make is that unrefined carbohydrates such as whole grains should provide a solid base to our diet. High-protein diets have absolutely nothing to recommend them. Protein should be taken as a condiment – for example, in pasta sauce. We should take very few of our calories in the form of saturated fats, such as butter and cheese, or sugar.

MIRIAM'S *golden rules* for exercise

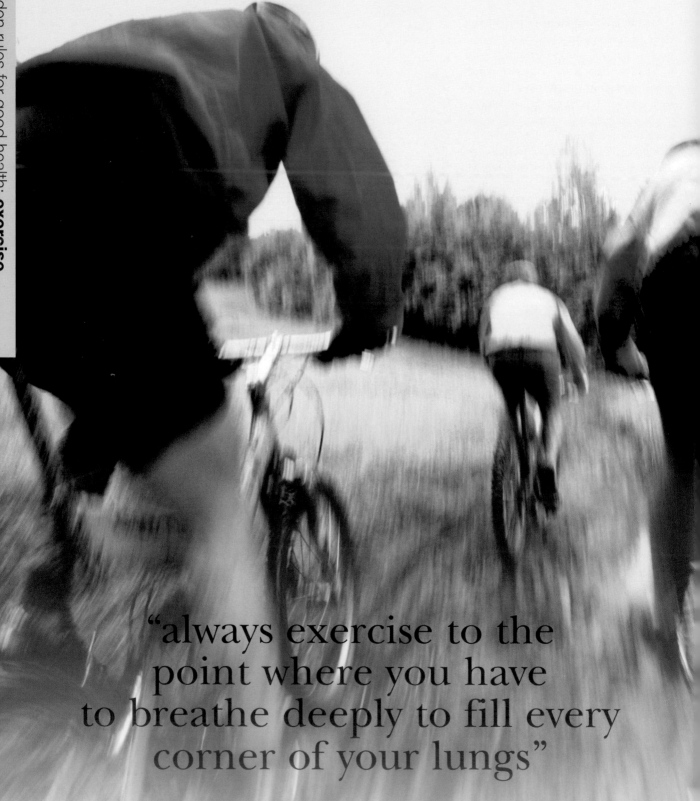

"always exercise to the
point where you have
to breathe deeply to fill every
corner of your lungs"

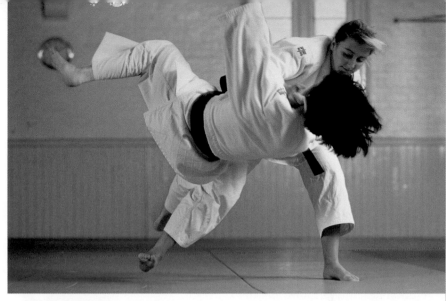

* **Do some physical activity for 30 minutes** at least five days a week. Brisk walking will do.

* If you're over 40, take any medication or have a chest or heart condition, **never start on an exercise programme without a medical check.**

* If you want to, wear a heart-rate recorder and **never exceed the maximum heart rate for your age.**

* **Always do warm-up exercises before you start** – 5–6 minutes. Cold muscles injure easily. The older you are, the longer you should spend warming up – 10–15 minutes if you're over 50.

* **Always spend five minutes "warming down"** after exercise. Do a few stretches to prevent stiffness and aching.

* **Swimming is excellent as we get older** because it supports stiff joints and exercises the whole body.

* **The most important muscles to keep fit are the quads on the front of the thighs** – without them you'll become tied to a chair because you won't be able to get out of it. Cycling is good for the quads.

* **If anything hurts, stop** – the saying "no pain, no gain" is rubbish – if a muscle is hurting it's dying.

"take up an activity or sport that you adore"

* You should always **exercise to the point where you have to breathe deeply** to fill every corner of your lungs – this alone protects your lungs from infection.

* **Increase the time and vigour of your exercise programme gradually**, say a week at a time.

* **Weight-bearing exercise is best** because it protects against osteoporosis (brittle bones).

* Exercises aren't just for strength and stamina, they **promote balance, agility and mobility** – very important as you get older.

* **Yoga is superb exercise** (though not for the heart and lungs) because it exercises muscles through stretching.

* To ensure the success of your exercise programme **take up an activity or sport you adore**, so it's never a chore.

Here's my list of the good things resulting from exercise. It:

* keeps your heart and lungs healthy
* promotes endorphins which give you an eight-hour high
* cures headaches, irritable bowel syndrome and migraine
* suppresses appetite
* can change your eating habits to healthy ones
* makes you take more exercise
* burns calories
* cures insomnia
* relieves anxiety
* cures panic attacks
* treats depression
* reshapes your body
* cures jet-lag
* reduces cholesterol
* lowers blood pressure.

In addition to these benefits, we now know that exercise also improves self-esteem, self-confidence, performance and mental health.

Benefits of exercise

Physical activity can boost mental as well as physical wellbeing and change your outlook on life. It could even prevent problems starting. As I know from personal experience, regular activity can lift your mood, help you deal with negative emotions like anger and bring you a general sense of mental wellbeing.

I've noticed that if I wake feeling a bit down, 30 minutes on my exercise bike cures the blues. That's because exercise floods my body with hormones that reduce tension levels and feelings of stress or fatigue. These changes happen straight after a session, particularly as I do six hill programmes. No wonder I'm addicted to it and can't miss a day. This kind of exercise can make a difference to anyone suffering from anxiety, depression or low self-esteem – and it has no side effects.

Self-image

Studies have shown that people feel better about themselves once they start an exercise programme. Changes to body shape – as you begin to lose weight and feel your muscle tone getting better – improve your self-image, which can boost mental wellbeing.

Exercise helps you to see just what you're capable of, giving you a sense of achievement. Learning a new skill or achieving a goal, however minor, boosts self-esteem and motivation.

Social life

Joining a local group, going to classes at a gym or leisure centre, or cycling with a friend or relative, for example, can give you a way to meet people and socialize. It gives you something

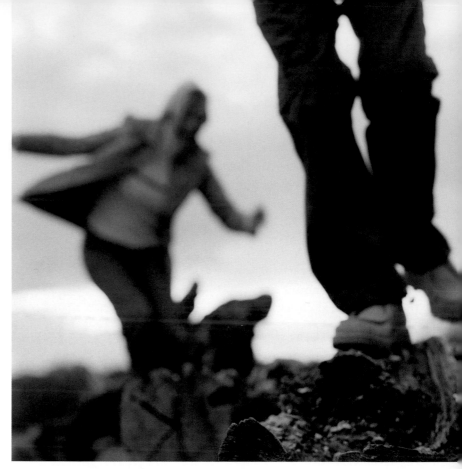

"regular exercise can lift your mood"

in common and helps to break the ice. If you'd prefer not to join in with others, there are many activities you can enjoy on your own, such as swimming or walking.

Health benefits

People who are active have half the risk of developing coronary heart disease of those who aren't. Regular exercise ameliorates common risk factors for heart disease such as high blood pressure, obesity and high cholesterol levels.

Keeping up an active lifestyle is good for bones, joints and muscles and it can help to delay the onset of osteoporosis and arthritis. It can significantly improve and maintain the strength and flexibility of your muscles, helping to prevent injury and reducing the risk of falling,

allowing you to enjoy life to the full as you get older.

It can also help control conditions such as diabetes and may reduce the risk of some cancers – in particular bowel cancer.

Staying active

Latest research on the longest-living people in the world, the Okinawans living on islands between Japan and Taiwan, suggests that beneficial physical activity can simply mean everyday pottering – gardening, cleaning and walking to catch a bus, as well as exercise such as cycling, swimming or working out, or playing sports such as football, golf or netball. It doesn't necessarily mean an intensive work-out in the gym, but it does mean being active for 30 minutes at least five days a week.

MIRIAM'S *golden rules* for not smoking

✱ **Giving up smoking is one of the best things you can do for your body.**

✱ **Stop smoking three months before trying for a baby** – men and women.

✱ **Don't smoke during pregnancy.**

✱ **Tobacco is the gateway drug to other drugs**, including cannabis.

✱ **No one who smokes should hold a baby** (to lessen the risk of cot death).

✱ **Don't smoke high-tar cigarettes.**

✱ **Never smoke right down to the filter**, this is where cancer chemicals are concentrated.

✱ **If possible smoke only five cigarettes a day.**

✱ **Don't smoke while drinking alcohol** – you'll find you can't have one without the other.

✱ **Most people find giving up much easier than they first thought** and wish they had done it earlier.

✱ Smokers with a young family **must smoke outside**.

✱ **Inflicting your smoke on other people is antisocial.**

Giving up smoking

Addiction to cigarettes is the most common and vicious of all the addictions, worse than heroin and more difficult to kick – and it's legal! Giving up smoking brings both short-term and important long-term health benefits.

Here are some of the dangers:

There are 3,000 dangerous chemicals in cigarette smoke.

Up to 5 percent is carbon monoxide – the same deadly gas that's in car exhaust fumes – and it stops your blood from absorbing oxygen properly.

The same tars that are used to surface roads are in tobacco smoke, and can cause cancer.

The most dangerous tar is a powerful nitroso chemical, one part per billion in food is a hazard: in tobacco smoke there are 5,000 parts per billion.

The other chemicals inhaled include ammonia, a chemical found in explosives, bleach and lavatory cleaners; cyanide, a deadly poison; and phenols, chemicals used in paint stripper.

Here are some of the reasons why people smoke:

When nicotine reaches the brain, it makes the head spin and people feel stimulated and alert.

Nicotine makes the heart beat faster, so more blood circulates

"giving up smoking is one of the best things you can do"

"within 5 years of quitting, the lung cancer risk decreases by half"

around the body per minute; people say they feel ready to get up and go.

Nicotine reduces tension in muscles, which makes people feel relaxed and seems to relieve stress.

Nicotine seems to help people work by improving concentration: it can stave off boredom and fatigue.

Effects on your health

Lung cancer: Smoking causes lung cancer, when it can be less than six months from diagnosis to death.
Fatal heart disease: Nicotine makes your heart beat faster and raises your blood pressure – the end result can be a heart attack.
Stroke: Smoking makes your blood thick and more likely to clot. A clot in the brain can mean permanent brain damage, paralysis, even death.
Gangrene: Your blood gets so sticky it can block the arteries in your legs, leading to gangrene and amputation.
Emphysema and bronchitis: Air passages become clogged, narrow and damaged until you're crippled by breathlessness.
Cancers of the mouth, throat, oesophagus, bladder, pancreas, kidney, cervix and breast are all more common in smokers.
Ulcers: You are more likely to get stomach and duodenal ulcers if you smoke.

Why quit?

Cigarette smokers look older than their age because smoking speeds up ageing of the skin.

The risk of premature death is double that of non-smokers.

Smoking-related diseases kill 40 percent of smokers before they reach retirement.

Non-smokers live at least six years longer than smokers.

What are the benefits of quitting?

Giving up smoking has instant benefits.
✱ Within 20 minutes blood pressure and pulse fall.
✱ Within 2 hours lung airways relax, making it easier to breathe, and the volume of air our lungs can hold increases.
✱ Within 8 hours carbon monoxide levels drop to normal and the oxygen level goes back up to normal.
✱ Within 24 hours the risk of a heart attack decreases.
✱ Within 48 hours damaged nerve endings start to regrow, so smell and taste become stronger.
✱ Within 1 to 3 months circulation improves; lung function improves by up to a third.
✱ Within 5 years the risk of lung cancer decreases by half.
✱ Within 10 years the risk of lung cancer is normal.

Helping yourself quit

Many people wonder if aids to quit smoking work and if they should try them. Most smoking experts agree, and I am with them, that there's no substitute for willpower, but you could try nicotine gum or skin patches, hypnosis, acupuncture and going to smoking cessation clinics.

Here are 20 tips for helping you to quit smoking:

Don't try to do them all at once. Choose three or four, never more, to begin with, then add one or two more each day. Good luck!

1 Never smoke in the car.
2 Refuse every cigarette that's offered to you.
3 Don't have a cigarette before breakfast.
4 Buy only one pack at a time.
5 Buy only 10 cigarettes, not 20.
6 Buy a different brand of cigarettes every time, not just your favourite.
7 Before you light up, count to 10.
8 Every time you take a cigarette, put the pack away in another room.
9 When you run out of cigarettes, never take one from someone else.
10 After each puff, put the cigarette down.
11 Never smoke out of doors.
12 Never smoke in bed.
13 Stop smoking at work.
14 Don't smoke in the house.
15 Stop carrying your lighter or matches with you.
16 Stop smoking a cigarette more than half way down.
17 After a meal, don't smoke until you've left the table.
18 Don't smoke while you're relaxing with a drink.
19 Only smoke if you're sitting in an uncomfortable chair.
20 Keep a rubber band around your cigarette pack as a reminder.

Smoking and pregnancy

✱ **Mothers:** Don't smoke when pregnant or you risk harming your unborn baby, having a miscarriage or giving birth to an underweight baby, vulnerable to infections.

✱ **Fathers:** The children of fathers who smoke 20 or more cigarettes a day have a higher risk of cancer than children of non-smoking fathers. Smoking damages sperm, so men should give up smoking at least three months before trying for a baby.

Smoking increases the likelihood of cot death.

MIRIAM'S *golden rules* for safe drinking

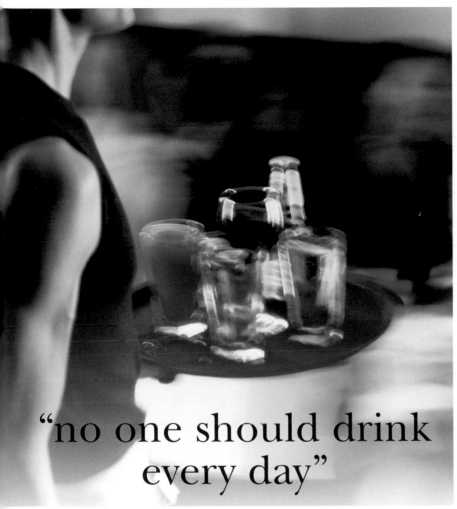

"no one should drink every day"

✱ Do drink twice as much still water as alcohol, and **a big glass of water before bed to avoid dehydration**.

✱ Avoid carbonated drinks. The **bubbles get the alcohol to your brain faster**.

✱ Remember that **alcohol has a greater effect on women than on men**.

✱ **Don't mix drink and drugs**, you won't be able to handle an emergency.

✱ Do **make a note of how much alcohol you get through in a week**. A diary can be a real eye opener!

✱ **No one should drink every day.** Have some alcohol-free days every week.

✱ **Stay off alcohol for a few days** after a party to let your liver recover.

✱ Do **eat food as you drink** to soak up the alcohol.

✱ Plan how you'll get home after drinking – **order a taxi**.

✱ **Don't keep pace with your mates** – drinking isn't a competition.

✱ For teenagers – **don't think that drinking alcohol means you're grown up**. It doesn't.

✱ **Being drunk at a football match could be an offence.**

✱ **Keep below recommended limits**. These are no more than 3–4 units a day for men and 2–3 for women. One unit = half a pint of beer, medium glass of wine or one measure of spirits.

✱ **Don't binge at the weekend** and drink a week's allowance in a short time; **it's bad for your liver**.

✱ Don't mix the grain (beer) with the grape (wine) if you want to avoid a hangover.

✱ **Always sip alcohol rather than gulp it.**

✱ Do eat first if you plan to drink: **even a glass of milk can help prevent a hangover**.

✱ **Don't drink and drive** and never ride in a car driven by someone who has been drinking.

✱ **Don't mix drink and sex** – you're more careless and could catch an STD or get pregnant.

"vitamins C and E can help accelerate alcohol detoxification"

Dangers of heavy drinking

Alcohol is intoxicating, and although it gives you an initial lift, it's a depressant drug. It slows down responses (affecting coordination) and the way the brain works (affecting judgement), so it makes people clumsy and dopey. It's one of the most widely used drugs, above and below the legal age limit. In large quantities over a short time, alcohol is a poison and will kill.

What happens to alcohol in your body?

Although it takes minutes for alcohol to reach the brain, it takes the liver an hour to break down the alcohol in a glass of wine or beer. The less you weigh, the more alcohol affects you, so there's a good reason for alcohol being illegal below a certain age. A slim teenage boy will get drunk far more quickly than a large adult male. A woman will feel the effects of alcohol faster and for longer than a man because women don't have enough body fluid to dilute alcohol the way men do.

Drinking too much always has horrible effects

Drinking too much can make you aggressive and violent. You're more likely to start arguments and pick fights.

You become uncoordinated and clumsy and you shouldn't try to use sharp instruments or machinery.

Too much alcohol gives you double vision and slurred speech.

Drinking when you're feeling down can make you more depressed.

Alcohol is loaded with calories. It can make you fat, and is bad for your skin.

A bad hangover makes you feel really fragile. Your head pounds and you have an upset stomach. You can't work or study.

Alcohol can damage a man's fertility and potency (lowers sperm count and brings on "brewer's droop").

It's difficult to get and maintain an erection if you've been drinking.

Avoid alcohol if you're:

✻ taking any over-the-counter medicines – even cold cures – without first checking the labels
✻ taking any prescribed or illegal drugs
✻ going to drive a car, ride a bike or operate machinery.

Check the dangers of drinking

If you drive after you've had only one drink, you're still five times more likely to have a car accident than a non-drinker.

Accidents are more common with alcohol because your reflexes slow down and you lose coordination.

You're more likely to be careless and have unprotected sex if you're drunk, thereby risking a pregnancy or a sexually-transmitted disease.

You can black out or forget what you did for whole periods. If you wander off alone you could pass out and choke on your own vomit.

Serious binge-drinking can cause you to fall over, injure yourself and even lose consciousness or have fits.

Alcohol has a high sugar content, so anyone with diabetes is advised to avoid it altogether.

Drinking during pregnancy can cause fetal alcohol syndrome in your developing baby. The baby could develop abnormally in your womb and behave abnormally as he or she grows up. Keep to one or two units a week or don't drink at all.

Long-term heavy alcohol use leads to physical dependence – which means you can't do without it – and seriously damages the heart, liver, stomach and brain.

Final stages of alcoholic dependence aren't pretty – DTs or delirium tremens (a state of confusion accompanied by trembling and hallucinations), swollen abdomen, cirrhosis of the liver, weak heart, coma and death.

Drinking and sex

Because alcohol lowers inhibitions, more than half of all teenagers have sex for the first time when drunk. This may have disastrous results.

Both sexes get careless about contraception and this can lead not only to unwanted pregnancy but also to HIV/AIDS, herpes and other sexually transmitted diseases (STDs).

It's harder to maintain an erection when you're drunk. Girls think boys' lovemaking is fumbling and shambolic when they're drunk.

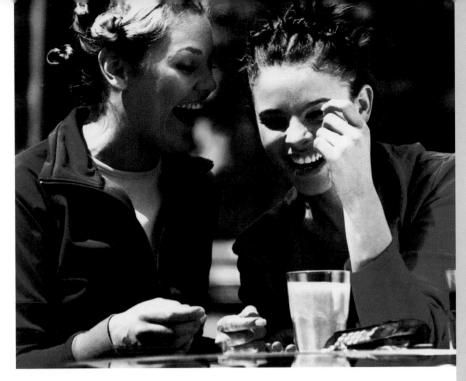

Stages in alcohol dependence

The first stage is when the heavy social drinker finds that he or she is able to drink more and more alcohol without noticing its effects.

Then come periods of memory loss, followed by the realization that they are no longer in control of their drinking. They can't be certain they can stop whenever they please.

The next and final step is characterized by prolonged binges and by serious physical and mental problems.

Treatment

Different methods of treatment – psychological, social and physical – are appropriate for different people and may be combined.

Psychological treatments involve psychotherapy and are commonly carried out in groups. There are various types of group therapy.

Social treatments include help with problems at work and in particular the inclusion of family members in the treatment process.

Physical treatment is needed only by some alcoholics. It generally includes the use of disulfiram, a drug that sensitizes the drinker to alcohol so that he or she is afraid to drink because of the unpleasant side effects.

Detox

Many alcoholics require medical help in getting over the physical symptoms when they stop drinking, and this may mean staying at a detox clinic for a few days or maybe longer. This has to be followed up by long-term treatment, which depends on individual needs. For example, some people benefit from psychotherapy, which is often carried out in groups.

"alcohol is loaded with calories. It can make you fat"

Alcoholics can also suffer from nutritional deficiencies. Studies have shown that supplements of zinc and vitamins C and E can help accelerate alcohol detoxification and prevent liver damage.

Naxtrexone

A new and revolutionary alcohol treatment, naxtrexone, has been launched that allows patients to continue drinking during and after treatment. Trials have shown it to be a powerful technique for patients who have not descended too far into alcoholism and who are sufficiently motivated to get well. In Finland, 78 percent of patients had still not relapsed after three years.

Naxtrexone is not yet licensed for use in treating alcoholism in the UK, but can be prescribed on a named-patient basis at a new chain of private clinics.

Alcohol and children

Over 1,000 teenagers a year in the UK get acute alcohol poisoning from not knowing the facts about the dangers of drinking. Here are some grim statistics.

Children – mainly girls – as young as nine are drinking themselves close to death.

The number of young people admitted to hospital with alcohol poisoning has grown tenfold in 10 years.

9 out of 10 boys under 13 drink secretly.

1,000 children under 15 are admitted to hospital with acute alcohol poisoning each year in the UK alone.

1 in 4 teenagers, especially boys, get into arguments or fights after drinking alcohol. This could result in the police being called in.

MIRIAM'S *golden rules* on drugs

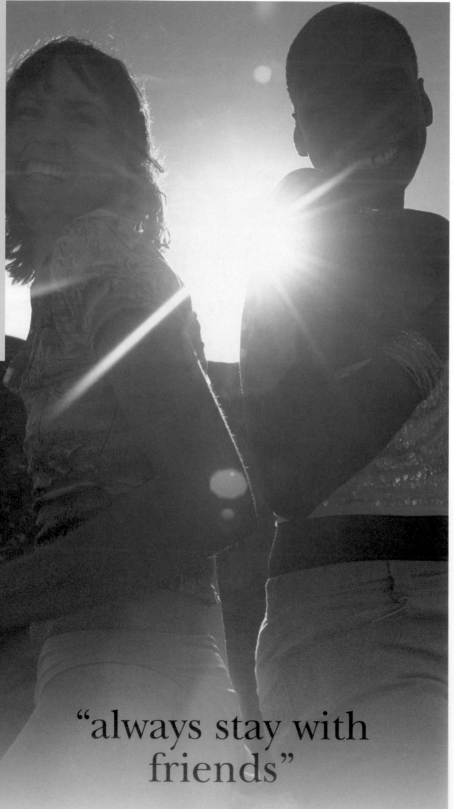

"always stay with friends"

My aim is to inform and educate children on the dangers of drugs, and certainly not to advocate their use. But I don't believe in scare tactics or moral indignation. I find it as unrealistic to imagine a society without drugs as one without alcohol or sex.

* **Don't mix alcohol and drugs**, the effects are addictive and dangerous.

* **Keep sipping water if you take drugs** – you need 300ml (½ pint) every half hour.

* **Keep your salt levels up** by eating salted crisps or nuts.

* **Learn CPR and basic first aid for emergencies.**

* **High-energy drinks are best,** then fruit juice.

* **Never wear a hat**, you need to stay cool.

* At a rave take frequent rests so you **don't overheat**.

* Memorize the **drugs helpline telephone number**.

* Never take drugs from someone you don't know.

* Always stay with friends.

* **Don't mix drugs**, all side effects are much worse, especially dehydration.

* **Know where to go for help.**

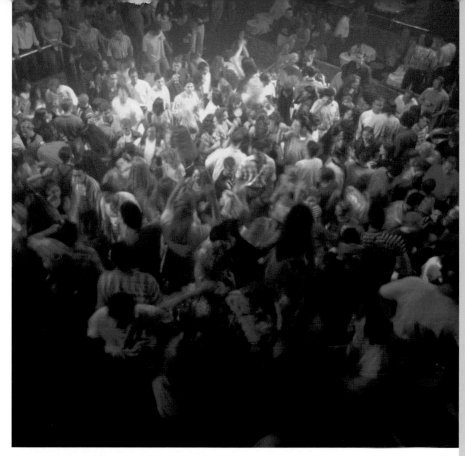

My main concern is the welfare of children and, although we may never eliminate drug use completely, I believe we can minimize the dangers by giving young people sound, honest, realistic information. Then the consequences for them and the community at large will be the least damaging.

What you need to know about drugs

The mere mention of drugs is enough to strike fear into almost every parent's heart. Parents fear that their child might want to experiment and ultimately pay with their life, especially when there seems to be no end to the tragic cases of young people who die after taking drugs.

But most young people today see occasional drug use in the same way as their parents see alcohol – as part of normal life. Most describe it as something that makes them feel good and gets rid of their inhibitions. In the main, I think they're as responsible about drugs as most of us are about alcohol.

The "just-say-no" approach to drug-taking is based on the belief that our sons and daughters are incapable of making decisions about drugs. And it implies that adults aren't interested in their opinions and experiences. Well, I do respect young people's ability to reason, and feel they should have reliable, accurate information on drugs. I discuss drugs in honest terms of harm to mind and body, without relying on the law to separate what's dangerous from what isn't.

My goal is to be scientific and even-handed, separating real from imagined dangers. I've been lecturing, making television

documentaries and researching drugs for more than 20 years. As a mother myself, I felt it was important to speak directly to concerned parents as well as to potential drug users as part of that research. It's not surprising that many teenagers reject all advice – good and bad – from adults on the subject of drugs.

The messages are often exaggerated or false, sometimes ridiculous, but nearly always inconsistent with their own observations and experience. I have tried to avoid exaggeration and pre-judgement and I have re-examined the assumptions that are too often made about drugs.

A realistic examination has to consider the following:

✽ Despite possible dangers, most drugs induce some pleasurable feelings.
✽ Total abstinence may not always be a realistic goal.
✽ The use of illegal substances need not mean abuse.
✽ One form of drug use doesn't

inevitably lead to other, more harmful forms.
✽ Understanding the risks of drug use will not necessarily deter young people from experimentation.

Heroin (street names: H, Brown, Gravy)

A depressant drug that numbs the brain and body and kills pain. It's highly addictive. Comes in three forms: brown (which should never be injected), China white, and pharmaceutical heroin, which can easily cause overdose. Brown is sometimes dissolved in vinegar or lemon juice and can cause sight problems if injected. Sores and open wounds can develop with heavy heroin use. On withdrawal, addicts suffer craving, panic attacks, cramps, nausea and diarrhoea.

Cocaine (street names: Charlie, Toot, Snow)

A powerful stimulant that brings on feelings of euphoria and wellbeing. It's highly addictive. Long-term users

"users can become psychotic, delusional and violent"

may become psychotic. Snorting can burn a hole in your nostrils. Injecting cocaine is highly dangerous because there is a real risk of overdosing. Mixing it with heroin (speedballing) is also very dangerous. Most street cocaine comes as a powder that is "cut" with glucose, lactose or even anaesthetics. Cocaine content may be as low as 30 percent.

Cannabis (street names: Grass, Draw, Spliff)

Often exaggerates the way a person already feels. Users become talkative and think they have a greater "insight" into the world. They often find everything hilarious. Some long-term, heavy users may get panic attacks, exaggerated mood swings and feelings of persecution. Mixing cannabis with speed or ecstasy can make you seriously dehydrated and cause other severe problems such as heart attacks. There are three forms: herbal, resin and hash oil.

Acid (LSD) (street names: Tabs, Trips, Blotters)

An extraordinarily powerful, mind-altering drug, causing hallucinations. Acid is unpredictable and should never be taken on the spur of the moment. If you are feeling down, you are more likely to have a "bad trip". There's virtually no risk of physical side effects and it's not addictive, but the mental effects can be very serious. It can unlock a mental illness of which you weren't aware, which can lead you to become depressed, paranoid or even needing psychiatric treatment. Bad trips can cause terrifying, uncontrollable flashbacks. Acid is almost always soaked in small squares of blotting paper. The average amount in an acid tab is

around 50 micrograms – enough to induce a fairly mild trip – but could contain as much as 250 micrograms, enough to cause the equivalent of a nervous breakdown.

Ecstasy (street names: E, Adam, Disco biscuits)

Releases mood-altering chemicals, such as serotonin and L-dopa, which generate feelings of love and friendliness. It's also hallucinogenic. Ecstasy can cause the body to overheat, resulting in potentially fatal heatstroke. It can also interrupt blood flow in the brain, leading to a stroke, and cause fatal kidney and liver failure. Tablets come in different designs, often with logos on them. Ecstasy may be "cut" with talcum powder or ketamine (a horse tranquilliser), giving horrible side effects.

Amphetamine (street names: Speed, Whizz, Billy)

A stimulant that makes you more energetic and alert. Users become very talkative and can stay awake for hours.

You can still be "wired" 12 hours after taking the drug. It can cause heatstroke and may also lead to a heart attack. Liver and kidney failure can occur if you mix it with alcohol. Injecting it is highly dangerous as the heart can't take the shock. Speed is least dangerous when it is swallowed.

Crack (street names: Rock, Wash, Cloud)

According to users the intensity of the hit can't be exaggerated. It comes within seconds but is short-lived. It can give an intense euphoria and an energy surge with an incredible sense of wellbeing and power. It's highly addictive. After the hit, users will often feel weak, tired, paranoid and depressed. The comedown can last for days. Crack use can lead to severe psychological problems. Users can become psychotic, delusional and violent. Combining crack with any other drug is potentially lethal. Crack is cocaine that has been processed and can be 80–100 percent pure, which makes it much more dangerous. It is generally smoked.

The penalties

Remember, above all, that if you get caught in possession of illegal drugs, or intend to supply them, the penalties are harsh. They are particularly severe for drug pushers, who get rich from peddling misery. Here are the maximum UK penalties.

Class	Possession	Intent to supply	Supplying
A (e.g. heroin)	7 years in jail	Life in jail, plus unlimited fine	Life, unlimited fine, plus seizure of drug-related assets
B (e.g. speed)	5 years in jail, plus fine	14 years in jail, plus fine	14 years in jail, plus fine
C (e.g. steroids)	2 years in jail, plus fine	5 years in jail, plus fine	5 years in jail, plus fine

MIRIAM'S *golden rules* for good sex

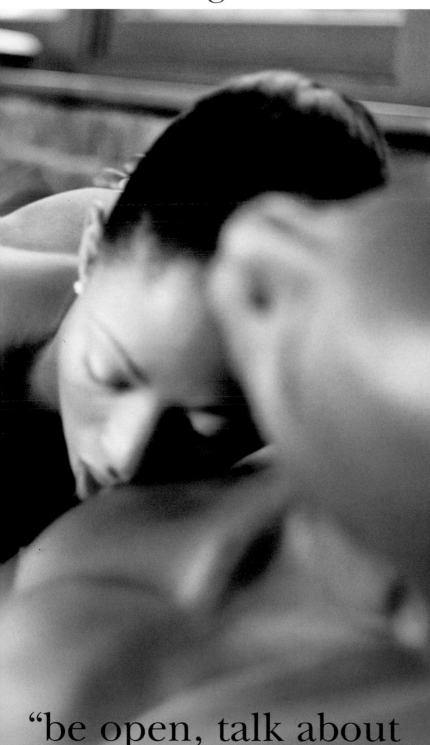

* Be open, **talk about what does and doesn't turn you on** and show reciprocity by asking for feedback.

* **Low, medium and high sex drives are all normal** so be generous when your partner's libido is different from yours.

* **Don't hold back sexual grudges**, get them off your chest – the longer you leave it the more difficult they become to discuss.

* **Anything is OK** between consenting adults.

* **Find out what pleases you** by masturbating, then show your partner how to please you.

* **Simultaneous orgasms aren't the holy grail of sex** so stop chasing them.

* **Multiple orgasms aren't either, one is fine**, so is one a night.

* **When a woman says NO, that means no sex**. Anything else means rape.

* **The G spot is a fiction**.

* **Sex isn't an athletic competition**.

* **Smoking, drugs and alcohol impair erection**, arousal and orgasm.

* **The female orgasm resides in the clitoris**. The penis is therefore not the best kind of stimulation, the tongue, finger or a vibrator often being superior.

"be open, talk about what turns you on"

MIRIAM'S *golden rules* for restful sleep

✱ Do whatever you have to do to sleep more – **have a hot drink, read a book or the paper**, watch television or do all three.

✱ Just as a bedtime routine helps children, so the body and brain of adults respond to bedtime cues and rituals, **so have a wind-down routine that you follow most nights**.

✱ Alcohol doesn't help you to sleep, it does the opposite, so if it's sound sleep you want, **avoid alcohol late in the evening**. You may fall asleep but you'll wake a few hours later and be unable to go back to sleep.

✱ Two drops of oil of clary sage or **lavender on the pillow can aid sleep**.

✱ Being either too hot or too cold can prevent sleep, so **spend some effort on making your bedroom temperature equable**.

✱ If you have a tendency to insomnia anything will keep you awake, so **turn off dripping taps, close squeaking doors and batten down anything that can flap in a draught**.

✱ **Learn some kind of self-hypnosis that induces sleep quite quickly** when you can't drop off – mine is counting backwards from ten, repeating "I'm falling asleep" with each number – I've never got beyond five.

✱ **Wear loose-fitting cotton sleepwear** or none at all.

✱ **Change your mattress every seven years or so**.

✱ If your partner likes music or television last thing, don't get worked up – **snuggle down with ear plugs and an eye-shade**.

✱ If you wake up in the early hours and can't get back to sleep, **don't lie there and fume; get up**, do the odd chore, make a cup of tea, do a crossword, read and when you're feeling sleepy go back to bed.

✱ **Only ever take sleeping pills in the short term to get you over a bad patch**.

✱ **Sex is the best prelude to sleep**.

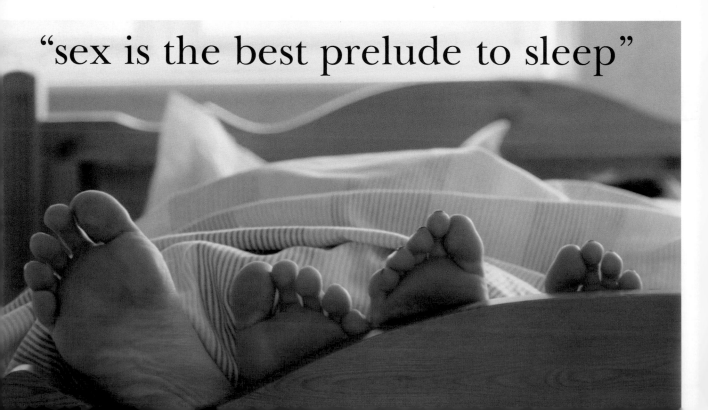

"sex is the best prelude to sleep"

miriam's golden rules for good health: **managing stress**

MIRIAM'S *golden rules* for managing stress

* **Some stress is good for us**. It increases productivity, so don't rule it out altogether – find your optimum level.

* **The body** *loves* **the stress of exercise** and releases hundreds of beneficial hormones as a result.

* **Desensitize yourself to excessive levels of stress** with instant relaxation, imagery training, activity of any kind and writing out an action plan.

* Instant relaxation is a quick, simple exercise that you can do whenever you can to **conquer stress in a few minutes**:

1 close your eyes
2 lower your shoulders
3 halve your breathing rate
4 count to five breathing in and to five breathing out
5 think of black velvet.

* **Simple breathing techniques can relieve stress**. Learn yoga breathing.

* **Exercise itself relieves stress** but it also increases your *resistance* to stress, so walk briskly when you can, climb stairs and incorporate some formal exercise into your life every day if you can. It needn't be excessive – 30 minutes of walking is enough.

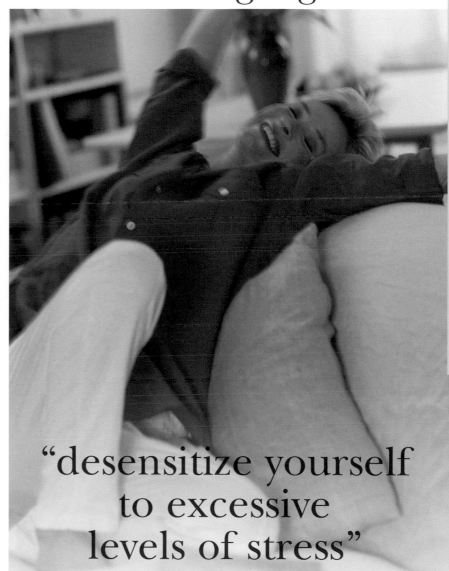

"desensitize yourself to excessive levels of stress"

* **Stress-relieving aromatherapy includes oil of clary sage and lavender** – a couple of drops on a handkerchief or pillow and in the bath.

* **Learn biofeedback to keep your heart rate and blood pressure down** when you feel stress taking its toll.

* **Learn deep muscle and deep mental relaxation techniques**. Then you can control stress.

* **Massage will relieve the muscle tension, aches and pains that result from stress**, so incorporate sessions into your life.

Life Stages

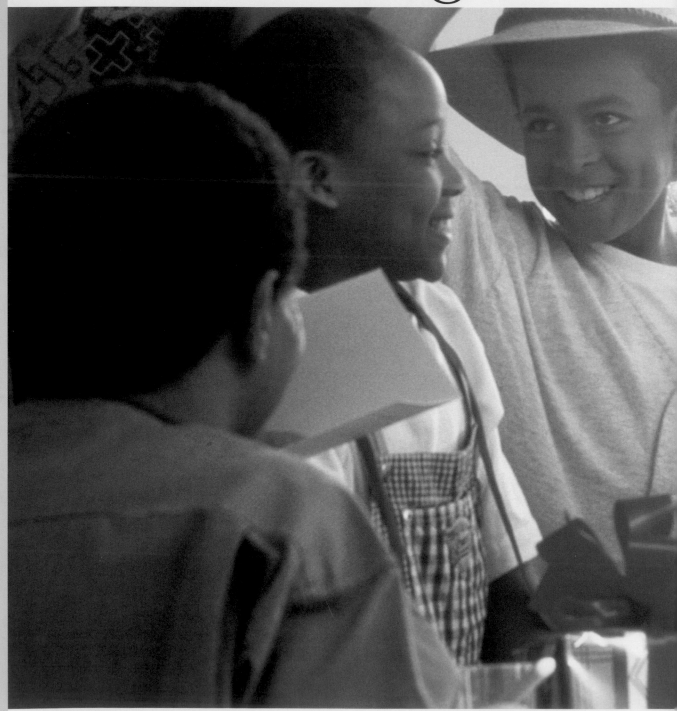

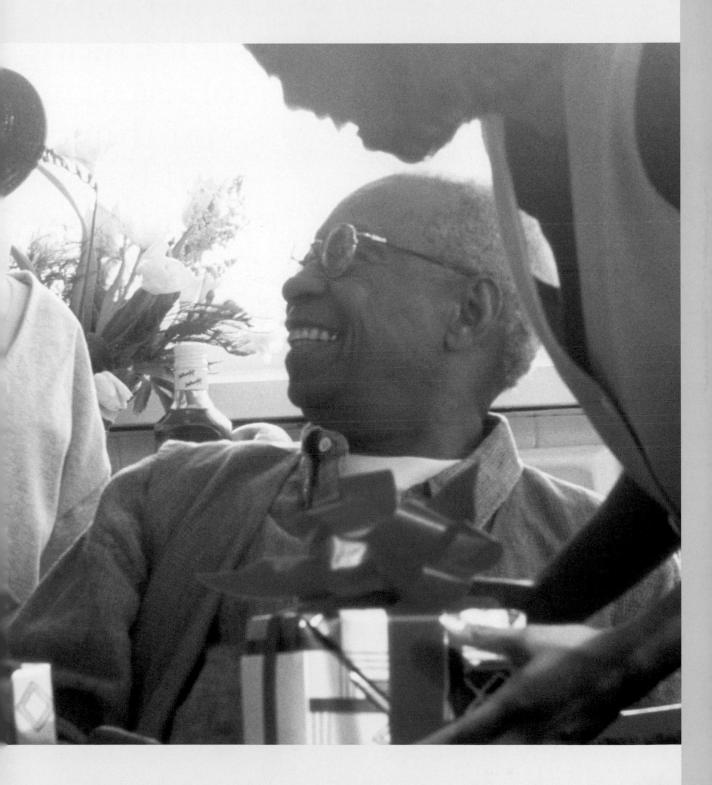

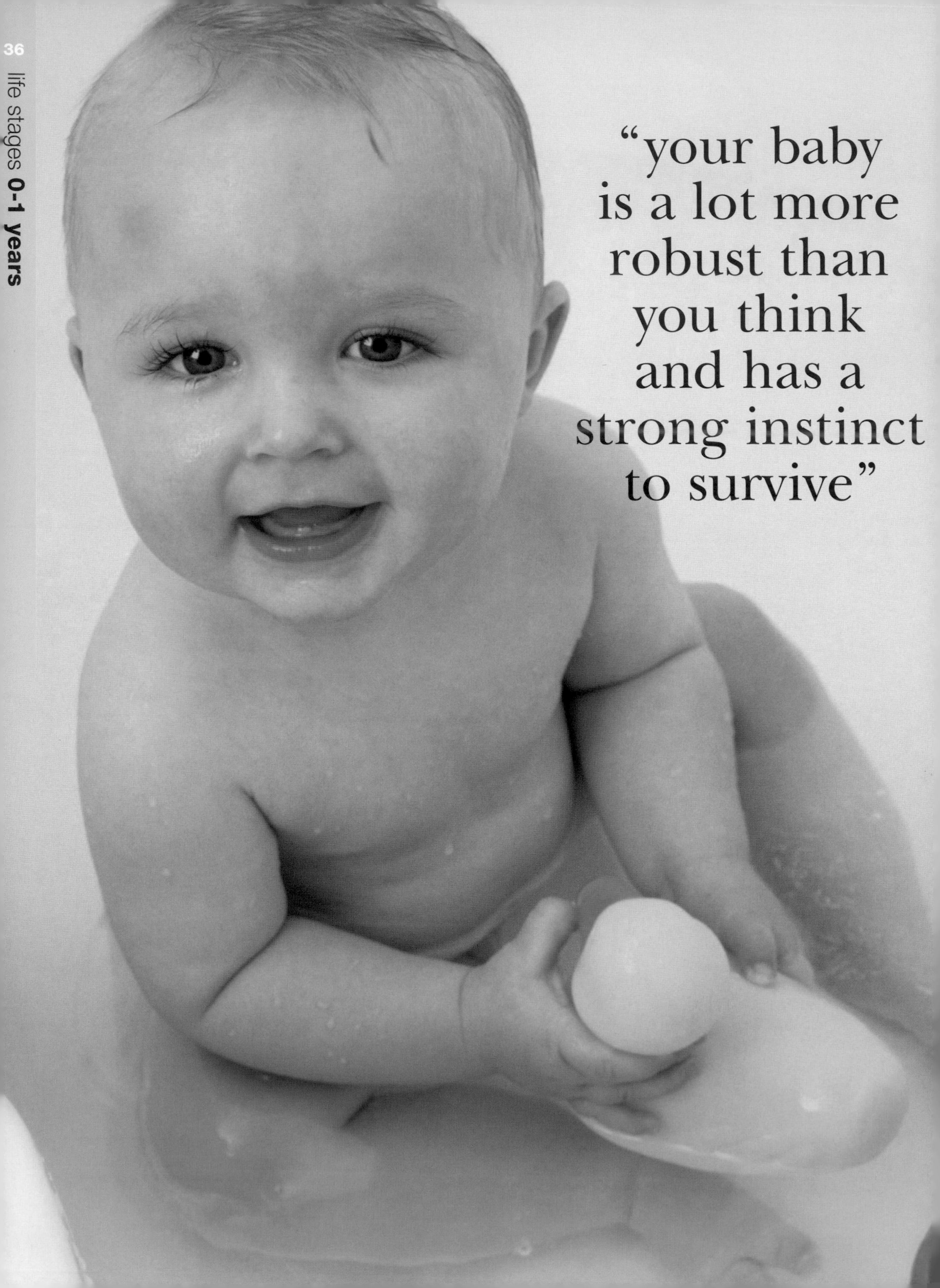

"your baby
is a lot more
robust than
you think
and has a
strong instinct
to survive"

life stages: 0 to 1 years

You're thrilled by the arrival of your new baby, and like most new parents you'll probably feel nervous about handling this tiny scrap of humanity who seems so weak and vulnerable. But, in fact, from the moment of birth your baby is a lot more robust than you think and has a strong instinct to survive.

The importance of bonding

A newborn baby sleeps for most of her first days, so try to spend all of her waking time together. Research has shown that physical contact with you, the sound of your voice and the smell of your body are very important during the first few days of life. During this time your baby forms a bond with you which, if encouraged, is unique and unbreakable.

To help the bonding process make sure your baby has frequent contact with your skin as this is critical for establishing bonding. Make feeding a time of physical intimacy; hold her close and talk gently.

Growth and development

In your baby's first year, growth and development cover three main areas:
● **Brain** – she will be using her brain to think and to develop language
● **Mobility** – she will be learning to stand upright and walk, starting with attempts to control her head as early as her first week
● **Dexterity** – she will be acquiring fine control of her fingers so that by around 10 months she can pick up a pea between thumb and forefinger.

All that you have to do to help a skill develop is take your lead from your baby. This is the golden and unbreakable rule of child development. And your baby will always show you with some sign that she wants to and can move on. It's important to follow her lead because if you do you'll hit exactly the right moment when it's essential for her to acquire the skill.

This makes her feel very pleased with herself (especially if you praise her) and you'll be building her self-confidence and self-esteem right from the start. Just think what a confident, balanced, affectionate child she'll grow into. And all the groundwork is laid in the first year.

Emotional continence

It is also vital for your baby to learn "emotional continence" in her first year. Emotional continence means being able to manage emotions, not letting them get out of hand. It involves being able to control strong emotions by turning them to good purpose.
● Babies learn emotional continence from you.
● If emotional continence isn't learned in the first year it's very difficult to acquire later.

Without this skill she finds it very difficult to cope with anything that thwarts her wishes or stands in her way as she grows up – in other words she becomes emotionally incontinent. The classic outcome of emotional incontinence is a pre-schooler who bullies, is disruptive, even destructive at home and at nursery school.

In the pages that follow I offer guidelines on what happens during your baby's first year and advice where I feel there may be a need.

Building emotional continence

It's not difficult to impart early lessons in emotional continence to your baby. There are three easy steps in any situation.

● *Legitimize* your baby's emotions. Tell her "I know it hurts" if she's fallen over or "That is annoying" if she's frustrated by something and becomes angry.

● *Defuse* your baby's emotions. Say "Mummy will kiss it better" or "Daddy gets annoyed with that too, you know".

● *Move on* from the emotion. Suggest "When it's stopped hurting we'll go out to play" or "Let's forget that and have a cuddle".

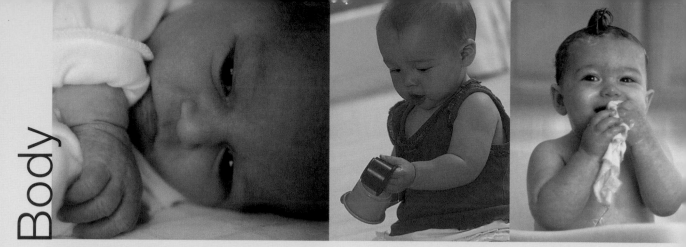

Body

Mind

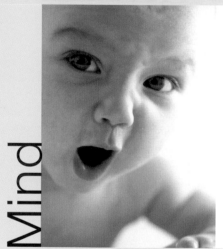

"a baby's bond with you is unique and unbreakable"

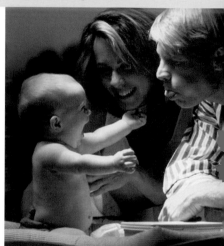

Social

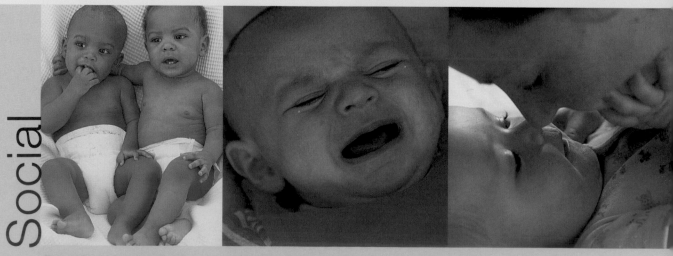

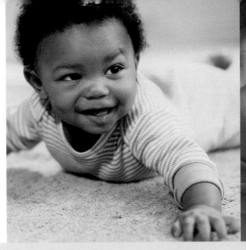

"your new baby has a number of amazing innate skills"

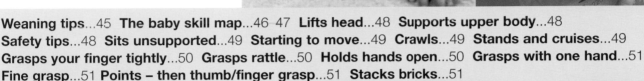

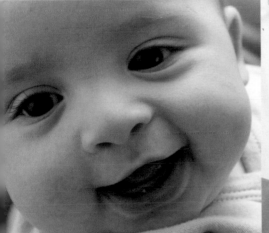
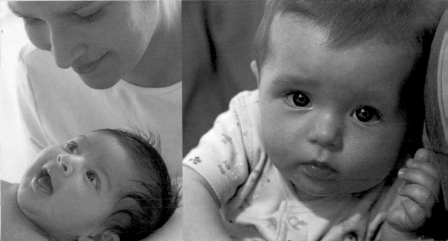

"she learns to be loving and friendly by imitating you"

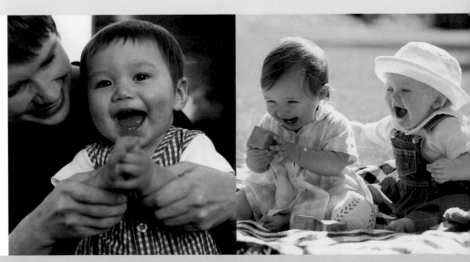

0-1 your new baby

Your feelings on the birth of your new baby are likely to be pride, wonder and exhilaration mixed with exhaustion. Your baby may seem smaller than you imagined and very vulnerable, but don't worry – your baby is equipped with reflexes and behaviour that help him survive.

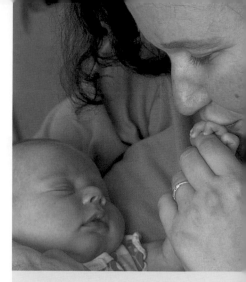

Premature babies

One in 18 babies born in Britain today is premature. The medical definition of a premature baby is one that is born at less than 36 weeks. All premature babies need special treatment but not necessarily in a special care unit. Premature babies are not well equipped for life outside the womb and may have the following problems:

● **Breathing** Due to the immaturity of their lungs, most premature babies experience difficulty in breathing, known as respiratory distress syndrome (RDS).
● **Immune system** An underdeveloped immune system and a body that is too weak to defend itself properly means there is a greater risk of infection.
● **Digestion** A premature baby's stomach is small and sensitive, which means he is less able to hold food down, and so is more likely to vomit. The immaturity of his digestive system makes it difficult for him to digest essential proteins so they have to be given in a pre-digested form.

● **Temperature regulation** A premature baby's temperature control is inefficient and he is likely to be too cold or too hot. He has less heat insulation than a full-term baby, as he lacks sufficient body fat.
● **Reflexes** Inadequate development of his reflexes, particularly his sucking reflex, creates difficulties in feeding. Premature babies usually need tube feeding.

Progress

The development of a premature baby can be slow and erratic. It can be a shock to see just how tiny your premature baby is, but he will have a great will to live. For a premature baby, every day can be an uphill battle. Periods of improvement may be followed by setbacks, and this uncertainty makes you and your partner very anxious. It is encouraging to know, however, that most babies born after 32 weeks will develop normally. Of those babies born at 28 weeks, 6 out of 7 will survive.

Baby skills at birth

Although your baby is physically helpless at birth, he has a number of amazing innate skills. Your newborn
● is wired to communicate
● is programmed to imitate the facial expressions and sounds you make when you talk
● loves eye contact and skin contact
● sees everything 20–25cm (8-10in) away clearly and responds eagerly to your face at this distance, looks intensely
● at 20–25cm (8–10in) can "read" emotions and may smile if he sees you smiling
● can hear your voice very clearly and recognize it.

What you can do to help
● Trust, warmth and sociability are developed in the first few months, and during this time you must teach your baby most of the basic ways to relate to people. So most importantly, be positive in all you do, and overt in all you express.
● Smiling is your most important tool to show pleasure, approval, love and joy. Voice comes next. Babies are sensitive to loving, approving, delighted and joyful tones of voice, pitched light and high.
● Body contact – the warmth, closeness and smell of your body – is important, too, as are touch and physical demonstrations of affection.

Preventing cot death

Sudden infant death syndrome (SIDS), commonly known as cot death, is the sudden and unexpected death of a baby for no obvious reason.

The exact causes of cot death are still unknown, and there is therefore no advice that can absolutely guarantee its prevention. There are, however, many ways in which parents can vastly reduce the risk. Recent surveys have proved that the routine immunizations reduce the risk, as does keeping your baby in your room with you at night for the first six months of her life. Falling asleep with your baby on the sofa greatly increases the risk of cot death.

A mother who smokes during pregnancy increases the risk of SIDS. The risk of cot death in babies born to smokers is twice that for babies born to non-smokers, and with every 10 cigarettes a day the risk increases threefold.

Reducing the risk

● Always place your baby on her back to sleep.
● Don't smoke, don't allow smoking in your house and avoid taking your baby into smoky places.
● Don't let your baby get too hot.
● When covering your baby, allow for room temperature – the higher the temperature, the fewer bedclothes your baby needs and vice versa.
● Avoid tucking in, so your baby can throw off bedclothes if she is hot.
● If you think your baby is unwell, don't hesitate to contact your doctor.
● If your baby has a fever, don't increase her wrappings; reduce them so she can lose heat.

Your new baby's appearance

When you hold your baby for the first time, her appearance will probably surprise you. She's undoubtedly a joy to you, but you may have expected a clean and placid bundle, similar to the babies that appear in baby-food commercials. Real life (as you'll now suddenly discover) is a bit different.

Skin

● **Vernix** – a whitish, greasy substance – may cover your baby's skin. This natural barrier cream prevented the skin from becoming waterlogged in the uterus. It may be removed at once, or left to give your baby some natural protection against minor skin irritations such as flaking and peeling.

● **Nettle rash** (urticaria) is quite common in the first week. There's no need for treatment; it will disappear quite quickly.

● **Milia** are small white spots seen mainly on the bridge of the nose but also elsewhere on the face.

● **Heat rash** – if she's too warm, your baby may get small red spots, particularly on her face.

Head

The soft spots on the top of your baby's skull where the bones are still not joined are called the fontanelles. The skull bones won't fuse completely until your baby is about two. Be careful not to press the fontanelles.

Eyes

Your baby may not be able to open her eyes straight away due to puffiness caused by pressure on her head during birth. This pressure may also have broken some tiny blood vessels in her eyes, causing harmless small, red, triangular marks in the whites

that need no treatment and disappear in a couple of weeks. She may have "sticky eye" – a yellow discharge around the eyelids. This is quite common, and although not serious should always be treated by a doctor.

Hair

Some babies are born with a full head of hair; others are completely bald. The colour of your baby's hair at birth may not be the colour she will end up with. The fine, downy hair that many babies have on their bodies at birth is called lanugo, and this will fall off soon after birth.

Genitals

The genitals may look swollen and enlarged.

Legs and arms

The baby's legs and arms are still bent, as they were in the uterus.

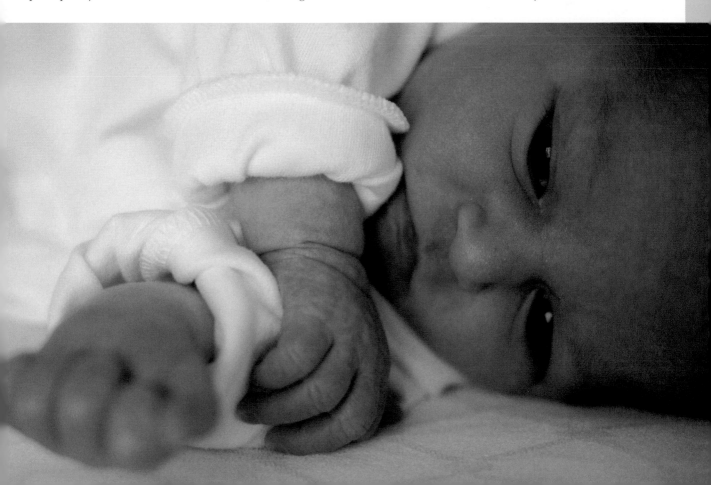

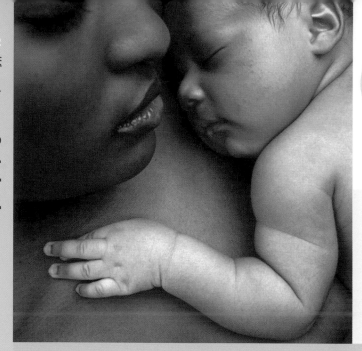

0–1 helping your baby to sleep

Some babies sleep through the night from early on, some do not. As a rule, the more active your baby is and the more energy she uses, the more soundly she sleeps – her sleep being divided between daytime naps and night-time.

Sleep patterns

The way babies fall asleep differs from adults; adults can crash suddenly, whereas babies sleep lightly for about 20 minutes, then go through a transitional stage before reaching deep sleep. **Nothing will wake them, until they've had enough sleep.** This means that babies who are simply "put down" will not necessarily go to sleep peacefully. You may need to nurse your baby to sleep for quite a while, so try to be patient, particularly if you are trying to get him back to sleep at night, when you are longing to go back to bed yourself.

Where should a baby sleep?

Where a baby sleeps isn't important to start with. He won't automatically fall asleep when put into a darkened bedroom; light doesn't bother him at all. He's much more likely to be disturbed by being too hot or too cold. Your baby will be happiest going to sleep hearing your voices and the household noises that he is used to in the background, so from the start, be kind to yourselves and the baby by letting him sleep in a Moses basket or carrycot placed in whichever room you happen to be.

Using a baby monitor

If you leave your baby in another room, set up a baby monitor so you can hear him as soon as he wakes.

Bear in mind that your baby may feel disturbed by the silence when you leave the room, and this could make him more fretful; leave the door open so he can hear you moving around the house – unless you have a cat which may climb into the cot. Avoid going back into the room once your baby is asleep; your smell could wake him, so resist the temptation to check on him too frequently.

Encouraging longer sleep periods at night

A young baby requires nourishment and calories at regular intervals, so he'll wake for a feed when his body tells him he needs it. The way to encourage your baby to sleep for a stretch (four, then rising to five or six hours) during the night is to make sure he's taken in sufficient calories to last that long. This means feeding him whenever he shows he's hungry during the day. As he steadily gains weight, he can go longer between feeds and by about six weeks he could be sleeping for at least one period of about six hours – hopefully during the night. **When he wakes for a night feed, make as little fuss as possible:** feed him in bed; if he needs changing, do it gently and quickly in a dim light. Don't make this a time for chatting and games and he'll begin to learn that waking at night doesn't bring any special privileges.

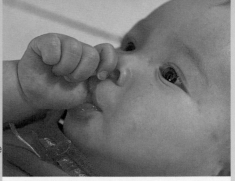

Dummies

Babies are born with a sucking reflex. Without it, they wouldn't suckle or be able to nourish themselves. **I feel it's important that babies are allowed to indulge their desire to suck.**

Some babies are more "sucky" than others. One of mine wanted to suck all the time, whether he was hungry or not. With all my sons, I used to put their thumb gently into their mouth so they could suck to soothe themselves. **But at the same time, I see nothing wrong with using dummies as comforters,** although very young babies will not take to them readily.

There are several types of dummy. Some are moulded to the shape of the baby's mouth; others are designed to move in and out like a human nipple when sucked.

Dummies for a very young baby should be sterilized in the same way as feeding bottles and teats. But once your child is being weaned and starts to use his fingers for feeding himself, it is pointless to sterilize dummies. Careful washing and rinsing are all that is needed. Have several dummies so that they can be changed for fresh ones when they get damaged.

Sleep tips for older babies

● Keep the time just before bed as happy and pleasant as possible.
● Try giving a comfort suck from the breast or the bottle just before putting your baby to bed.
● Develop a routine and stick to it. Don't just put your baby straight to bed: work out a routine of play, bath, bed, story, song and then say goodnight. But don't leave the room; quietly tidy up so that your baby learns that she can drift off to sleep without actually "losing" you.
● Let your baby develop comfort habits such as using a blanket, a muslin square, a handkerchief, a doll or her own thumb. There is nothing wrong with any of these. There's no particular age at which comforters should or shouldn't be used and, like bed-wetting, children grow out of them.

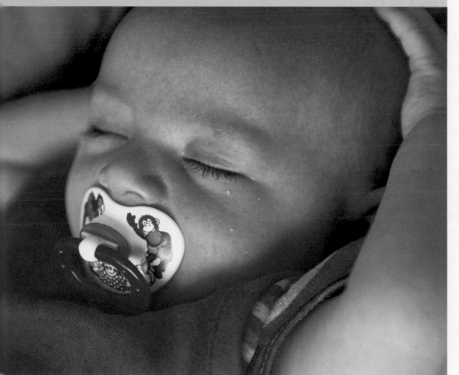

Soothing and settling your baby

There are numerous ways to soothe and console your baby if she's crying. As a general rule, most babies respond to either movement or sound, or both.
● Any movement that rocks her, whether it is you holding and rocking her in your arms, going gently back and forth on a swing or rocking her in a cradle or rocking chair.
● Walking or dancing with an emphasis

on rhythmic movement, since it will remind her of the time when she was being jogged inside your uterus.
● Bouncing her gently in your arms, the cot or on the bed.
● Putting her in a sling and walking around with her. If you're on your own, just get on with whatever you want to do and try to ignore the crying.
● Taking her for a ride in the car or in

a pram, or for a walk in a sling, even at night (you may want to take a mobile phone with you).
● Any form of music as long as it is calm, rhythmic and not too loud; special CDs are available.
● A steady household noise, for instance the washing machine.
● Your own soft singing voice, especially if you sing a lullaby.

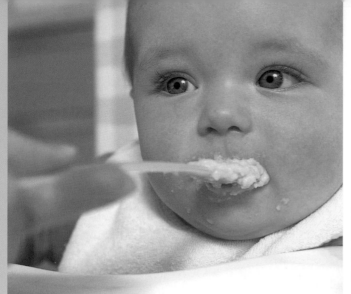

0-1 caring for your baby

Looking after your baby does not require any specialist skills – just some basic knowledge, plenty of common sense and a willingness to ask for help and advice.

Immunizations

Immunization is vital to every growing child to make sure the immune system is strengthened. **Most parents don't realize that when we vaccinate our babies we don't just protect our own, we protect all other babies.** If the number of babies vaccinated against measles drops below 75 percent, measles can escape into communities. For a community of babies to be protected, 95 percent must be vaccinated.

● Before the addition of mumps vaccine to create the MMR, mumps caused 1,200 hospital admissions a year in the UK and was the most common cause of viral meningitis in children under 15. Mumps can also cause permanent deafness.

● Measles has nasty complications including encephalitis, ear infections and pneumonia.

● Fifteen percent of children who suffer from measles encephalitis will die and 20–40 percent of survivors will suffer brain damage.

● I sincerely do not believe there is any scientific evidence to support a connection between the MMR and autism.

● Nor is there any evidence that giving the vaccine in three separate doses is safer than giving it in a single dose.

How effective is MMR vaccine?

Following the introduction of MMR vaccine in 1988, there have been only 11 deaths due to measles in the last 10 years compared to an average of 13 per year from 1970 to 1988.

Why immunize if the diseases are so rare?

There are several important reasons.

● The diseases are now rare but will only remain rare because of vaccination.

● These diseases can have serious consequences. As the uptake of the vaccine has fallen in the UK, there will be infant deaths.

● These highly contagious diseases can be brought into the UK by visitors, putting unimmunized children at risk.

● There will always be some susceptible children who cannot be vaccinated, so high immunization rates must be maintained to prevent epidemics.

Breast-feeding

Breast-feeding has to be learned and you should seek support and advice from your family, from friends with babies, and from your midwife or health visitor. Above all you will learn from your baby, by understanding his signals and discovering how to respond to them.

Colostrum and breast milk

During the 72 hours after delivery, the breasts produce a thin, yellow fluid called colostrum, made up of water, protein and minerals. Colostrum contains antibodies that protect the baby against a range of intestinal and respiratory infections. In the first few days, your baby should be put regularly to the breast, both to feed on the colostrum and to get used to fixing on the breast.

Once your breasts start to produce milk, you may be surprised by its watery appearance. When your baby sucks, the first milk that he gets – the foremilk – is thin, watery and thirst-quenching. Then comes the hindmilk, which is richer in fat and protein.

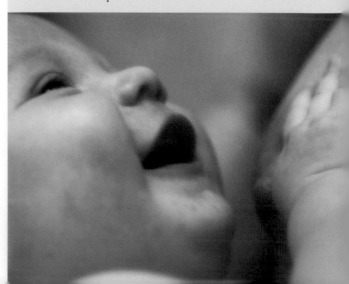

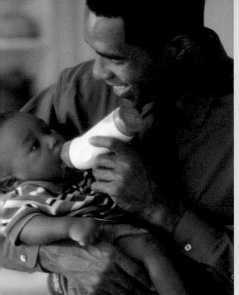

Vegetarian weaning

A growing baby can get all the nutrients necessary for health and vitality from a diet that excludes meat, fish and poultry, provided a proper balance of the different food groups is maintained.

● Your baby's main source of calories will still be milk, so give this at each feed.

● Cereals and grains provide carbohydrates and some protein for energy, while vegetables and fruits supply essential vitamins and minerals. Pulses (puréed or mashed beans or lentils), eggs, cheese and cheese sauce provide protein and minerals for growth and development.

Hard cheese, eggs, nuts and gluten should not be given to your baby before he is six months old.

Foods for teethers

When your baby is teething, she will like to chew and suck to soothe her gums. Any piece of raw vegetable or fruit that is large enough to hold easily and can be sucked or chewed makes a good teething food, particularly if it is chilled but not frozen solid. The following are all suitable:

● green celery stick
● Italian breadstick
● oven-baked rusks
● peeled cucumber
● peeled raw apple
● plain oat biscuit
● teething biscuit
● carrot stick.

Never leave your baby alone while she is eating in case she chokes.

Bottle-feeding tips

Bottle-feeding is straightforward, but you will need to make sure that your baby can swallow properly, and that she is not taking in air with the milk.

● Before you start feeding, test the temperature of the milk by dropping a little on to the inside of your wrist. It should feel neither too hot nor too cold.

● Never leave your baby with the bottle propped up on a pillow or cushion; this can be dangerous. She could become very uncomfortable if she swallows a lot of air with the feed, and could choke. She will also miss the cuddling she should enjoy while she feeds.

● Tilt your baby on your arm. It is very difficult for your baby to swallow when she is lying flat so don't feed her in this position; she may gag or even be sick.

● If your baby has a blocked nose she can't swallow and breathe at the same time. Your doctor can give you nose drops to be used before each feed.

● Don't change your milk formula without first consulting your midwife or health visitor, even if you think your baby doesn't like it. It is very unusual for a brand of milk to be responsible for a baby not feeding well; very rarely cow's milk causes allergies in babies and your doctor may advise you to use a substitute soya formula.

● Your baby knows when she's had enough, so don't try to force her to go on feeding and finish the bottle after she has stopped sucking.

Keeping baby teeth healthy

Make toothbrushing fun for your baby.

● Start brushing your baby's teeth as soon as the first one appears in his mouth.

● Babies are born mimics and one way your baby will learn is by watching you brush your teeth, so make sure he sees you.

● Use a small baby brush and a tiny smear of fluoride toothpaste.

● Make toothbrushing part of a baby's morning and bedtime routine.

● Baby toothpastes may have a milder taste but do not give as much fluoride protection. Check with your dentist whether they provide enough fluoride for your baby's needs.

● Sing a song as you brush his teeth. Make up a toothbrush song to a favourite nursery rhythm.

Weaning tips

Somewhere towards the end of five or six months, according to her size, is a good time to start to wean your baby on to solid foods. By this time she's drinking milk to full capacity at each feed but still doesn't have enough calories for her needs.

Have a small amount of prepared food to hand. Start by feeding her from one breast or giving half the usual bottle, then give one or two teaspoons of food. The midday meal is ideal because your baby will not be ravenous but will be wide-awake and cooperative.

● Your baby may be reluctant to try new foods, so give her time to get used to each food and don't persist if she seems to dislike something.

● Use unprocessed infant cereals rather than ones that are ready mixed and make them up in small quantities.

● Don't give foods containing nuts, gluten, whole cow's milk or egg until at least six months, to minimize the risk of your child developing allergies later.

● Give one new food at a time. Try it once and wait a few days before giving it again to see if there's a reaction.

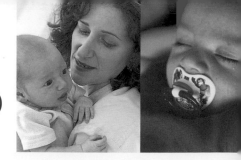

0-1 the baby skill map

0-1 months   1-2 months   2-3 months   3-4 months   4-5 mont

In developing skills such as language and movement all babies follow the same path, but the time it takes to reach each milestone varies from one baby to another. The ages given below are only a rough guide. All you have to do to help a skill develop is take your lead from your baby.

gets excited at sight of breast or bottle

looks at own hand

spontaneous smile

mind
listens and is alert

supports upper body

moving
lifts head to 45°

blows raspberries and bubbles

squeals

talking
mouths

grasps rattle

holds hands open

hands
grasps your finger tightly

cries at disapproving tone of your voice

friendliness
jigs whole body when sees you

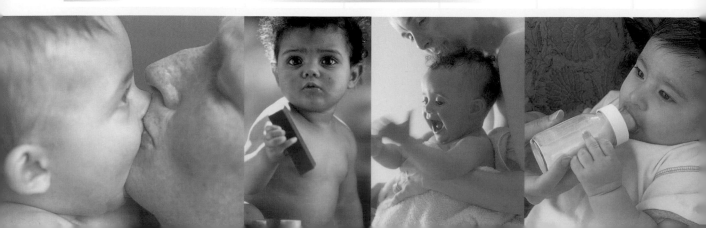

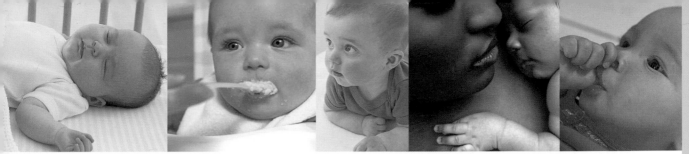

-6 months 6-7 months   7-8 months   8-9 months 9-10 months 10-11 months 11-12 months

shows you things in a book and shakes head for "no"

waves goodbye

holds arms out

understands "no"

stands and cruises

crawls

sits unsupported

"dada" and "mama" with meaning

single syllables "da" and "ma"

stacks bricks

bangs cubes together

points – then thumb/finger grasp

grasps with one hand

reaches out

loves theatrical show of emotions, laughs at "jokes"

plays clapping games

touches your face and touches other babies

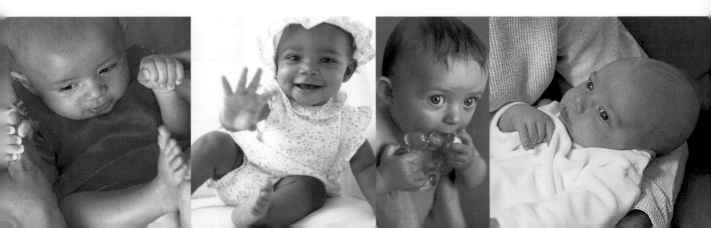

0-1 how your baby learns to move

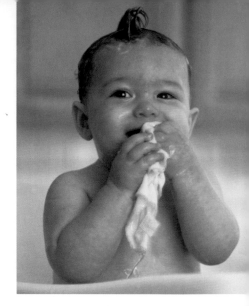

Movement begins with head control. Your baby cannot sit up, stand up or crawl without being able to control the position of her head. Development of any kind goes from head to toe.

Lifts head

By two to three months your baby is really learning how to use and control his body. This means that he
● has stronger neck muscles so there's much less head lag when you pull him into a sitting position. His head is steady for several minutes when he's held in a sitting position or is propped up, but his back is curved
● can raise his head and hold it up when lying on his tummy and he's learned to lift his chest off the horizontal by supporting himself a little on his hands, wrists and arms
● practises bending his knees while lying prone
● enjoys the control that he now has over his movements and kicks and waves his arms about when he's lying down – for this reason, never leave him unattended on a changing table or bed.

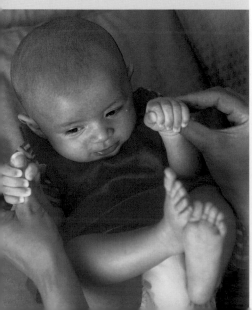

Supports upper body

By four to five months your baby's muscles are developing fast. She's gaining all-important head control and so she can
● move her head from side to side easily, without it wobbling
● keep her head in line with her body when she's pulled to sitting without it lagging behind – a major milestone in her development
● keep her head steady when sitting up, even if gently rocked to and fro
● raise her chest off the floor when she is lying on her tummy and look forwards steadily, supporting herself on her arms.

Now that her upper body is strong and mobile and head control is complete you can play bouncing games on your knee. She may also start to roll from her front to her back, so play floor games and roly-poly.

Safety tips

Before your baby starts walking make your home childproof.
● Never leave your baby alone.
● Remove all furniture with sharp edges and corners from the room.
● Remove anything breakable from a surface that is less than a metre (3ft) from the floor.
● Make sure there are no electric wires trailing across the floor.
● Make sure all electric points are covered with safety plugs.
● Make sure that there are no switches less than a metre (3ft) from the floor.
● Make sure that all doorways and stairways have adjustable safety gates.
● Try and keep the floor clear of small, sharp toys.
● Make sure all fires are guarded.
● Don't leave any cloths hanging from tables that a baby could reach and pull.
● Make sure that all furniture and fixtures are sturdy and safely attached.
● Never leave anything hot on a table in the same room as your baby.
● Make sure that stair banisters are too narrow for a small child to squeeze through.
● Make sure that all cupboard doors are closed firmly and that the handles are out of a crawling baby's reach; if they aren't, lock them or seal them up with masking tape.
● Make sure there are no containers of poisonous substances on the floor or within reach.

Sits unsupported

At six to seven months he'll make great strides in the way he moves. Now he
- can lift one hand off the floor in the press-up position and take all his weight on one arm
- can sit quite safely without support
- is strong enough to lift his head to look around when he's lying on his back
- can roll over from his back to his tummy (much harder than the other way round)
- can use his muscles to straighten his legs without wobbling so that he can take his whole weight steadily when you stand him on your lap
- bounces by bending and stretching his ankles, knees and hips.

Now he can roll over from his back to his tummy, try some floor games. Don't be afraid to be a bit silly – he's developing a great sense of humour and it's good for you too. On his tummy he can rest on one hand so give him things to reach when in this position to improve his balance and strength.

Starting to move

By eight to nine months your baby is discovering that sitting up isn't enough – she wants to propel her body and to try to bring herself upright. Encourage her to pull herself up by placing furniture that will give purchase and hold her upright yourself. Her muscles have developed to the extent that she
- can sit for up to 10 minutes before she gets tired
- can lean forward without falling, although she can't lean sideways or swivel at the waist
- won't give up if she wants to reach an object, she'll try various ways of moving to reach it, but she still over-balances
- may roll over to get to a sitting position and may move around this way
- may try crawling movements if you lie her on her tummy and ask her to come towards you; don't be surprised if she goes backwards though – her brain can't yet sort out the correct muscles for forwards and backwards
- may pull herself to standing in her cot or by holding on to furniture, but she flops down because she hasn't the balance or coordination to sit down in a controlled way.

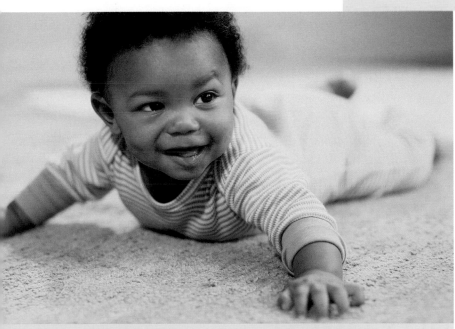

Crawls

By nine to ten months your baby may really be on the move and he
- can pull himself up to standing with ease, confidence and good balance
- crawls or shuffles on his bottom, pulling himself forwards with his hands, but his tummy may still not be completely off the floor when crawling
- may miss out crawling or shuffling altogether, but however he moves, he's confidently mobile and moves forwards on to his hands and knees when he's sitting
- loves his movement skills – he'll roll over and over, get himself into a sitting position, pull himself to standing, then sit down again
- can nearly control the movement from standing to sitting without toppling over. **He's learning to balance his body now because he**
- is beginning to twist his trunk around in an attempt to swivel, but is still unsure
- can move from his tummy to sitting up and from sitting up to lying on his tummy
- has perfect balance when seated. He's so good at crawling you'll be worn out if you try to crawl at the same rate! Create play tunnels and play crawling chase games on the floor or out on the grass in the garden.

Stands and cruises

By ten to eleven months, your baby is striving to get upright most of the time and she
- tentatively practises lots of pre-walking movements, so when she's standing holding on to the furniture or your hands, she'll lift her foot off the ground in a stepping movement and may stamp her foot a few times
- can scamper about swiftly on all fours if she's a crawler, with her tummy well clear of the floor

- can lean over sideways when sitting without toppling over
- can twist her trunk right around to reach something behind her and still keep her balance
- will cruise around the furniture to reach something she particularly wants. Now she'll start to pull herself up and cruise around the furniture, so help her with a treasure trail or an obstacle course or hold her hands to encourage her to walk. Be adventurous!

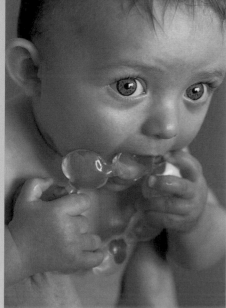

0–1 learning how to use her hands

Your baby was born with the reflex to grasp anything that is placed in her palm – such as your finger – and not let go. At first your baby has little interest in her hands, but as she becomes more aware of her body they'll begin to fascinate her more and more, and she gets more dextrous.

Grasps your finger tightly

It will be a while before your baby realizes his hands are a part of him or that he has any control over them. His fingers remain tightly curled for at least the first three weeks of his life.

Once the grasp reflex that he was born with is lost, his hands relax and they will begin to open. Meanwhile your baby will hang on to your finger even when he's asleep. Play with his hands and fingers to encourage him to open his fists.

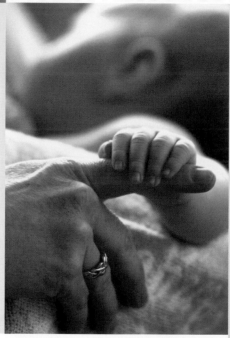

Grasps rattle

At four to five months your baby is beginning to realize that his hands are great tools and he
● has found his toes and discovered he can pull them into his mouth
● puts everything, including his fists, into his mouth as it's his most sensitive area
● tries to grasp his toys for the first time with his hand wide open, palm down, and mainly by curling his little finger in to his palm – he can only do this with quite large objects because he hasn't any fine finger movements yet
● reaches out for everything, grabbing and hitting, but beware – he loves to grab hold of long hair!
● loves crumpling paper, clothing or blankets.

Holds hands open

At one to two months your baby will soon be fascinated by her hands. In preparation for this, she
● has completely lost the grasp reflex she was born with by the end of the second month – her fingers are hardly ever curled in a fist now, they remain wide open most of the time, ready for clasping things she wants in her palm
● is becoming aware of her fingers and she'll begin to study them intently by the end of the second month
● has very sensitive fingertips and enjoys having them held, tickled and massaged by you
● may take a swipe at a toy which is held out to her. She'll miss at this stage – even though her arm movements are becoming more purposeful, her ability to judge the distance between the object and her hand (known as her hand-eye coordination) is still quite poor, as is her muscle control.
Increase her awareness of her hands by using all kinds of tactile stimulation. Open her hands and tickle her palms.

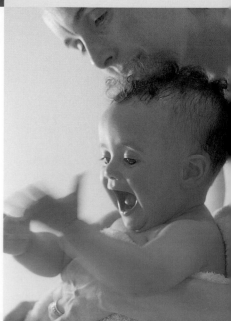

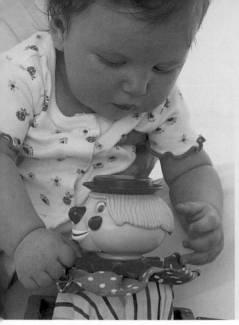

Grasps with one hand

By six to seven months your baby's grasp is becoming more and more precise – it's the key to so much future learning and independence. He's also putting things expertly in his mouth to explore so don't let him hold very small objects that he can swallow. He has so much more control over his hands and arms now and he

● can easily pass a toy from one hand to another

● reaches for a toy with one hand and not two as previously

● reaches for a cube with his fingers instead of palming it with an open hand

● holds on to one cube in one hand and takes another cube offered to him in the other.

Help your baby practise his grasping and improve his coordination by giving him finger foods and his bottle to hold, and introduce him to a two-handled cup for drinking. Give him small objects to hold between his fingers (but not so small he can swallow and choke on them). He loves to make a noise so show him how to bang with the flat of his hand and play "Pat-a-cake".

Fine grasp

By nine to ten months, your baby will be able to do a lot more with her toys now that she

● reaches out for small objects with her forefinger guiding her hand accurately to them

● has entirely mastered her fine grasp between finger and thumb

● has excellent hand-eye coordination so she can pick up a small object with ease (but be careful what you leave lying around)

● loves dropping and picking up games now that she can release her grip – she'll drop toys endlessly from her highchair and she'll watch them fall, she knows exactly where they've gone even if they roll out of sight and she'll shout and point for you to pick them up again

● loves rummaging in bags and boxes and will repeatedly take things out and put them back.

The finest movement she'll ever learn – the pincer grip between thumb and forefinger – is perfected at this time, so give her small, safe objects to pick up on her highchair tray or give her a treasure basket to sort.

Points – then thumb/finger grasp

At eight to nine months your baby's grasp is getting finer. His ability to handle small objects is improving and he demonstrates this perfectly when he

● tries to turn over the pages of a book, although he often turns several at a time

● holds a brick in each hand and can bang them together

● holds an object between his thumb and fingers

● "rakes up" small pieces of food, like raisins, with his fingers and thumb.

Pointing is an important milestone in his development. Control of the index finger is the first step towards mastering the very fine skill of bringing together the thumb and forefinger to nip or pinch small objects, which happens between 10 and 12 months. Give him small objects such as raisins and cooked peas to pick up to practise his grip and hand-eye coordination.

Encourage him to point at things by asking, "What do you want?" and "Show Daddy". Point at the pictures as you look at books together to encourage him to copy.

Show him how to stack bricks one on top of the other because he can release his grasp now.

Stacks bricks

By eleven to twelve months her wrist bones have grown so her hands are more manoeuvrable and she

● is much more accurate at getting food into her mouth with a spoon

● has stopped mouthing everything she picks up – how an object feels in her hands is more important now

● is quite good at throwing

● can hold two bricks in one hand

● is able to build a tower of two blocks, thanks to her improved hand-eye coordination and steadiness

● will hold a crayon and may try to scribble if you show her how.

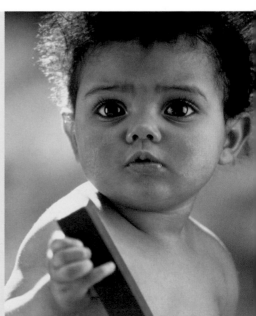

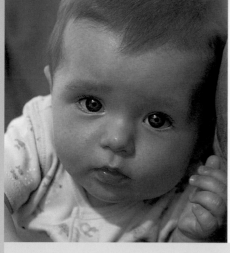

0–1 your baby's mind

Your baby's world is a confused blur of sights and sounds at first, and in the early weeks he is fully occupied with sorting out the things that have significance. Your face and voice will be among the first things he recognizes.

Listens and is alert

Your baby "understands" from the moment of birth – he's not inanimate. You can chart his progress in the first month. For example:

Day 1 He "stills" when he hears your voice – he becomes quiet and alert, his body stops moving and he concentrates on listening.

Day 3 He responds when spoken to and his gaze becomes intense.

Day 5 At 20–25cm (8–10in) he's attracted to things that move so will watch your moving lips or your gently fluttering fingers with interest.

Day 9 His eyes will "dart" at the sound of a high-pitched voice, indicating that he can hear you.

Day 14 He can tell you apart from other people.

Day 18 He turns his head to sounds.

Day 28 He's learning how to express and control his emotions and will adjust his behaviour to the sound of your voice: he'll get upset if you speak roughly or loudly and quieten if your voice is soothing.

Play your baby some classical music. As well as soothing him it will encourage him to listen, make sounds and, believe it or not, add up numbers later.

Spontaneous smile

By one to two months your baby is taking more of an interest in her surroundings and soon she

● knows who you are and recognizes you, she's very interested to see you and shows her excitement by jerking her whole body with pleasure, kicking and waving her legs and arms

● smiles readily as soon as her eyes can focus at any distance, usually around six weeks

● watches what's going on around her; if she's propped up on cushions or in a bouncing chair, she will look in the direction of any sounds and movements

● stares steadily at things that interest her as though she's "grasping" them with her eyes.

When she smiles, smile back and tell her she's clever. Smiling means she's happy so let her know you're happy too. She loves looking at things so make sure she has plenty to look at – frequently change pictures or mobiles hanging over her cot to give lots of interest.

Looks at own hand

Even at two to three months she's a keen thinker and she

● is fascinated by her own body and is beginning to understand that she can make it move – the first step in understanding the concept of cause and effect

● enjoys looking intently at her hands and fingers while she moves them in front of her face

● is attracted by moving objects and has sufficient control over her head to follow a slow-moving object with her eyes – if you hold a brightly coloured toy in front of her, she'll take a moment to focus on it and then her eyes will follow it to either side as you move it (in a week or two she'll be able to focus instantly and follow the movement easily)

● is very curious about what goes on around her and watches everything with interest – sit her propped up so she can see better.

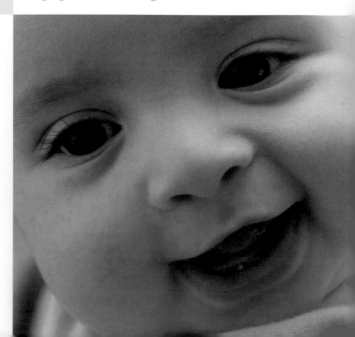

Gets excited at the sight of breast or bottle

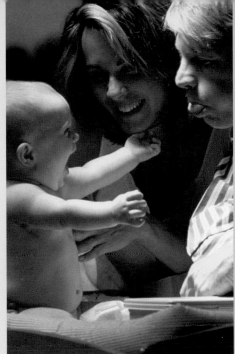

At four to five months he is asserting his personality and relating more to other people. He
● loves the breast or bottle and shows this by patting it when feeding
● has a repertoire of emotions such as fear, anger, disgust, frustration, sadness and pleasure to which he wants you to respond sympathetically – and you should because it makes him feel comfortable with his emotions
● loves all games because this is the way he learns and as he wants to learn he'll join in anything you suggest. He'll even make up simple games like

splashing the bath water and he studies intently the effect of his hands and feet in the water
● is learning to concentrate, and spends a long time just looking at something he holds in his hands, although he often drops it
● smiles at his reflection in a mirror, although he doesn't yet realize it's actually himself
● moves his arms and legs to attract your attention and makes noises to call you to him
● is desperate to learn and to imitate, so try new games with rhymes and actions.

Understands "no"

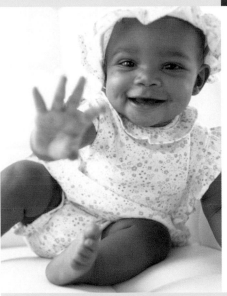

By seven to eight months you'll notice signs that your baby understands what you say even though she can't speak words with meaning. At this time she
● can remember opposites through touch (hot and cold; hard and soft)
● understands some differences – for example, "Mummy's coat", "Baby's coat"
● can begin to judge the size of objects up to a metre (3ft) away
● understands phrases if they're part of routines so when you go into the bathroom she understands, "It's time for a bath"
● understands that "no!" means stop, don't do it or don't touch
● shows determination and reaches for a toy she really wants – she's persistent and may cry with frustration if she's unsuccessful
● plays for a long time with her toys, examining and concentrating on them
● is becoming very assertive about showing she wants to feed herself. Now that she understands the words "yes" and "no", use them all the time. Be extra positive about "yes" and be careful about saying "no".
     Try not to make "no" an automatic reaction because she'll soon figure out you're just pulling rank. Always make "yes!" a celebration.

Waves goodbye

By nine to ten months your baby enjoys showing off her understanding. See how she
● is becoming very familiar with routines and enjoys them
● puts her foot up when you hold out her sock and holds her hand up to go into the sleeve of her coat
● waves "bye-bye" when you say it
● knows her favourite soft toys and pats and strokes them when you say, "nice teddy".

Shows you things in a book and shakes head for "no"

By ten to eleven months his recognition skills and his understanding of concepts are sharpening so that he
● points to familiar things in a book that he likes
● understands that the cat and kitten in his book, his toy kitten and Granny's cat are all cats, even though they're so different
● enjoys playing games that involve opposites – hot/cold, rough/smooth, round/square, big/little – especially if you act them out

● still has a short attention span when looking at books and will want to turn the pages quickly
● is learning about cause and effect – drop the brick and you pick it up, bang the drum and it makes a noise, shake the rattle and it rings a bell
● enjoys putting things into a container and taking them out and pouring water into and out of containers in the bath
● nods or shakes his head to indicate "yes" and "no" to simple questions like "Do you want a drink?"

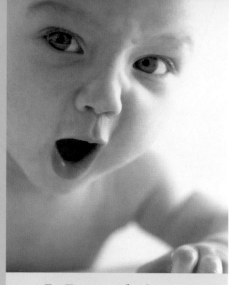

0-1 how your baby learns to talk

Babies need and want to communicate from the very earliest days, and even before they begin to talk to you they will listen and try to imitate sounds.

Mouthing

Your baby was born wired for sound and is longing to talk. He's a natural conversationalist.

● From birth he'll respond if you speak animatedly to him with your face 20-25cm (8-10in) from his by "mouthing" with his lips and tongue, like a fish.

● From two weeks he makes his own non-specific sounds.

● From three weeks he has a baby sound vocabulary.

● From four weeks he understands the interchange of conversation and knows how to respond when you talk to him. From early on he leads the conversation and *you* follow *him*.

The more your baby is talked to and encouraged to respond, the earlier he will learn to speak and the better will be the quality of his speech. Start talking to your baby the instant he's born and never stop. Say his name over and over (and watch his eyes dart in response).

Squeals

By two to three months he's found his voice and takes every opportunity to practise his full range. In doing so he

● makes all kinds of noises to indicate pleasure – you'll hear squeals, gurgles, shouts and cooing sounds

● may be starting to add consonants to his vowel sounds, the first normally being "m", then the explosives – you can help him by showing him how to blow raspberries

● tends to use "p" and "b" when unhappy, and then by three months he'll use more guttural sounds, "j" and "k", when happy.

Speak rhythmically in a sing-song voice and laugh a lot; jog him in time to your rhythmic speech. Respond to the many different kinds of noises your baby is now beginning to make by talking as much as possible to him while making full eye contact. Repeat every sound your baby makes.

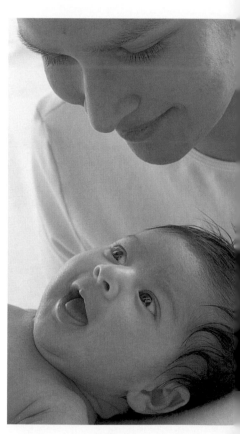

"Dada" and "Mama" with meaning

At nine or ten months your baby understands language as more than just vocal patterns. As proof of this new skill she

● understands the precise meaning of quite a few words, although she can't say any yet

● may say one word with meaning by about this age, but don't worry if she doesn't do this, just

understanding the meaning is more important for now

● develops the word "Mama" soon after "Dada", which she says more often when Mummy is present than when she's not

● might begin to sound the beginning of words like "do" for "dog" – help her hear the "g" on the end of the word by emphasizing it with another

syllable, as in "doggie", "horsey", "Mummy", "Daddy".

She's babbling away so babble with her. Ask lots of simple questions and recite nursery rhymes to promote her understanding of words. Repeat her words, such as "Dada" for Daddy, "doe-doe" for dog, but with meaning – say, "Yes, there's Daddy" or "Look at this picture of a dog."

Single syllables

At five to six months she's getting the hang of taking turns in conversation and trying new sounds. Listen as she

- attempts to converse with her mirror image and has a "conversation" of gurgles with herself
- has a growing repertoire of speech sounds, especially the blowing and raspberry sounds that she practises all the time
- makes special sounds to attract your attention, even trying a cough
- starts to join real vowels and real consonants together in a simple way, saying "ka", "da", "ma" and "ergh"
- is intent on imitating your conversation and uses her tongue a lot, poking it out and playing with it between her lips
- begins to respond to her name – use it at every opportunity so she'll achieve a sense of self and feel important
- understands bits of what you say, such as, "Here's your bottle", "Daddy's coming," "yes" and "no"
- begins to babble – repeats sounds over and over, listens, then tries them out again.

Talk to her all the time – tell her what you're doing all the time, point out interesting things, especially animals, when you're out and about. Repeat phrases and praise her when she appears to understand you. Sing songs and say rhymes to her. Play clapping games together. Read books together, pointing, naming and making the sounds of animals.

Blows bubbles

At three to four months your baby will start trying to hold a "conversation" with you now that he

- makes more than simple vowel and consonant sounds
- tries to imitate sentences like yours by stringing sounds together or coming out with "words" like "gaga" or "ahgoo"
- can blow through his lips – he shows off his new skill by blowing bubbles
- uses quite a repertoire of sounds, and by 16 weeks he'll express his feelings, many of which signify delight, by chuckling, laughing and squealing. All babies love to make someone laugh – it's instant feedback.

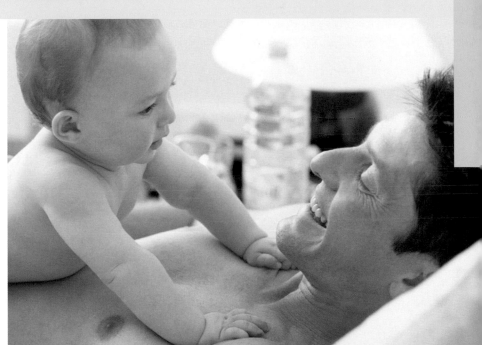

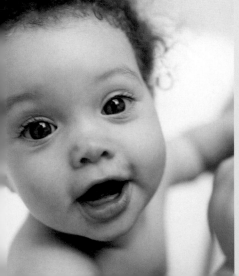

Starting to talk

At eleven to twelve months her speech is really taking off and she

- can say two or three words with meaning and make animal noises
- starts "jargoning" – an imitation of what she hears you say to other people or an attempt to copy the running commentary you keep up when you're with her – you'll notice long ramblings of sound and, here and there, the odd intelligible word
- has completely mastered "yes" and "no" while nodding and shaking her head
- understands simple questions like "Where's your shoe?" or "Where's your book?" and will search for them
- doesn't dribble much any more, a sign that she's gaining control over her tongue, mouth and lips ready for speech. Encourage those first words she uses with meaning by repeating stories with her, repeating nursery rhymes, call and response games, clapping games, music and puppet play.

0–1 your friendly baby

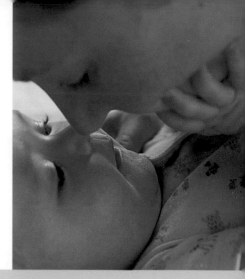

Your baby needs to exchange love and friendliness, especially with you, her parents. She learns to be loving and friendly by imitating you, first with facial expressions, then with gestures and movements, and finally with a whole range of friendly behaviour.

Jigs whole body when sees you

From the moment of birth your baby is a highly developed person with many accomplishments. He is born friendly and longs for company so he
● wants to respond to you and listens and looks intently even at birth
● demonstrates this with whole-body jerks, mouthing, sticking out his tongue, nods, bobs, throwing out his hands and spreading his fingers
● smiles from birth if he can see you talking and smiling at him from a distance of 20–25cm (8–10in)
● loves to have eye contact and skin contact, especially when he's feeding
● can show emotions by using the correct face muscles to smile and grimace – he'll be upset if he hears a harsh-sounding voice.
Cuddle him when he's awake. Try to give him skin-to-skin contact with both parents whenever possible. By stroking, caressing and massaging him you'll make him feel loved and secure.

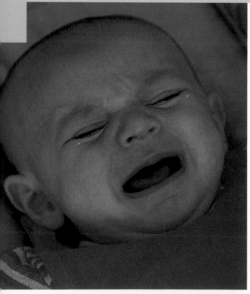

Cries at disapproving tone of your voice

By four to five months your baby is learning how to express his feelings in a variety of ways. By the end of the fifth month he
● knows your voice and its modulations very well and doesn't like the different tone of voice you use when you say "no", although he doesn't yet know what it means
● eagerly smiles at people he knows
● uses body movements, facial expressions and sounds as well as crying, to show his different moods.

Tone of voice

Because your baby is disturbed by an angry tone of voice he'll stop when you sound displeased to see if you really disapprove of him. This response is the basis of all future discipline – all that's needed is a change in the tone of your voice. He loves a friendly voice and will do almost anything to hear one, even refraining from doing what he wants.

Touches your face

By five to six months she's showing love for the first time. Get her to touch your face and say "Hello" as she does so. Put a mirror in a position where she can see herself and help her to pat her image. There are many games you can play with reflections. Teach her to show love with lots of patting and stroking of pets and cuddly toys and show her books with pictures of mother animals and their babies. You'll notice that she
● makes lots of advances to you and wants to touch you, but because she hasn't developed refined movement, she tends to pat you roughly
● loves your face – she'll nuzzle and stroke it and she may also grab a handful of hair!
● may begin to be shy with strangers towards the end of the sixth month – she'll bury her head on your chest if someone she doesn't know speaks to her or to you, and may cry if a stranger picks her up.

Naturally outgoing

At three to four months she's naturally outgoing and at this stage not at all shy. This is clearly seen in the way she
- looks, smiles, grunts and coos at anyone who speaks to her or pays her attention
- knows you and the rest of the family and recognizes family pets
- gets lonely and lets you know she doesn't like being alone for too long when she's awake
- stops crying when you go to her, showing pleasure at your presence
- jigs her body when she sees you
- uses laughter to charm you.

Pats other babies

At six to seven months your baby may like company but he's becoming more self-contained and happy with his own company too. He
- recognizes other babies as being like himself and reaches out to them in friendship
- pats other babies or his own reflection, just as he pats you
- vocalizes to himself and other babies, just as he does to you
- joins in games like "Pat-a-cake" and "This little piggy"
- is very sociable and wants you to understand him so he laughs, coughs, cries, squeals, blows bubbles, smiles and frowns to converse with you.

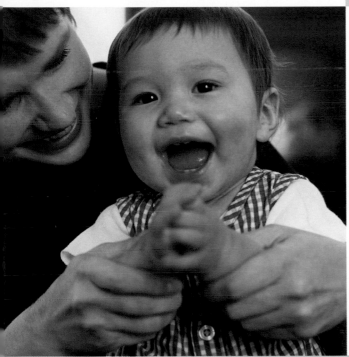

Plays clapping games

By eight to nine months your baby's personality is emerging – he may be serene, a fusspot, noisy, determined, irritable, sensitive. Whatever he's like, he
- loves to join in everything that you do, although he's quite good at playing on his own
- enjoys playing with you – batting balloons or playing clapping games like "Pat-a-cake" – and anticipates actions involved
- understands when someone is going and may start to wave "bye-bye"
- enjoys having a joke and teasing games.

Try some cooperative games like rolling a ball backwards and forwards, Incy-wincy spider and Peep-bo.

Friendliness

By eleven to twelve months your baby knows the power of her affections and will give them or withhold them for effect. For example she
- kisses on request, but won't if she doesn't feel like it
- shows many emotions, especially affection, and will pat the dog, kiss Mummy or hug Daddy
- is apt to be shy with strangers but loves family gatherings and outings in the car or in her buggy
- loves being in a crowd, especially with other children, but she'll hold on to you until she's confident enough to join in – even then she'll keep checking that you're close by and may cry if you leave the room unexpectedly.

She loves babies of her own age so invite little friends to play at your house and go to parent-and-toddler groups where she can meet other babies.

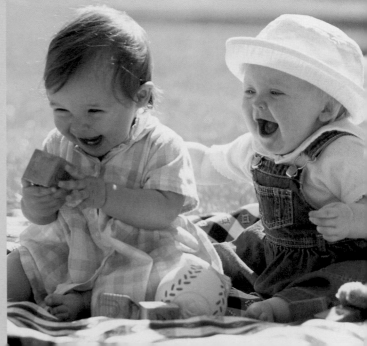

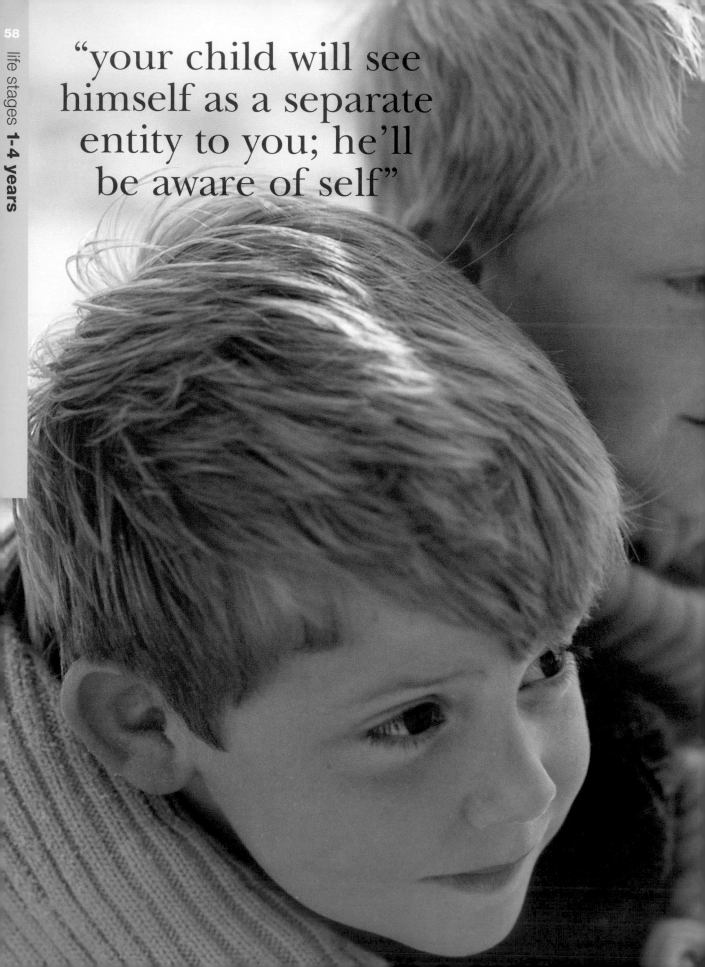

"your child will see himself as a separate entity to you; he'll be aware of self"

life stages: 1 to 4 years

During the first year of your baby's life the accent is on learning physical things: he learns to crawl, to stand up and possibly even to take a few steps. The ability to do these things brings with it a sense of physical achievement and a sense of independence. He is able to go and explore the world without having to wait for you to bring it to him.

During the next few years he'll not only consolidate all the physical skills he acquired in his first year, but he'll also master one of the most difficult intellectual ones – speech. Your child will be struggling to express his thoughts and desires through speech and with his increasingly able brain he'll now see himself as a separate entity to you; he'll be aware of "self". He'll probably be quite frustrated at times and you may notice more tantrums. He'll need a lot of affection, much encouragement and constant support.

Learning spurts

Your child doesn't grow, develop and learn at a constant rate. Learning spurts are well known and every child has them. During a learning spurt, your child will gobble up new ideas, acquire new skills and put them into practice immediately. However, while he's going through these learning spurts some activities, and possibly certain skills that he's already learned, may appear to slip. Don't worry. They won't have gone for good. It is just that your child is using all his concentration to learn something new, but once it is learned he'll regain all the other skills he'd mastered previously.

During a learning spurt try to make your child's life as interesting as possible. Of course if he shows that certain things are enjoyable then you should do them as often as you can, but don't hesitate to introduce him to new things; he is ready to learn and absorb information very fast. And don't be too discriminating about the kind of entertainment you give. Young children simply sieve out what they prefer and understand and let the rest go by.

Such spurts are invariably followed by periods when development appears to slow down. Treat them as recovery periods during which your child can consolidate newly learned skills and prepare himself for the next spurt. Don't get anxious about this – just let him practise the skills that he has already learned. You can help during these slower learning times by playing and practising with him, saying something like "Let's sing that song again", or "Why don't we try to push the peg through the hole again".

Let your child guide you

All the way through life, teachers who succeed do so by helping us to develop and reach our full potential. They maximize our strengths and minimize our weaknesses. As your baby's teacher you should try to make the best of his good points and play down his bad ones.

You also have to give your child the kind of help he needs when he needs it. Giving help is worthless if the person who is being helped doesn't really require it or like it, so while you have to be an active helper, you mustn't be an interfering one. Your baby should not be learning what *you* want him to learn, he should be learning what *he* wants to learn, and this should be your first priority.

You have to suppress any ideas of what you think a child of his age ought to be doing and respond to what he wants to do. This means that you have to be guided by your child and respond to his needs. While it is your job as a good parent to introduce him to as wide a range of interesting things as possible, it isn't your job to decide which of those things he should find interesting. In other words, having presented the menu, you must let him choose the dishes.

In the pages that follow, I offer guidelines where appropriate, advice where I feel there may be a need and strategies for dealing with potentially difficult situations.

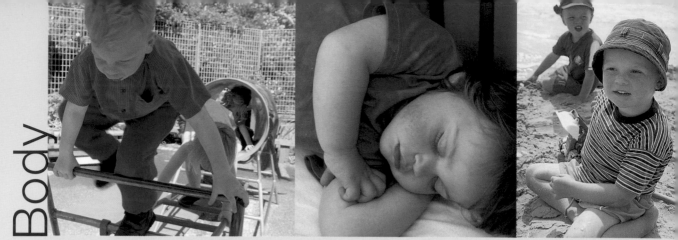

Body

Social

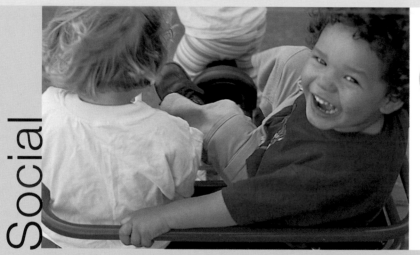

" *be guided by your child and respond to his needs* '

Mind

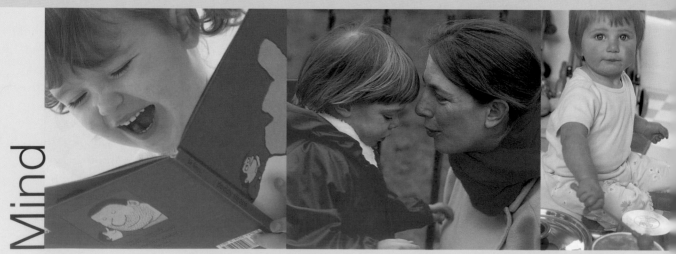

"toddlers need almost constant activity to develop normally"

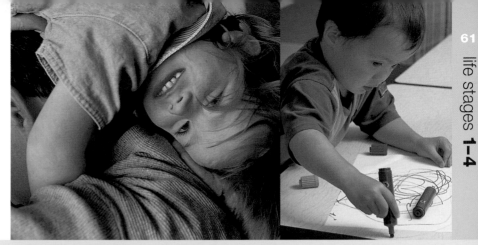

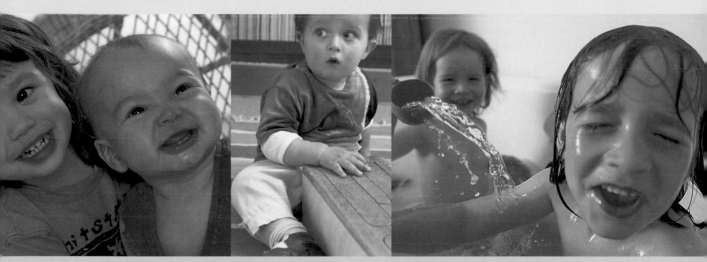

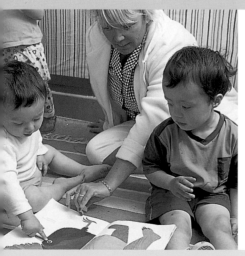

"she is ready to learn and absorb information very fast"

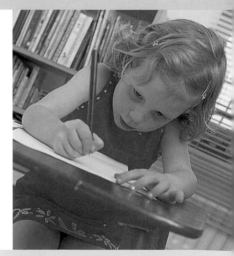

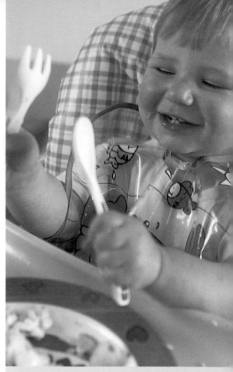

1-4 your growing child

Watching your child grow and develop is one of the most exciting aspects of being a parent, and during the early years you'll be astounded by how quickly he changes.

Why your child should exercise

Human beings were born to be active, not sedentary. Toddlers are so named because they toddle almost ceaselessly. And so they should. Their bodies need almost constant activity in order to develop normally. Woe betide the toddler who isn't encouraged to run around or, even worse, is left parked with a snack to be baby-minded by the Teletubbies. This toddler will be fat because he isn't burning off enough calories with natural exercise. And a fat toddler means a fat child. A fat child may develop diabetes in his teens and be a candidate for heart disease by the time he is in his 20s.

The human race has evolved very efficiently to survive without food for a period. It has never had to accommodate a sedentary life. A sedentary life that starts in infancy can be fatal, so exercise is crucial for your baby and child. Encourage it whenever you can. Join in. Play a family sport even if it's only chucking a ball around.

Encouraging your child to eat

As with all feeding, the key word is flexibility. You and your child should enjoy yourselves, so give a little thought to making mealtimes entertaining.

● If she wants to use a knife, give your child a plastic or blunt-ended one.
● Let her use a straw for drinking sometimes. So that she won't tip the drink over, cut the end of the straw so that there is not too much projecting above the cup.
● Ice cream cones don't have to be used just for ice cream. Fill one with cheese and tomato chopped together or with tuna fish salad and give your three-year-old a snack on the move.
● Be open to innovation and occasionally serve your child's meal on a doll's plate or on a flat toy.
● Fill a cake tin with lots of different finger foods such as cheese cut into cubes, bits of cold meat, raw vegetables, fruit, potato crisps and tiny peanut butter sandwiches and let your child pick out what she wants.
● Let your child "build" her meal from sandwiches, cubes of cheese and vegetables. She could make a house or a car, and eat it when it's finished.

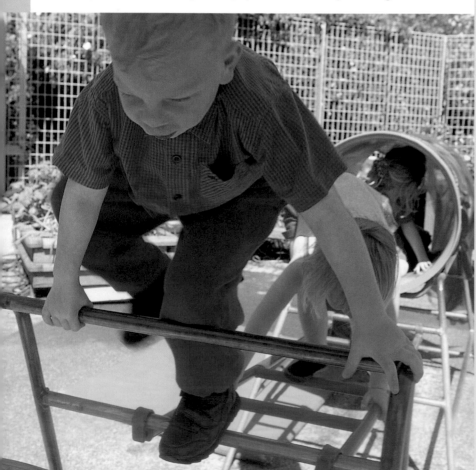

Physical milestones

Remember that every child develops at his own rate. Don't force your child to go more quickly than he wants to – it will serve no purpose. Let him go at his own pace, while still providing all the help and encouragement you can.

13 months

Let him practise standing alone. If you place furniture close together, he'll "cruise" around and may even take his first independent step. Stable toys or pieces of furniture with rounded edges are ideal for holding onto and help independent stepping and cruising. Once he is mobile, keep an eye on him at all times.

15 months

Provide him with a sturdy chair so that he can kneel and lower his body to sit without support and enjoy getting in and out of the chair. You'll be helping him to practise bending and flexing his hips and knees. Make sure the chair will not tip over if he uses it to hold on to when he stands up. His steps are high, unsteady and of unequal length and direction. Use stairguards – he can creep upstairs now.

18 months

Show him how to squat to accelerate his muscle development. Encourage him to imitate you. Climb the stairs with him until he can do so unaided, both feet on each step, though he'll need to hold on. He walks with a steadier, lower-stepping gait, runs, walks backwards, and seldom falls.

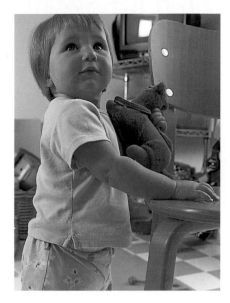

21 months

Let him join in your daily activities because he's fascinated by everything you do and he'll want to imitate your every move. He can pick up objects without falling over now. Encourage games such as football so he can show you how fluent his movements are – he walks backwards easily; he can also walk up stairs, both feet on each step, but without holding on, and can stop quickly and turn corners.

2 years

Encourage dancing and singing because your child is starting to get rhythm, and making movements to rhythmical music is something he'll enjoy. Dance with him – it will also give

him practice in making a wide range of movements. He can run, but not slow down, and can squat with ease so get down on the floor with him.

2½ years

Provide him with a moving toy with wheels that he can sit on and use his feet to propel. He is probably too young for a tricycle, but there are many simpler, suitable moving toys you can get. He'll love to jump with his feet off the ground and walk on tiptoe. He's steady enough on his feet to carry a breakable object and he can sit and hold a baby brother or sister on his knee for a few moments.

3 years

Play hopping games. He's much more nimble so show him jumping games, such as hopscotch, which are also good for working off excess energy. Include hopping in other games such as "Simon says". He can walk up stairs with one foot on each step, stand on one foot for a second, swing his arms like an adult when walking and ride a tricycle.

4 years

Show him how to use a skipping rope because he's now very active and should be well coordinated. All his muscles are working together and play such as this gives him a workout for a wide range of movements. Make sure he has access to outdoor apparatus. He races about, hopping, jumping, climbing and goes downstairs rapidly one foot per step. He can even carry a cup of liquid without spilling any.

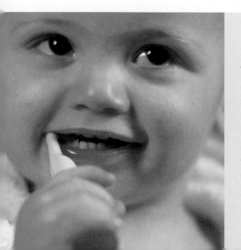

Visiting the dentist

Take your child for her first dental check-up around her second birthday, and make sure this visit is as pleasant as possible. Get your child used to the sight of instruments and the smell of the surroundings by taking her with you when you go for your own check-up. If she can be trusted, and your dentist has no objections, let your child sit on

your lap while the dentist examines you. She'll watch with fascination and will be delighted to copy your example. Just before your child's first visit, play a game of going to the dentist and look into each other's mouths. Then, when you get to the surgery, pre-arrange for the dentist to look at your mouth just before he looks at your child's.

1-4 learning hand skills

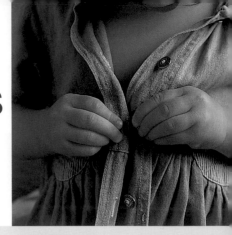

Between the ages of 1 and 4 hand and finger skills really flower. Given how crucial they are for writing, encourage your child all you can.

Hand-eye coordination

Your child's first attempt at hand-eye coordination is feeding herself. She learns how to steer food to her mouth with her hand and eye very quickly and from then on her skills develop rapidly. You can start a one-year-old with stacking blocks and fingerpaints, and go on to materials like Lego and games with a bat and ball.

13 months

Offer food to eat with a spoon. If you give her more solid food that sticks to the spoon, and doesn't slide off easily, she'll be encouraged to feed herself. As she learns to rotate her hand to get the food to her mouth she will become more and more accurate. Throwing things is a favourite game and she can also make lines with a pencil and hold two blocks in her hand. Having mastered relaxing her grip to release objects, she can build a tower of two blocks.

15 months

Help her build towers to increase her hand skills. She can now manage putting three blocks on top of one another. She also tries to turn over the pages of a book, so read with her often. Let her try to put on some of her clothes herself, too. Feeding herself with a spoon, and getting it

to her mouth before anything runs off is quite easy now.

18 months

Give her an activity board or similar toy to practise turning, twisting, spinning, dialling and sliding movements. She's good with zips and other fasteners and they fascinate her. Her fingers are dextrous, so provide the materials for fingerpainting and making scribbles. She'll read a book with you, turning over two or three pages of a book at a time. Give her the chance and she'll feed herself completely and use a cup without spilling anything.

2 years

Encourage her to dress and undress herself and put on her own socks, shoes and gloves as much as she can – plenty of scope for fine finger movements. As she's mastered a screwing movement, she can turn a door knob and unscrew loose lids from jars, and undo and do up a zip, so get her to show you. She can use a pencil more deliberately, so draw together. Let her show you how she can build a tower four cubes high.

2½ years

Give her blocks and toys to build models that require pressing and

fitting pieces together and use the small muscles of the hand. Let her thread beads and show you how she can fasten an easily placed button into a slack buttonhole. Drawings are more representational; she may also build a tower that is eight blocks high.

3 years

Ask her to help with simple tasks that involve a number of coordinated movements, like setting the table. Encourage her to fasten and unfasten buttons by herself, so she can dress and undress herself completely, if she wishes. She'll draw a recognizable image and her towers may now be nine blocks high. Help her start to try to use scissors – a huge step forwards in brain/muscle coordination, and in manual dexterity.

4 years

Give her lots of practice with small movements, such as arranging small toys. She's getting much better at fine tasks, so ask her to set the table properly, wash her own face and hands, make her bed and put her clothes tidily away. Show your four-year-old how to draw a circle and she will. She can also copy two straight lines crossing at right angles, though imperfectly.

Suitable toys

Give your child toys to help her develop coordination and manipulative skills. Toys that make use of both of these will provide the most enjoyment, but be prepared for your child to be a bit hamfisted at first and give her quite large, straightforward items. Household objects are popular, but other toys may stretch both coordination and mental processes further:

- posting box
- stacking blocks
- building blocks
- hammering table
- push/pull toys
- dolls
- cars
- frame
- crayons and felt tips
- paints and brushes
- blackboard
- books
- plasticine
- sand pit
- slide
- paddling pool
- trolley
- swing.

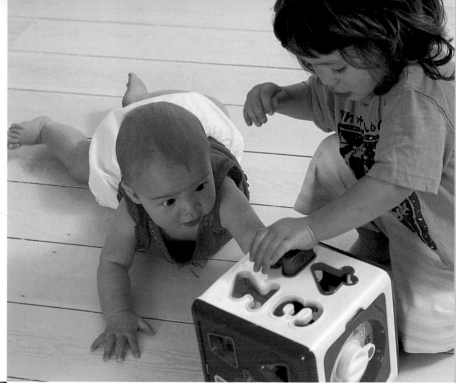

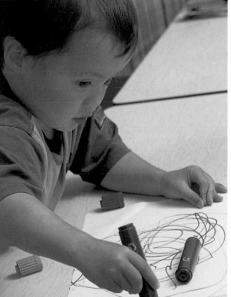

Right- or left-handed?

If both you and your partner are left-handed, 1 in 3 of your children will be too; the chances of this happening with two right-handed parents is 1 in 10. **There is no natural law that states that one hand is superior to the other** so it should never bother you if your child is left-handed.

Your child has no control over which of his hands is dominant; dominance is decided by the developing brain. Think of the brain as two linked halves, each of which controls different activities. One of these sides becomes dominant as your child's brain develops. If it is the left side of the brain that dominates, the child is right-handed. If it is the right side, the child is left-handed. In the first few months your

baby may seem to have no preferences but in fact most newborns turn their heads more to the right than to the left.

As your child's coordination improves and he starts to acquire manual skills, you may find that he starts to use one hand more than the other. Don't be worried if he doesn't do this. Your child will develop at his own speed. Never, ever, try to dissuade your child from being left-handed. You may think that by "encouraging" your child to use his right hand instead of his left you're doing him a favour for later life. You are not. And, what's more, you could well risk causing psychological side effects like stuttering, as well as reading and writing difficulties, by altering what his brain naturally wants to do.

Is my child stimulated enough?

If you provide the right environment and the right equipment, you needn't worry about whether your child is being stimulated enough. At this stage your child is developing his thinking about playing, and what he needs is freedom to allow his thought processes to expand so that he can follow new ideas as they occur to him, and see play though to its conclusions. It is your job to provide the floor space, the tools and uninterrupted time.

You can't teach your child to use his imagination, but you can encourage his natural gift for fantasy by doing the following.
- Play make-believe games with your toddler.
- When you tell a story, act out the character's parts and make up all the various characters' voices.
- Play "What's this?" games. Get your child to shut his eyes then gently stroke

an object across his skin. Ask him to guess what it is.
- Help your child in his imaginary world by giving him some glove puppets – either bought ones or brown paper bags with faces drawn on them.
- Start to stock a dressing-up box. Put in old shoes, shirts, skirts, dresses, hats and scarves. Add some special cheap jewellery as well. Make a cloak from a length of fabric and attach a clasp at one end.

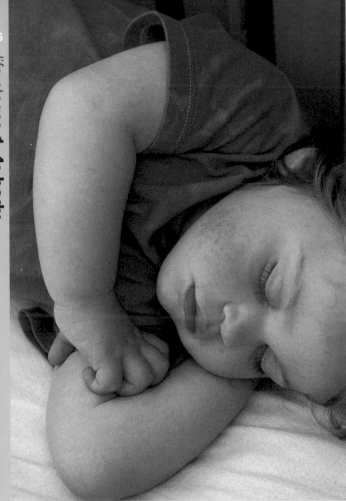

Bedtime routines

Bedtimes should be happy times and even if you're worn out, try your best to be calm and relaxed. If you're not, your child will pick up your anxiety and be fretful, and you may have to spend twice as long trying to get him to go to sleep than if you had given him an extra five minutes of your undivided attention in a quiet, direct way.

Helping your toddler to sleep

● Don't put your child to bed immediately after an exciting game or rough-and-tumble play – he will have great difficulty settling which will be frustrating for you. Give him time to quieten down, sitting with you watching television or looking at a book.
● Even a small child likes looking at a book in bed, so if yours is quite happy, leave him with a favourite non-scary book.
● Put a dab of your perfume or aftershave on your child's pillow and suggest that he breathes it in deeply. Deep breathing is relaxing and calming and will help your child go off to sleep.
● Give your child a bath before bedtime and follow this with a warm drink and a story in bed.
● There is nothing magical about bedrooms. Let your child go to sleep where he is most comfortable: at your feet on the floor, on a couch, in your lap.
● Be flexible about bedtimes. Left to themselves, most children go to sleep at around seven or eight o'clock in the evening, whether you put them to bed or not. Why should they be unhappy in a room on their own, instead of happy in your company?

1-4 daily care

Keep your child healthy by looking after her hygiene and sleep needs and making sure she has a safe environment.

Safety

Once your child starts to move around the house easily, your main concern will be to keep her safe. Here are some guidelines:

Indoors
● Block open stairways and other unsafe areas with gates. These should be made of a rigid mesh with a straight top edge and should be swung open from a fixed surround.
● The bathroom and kitchen may contain poisonous and dangerous substances, and children should never be allowed to roam free in either room. Many house plants are also dangerous to young children.

Outdoors
● Keep garden gates locked with child-resistant locks.
● Install swings, slides and climbing toys on grass or sand, never on concrete or paving. Check equipment regularly for strength, stability and signs of corrosion.
● Check all play equipment to ensure that there is no risk of scissoring, shearing or pinching injuries and that surfaces are free from snags and splinters.
● Instruct children carefully on what they can and can't do on play equipment.

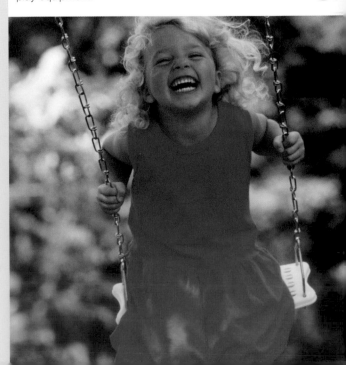

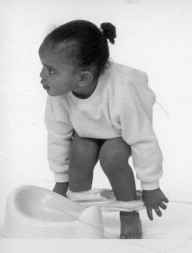
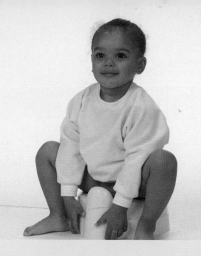
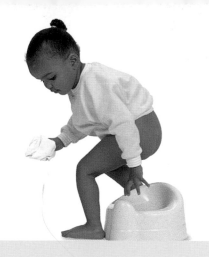

Toilet teaching

I am whole-heartedly against anything that resembles toilet training. For me there are no arguments in favour of it, only against. I believe that toilet training and the attitudes that advocate "training" a child's bowel movements and bladder function should be expunged from child care and child development.

There are good reasons to feel this way: it is impossible to train children to do anything unless their bodies have developed to a point where they are anatomically and physiologically able to perform the tasks that you demand. Applied to bowel and bladder control this means that it is impossible for your child to control either of these functions unless the bowel and the bladder muscles are strong enough to hold urine and faeces, and that at a given order from the brain the nerves to the bowel and bladder are mature enough to obey the order and evacuate.

If this level of development has not been reached, there is nothing that your child can do to meet your expectations. You can see immediately what a dreadful position this puts your child in. She is aware of what you want, but her body is unable to perform the task. Your child's desire to please you overrides almost all other desires and in this she is frustrated. She becomes unhappy at not being able to do what you want and may then feel inadequate, ashamed, guilty and finally resentful.

If you insist on a toilet programme when your child is not ready for it, the end can only be sadness. Your relationship with your child will deteriorate. You will become a source of unhappiness, and bowel movements and potty training will become a battle ground of your child's will against your nerves – and you will always be the loser. You cannot make your child pass a stool, or keep a nappy dry, and if you try to do either of these things you'll make her suffer every time the inevitable accident occurs.

Toilet teaching tips

● Do let your child develop at her own pace. There is no way that you can speed up the process, you can only be there to help your child along.

● Let your child decide whether or not to sit on the potty. You can suggest that she does but you should never force the issue.

● Do treat your child's faeces in a sensible manner, and never show any disgust or dislike for them. They're a natural part of your child and initially she'll be very proud of them.

● Do not delay once your child has signalled that she wants the potty as control is only possible for a short time.

● Praise your child and treat her control as an accomplishment.

● Whenever you travel, make sure that you have a potty with you so that your child can go under any circumstances without having to wait.

● Tell your child quite firmly and sympathetically that accidents will always be ignored and forgiven and that she's not to worry about them.

● Some children acquire bowel and bladder control much later than others and in nearly all cases it is wrong to blame the child. Most doctors feel that there is no need to investigate this difficulty before your child is three years old, and if she is only wet at night your doctor may feel that these investigations can be put off until she is five.

1-4 a loving child

To help our children grow up into generous, loving adults we must respond to their social demands from the very outset. In doing so, we make them responsive, friendly, outgoing and affectionate.

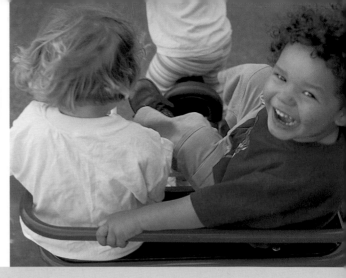

Sociability milestones

12–15 months

Include your child in as many activities as possible, and make certain she has a ring-side seat. Social gatherings are fun and she will follow conversations, making noises in the gaps. She can say one or two words with meaning, ask for things, indicate thank you, and will stop doing something at the word "no". But she's not so independent that she doesn't want to hold your hand for security.

15–18 months

Encourage your child to express love. Praise her when she shows affection and care towards others – siblings, relatives, pets or toys.

Encourage helpfulness, both with chores and dressing and undressing. Keep her with you because she loves being with adults and wants to imitate them, but don't expect too much. At social gatherings, she'll play next to, but not with, another child.

18 months–2 years

Help her to understand sharing. Invite her friends to the house so that she can start to play group games and share out play materials. Attention-seeking devices such as grabbing your arm, hitting you and doing forbidden things are common and she will often refuse to obey. But there is much less fighting and more cooperation with other children so she'll modify selfish behaviour to accommodate a playmate.

2–2½ years

Make sharing a game. Initiate games that involve giving things to others and she will learn to share with them. Sharing is hard for her and she'll show feelings of rivalry and will try to force her will on other children. She wants to be independent but also seeks your approval, so give it often. She may react to frustration by having tantrums, which are best ignored.

3 years

Encourage her to play with others. Sharing leads to social acceptance, and this leads to generosity. Have her friends to play and stay at your house. Independence is flourishing and she's more outgoing towards other children. Unselfishness starts to blossom, and firm friendships with other adults and children form. She will show signs of sympathy when someone is distressed and be more generous – share that with her.

4 years

Talk to her about her feelings as much as you can. By the age of four your child is showing signs of being a fledgling adult in terms of her emotional development. She loves animals, may cry if they're hurt and rushes to help and heal them. She's very fond, too, of her family and friends who are clearly special to her.

How to help a shy child

Shyness is something that affects many children. Common types of shy behaviour include disliking new experiences, reluctance to join in social gatherings, unwillingness to talk to unknown people and difficulty in making new friends. Don't think of shyness as something wrong with your child; many well-adjusted adults are quite shy. The best way of dealing with it is not by criticism or forcing change but by preparing your child for any situation he's likely to find difficult, perhaps with stories or role playing. In most cases, time and patience are all that is needed.

If your child has poor social skills there are various ways that you or your child's nursery school teacher can help:

Opposite pairing Pairing a neglected or unsociable child with a child who is outgoing and sociable. By being seen as the friend of a popular child, the shy child will gain a significantly higher level of social acceptance in a short time – in some cases as little as three weeks.

Younger pairing Pairing a child with poor social skills with a younger child can be another way of conferring status. A study carried out in the 1980s showed that when unpopular children between the ages of four and five played with children younger than themselves, their level of popularity increased by at least 50 percent. Younger playmates offer friendship which helps build self-esteem and assertiveness.

Clique activities Although it might seem bad for children to form small, exclusive groups within a large group, allowing them to mix in their preferred clique motivates them to get on with their peers outside the clique. Clique-based activities give children a sense of security and confidence about all social relationships.

Small groups It is sometimes mistakenly assumed that an unsociable child will become sociable when surrounded by a big group. In fact, small groupings are better at facilitating friendships because in a large group the unsociable child can remain very much in the background; in a small group he can't be ignored. A nursery school teacher can help by placing an unsociable child in a small group – say of three or four children – then gradually extending the size of the group.

Star responsibility Establishing definite roles, such as giving the most popular children responsible tasks to do, appears to have a settling effect on all children of nursery school age. Tasks could include giving out the straws for milk or organizing tidying up. Unsociable children appear to benefit from this strategy as much as other children.

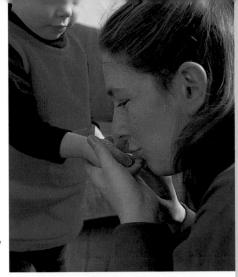

Leaving your child

Children in this age group dislike being separated from their parents, even if you are only going to spend the evening out of the house. It is quite usual for a child to shed a few tears until she is reassured about some of the details of the evening. These might include what time you are leaving; how far away you will be going; who you will be with; what you will be doing and what time you will return.

● Start getting dressed 15 minutes early so that you can spend a few moments with your child quietly doing something nice before you leave. Never rush off without proper leave-taking.

● If you make a promise that you will be back by a certain time, keep this promise and, as you are going, remind your child that you will always come back.

● Have a goodbye ritual – tell a story or play a game, give a hug or blow a kiss as you get into the car.

● Think up a few games – kiss her palm, fold her fingers around it and say that if she needs a kiss while you are away there is one for her to have.

● Never keep the fact that you are going to go out a secret from your child. In fact, talk about it well ahead of your absence. Try to do it very casually the day before and once or twice during the day.

● When your child is very small, don't use time scales that she can't grasp; instead, compare the time with some of her favourite activities. For example, say, "I'll be gone half an hour – that's four cartoons' worth".

● If you are going to have a babysitter, ask her to come a good half hour before you leave so that she can get involved in a game with your child before you go.

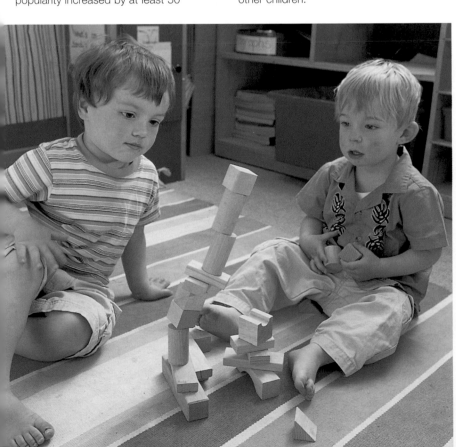

1-4 learning to fit in

One- to four-year-olds face many changes as they
mature and may feel "hurried". Be patient with problems
and allow your child to develop in her own good time.

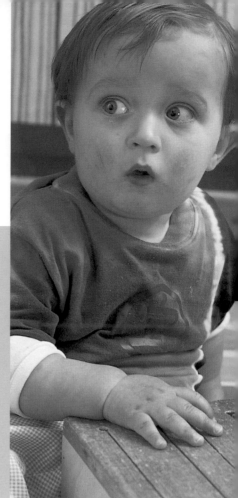

Right and wrong

Your child will only learn the difference
between right and wrong if it's clearly
pointed out. If your child understands why
you want her to do or not do something
she is much more likely to do it willingly,
so try to explain and then ask her opinion.

But there are situations that are non-
negotiable: when your child's safety is
threatened, when the thoughts and
feelings of others should be considered,
and when your child is tempted to tamper
with the truth. You should be very firm on
these points and she will gradually learn
a sense of responsibility for disciplining
herself as she grows up.

Cheekiness can often be mistaken for
impertinence, but unless your child is
imposing on the feelings of others, she
may be displaying nothing more than a
healthy resistance to authority which can
be useful, if sensibly directed.

A spoilt or over-indulged child will
behave in a self-centred way and this may
be the result of the over-protectiveness,
favouritism or the high expectations of her
parents. The best cure is to let her go to
playgroup or preschool at two-and-a-half
to three as a leveller. She will get used to
mixing with other children and start
learning how to get on with them.

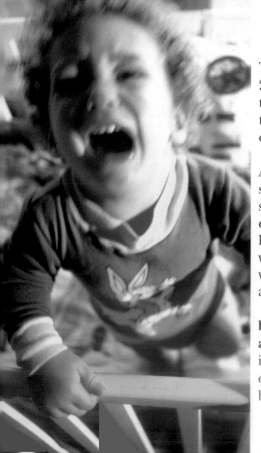

Tantrums

Toddlers between the ages of
2 and 3 may often have temper
tantrums as a means of giving vent
to frustration when they can't do
or get what they want.

This is quite normal behaviour.
At this age your child will not have
sufficient judgment to control his
strength of will or the language to
express himself clearly, but as his
knowledge and experience of the
world broadens, so the occasions
when his will is pitted directly
against yours become less likely.

**A tantrum may be brought on
by such feelings as frustration,
anger, jealousy and dislike.** Anger
is brought on by not getting his
own way and frustration by his not
being sufficiently strong or well

coordinated to do what he wants.
A tantrum usually involves your
child throwing himself on the
floor, kicking and screaming.

**The best thing you can do
during a tantrum is to stay calm**,
since any attention on your part
will only prolong the attack. If he
has a tantrum in public, take him
away from too much attention,
without making a fuss.

At home an effective technique
is simply to leave the room.
Explain to your child that, while
you still love him, you have to
leave the room because you are
getting upset. Never confine him
in another room because this
denies him the option of coming
back and saying sorry.

Your child's position in the family

No position in the family can be regarded as best. First-born children grow up in a more child-centred environment where the family activities concentrate on the child more than is possible for later-born children. First-born children have more guidance and help in their development, receive more complex language from their parents during infancy, and because of parental pressures on them, they usually achieve more than later-born siblings. First-born children tend to be better accepted by grown-ups and are more likely to take up leadership roles because they conform more closely to social expectations.

On the other hand, parents are less skilled at parenting with the first child and tend to intervene, intrude, restrict and use more coercive discipline and more punishments of all kinds than they do with later children. This can lead to first children receiving more feelings of anxiety from their parents, in other words, "Am I doing right?" However, there is little doubt that if children born later in the family were given the same guidance and attention as first-borns, they would probably achieve as much and be as well accepted socially.

The effects of family position become persistent very quickly and greatly influence the personal and social adjustments children make as they grow up. For instance, there is evidence that first-born children are more health-conscious than their younger siblings and as adults consult doctors more often. They also tend to be more cautious and take fewer risks.

The number of small children in the family greatly affects a child's development. Children with several younger brothers and sisters must share their parents' attention. If one child is needy, he is likely to get the lion's share of parental attention, leading to sensitivity about favouritism in the others. Rivalry between siblings, competition, bad feelings and resentment will be heightened. In addition, a needy child is likely to develop a "follower" personality pattern, and feelings of inadequacy and martyrdom, while the stronger may feel discriminated against and learns to play the leader.

Fantasy and reality

In order for a child to tell a lie he must have reached a stage in his psychological development where he can distinguish fantasy from reality. For example, if a 15-month-old baby is chastised by his mother for daubing poster paint on a wall, and he shakes his head vigorously in denial, he is not lying – it may be that he has genuinely forgotten the action, wishes that he hadn't done it or simply cannot recognize the difference between fantasy and reality. Only when a child reaches the age of 3 or 4 years is he capable of lying, and most children will lie if they find a situation sufficiently threatening. So to encourage a truthful child, avoid a threatening atmosphere and reward the truth.

How serious is lying?

Children lie for many different reasons and some types of lying are more serious than others. For instance, a make-believe lie is a natural part of a child's fantasy life, whereas a cover-up lie is a conscious attempt to avoid punishment. Because children lie for different reasons, every child and every lie must be treated individually.

do

✔ Act calmly – your child may simply be confusing reality and fantasy.

✔ Try to understand the motive for a lie. Your child is not lying because he wants to be malicious, but because he is afraid of punishment.

✔ Explain why it is wrong to lie. Use examples that he can understand.

✔ Make your child aware that, although you are upset by the lie, you still love him.

don't

✘ Ridicule the child who persists with bragging lies. Bragging indicates low self-esteem and you should work to increase your child's self-confidence with praise and affection.

✘ Use physical punishment on a child who lies. Research shows that constant smacking for lies only encourages children to lie more, because they are afraid of being smacked again.

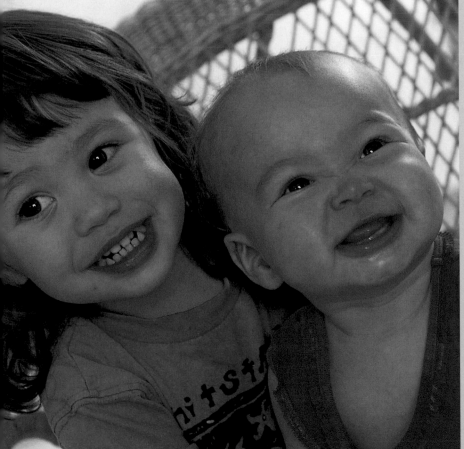

1-4 open attitudes

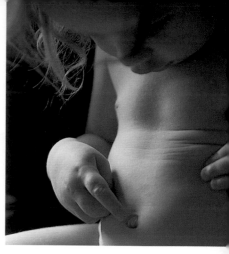

Children who grow up in a secure, loving home, able to discuss anything with their parents, are likely to become well-adjusted, responsible adults, but most will have a few worries along the way.

Answering children's awkward questions

Parents whose responses are shifty or furtive when faced with controversial questions not only make it difficult to raise subjects like race, sex, religion or drugs within the family, but also encourage their children to be furtive themselves. Parents who are open, responsive and frank encourage self-esteem, balance and fairness in their children and give them the space to think, weigh up options, make decisions and act responsibly. This healthy

dialogue between parents and children has to begin early – from the very first question – and should continue throughout the time they are at home.

● Treat your child's questions seriously and always try to give the most accurate, truthful answer you can.

● Think about the point of questions. If a child asks what a ruler is, for example, he may want to know more than just the name. Explain what it is used for and try measuring something together.

● If you don't know an answer to a question, be truthful and say that you don't know but suggest that you look it up or ask someone else together.

● Don't shy away from giving truthful and accurate answers to children on difficult topics. Always answer questions on matters such as death and sex truthfully. But don't feel you have to give the whole truth. Supply as much as you feel your child can cope with and understand at that time.

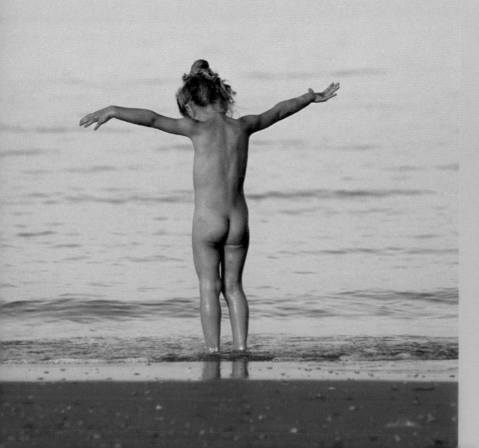

Make her proud of her body

A child's sex education begins with the first cuddle. All children take pleasure in physical contact and joy in their parents' reciprocity. They grow up realizing that people touch one another as an act of friendship as well as an act of love.

As your child gets older she will become pleasantly aware of her body, without being at all self-conscious about it. **You can encourage this by having an open attitude to nudity within the family**. Like everything else, a child learns patterns of behaviour and attitudes from you. The child who sees her parents unclothed and unembarrassed will take nudity as a matter of course and is unlikely to grow up concerned about nakedness. But if you are worried about it she will almost certainly worry too; if you're embarrassed she is likely to be too.

Childhood emotions

Your toddler's emotions develop very rapidly. She can feel guilt, shame, jealousy and dislike, and be so upset that these emotions make her cry. Even in the most loved, secure child, fear, too, is quite near the surface and will provoke tears.

Dealing with fears

The commonest childhood fears are of the dark and thunder. One of the best ways to dispel fears is to talk about them, so encourage your child to be open and frank about what frightens her. Give her your full attention and ask questions, so that she knows that you are taking her seriously. Quite often fears are difficult to put into words, but hear your child out. Help her to explain by supplying a few examples and confess that you have similar fears too. Never scold or ridicule your child about her fears. Do something simple and reassuring, like demonstrating to your child that it is fun in the swimming pool and the water is nothing to fear. Your child will trust you and her fear will gradually diminish. When she's old enough, try to explain how things work: for instance, that lightning is just like a giant spark of light, like striking a match.

A new baby in the family

Your child is bound to feel pretty distressed at the thought of a new baby brother or sister and the "dethronement" that she thinks will follow. Take all the precautions you can to make her feel good about the baby. When you talk about the baby, refer to it as her new sister or brother, and let your child feel your tummy as the baby grows and kicks. Show her where the baby is going to sleep, and teach her all kinds of helpful things she can do to look after it. If you are having the baby in hospital, make sure your child is at ease with the person who is going to look after her while you're there. When you come home, have someone else carry the baby; you should have your arms free to scoop up your child and give her a big cuddle. Don't turn to the new baby until she asks to see her. Make sure that you bring home a present from the baby for her. If you have to stay in hospital, let her visit you as often as she likes and when she does, make sure that the baby is not in your arms but in a cot, so you're free to hold your child.

Over-tiredness

A child of this age very often becomes over-excited and over-tired towards bedtime. She'll try to put off going to bed for as long as she possibly can and simply become more and more distressed. Your child might become so fragile that the slightest discomfort or frustration will make her cry inconsolably.

If you are expecting your child to have a late evening or a special treat such as a birthday party or a school play, make sure she has a nap during the day so that her energy will last. If she does become over-excited and over-tired, it is especially important that you remain calm and quiet. Talk to her gently, give her lots of cuddles, be infinitely patient and take her gently to her bedroom. Sing her a song or read a story until she has become calm and quietened down, ready for sleep.

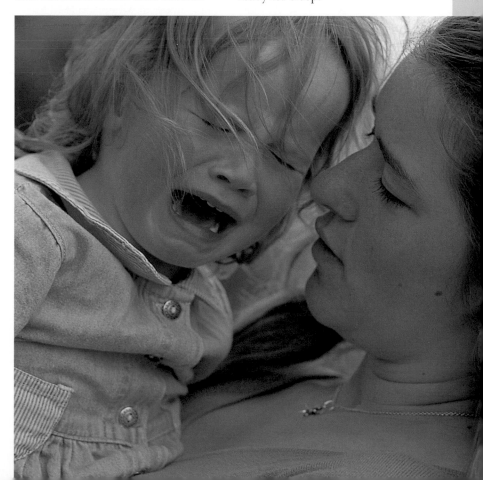

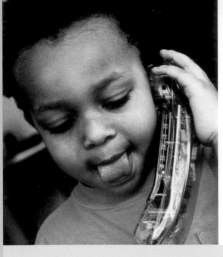

1-4 learning to talk

During these years your child's language will progress rapidly. She'll be able to talk to you and ask for what she wants and, equally important, understand what you are saying to her.

Talk to your child

If you want your teenager to feel free to talk to you about anything, then you have to set this up early in your child's life and talk about anything to him. **So talk endlessly to your toddler, and go on introducing new words and making your meaning clear with gestures and facial expressions.** It is just as important, however, that you give him space to respond so that he learns that conversation works two ways. If he initiates a conversation by showing you something or asking you a question, always make eye contact and give him your full attention. If you are impatient, or just respond with "That's nice" without even looking at him, he'll become discouraged and give up trying to talk to you.

Talk about everything you are doing in detail. When you are dressing him, give a running commentary: "Now we'll do up your buttons... one, two, three". Describe objects you are using: "Let's put the apples in the glass bowl". "Would you like a yellow sweet or a red sweet?"

While you shouldn't correct your child when he makes mistakes, there is no reason why you should talk to him in his own baby language. If he makes a mistake in grammar or pronunciation – "Granny goed" – just repeat his words giving the correct form: "Yes, Granny went home".

Developing language

Your toddler learns new words all the time and she starts to put them together, even if it's only two at a time, "Teddy fall". Her pronunciation will be indistinct, but this is no cause for worry; if she is using words with meaning and putting them together, then her language is developing. Mild speech defects, such as lisping, are very common in children, and usually disappear without any intervention.

Language in girls
● Right from the moment of birth, girls are more responsive to the human voice than boys, and they have better verbal skills throughout childhood.
● Girls talk earlier than boys, and begin to string words into sentences earlier. They have better articulation, pronunciation and grammar, and are better at verbal reasoning. They also learn to read earlier than boys.
● The structure of the female brain is believed to be the reason for girls' superior verbal skills: the speech centres are more tightly organized in the female brain than in the male brain and have more and better connections with other parts of the brain.

Language in boys
● Boys are almost always slower than girls at developing language skills and this discrepancy lasts right through childhood.
● Boys are later in talking than girls, are slower to put words together in sentences and take longer to learn to read. Speech disorders such as stuttering are far more common in boys than in girls, and boys outnumber girls in remedial reading classes by four to one.
● Although this difference in linguistic ability levels out somewhat during the teenage years, you can help your son's language skills in the preschool years by reading aloud to him and playing lots of word games.

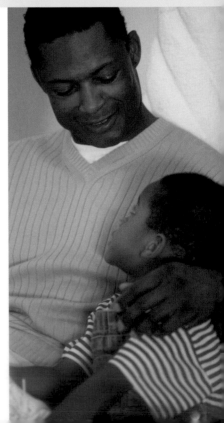

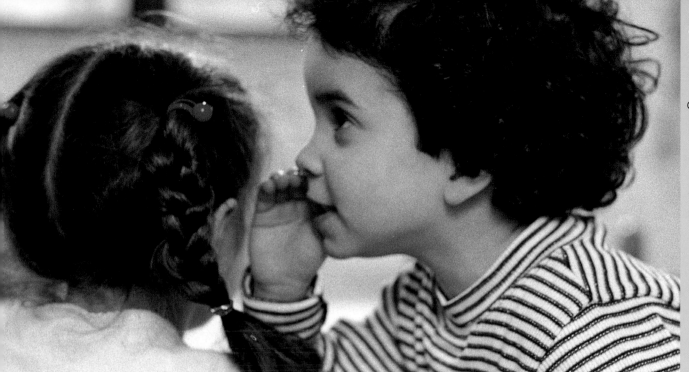

Speech and language milestones

There is great variation in the speed at which children learn to talk, so don't feel the need to compare your child with others of his age and don't worry if his development doesn't match the timetable given here: I give these dates merely as average guidelines, and no child corresponds to the average.

12–18 months

● Your toddler's comprehension is miles ahead of his ability to express himself, e.g. "Mama" can mean lots of things, including "Mummy, give me a drink". When you discover what he means, say "Mummy will get you a drink" and say the word "drink" again. Soon he'll say, "Mummy, dink".
● Introduce your toddler to all kinds of noises, such as those made by animals, vehicles and music. He is very switched on to sounds, so point them out: doors squeak, taps drip, paper rustles.
● Read books as often as you can, going over and over favourite ones, repeating names and objects. Point to familiar objects. Give their names. Ask him to repeat the names. Show pleasure when he remembers.
● Name everything, everywhere. Name colours, textures and other properties.
● Start counting and use numbers whenever the opportunity arises.

18 months–2 years

● Start to use adjectives whenever you can. The first are usually "good", "bad",
"nice", "nasty", "hot", "cold". Couple them with nouns ("cold milk", "nice girl", "good teddy") especially when you are describing food, people and toys – your toddler's favourite subjects.
● Use adverbs, too, such as "here" and "where". Emphasize all verbs and add actions to promote understanding.
● Prepositions are understood long before your toddler uses them, but always stress them and show what you mean. Always indicate where "under", "on top of" and "behind" are.

2–3 years

● Your child will talk more to children of his own age than to adults, so exposing him as often as possible to the company of other children will help develop his linguistic abilities. This is one of the reasons why nursery school becomes important. At this age, speech ceases to be egocentric and becomes more social, so contact with other children is essential if your child is to develop social language.
● Repeat favourite stories, so that your child can work out his feelings about the world around him.
● Read more complex stories and introduce new words, explaining them by using them over and over in your speech.

3–4 years

● Never overtly correct your child's mistakes; just repeat what he has just said, but correctly. If he hesitates over a
word, supply it instantly, to maintain his momentum and interest.
● Your child responds well to reasoning, so include him in simple problem-solving, with questions, options and solutions – openly discussing each step. Ask his opinion about something you know you can agree with, so that he feels he has made a decision.
● Make sentences longer and more complex. When your child speaks to you, turn to him and listen attentively. Nod, and incline your head to show you are listening.
● Always answer questions. There is no need to tell the whole truth, just the amount that he can handle, but never lie or dissemble. Your child will find you out and mistrust you. Your child will ask the same question over and over; just give the answer again, never become impatient.
● Children like whispering, so play whispering games to aid expression.
● In your child's list of reading include fairy stories, because they help your child to come to terms with his own world without it hurting him, and because they improve his concepts of real and unreal; past, present and future; fairness and injustice; good and evil; kindness and brutality, and so on.
● Language acquisition is not smooth, it stops and starts, so follow your child's lead and don't press. Don't compare your child with anyone else; language is learned at different rates by different children.

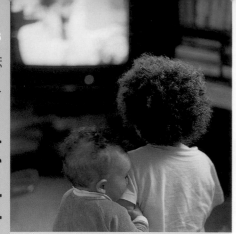

1-4 a growing mind

Sharing your child's pleasure in new skills and achievements is one of the great joys of parenthood. Help your child by giving lots of praise and encouragement.

Television

Some parents see television as a built-in babysitter because it keeps children amused when there is no-one who wants to look after them. For quite a lot of children, television is more popular and consumes more of their playtime than all other play activities added together.

Television is at its least useful when a child is left to watch alone. Even if she's watching a highly educational programme she'll get less out of it if she watches it in an entirely passive way. If she watches it with other children who comment on it, or with an adult who asks questions and makes observations, the programme acts as a springboard for ideas and discussion rather than one-way, non-participatory communication.

Television prevents your child from:

- scanning, sifting and analysing information and then applying it to everyday situations
- practising motor skills
- using more than two senses at a time to expand the appreciation of her environment
- asking questions and receiving helpful educational answers
- exploring and using her curiosity
- exercising initiative or motivation
- being challenged and solving problems
- thinking analytically
- using her imagination
- having conversations with the rest of the family and improving verbal skills
- writing and reading
- being either creative or constructive
- developing the ability to concentrate for long periods because of the flicker of the television screen
- developing logical, sequential thinking because the action in programmes constantly shifts backwards, forwards and laterally in time.

Mental development milestones

Many brain and body skills advance on a tide of growth and expansion as general understanding increases. The determining factors are your child's sociability and personality, and the environment you create for him.

15 months

Let him help you as much as he can with simple tasks like tidying up that are well within his abilities and encourage feelings of pride. Get him to point to parts of his body, make animal sounds and help to take off his clothes – he loves it. He understands the concept of "cattiness" – he knows that a picture of a cat, a toy cat and a real cat are all cats, even though very different, so keep pointing out to him the defining features of things.

18 months

Use repetition for learning. Whenever you do something, repeat certain key phrases over and over. "Jack has an apple. Yes, Jack has an apple." Help him recognize a few items on a page and ask him to point to them if you say their names. Give him a few chores – he's dying to have a go and will try to imitate your actions. He'll carry out a request that requires assessment and memory: "Go and bring me your teddy".

21 months

Describe the character of things. When showing something to your child, point out whether it is hard or soft, its colour, if it makes a noise and so on. Introduce opposites such as rough and smooth. Encourage him to ask for food, drink, toys and about going to the potty. He's beginning to understand more complicated requests: "Please get your hairbrush from the bathroom". He may grab your arm or use other gestures to get your attention.

2 years

Stimulate his spatial sense by helping place the various cubes, rectangles and squares into their correct receptacles in a shape-fitting toy or box. Use names all the time to stimulate a rapidly increasing vocabulary of names and objects and so that he can describe the properties of familiar items and identify them. Give him quite complicated orders, and ask him to find an object played with previously to encourage a good memory. Stimulate him to talk non-stop by answering his questions and asking him questions too.

2½ years

Play lots of number games. Incorporate numbers into everything you do. Count items when you shop, get dressed or say what you have to do. A toy farmyard is a good toy at this age – use it to count cows, sheep, pigs and chickens. He's starting to add detail to broad concepts – a horse has a long tail – and he knows one or two nursery rhymes, so ask him to find them in his book. He's starting to ask "Why" and says "No", "Won't", "Can't" in answer to everything.

3–4 years

Add to his sense of self. Encourage independence and self-reliance by involving your child in simple decisions: ask him to choose his clothes and food. Your child asks questions incessantly – "What?", "Where?", "How?", "Why?" Always answer them. Encourage a good memory by referring to the past and reminding him what you did the day before. He knows his own gender now so point out differences with girls.

Books and reading

If I had to choose a single way in which a parent could enrich their children's environment and help them to develop well, I would suggest having books in the house. If you enjoy reading, make it obvious and talk about it, your child will too. Words are crucial to the way our brains function: reading is therefore very important and there is a correlation between how many books you have in the house and how much your child will read as he grows up and later in life.

Books are one of the great pleasures of life and are vital in providing your child with the words to express feelings, ideas and thoughts. Moreover, books can help to explain the world he lives in – describing relationships, depicting situations and introducing personalities.

Books provide the impetus for imaginative play, they introduce ideas and they are fun. In our house, books were given to the children as soon as they were born, and reading was a shared experience up to the age of 10.

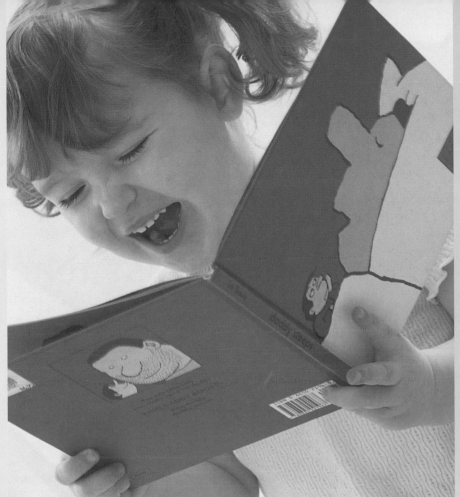

Bad dreams and nightmares

Nightmares Three- and four-year-olds quite often have bad dreams. Your child may walk or talk in her sleep, or have night terrors. They're normal because while her understanding of the world is growing, she cannot make sense of it, and so she goes to sleep with unresolved questions. She's also getting more in touch with her feelings and she knows what it is to be afraid or feel something is not quite right. These feelings come out at night.

Often a child cannot explain her dreams and has difficulty in going back to sleep. Animals, especially wolves and bears, may chase your child during a nightmare, or she may dream of strange, bad or odd-looking people, fires and deep water. Only if your child wakes up should you try to console her and take her in your arms. If she remains asleep, don't do anything to wake her; simply stay by her. If you find that she is sleepwalking periodically, put a gate across the stairs to prevent falls.

Night terrors Sometimes you will find your child in bed, apparently awake, terrified, and possibly thrashing about and screaming. She may be angry or desperately upset. This is a night terror rather than a nightmare, and it can be very alarming. You will feel quite anguished at your child's fear and pain, but all you can do is stay close and wait for the terror to pass. There is no point in trying to reassure your child specifically, because she is beyond reason. Don't leave or scold her; that would simply make the terror worse. She won't remember anything in the morning.

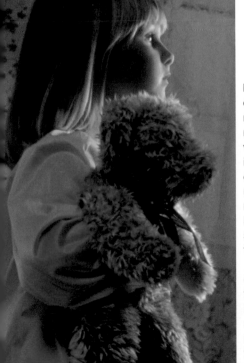

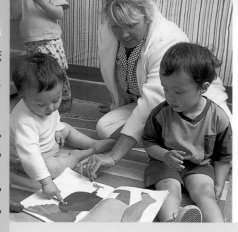

1–4 learning by play

Play is crucial to your preschool child's development. Once she has practised her creative talents during play, she can apply them to the real world.

Parent as teacher

A child starts to absorb information from the moment she is born, and it is from her parents that she gets most of this information. A parent is responsible for encouraging a child's imagination and teaching helpfulness and self control, among other things, and there are simple ways to approach all these lessons.

Set appropriate goals

Never pursue perfection as this will lead to frustration and you will end up with an unhappy, demoralized child who simply cannot thrive and develop well. Never fall into the trap of expecting too much too soon, but be aware of the small successes that your child achieves every day. Try not to focus on deficiencies; concentrate instead on noticing and praising every single positive act or achievement.

Always join in

One of the jobs of being a teacher to your child is that you actually have to DO THINGS. Your child learns through example and imitation until she is over eight years old, so get up and do something in front of her or with her. This means that you do not rely on just giving your child orders or directions. Instead of telling her to "Go and tidy up your toys", you need to get down on your knees with her,

and make a game of tidying up the toys together.

Repeat, repeat, repeat

With all children, but especially young children, it is frustrating but necessary to tell them over and over again to do the same thing. For example, a young child will not sit calmly while she is eating lunch or waiting for anything. So you may have to repeat certain messages like "We don't swing our legs and kick the chair while we are eating" for months

Know when to forbid

I found only three situations in which it was absolutely necessary to say "no" to a child:

● When my child might harm himself; for instance, reaching for a cooking pot on the stove.
● When my child's actions could have been harmful to others; for example, something as simple as playing noisily or banging toys near a sleeping baby.
● When my child's action would result in real damage; for example, trying to use crayons on the sitting-room wall. Even when you say "no" it does not have to be a head-on confrontation. The best way to do it is to distract your child with something interesting.

and months until your child's body gets the message as well as her mind.

Give positive examples

Remember, whenever possible, to state something in a positive way. Say, "Yes that is a nice little dog; let's pat the dog" and show your child how to do it. Don't shriek, "Don't hurt the little puppy". Sentences that begin with "do not" communicate displeasure from the moment you start to speak. An infant's brain does not necessarily process every word, so in the case above, your message may come out as "… hurt … puppy!" – your opposite intention.

Don't interrupt

A lot of children have difficulty with concentration span, and it is hard to foster because a small child simply cannot concentrate as well as an adult. One of the major things you can do to help your child sustain attention is not to interrupt when she is clearly absorbed in something.

Give attention

A child only feels that she is being listened to if you make eye contact and stop what you are doing in order to listen. If you do this from a very early age, your child will know that she has a voice, and that you respect her as an individual.

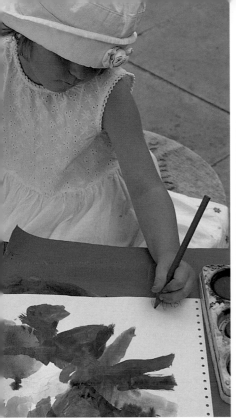

Drawing can help him understand his ...

...Emotions You can help your child to become in touch with his feelings and to recognize emotions in others by getting him to draw happy faces and sad faces, first with a guiding hand from you. Then move your child on to looking at photos of people he knows and deciding how they are feeling in the picture. This not only helps your child to recognize emotions but to empathize, and to relate closely to them. Later, you can show your child pictures in newspapers and magazines. When your child is a little older, you can draw stick figures and ask what the various postures mean in terms of feelings. Then get your child to draw stick figures and to express the various emotions that they feel.

...World You can also use drawings to expand your child's view of the world. A very simple idea would be what happens when you spill water. You and your child could do a drawing of knocking over a jug of water and it spilling onto the floor and making a puddle, perhaps running off the edge of the table onto the floor in big drops and splashes. This kind of exercise reinforces your child's memory and provides him with his own experience.

Whenever you are telling or writing a story, or when your child is old enough to do either of these things, always ask if there is any part of the story that could be illustrated. At first, help your child draw some kind of picture, so that he can visualize what is in his imagination and express it in pictures, not only words, then ask him to do one by himself.

Even in conversation you can introduce the idea of mind pictures and get your child to describe the picture in his mind's eye in words, not just in drawings.

Ideas for play

Sometimes your child will be absorbed in a make-believe world of her own and won't need your involvement. At other times you can add to her enjoyment by suggesting new games, or new ways to play with her toys.

Make-believe play Your child will create a little world of her own as part of her imitation of adults. An instant tent or playhouse can be made from a couple of chairs or a small table draped with a blanket. Children love playing with cardboard boxes as long as they are big enough to climb into. Small ones become boats and cars; piles of them turn into castles and houses. Dressing up is a favourite game at this age: a few simple props can transform your child into a doctor or fire-fighter and, in her fantasy world, she is the adult, and a teddy bear or doll serves as a child.

Messy play Any play involving water, sand, mud, or dough will stretch your child's intellect. To make your supervision easier, set aside a time when messy play is allowed and a place where the mess can be contained, and encourage your child to look forward to it.

Domestic play Helping you around the house is play rather than work because she's so keen to copy you. She helps in the kitchen by tearing salad leaves or arranging bread on a plate, and will enjoy laying the table, so improving manipulative and counting skills as well as independence and self-worth.

Musical play All children are born with perfect pitch so any child with normal hearing adores musical sounds. She probably won't be able to play melodies, but she may be able to hum them and will enjoy banging out a rhythm. Rattles, wooden clappers, trumpets and drums are all very good for this purpose, as are old pans or baking tins and wooden spoons. A xylophone will enable her to identify musical sounds and experiment with high and low notes.

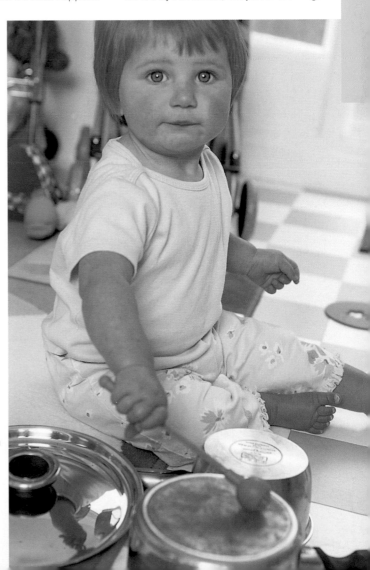

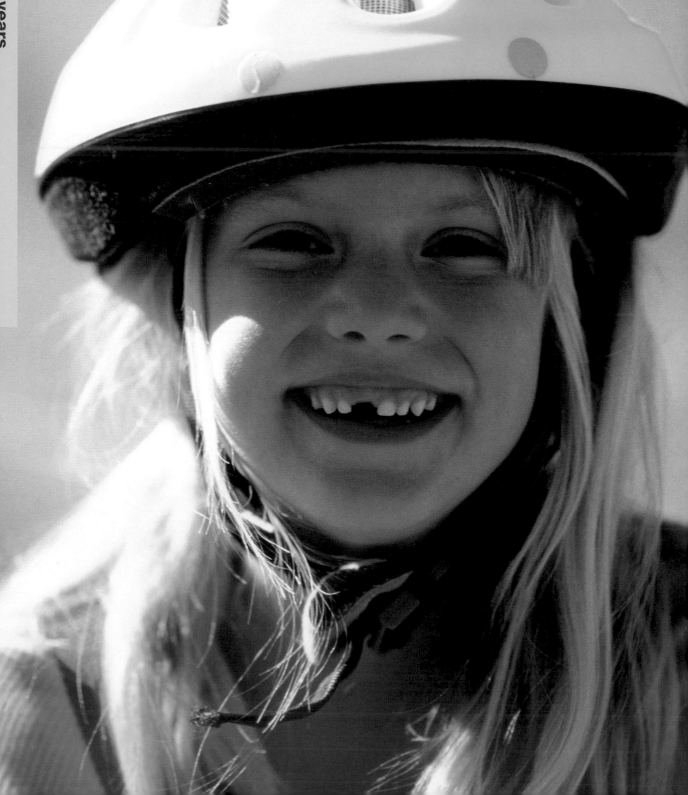

"a child needs self-belief
if she is to fulfil her potential"

life stages: 4 to 11 years

Between the ages of 4 and 11 your energetic, loving, mischievous pre-schooler is going to grow and develop into a reflective, kind, industrious, cooperative adolescent with whom you can have a serious conversation, on whom you can rely and whose company everyone enjoys. That's a tough assignment for any 4-year-old and there are many complex skills to acquire along the way, not the least of which are self-control and self-discipline.

Most important, milestones can only be achieved if parents show loving care to their children. Children can't survive let alone thrive without close parental interest. They can get by of course and most do, even if parental care isn't forthcoming.

Achieving self-belief

But there are some milestones that are exceedingly difficult for a child to master alone and they can go astray without feedback and guidance. Let me give you just one example of a milestone that involves an important step in personal development – achieving **self-belief**.

Call it self-confidence, call it self-assurance, but without it a child will not only fail to fulfil her potential, she could get into all kinds of trouble because she won't know how to control her emotions or how to rechannel her frustrations and anger to gainful purpose.

You may think, well, she'll grow into a shy child, unsure of herself. That would be bad enough, but you're wrong, it's worse than that.
● She grows into a child who becomes a loner without friends, which is heartbreaking for any parent to see.
● She may seek attention and affection to bolster her waning ego with all kinds of inappropriate behaviour, sometimes being labelled as **hyperactive**.
● And then, if no one helps her to build belief in herself, she resorts to lying, stealing, bullying, even to drinking and taking drugs to feel good about herself.

You can see that without achieving **self-belief**, there are problems ahead. So important is this milestone, and several other crucial milestones, that I call them **islands of development**. If a child doesn't reach the haven of these islands, there can be disastrous fallout later.

Think of your child as bobbing along on a river of development trying to negotiate the equivalent of white water, the flow sometimes fast as she goes through a spurt of skill acquisition, or slower and more placid as she consolidates her achievements.

These islands make the river navigable. They're places where your child can rest up, so to speak, take stock and move on to the next milestone – with lots of encouragement and praise from you of course.

The islands are also an insurance policy. If you can help your child to reach one she'll tackle the next stretch of white water with determination, courage and good sense. And, having enjoyed the security of reaching one of these islands, your child can safely be given responsibilities of increasing gravitas both for herself and others.

In the pages that follow, I offer guidelines where appropriate, advice where I feel there may be a need and strategies for dealing with difficult situations.

The right age to…

● A child is ready to learn to tie her own shoelaces at about 4 years old.

● A child may be able to cope with moving into a proper bed at about 5 years old.

● A 6-year-old is probably ready to receive pocket money and decide how to spend it.

● At 7 a child can learn to cross the street alone.

● A child of 8 can sleep over at a friend's house.

● A 9-year-old is ready to learn about puberty.

● A child of 10 may enjoy the responsibility of looking after a pet.

● An 11-year-old can be left at home alone for short periods.

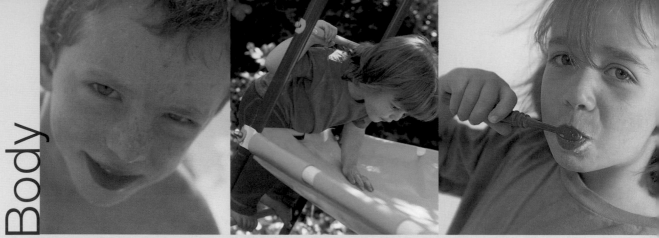
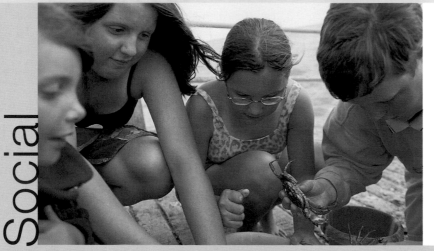
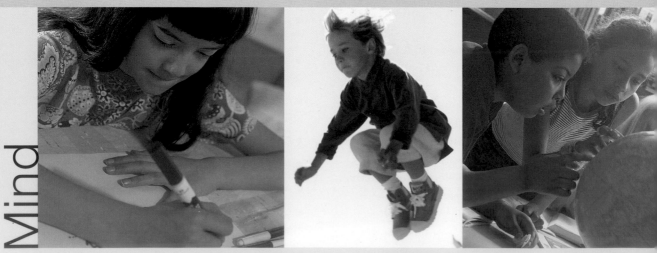

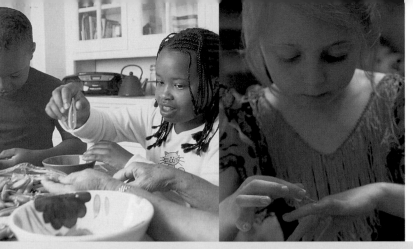

"encourage physical activity in your child as early as possible"

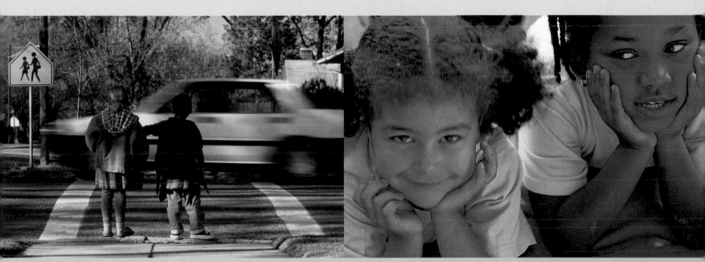

"tell your children the facts of life as soon as they begin to ask"

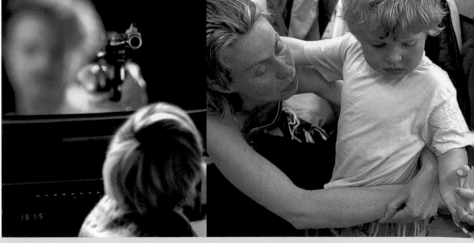

4-11 feeding children

The best way to make sure that your children eat a healthy, balanced diet for the rest of their lives is to help them develop good habits from the beginning.

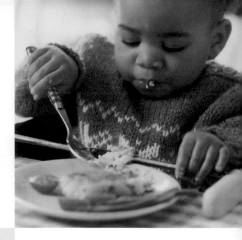

Happy mealtimes

do

✔ Make mealtimes an important family ritual so your child can learn how to be part of a group.

✔ Set up some basic ground rules for meals so that everyone knows they can't throw tantrums or just grab and run.

✔ Have meals at regular times so that you set up a rhythm for family life – children love this.

✔ Encourage thoughtfulness for others – never take the last portion without offering it to everyone else.

✔ Foster chat and discussion and make sure each child is listened to, including the youngest.

✔ Trivialize accidents and spillage so that the conviviality isn't broken.

don't

✗ Let meals become battlegrounds. You can't force a child to eat. Let them refuse food, they'll ask for it soon enough if you don't insist.

✗ Let a child spoil family calm and harmony at the table for everyone else; remove them to another room.

✗ Exclude children from your conversation – they become naughty to attract your attention.

✗ Let meals tail off without a formal ending. Each child should say they've had enough and ask to go and play.

✗ Leave the youngest until last to get her food. Give it to her first – her patience is shortest.

✗ Have the television on or music playing during meals.

Veggie child

It's quite safe for a child to be a vegetarian from the age of weaning, but think about the following points.

● Their diet should contain dairy products and eggs and be planned carefully to contain all essential ingredients.

● With dietary supplements, and ingenuity on the part of parents, even a vegan diet excluding dairy, eggs and meat can be OK.

● Children weaned onto a vegan diet tend to be smaller and lighter than average. While their height does "catch up", vegan children usually remain lighter and leaner.

● The slow growth is because a typical veggie diet contains fewer of the high-energy foods needed for growth.

● Children need high-energy foods for growth and play so nut products, cheese and avocado are useful. Veggie children should be given full-fat milk to provide crucial calories. Go easy on bulky foods such as lots of fruit and vegetables and high-fibre cereals, which reduce absorption of iron and zinc.

● Variety is key. All four food groups should be included in these daily ratios. Cereals and grains: 4–5 helpings; fruit: 1–3 helpings; vegetables: 2 helpings; pulses, nuts and seeds: 1–2 helpings; animal protein (milk, cheese and eggs): 3 helpings.

● Veggie children should have some vegetable oil/butter/yeast extract.

● Good sources of veggie protein are nuts, pulses, tofu and soya in any form. Milk and dairy products and eggs are "complete" proteins.

● To keep up intake of calcium, iron and vitamin C, children need to eat plenty of fortified foods – for example, breakfast cereals and wholemeal bread – diced fruit, dark green vegetables and dairy.

● Vitamin C promotes iron absorption so food containing these nutrients should be eaten together.

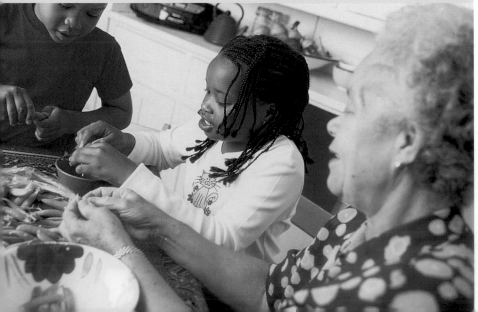

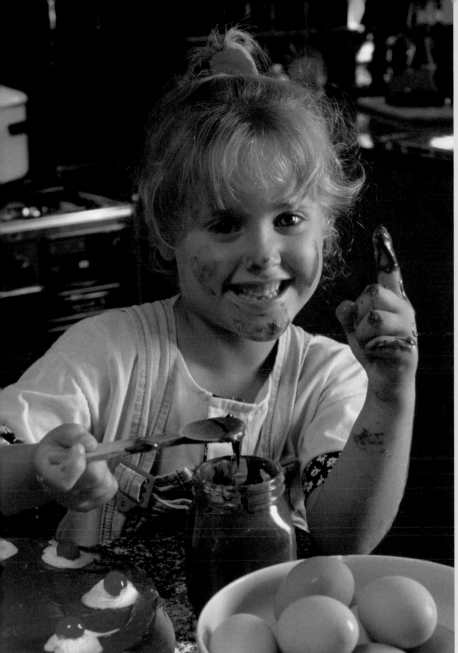

Junk foods

■ **How many times a week does your family eat fast food?**
Rarely (0)   Once (2)
Twice (3)   More (4)

■ **Do you serve chips with food?**
Never (0)   Occasionally (1)
Frequently (3)   Very frequently (5)

■ **Do you give in if your child whines for a Big Mac?**
Never (0)   Sometimes (1)
Often (3)   Always (4)

■ **How often do you use junk food as a bribe?**
Never (0)   Now and then (2)
Quite often (5)   All the time (7)

■ **Do you put hamburgers and fishfingers in the weekly shop?**
Never (0)   Once a month (1)
Every two weeks (3) Every week (5)

■ **Do you have sweet fizzy drinks in the fridge?**
Never (0)   Sometimes (1)
Often (3)   All the time (5)

■ **Do you finish off meals with a sweet pudding e.g. ice cream?**
Never (0)   Now and then (1)
Every day (5)   Every meal (7)

■ **Is there ketchup on the table?**
Never (0)   Occasionally (1)
Often (2)   Always (3)

■ **How often does your family eat take aways?**
Never (–5)   Now and then (1)
Weekly (2)
More than once a week (4)

■ **Do you serve much fried food?**
Never (0)   Sometimes (1)
Often (5)   Very frequently (7)

Now add up your score.
Up to 15: OK – your family's diet slips occasionally but is generally good.
Up to 25: Too much – the junk food level is creeping up. Try to cut it down.
More than 35: STOP! Your family is eating far too much junk food and it will damage their health.

Sweets

I don't believe in giving sweets freely nor in placing a total ban on sweets – that only encourages children to be secretive and dishonest. What I do believe in is rationing sweets, and this always worked with my own children. If you let your child have a few sweets after a meal and encourage him to brush his teeth afterwards, you'll be helping him develop good eating habits, self-control and good oral hygiene. Sweets might seem like a suitable reward for children and they are, but not all the time. There is no hard and fast rule on this, and no reason why you shouldn't occasionally reward your child with sweets as long as you make it clear that this is a one-off treat. It's worth making an effort, though, to devise other forms of reward, such as a favourite yogurt flavour or a small toy.

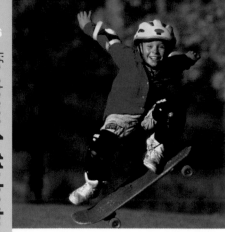

4-11 active children

Healthy, happy children have boundless energy. Encourage their adventurousness and allow them to be independent.

Importance of physical activity

There is a great deal of medical evidence to show that physical activity in children favourably affects efficient action of the muscles and the heart and lungs, a tendency to leanness rather than to fatness, and the strength and growth of bones. Since the benefits of physical activity depend on its intensity and duration, it follows that children who play hard and exercise hard are likely to be fitter adults. Active children are generally leaner and show greater physical capacity at all ages than their less active contemporaries.

Just how much exercise is necessary during the growing years is not known and individual variation is great, but it is a good idea to encourage physical activity in your child as early as possible. Promote the taking up of hobbies and sporting activities that involve strenuous exercise and do not be overprotective, preventing your child from being physically active and adventurous. The more the whole family can join in, the better – and it won't do office-bound parents any harm either.

A sedentary child is nearly always a fat child and a fat child is in danger of developing diabetes, simply as a result of being overweight. Obese children are also in danger of developing conditions of "old age", like heart disease, in their 20s. Another persuasive reason for encouraging your child to be active.

Healthy feet

Children are born with soft, pliable feet. As their feet grow, the toe bones are the last to harden so they are easily bent out of shape. Let small children go barefoot around the house so that toes have room to move.

When you buy shoes for your child it is important to have his feet properly measured for width and length by a trained fitter, so go to a shop that specializes in children's shoes. There should be plenty of room for the child's toes in the front of the shoe when he is standing up: half your thumbnail between the top of the shoe and his toes is a rough-and-ready guide. Choose shoes with an adjustable strap across the instep and with supple uppers which give support but bend easily during walking. Remember that your child's feet will probably increase by at least two sizes a year until he is 6 or so, so keep an eye on how his toes are growing.

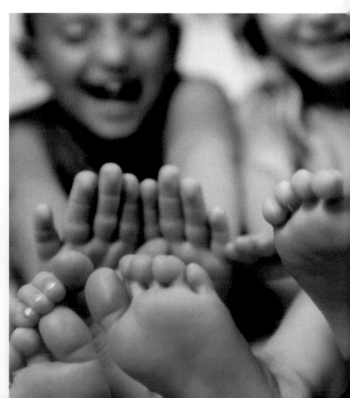

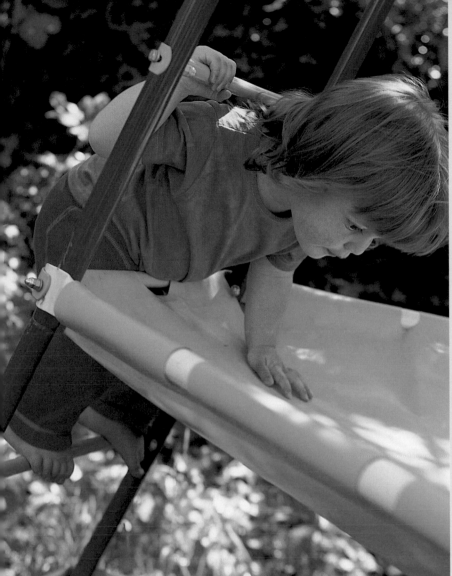

Teeth

The first of your child's 32 permanent teeth will probably come through around the age of 6. These are the first molars, one each side at the back of the upper and lower jaw. They appear before any of the baby teeth are lost. Then, between the ages of 7 and 9, come the incisors, the sharp teeth at the front of the mouth, which we use for cutting food. After that come the premolars or bicuspids, the square back teeth we use for gripping or tearing food.

Your child will usually have her new set of permanent teeth by about 13 or 14 years of age, with the wisdom teeth coming through several years later. There is no difference between the time teeth come through on the right and left sides of the mouth but there is a marked difference between boys and girls: every tooth appears earlier in girls, by two months for the first molars and as much as 11 months for the canines. Do not worry if your child's teeth seem to be slow in coming through. The timetable for dental development varies from child to child, just as the timetables for height and weight vary.

Brushing teeth

Until your child is about 8, you will probably have to help her to brush her teeth efficiently. Some children can manage earlier than this, but you will need to keep a check on how well they are brushing their teeth until you are sure they can be trusted to do it properly.

Adventurousness

Encouraging your child to be adventurous has countless pay-offs, not least that you'll help her to push herself to the limit and develop her full potential. It's the quickest way to self-confidence.

● Good parents separate their fears from their children's. Her own fears are sufficient to make her sensible and circumspect. Your fears cripple her curiosity and spirit.

● Overprotective parents don't allow their children to test their abilities, master new skills and move on to new feats. They hold children back so that they lack the coordination and confidence that gives them pride and trust in their own bodies and their own abilities.

● By the age of four your child has a clear sense of self and her abilities and can experiment to find out what's feasible and safe on her own without danger. Play equipment such as a climbing frame allows such experiments, and research shows that children, left to their own devices, rarely overstep the limits.

● Your child has boundless energy and can tackle demanding activities like climbing, pedalling and skating. Your role is to provide the tools within sight of the house for easy supervision.

● If necessary, guide her through the most difficult tasks or add stabilizers to her bike, but don't stop her. This way you'll lay the foundations for a lifetime of enjoyment and give her the desire to further her skills and the confidence to venture into the unknown. And you'll help her to become a well-balanced, confident person.

Encourage girls to be adventurous

● Never fuss about her getting dirty.
● Encourage games with energetic movements.
● Think of her as a boy; encourage all "boy's" games – climbing, swinging, balancing, kicking a ball.
● Get her physical toys like a bike early rather than late.

Encourage boys to be adventurous:

● Start physical games on large soft floor cushions early.
● Introduce "spatial" toys like Lego early to stimulate adventurous thinking.
● Help his imaginative curiosity by giving him items like toilet roll tubes and old egg boxes to make anything he can think of.
● Provide him with physical apparatus – rope ladder, swing, bike, skates, football.

4-11 growing up

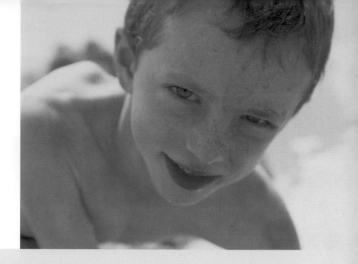

Children in this age group grow fast. Parents should make sure that their children are prepared for the changes in their bodies and what they mean.

Guiding principles

There are certain well-established guiding principles about the growth and development of children which are useful for parents to bear in mind:

● Each child is an individual. His growth and development will be different from other children and will differ at different times of his life. These variations are partly due to the tendencies he inherits from his family and partly to the environment in which he is brought up – for instance, how well nourished he is. Parents should never expect the same growth and development, or behaviour for that matter, in each of their children.

● A child's happiness varies and this can affect development. Happy children are normally healthy and energetic, whereas unhappiness tends to sap strength and energy and reduce wellbeing. Happy children use their energy purposefully, while unhappy children tend to dissipate their energy in brooding and self-pity.

● There is no point in parents trying to plot their child's size and weight on a complicated graph to see if he is "correct" for his age. Averages in the physical growth of children mean very little in relation to your child. The most important index of your child's normal development is his health and happiness, rather than his size.

Height

In the first year after birth children increase their length by about half. During the third, fourth and fifth years height gain falls off but is relatively steady at about 6–8cm (2½–3in) per year. Between then and the growth spurt at about 11 years in girls and 13 years in boys, weight remains fairly constant with a height gain of about 1cm (½in) per year.

Weight

During the second and third years of life a child gains from 1.4–2.3kg (3-5lb) a year. After this, weight gain tends to slow down. During the third, fourth and fifth years weight gain is fairly steady at about 2kg (4½lb) a year. In addition, most children become relatively lean in comparison with their early body shape.

The early school years are a period of relatively slow but steady gain in weight, on average about 3.2kg (7lb) a year. By the time a child is five years old he typically weighs about five times his birth weight and by adolescence he is between 36 and 40kg (80 and 90lb).

Towards sexual maturity

The age for the onset of puberty varies but is quite often around 10 or 11 for girls and around 12 years for boys. Apart from growing faster, children will notice changes in their bodies. For a girl, this begins with the dark area around the nipple (the areola) growing larger or puffing up slightly. Then the breasts begin to develop, becoming slightly conical in shape at first, then rounding out as her menstrual periods start.

For a boy, puberty means that, besides growing taller, his penis and testicles enlarge and pubic hair begins to grow. Later his voice will crack and deepen. Though puberty comes later in boys than girls, in some early developers it can begin as early as 10 years of age.

An explanation before the event of what will happen, in a calm and reassuring manner, is the best way of preparing your son and daughter. If a girl's first period comes without warning it can be a frightening experience, particularly as at this stage the discharge will not be bright red, as she might expect, but brownish black. Girls are menstruating, on average, nine months earlier than their mothers did. An increasing number of girls begin their periods at 10 or 11, which may be before they begin secondary school. And 1 in 6 girls now begins her periods at 8 years old, and 1 in 14 boys of 8 years old has pubic hair. For the first time, we have 8-year-old children who are sexually aware. They must have good sex education, and parents are the adults who must give it.

Menstruation

Periods start because hormones from a gland in the brain (the pituitary gland) tell the ovaries to manufacture the female sex hormones, oestrogen and progesterone. The ovaries begin producing a monthly egg and you begin to menstruate (have periods). Although 12 is the average age for periods to begin, anything between 8 and 16 is normal.

The start of menstruation is called menarche. Even before your first period you may be fertile, which means that you can get pregnant if you have unprotected sex. Menstruation ends at menopause, when you're about 50 years old. Some pain during a period is common but if you have very painful periods, see your doctor.

Calculated from the first day of blooding, the cycle is about 28 days.

Hormones make the ovaries produce an egg, and the lining of the womb grows. The egg travels to the womb through the fallopian tubes. If the egg isn't fertilized, it is shed with the womb lining.

Days 1–5 Menstruation: the lining of the womb is shed and flows out through the vagina.

Days 1–12 Pituitary hormones stimulate growth of an egg follicle; oestrogen from the ovaries causes womb lining to thicken.

Days 12–16 Ovulation: an egg is released. Ovary starts to produce progesterone.

Days 17–24 Egg travels along the fallopian tube to womb.

Days 24–28 If conception does not occur, your ovary stops producing progesterone, triggering menstruation.

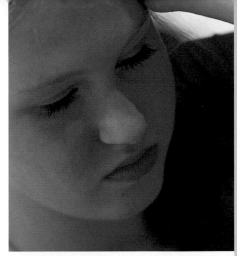

Coping with periods

Your choice of pads and tampons

Ordinary towel Bulky pad that fits inside pants, usually with self-stick panel.

Shaped towel Fits inside pants. Held in place by self-stick panel.

Towel with wings Self-stick "wings" anchor the pad more securely within pants.

Panty liner For light bleeding. Has self-stick panel.

Tampon Small, convenient, but requires manual insertion.

Tampon with applicator Applicator pushes tampon into vagina.

How pads and tampons work

Sanitary towel Worn externally inside the gusset of the pants.

Tampon Worn internally in the vagina. String through vaginal opening allows removal.

Sanitary hygiene during your period

● Change a sanitary pad or tampon 3–4 times a day.

● Wash your hands before and after changing towels and tampons.

● Wash your vulva daily from front to back, using baby soap and water. Don't use talc or deodorants.

● To minimize risk of infection, don't wear tampons overnight. Use a pad.

● There is a very rare infection called toxic shock syndrome (TSS), which is thought to be linked with wearing tampons. To avoid this, always use the least absorbent type of tampon to meet your needs and never leave a tampon in for longer than eight hours.

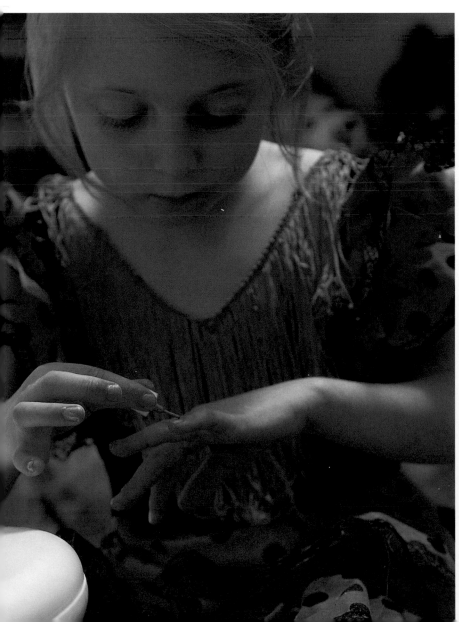

4-11 gaining confidence

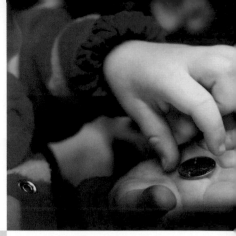

More than anything, children need caring, interested parents who will help them learn to make their way in the world and build self-confidence.

Holidays away from home

Your child can gain a good deal of confidence and independence from being away from home, helping with the chores and taking responsibility for keeping his own things neat and tidy. For many children, their first experience of going on holiday with people of their own age, instead of their parents, is a short camping trip with the Cubs or Brownies. The cost is quite low and the camp leaders are trained and experienced in looking after children. Any early homesickness usually disappears as soon as the fun starts, but only you can judge whether your child is ready, at the age of nine or so, to take the step towards independence. It is probably best to be guided by the child's enthusiasm; don't push him into it because you think it will do him good.

Camps often have open days for parents, when it is important to go along if you possibly can. A child can feel let down and isolated if all the other parents are there and his are not.

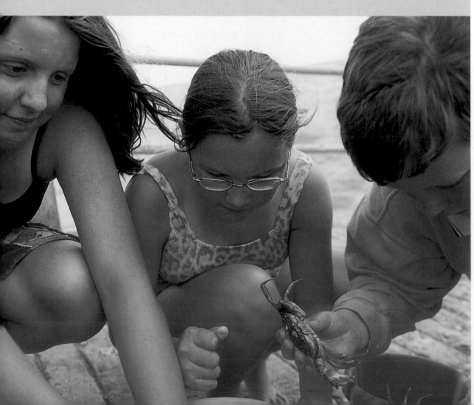

Pocket money

The ability to manage money is not something that comes naturally, it has to be learned. Most of us have less money than we need, or would like, so we are always having to choose between different kinds of spending. For a child, pocket money is the first chance to learn how to manage money.

● For children under six, give a small amount to spend when you are out shopping together, so that she gets used to handling money and realizes that she can choose between buying herself a lolly or a comic.

● When you are deciding on the amount of her weekly allowance, ask around other parents to get an idea of the going rate so your child has about the same as her friends.

● By the time she is seven or so, sit down with your child and draw up a "balance sheet", so that you can work out how much she will need and she will know what her pocket money is supposed to cover: for instance, is she only expected to buy sweets and ice cream or does it cover her Brownie subscription and her bus fares as well?

● Encourage your child to put something in her piggy bank each week to save up for special extras or holiday money.

● When relatives who are visiting hand out cash presents, it is reasonable to allow the child to spend them as she likes, as a treat. If large sums are involved, then she could spend some and have the rest put into a savings account in her name.

● Most children enjoy earning a little extra for jobs around the house. This does not mean that they should be paid any time they lend a hand, or they could soon become mercenary, but if they undertake a real job – like cleaning the inside of the car – then small payments can be put towards something they really want.

Self-confidence

A child is not born with a sense of "self-awareness". He develops it gradually through his dealings with other people – parents, brothers and sisters, friends and teachers. His self-image is moulded by the way they see him and the way he wants them to see him. If his immediate circle of family and friends is a happy, relaxed and outgoing one, which loves and accepts him as he is, he will have a good self-image, adjust well to the world around him, develop his independence and get along well with others. If, however, they are always tense and critical, so that he feels he is constantly letting them down, he will have a poor view of himself, be over anxious and defensive and find it far more difficult to form relationships.

As he grows he has to master all sorts of skills, from getting dressed and learning to read to social skills, the making of friends and talking easily with members of the opposite sex. He needs sufficient confidence to know that he can cope. If he has never developed that confidence, he may feel inferior and inadequate. The more inadequate he feels, the more likely he is to fail.

If your child sees that you notice and care when he makes the effort to master a new skill, or when he tries hard with his schoolwork, he will want to step up his efforts. Make sure you encourage any progress he makes, even if he happens to be slower at learning to read than your friends' children or has difficulty keeping up with the rest of his class. You can easily destroy a child's confidence if you only seem to notice when he makes mistakes or does badly and go on nagging or criticizing about it. Of course, you are only trying to spur him on, but it doesn't look like that from his angle.

Parental interest is vital in helping a child develop his abilities to the full – providing it is not too intense or demanding. Then it can do more harm than good. If parents have unrealistically high expectations, so that the child can never quite meet them, his self-esteem will suffer. Then he may opt out and stop trying altogether. A confident child may be spurred on to try harder by a failure. A child who already feared he was "no good" may see the failure as confirming his worst fears and simply give up. There are children who never reach their full potential because they are so afraid of failing that they avoid any situation where they might be tested.

Road safety

It is never too early to start road safety drill. Every time you are out with your child, holding her hand so that you stay close together, give a running commentary on what you see, so she learns to judge the speed of an oncoming car, knows that she should never run across the road but always walk at a steady pace and so on. Children under the age of 6 should never be allowed on the road alone, and children between the ages of 6 and 10 are not mature enough to be completely safe on the road. Once your child is old enough to be out on her own, teach her several unbreakable rules:

● Never dart into the road after a ball or a pet.
● Never walk or play along the kerbside, particularly near a blind corner.
● Stop, look and listen for traffic before crossing a road, or even crossing a gateway whose opening may be obscured by walls.
● Never cross the road between parked cars if you can avoid it.
● Whenever you have to cross the road, choose a place where you have a good view of the traffic in both directions. Always use a zebra crossing if you can.
● Treat a zebra crossing as if it were not there – approach the kerb, stop, look and listen. Always walk across, never run.

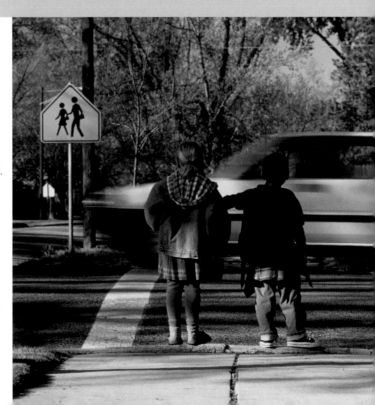

4-11
learning to live with others

Parents have the daunting task of turning infants into sensible, sociable children and eventually into responsible, loving adults who relate well to others.

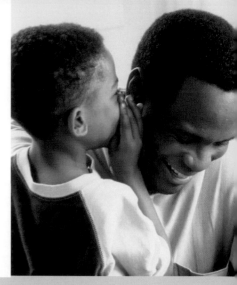

Knowing where to draw the line

At some time, most parents are filled with self-doubt about when and how to discipline their children. Naturally they want to strike a balance between constantly nagging them and being too lax. We all like to think of ourselves as positive encouragers, not punishing dictators. The last thing we want is for our children to fear us and we'll do anything to keep channels of communication open. However, day in, day out, there are times when we don't know quite where to draw the line.

The aim of teaching children discipline should be to help them exercise self-discipline. It isn't about exerting control over them or pulling rank. Most harm is done by being too rigid. A classic study from Berkeley in California examined three disciplinary styles and how they affected kids.
● Authoritarian parents (controlling, cold and detached) had children who were discontented, withdrawn and distrustful.
● Permissive parents (warm but non-demanding) at the other end of the scale, had the least self-reliant, inquisitive and self-controlled children.
● Authoritative parents (setting firm limits but warm, rational and receptive), however, were the most likely to have self-reliant, self-controlled and contented children.

Strike a balance

Your child begs to stay up past her bedtime to watch television. What's your response?
● Too hard: "Bed! Now! Or I'll ban television for a month."
● Too soft: "Oh, all right, but just this once."
● About right: "Come on now. You know the rules. You can watch television late Friday and Saturday nights only."

Your child wants to wear tattered jeans to her granny's birthday party.
● Too hard: "Put on your best trousers. That's final!"
● Too soft: "Well, all right, but put on a nice sweater."
● About right: "I don't want to upset granny and you should look nice for her. I'll help you choose some smart clothes if you like."

As a parent, I wanted to keep rules for my children to a minimum, but those that were important weren't negotiable. For instance:
● activities that were dangerous to my children or others were banned
● respect for, and kindness to, others were the order of the day
● cruelty in life and on television had no place in our family
● the truth would always be rewarded (no matter what was confessed).

Children and the too-friendly stranger

When children are out alone, it is possible that they will meet an undesirable stranger and, because most children are trusting, they may put themselves in danger. It is every parent's duty to inform their children of the risks of being out in public places. There is no need for this explanation to be alarming, but all children should be on the alert for friendly strangers who talk to them, offer them sweets or a treat or a ride in their car when they are in parks or on waste ground, on playing fields, in public lavatories or even walking down the street.

It is always better to be as honest as you can with children, and your warning words in this instance may be life-saving. Be perfectly frank and tell your children that adults who are mentally sick may do more than just try to speak to them, but may touch them, invite them to look at pictures, try to undress them or handle their genitals. These adults may also undress or touch themselves.

Be very clear in giving instructions about what your child must do if this ever happens. The priority is to get help. They should not worry about where they get it from – they should go into a shop, stop a passer-by or knock on someone's door. Also warn your child that he should never go off to play with another child without first asking your permission.

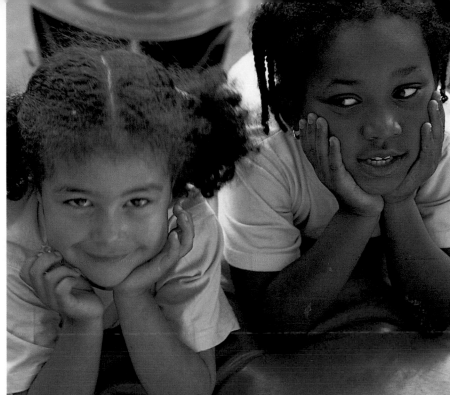

Being considerate

Good manners and consideration for others – saying "please" and "thank you", offering a helping hand, giving a seat to an elderly or infirm person, waiting our turn in the queue – are the outward signs that we feel that other people and their rights matter. The actions themselves may be trivial but what they show about our concern for others, whether they are friends or strangers, is very important. Without a generally accepted code of manners, life would become thoroughly brutish and unpleasant, so parents need to pass them on to their children.

The best way to teach your child good manners is by consistent example. If you see a mother yelling at her child: "hey you – get in here!" you won't be surprised to find the child has obnoxious manners. A father who elbows his way to the front of the queue, dragging his young son behind him, is likely to produce the sort of child who pushes others out of the way to grab the best cake for himself.

If you treat other people, including your child, with consideration, you will need very little in the way of formal manners teaching. Of course, you will have to prompt, remind and explain occasionally. A child starts off as a self-centred little being and he does not naturally think of the other person. As he gets older and identifies with you, he will want to copy your style of behaviour and if you are considerate to others, so will he be.

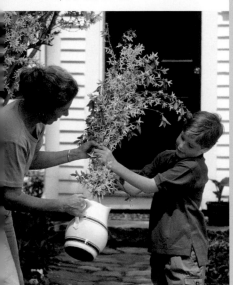

Changing patterns of friendship

Friendship patterns change dramatically with age and the factors which govern friendship in young children are quite different from those which apply among teenagers or adults.

The relationships of preschool children are normally friendly and cooperative rather than hostile or competitive, even among the most aggressive youngsters. They tend to have a number of friends, none favoured above the others. Don't worry too much if your child is not very popular at this stage. Friendships among this age group are casual and unstable, here today gone tomorrow, so they are not likely to have important or lasting effects on the child's personality.

Studies of nursery school children show that it is the girls who seek to make friendships, spending more of their time playing with friends, while boys prefer some sort of physical activity like running and chasing.

Once they are established at school, around the age of 5 or 6, individual friendships are more likely to develop and they attach themselves to a few special pals. They choose friends of the same age, perhaps the child who sits next to them in class or at meals or is in their group when they take turns at playing in the Wendy house. It is unusual for a child of this age to be playing alone most of the time.

Sex differences seem unimportant in small children's play but by the age of 8 or 9, they are playing in single-sex groups. Boys of 9 to 13 probably belong to a group or gang, though they may have one particular friend in the group. Girls usually have a best friend – though not always the same best friend – and if they belong to a group or "club" it is less tightly knit and less important to them. Both boys and girls are now forming friendships on the basis of interests rather than proximity.

Children's temperaments vary and so do their social needs. You may have one child who sticks to the same close friend for years and takes little interest in other children – another who has such a wide and changing circle of friends that you can hardly remember their names. So long as your child is content with the way things are, there is no reason for you to interfere.

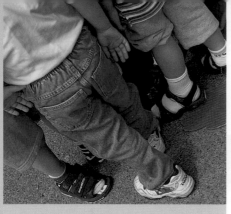

4-11 sensitive issues

At some stage in nearly every child's life, problems and questions arise that need careful handling from parents.

Bullying

Bullying is one of the most insidious problems within schools – and it can exist in any school, no matter what the system or age of the children. Vigilant teachers in a school with a positive policy on bullying will be keen to nip it in the bud, so if your child's questions hint at bullying, see your school's headteacher immediately.

● Bullying is always wrong and must be stopped. Convince your child of this fact in whatever way you can. She will find it easier to tell you about bullying if she is clear about this basic belief.

● Boys are particularly conscious of the ridiculous code that they mustn't tell on bullies, even if they are the victims. Convince your children that this code is wrong and that they must seek help if they are being bullied.

● You may wonder whether your child should retaliate if faced with bullying. Under the age of nine, I used to tell my son to give the bully one warning and then hit back, but a child shouldn't do this if faced with several others. A child can ask a trusted older child to help deal with bullies, but you should always report bullying to the school, even if it is happening outside school premises. Ask for the staff's help to bring bullies to book, but in a discreet way to protect your child.

● Girls are just as capable of bullying as boys, and very often it takes the form of a cruel, whispering campaign, or excluding a child from a group of friends. If prolonged, this can be just as wounding as physical violence and should be taken seriously.

● Children aren't born bullies but they often learn a pattern of selfishness, victimization and bullying from adults in their own homes. This may be due to excessive strictness from an authoritarian parent or arise in a home which is disorganized, where a child is neglected.

● Bullying is a child's response to pain and lack of love. While bullying can never be condoned, these children need help to change their pattern of behaviour.

Problem behaviour

When should we begin to worry that problem behaviour goes beyond the bounds and becomes abnormal? There is no simple answer. The point about real "problem" behaviour and emotions is that they are too intense and too frequent, so that they lead to unhappy consequences for the child and the people around him. It is one thing to wet the bed at two and half, but think what a terrible time an 11-year-old who could not control his bladder at night would have.

Several criteria are helpful when considering whether problem behaviour has overstepped the bounds. The first three concern the frequency, persistence and intensity of a particular symptom. Many children have fears, tell lies and steal, but for most of them it is simply a bad patch and they soon leave it behind. But occasionally a child may be so full of fears that as soon as one disappears, another takes its place, or he may go on making up fantastic stories which seem totally real to him long after most children have learned to distinguish fact and fiction. Then he could be having psychological difficulties in adjusting to the world he lives in and may need help.

Most children bite their nails at some time or other. However, few do it so fiercely they draw blood. Such intensity suggests emotional disturbance rather than just a bad habit. Another example is the child who seems unable to tell the truth, even when it would be better for him if he did.

The fourth criterion is age. We need to measure the child's behaviour by the norm for his stage of development. It is common for a four-year-old to have lots of temper tantrums, but they are so rare in an 11-year-old that they are likely to be a sign of emotional disturbance.

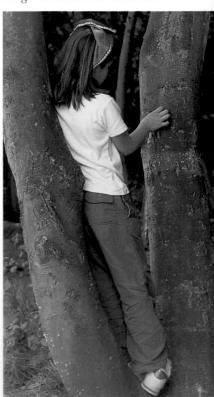

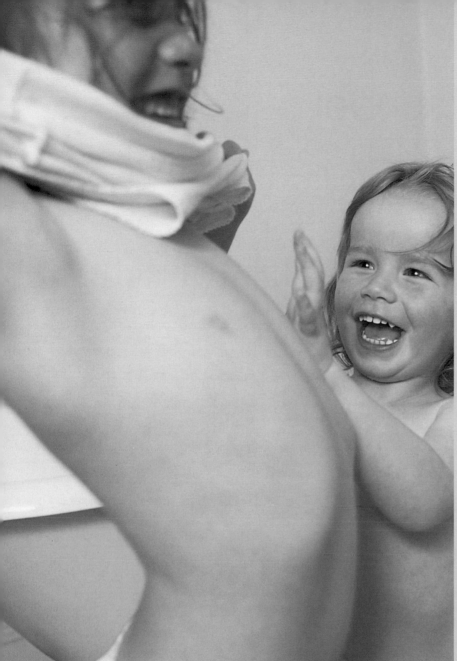

A healthy attitude to nudity

The subject of nudity is unfortunately often surrounded by taboos, but there needn't be any inhibition within a family with children under 11.

● Try not to programme your children with your own hang-ups about nudity, if you have them. Your younger children will be naturally unembarrassed; take your lead from them.

● At around eight or nine, however, some children (particularly girls) may give you very clear signals that they are no longer comfortable about exposing their bodies. You may find that your daughter starts to bolt the bathroom door for the first time, and cover herself up when changing for swimming or sport. When this happens, respect her need for privacy.

● The fewer limits set, the better. My own children followed me into the lavatory until they were five or six years old and felt free to come into the bedroom at any time while I was dressing. Some parents may well feel shy about this. but my primary concern was to make myself available to my children at all times, as well as to make them feel comfortable with nakedness and therefore with their own bodies.

● Of course, your child also will have to learn that outside your home others may not be so open about nudity and some, particularly older people such as grandparents, may see things differently; you may need to explain that it's good manners not to embarrass other people. What is perfectly acceptable at home may not be possible or advisable elsewhere.

Masturbation is normal

Masturbation can be a difficult question for parents to face – not because the subject is in itself complicated, but because of their own attitudes to it. Your child has the right to be relaxed about masturbation. Being clear in your own mind that masturbation is normal and beneficial will help to dispel the myths that surround it.

● Many parents feel very confused about masturbation because of misunderstandings starting in their own childhood. Masturbation is not bad in itself; treat it as a normal part of growing up and don't plant the seeds of shame.

● Tolerate or ignore masturbation; if questions arise, answer them; agree that "It feels nice to touch your penis", but set limits: "This is something we do in private." If your child masturbates in public, treat it as you would bad manners or lack of thoughtfulness.

● Up to the age of 5, one child touching another is nearly always innocent. Make sure that one child is not an unwilling victim and that they are not trying to put things into themselves. The exception to this would be a child who has been abused when very small.

● If a child talks about someone who is significantly older and more developed touching him, you should treat this as a danger signal. Calmly ascertain exactly what has happened (if anything) and be vigilant when he's with that person.

● Masturbation is a healthy and natural way to release tension. The only time I would be concerned is if a child were masturbating habitually to escape from a horrible world, because he was being emotionally deprived. A child like this needs help; the way to correct it is to give love, not punishment.

4–11 starting school

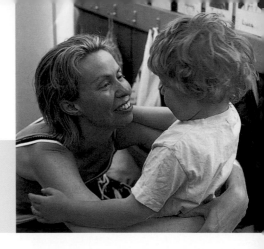

If you prepare your child gently and carefully, she should take starting school and learning to read and count in her stride.

Preparing your child for school

It will help your child to cope with her first few weeks at school if she can
● say both her names and her address clearly
● handle a knife and fork to cut up her food
● ask for the toilet without using special "family" names for it
● deal with buttons and zips
● use taps, towels and flush toilets.
It is natural enough for parents to feel anxious as the day approaches for their child to take her first big step into the outside world, especially if she is the first or only child. Parents who have been cementing a close relationship with a child

for four or five years sometimes see school as taking their baby away and destroying something of that precious relationship.

If your child has been to nursery class or playgroup, she is already used to the idea of school and being away from home for part of the day, so she should settle in without problems. If she is the second or third child in the family, she may already be quite envious of her older brother or sister, who seems so much more sophisticated.

If your child has not spent any time at playschool, particularly if she is an only child, then make sure she is used to being parted from you for short periods, perhaps spending an afternoon playing with a

neighbour's children, knowing you will collect her at a set time. A regular walk past the school at playtime can help, too. This gives her an opportunity to look in and see what is going on. She will see other parents near the railings, perhaps waving to their children and you might promise that you will come and wave to her from time to time, when she is one of the children in the playground. Most schools encourage new parents to visit the school with their child at least once before the actual starting date, so that she can see the other children working happily and know there is nothing frightening awaiting her.

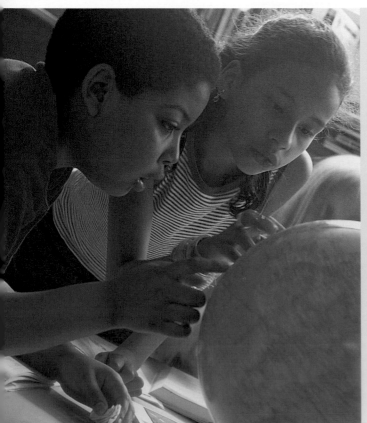

Project work

Project work has been devised to use children's natural curiosity to explore a wide range of subjects. Instead of learning to recite lists of dates or capital cities, they develop a real feeling and understanding for history, geography and the other subjects that make up the formal curriculum.

If they are working on a project about the Romans, for instance, they might make a map of Roman settlements in Britain, discuss the reasons behind the choice of site and study how they built roads. They could plan out how they might have fought a battle, investigate their religious beliefs, make a model of a Roman fort, write and act a play about Julius Caesar, making their own costumes, and visit a museum to see objects made by the Romans. By the end of the project, each child should have a personal folder of written work, pictures and charts and will have learned a good deal about collecting, recording and presenting information.

How parents can help with reading

If your child seems to be making little progress with the first stages of reading it may be that his whole approach is wrong and he is relying too much on his eyes, instead of using his brain. Settle down with him one evening and ask him to read a little from his school reading book. If, as he reads, he struggles from one word to another and comes out with a sentence which is a nonsensical jumble, it is because he is trying to interpret a string of shapes, instead of thinking about the meaning of the words. Without taking the meaning into account, he cannot check whether he has got it right or not. Yet when his mother talks to him, he understands without needing to identify every word or syllable. For some reason he is not applying the same technique in reading. He is not using his knowledge of language to guess what is coming next, so that interpreting the symbols becomes much easier.

You can use a simple reading game to help him. When you read him a story, move your finger along the line of words, so that he follows it with his eyes. After two or three sentences, suddenly stop and let the child guess the next word. If the sentence was: "Mum said Jenny could go out and play but she had to be home by…", the child might guess five o'clock. He might be wrong, but he knows it must be a time that is missing and he knows children have to come in from play around teatime. Soon he will realize that he only needs to identify the first one or two letters of the unknown word to get the answer right. If you repeat the game over and over again he should eventually get into the habit of using his brain as well as his eyes as he tries to read.

Reading for information

If children can be encouraged to see reading as a useful and necessary part of life in dozens of different ways every day, then they will accept the written word easily and naturally instead of being slightly nervous of it all their lives, like many adults. Help your child by putting him in charge of the shopping list, for example, and asking him to read out the items one by one as you go round the supermarket. Or ask him to read out a recipe as you cook or to look up the time of a film in the paper.

Helping with numbers

Many parents still teach their child to count to 10 by heart or by pointing to her fingers one at a time, but it will be far more useful to her if she learns by moving her counters or raisins or pennies into groups. Then she won't begin with the idea that four means the fourth in a series, rather than all four in a set of objects.

Once she has grasped the idea, you can practise by spotting men with umbrellas or dogs on leads when you are out walking: this aids concentration as well as counting. Instead of threading big wooden beads on the laces just as they come, she can try threading two red ones together, then three green ones, and so on.

Sorting games can be an excellent path to learning. You could ask your child to sort out household items, such as different types of nuts from one large bowl into four smaller ones.

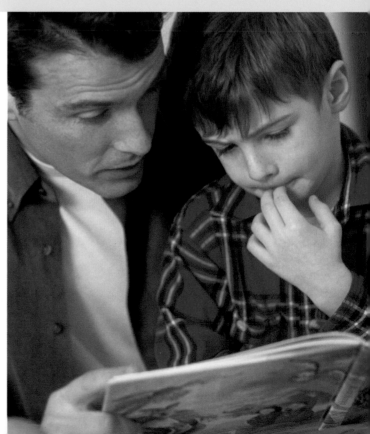

4-11 problems of growing up

All children go through phases of "problem behaviour" that worry their parents. Most are solved in time, but children may need understanding and sensitivity meanwhile.

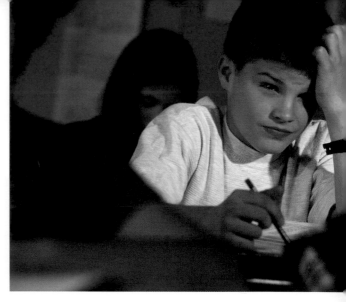

Why does a child cheat?

Parents are usually horrified if their child, who has been brought up to think that honesty is very important, is found to be cheating at school.

A normal child cheats when he wants to cover up a real or imagined weakness. If he is self-confident and secure, he will seldom feel the need to cheat. If you find your child is persistently cheating, ask yourself why he feels he cannot stand on his own ability. Often

the trouble comes from putting children in fiercely competitive situations and only praising those who come out on top. Perhaps your child feels he cannot keep up with the rest of the class, in which case his teacher may be able to suggest a way round the problem. It may be that you are pushing him too hard and expecting too much, so that he cheats in a misguided attempt not to disappoint you.

Why does a child lie?

Children often try to boost their prestige in a world where they feel small and insignificant by telling their friends tall stories about the family's gleaming new sports car, which is really a battered old saloon, or father's important jet-setting lifestyle, when he actually has a routine office job. They only do this because they have learned from the adults around them that these are the things that will bring them admiration and esteem.

But sometimes children who "lie" simply are not seeing things the way you do and feel thoroughly misjudged if you call them untruthful. When two brothers fight, it is always the other one who started it. It is always the other sister who suggested climbing onto the toolshed roof or picking all the flowers in the garden.

When you judge whether or not a child is lying, take into account the way she sees the world. Childhood is a period of vivid imagination, make-believe and

fantasy. For a child with an active imagination, the borderline between fact and fantasy is not clearly defined. What she has wished and dreamed may sometimes be more real to her than mere fact. So if she comes and tells you she has been talking to a little green man in the garden – "he was there, honestly Mummy, I'm not making it up" – why not join in the fun, at the same time making it clear that you know it is all a fantasy.

As a child gets older and gains more confidence she normally finds she no longer needs all the little lies that bolstered her self-esteem. But of course some children go on lying into adulthood and, in the end, have trouble distinguishing truth from untruth.

Persistent lying is a danger signal. Parents need to make sure they are not aggravating the problem by being too strict. If the punishment for breaking the rules is too severe, the child will go to

great lengths never to admit she has broken them. If a child accidentally breaks a treasured ornament and owns up, only to find you lose your temper and give her a good smack, she is far more likely to blame it on the cat next time. The main step in teaching a child not to lie is to reassure her sufficiently, so that she does not feel she has to lie.

If she feels that lying is the only way to keep her end up with her playmates – perhaps they come from a more expensive part of town, so she pretends her home is as grand as theirs – teach her that possessions are not all-important and that people will like her for what she is, not what she brags about.

Finally, make sure you set her a good example. You may tell her fibs for the best possible motives, saying that there are no sweets left when there are plenty hidden away, but she will have trouble seeing why her lies are wrong and yours are not.

Hyperactivity

For want of a label, some difficult but completely normal children are said to be hyperactive. To my mind this is unjustified. The word "hyperactive" is the broad term formerly used to describe children who have Attention Deficit Disorder (ADD) and Attention Deficit Hyperactivity Disorder (ADHD) – behavioural conditions that include disruptive behaviour, poor attention span, sleeplessness, and excitability (see p.529). Contrary to parental belief, certain food colourings and flavourings have never been proven to contribute to hyperactivity, and sympathetic handling by parents can improve the behaviour of most children. There are only a few degrees of hyperactivity in children that are abnormal, serious or need medical treatment. I, personally, am against the use of drugs such as Ritalin without very careful assessment by several doctors, especially as so many children respond to kinder cognitive and behavioural therapies.

Genuinely hyperactive children will probably need specialist help in retraining their habits, known as "behaviour therapy". However if your child's boundless energy leaves you limp and exhausted by the end of the day the chances are that he is simply overactive, **not** hyperactive. If your child is always "on the go" and never wants to go to bed, make certain that he has plenty of opportunity to work off his energy through boisterous outdoor play, then use the basic training rules which work with a toddler who is testing out the limits you have set for him. Ignore "bad" behaviour as far as possible, provided he is not likely to injure himself or others. But never overlook "good" behaviour and always praise him when he is calm and cooperative. Instead of telling him off when he knocks things flying as he charges into the room, make him feel he has done well when he walks in normally. It will take plenty of patience, but it will gradually get results.

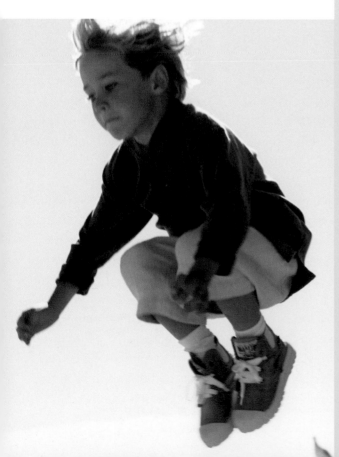

Why does a child steal?

A child of four or so takes things because she has no clear idea of what is rightfully hers and what belongs to someone else. She is always being urged to share her toys, so if the little girl next door has something she likes, she sees no reason why she shouldn't take it home with her.

She soon begins to learn that it is wrong to steal or use other people's possessions without their permission. But the way children see stealing varies at different ages. Younger children tend to see stealing as a bad thing to do because they fear the punishment that follows. Older children are more likely to see stealing as undesirable because it injures others.

How to deal with stealing

Most parents are alarmed when a child steals because, as adults, we have learned to look on theft as a serious crime. Yet research shows that stealing is common among older children. Punishment is not a very effective way of stamping it out. Try to avoid sermons and melodramatics, making your child feel she has done something unforgivable so that you will never love her in the same way again. Talk to her calmly and firmly, making her see that she is hurting someone else by taking their property. If she has stolen from friends, see that she pays them back. If she has taken goods from a shop, take her back there and explain to the shopkeeper that she took something without paying and wants to apologize and return it.

A child may steal from her mother if she feels she is not getting enough love and attention from her – perhaps she thinks that, once the toddler stage with all its cuddles has passed, you do not love her so much, so you need to show her that she is mistaken. Sometimes a child steals objects she does not need, or even want, to prove herself in some way – perhaps the discipline at home is over-strict or her mother is too fussy and protective, so she needs to break out.

Children who go on stealing do need professional help, but if they are seriously disturbed, stealing will not be the only symptom. They are often playing truant from school and showing other problems.

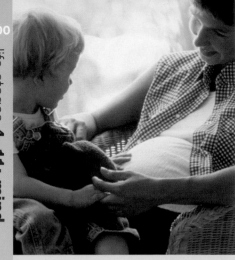

4-11 keep talking together

Stay in touch with your child on everything – from the facts of life to what he sees on television.

Sex play is normal

The way you deal with sex play is important because it can influence the way your child feels about sex later. Sex play becomes far more common once children start infant school. By the age of 13 as many as two-thirds of boys have taken part, though sexual activity among girls of this age is less common.

Homosexual play

Homosexual play, with youngsters handling each other's genitals, is also more common as children get older. It is far more likely to happen in single-sex boarding schools than in day schools, for obvious reasons, but there is no hard evidence to show that this passing phase of homosexual activity has any bearing on long-term adult homosexuality.

Sexual interest and behaviour in children is intermittent, casual and not at all intense. So why not treat it in the same way? Don't get excited and tell children they are being "naughty" or "dirty". The child may begin to feel guilty and furtive about his sexual feelings

or he may become far more interested and excited because he feels it is forbidden. If you make a great issue of it, you are implying that sex is unnatural. Treat sexual curiosity as normal and natural, but gently insist that there are conventions of behaviour that must be followed.

Many problems can be avoided by an open attitude towards sexual subjects from the time children become aware of the difference between the sexes. If your small son wants to compare the size of his penis with his father's, then there is nothing more likely to allay his curiosity than a good look. It will do much to prevent him from being neurotic about his own body.

The facts of life

You can also encourage a sensible outlook on sex by telling your children the facts of life as soon as they begin to ask, so that they know there is nothing to be furtive about. So explain clearly to your children about how a baby grows

in the mother's uterus. Once you have dealt with this point, it is important to go on to say how the baby is actually born, so that children do not grow up thinking that the abdomen simply splits open and delivers the baby like a pea from a pod.

Be guided by your child

If possible, separate the account of the growing embryo from a discussion on intercourse. Parents can be guided by a child's questions, so that they give him all the information he wants at the time without launching into a full lecture on sex before he is ready to understand fully.

Try to use simple accurate language, so that words like penis, vagina and sperm are never something to giggle over. If you are worried about putting the information over properly, there are plenty of simple books in the library that will help – but don't just hand over the book to your child to look at by himself, sit and read it together.

Answering questions about sex

Answering questions such as "What is making love?", "What is a penis?" etc., provides an opportunity to emphasize to children that sex should come from love and that with love comes responsibility: the responsibility to put the other person before themselves, never to coerce, pressure or force and to have respect for others and for themselves.

● Don't shrink from telling your child the truth. You owe your child an honest and open answer without any fear of being embarrassed.

● Don't feel that you have to give every single detail to a young child: it's neither necessary nor good for your child, who may be frightened by what she can't grasp. Remember there's rarely need for detailed information about the mechanics of sex for a child under 8.

● Think of each question your child asks as an opportunity to convey your standards and values and to help your child feel loved and well informed.

● Try to anticipate your child's concerns. Remember that sex is also about self-control and abstinence and you should school your child about these qualities.

● Don't ever scold your child for being sexually curious about people of the opposite sex; satisfy that curiosity by answering questions frankly and honestly.

● Talk to sons and daughters together. Boys need to know about girls because knowledge and understanding will help to instill in them a sense of responsibility and understanding of girls' and women's needs from an early age.

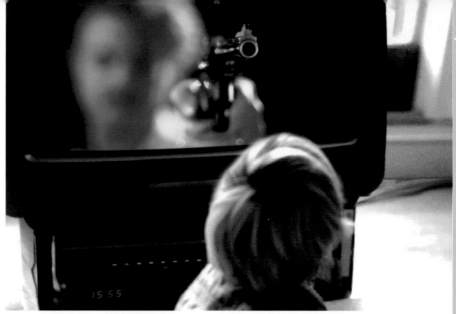

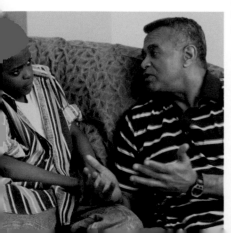

Television?

Most of us have our own firm opinions about whether the overall influence of television is good or bad. But, like it or not, television is here to stay. Many parents find it difficult or impossible to cut down their children's viewing but they worry what effect the frequent scenes of violence will have on their children and about the amount of time being "wasted" when it could be used for reading, hobbies, music and so on.

Violence on television

Research evidence shows that the effect of television violence on young children is likely to be rather small. This is probably because much of the violence they see is in cartoons or action films, full of characters who are part of a fantasy world quite different from their own. Children imitate people like themselves – other children, brothers and sisters or their parents and teachers. They are well aware of the difference between real people and Tom and Jerry or a character in *Star Wars*.

"Cops and robbers" films may have slightly more influence, but even then many children, perhaps most, realize that there is a strong element of fantasy. They know that their fathers and brothers do not drive fast cars and spend their time in expensive nightclubs and they know that when someone punches you, it hurts. The evidence shows that it is young adults, rather

than children under 12, who are most likely to be affected by the violence in films, because it is often committed by people from their own age group whom they may be tempted to copy.

Surprisingly, it is the real-life news film or documentary that is most likely to affect a child, because there he can see children throwing stones at soldiers in Ulster or youngsters just like his brother fighting on the terraces at football matches. These are real people behaving violently in real situations. Whether we own a television set or not, our children are likely to be influenced by the attitudes and actions of the society around them. Parents cannot protect them from all that is ugly in life.

Probably one of the most useful things parents can do is to watch news programmes with their children, so that they can talk about what is going on and the way they feel about it. Discussion after programmes meant purely for entertainment can be useful too, helping children to form and put across their thoughts about the "goodies" and the "baddies" and the way the characters treat one another.

You can be reassured that the behaviour of family and friends, seeing them treating one another with gentleness and consideration, will exert a much more powerful influence on your child than anything he may see on television.

"teenagers need to experiment and test limits – their own and other people's"

life stages: 11 to 18 years

Until a child is about 10, most parents can confidently say they know them well, as young children mirror what they're taught. This changes when youngsters reach adolescence. Those years of adolescence are often described as "normal insanity" because, in most cases, things do eventually settle down.

Rebellion is normal

Teenagers are natural risk-takers. They need to experiment and test limits – their own and other people's. Rebellion is a normal part of dealing with the emotional changes of adolescence. Teenagers may feel rebellious about the rules and regulations that society tries to impose on them or that their parents expect them to live by.

Much of the natural rebelliousness of adolescents stems from their need to be different from their parents and to establish their own separate identity. This rebelliousness may not be particularly comfortable for the adolescents themselves, and they may make decisions or act in a particular way precisely because they know their parents won't want them to do it.

But remember, most bad behaviour is a sign that your child is finding life difficult. In my experience, it makes things easier for everyone if parents:

● **overlook** what they can
● **avoid** too much confrontation and look for ways to compromise
● are **tolerant**.

I'd very strongly advise against fighting fire with fire. It only makes things worse and heightens a teenager's resentment against everyone. That's why it is so important to try to understand the cause of problem behaviour, not just concentrate on the fallout from it.

For instance, if your children are having trouble at school, encourage them to explain what their motivation is for behaving badly. Are there any teachers or lessons that cause them particular difficulties? Low self-esteem often lies at the root of problem behaviour, so give your teenagers praise when they do something well to give their confidence a boost.

No problem should be too serious for them to share with you. If it seems impossible to talk to your teenage children because you meet a blank wall or tempers flare on both sides, it's worth asking a third party like a friend or relative to talk to them.

The teenager's point of view

Your teenage years are a very precious part of your life; your horizons broaden in a unique way and new choices constantly present themselves. This time is also unique because of how much you grow mentally. You enter the teenage years feeling awkward, clumsy, shy and bewildered and you emerge from them with clear opinions and ideas about your career, the kind of relationships that you're looking for and possibly the sort of life that's going to make you happy. Probably at no other time in your life will you grow at such a fast rate, both emotionally and intellectually.

Do try to talk to your parents – you need them and their support, and you're unlikely to find anyone else who's as interested in you as they are. What's essential is to persuade them that you have important things to talk about while you're growing up and you need their help. Few parents can resist such a request.

There are few periods in our lives that seem as difficult as our teenage years, and when they're over, you'll probably look back and feel that you did very well in negotiating them. If you manage this, your achievement will be enormous. If you come to the end of this time feeling fairly contented with a positive outlook on life, it's a triumph and you can be very proud of yourself.

In the pages that follow, I offer guidelines where appropriate, advice where I feel there may be a need and strategies for dealing with potentially difficult situations.

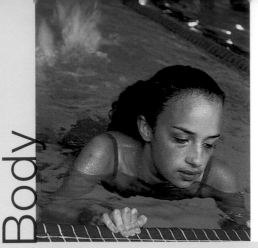

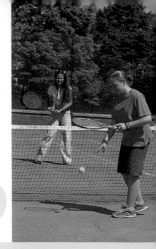

" the key to a smooth passage through adolescence is self-esteem "

Body

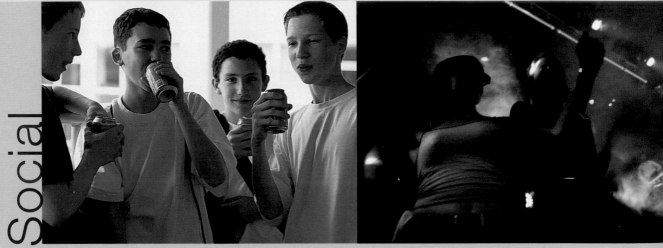

Social

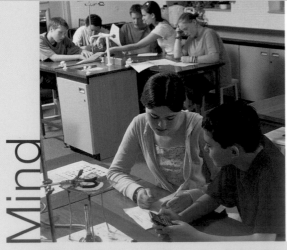

" your teens are a very precious part of your life "

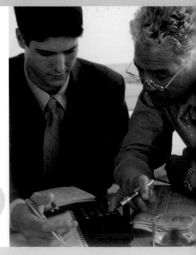

Mind

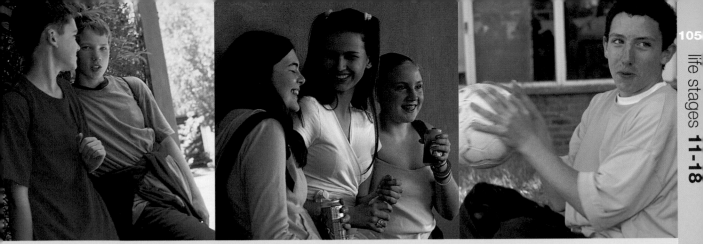

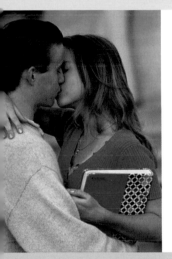

> ❝ the only
> reason to
> have sex
> is because
> you
> want to ❞

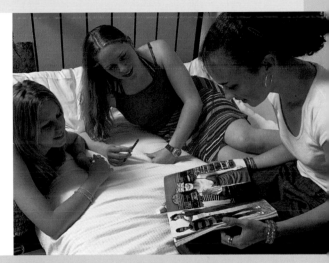

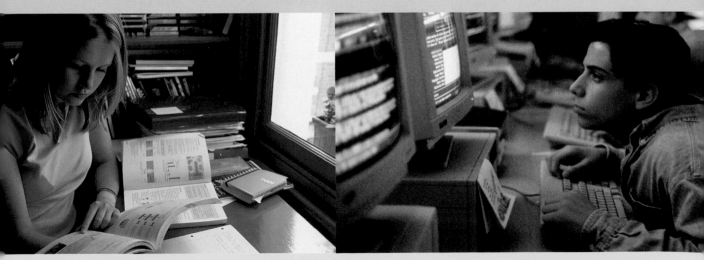

11–18

a girl's body

Between the ages of about 8 and 18 a girl's body changes, under the influence of the female hormone oestrogen, from that of a child to a woman.

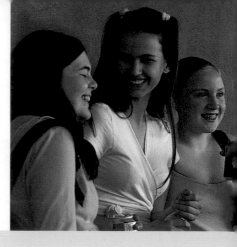

Physical growth

At around the age of 8, a year or so before puberty for most girls, the pelvic bones begin to grow and fat is deposited on the breasts, hips and thighs. In the adolescent phase, which generally starts between 10 and 16 years, your nipples start to bud, and pubic and underarm hair appears. At this stage, the genital organs develop and your periods start. More fat is deposited on your hips, breasts and thighs. By the time you are 18 or so, bone growth will be complete and you'll have reached your adult height.

The speed at which your body changes depends on many factors and it varies enormously from individual to individual, so don't worry if your friends are developing more quickly or more slowly than you.

Armpit hair At about 14 years, hair starts to grow in the armpits and the sweat glands become active.

Skin The hormone androgen affects the skin, causing more oil to be secreted. Pimples may appear.

Waist In contrast to broadening hips and breasts, the waist begins to look much more slender and defined.

Pubic hair Hair first appears when you are about 12 years old and then gradually becomes thicker and curlier, spreading up to form a triangle shape. It may not match the colour of the hair on your head at first.

Thighs The inner and outer thighs develop pads of fat from about the age of 14, giving the body a more curvaceous, womanly outline.

Hips As the pelvic bones grow, the hips begin to broaden. Fat is then laid down on the hips, helping to give the body its characteristic female shape.

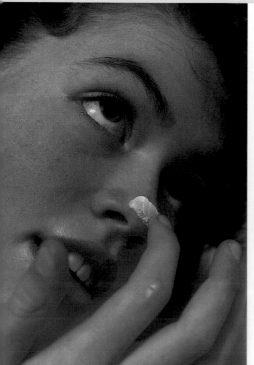

Take good care of your skin

Really great-looking skin is a big plus and one of your most important assets. So whether you were born with a perfect complexion, or one that is not so good, you should make an effort to take care of it properly. When you are going through adolescence, your body is trying to adjust to a change in hormone balance, and this affects your skin.

Pimples Never squeeze pimples because this spreads the infection into the deeper layers of the skin. You can squeeze uninflamed blackheads after a hot bath or shower, when all the pores are open, but afterwards apply a small dab of antiseptic cream to keep the skin clear. Don't use over-the-counter pimple cream,

and if your skin is very oily, refrain from using an abrasive cleanser – this simply spreads the bacteria.

Acne Nearly every teenager has acne at some stage. During adolescence, high levels of sex hormones are produced, which lead to the production of large quantities of sebum in the skin. Sebum is an irritant that may block the pores, causing a purplish lump which may become infected and form a pustule. An occasional pimple is normal at this age, but severe acne does tend to scar, so ask your doctor for advice on how to clear it. There are many good acne preparations available, but the best need a prescription.

Breast development

Breasts come in every shape and size. Remember that it's not true that boys prefer girls with big breasts or that small breasts mean you can't feed a baby.

It's normal for your breasts to feel tender as they grow during puberty, and in the week before your period. You may find that wearing a bra helps to relieve any tenderness. A good bra will support heavy breasts and stop them from wobbling.

Buying a bra

There's no need to wear stiff, heavy bras with under-wiring. Today there are plenty on the market specially designed for girls who lead active lives, who need support and who want to look as natural as possible. Cotton is the best fabric to choose if you can, particularly if you play a lot of sport. But there are good bras made of synthetic fabrics, too.

Measuring for a bra

Measure yourself under the bust and round up to the nearest size. For instance, if your measurement is 84cm (33in), you'll need a 86cm (34in) bra. For your cup size, measure around the largest part of your breasts and take the first measurement away from this. If the difference is less than 12.5cm (5in), you are an A cup, less than 15cm (6in) you need a B cup, 15–22cm (6–8½in) a C cup, 23cm (9in) or more, a D cup.

Many stores offer a fitting service with trained assistants and the chance to try on different bras before you buy. This will help you establish what kind of bra suits you.

Problem periods

Girls often experience actual physical distress during their periods, the causes of which have been investigated and treatment is available. Painful periods (dysmenorrhoea – see p.247) can be quite disabling, needing time off school and work.

Dysmenorrhoea means menstrual cramps, which can range from very mild to completely disabling. Once thought to be a neurotic condition, it is now known that it's all in our hormones – not in our heads. A girl who has very painful periods either makes too much of the hormone prostaglandin, or her uterus is more sensitive than usual to normal amounts of it.

Drugs containing antiprostaglandins such as ibuprofen, which get to the root of the problem and bring relief in more than 80 percent of cases, are on the market in the United States, Britain and most European countries. The use of antiprostaglandin has proved to be enormously helpful to many girls. It can shorten the time during which you feel pain and this can reduce how long you have to stay in bed, so that you can continue working at your studies or doing your job. Start taking medication the day before your period.

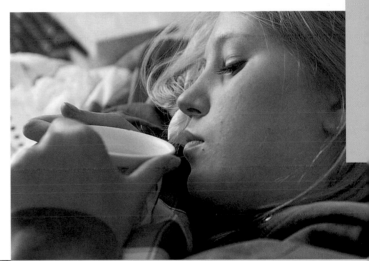

Sharing worries

Many girls worry about how their bodies look and feel, and find their growing sexual awareness disturbing. The "supermodels" used in fashion magazines promote an unrealistic "ideal" image of how girls should look, and it can be hard if you think that you don't match this ideal. Girls may feel that they lack control over their bodies. From time to time they also feel out of tune with their families, school mates, friends and especially their boyfriends. A lot of girls (and increasingly boys) blame the way they look for their low self-esteem, which in turn may lead to more serious problems. If you feel bad about yourself, have the courage to ask for help before things get worse.

Talking about it

● Your mother is the best person for advice but if you can't talk to her, ask another older female relative who is sympathetic.
● Talk to a biology teacher, school nurse or counsellor or see your doctor, and read as many books as you can.
● Compare notes with your best friend. Nearly everyone wonders if other girls are like them and the answer is often a reassuring "yes". Most girls experience the same anxieties.

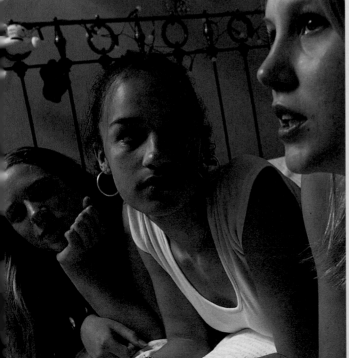

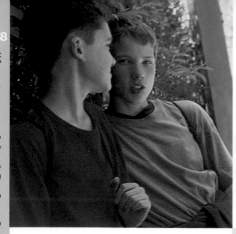

11-18 a boy's body

Boys' bodies start to change at 11 to 12 years. Their voices "break" and they begin to grow body hair at 14 to 15. Most boys will have to start shaving at 16 or 17.

Talking over problems

● Like many boys, you may find it difficult to talk about the problems of adolescence with friends or family for fear of losing face. But try to overcome this.
● Read books on the subject or ask your doctor for information.
● A teacher or school counsellor will help on matters of fact, and can advise you where to go for help.
● If possible, talk to your dad, an older brother or a male relative. Ask him about his adolescence, and how he dealt with any problems he had.

How your body changes

● Shoulders and chest grow wider.
● Muscles develop.
● Soft hair, which becomes coarse and curly, grows around the penis.
● Penis grows larger and longer and skin of scrotum darkens.
● Arms, hands, legs and feet grow bigger and longer.
● Larynx enlarges and becomes an "Adam's apple".
● Voice breaks.
● Hair grows in armpits, chest and on arms and legs.

● Testicles grow larger and fuller and become sensitive.
● Wet dreams and erections start to occur.
● Sperm are produced.
● Weight and height increase.
● Body sweats more.
● Face matures as the bones in your face grow.
● Skin becomes oily and pimply.
Be aware of how your body is changing. Boys are affected by hormones just as much as girls.

Worries and questions

The speed at which your body changes at puberty may take you by surprise. The changes take place when your testicles begin making the male sex hormone testosterone. Testosterone also triggers sperm production and makes you sexually aware. You'll begin to get erections because your penis is more sensitive to touch, or because you become excited by something you think about or someone you see.

Penis size

Most boys worry about the size of their penis, but the size of a person's body parts has nothing

to do with how well they work. Also, size when soft has no relation to size when erect. In fact, it is often the opposite: small penises seem to get bigger when erect than large penises. The most important thing to remember is that girls aren't really interested in size, because a big penis doesn't make you a better lover. Just remember – once you start to produce sperm, you are fertile, which means you could father a child if you have unprotected sex.

Wet dreams

When sperm production begins, sperm collect in the seminal

vesicles. Wet dreams act as a safety valve; the pressure builds up to the extent that you may ejaculate in your sleep – that's why it's called a "wet dream". You may be embarrassed when you have a wet dream, but it's totally normal – all boys have them – and they usually stop as you mature physically.

Circumcision

Removal of the foreskin, the protective layer of flexible skin on the penis is called circumcision. It is a simple operation and may be done for religious or medical reasons, but it doesn't affect the way the penis works.

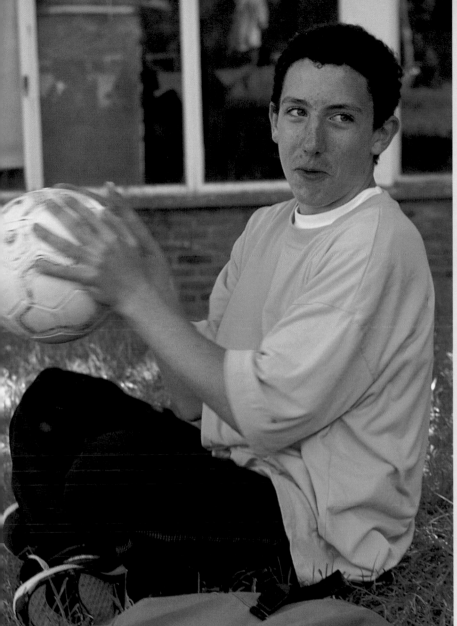

New feelings

Hormonal changes can affect your mood. All young people experience these changes and you feel miserable and confused, but it's normal.

As your body changes, you'll also start to experience new feelings. Your moods swing up and down like a yo-yo – you're laughing one minute and crying the next. **Sexual desire makes such an untimely entrance in a teenager's life**. Just as you begin to feel attracted to the opposite sex, you find that your emotions are all over the place, and you're feeling really anxious about your body. Your mixed emotions are not the end of the world, even though they feel like it at times. You're learning to cope with life's ups and downs, and this is a valuable lesson. It helps to compare notes with a close friend; someone you can confide in.

do

 Be positive
Think about the times when you've triumphed.

 Be active
Try to take the initiative.

 Take care
Make sure your actions don't hurt anyone along the way.

 Be cautious
Don't expect everyone to return your feelings.

Going it alone

Touching yourself "down below" is a perfectly normal habit, no matter what age, gender or sexual orientation you happen to be. **Everyone masturbates, boys and girls, men and women, and for most of us, it is our first experience of sex**. Masturbation never does any harm, unless it turns into an obsessive occupation, when it may indicate problems to do with poor self-esteem.

Although it's common for boys to masturbate more frequently than girls, masturbation is more important to girls because it allows them to explore and experiment with their bodies long before they have sex with another person. A girl can stimulate her own body to find out what her responses are and what she likes and prefers.

Although they may not often admit it, a lot of boys and girls achieve their best orgasms by masturbating. Nowadays, I am pleased to say, most young people believe that it is acceptable and harmless to do this, and of course they are right.

Masturbation will not make you go blind. Nor will it give you acne, insanity or hairy palms – these are all myths. It is also quite normal to fantasize about somebody while you are masturbating and these fantasies are almost always innocent. Most people have no difficulty in drawing a line between fantasy and reality, and do not want to act out their fantasies.

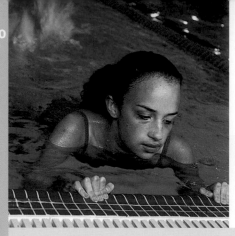

11-18 teenage troubles

A key factor influencing how teenagers feel about themselves is the way they look. Worries about weight, for example, can affect self-esteem.

Maintaining a healthy weight

Many teenagers go through phases of being very worried about their weight. They may feel that they're too fat all over, or that they're too fat in some places.

Also, at your stage of life, your weight may fluctuate – you may well still be growing, for one thing – and a girl may also weigh more when she is premenstrual. So it's not a good idea just to focus on your weight, but to look at your overall shape and the fact that it does change as you mature and develop breasts and hips. If you are at all concerned about your weight, talk to your school nurse or doctor so they can assess it properly for you.

Some fat is good!

We all need some body fat to stay healthy. Females need more than males – especially once periods start – to make enough of the female hormone oestrogen, to be fertile and to build strong bones. So some fat is good!

When, for whatever reason, your food intake is higher than your energy output, you have an excess that is stored as extra fat. The reverse happens when output outstrips intake; fat becomes a source of energy, it is burned up and weight is lost. If you want to stay a healthy

weight, then the best way to do that is to stay active and to enjoy a healthy diet. No need for drastic diets or to be "model" thin – these are unhealthy and unrealistic measures.

The energy balance

The aim is to stay in energy balance. There are certain influences that can affect the balance of the energy equation. One of these is your basal metabolic rate (BMR), the measurement of the amount of food energy that your body uses to fuel all the functions essential for life and health, such as breathing and

digestion. This accounts for about two-thirds of the body's energy needs and is linked to your weight and how much muscle you have. The heavier you are the higher your BMR.

When planning to lose weight, most people opt for cutting down the amount of food they eat because they think they can lose weight quickly this way. In fact, it's much more beneficial to increase the amount of exercise you do, because this can affect the energy equation just as quickly, and more effectively, in the long term.

Crash dieting

Crash dieting is a very bad way of losing weight in the long run. Although the amount of weight you lose right away is likely to be impressive, and may be as much as 4kg (8½lb) in the first week, less than half of this will be fat, which is what you're aiming to lose. If you reduce your food intake to, say, 400 calories a day, more than half the initial weight reduction will be because of water loss.

Cutting down your food like this is really low-grade starvation; all you'll do is gradually put your body into a state of hibernation – it will turn down the fuel burners to conserve energy and to stay alive. You will also feel hungry, bored, irritable and likely to binge, which just makes you more miserable, especially as the weight goes back on.

Crash dieting does nothing to retrain your eating habits. If you want to lose weight and keep it off permanently, you must revamp your whole style of eating and adjust your activity levels.

Exercising to stay slim

Exercise not only affects the energy equation in a more subtle way than through direct expenditure of energy, but it is also the only way we know to alter our BMR. If you exercise enough to become fit – that is, four times a week for 30 minutes or longer, over a period of months – muscles become stronger and body fat is better regulated. Exercising muscle has about twice the BMR of fat and resting muscle, so the body adapts and prepares for the increased work done by the heart, lungs and muscles by working, or metabolizing, at a slightly higher rate, thereby using more energy even on days when you don't exercise.

This makes exercise one of the most valuable of all weight-control aids. Research shows that regular activity is the most effective way to control weight in the long term.

Your weight loss depends on how many calories you go without or burn off. If your average calorie needs are 2000 per day, even a fairly generous diet of 1500 calories creates an energy deficit of 500 calories per day or 3500 per week, which is the equivalent in energy terms of 0.5kg (1lb) of body fat. You can double this by taking a moderate amount of exercise.

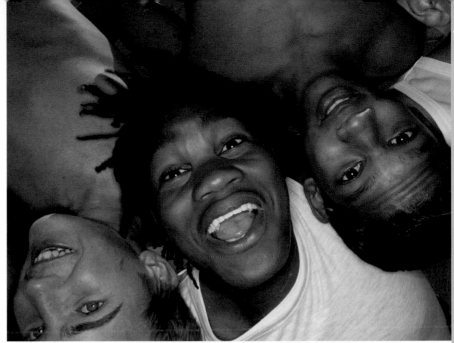

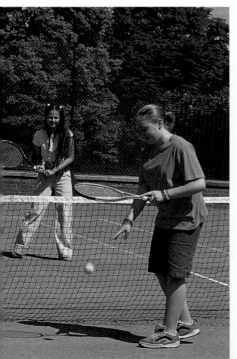

Self-esteem

The key to a child's smooth passage through adolescence is high self-esteem. Without it, teenagers can fall foul of eating disorders, get into bad company or even injure themselves. Most people will not have just one idea about their self-worth, but will have a number of views depending on the arena they find themselves in.

An adolescent may report high self-worth around friends, who think he is "awesome"; lower self-worth around parents who think he is "lazy" and "irresponsible"; and the lowest level of self-worth around strangers, who he feels may see him as "a total dork".

By and large it is parenting styles that contribute most to a child's self-worth. But while the behaviour of parents continues to be important during the teenage years, the views of peers come to play an increasingly crucial role as young people move towards adulthood.

Another key factor affecting self-esteem, particularly during the early teenage years, is physical appearance. For young people in this age group, it is body image satisfaction that correlates most highly with global self-esteem. In early adolescence girls have much higher levels of dissatisfaction with their bodies than do boys, both during and after puberty. Girls are more dependent on peer approval at this stage in their lives, and more sensitive to the opinions of their friends.

Self-esteem doesn't remain constant during childhood and adolescence. A range of factors will operate to determine the way in which self-esteem varies, depending on things such as success at school, family circumstances, the behaviour of friends, and so on. Research in this area has provided some important new insights into the way adolescent self-esteem alters. Researchers identified four different groups: one with consistently high self-esteem; another showing rising levels of self-esteem between the ages of 12 and 16; a third group showing consistently low self-esteem; and a fourth whose self-worth actually declined during the adolescent stage.

Young people in the third group might be helped by exercises that encourage them to feel better about themselves (for example, write a list of all your good points or write down every positive thing that's happened to you today). In the fourth, the aim might be to identify skills – whether academic, social or sporting – and then work to improve them in the expectation that better performance in some important areas will lead to a greater sense of self-worth in others.

11-18 relationships

Friends become more important in your teens; they help you broaden your interests and give you loyalty and support. Some friendships may even blossom into deeper relationships.

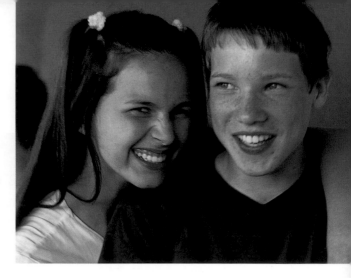

Deeper relationships

As you grow older and start thinking about having deeper relationships (which may involve sex eventually), you have to start paying attention to your responsibilities. Not only to your girl- or boyfriends, but to your family, your friends and yourself. Responsibility involves morality, which doesn't mean you have to be a prude, it means having a clear idea of the boundaries of fairness and kindness in your behaviour to others. It's sensible to approach relationships responsibly – irresponsibility leads to trouble in the long run. You'll know when you're being irresponsible, because the consequences are hard to live with. And when you feel shame and guilt, all this does is create unhappiness, because you're bound to take it out on others. Try to be honest and true to yourself. People will respect you for it.

Good relationships

A good relationship is personally enriching; it provides you with comfort, understanding and support. You'll feel that you are being loved – you'll get pleasure from giving, too. While your values may be similar to your partner's, any differences are exciting, and you should be able to respect each other's views without any real friction. Good relationships aren't too "exclusive". They don't block off your involvement in other things that are still important.

Thinking about sex

Sex, particularly good sex, is fun and it gives a great deal of pleasure in many contexts. It can be thrilling, exciting, moving, comforting, even consoling. All of these are positive reasons for having sex.

But then there are the questions of safe sex and contraception. Sex is a minefield and you must reflect deeply before stepping onto it.

How old should you be?

For all teenagers, this is the ultimate question. Does age matter anyway, you may ask? I think it does.

For purely medical reasons, I'm against very young girls having sex, because as a doctor I know that if you begin sexual activity, especially with several partners, early during your teenage years, it can make you more vulnerable to cancer of the cervix. I am also against any

teenagers having sexual relationships before they are emotionally mature and have established their sexual feelings and sexual values. For most of us, this is quite a problem and it takes years to do; even adults find it difficult.

In addition to these personal issues, I think you would be unwise to ignore the very strong opinions that are held by society in general. Although conventional thinking doesn't matter as much as the opinions of your parents, teachers, friends and relatives, it does matter a little and you can't ignore it. Everyone has strong opinions about teenage sexuality and you're almost certain to find that your opinions conflict with those of someone who matters to you. Don't ignore this situation completely because your relationship with that person can only deteriorate if you go against their views.

No one can tell you when sex is OK, but there are a few things you should bear in mind. The first is the law. The law varies on the age of consent (the age under which it is a crime to have sexual intercourse) in different parts of the world, but it usually ranges between the ages of 16 and 18. Therefore you would be breaking the law if you had sex before the age of consent. In any case, coping with sex is difficult under the age of 16.

Another basic requirement when thinking about having sex for the first time is to make sure that there is no risk of an unplanned pregnancy. In other words, both of you should investigate, decide on and use a method of contraception with the lowest possible failure rate (see p.118). Finally, it is vital that you feel confident that you will not expose yourself to a sexually transmitted disease, including AIDS.

Friendships

Friends of your own age matter a lot and you want to spend as much time as possible with them. You may begin to feel there's a growing rift between you and your parents and that they often cannot see your point of view. You turn to your friends instead – they know what you're experiencing, they're sympathetic with your views and they make you feel you belong.

Straightforward friendships with other people of your own age are just as important as those that involve sexual attraction. In fact a relationship that isn't also a friendship won't work. But making friends is difficult for a lot of people. Joining a club or group is a great way to meet friends, but you may find you haven't got the self-confidence to take the first steps. It helps to know that others are having the same problems.
● Don't judge people too hastily; appearances can be deceptive.
● Do be yourself rather than trying to imitate others or be top dog.
● Do ask others about their interests, such as music or sport.
● Do compliment someone on doing something well.
Friendship means giving and taking. Concentrate on your contribution to a friendship, not what it gives you, and you'll get more out of it.

Remember that each partner in a relationship has the right:
● to have opinions
● to respect
● to see family
● to be trusted
● to show feelings
● to time alone
● to support
● to talk
● to religious beliefs
● to faithfulness
● to make mistakes
● to see friends
● to affection
● to tolerance
● to be listened to
● to security
● to ask for help
● to say "no"
● to have fun
● to be cared for
● to patience.

Use the following as a starting point for your own lists, then, once you have established a relationship, look back at your list of "likes", and see just how close you've come to your ideal.

What I can offer

Fun	Understanding
Support	Respect
Happiness	Togetherness
Love	Company
Trust	Patience
Help with problems	Sense of humour

What I would like

Someone I can have a good laugh with
Someone to go out dancing with
Someone I can really talk to
Someone to lean on
Someone to care for
Someone who won't mind me crying
Someone who really understands me
Someone who won't get jealous

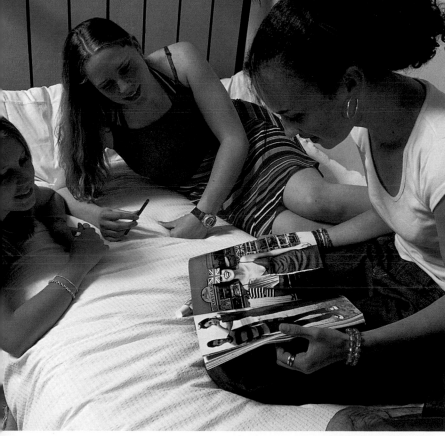

The risks of promiscuity

By far the majority of people decide to have one lover at a time. A few decide to have several at the same time, and if they do, they are behaving in a way that some people would call promiscuous. This may be your choice, but there are certain issues you should consider because, quite beside any moral and religious judgment of what is right and wrong, there are problems and quite a few risks attached to having sex with more than one person.
● The chances that you could catch a sexually transmitted disease (STD) and, for girls, the risk that you will develop cancer of the cervix, are greatly increased.
● If you or your lover have had other partners, there is a risk of contracting HIV, leading to AIDS. It is therefore crucial for all young couples to use condoms and spermicides every time they have intercourse to reduce the risk, regardless of whatever other contraceptive they use.
● By squandering time and emotional energy on more than one relationship you may find that you don't have enough time or energy to make any one of them work.
● You are greatly increasing the risk of hurting other people who don't approve of what you're doing.
● You may not think so at the time, but you are running the risk of losing your self-respect if you have even the slightest suspicion that what you're doing isn't right.
● People who disagree with your values are quite likely to label you, and you may get a bad reputation.

11-18 deciding about sex

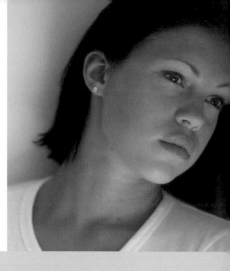

Girls and boys need courage to withstand the pressure of the moment: to realize they can say "no" without losing face. There are many reasons why you may feel unsure or uncomfortable about sex.

Saying "no" to sex

The only reason to have sex is because you want to. Deciding to have sex should never be taken lightly. No-one should ever make you have sex. Young people are presented with many difficult choices and pressures to do things that they feel uncomfortable about – taking drugs, drinking alcohol, smoking and sex.

For your own sense of self-respect, don't be pressured into having sex because you think your boyfriend or girlfriend will leave you or be disappointed. You and nobody else, decides whether you want to enter a sexual relationship. If you haven't managed to sort out your sexual values yet, then you really should say no.

No means no

People can come up with lots of apparently plausible reasons for persuading their partners to have sex when they don't really want to.

Typical ploys include saying things like "If you don't, I'll tell everyone you're a tease" or "You know you want to really" or "I'll leave you if you don't". It's not acceptable to trick your partner in this way – if a person says "no" then you should respect his or her wishes.

Why girls find it hard to say "no"

Almost every girl has difficulty in saying "no" at some time and finds herself on a date having sexual contact when she doesn't really want it.

There are lots of reasons why girls find it difficult to come out and say "no" firmly, the most common being that they don't want to hurt the boy's feelings, or they're afraid of being thought a prude.

Some girls worry that they're not going along with what other girls appear to be doing. With all these pressures, it takes a

brave girl to say "no", but you must say it if that's what you feel. If your boyfriend really cares for you, he'll agree. On the other hand, you'll lose a lot of self-respect if you say "yes" when you really mean "no".

Ways to say no

If you're really concerned about refusing sex, you can practise these replies:
● No, I hate being forced to do anything.
● No, I don't feel ready for it.
● No, I'm really too scared.
● No, I don't think I know you well enough yet.
● No, do you really want to have sex with someone who doesn't want to?
● No, I want to have time just being friends. Then I can decide if I want to have sex with you.
● No, you're hassling me. I'll know when I'm ready.
● No, I don't feel I trust you enough yet.
● No, I believe I should wait until marriage.
● No, I only want to have sex as part of a long-term relationship.
● No, not until we've discussed contraception.
● No, not until we know there are no risks at all.
● No, I don't want to and if you make me that's rape.
● No, you're giving the impression you don't really care about me.
● No, you're making me think that you'll leave me if I don't.
● No, you're moving too fast for me.
● No, you're making me feel really frightened of you.
● No, you're acting like a person I don't really want to know.
A question that will really bring things to a jolting halt is: "Are you ready to be a father yet? "

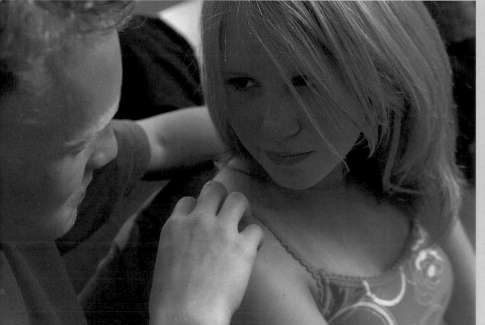

The risks – STDs

While sex is one of the ways of showing affection, if you don't wear a condom it is also a way of spreading certain sexually transmitted diseases, most of which are very unpleasant and some of which are incurable. They are nearly always infectious and are contracted only by having sex with another person. Here are some of them:

● Genital warts and genital herpes are viral infections; warts are curable, herpes is not, but the symptoms can be treated. The warts virus can also lead to cervical cancer.

● Gonorrhoea, syphilis and chlamydia are bacterial infections, which are treatable with antibiotics. However, chlamydia is difficult to diagnose since it's often symptomless. It can also cause pelvic inflammatory disease (PID).

● HIV/AIDS and hepatitis B are incurable viral infections; AIDS is fatal, although hepatitis B is not.

● Pubic lice ("crabs") and scabies are parasites, which are treatable with insecticides.

● Candidiasis ("thrush") is a yeast infection, which is treatable with a fungicide.

● Trichomonas is a single-cell parasite, which is treatable with antiparasitic agents.

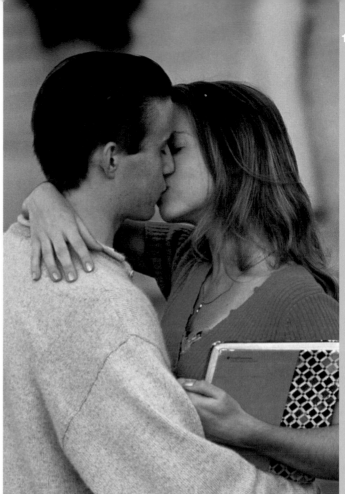

How to tell if you have an STD

Some STDs are symptomless in the early stages or have very vague symptoms, but if you suspect that you may have contracted an STD and have any or all of the following symptoms, you should seek medical advice immediately:

● pain when urinating or moving your bowels
● a smelly, discoloured vaginal discharge that is greater in quantity and with a worse odour than usual
● any vaginal discharge accompanied by a rash or that makes you sore and itchy
● lower back pain or pain in the pelvis or in the groin
● pain when having sex
● a sore lump or spot on any part of the genital area, including around the anus
● a fever combined with any of these symptoms
● oral sex may lead to symptoms around the mouth, including a sore throat
● anal sex may result in symptoms around the anus.

Where to get help Most people who think that they've got an STD are too embarrassed to visit their own doctor. This need not cause you any delay. There are special clinics – called STD or GUM clinics – in every major city that are well advertised and guarantee confidential treatment. If you want to find the clinic nearest to you, ask at your local health centre, call the hospital or look in your phone book.

Satisfaction without sex

In a good sexual relationship, there are masses of ways to explore each other's bodies without having actual sexual intercourse. Sex is the iceberg of which intercourse is only the tip – the one-eighth that's showing above the surface. Foreplay is the seven-eighths beneath the surface and can help you to overcome any anxieties that you may have about sex. It can often lead to orgasm and may even be more fulfilling than full sexual intercourse, particularly for girls who may find it easier to have an orgasm with foreplay than with penetrative sex, because foreplay concentrates on the clitoris.

Different kinds of stimulation

● Mutual masturbation is when you stroke and rub each other's genital organs. A girl strokes or rubs her boyfriend's penis while a boy strokes his girlfriend's clitoris.
● Oral sex is when you kiss, lick, nuzzle and suck each other's genital organs; girls do it to the penis (called fellatio); boys do it to the clitoris (called cunnilingus).
● 69 is when a boy and girl perform fellatio and cunnilingus for each other at the same time (stimulates orgasm).
● Simultaneous orgasm is possible if a boy rubs a girl's clitoris with his penis; he should still wear a condom as semen can enter the vagina even without penetration.

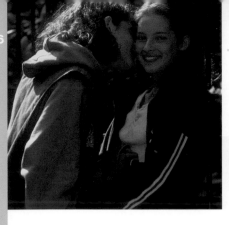

11-18 your sexuality

Whether you're heterosexual or gay, practise safe sex. That means always using a condom.

Making sure sex is safe

In order to be safe from STDs, you should use a condom for all forms of penetrative sex – anal and oral as well as vaginal. Make sure that you know how to use one properly, and never use condoms from out-of-date packets. Practise safe sex; think carefully about your sexual behaviour. While condoms are great for safe sex, don't rely on them alone to prevent pregnancy. Semen can leak if you haven't managed to use the condom correctly, or if you've used an out-of-date one. It's best for girls either to be on the Pill, or to use a diaphragm as well.

Getting help

● Your doctor, family planning clinic or advice centre will gladly give you information on condoms.
● A whole variety of condoms are available, and some of them have been designed to make sex a little more interesting! Condoms are available from retail outlets, supermarkets, pharmacies and even public toilets.
● Safe sex also means that you must report a suspected STD immediately to an STD clinic where you can get confidential treatment and also say who your suspected contacts are. If you contract a contagious STD such as genital herpes, you must always be honest with subsequent partners.

Safe sex guidelines

Carry a condom
Do carry a condom with you at all times, girls as well as boys.

Practise first
Do make sure you know how to use a condom before you have sex with someone.

Condoms every time
Do use a condom until you're absolutely sure there's no risk of sexual infections to or from your partner.

Once only
Don't ever try to use a condom more than once.

Be frank
Do be open about previous sexual experiences when you start a relationship, and tell your partner about any chronic infections, such as herpes.

No casual sex
Don't have sex with someone at a party, or on holiday, who you hardly know and may never meet again. Be especially careful after drinking a lot.

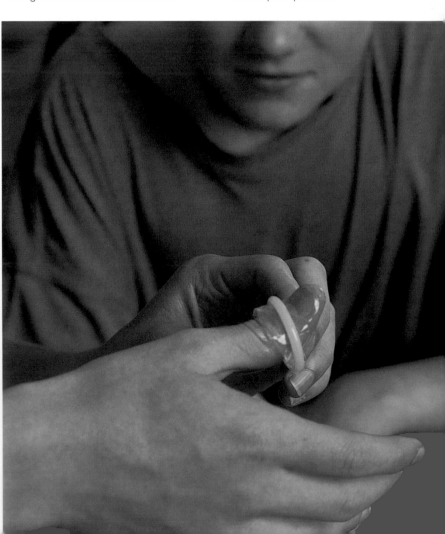

Accepting that you're gay

Feeling fundamentally different from one's family and friends can be an extremely isolating and unhappy experience. What can make matters even worse is hearing friends and family make despairing or abusive remarks about gays. Experiences like this can lead many young gay people to feel guilty and ashamed and, as a result, forced to keep this secret about themselves for a very long time. A great many have no idea that there are an enormous number of people who are sexually attracted to members of their own sex just as they are. **In fact, a significant number of the population are gay.** Nobody knows the exact figure because there is a wide gulf between being exclusively heterosexual and exclusively homosexual. Many young people have homosexual feelings or experiences but this does not necessarily reflect their adult sexuality.

A gay person can't help the way they are any more than a blond person can help having fair hair. Medical evidence suggests that a person's sexual orientation is formed before the age of five. So it's highly unlikely that an adolescent could be "turned" homosexual or lesbian simply by contact with another gay person – although such a contact could bring to the fore an orientation which was previously unrecognized.

Be proud of who you are
Accepting the fact that you are gay is the first and most important step in the process of coming to terms with your identity as a gay person. You can't, and shouldn't, live in the shadows, and have every right to be proud of who you are. However, it's important that you shouldn't feel

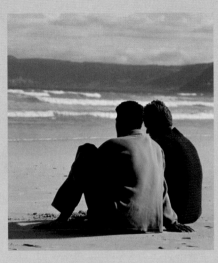

pressurized into announcing yourself to the world at large. Sexuality is a private matter and if you'd prefer to keep yours under wraps for the time being, that is your choice. The point is that you feel comfortable about yourself – "confessing" to friends and family won't necessarily make this so.

Knowing you are not alone
Meeting other members of the homosexual community should be your next step. Talking to young people who are or have been in a situation similar to your own will help build your confidence and reduce feelings of alienation. You may, at first, prefer not to meet anybody face to face. If so, you should telephone the Gay Switchboard (see p.567), which is run by gay people to give help, support and counselling to other gay people. Knowing you are not alone will help you feel stronger and help you to cope with the challenges that lie ahead.

The last and probably most crucial step is sharing what has been a secret part of your life with those whom you love most in the world – your family. This last stage can be especially daunting because the parents of most

gay people are heterosexual with entrenched ideas and expectations for their offspring usually revolving around marriage and a family of their own. You may believe your family and friends will hate you if and when they discover that you're gay. But this need not necessarily be true. **Many people now realize that being attracted to a member of the same sex is absolutely normal for a gay person.**

But it must be accepted that some people are still anti-gay. These people usually have never met a gay person in their lives and are content to agree with what their friends say because they don't want to be thought of as different. They haven't had the chance to realize that people are people and should be liked or disliked for their personality, not for their sexuality.

It would be wonderful to say with confidence that your family and friends won't desert you once they discover you are gay, but this is impossible to predict. But it's highly unlikely that they will turn against you. Once they've allowed the news to sink in, I'm sure they will realize that you are still the same person they have loved all these years. That's what you must try to remember. **If they love you now, why shouldn't they love you once they know that you're gay?** After all, nothing will have changed except their false impression of the truth.

As I said, there's no rule which says when you should tell your parents or if you have to tell your parents. It's entirely up to you. Once the news is out, nothing can hide it so it's not something you should do unless you feel completely ready. Good luck!

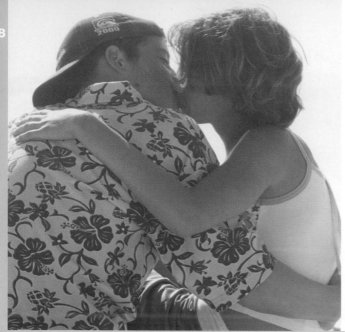

11-18
preventing pregnancy

Once you decide you want to have full sexual intercourse, it is crucial that you don't have an unplanned pregnancy. If you do get pregnant, never keep it a secret. Tell your parents or your doctor at once.

Contraception

If you are thinking of starting a sexual relationship, first make absolutely certain that you want it. Talk over your doubts together and make your own decision. Once you decide you want to have full sexual intercourse, it is crucial that you don't have an unplanned pregnancy. Before you start having sex, the most responsible thing to do is to seek advice on contraception from a family planning clinic or your doctor.

As the law stands, a girl under the age of 16 can seek contraceptive advice and receive it without the doctor telling her parents. This is one of the rights of every teenage girl.

Natural methods

These methods include the oldest forms of contraception.

Periodic abstinence Abstinence from intercourse during the time of ovulation. This method is based on calculations using the calendar, plus the rise and fall of the woman's body temperature and an ovulation-predictor kit. Using these indicators, you can decide to abstain from penetrative sex during ovulation. Failure rate is high because ovulation is difficult to be certain of.

Withdrawal Another ancient method with a very high failure rate. The penis is withdrawn just before ejaculation. It doesn't require discussion about methods at clinics and there's no financial cost, but it also leaves much of the responsibility with the man. The failure rate is very high

because often men wait too long to withdraw.

Barrier methods

These methods physically block the sperm from reaching the ovum.

Male condom A latex rubber or plastic sheath placed over the erect penis before penetration. It should be lubricated with a water-based lubricant – never use anything oily or greasy – and freed from air so that it doesn't burst inside the vagina. It prevents transmission of sexually transmitted diseases, especially AIDS.

Female condom As effective as the male condom, it's designed to line the inside of the vagina. Consists of a lubricated plastic sheath with an anchoring ring to keep it in place within the vagina and an outer ring that holds the sheath open to allow insertion of the penis. Cumbersome.

Diaphragm and cervical cap
A diaphragm is a dome of rubber with a coiled metal spring in its rim. It fits diagonally across the vagina and is used with a spermicidal agent. It must be left in place for six hours after intercourse. The cervical cap is smaller and more rigid and fits over the cervix, where it is held in place by suction. Very efficient.

Hormonal methods

These use hormones (synthetic oestrogen and progesterone) to suppress ovulation; they are practically 100 percent effective used properly. They interfere with the

cervical mucus, making it thick and impenetrable to sperm, and thin the uterine lining so that conception cannot occur.

Pill forms include the combined pill, low-dose minipill (no oestrogen, only progestogen) hormonal injections and implants and the post-coital pill. The combined pill must be taken for the full course of 21 or 28 days to be effective. The low-dose mini pill is taken continuously.

Injectable contraceptives, ideal for women who have difficulty remembering to take the pill regularly, contain only progestogens and are administered every two or three months.

What are the risks?

A pill containing oestrogen may not be suitable for you if you are overweight, if you smoke or suffer from diabetes, high blood pressure, a heart condition, deep vein thrombosis or migraine.

After-sex methods

There are two means of preventing conception after unprotected sex and they must be started within one to five days of intercourse, but they are not recommended as a routine form of birth control.

The hormonal method involves a short high-dose course of the combined pill – "the morning after pill". For women who cannot take the high-dose pill, a copper-bearing IUD an be inserted within five days of unprotected intercourse; this prevents a possible pregnancy.

Teenage pregnancy

Once you've begun a sexual relationship, there is always a chance of you becoming pregnant, even if you use contraception.

How to tell if you're pregnant

If you have any of the symptoms below, go straight to your doctor or family planning clinic and ask for a pregnancy test. You'll need to give them a small sample of your urine. For a quicker result, home pregnancy testing kits can be bought from any chemist.

● A missed period, if your periods are regular.
● A short, scanty period at the correct time.
● Swollen tingling breasts and darkening nipples.
● Wanting to pass urine more often.
● More vaginal discharge than usual.
● Feeling really tired.
● Disliking food you liked before.
● A strange taste in your mouth.
● Feeling sick, particularly after a long time without food, such as early in the morning.

Telling your parents

● If you find it easier to talk to your mum, tell her first, and ask her to tell your dad.
● It can help if you tell a close relative – someone your parents trust – and take the person along.
● Consider your options before talking to your parents; let them see how responsible you can be.

Girls: telling your partner

If the father wants to be involved but disagrees about the course of action, listen, but explain that the final decision is

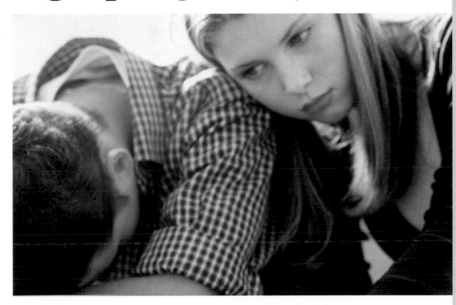

yours. If he won't support you, try to get by without him for now; you have enough to worry about.

Boys: getting the news

Try to remember that while you're equally responsible, your girlfriend's burden is infinitely greater. Ultimately you cannot control events, but you'll never have a better opportunity to give your partner your full support.

If you're still at school

If you've not completed your education but decide to have the baby, you need to consider carefully what your options are.
● Are you above or below the legal age for compulsory schooling? Your school or education authority can advise you on how to continue your education throughout your pregnancy and after the birth.
● You may feel tempted to leave school straight away, but try to think of your long-term future before making any rash decisions. You still need qualifications for your career and your self-esteem.

If you're a father

If your girlfriend's pregnant, you'll certainly have views about what your partner should do, even if they're negative.

In most countries you have no legal right to a say in whether she goes ahead with the pregnancy or not. However, this doesn't mean you should be excluded from the discussions. Your attitude and support will count for a lot in helping your

partner to make up her mind. Fathers have rights once the baby's born, and with those rights come all the responsibilities of having a family.

Girls: some of your options

● Getting married: get married to the father and have the baby.
● Live together: live with the father and raise the child together.
● Be a single mum: bring up the child on your own as a single parent.
● Start over: sometimes an abortion is the only answer.
● Family affair: have the baby and stay with your parents, who may be only too glad to help you look after the child.
● Another home: get the baby fostered or adopted by a loving family. It's a relief to know your baby will be well cared for.

The right choice for you

As well as your partner, parents and a close relative, try to talk to a doctor, or a minister if you have a religious background.

But in the end, whatever anyone else says, you have to weigh up your future, your strengths, your weaknesses, your ambitions and the strength of your maternal drive. Only you know how you want your life to be, so only you can make the right decision.

Warning

Don't allow yourself to be forced into a decision you're unhappy with because it seems to be the easiest. You'll always regret it.

Cervical smear tests

Cervical smear tests are important for girls who start having sex in their early teens because the young cervix seems vulnerable to cancerous changes when exposed to semen early in fertile life. The test is simple and quick and results should be available within six weeks.

Cancerous change is even more likely if you have several partners. Promiscuous sex also increases the chance of being infected with genital warts, the virus that also promotes cervical cancers.

11-18
alcohol and drugs

More teenagers are drinking and experimenting with drugs, and more and more are battling with drink and drug problems. Never be afraid to admit that you need help.

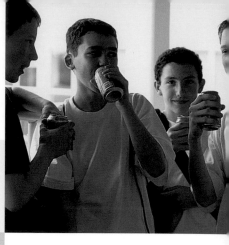

Drugs

When parents ask their children if they take drugs, they're looking for one answer – NO. Some parents don't even get as far as asking. They're not prepared to have any kind of discussion about drugs, except possibly to condemn them out of hand. This is a pity because there could well be a time when you need to talk about drugs to your parents, and not just because they've found out that you've been taking them. It may be that a friend has been taking drugs and you're worried about her health; or another friend may have been caught with drugs and you're frightened about what may happen to him.

The strict approach doesn't work. Being really strict simply means people go to greater lengths to conceal what they're doing. It's human nature – anything that's forbidden is immediately attractive.

Take the initiative

Drugs may be the last thing you want to talk about with your parents, especially if it means admitting that you've taken them yourself. But for your sake and theirs, it's a good idea to try to take the initiative in starting a dialogue with them about drugs before there's a crisis. Your parents are concerned about your welfare so tell them what you know. Many parents only know scare stories about widely publicized drug-related deaths and jump to the conclusion that so-called soft drugs inevitably lead to hard drugs or believe that all illicit drugs are more harmful than tobacco and alcohol. If your parents are very rigid in their thinking, you may feel inclined to abandon attempts at reasonable discussion and honest behaviour. Try to resist this because you'll both lose out in the long run.

Parents and drugs

Some adults are probably as confused and ill-informed as some young people.
● Show your parents the drugs education material you get from school.
● Show them books about drugs.
● Give them leaflets about drugs from nationally recognized agencies such as the Health Education Authority.

What parents can do

Rather than being judgmental and heavy-handed, there are practical things you can do to help your children:
● Learn about drugs and help your child to learn about them too.
● Think carefully about your views on drugs, and be honest with yourself and your child about your own drug use past and present – be it alcohol, nicotine, tranquillizers or cannabis.
● Don't be authoritarian; you'll lose your child.
● Know where to get help if it's ever needed.
● Keep drugs in perspective.

Teenage drinking

Alcohol is an intoxicating substance made from fermented starches, and although it gives you an initial lift, it is actually a depressant drug. It slows down responses (affecting coordination) and the way the brain works (affecting judgment), so it makes people clumsy and dopey. It's one of the most widely used drugs, above and below the legal age limit.

The alcohol effect

Drinking alcohol makes people:
● feel like they're having more fun
● feel confident
● feel relaxed and calms their nerves
● feel able to open up and talk more
● let go and lose their inhibitions
● feel they fit socially
● feel really happy and laugh more
● think they have the courage to overcome their fears.

The downside

Drinking too much alcohol always has horrible effects.
● Drinking can make you aggressive and violent. You're more likely to start arguments and pick fights.
● You become uncoordinated and clumsy.
● Too much alcohol gives you double vision and slurred speech.
● Drinking when you're down can make you feel even more depressed.
● Alcohol is loaded with calories. It can make you fat, and it's bad for your skin.
● A bad hangover makes you feel really fragile. Your head pounds and you have an upset stomach.
● Alcohol can damage a man's fertility and potency (brewer's droop).

Warning!

Alcohol is responsible for many, many more deaths than hard drugs.

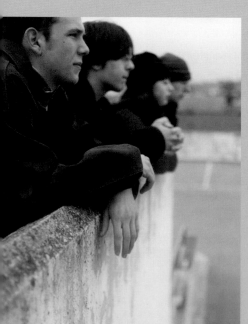

Drug emergencies

Drugs are unpredictable – the same drug can affect different people in different ways. In an extreme case a friend may collapse unconscious after taking a drug. But a drug can also cause a person to become dangerously hot or very drowsy or to have terrifying hallucinations or even a fit.

Take action

If a friend suffers adverse side effects from taking drugs, it may be frightening for you, but it could be life-threatening for your friend. It's vital to be able to recognize that something is going wrong as well as to know what to do in an emergency – quick action can save lives.
● If you see someone you think has had a bad reaction to a drug, don't hesitate to get help and don't panic.
● If you're in a club, shout for the security staff and ask for the qualified first aider.
● If you're not in a club, call an ambulance or, better still, get someone else to make the call while you look after your friend.

Calling an ambulance

Call the emergency services, ask for an ambulance and give the following information as clearly as you can:
● the telephone number you are calling from
● where you are – the name of the club, for example
● what's wrong with your friend: she's very hot or she's collapsed; she's unconscious. Don't be afraid to say that your friend has taken drugs, and preferably name the drug; the information could save her life.
    If someone else makes the call, ask him to come back and confirm that it's been done.

Kicking a drug habit

Coming off drugs is difficult and you shouldn't attempt to do it by yourself, but as long as you want to come off you can. Many people before you have come off drugs and if you go about it the right way and with the right help you'll succeed too.

Getting help

Find out from the National Drugs Helpline (see p.567) what services are available in your area; they can advise you on what type of help would be most appropriate. Alternatively, ask your GP to refer you to the most suitable organization. Whatever you choose, remember that all drug agencies and medical services are duty bound to treat your case in complete confidence.

Coming off

Clearing your system can take anything from a few days to a few months, and for safety's sake it must be done under medical supervision. Some drugs can be stopped straightaway; others, such as barbiturates and tranquillizers, have to be cut down gradually – to stop them suddenly is very dangerous. The first few days are the hardest, so once you're through them hang on in there – it will get better, but it takes time.

Staying off

Withdrawal is only half the battle: the toughest part is staying off the drug. Give yourself the best chance:
● Keep yourself busy.
● Stay away from all drugs, and that includes alcohol.
● Avoid situations where there are drugs, and places where you used to go to take drugs and avoid people who take drugs.
● Get support when you feel you might slip back.

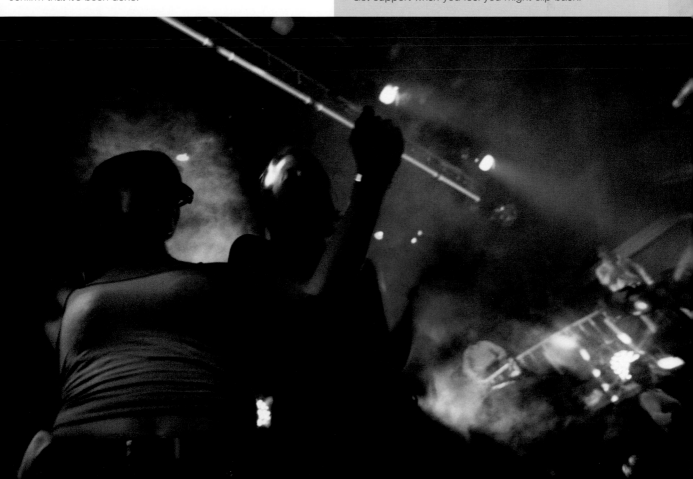

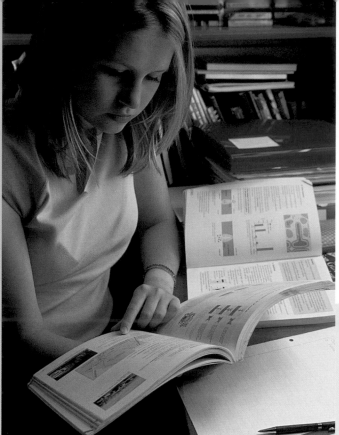

11-18
a good education

Education should be a priority in life – it is the best tool a person can have to help them manage their lives, achieve happiness and enjoy some freedom.

Why homework helps

When you do homework, you are understanding and consolidating what you have been taught during the day. Although you may think homework is a chore, it can be the road to great achievements because, as well as providing the information to do well in exams, it teaches you many personal skills.

● Homework teaches you how to study independently without guidance and how to use your own judgement.

● It teaches you discipline – not only the discipline of routine, but also discipline in the way you have to tackle your work, plan it, present it and write it out.

● When you have a difficult or long assignment to complete against a deadline, it teaches you persistence and determination – qualities that you need in ample supply if you are to follow a demanding career.

● Learning to manage your schoolwork alongside outside interests and the normal social life that all teenagers need and enjoy actually prepares you for the world of work later. It instills such skills as time management and the ability to handle pressure.

● All of these achievements will bring you a sense of self-respect and confidence, not to mention the pride that your parents and teachers will feel in your successes.

Schoolwork away from school

Most people have to do a great deal of hard work and study for many hours to prepare for exams. You often have several subjects to study, and this work can seem a real chore. If you don't love information for its own sake, then the most practical way of looking at this work is that it has to be done to give you the freedom to do what you want later on. It's a grind that you just have to go through.

It's good for you to learn determination and develop staying power early in your educational career because you will need a great deal of these qualities later on if you're going to hold down a job successfully in a competitive world. Life beyond school is perhaps not as straightforward as it used to be – even some college graduates with good degrees have difficulty in finding jobs.

Fitting it in There's no doubt that while you're having to study in the evenings, you'll sometimes feel jealous and resentful of those of your friends who may have left school, have jobs and money and go out every night apparently without a care in the world. You're not unique; everyone who studies has experienced this, and many before you have ignored it, continued to study and become successful.

The right amount of homework Most young people are expected to do about two hours' homework an evening during the week, plus three to four hours on weekends as well as some extra project work during vacation periods. Your school should guide you as to the amount of homework you are supposed to do. If very little homework is being given to you, or you're finding that you can do what you're given on your trip home, it's not going to do you much good in the long run. However, if you suddenly realize that you're doing three or four hours a night and more on weekends, you may be overloading yourself or working too slowly. Talk to your parents and teachers about maintaining a balance or possibly learning how to work faster.

What an education can offer

It wasn't until I was through my adolescent years that I realized that continuing my education offered me the kind of freedom that nothing else in my life possibly could. With qualifications, it was possible to apply for jobs that paid enough so that I didn't have to worry about paying for basic needs like a roof over my head, food and clothing. **My education made me strong and independent, not just financially, but also emotionally and intellectually**. With it, I had the ability to follow my preferences and exercise my options.

Having an education also means that you will always have interests to fall back on during low or lonely points in your life because it will give you a vast fund of inner resources. It should also mean that you will be able to analyse problems, sort out solutions and expedite actions at work, in the community and in your social life.

Making space for home study

Your studies are important and if domestic arrangements allow, you should make sure that the rest of the family understands that keeping up with your schoolwork is one of your main priorities.

You will need:

● **A quiet space**. If you're going to study for long hours alone, it's only fair that you have a room, or at least a space, in your home where you can study, that is quiet, comfortable and well heated. This room will probably be your bedroom, but wherever it is, it should be a calm place that is recognized by everyone as being yours and where disturbances from the rest of the family are minimal.
● **Adequate furniture**. You need a minimum of furniture such as a desk, a few drawers or shelves for your files and equipment and some shelves for your schoolbooks and reference texts.
● A good **reading light** and a **comfortable chair** that gives you good support.

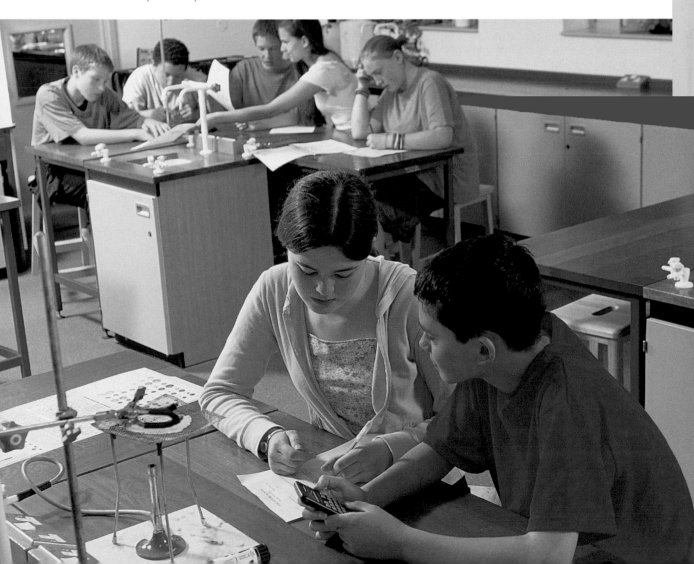

11–18
school pressures

Coping with the demands of school and resisting other temptations is not always easy, but if you persevere you will find it really worthwhile.

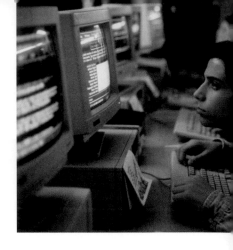

Bunking off

Some people absent themselves from school because this is their way of rejecting the monotony and the seemingly stupid rules to which they have to conform there. But it can also be the case that you're pressured into staying home by one or both of your parents because there's no one else to do the housework or look after small children while they are at work. If you do start to stay at home, you'll fall behind in your schoolwork and going back will become more and more difficult. Once you drop out, it's an easy step to avoid school and spend your time going out or just staying at home playing music. So if you are getting pressure from your parents, rather than pressure from your own friends, remind your parents that it is actually against the law for them to keep you at home. But if you're staying away from school because you want to, and your parents don't know about it, remember that the school will soon contact your parents and you will be called to account for your absence.

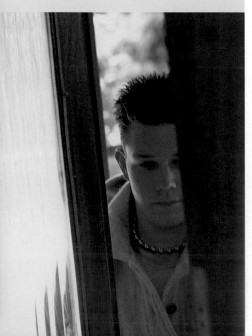

Computers and the Internet – a parent's guide

A research team of psychologists and educationalists in America found that over-exposure to computers can lead to obesity and long-term emotional damage. Youngsters only really learn through human interaction. Computers simply present them with a huge amount of information they can't properly digest.

The report, which concludes that computers should only be used at secondary school level and not by younger children, also warns that there's no real evidence to suggest computers or the Internet help with academic achievement.

Safety and the Internet

Most parents are concerned about the safety of their children using the Internet. Prevention is always better than cure, so parents should look for approved Internet service providers that will carry family friendly kitemarks. That way you can ensure your children are logging on in safety. Some, for example, offer a range of censorship levels on the Internet catering for the under-12s, young teens and older teens. Others automatically filter swear words and sexual references and have an adult to vet messages in the chat room.

Then there are children's e-mail services that come with similar restrictions, including one that only sends e-mails that are first approved by parents.

Everyone knows that teen chat rooms are used by paedophiles. I'm not sure why they are allowed at all.

An educational tool?

Your child may insist that she needs the Internet for school, and there's no denying that it can be a good educational tool. Much is made of the Internet's educational efficacy. She may even claim she can't do her homework without it. But, as one survey found, when children get that much-needed computer, a quarter of under-17s log on and head straight to gambling or porn sites. Of the 5 million under-16s who use computers regularly, 1.15 million spend most of their time on-line in chat rooms. So parents are right to be concerned and right to exert some control.

If your child does use a computer at home, make sure that the keyboard and screen are correctly positioned to avoid repetitive strain injury and back strain. Try to limit the hours she spends at the computer and encourage her to take breaks.

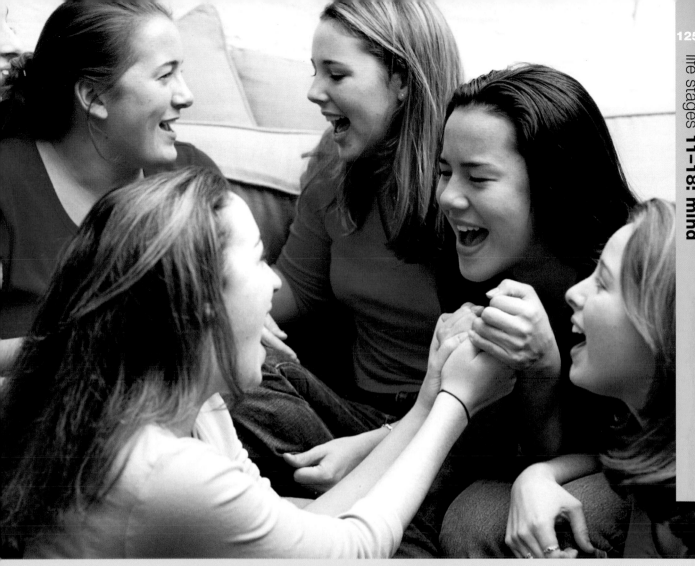

Surviving school

Everyone has a few problems at school. There may be teachers you don't get along with and subjects that you don't like. It's possible you may find that certain subjects are beyond you. You may also find that worries about your appearance, social life and popularity distract you from your schoolwork and sometimes seem more important than your academic abilities.

As you progress through school, and possibly go on to further education, it's sometimes tempting just to give up and have time to enjoy yourself. **Try not to be influenced by friends who've given up studying, who've left school early to get a job**, or feel that marriage and a family at 18 is what's right for them. Remember that they, not you, are the ones who may be narrowing their options for the rest of their lives.

There's no point in saying that it's easy for a young person to survive hard days at school and long hours working at night, especially when the rewards aren't immediately forthcoming or easy to see. It isn't. It takes a lot of staying power, a lot of grit, guts and determination. It also takes resilience. There will be times when you'll feel depressed and think that it's just not worth the effort. Well, no one can give you the will to carry on and the will to succeed. You're going to have to find that somewhere inside of yourself.

If you feel that your willpower is cracking, have a chat to the teachers you most respect and ask them for tips. Most schools nowadays know that examinations can be especially stressful and will provide revision classes and advice on how to cope.

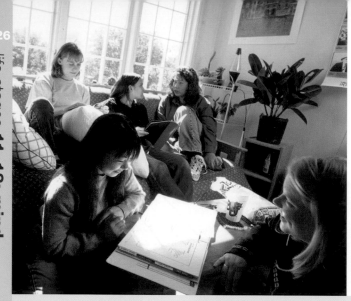

11-18 after 16 – what then?

I believe that staying on at school or college after 16 gives you far better career opportunities. But if you do decide to leave, do your best to find a job that interests you.

Carrying on with your education

Like many other teenagers, I wanted to leave school at 16. I felt a great desire to be independent, to be working and to be earning money of my own. I wanted to stop studying and start enjoying myself. Fortunately for me, my parents and teachers persuaded me to do otherwise. I went to college after the summer holidays and continued to study for A levels, and then went on to medical school. Thank heavens my parents and teachers won me over.

If you are a teenager who has academic ability, it would be a great shame if you didn't go on to further study, because it's then that you can really start to enjoy complex and more specialized work. Besides

this, your relationships with teachers will become easier, friendlier and more informal, **you're given responsibility and you're treated as an adult.** In further education you have more choice – you may stay on at your own school, or transfer to a designated sixth-form centre or to a further education college, where you may be studying alongside adults. You should also be aware that by staying on you're possibly preparing for a university career and university life, which will offer independence, living away from home, a new social life and an open academic curriculum. Don't, therefore, be tempted to leave school on a mere whim.

Thinking about a career

If you know what sort of job or career you want to pursue, get career advice early, and this means usually at around the age of 14 or 15. Most schools begin careers guidance at this age, if not earlier, and increasingly there are opportunities for useful work experience with local businesses and professionals organized through the school.

Career guidance will help you choose the right subjects to study so that a particular career will be open to you. **However, beware of closing off any future options by specializing too early**. You may change your mind later and it will be harder to go

back – although you can take certain extra GCSEs while doing your A levels.

The aim of most modern education systems is to provide a rounded education for as long as possible and to keep you studying the broadest possible range of subjects. Make sure that your career counsellors know what kind of career you want to pursue, so that they can put you in touch with recruitment departments in different professions and industries. They can also point you in the direction of the different training or college courses that you should be aiming for.

Preparing a CV

If you decide to look for a job, rather than going on to college or a technical training institute, get as much help as you can on how to apply for jobs and handle interviews. Some guidance counsellors will set up mock interviews, often with professionals or local business people, to help you with the technique. They should also show you how to write good application letters and fill in application forms. Putting together a lively CV is an important part of this.

Writing your CV

Draft your CV on a computer, if possible, before you even need to think about applying for jobs, and then all you have to do is adapt it to suit your prospective employer.

Obviously, you're not going to have much of a record of employment, although vacation or weekend work is relevant because it shows that you've got some experience of workplace routines. Give the names of two people as referees. Most employers ask for this anyway, but line them up beforehand. They need to be people in responsible positions who know you, such as teachers, youth workers, church leaders or past employers. You should ask their permission first, and let them know that they may be contacted by potential employers.

What goes into a CV

Your CV should include the following in this order:
● Your name, address and telephone number.
● The names of schools and colleges attended and the dates you were there.
● Qualifications – subjects (with grades), plus any other certificates such as music, drama, sports, youth awards.
● If you're looking for a short-term position for a few months before going to college, give details of the course you're going to study and where you'll be studying as well as the starting date, so that your employer knows exactly how long you're going to be available for work.
● Previous temporary employment, such as weekend, evening or vacation work, with dates and names of employers.
● Volunteer work, including any community work, fund-raising or amateur arts involvement, such as membership of a drama or dance group or orchestra.
● All your interests – don't leave any out. Even playing computer games can count because it shows that you're familiar with computers and probably have quick reflexes.
● Future training or education plans. If you're taking a year off before going to college, explain this.

Going to interviews

It's exciting but nerve-racking to go to your first job interview, but you can feel confident by following a few simple rules. (These apply equally to going for an interview at a college.)
● When you get invited for an interview, write as soon as possible to confirm that you can be there on the day and at the time requested. If it's difficult, be open about it, and ask for another appointment. Employers and colleges realize that people may have commitments.
● **Find out as much as you can about the company (or college) beforehand** so that you can tailor your answers. Almost all interviewers will ask why you want to join their organization.
● Go to bed early the night before, and work out what you're going to wear in advance so that you're not overtired or rushed in the morning. Aim to look smart, but not flashy.
● Plan how to get to the interview in time, and leave plenty of time so that you're not late – this gives a bad impression from the start. However, in case you're let down by public transport, make sure you have the telephone number so you can let them know.
● Don't worry about being on edge; the interviewer will expect it and a good one will try to put you at your ease. Sit down when you're asked. Always refer to your interviewer as Mr A, Mrs B, Ms C or Miss D unless you're invited to use first names.
● When you answer questions, don't just answer yes or no. Enlarge on what you're asked. Speak clearly and look the interviewer in the eye. Don't forget to smile.
● **Don't be afraid to ask questions** – most interviewers will ask you if there is anything you want to know, usually towards the end of the interview. If it hasn't been made clear or you're not sure, ask the interviewer to confirm the salary, and inform you about possible overtime or weekend work, as well as about vacations.
● You may be offered a job on the spot. If you're undecided, ask for time to think about it, even if it's just overnight. Go home and talk to your parents or teachers so that you can decide calmly.

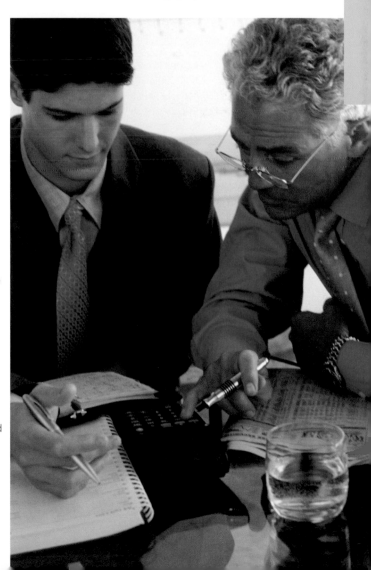

FOCUS *on* pregnancy and birth

If you are waiting for everything to be just right before you have your baby, you may as well give up now and take up a hobby instead. It's rare for a couple to feel that the perfect moment has arrived to have a child, but now that men and women have control over their fertility, it gives time for consideration.

WHAT AGE IS BEST FOR HAVING A BABY?

Many women are delaying pregnancy until their 30s and even 40s. This is no more hazardous than being in your 20s as long as you are fit and healthy. Whatever your age, you are likely to have a normal pregnancy and birth, although problems such as infertility and chromosomal defects – for example, Down's syndrome – do become more frequent with the increasing age of both parents. Tests for chromosomal abnormalities are always offered to older women.

WHEN DO I STOP CONTRACEPTION?

If you use barrier methods, such as condoms or a diaphragm, you can safely conceive as soon as you stop using them. But most doctors prefer that you have at least one normal period after ceasing other forms of contraception before you start trying to conceive. This allows your

metabolic functions to return to normal.

If you've been on the pill, the best plan is for you to stop taking it three months before conception. A month would do, as long as you have a normal period before you conceive.

If you have an intrauterine device (IUD), the same timescale applies – have it removed three months before you intend to get pregnant. Have at least one normal period before stopping all contraception – use a barrier method in the meantime.

DO I NEED GENETIC COUNSELLING?

Seek advice and have tests in advance if a genetic disorder runs in your family. Examples of heritable conditions include cystic fibrosis, muscular dystrophy and haemophilia.

What happens in counselling?

The counsellor explains the condition and your family background and shows you the pattern of inheritance through past generations. Not all carriers of a defective gene get the condition: if it's recessive it can be masked by a healthy version, whereas a dominant gene will always show up. With a dominant gene the chances of your baby being affected are one in two, with a recessive gene they are one in four.

HOW DO I PREPARE FOR PREGNANCY?

When you make the decision to become parents, it makes sense to prepare yourselves in advance. To have a healthy baby, research shows that by far the most important factors are your own fitness and nutrition. As a prospective mother, the fitter you are, the more easily your body will be able to cope with the stresses and strains of pregnancy. But fitness and lifestyle may also change a man's ability to father a child, by affecting sperm production. It's best if you both try to think about your general health and lifestyle at least three months before you're planning to stop contraception.

I'm not in the business of using scare tactics to get a message across, but there are facts you should know for the sake of your baby.

Must I stop smoking?

Smoking is one of the greatest threats to the health of your unborn baby and the major cause of avoidable health problems. The associated risks include miscarriage and stillbirth, damage to the placenta, a low birthweight baby who fails to thrive and an increased chance of fetal abnormalities. Smoking can cause a low sperm count, and a man who continues to smoke while his partner is pregnant risks damaging the health of his unborn baby via passive smoking.

What about alcohol?

Alcohol is a poison that can damage the sperm and ovum (egg) before conception as well as harm the developing embryo. The main risks to the unborn baby are mental retardation, retarded growth and damage to the brain and nervous system – well documented as fetal alcohol syndrome. Alcohol can also cause stillbirth. Research suggests that the effect of alcohol is variable – the only certainty is that there will be no effect if alcohol is avoided.

And drugs?

Over-the-counter medicines should only be taken when necessary and social drugs should **definitely** be cut out before you conceive. Marijuana interferes with the normal production of male sperm, and the effects take three to nine months to wear off. Hard drugs such as cocaine, heroin and morphine can damage the chromosomes in the ovum and sperm, leading to abnormalities. It is best to avoid taking anything during pregnancy unless your doctor determines that the benefit to you outweighs any risk to the fetus.

SHOULD I CHANGE MY DIET ONCE I'M PREGNANT?

Your body uses up a lot of energy during pregnancy, and you need to eat well to fuel your requirements and those of your growing baby. Pregnancy is not the time to go on a diet, but you should also forget the myth about "eating for two"; the rule is to eat to satisfy your

First signs of pregnancy

If you are planning a pregnancy and miss your period, you may suspect that you are pregnant. You may not notice any other changes apart from the missed period at first, but an increase in hormonal activity will confirm your pregnancy with one or more of the following physical signs.
• A feeling of nausea at any time.
• A change in taste – you may suddenly be unable to tolerate alcohol or coffee, for example.
• A preference for certain foods, sometimes close to a craving.
• A metallic taste in your mouth.
• Changes in your breasts; they may feel tender and tingly.
• A need to urinate more frequently.
• Tiredness at any time of the day; you may even feel faint or dizzy too.
• Increase in normal vaginal discharge.
• Your emotions swing unpredictably.

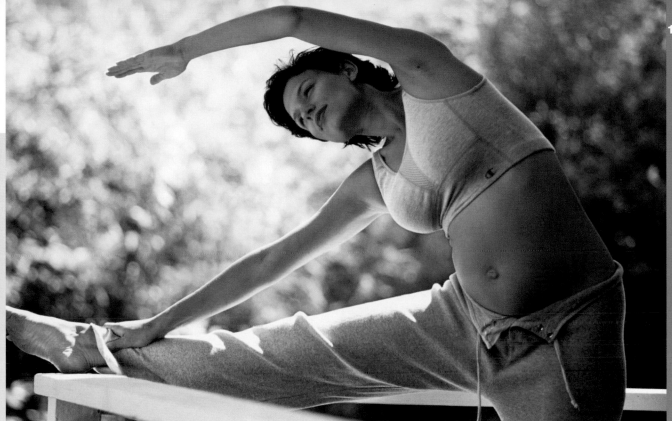

hunger and no more. Later in pregnancy you may find you simply can't take in much food at any one time, so eat little and often. Keep supplies of healthy snacks such as dried fruit, rice cakes, crispbreads and hard fruits in your bag, car or office, and low-fat cheese and yogurt, raw vegetables, fresh fruit and unsweetened fruit juice in the fridge at home.

What should I eat?

To provide for your baby's needs as well as your own, note the following tips about diet.

● Complex carbohydrates such as pasta, potatoes or pulses (beans and lentils) are needed for energy.

● Protein is needed for your baby's growth. Eat fish and poultry, dairy products, wholegrain cereals, seeds and pulses.

● Don't cut out fats altogether, but don't eat too much of them. You'll get enough from dairy products and normal cooking methods.

● Get vitamin C daily from raw fresh fruit and vegetables, and the B complex from wholegrains, nuts and pulses, green vegetables, dairy products, eggs, oily fish and meat.

● Iron maintains red blood cells; it's found in red meat, fish, egg yolks, apricots and cereals.

What about morning sickness?

Though called morning sickness, nausea can occur at any time of day. To combat it many women find that small, frequent snacks help

Is it safe to exercise?

Both you and your baby benefit from exercise: your blood starts circulating freely, there's a blast of oxygen to your baby's brain, exercise hormones such as endorphins give you both a wonderful high and your baby loves the swaying motion. Exercise increases your strength, suppleness and stamina, which will make pregnancy easier and equip you for the rigours of labour.

But exercise in pregnancy is not just about fitness. It helps you to understand your body, to believe in its power, and it gives you the key to relaxation so that you can cope with fatigue and prepare yourself for the birth.

Whole-body exercise

Try to incorporate some exercise into your day, beginning gradually, at a pace that is comfortable. Always stop if you get out of

breath or feel pain. Whole-body exercise is best as it tones up your heart and lungs, so walking and swimming are excellent. Dancing is good, too, as long as it's not too energetic. Yoga is ideal because it stretches tight muscles and joints and also relieves tension. Yoga methods can also help with labour and pain relief.

Exercises to avoid

Pregnancy is not a time to start learning an energetic contact sport. However, you can continue sporting activities for a while if you're already fit and play often. Don't engage in sports like skiing, cycling or horse riding after 20 weeks because balance may become a problem from that time. Take it easy with very energetic sports like tennis or squash, and don't do heavy workouts at the gym, especially tough abdominal exercises.

during the difficult weeks. Here are some snack foods that you can prepare at home or have at your workplace to damp down the rising nausea during your working day.

● Raw vegetables such as carrots, celery, tender young beans, peas from the pod, tomatoes.

● Slices of wholemeal bread dried in the oven.

● Sandwiches made with wholemeal bread and hard cheese.

● Nuts, raisins and dried apricots.

● Fruit cake (preferably made with wholemeal flour and added wheatgerm).

● Green crisp apples.

● Water biscuits and cottage cheese.

● Fresh fruit juices.

● Commercial muesli bars.

● Unflavoured natural yogurt with honey.

● Herbal teas.

● Milkshakes made with skimmed milk.

● Juicy fruits such as peaches, plums and pears. ▶

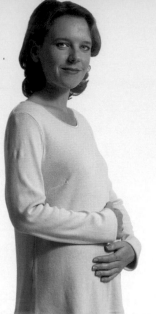

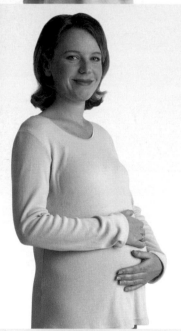

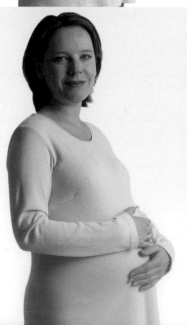

Growing bigger

Having a baby growing inside you is like being part of a real-life miracle. Sometimes you'll pat your bump and feel you can hardly believe your child is in there – it seems so amazing and extraordinary. Find out as much as you can about how your baby develops. It will help you both to understand the minor discomforts and ups and downs that a pregnant woman feels.

FOLLOWING YOUR PREGNANCY
No part of a woman's body escapes when she's carrying a baby, and you and your partner need to keep that in mind. For instance, tender breasts that are getting ready for breast-feeding need to be treated gently by a father when he caresses them; the growing uterus pressing on your internal organs means that you must never be too far from a toilet during the last three months of pregnancy. The guide that follows is a brief outline of the complex changes going on inside your body.

What's happened by three months?
The first three months of pregnancy (the first trimester) are tremendously important in laying the foundations of your baby's healthy development, although there are few visible signs of your baby's phenomenal growth.

You
- You'll really start to gain weight; any morning sickness will soon disappear.
- The uterus is rising out of the pelvis and can be felt.
- The risk of miscarriage is almost zero now.
- Your heart is working flat out and will continue to do so right up to labour.

Your baby
- She has a fully formed body, complete with fingers, toes and ears.
- Her eyes move, though her eyelids are still closed.
- Her body is covered with fine hair.
- She wriggles if poked – her muscles are growing.

What's happened by six months?
The period from about the third to the sixth month (the second trimester) is when pregnancy sickness ends, your baby really grows and you begin to feel her move. You're brimming with energy, vitality and wellbeing.

You
- You're putting on about 0.5kg (1lb) of weight a week.

Sex in pregnancy

Many women say that sex when they were pregnant was the best they've ever had. There are lots of reasons for this.

- Physical factors: the blood supply to all the pelvic organs increases and pregnancy hormones make the vulva more erogenous.

- The breasts are more sensitive as they prepare for lactation and become more easily aroused.

- A woman who's relaxed and happy about her pregnancy may feel such a surge of love for her partner that she becomes passionately responsive to him.

You can have sex all the way through pregnancy as long as you're comfortable. By the way – you might like to know that your baby feels your orgasm with you and enjoys it just as much.

Some women are scared that sex will crush the baby. This is not possible because the baby is suspended in the amniotic sac and surrounded by amniotic fluid, which cushions it from any kind of bumping and bruising.

On the other hand, it is not safe to have sex if you experience either of the following symptoms:

- If bleeding occurs – in such a case, consult your doctor.
- If you have blood-stained vaginal discharge, heralding the onset of labour, or if the waters break.

Also, if you have had a miscarriage in the past, seek medical advice about having sex. You may be advised to abstain during the early months of pregnancy.

• Your uterus is a good 5cm (2in) above the pelvis.
• You may have bouts of indigestion.
• From 16 weeks or so, you'll feel the baby move.

Your baby

• Her hearing is acute, she can recognize your voice.
• She's becoming better proportioned – her body is catching up on her head.
• She's well muscled but thin.
• Her lungs are maturing fast.

What's happened by nine months (full term)?

The final 12 weeks or so of pregnancy (the third trimester) are when the baby puts on fat in preparation for birth, and the brain and lungs mature in preparation for independent life.

You

• You may feel a "lightening" as your baby's head drops into the pelvis.
• It's more difficult to find a comfortable position for sleep.
• You visit the antenatal clinic every week.
• Your breasts secrete a clear-coloured nutritious liquid – colostrum.

Your baby

• She weighs about 2.7–3.5kg (6–8lb) and she measures 35–38cm (14–15in) from crown to rump.
• Her head is "engaged", lying just on top of your cervix.
• The placenta is 20–25cm (8–10in) across and there are 1.1 litres (2 pints) of amniotic fluid.
• Her breasts may be swollen due to the action of your hormones.

COPING WITH FATIGUE

Fatigue is a periodic problem during pregnancy, especially during the first three months and the last six to eight weeks. Its extent may take you by surprise – it's the kind of tiredness that makes you feel you don't even have the energy to blink, but just stare straight ahead. You're sleepy in the early stages of pregnancy because you're sedated by the high levels of progesterone. Your metabolism speeds up to deal with the demands of your baby and the extra work all your organs are called on to do. Later on in pregnancy you're tired because your whole body is working flat out 24 hours a day, and you're having to carry extra weight around that puts a strain on your heart, lungs and muscles. Help yourself by resting when you can, putting your feet up when you sit, and going to bed early at least three times a week. ▶

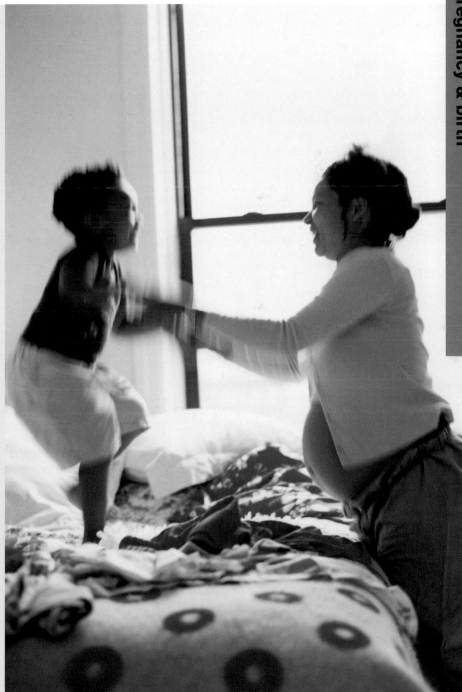

The birth

These days it's possible to plan exactly the kind of birth experience you want because most doctors, obstetricians and midwives are well aware that a relaxed, confident, informed mother is more likely to have an enjoyable labour and a successful delivery.

MAKING A BIRTH PLAN

Making a plan for your baby's birth will help to ensure you are actively involved in the way he is born and what happens to you as a family after the birth. By carefully considering all your preferences, and by discussing them with your birth attendant and partner, you will be able to establish a bond of trust and so create a happier and more comfortable birth environment. The following are some of the issues you might want to think about.

BIRTH PARTNERS

Every woman going into labour should have with her someone other than medical and nursing professionals to offer support, comfort and encouragement. The best assistant is your

partner, especially if he has attended your antenatal classes with you, and knows how to help you through each stage of labour, but it doesn't have to be him. Your mother, sister or best friend would be an excellent choice, particularly if she's had children of her own and can stay calm if things do not go quite as planned. Whoever you choose should be someone that you trust to make decisions on your behalf, if necessary, so make sure they know your views inside out. It can be a help for your birth partner to deal with hospital staff – you may not want your concentration disturbed.

STAYING ACTIVE

The most important thing for a mother in early labour is to keep active. Moving around is a great help in getting and keeping labour established, and most women find it easier to cope with contractions if they're upright. If you have a contraction, just stop and breathe through it. As labour progresses, keeping upright as much as possible helps the contractions work with, not against, gravity.

PAIN RELIEF

For many women, particularly first-time mothers, anticipation of their baby's birth may be overshadowed by worry about pain during labour. Labour invariably involves some level of pain, but you can build up your confidence by preparing for the intensity of contractions, trying to understand your own limits of pain tolerance and by learning about different methods of pain relief. View the pain as a positive element of labour – each contraction brings the birth of your baby nearer.

Find out as much as you can about the types of pain relief available. Have a discussion with your doctor or midwife and then outline your choices in your birth plan. Be prepared for your plan to change if any complications arise.

Regional anaesthetics

These remove sensation from part of your body by blocking the transmission of pain from nerve fibres. The most widely used form of this type of anaesthesia is the epidural. This prevents pain from spreading out from your uterus by acting as a "nerve block" in your spine. After an injection of local anaesthetic in your back to numb it, the anaesthetist inserts a fine, hollow needle into the epidural space – the region around the spinal cord – and the anaesthetic is injected through this.

A well-managed epidural removes all sensation from your waist to your knees, but you remain alert and it does not affect your baby. It is recommended if you have pre-eclampsia or severe asthma, or if labour is difficult or a forceps delivery is likely.

Inhalation analgesic

Entonox is a gas that you administer yourself using a face mask. It consists of nitrous oxide and oxygen. You inhale the gas deeply as the contraction starts and carry on until it peaks or you have had enough. You then put the mask aside and breath normally. Entonox works by numbing the pain centre in the brain, and can make you feel as though you're floating.

Narcotics

The most commonly used is pethidine, which is derived from morphine and is given by injection in the first stage of labour. It dulls the sensation

Stages of labour

Labour can start in a variety of ways, but once it's really under way, you will know all about it. If you're unsure, you probably aren't quite in labour.

There are various signs that labour is starting.
• **The show** – brownish/pink discharge that indicates that the mucus plug that has sealed the cervix during pregnancy has come away in readiness for labour.
• **Waters break** – sometimes the amniotic sac ruptures before labour starts, causing fluid to leak slowly or in a gush from your vagina.
• **Contractions start** – the muscular tightenings of the uterus – contractions – gradually start to pull open the cervix. If they're coming regularly every 10–15 minutes, you're in labour.

There are three stages of labour.
• **First stage** – during this stage the cervix opens out (dilates) to allow the baby's head to pass through. Before it dilates, the cervix becomes thinned and softened and is gradually pulled up by the contracting uterine muscles. When the cervix is about 10cm (5in) in diameter it is said to be fully dilated. This is the completion of the first stage of labour.

• **Second stage** – this is the expulsive stage, when you push your baby out through the birth canal. It lasts from the full dilation of the cervix until the baby is born. The uterine contractions are 60–90 seconds long at this time and occur at two- to four-minute intervals. As your baby is gradually pushed down your birth canal, you should try to use gravity as much as possible to help, so keep as upright as you can. The first sign that the baby is coming is the bulging of your anus and perineum. With each contraction, more and more of the baby's head appears at your vaginal opening, until the head doesn't slip back at all between contractions. This is known as crowning. If you take your time and let your vagina stretch slowly, you may avoid a tear. As the head emerges, the midwife will ask you to pant, not push. With the next contractions, she will gently turn the baby so that the shoulders can be born one at a time and the rest of your baby's body can slide out. Now is the moment for which you've waited nine months.
• **Third stage** – once your baby has been born, your uterus will rest for about 15 minutes. It will then start to contract again in order to expel the placenta.

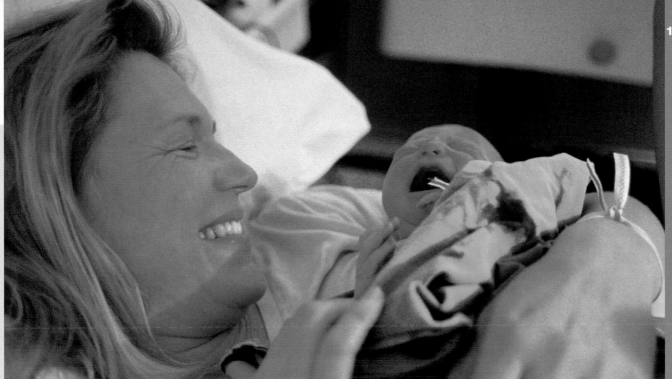

of pain but also reduces consciousness and tends to make the labour longer.

TENS

TENS stands for transcutaneous electrical nerve stimulation and is a means of relieving labour pain by stimulating production of the body's natural painkillers – endorphins – and by blocking pain sensation with an electric current. The electrodes are placed on the woman's body and she is able to regulate the intensity of the current herself. TENS has been used successfully but it does not help everyone. A try-out before labour is advisable.

Acupuncture

I would recommend using acupuncture for pain relief in labour only if you have found it successful in the past. For some women it will

undoubtedly work, but the acupuncturist must be practised at giving pain relief in labour.

Massage

This is a wonderful way of getting reassurance from your partner while relieving discomfort, whether you're lying, standing or squatting. It can be particularly helpful if you have backache during labour, which most women do.

Breathing

Relaxing your body and focusing on your breathing will help alleviate your anxiety and let you ride out your contractions. Practise before the birth with your birth partner.

EPISIOTOMY

This is a surgical cut to enlarge the vaginal outlet at delivery and is the most commonly performed

operation in the West. Episiotomies are used in order to avoid tears, which have ragged edges and are difficult to stitch together and were believed to heal less well. This is not the case. Tears can be avoided if a woman is encouraged to stop pushing while the head is being born, and is allowed to let her uterus ease the head gradually rather than quickly. When the head delivers too fast, an episiotomy may be performed because the perineum is thought to be under stress. If you wish to avoid an episiotomy, note in your birth plan that you don't want one unless absolutely necessary.

Help yourself through contractions

● Relax as much as possible, especially during contractions; concentrate on the out-breath as you exhale, and drop your shoulders.
● Keep moving about between contractions, then get into a position that feels right for you. These may include a supported squat, leaning against your partner, on all fours, or kneeling down and leaning forwards on a pillow placed on a chair.
● Try counting backwards from 100 through a contraction – the concentration needed takes your mind off the pain. Keep your eyes open to externalize the pain; focus on something in the room such as a picture.
● Take sips of still mineral water from a sponge if your mouth is dry, and ask your partner to massage your back during a contraction.
● Don't be afraid to say – or shout – anything you like during labour; no one will hold it against you after the birth.

Water birth

Using a birthing pool during labour can help to relax you and reduce the pain of contractions. You are less likely to be subjected to interventionist procedures because of imposed time limits. This in turn means that you will have the time needed for your tissues and muscles to open and stretch. Your partner can share in the intimacy of a water birth, and your baby can be welcomed with a skin-to-skin cuddle from both of you right after the birth.

Birthing pools are a method of pain relief; the birth isn't necessarily under water. There can be some danger to the baby if she is delivered under water and her head is not lifted out right away. Water births must always be supervised by a qualified attendant. Many hospitals now offer birthing pool facilities, and there are companies that have portable pools for hire. These can be taken to hospital – check with them first – or used at home.

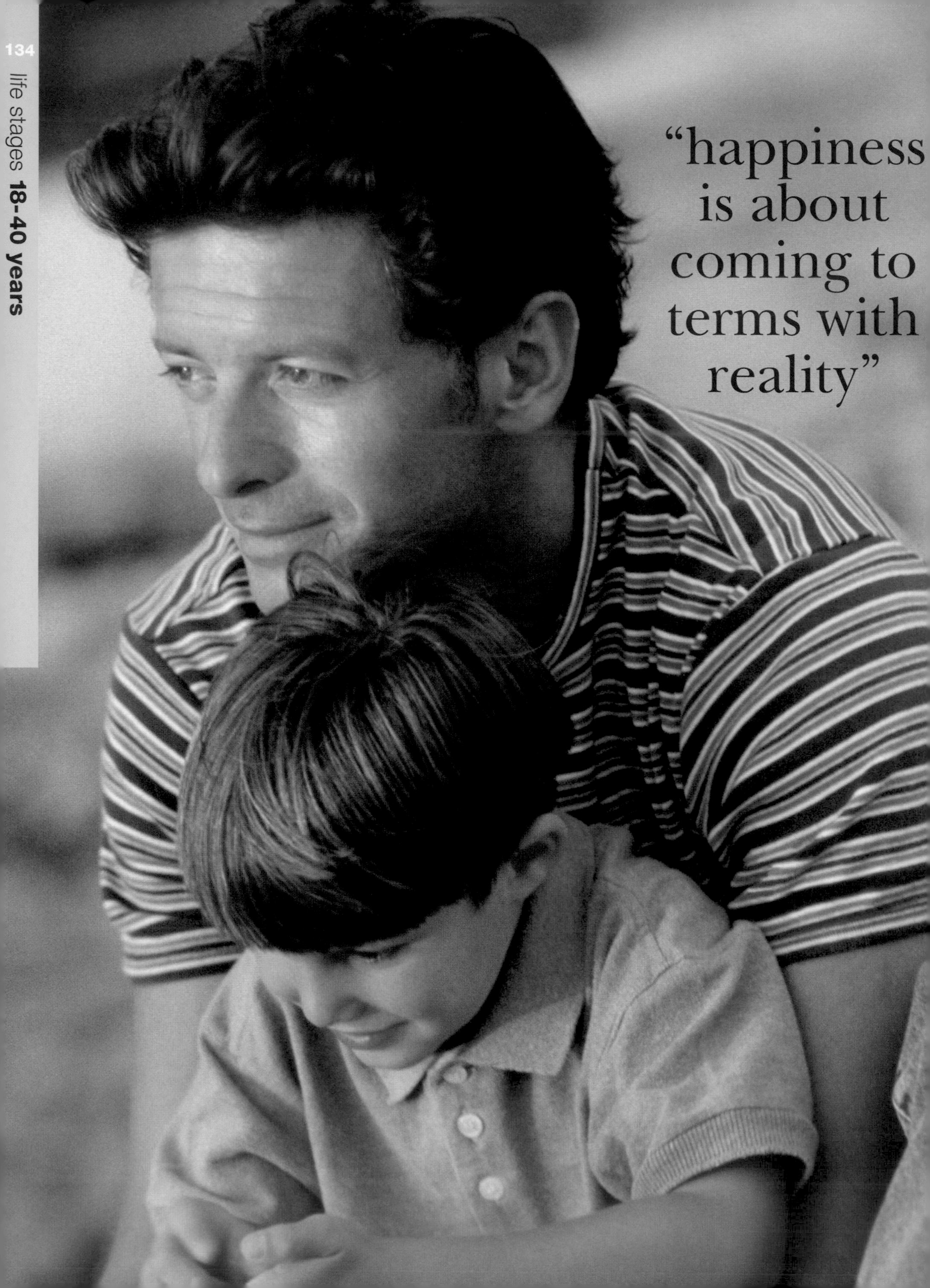

"happiness
is about
coming to
terms with
reality"

life stages: 18 to 40 years

Living in the 21st century is about as stressful a form of life as you can think of. Human beings are not very well designed to live under such conditions, for every aspect of modern life has an element of stress. We live in a success-orientated society in which it's impossible to escape from competitiveness and the desire to succeed. And during our 20s and 30s we may be particularly exposed to stress as we struggle to establish ourselves in careers and relationships.

Although many people still think of stress as wholly negative, it can, in fact, be either positive or negative. There is evidence to show that a moderate degree of stress can be good for us – it improves performance, efficiency, productivity and many of us thrive on it. Indeed, there are some people who *need* stress and function at maximum efficiency when they are under stress. But they are rare. For most of us, if stress goes beyond a certain point, everything disintegrates and this can lead to both mental and physical illness. It is, therefore, very important for all of us to come to terms with what causes us stress, to recognize the part that it plays in our health or, conversely, ill-health, and finally to try and find out how we can get rid of it or cope with it.

Coping with stress

Actually taking action is one of the best ways of coping with stress; doing something, doing almost anything. I have found one of the best ways to manage stress is to start analysing the problem on paper. Define it, write down as many solutions as you can think of and select the most realistic two or three. Opt for one of these if you can and write down an action plan, taking into account each step you need to take to bring about a solution. Even just the act of writing everything down should help you see your problem in proportion and will scale down the stress-producing difficulty. Follow your plan through and you should feel less stressed. If you don't or it doesn't work, you can always try one of your other options.

Learn to love yourself

One of the greatest causes of stress and mental ill-health can be a disparity between expectation and achievement, between hope and actual result. Happiness and mental wellbeing are not about playing out a fictitious role conjured up by authors and journalists. Happiness is about coming to terms with reality. One of the most important parts of that is learning what you want to do, deciding to do it to the best of your ability, and not feeling inadequate because it doesn't happen to coincide with what you think you ought to do. Forget what you ought to do. Learn to live with yourself. Most important, learn to love yourself for who you are.

We don't stop developing at the age of 18. Most adults learn that the real growth period for us as people only begins after this age and that the achievement of true happiness may take another three decades of hard work. Going through a period of self-analysis, choice and possibly change of lifestyle requires courage, so brave you must be. In the pages that follow I offer guidelines where appropriate, advice where I feel there may be a need and strategies for dealing with potentially difficult situations.

Beating stress

● Make a list of your three best attributes. Do people describe you, for example, as generous, affectionate and trustworthy? Carry the list with you and read it to yourself whenever you find yourself thinking unpleasant thoughts.

● Keep a list of affirmations to say to yourself when under stress. It's amazing – chanting simple phrases such as "I really can handle this" can divert the stress response.

● Keep a daily diary of all the small, pleasant events that happen and talk about them with your partner or a friend each day. Write down what you did for enjoyment or fun. Look back at your diary every week to see what progress you have made and to make plans for what you intend to achieve next week.

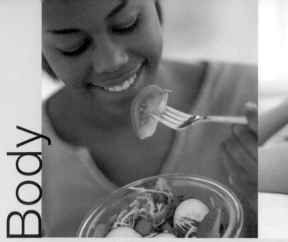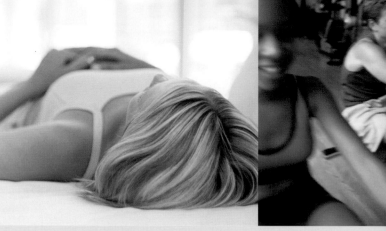

Body

Social

> "few couples realize the impact a new baby will have on their lives"

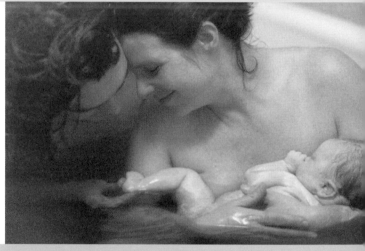

Mind

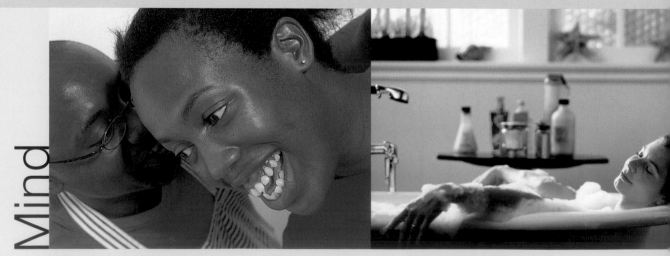

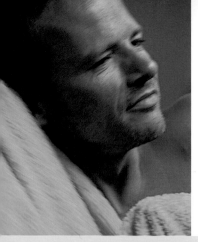

"it's never too early to start looking after your heart"

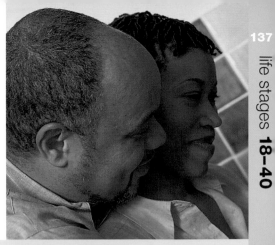

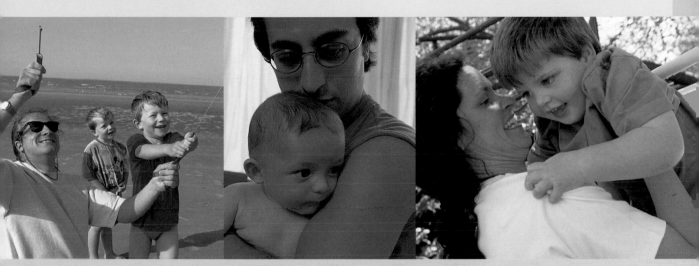

"mental fitness is just as important as physical fitness"

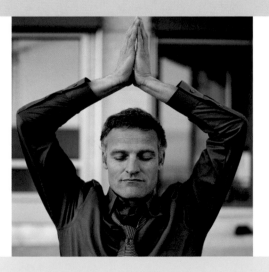

"realize you can't totally control the world around you"

18-40

healthy heart, healthy body

It's never too early to start looking after your heart. Take action now to improve your general level of fitness and control your weight and you will have fewer health problems later in life.

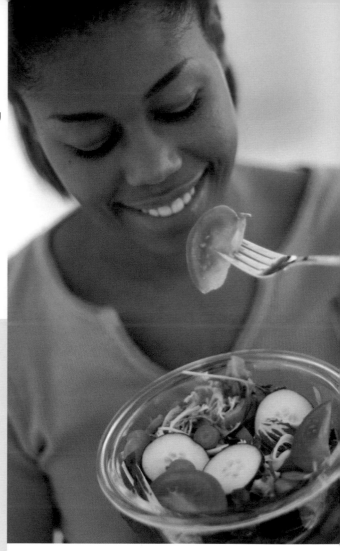

Stop drastic dieting and start eating

The amount of energy you burn daily, apart from any specific activities you undertake, is variable and you can make a positive impact on it. You can also do the opposite.

The popularity in the last few years of microdiets (diets where you consume only some 350 calories a day) has prompted concern that you end up losing too much lean muscle mass rather than mainly fat. But the most striking argument against them is their effect on your basal metabolism. If you put your body on a starvation diet, it thinks it really is starving and takes appropriate action. This is akin to hibernation, although not quite as drastic. The body simply slows down and burns about 15–20 percent less energy. You will still lose weight on these diets, but not in a healthy way. Nor do you learn anything about making the important lifestyle and behavioural changes needed to lose weight and keep it off in the long term.

A sensible eating pattern

Instead of starving yourself, eat a sensible amount each day of different kinds of foods – that is, very little fat, salt, sugar, red meat and processed foods, but moderate amounts of poultry, eggs and fish, and lots of fresh fruit and vegetables, beans, pulses, wholegrain rice and oats. By eating your food in six smaller instalments, you will find that you burn off more calories than if you ate the same food as three larger meals. Eating little and often can also help regulate your blood glucose levels and appetite. And remember that if you don't exercise, you will lose weight more slowly, so take regular exercise.

Health checks

Women
● There are national screening programmes for cervical cancer and breast cancer. Every woman from age 20 onwards should check her breasts daily (see p.243).
● To help prevent cervical cancer, any woman who becomes sexually active should be having regular smear tests.

Men
● Testicular cancer is the most common form of cancer in young men in the UK and it is the biggest cause of cancer-related deaths in males aged 15–35.
● The number of cases has trebled in the past 20 years.
● It's easily treated and if caught at an early stage, testicular cancer is nearly always curable. Every man from 15 onwards should be doing regular self-examination of the testicles to make sure everything is normal (see p.264).
● More than 50 percent of sufferers consult their doctors after the cancer has started to spread. This makes it more difficult to treat successfully and the side effects of the disease and the treatment become more unpleasant.

Keep your heart healthy

Heart disease is the UK's biggest killer. It's never too early to start looking after your heart. Lack of physical activity is probably the most common risk factor for heart disease in the UK. Seven out of 10 people in the UK don't take enough regular exercise to achieve health benefits to protect their heart. You should aim for at least 30 minutes of activity that makes you slightly breathless three times a week.

Exercise has direct benefits for your heart.
● It helps to improve your blood cholesterol levels.
● It helps to prevent blood clotting.
● It helps to lower blood pressure and prevent high blood pressure.
● It helps you to reach and maintain a healthy weight.
● It helps your recovery after you have had a heart attack.

The risk raisers

● Physical inactivity.
● Smoking.
● High blood pressure.
● High blood cholesterol.
● Obesity.
● Drinking too much alcohol.

Cut out: smoking

Giving up smoking has immediate benefits for your heart.
● Within 20 minutes blood pressure and pulse rates fall.

● Within eight hours carbon monoxide levels drop back to normal and the oxygen level goes back up to normal.
● Within 24 hours the risk of a heart attack decreases.
● Within 72 hours lung airways relax, making it easier to breathe and the volume of air the lungs can hold increases.
● Within one to three months circulation improves and lung function improves by up to a third.

Cut down: alcohol

Too much alcohol can damage your heart muscle, increase blood pressure and also lead to weight gain. Heavier drinking can contribute to heart ailments, including high blood pressure and stroke. Professional women are particularly prone to drinking too much – they're three times as likely to drink more than the recommended amount than women in unskilled, manual jobs.

Cut down: salt

People who have a high salt intake seem more likely to have high blood pressure. Most people eat more salt than they need. On average we eat nine grams a day and the recommended maximum is six grams. The body only needs one gram.

Choose low-salt or reduced-salt foods, limit smoked foods and try to eat as much unprocessed food as possible. Around three-quarters of the salt we eat comes from processed foods.

To cut down on salt, first try not to add it to your food at the table. Later, try cooking without adding any salt. Within a month your palate will have adjusted and you won't like salty foods.

Cut down: cholesterol

Lowering blood cholesterol levels by just 1 percent reduces the risk of coronary heart disease by 2 to 3 percent. To reduce your cholesterol level, cut right down on saturated fats such as fatty meats and dairy produce and replace them with small amounts of polyunsaturated fats and monounsaturated fats – for example, olive oil, rapeseed oil, nuts, avocados. Base meals on starchy foods (bread, pasta, rice, cereals and potatoes) and remember to eat five or more fruit and veg each day.

● Foods such as oats, lentils, beans and fruit contain soluble fibre and this is useful for mopping up cholesterol.
● A bowl of porridge every morning made with skimmed milk can help reduce your cholesterol levels.
● Garlic is useful too. Large doses of garlic (seven cloves a day) may help to prevent blood clots forming. It may also lower total cholesterol levels.
● A portion of oily fish – mackerel, salmon, sardines – at least once a week won't help lower cholesterol but can reduce your risk of a heart attack.

Fit muscles help weight loss

When you are overweight, the problem is not as simple as you may at first think. Not only are you over your ideal weight, but you also probably have a disproportionate amount of fat instead of muscle. The point is this: when you diet, the more muscle you lose as a percentage of your body weight, the less energy you need and this leads to a further imbalance between fat and muscle.

However, if you combine a sensible diet with exercise, you will not only build up your muscle mass and tone up muscles that are out of condition,

you will also raise your metabolic rate and so burn up more energy regardless of what you are doing. And by exercising, whether it's brisk walking, dancing or marathon running, you will burn up energy over and above your basal metabolic requirements, which means that, once your weight is satisfactory, you can consume more calories and still stay at your ideal weight.

Exercise is therefore the key to weight loss. None of this is new information but it's surprising how easily it can be overlooked.

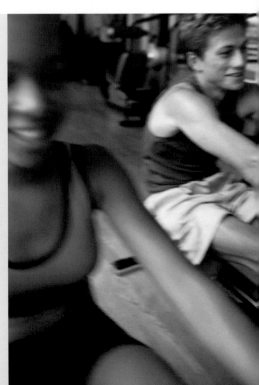

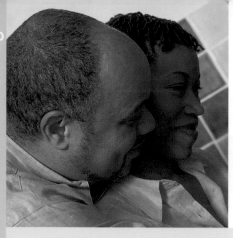

common worries

Both men and women in this age group may suffer anxieties about their appearance and their sexual performance, but there are ways you can help yourself.

Hair loss in men

Thinning hair can be a major cause of anxiety to men in this age group. Male baldness is an inherited condition and the most common form of alopecia (hair loss). The process starts when normal hair at the temples and crown is replaced by fine, downy hair. The hairline then gradually recedes. Only a trained dermatologist can determine if the hair follicle is so badly damaged that hair loss is permanent.

Over the years a number of different strategies have been used to help balding men with varying degrees of success. Here is a brief summary of those currently available.

Hairpieces

This is the safest and least painful way (in terms of health and money) to camouflage hair loss. Some hairpieces can be permanently attached to the head, either by being tied to existing hairs or by being sewn on to the scalp. The latter can cause infection and are not recommended

for that reason. The only possible side effect of hairpieces is that people may be sensitive to the adhesive that is sometimes used.

Hair weaving

This is a non-surgical procedure that adds replacement hair to existing hair in order to cover bald patches. The new hair is braided strand by strand on to the edges of the hair *in situ*. Hair weaving requires maintenance and careful cleansing.

Hair implant

This is a quasi-surgical procedure where strips of hair are attached to the scalp in the form of surgical threads implanted in the balding area. The implants are usually synthetic so a hairdryer mustn't be used.

Hair transplant

This is a surgical procedure that generally results in the permanent replacement of hair – though even when well established it is not as luxurious as the hair you've lost.

Plugs of hair are cut from remaining healthy hair on the sides and back of the head and implanted in bald spots. This hair normally falls out after transplant but is replaced by new hair. Quite a few hair follicles must be transplanted at the same session and the process needs to be repeated for bald areas to be covered.

Medication

During research on drugs to control high blood pressure, it was discovered that minoxidil promoted hair growth, and it is now available for this purpose. It has to be applied to the scalp twice daily for a minimum of four months for any effect to be noticeable. Treatment has to be continued or hair loss will recur.

A second drug, finasteride, used for treating benign enlargement of the prostate gland, has been found to help male baldness by reducing the effect of the enzyme alpha reductase which is thought to cause baldness.

Choosing celibacy

There is so much emphasis on sex and having successful sex, but it must be said that there is nothing wrong in not wanting sex at all. Sexual desire varies from none to

a lot, and all variations are normal. **There is absolutely nothing wrong with you if you don't want to have sex**. If you really don't want it, and are upset by having sex, be plain-

spoken about it and let it be known. Sex is supposed to be a pleasure, not a burden. If it is onerous and distasteful, don't have sex and don't feel guilty about it.

A woman's failure to orgasm

Probably the most common sexual problem seen in women is that of difficulty in reaching an orgasm (climax). There are two main groups: the first group consists of women who have never achieved orgasm, while the second group are women who have had orgasms but only in special circumstances.

Just because a woman is unable to reach a climax does not mean that she is frigid. She may well have a strong sex drive and be capable of falling in love. If a woman often fails to reach a climax, she is likely to become disappointed and eventually may lose interest in sex altogether.

A woman may find difficulty in reaching a climax if she is uncertain about her commitment towards her partner, or if she is frightened of losing control. If a woman has never reached a climax, this may just be due to the fact she has not had sufficient sexual stimulation for orgasm to take place. If she has had a lot of stimulation and she is still unable to reach a climax, either during sexual intercourse or by stimulation of the clitoris, then this is a problem which needs attention.

It has been found that it is easier for a woman to reach a climax on her own than when her partner is present. So to begin with, having ensured that she is alone and will not be disturbed, she should stimulate her clitoris by masturbation. She may well feel that it is wrong to reach an orgasm this way, but it is important that the woman should reach her first climax by whatever means possible. As soon as she is highly aroused she should contract her stomach muscles, as this will help her to reach a climax.

Achieving orgasm

She should continue with these masturbation sessions until she is able to achieve an orgasm fairly easily. At this stage, sexual intercourse may take place, but the woman should on no account make any attempt to achieve orgasm while the penis is in the vagina. Once the man has ejaculated, he should stimulate her clitoris so that, in her own time, she too can reach orgasm. She should concentrate only on her own sexual sensations.

There are many women who can reach orgasm by direct stimulation of the clitoris but, in spite of finding sexual intercourse an enjoyable experience, are yet unable to reach a climax with the penis in the vagina.

When there is a problem of this type, the couple should enjoy some foreplay until the woman is aroused, and at this point the man inserts his penis into the vagina and starts thrusting slowly. Then he withdraws the penis, and after a few minutes, he penetrates the vagina again.

If the woman is still unable to achieve orgasm by this method, then the man should stimulate his partner's clitoris with his finger between one insertion and the next. Again the man should wait until the woman is strongly aroused before penetrating again. As she comes closer to orgasm, she quickens her thrusting movements to help her reach climax.

Self-stimulation

If all these measures fail, then the woman should stimulate her own clitoris during sexual intercourse. She stops stimulating herself as she nears orgasm and finishes off by thrusting. Provided that care is taken in following these instructions, there is every likelihood that there will be a successful outcome. In a small number of cases where this is not sufficient, it is recommended that the couple consult an experienced therapist after discussion with their general practitioner.

It is a tremendously rewarding experience for a woman to reach a climax with the penis inside her vagina. This may well lead to a great improvement in the couple's relationship as a whole.

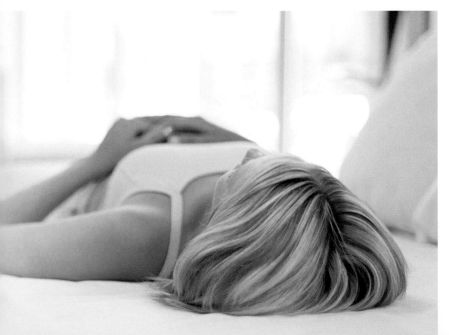

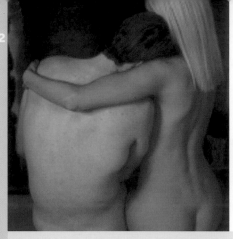

18-40 sexual problems

Premature ejaculation and anxiety about the size
of his penis are common worries for a man and few
manage to escape them altogether.

Penis size

A great many men worry about the size or shape
of their penis, usually because they believe the size
reflects their masculinity and manliness. The bigger
the penis, the better the man. This is, of course,
nonsense and is based on emotional responses rather
than on hard fact. It compares with judging a woman
by the size of her breasts and is just as senseless.

Besides its sexual function, the penis, like the
breasts, has a physical job to do and, while it has
to be big enough to get the job done, there is no
advantage in hugeness. Penile size is not related to
sexual potency – in fact, an overly large penis could
cause a woman pain and this defeats the whole object.

What is the real problem?

It's hard to say if a lack of self-esteem causes anxiety
about penis size or if penis size itself is the culprit.
Either way, a loss of self-esteem is always present in
those men who suffer from anxiety about the size
of their penis.

Who really cares?

Penis size matters far more to men than it does to
women. When it comes to being attracted to a
member of the opposite sex, penis size is low priority.
Women are more likely to seek kindness, warmth,
generosity and a sense of humour. Furthermore,
most of a woman's sensations from intercourse come
from the clitoris and from the nerve endings that are
mainly in the first part of the vagina, so the length of
the penis really is irrelevant. It is a man's skill and
patience as a lover, not the size of his penis, that is
responsible for giving his partner sexual satisfaction.

Is there any treatment?

There is no operation that will make a penis longer,
but there is one that can increase the girth. Fat is
taken from other parts of the body and used in a
process called liposculpture. It is painful and is not
available on the National Health but only from the
private sector. You would have to ask your GP for a
referral to an appropriate specialist.

It's more than possible that your doctor will be
reluctant to make the referral for this operation. You
can, if you wish, visit another doctor for a second
opinion. However, you should think closely and
deeply about the risks associated with any surgical
procedure and ask yourself if the end result is worth
taking these risks for.

What is the outlook?

Everybody cares about the way they look and
most of us try to make the best of our appearance.
But if concern about a particular aspect of bodily
appearance prevents a person from enjoying their life
to the full, it is a symptom of a lack of self-confidence
and self-esteem.

Sadly, some men allow their fear of failure to
become an obsession and this can actually ruin their
life. Penis size makes no difference at all to a man's
personality and character and it is wrong to think
that a bigger penis would, or even could, make a
man better and more desirable than he already is.
It simply wouldn't happen. If worrying about the
size of your penis is a problem for you, it is your
self-esteem that needs a boost.

Premature ejaculation

Premature ejaculation is the release of semen before or just after penetration. The most important aspect of premature ejaculation is that the man is unable to have any control over his ejaculation, so that once he is sexually aroused he reaches orgasm very quickly. The time between inserting the penis into the vagina and reaching orgasm is short – often less than 30 seconds. This does not allow the female partner sufficient time to become sexually aroused, especially if there has been no clitoral stimulation. This can lead to frustration in the woman and guilt in the man, and may well have a damaging effect on their relationship.

If premature ejaculation has always been present in a healthy man, then the cause is almost certainly psychological. But if a man develops premature ejaculation out of the blue, his doctor should exclude any physical disease. This latter type of premature ejaculation is rare.

What causes it?

Most men will experience premature ejaculation at some time in their lives, probably more than once, and for no apparent reason. Most will find that difficulties pass spontaneously as quickly as they appeared. Men who are young or inexperienced, who have abstained from sex for a long period of time or who are anxious and lack confidence are more likely to experience premature ejaculation.

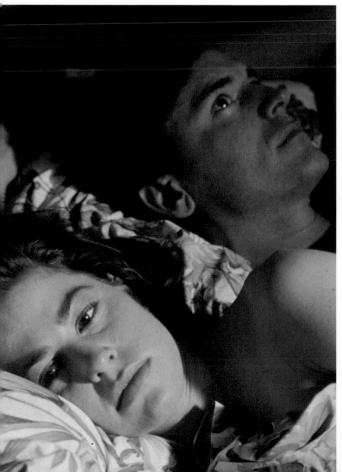

What can I do about premature ejaculation?

When premature ejaculation is the result of a psychological problem, it is important that the man focuses all his attention on his own sexual sensations before orgasm is reached, using the "stop-start" method.

Try the following steps

1 First, the couple should engage in some foreplay so that the man gets an erection. He should then lie on his back and his partner should stimulate his penis with her hand. During this time, he should concentrate only on his own sexual sensations.

2 As soon as he feels that he is near to orgasm, he must tell his partner to stop stimulating him until the sensation disappears again. Before the erection is allowed to disappear completely, he asks his partner to stimulate him once more.

3 This cycle is then repeated, and ejaculation is only allowed on the fourth occasion. It is up to the man to signal to his partner when she should stop stimulating him and when to begin again.

4 Once the man is able to focus his attention on his own sexual feelings, and he is able to recognize the intense sensations immediately before orgasm, the couple can go on to the next stage.

5 This involves repeating the previous instructions but this time using a lubricating jelly, as orgasm occurs more rapidly in a moist situation. This is due to the similarity of the lubricant to the vaginal secretions.

6 The third stage is sexual intercourse. In the first instance the man lies on his back and his partner should sit astride him. He then lowers her onto his erect penis.

7 Again the "stop-start" method is used, and just before he reaches orgasm, all movement is stopped but the penis remains inside the vagina. When the sexual sensation subsides, but before the erection has gone, they begin to move again. As before, orgasm is only permitted on the fourth occasion.

8 As soon as the couple find that sexual intercourse is successful in this position, they then repeat the whole procedure in the side-to-side position, and finally with the man on top of the woman. You continue the stop-start exercises once every two weeks until he has fully recovered.

Outlook – good!

Provided that the couple follow these instructions carefully, practically all men with premature ejaculation are likely to make a complete recovery.

If the treatment is not successful, this may either be due to deep-seated emotional problems in the man, or because his partner finds difficulty in cooperating. It may help for the couple to seek expert advice from an experienced therapist, after first discussing this with their own doctor.

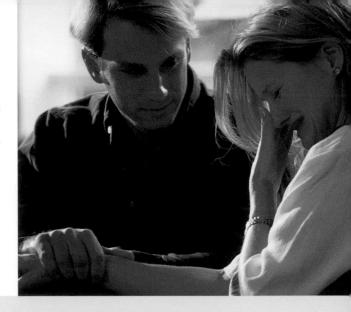

18-40
miscarriages and infertility

Both these problems are surprisingly common. One in five pregnancies ends in miscarriage. One in six couples have difficulty conceiving.

Miscarriage

Miscarriage is the spontaneous loss of a baby and can happen at any time from around the date of a missed period up to the 24th week of pregnancy. The anguish of the bereavement is more intense because all the hopes and expectations built on the arrival of a new baby are suddenly dashed.

What causes a miscarriage?

A miscarriage can result because of parental factors, fetal factors or a combination of the two. These are the main things that can go wrong:
● A defective egg or sperm forms an abnormal fetus.
● An abnormally shaped uterus can't sustain a pregnancy.
● Fibroids in the uterus disturb the growing fetus.
● A weak cervix may open during pregnancy.
● A weak placenta may not develop properly.

● Diabetes or very severe high blood pressure may not be fully controlled by medication.
● Rhesus incompatibility.
● Maternal infections by bacteria or viruses damage the fetus.
● Pregnancy hormones aren't in balance and the fetus can't grow.

Should I see a doctor?

If you know you're pregnant, or think you might be, and experience any vaginal bleeding and/or cramping pain, ring your doctor immediately.

While you're waiting, go to bed and keep your feet raised. Wear a sanitary pad if necessary. Don't flush away any of the discharge as your doctor will want to examine it.

What is the surgical treatment?

● If you have an incomplete miscarriage (when the fetus is expelled but parts of

the placenta remain) an ERPC (evacuation of the retained products of conception) will be essential to prevent infection. Infertility can result from such an infection if it is not treated.
● If the fetus dies in the uterus but remains there, the fetus will have to be taken away surgically.
● If you miscarry several times in a row, your doctor will carry out tests to try to find the specific cause and prevent it happening again.
● You may be given a hysterosalpingogram to check out the condition of your uterus and fallopian tubes.
● Your doctor will examine the aborted fetus and placenta to make sure they're normal and treat you accordingly. In some cases, you may be referred to an infertility expert for advice.
● If you have a septic miscarriage (your internal organs have become infected) you'll be given antibiotics in large doses to deal with the infection.

Coping after a miscarriage

Whatever the reason for the miscarriage and whatever the treatment your doctor prescribes, the emotional effects can be devastating. As well as the natural feelings of grief, you'll probably feel angry that your body has let you down.

The one emotion you must try to quell is guilt. It's not your fault and, although you may be feeling like hiding yourself away and perhaps punishing yourself, this isn't the way to get back to normal. Try not to

isolate yourself and try to be positive about what you can do in the future.

Anxiety is one of the emotions that can prevent conception. Your doctor should give you an honest answer as soon as possible about whether you can carry a baby to full term without medical treatment. If he says it's possible, keep trying, but try not to become obsessive. If you have a problem that can be treated, don't waste time – seek treatment.

A miscarriage is a true bereavement and is difficult to cope with. Counselling might help and is available. If you think you'd benefit from it, ask your doctor to put you in touch with a counsellor.

You can usually resume sexual intercourse within about three weeks, when the bleeding has stopped and the cervix has closed. But you'll probably be advised to wait about six months before trying to conceive again.

Difficulties in conceiving

Having problems conceiving doesn't always mean you are infertile. Most couples who think they are infertile are only subfertile and with help can conceive successfully.

What is infertility?

To most people infertility means the inability to have children but it's more complex than that. A couple may have no difficulty in conceiving their first child but find they cannot have a second; this means that they are suffering from secondary infertility. Another couple, who have both had children by their previous partners, may now find that they cannot conceive together. This is known as subfertility and happens because the fertility of a couple is the sum of their individual fertilities.

If both partners' fertilities are marginal, conception may not occur. But if one partner's fertility is strong, it still may be possible for the couple to conceive. Only 50 percent of couples conceive within three months; if a couple hasn't conceived within six months and then approaches their doctor for advice, he or she is most likely to send them away with encouraging words but advising them to come back if nothing has happened after a year.

Women produce lower-quality eggs as they get older, so age is undoubtedly a factor. Statistics show that around 90 percent of women in their 20s will become pregnant within a year of trying, and the remainder still have a high statistical chance of becoming pregnant naturally within a further year or so. But women in their 30s have a much lower statistical probability of becoming pregnant after a year of trying, so should seek help after that time has elapsed.

There are now many different ways in which a couple can be helped to conceive a child. These range from simple advice on sexual technique to drug treatment, surgery and, ultimately, to the new assisted reproductive technologies (ART).

The importance of counselling

Given the tensions that surround the treatment of infertility, couples deserve and should get psychological support. When you decide to embark on investigation and treatment, ask your doctor to refer you to a counsellor trained in dealing with the stress of infertility at all stages of its management. You shouldn't have to wait until you find yourselves well on into secondary referral; you both need help and advice right from the start. Some procedures require a good deal of deep self-questioning and a couple will need a great deal of support because of the lengthy and invasive nature of the treatment, and especially the ethical issues surrounding assisted reproductive technologies, insemination, and any technique involving donors.

Psychological factors affecting fertility

The way you feel can in itself affect your fertility by causing a hormone disturbance or impotence. So, without proper support, fertility treatment may make matters worse. On the other hand, doctors have plenty of anecdotal evidence that couples suddenly conceive very soon after making the decision to have their infertility investigated, as if initiating an investigation releases the psychological tensions that may have been affecting fertility all along.

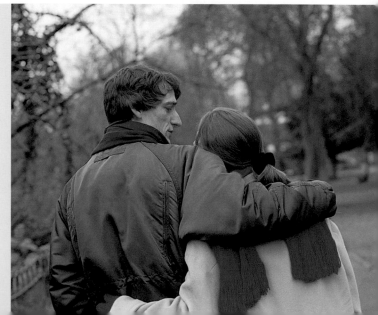

Issues to consider about fertility

Even before you have counselling, it's worth asking yourselves some questions, so that some of the issues are out in the open.
- Would you tell friends and family, or would you attempt to keep your fertility treatment a complete secret?
- If you intend to keep it a secret, can you be sure that the truth won't come out, perhaps destructively, at a time of crisis?
- Could you cope with a multiple pregnancy?
- What if one, some, or all of the babies died?
- Having committed so much time and money to having a baby, how easy will you find it to let her go once she grows up?
- How long would you persist with infertility treatment?
- Would you consider donor eggs or sperm?
- Is adoption an option?

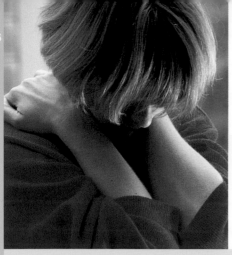

18-40 abortion

Opting for an abortion is never an easy decision. Some people feel that it is morally, religiously and biologically wrong to interfere with a pregnancy and they are fervently opposed to abortion. Others are just as strongly in favour.

Deciding to have an abortion

Most of us would probably suffer a mixture of feelings were an unwanted pregnancy to be confirmed. We may be fearful that our families and friends will find out and that we may be punished. We may be fearful that we won't be able to decide what to do, and this indecision increases the circuit of anxiety. We are afraid that we will be alone in trying to decide what to do, and, of course, we are afraid of the prospects of motherhood.

We may also be afraid of abortion, even though we know it's legal and safe. "Will it cost more than I can pay?", "Can I have it on the National Health?", "Will it be painful?", "Will I be punished by suffering post-operative complications?", "Will I be sterile afterwards?", "I feel guilty now but will I carry around guilt feelings for the rest of my life?", "Will I regret what I have done and wish that I had had the baby?", "Will I fear sex and never be able to have a proper relationship with a man again?".

Seek help and support

It is quite normal for you to feel all of these fears and to be, in some instances, profoundly affected psychologically. But the reassuring news is that the majority of women feel relieved after an abortion although they may feel sad as well. You are going to have a fairly hard time and you need support, so establish it before you go into your abortion. Seek the help of a friend, make sure that your friend will stand by you and comfort you during and after the abortion. If this friend can be your doctor, that is even better; if it is one of your parents, you are very lucky; if it's your partner, you have the best of all worlds. Whoever you find, find someone because you are going to need them and you will pull through the post-abortion upset faster by having them close to you during this time.

Where can I go for advice?

First go along and see your family doctor (who should be well acquainted with your medical history), or go to an organization that specializes in giving help to people in your position. They offer a full, non-pressurized counselling service. You will have the opportunity to ask all the questions you want to. You will be reminded about anything you have forgotten, all the various alternatives other than abortion will be discussed with you, and your personal domestic and financial commitments will be carefully considered.

Once you have decided on an abortion, your own general practitioner will need to make a second appointment, usually with a gynaecologist or a psychiatrist. This can be done within a day or two. Having seen the second physician, the abortion will be arranged as soon as possible. About the earliest would be a week, the average two to three weeks.

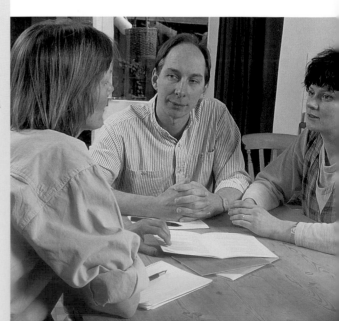

Legal requirements for abortion

In the UK, in theory at least, two doctors must testify to one of the following before you can have an abortion:

● Continuing the pregnancy involves a greater risk to the woman's life than abortion.

OR

● Continuing the pregnancy involves a greater risk of injury to her physical or mental health than an abortion.

OR

● Continuing the pregnancy involves a greater risk of injury to the physical or mental health of the existing children in the family than an abortion would do.

OR

● There is a substantial risk that the child will be born seriously deformed (e.g. spina bifida, Down's syndrome).

The time to have an abortion

If you do decide on an abortion, you should arrange it as soon as you possibly can because the earlier it is done the safer it is. The later you leave it, the greater the chances are of complications.

There is no question that abortions are best performed before 12 weeks. After that time, and certainly after 16 weeks, it becomes not only more difficult, but also more dangerous to procure an abortion through the vagina. After this time, an abortion is usually completed by injecting prostaglandins into the uterine cavity itself, which stimulates the uterus to contract. The abortion may take 12 hours and can be painful.

Late abortions

Only 1 in 100 abortions is undertaken after 20 weeks, and nearly all of those are done because a very severe abnormality of the fetus has been discovered or because of extreme distress or illness of the mother. In these instances, abortion is performed by hysterectomy – that is, an operation through the abdominal wall to open up the uterus similar to a Caesarean section – or by medical induction.

After an abortion

If you have your abortion performed within the first 12 weeks of pregnancy, you will be physically back to normal within a week.

Psychologically, though, it may take considerably longer for you to feel your usual self. It varies from individual to individual. Most women take three to four weeks to get over the psychological effects of an abortion. Some take several months. After an abortion it's common to feel withdrawn, tearful, and be unable to make decisions. But take heart; along with the sadness will come a sense of relief.

If your sadness persists, see your doctor. Most abortion units have a counsellor you can confide in, and the right professional support can really help you to start feeling better about yourself.

How soon can I have sexual intercourse?

Provided you are using contraceptives, you can have sex again in about two to three weeks if you feel up to it. Do not have intercourse any earlier than this, because you are somewhat more prone to having an infection introduced into the genital tract immediately after an abortion.

do

 Take it easy
Do look after yourself by taking things very easy and resting for at least a day.

 Check-up
Do have a proper medical check-up within a week of the abortion, even if you feel fine.

 Symptoms
Do consult your doctor immediately if you start to vomit or bleed heavily, if you have a prolonged or smelly vaginal discharge, or if you develop severe pain or fever.

don't

 No exercise
Don't take any strenuous exercise for at least three days.

 Tampons and towels
Don't use any tampons for two or three weeks to avoid the risk of infection; use sanitary towels instead.

 Next time...
Abortion is a tragedy, so make sure that there isn't going to be a "next time". Get advice on contraception now (see p.118). And think of the results of all of your actions.

18-40
adjusting to parenthood

It's a huge leap from being a couple to becoming a family. Few couples realize how much impact their new baby will have on their lives, their work, their emotions and their feelings for one another.

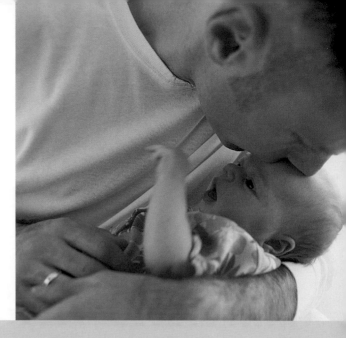

Tips for new dads

As a new father you may feel rather cut off from your partner. The best antidote is to get involved with the baby and to offer help at every opportunity. Even if at first your partner may seem a bit distant, your understanding and help will break down any barriers.

What you can do to help

● Take the initiative; don't wait to be asked to share your baby's care. Learn while your baby's still a newborn.

● Get to know your baby. Use these early days to establish a close relationship with your baby by changing her and learning to handle her. Hold your baby close to you so that she can focus on your face. Carry your baby around in a sling whenever possible, try to be there for the first bath and do regular feeds, changes and bathtimes.

● Be ready for your partner's mood swings. At some point during the first week your partner will probably experience the so-called "baby blues" that come as a reaction to the sudden withdrawal of the pregnancy hormones and exhaustion after the labour. These "baby blues" are temporary; they subside after a week to 10 days.

● Never belittle or make light of your partner's feelings; she has a lot to cope with. Be sensitive to her needs and talk to her about them. If her depression lasts more than two weeks make sure she sees her doctor.

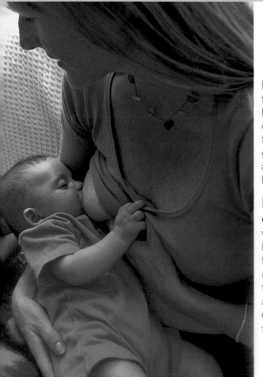

Tips for new mums

Even though you're longing to be home, try to take advantage of your time in hospital to regain your strength and lean on your midwife, health visitor and doctor for advice. Don't feel shy about asking – get as much help as you can. And friends and relations are also usually only too happy to help.

How you can adjust

● Share any aspect of your baby's care with your partner that you've been shown by the midwives. If you learn how to care for your baby together, you'll start out on an equal footing and he'll be more likely to take the initiative to help you once you are home.

● Prepare for time on your own. Build on the network of support that you have set up through antenatal classes before the baby was born. Within a week or two of the birth, your partner may have gone back to work, and friends and family will have withdrawn back to their own lives.

● Be ready for mood swings. At some point during the first few days you may experience tearful moments – and it often happens just as your milk comes in, three or four days after birth. The so-called "baby blues" are your normal reaction to the sudden withdrawal of pregnancy hormones and usually subside in a week to 10 days. Don't try to hide your feelings from your partner – be open about them.

● Make time for your partner. The baby may be time-consuming but it's good for your relationship to reserve some time and attention for each other.

New parents

What a new mother wants from her partner

● Recognize her vulnerability. A father needs to recognize how vulnerable a new mother feels, both physically and emotionally, in the days after the birth.

● Appreciate the depth of her feelings. A father needs to accept the strength of his partner's overwhelming involvement in the baby and not to construe this as a rejection of him.

● Protect her privacy. One of the most important roles for a new father is to make sure that his partner isn't overwhelmed by visitors and to give her time and space to establish breast-feeding and recover from the physical stresses of labour and birth.

What a new father wants from his partner

● Recognize his difficulties. She should be ready to accept that this is also a confusing and emotional time for her partner.

● Allow him to make mistakes. After a hospital birth, a new mother necessarily has more time to get used to the baby, but she needs to allow her partner to handle and care for the baby, and not to criticize if he fumbles.

Sex and parenthood

There's no magic date when you can start to have sex again. One of the things that will help is to start your pelvic floor exercises immediately after delivery, even though your genital area may be a bit sore. Take it slowly and gently.

● The ideal time to start making love again is when you and your partner want to, so discuss it and try it out tentatively.

● If you both feel like it, there's no reason why you couldn't try sex that's non-penetrative but nonetheless entirely fulfilling and satisfying within a few days of delivery. Some women want to have orgasms a few days after birth. Having an orgasm can be beneficial because it seems to help the uterus to shrink.

● You may find that you're a bit sore or tight, but waiting will not make you stretch. It helps, too, if the vagina is well relaxed before penetration, so concentrate on foreplay before entry.

● Try a different position from the woman lying on her back as the penis can press on the sensitive bruised rear wall of the vagina. Your partner can help by gentle manual dilatation if your vagina seems to be too tight. Don't be concerned about set backs, they're normal; try again gently.

● Many couples resume sex at six weeks – the time of the post-natal check-up. If you've had an episiotomy you'll be sore and tender for longer and your partner should not attempt penetration until you feel comfortable. However, this doesn't disbar gentle exploration. In fact, get your partner to feel your episiotomy scar. It's huge and he'll be sympathetic immediately.

● While you're breast-feeding, your breasts may feel sore and heavy and if you have cracked nipples fondling will be out of the question.

● The most important thing is to talk about your feelings and keep the channels of communication with your partner open.

● If, after several months, one of you is still feeling reluctant to resume your sexual relationship, do ask for help. You'll be surprised how much easier it is once you've talked to someone.

Episiotomy after effects

An episiotomy scar is often painful and, particularly if large, can make sex so uncomfortable that women shrink even from an embrace that might lead to other sexual activities. Women may feel aroused and ready for sex but the scar hurts so much that penetration is impossible, often for up to six months after delivery.

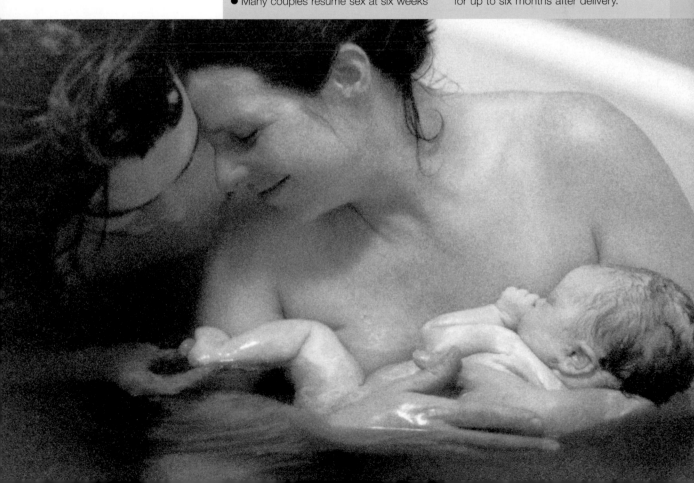

18-40 new responsibilities

Parenthood is full of ups and downs, especially at first. Having a positive and equal relationship with your partner, or a good support network if you are a single parent, can make the transition that much easier.

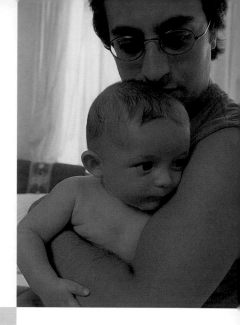

Fatherhood

Be aware that barriers between you and your partner are likely to spring from the fact that, as one psychologist put it, "although men and women become parents at the same time, they don't become parents in the same way". There are many sociological, financial and environmental reasons for this, but the result is often straightforward resentment or jealousy.

Jealous feelings

A man can quickly feel isolated within the family unit. He suddenly finds his partner's time monopolized by the new addition, and unless he is taking an active role in caring for the baby, he's no longer sure where he fits in. It is quite common to find a father becoming jealous of his own child. This situation may be exacerbated if there were differences of opinion about having the child in the first place (men often complain of being "pressurized" into having a baby).

A father may find these feelings particularly difficult to deal with if he also feels rejected on a sexual level. Often men take a new mother's diminished sex drive as a personal rebuff. If it's not too late, discuss the effects this may have on your relationship before the baby arrives.

Many of us remember our fathers seeming more unapproachable and distant than our mothers, but there is

no reason why a child cannot enjoy an equally close relationship with both parents. A baby's relationships do not operate on an either/or basis and parents should never worry that if a baby spends an equal amount of time with his father, he might love his mother less. All young children need as much love as they can get, and both parents should do their utmost to provide it.

For a father to take on an equal role as a parent, he will have to overcome cultural pressures, and perhaps change his own attitudes too. He will also have to recognize his role as a carer rather than just a provider. Some men confuse parenthood with taking care of the bills, because that is what they saw their own fathers doing.

Who's left holding the baby?

Today it may be economic factors that determine who is left holding the baby. If a woman earns more than her partner, or if he is unemployed, many couples can't afford to let misplaced male pride reduce their weekly income. While the rise of the house-husband has undoubtedly benefited lots of families, it is important to bear in mind that the man left at home with a small child may suffer from the same problems as a woman: isolation and boredom. Whatever your arrangement, when you're together try hard to talk about how you feel.

Single fathers

There are very few men who are the sole carers of a young baby, but for those who are, the pleasures and most of the problems will be the same as those of a single mother. Single men are at no more of a disadvantage in the practical care of their baby because they are male; the only thing they can't do that a woman can is breast-feed.

The benefits

Although it's not an ideal situation to be caring for a baby alone, a single father may benefit in ways that would not have happened had he been sharing the care with his partner. Research has shown that single fathers are more satisfied parents, feel closer to their children and are more confident and effective than the average father.

The problems

The main problem that may occur for a single father is that of isolation. He may find that he has to battle for recognition in female-dominated environments and, sadly, there will be those who question his ability to bring up his baby properly. But over time, a full-time father will stop being the token male and become just another parent, who shares the same pleasures and problems of parenthood as his female friends.

Lifestyle changes

The arrival of a child means that choices become stark: beforehand, for instance, if neither partner wanted to clean the bathroom floor, it could be left until later. But a baby can never be left until later. His needs take priority and somebody has to take immediate responsibility for meeting them. Time that was previously spent on other things must now be given to the baby.

Ideally, these lifestyle changes are shared equally within a partnership, but in practice women very often end up taking on the main burden. Depending on individual expectations, this can lead to deep resentment within a relationship, causing a couple to move apart following the birth of their baby.

Increasing conflict

Research in America has shown that 1 in every 2 marriages goes into decline after the birth of the first child. All of the couples in the study, no matter how well-adjusted, experienced on average a 20 percent increase in conflict within their marriage during the first year of parenthood. Although conflict can sometimes be healthy, it is often not what new parents expect. To reduce the stress placed on a partnership, it is vital that each partner has at least some idea of what to expect and is able to compromise. Having a baby means rearranging your life.

Lone parenting

Being a single parent, you won't have the luxury of a partner to share the day-to-day care of your baby or the joys of watching him develop. Without a good support network, it can be physically and emotionally exhausting, but the knowledge that you've done it alone can also be hugely rewarding for you and beneficial to your baby.

Single parent by choice?

If you've chosen to be a single mother, you may be more prepared emotionally, practically and financially for looking after a young baby and look forward to the prospect. If you've split with your partner during the pregnancy or soon after the birth, you may have more difficulties. Coping with the emotional problems of separating from someone while looking after a young baby is bound to have an impact on your ability to cope. In this situation, it's more important for you to ask for and accept help.

Lone parenting can be positive

Being a single parent is by no means all doom and gloom. You and your baby can benefit in many ways from the special relationship you'll form.

● Single parents tend to develop a much closer bond with their babies; they do not have to share their love between a partner and a child.

● Extended family – grandparents, aunts and uncles – often get more involved when there's only one parent. The baby can greatly benefit from this network of support and love.

● Looking after a baby alone is a great achievement. You'll strengthen as a person as you watch your baby develop.

● If you're single because your relationship has broken down, you have made the right decision; it's better for the baby to live with one fairly contented person than two people who are at war.

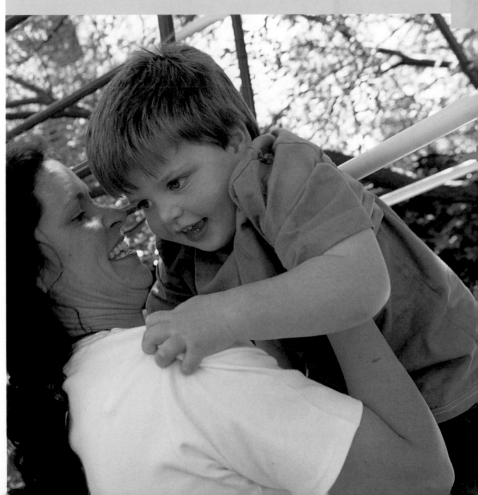

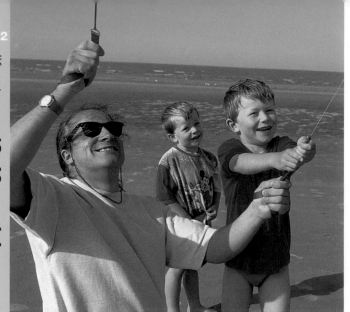

18-40 partnership problems

At some stage in every relationship, difficulties arise. In some cases couples live happily ever after, but many don't. Some problems can be overcome, but for others separation is the only answer.

Effects of divorce on your children

Research suggests that children are better off with two unhappy parents than with divorced parents. But the research gives no indication of the different divorce situations, which are critical in determining the effect on the child. An amicable divorce may be barely damaging and its effect entirely different from that of a bitter, acrimonious divorce. The main reason for this is that in an acrimonious situation, each parent usually does his or her best to turn the children against the other parent. This has a very negative and damaging effect on children, and should be avoided at all costs. Remember that a child has the right, indeed the need, to love and respect both parents, even though they're living apart. No child can split themselves in two.

Explaining to your children

A young child is like a sponge that soaks up emotional signals, whether or not they are directed at her. If you are happy, the chances are your child will be happy; if you are sad, she will be sad. Although it is always worth making an effort "for the sake of the children", don't fall into the trap of thinking they won't know what is going on. They usually sense when something is wrong, whether or not you have a smile on your face.

Because of this it's always best to explain, at least partially, what is going on. If you don't, children will invent their own explanations, mistakenly blaming themselves for problems in the family. This is because children under 5 only conceive the world in relation to themselves. If you don't give a plausible explanation of why you and your partner are arguing or splitting up, they may come up with explanations that are inconceivable to an adult, but make perfect sense to a child, such as: "Daddy has left because I don't clean my room properly", or "Mummy is upset because I wet the bed".

Feelings of guilt are severely damaging, especially for a child already struggling to come to terms with the emotional turmoil and insecurity that marital break-ups can trigger. Doubt is one of the worst fears in a child's mind, so never leave your child in any doubt that you love her and that you will look after her.

Access

Whatever your feelings are about your partner, it's best for your child if you're easy-going about access.

● Don't be stingy and don't be confrontational – it causes your child such anguish. Hand her over somewhere civilized like one of your homes, not somewhere like a park or shopping centre, or your child will feel like a commodity.

● Plan well ahead, don't break promises at the last minute, and if your partner is late, be breezy about it, otherwise your child will worry about both of you. Don't make it an opportunity to denigrate her other parent; be offhand, and keep your child calm: "Shall we have a game of snap till he gets here?"or "Oh, I expect the traffic's bad".

● If your partner is consistently late or unreasonable, arrange a separate meeting to discuss this, out of earshot of your child. The only time to consider preventing your ex-partner having any access to your child is if you think she's at risk of being kidnapped or otherwise harmed. In such cases seek professional advice.

Separation and divorce

More and more couples are experiencing problems with their relationship. This doesn't necessarily reflect a lowering of moral values; it is more an indication of the complexities and pressures of modern life. Support systems are weaker and expectations higher.

Statistics show that today 2 in 3 divorces are initiated by women, many of whom feel they are asked to do too much without adequate support from their partners. The average marriage lasts eight years – a depressing fact of life for growing numbers of children brought up without two parents.

Periods of change

The problem for nearly all couples is that in the long term people change. Although this can be difficult, it can also be invigorating and constructive. If you learn to develop together, you will prevent boredom building up in your relationship.

At the end of periods of change, which are often fraught with emotional insecurity, you will either grow together or grow apart. Whatever happens, it is vital that your children always feel secure of their future. For young children, change within a family unit (or fear of that change) is very damaging. Children do not have the defence mechanisms to protect themselves from the severe emotional insecurity that a break-up can cause.

Domestic violence

Many women live with a partner who resorts to physical violence when he can't win an argument. He uses threats to control her freedom of speech and movement, and invades her privacy by spying and snooping. To the outside world he appears to be the ideal husband but behind closed doors it's a very different story. As the latest report shows, such attacks happen every six seconds in the UK.

Making the break

Starting a new life alone is undeniably difficult. In ridding yourself of one set of problems, you'll inevitably find yourself with others you may not have expected. But you'll be in control of your own future and you may find that this more than compensates for the hardships you'll encounter. It may help to strengthen your resolve if you visualize the rest of your life as carrying on the same as it has been over recent years, then comparing this with how content you could be if left to your own devices.

There are no easy steps to changing one's life and little can be done to prevent the showdown you fear with your violent partner. The obstacles you have overcome to achieve your independence are very similar to obstacles an addict has to overcome. It's a matter of mustering the willpower and determination and once your mind is set, the rest will be surprisingly easy.

Your children

If you're a battered mother your first concern has to be the emotional well-being of your children, and how well they cope depends to a large extent on how you behave.

Brought up in a violent home, children rapidly come to think of masculine behaviour as violent and women always appear weak and powerless. In a violent home, children desperately need a parent who's strong enough to carry on, even when she's at her most vulnerable – a parent who still has the emotional capacity to love. Most women are strong and brave enough to do that, though they don't always see themselves that way at first.

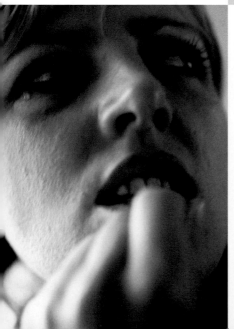

Getting out of a violent relationship

● Acknowledge that it's happening to you and stop playing down the abuse you're experiencing. It's not unusual for some women to minimize or justify what's happening to them.
● Recognize that you're not to blame. No one deserves to be assaulted, humiliated or abused, least of all by their partner in a supposedly caring relationship. Women often blame themselves because they have consistently been told it is their fault. Prolonged exposure to violence may convince you that you deserve to be hurt. But there is no justification for violence, ever.
● Begin seeking the help and support that's available. This step includes gaining emotional support and practical help. You can even start by talking to a friend you trust or calling an organization such as the Women's Aid National Helpline or your local Women's Aid refuge.
● You may want to think about moving somewhere safe, away from your abuser, or taking legal action that will protect you and stop the violence against you.

18-40 mental fitness

Many of us spend a great deal of time, energy and even money trying to do something about our physical fitness. Unfortunately, the same does not always apply to mental fitness, although it is just as important.

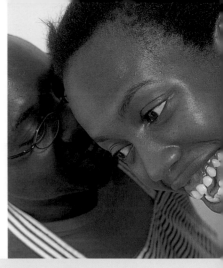

Women and mental fitness

For women especially, mental fitness should be as important, if not more important, than physical fitness. Why? Because there is no doubt that women, regardless of marital status, suffer from more mental illness than men: they outnumber men at psychiatric clinics, and they are more likely to have mental treatment in hospital. Women take more drugs that affect mental activity than men do and are more often diagnosed by doctors as suffering from mental health problems.

The reason for these phenomena is twofold. First, our physical condition makes us more vulnerable. Women are prone to psychological disturbances relating to hormonal

behaviour, not only monthly, but especially after pregnancy and childbirth, and we live longer to experience mourning, loneliness and the depression of old age. Second, the status of women has meant that we haven't always been given sufficient freedom of choice in our lifestyles, which leads to frustration. No matter what lifestyle we choose, there are conflicts that can breed unhappiness such as balancing a family and a career – even marriage itself may be an ongoing mental trauma for us, much more than for men.

This remarkable bombardment of mental trauma means that we must strive to maintain a basic state of

mental health – so that we can take knocks and not go under; so that we can rise to emergencies and cope well with them; so that we are resilient enough to survive long-term, stressful situations, so that we can deal with the possible loss of those closest to us.

Maintaining psychological equilibrium, however, requires a different sort of self-knowledge from physical fitness. It also requires supreme realism. It is essential that we realize our difficulties are not unique. We all go through periods of stress and, no matter how unpleasant, most of us survive. Adversity is normal, indeed it is a condition of living, and we must not over-react to it or feel that we've messed up our lives irretrievably and are failures because we're experiencing it.

When things go wrong, it is natural to think that we are to blame. **But we should bear in mind that difficulties in our environment, over which we have no control, might be a major factor.** Things such as overcrowding and violence in society are factors we can do little about. Poverty is a particularly powerful exacerbating factor and, as with physical illness, mental illness is much more common among poorer people.

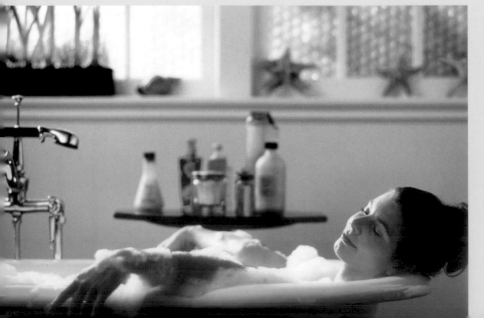

Ways of coping

It is important that we achieve a certain measure of emotional growth. Coming to terms with the way we feel about things, being able to work with our own emotions, as well as other people's, in a non-destructive but helpful, even affectionate, frame of mind is a goal we should all try to achieve. Accepting ourselves for what we are and permitting ourselves a proper measure of self-esteem means that we can take responsibility for our own actions and seek and accept forgiveness from others, when

necessary, without damage to our self-image. This process of independence is a long one and may even continue through life but is necessary to seek out the goodness within ourselves.

Another effort to make is not to set our standards too high; it's not necessary and it can be a great strain. It is acceptable for anyone to give way now and then, to have a good cry, to pour out troubles to a friend, or to rant and rave and let off steam. Better that than burning out your fuse wire and becoming ill.

But it is possible to prepare for catastrophes and the answer lies in yourself – you have to have the desire to cope and survive a bad patch. If you practise on manageable "disasters", you'll find the major ones cause you much less stress, bearing in mind that once your mental fitness is jeopardized it will take time to come back to normal. There are, however, two ways in which you can control your body and mind immediately: relax and breathe calmly and slowly (see p.292 for relaxation techniques).

Combating stress

Dissociate

This means putting your worries out of your head. Try to ignore your problem for as long as possible. The longer you keep it at bay and remain calm, the more time there is for the body's fight and flight reaction to lessen, thereby reducing stress and anxiety.

Have fun

Enjoy yourself; go out for dinner with a friend, or simply take the afternoon off to go shopping, or snatch a weekend away in the country. While you are having fun, and even after it, notice how most problems diminish in size.

Physical activity

Work off stress through any kind of exercise that you enjoy and are physically able to do. Physical activity of almost any kind counteracts the effects of stress and nearly always leaves you feeling more relaxed and rational about your problem.

Get another opinion

Most problems which to us seem so overwhelming and individual are not uncommon. Getting advice from someone with experience in the situation, with no personal connection, can help to throw new light on the problem. A problem shared is a problem halved. Groups such

as Weight Watchers, Alcoholics Anonymous and the Samaritans are specially set up to deal with particular stressful situations.

Look at the way you manage your time

Stress is often caused by mismanagement of time such as getting behind in our work or jobs at home. Assign priorities to tasks and do the important ones first. Look at the way you spend your time. For a few days write down all your activities, the relevance they have to sorting out your problem and the result they achieved. At the end of this period it's astonishing to see how your time was spent – how much of it was wasted and how much of it was put to useful purpose.

Scale down your expectations

Recognize your own limitations and take on only what you can accomplish in the time you've allowed yourself. Realize that it isn't possible for you totally to control the world around you. Setting up and meeting realistic goals can lessen stress, while failing to live up to your expectations can bring it about.

Withdraw

A more radical alternative is to cut yourself off from the situation that is causing your

stress. Withdrawal, however, may involve substantial effort. If, for instance, you find you cannot get on with your boss, you may have to change your job. If you hate the house you live in, you may have to consider moving to a new one, possibly in another area.

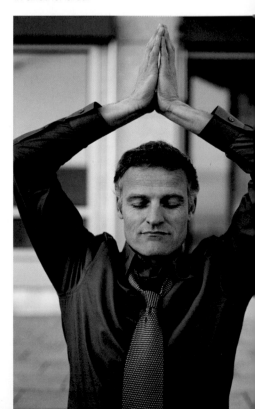

FOCUS *on* cosmetic surgery

Few people regret having cosmetic surgery, though many regret not doing so. If you want, a good surgeon can change your appearance. But beware. Such an operation requires that you be well motivated or you could be unhappy with the result.

You'll have to bear quite a lot of discomfort and may be somewhat depressed until the effects become apparent. It's important that you have the operation for the right reasons and not because a critical partner pressures you into having surgery.

If you have serious psychological problems, cosmetic surgery isn't going to put them right. If a relationship is disintegrating or a marriage falling apart, plastic surgery isn't going to remedy the situation. On the other hand, if you've suffered severe psychological stress because of your appearance, cosmetic surgery can have long-term benefits that will affect all aspects of your life. Nowadays, a good reason for having surgery may simply be that your body looks older than you feel. You need seek no further justification.

After cosmetic surgery, people are often more at ease with themselves and feel more self-assured. That alone makes you look better.

CHOOSING A SURGEON

First step is to find a good cosmetic surgeon with whom you get on well. Don't be afraid to shop around. Here are some tips to help you find one:
● Get a sound recommendation from a doctor or a good friend.
● As a rule, don't follow up an advertisement in a newspaper or magazine. Advertising is against the ethical code of doctors in the UK.
● A surgeon who is trustworthy will advise you on which operation will give you the best results. Be suspicious of a surgeon who agrees to perform exactly the operation you request without giving you a professional opinion as to what you actually need.
● No good surgeon will give you a 100 percent guarantee of success. He should take time to explain in detail exactly what the operation involves and what can be achieved, and give a realistic estimate of the chances of success. Be sceptical about a surgeon who's not realistic.

● Only entrust yourself to a surgeon if you get on with him or her from the beginning. If you don't like the surgeon at your first visit, you're unlikely to later.

REMOVING THE SIGNS OF AGE

Cosmetic surgeons say that typical face-lift patients are not vain, rich women with nothing better to do with their money, but energetic, active people who are less interested in hiding their age than in looking as youthful as they feel. These patients think that an obviously ageing face erodes self-confidence and may even cause panic. A typical question such a patient should ask herself is "Why should I go on looking like this when every other part of me feels young?"

Many women in their 40s and 50s are not ready to resign themselves to being thought of as ageing. They feel that growing older would be easier to bear if they could avoid looking old in the process. Furthermore, they often feel it is unjust that they should start to show signs of deterioration when they are just beginning to reach intellectual and emotional maturity. Consequently, when fine lines, wrinkles and sags appear on their faces, they decide to fight back.

A woman having a face-lift does not want friends and relatives to gasp with surprise at their first sight of her afterwards. She would prefer a natural look, an almost indefinable improvement in her appearance. For this reason, a totally smooth skin is not the desired outcome. If the skin is overstretched, a false oriental look around the eyes may rob the face of much of its expressive quality. The best advertisement for a good cosmetic surgeon is a patient who looks naturally young for her age, not one whose smooth skin seems artificial.

IMPROVING THE FEATURES

In some instances, the decision to have cosmetic surgery has nothing to do with ageing. Sometimes an obvious facial peculiarity, such as a long or bulbous nose, can have profound psychological effects that begin as early as adolescence. A teenager may find that no matter how she arranges her hair or puts on make-up, the flaw is still apparent. This situation may make a good student feel inadequate and too restless to continue education, or lead the school-leaver to a succession of jobs.

Facial operations

Face-lift – removes major wrinkles and lifts sagging skin.

Blepharoplasty – removes sagging skin that makes the eyes look puffy, raises drooping eyelids or reshapes eyebrows.

Cheek or chin augmentation – inserts moulded implants to reshape chin or cheekbones.

Otoplasty – takes back protruding ears.

Double chin reduction – removes the sag of fat and loose skin under the chin.

Chin reduction – removes bone and cartilage to reshape the chin.

Lip augmentation – reshapes the lips, using fat cells to make them fuller.

Rhinoplasty – reshapes, smoothes out or straightens the nose.

Before a face-lift

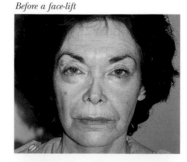

After a face-lift

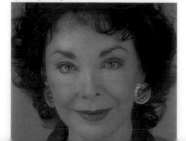

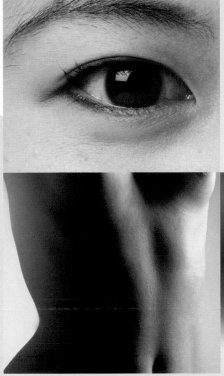
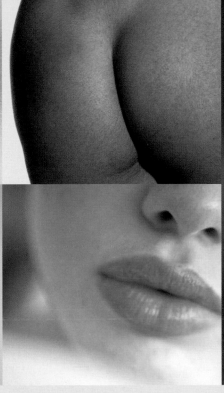
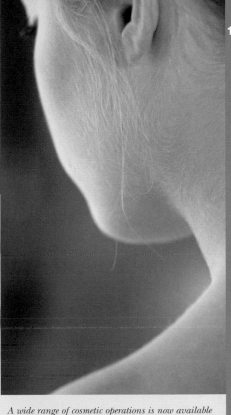

At some point, matters reach a crisis: the patient may resort to psychotherapy, for example, because of her problems with self-confidence, indecisiveness and inability to enjoy sex. She may find it impossible to relax with people because of her consciousness that she is not looking attractive. Very often there is not so much an intense desire to have the offending feature improved as a continual feeling of depression caused by the knowledge that she is not looking good. It is not unreasonable to expect many of these feelings to diminish sharply, if not to disappear, once the deformity has been corrected by cosmetic surgery.

The same feelings, of course, may arise from a flaw so trivial that scarcely anyone else is aware of it. Even in these cases, cosmetic surgery can bring about a dramatic psychological improvement – although it is always possible that the patient's own feeling that her appearance has been altered for the better may vanish when no change in other people's reactions to her is apparent. The inner quality that makes some people attractive is something no surgeon can give, and it is not necessarily linked with having beautiful features.

LIPOSUCTION

Liposuction is one of the three most popular cosmetic surgery procedures, along with breast enlargement and removal of bags under the eyes. But liposuction is not to be taken lightly. You should investigate the implications before going ahead.

The number of obese people in the UK increases all the time, and with magazines full of tall, thin models many women are tempted to strive for that kind of slender perfection. Not satisfied with dieting, you may be tempted to turn to a surgeon to give you a flat stomach and slim thighs. Liposuction may sound like a minor procedure but there are risks involved.

What is liposuction?

Liposuction is a way of removing fat from areas of the body such as hips, thighs, buttocks, chin and male breasts. It was designed, not as a cure for obesity, but to remove pads of fat that don't respond to diet and exercise.

How liposuction is performed

● Liposuction is not a gentle procedure. Initially, a cold salt solution, which also contains adrenaline, a local anaesthetic and a chemical to break down fat cells, is injected into the fatty area of your body.
● Next, a large, hollow needle, usually about 3mm in diameter, attached to a powerful suction machine, is inserted through several small cuts in the skin. It is passed into pockets of fat, where it is moved around with considerable force. Fat is quite solid, and it needs some liquidizing to be sucked into the draining tube. The saline solution helps to loosen and liquidize the fat.
● It's dangerous to remove too much fat. All body fluids are in equilibrium and the body responds to loss of fat as it does to loss of

A wide range of cosmetic operations is now available to improve features such as brows, eyelids, chin and lips, and to reduce fat on buttocks and stomach.

blood; if too much fat is removed, you'll go into surgical shock with very low blood pressure.

Recovery

There can be considerable discomfort and stiffness after the operation and the wider the needle used, the worse the pain and the longer it lasts. You can expect to resume normal activities within two to three days for minor liposuction, but it may take up to two or three weeks after major fat removal.

The operation can cause severe bruising so, to minimize this, special elasticated garments that compress the skin must be worn for two to three weeks after the operation to help skin contraction and support the operation site to prevent fluid collecting.

Side effects

Liposuction results do vary. The procedure works best on women under 40, whose skin is elastic and springs back into shape relatively easily. Older women can be left with unsightly sags and folds. If too much fat is removed from one place, or if it's removed unevenly, ridges and dimples are the result. Common complaints are stretched skin not shrinking back to its former size, numbness in muscles surrounding the area operated on and uneven fat removal, leaving lumps.

▶

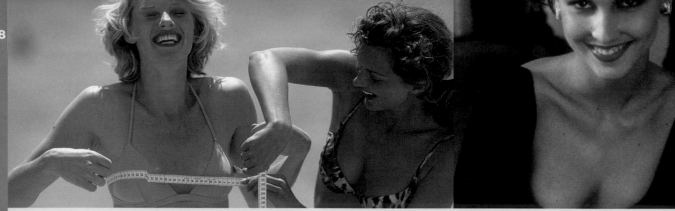

Breast surgery

There are several different ways in which cosmetic surgery can change the size, shape and uplift of your breasts. These include breast lift (mastopexy), breast enlargement and breast reduction. Do make sure you understand exactly what your operation involves before you take the plunge.

MASTOPEXY

A breast-lift operation is usually for sagging breasts – it removes excess skin and raises the nipple. The smaller the breast the better the result. It can be combined with augmentation if your breasts are small, or reduction if your breasts are very large. Without reduction, mastopexy is not very effective on large breasts because gravity will pull them down again.

Be realistic. Mastopexy can't give you the pert breasts of a teenager, and it will leave scars. Discuss the operation with your surgeon in some detail before proceeding.

As with all breast operations, make sure you see before and after photographs so that you can check good, moderate and poor results. Ask for a description of the kind of cuts that will be made, and even get the surgeon to draw on your breasts where the scars will be.

You should bear in mind that your breast-lift, just like a face-lift, is by no means permanent. Your breasts will continue to age and eventually sag all over again.

Ask your surgeon if the technique to be used gives you the option of breast-feeding if it's important to you. It's advisable to have a mammogram before you go ahead with any type of breast surgery.

The operation

A general anaesthetic is usual. Your surgeon will remove excess skin and fat from under the breasts and move the nipple upwards by pushing it through a hole in the skin higher up your chest.

After effects and follow-up

Mastopexy is usually very successful and there are few side effects, although you may notice loss of sensation in your nipple and areola. There's a 50–50 chance you'll be able to breast-feed after the operation, as long as the milk ducts aren't cut. You can expect to have all the stitches removed after two weeks and, if you're an active person, you'll have full movement of your arms and shoulders and be able to take up sports after about three weeks.

Although it may be slightly uncomfortable, it's advisable to wear a good supporting bra after the operation to support the inflamed breast and skin and help healing. You should be prepared to wear your bra day and night for at least three months after surgery.

BREAST REDUCTION

There are two groups of women who look for breast reduction. The first group dislike their large breasts because of the inconvenience and social embarrassment. The second group want cosmetic breast reduction to achieve firm, well-positioned breasts, and are happy with C or D cup as long as the breasts look good.

The operation

While different surgeons have slightly different techniques for reducing the size of breasts, the basic operation is very much the same no matter who does it. It requires a general anaesthetic and it'll probably take as long as four hours. The nipples are important. Ask whether your surgeon's going to simply move your nipples up, or remove them and then graft them back in a different position.

You can request that your nipple is preserved on a stalk of tissue – called a pedicle – so the tissue is taken from the sides and the underside of this stalk. This is essential if you want to breast-feed in the future.

If you wish to know exactly what's going to be removed, ask your surgeon to draw the shape on your breast with a pen. The nipple can be lifted up and stitched into the breast at a higher level. The flaps of skin underneath are stitched together, resulting in reduction and some uplift.

You'll be left with scars around the areola, in a line from the nipple to the underside of the breast and in the skin fold where the breast joins the skin of the chest.

After effects and follow-up

The results of the operation are usually extremely good, but this is major surgery, so you can expect to have some discomfort for several weeks after. By the time you go home two or three days later, however, the pain should have subsided. Wear a bra day and night for support and to aid healing. The stitches should be removed within about two weeks, after which you could restart work. After a month you'll virtually be back to normal.

BREAST ENLARGEMENT

Breast enlargement can only be accomplished with the aid of implants, which are inserted in front of or behind the muscles of the chest wall – the pecs – underneath the actual breast. Implants have received a lot of medical attention in recent years and their safety has been questioned. If you're considering breast augmentation, you owe it to yourself to become informed about these issues.

● Breast augmentation can have complications, so read as much as you can about it. Ask your surgeon if he can put you in touch with someone who's had the operation so that you can go into it with your eyes open.

● Have a detailed discussion about the size you'd like your breasts to be. Be realistic. If your frame is small and you already have tiny breasts, think twice before going for a D cup. Your surgeon will probably advise against it anyway. The best prostheses now are shaped and are of standard width. You will be measured for the appropriate size and shape of these biodimensional prostheses.

● Make sure that your doctor checks for cysts in the breast that might require treatment in future. It's difficult for a surgeon to interfere

with the breast once an implant is in place.
- Ask about the possibility of contracture (see below) and ask where the scars will be.
- Ask whether the incisions will interfere with breast-feeding or sensation in the nipple.
- Make sure that your surgeon tells you the size and the manufacturer of your implant in case it needs replacing at a future date.

The operation
The length of the operation is largely determined by where the implant is placed. If it goes underneath the muscles of the chest wall, the operation will take less time than if it is placed underneath the breast tissue but on top of the muscle layer, because there's less bleeding in the former operation. You might want to stay in hospital for 24 hours to recover from the anaesthetic, but then you can go home. You'll be asked to return to hospital in about 10 days to have any stitches removed.

The incision for an augmentation operation may be made in the armpit, around or across the areola, or under the breast. Scarring may occur in any of these areas depending on which incision your surgeon uses.

After effects and follow-up
Make arrangements to be off work for at least 10 days to a fortnight. Don't attempt to drive a car for a full two weeks and avoid overhead lifting for about four weeks. You should be back to normal in about three weeks, but it's best to avoid sports for about six weeks.

POTENTIAL WORRIES
Breast cancer
There's no proof of a link between silicone implants and cancer. The Food and Drug Administration (FDA) in the US concluded in 1989 that a carcinogenic effect in humans could not be completely ruled out, but if such an effect did exist, the risk would be very low. Breast surgeons around the world have found this statement reassuring enough to continue using silicone implants.

Mammography
Implants can make it difficult to read mammograms precisely. This means that women who have a strong family history of

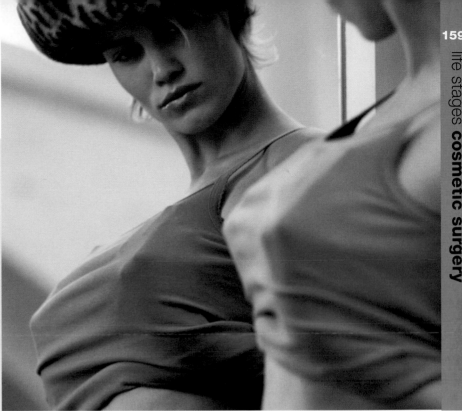

Types of implants

Silicone gel implants feel more natural than saline-filled ones and they're still the first choice of most surgeons in the UK. The likelihood of contracture is about the same with both types, but obviously there's no risk of silicone leakage with saline-filled ones. If silicone implants leak, they'll deflate and will need to be replaced. All implants used to be smooth, but nowadays a textured surface is preferred as this seems to reduce the frequency of contracture. Alternative implant-fill materials are being researched. It's hoped that these new materials will be absorbed by the body if leakage occurs, won't react with breast tissue and won't obscure mammography X-rays. One new implant available in the UK contains triglyceride, which is similar to body fat, and has a built-in electronic chip with a unique code to identify it.

breast cancer should probably not use silicone implants. It's a good idea for all women to have a mammogram performed before any breast surgery. It's possible to get a good mammogram of a breast with implants, but more than one view will be needed.

Contracture
The capsule of scar tissue that forms naturally around any implant can be quite thin and pliable but it may contract and become as hard as wood. One research study puts the possibility of contracture as high as 7 out of 10 at two to four years after surgery. Massaging the breasts may reduce hardness, but if they're very hard, treatment can be quite complicated.

Your surgeon can ease the tension by cutting a wider space around the implant. Or, if the implant lies above the chest wall muscles, it can be removed and a new one inserted below the muscle, where contracture is less likely.

Other complications
Breast pain, loss of sensation in the breast, difficulty with breast-feeding, infection and movement and leakage of an implant are all well-known complications. A more uncommon one is rupture of the implant, which can occur spontaneously or through physical force such as a blow. You'll need immediate surgery if this happens to remove all traces of silicone from the breast.

Some authorities say half of all breast augmentation patients will have some side effects by 10 years after the operation; others estimate a one-in-three chance. So it's not plain sailing, though none of the above side effects is life-threatening.

"life becomes fulfilling, satisfying and, perhaps for the first time, contented"

life stages: 40 to 60 years

Adults have a series of milestones in their lives just like children. But whereas in your younger days you may have rushed past the markers with your eye constantly on the lookout for the next, as you grow older, you tend to look back, reflect on what you have done, and you may find that it is time to choose a new lifestyle.

The saying goes "life begins at 40" and so it does for some. However, many of us reach a crossroads around 35 when we take stock, and it may take two or three years before life restabilizes. The mid- and late 40s, therefore, can be looked forward to as a period of equilibrium. The major problems of life and your place in it, and the adjustments you have to make to feel at one with yourself, have been largely sorted out and life becomes fulfilling, satisfying and, perhaps for the first time, contented.

Whether you feel renewed or resigned will depend on the choices you made at your crossroads. If you refused to make any changes, then a sense of staleness may progress into resignation and a feeling of discontent. You will not be growing and you will be aware that you're standing still. What happens is that things in your life that have made you feel safe, and that have supported you, will be gradually withdrawn. Your children will grow up and leave you, your partner could develop faster than you and grow away from you, your career may seem less satisfying and merely become a job that has to be done.

What is more, each of these events will gradually become less and less tolerable and a crossroads will probably emerge again around the age of 50, and, be assured, it will hit you much harder than it did at 40.

A renewed sense of purpose

If, on the other hand, you faced up to your 35-year-old crossroads and made the necessary adjustments, you will find a renewed sense of purpose, and from within yourself a drive and energy to build a good lifestyle, and the knowledge that you are looking forward to the best years of your life. For most people who are prepared to take on this difficult passage, personal happiness soars. A self-confidence that you never suspected emerges, and you can take on problems and difficulties calmly and rationally. You become less possessive about your children, you become less possessive about your partner, you find yourself warming and mellowing towards life and other people. Priorities suddenly become clear and decisions easier to take.

Facing the 50s

The 50s are a time when, once again, people take stock of their lives. We may feel increasingly aware of the importance of remaining as physically and mentally fit as possible. For women, the menopause is undoubtedly the period's most significant biological and physiological event, but there is no reason why we shouldn't feel as healthy, if not even healthier, as ever. Our increased physical awareness can lead to increased emotional awareness and we become more reflective. We become more tolerant of our own abilities and those of others; our outlook becomes increasingly philosophical and by the end of our 50s, if we've managed to remain married, we're often closer to our partner than at any other time in our life.

Planning for the future

Making plans for the years ahead is like planning a trip. Remember your last big holiday. Half the fun was thinking about it a long way in advance. The further ahead you made your plans, the more you looked forward to going and the more you enjoyed the trip. There may have been some unexpected adventures along the way, but because you had prepared yourself thoroughly you were able to cope with any eventuality.

Life can be much the same. In the pages that follow I offer guidelines where appropriate, advice where I feel there may be a need and strategies for dealing with potentially difficult situations.

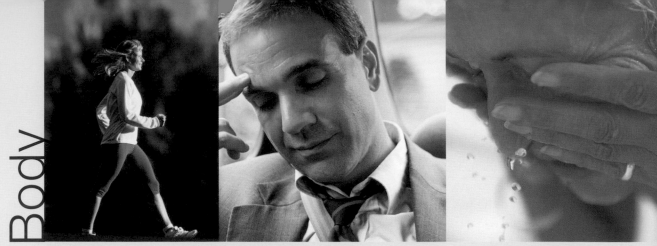

Body

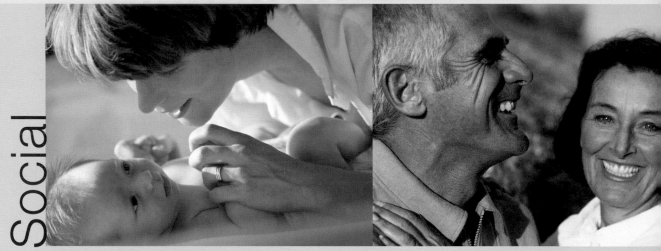

Social

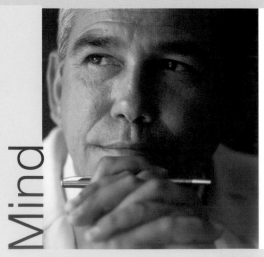

> "as we grow older we should be prepared to change our attitudes"

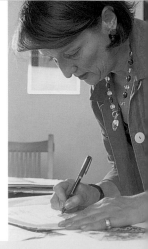

Mind

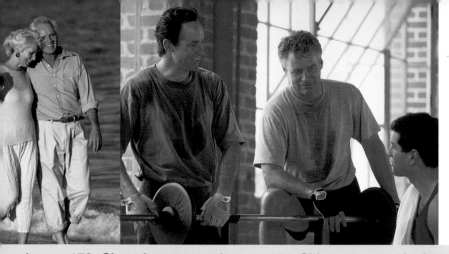

"exercise is particularly valuable as you get older"

"balancing work and family is a major issue for many people"

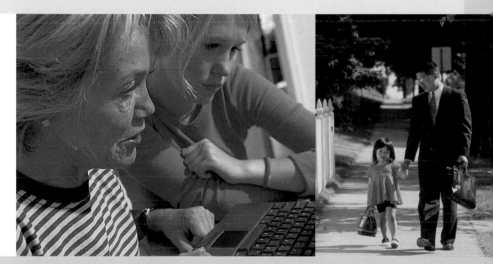

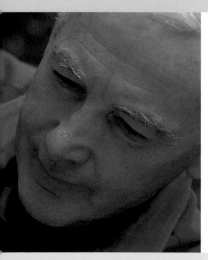

"if you don't think, your brain will slow and become feeble"

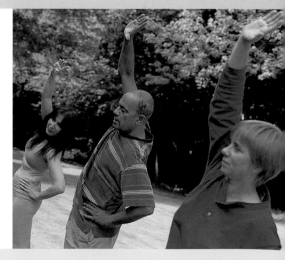

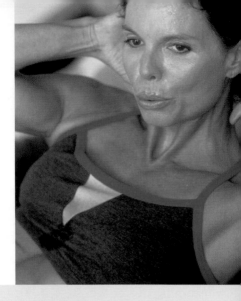

40-60
your changing body

Telltale signs such as wrinkling and changes in body shape may start to appear. But take good care of yourself and you can be as healthy as ever.

Increase in weight

Being very thin at any time of life means that a woman is unhealthy. Some fat is essential for true health and this is never more true than at the time of the menopause. Being too thin can increase your risk of osteoporosis and gives you no "reserves" in case you fall ill.

Slowing metabolic rate

Weight increase is gradual in both men and women as they age, but for women it may become especially noticeable during the menopausal and postmenopausal years. There are at least two factors involved here. First, lack of oestrogen leads to a change in body shape and fat distribution, so that the waist thickens and fat is deposited on the front of the abdomen (fat cells all over the body also increase in size). Second, the metabolic rate gradually slows down as we mature (by about 5 percent or 100 calories a day per decade) and, by the age of about 55, we need fewer calories.

Regular exercise

The main reason our metabolism declines with age is because we lose muscle strength through being less active. Unless we have a regular and frequent exercise regime incorporated into our lives, continuing to eat at our usual rate will lead to weight gain. To combat this we need to eat sensibly and take regular exercise.

Although we need fewer calories, our body's nutritional needs remain the same. Calorie counting may be too time-consuming for anyone to maintain in the long term, so it's much better to eat a diet that is well balanced and contains few "empty" high-calorie foods, such as sugar and fat.

Changing your eating patterns

It's within your power to change not only what you eat, but how you eat. As we get older, many of us find we can't manage three main meals a day. Try eating five or even six small meals at regular intervals so that the nutritional load is spread. This eating habit is very effective in terms of weight control because small frequent meals prevent troughs of low blood sugar, which are accompanied by cravings for food. By eating little and often you will gain confidence in your ability to control your appetite.

Many studies have been carried out to show the differences between people who eat small, frequent meals and those who eat fewer and larger meals. The latter invariably have more body fat than the former. Some slimmers find that a diet designed on a nibbling pattern helps to prevent hunger pangs, and there is evidence that this may speed up weight loss. Your digestive system will prefer a nibbling pattern, particularly if you suffer from indigestion or peptic ulcers.

Reducing the saturated fat content in your diet will also greatly help you to maintain your weight, and it will protect you from a range of diseases.

Avoid crash diets

Try not to attempt crash diets or long-term diets that are little more than starvation. The initial weight loss may be impressive – as high as 3–5kg (6–11lb) in the first week – but less than half of this will be fat; most of it will be water, and it could even include some of your precious body protein. A diet that restricts total calorie intake to below a thousand calories is only just adequate. Very strict diets, those around 500 calories, cannot provide all the required nutrients for an adult. You will even struggle with 1000 calories. There is much research to show that towards the end of a long period of this kind of dieting, the rate of weight loss not only decelerates, but the weight starts to go back on.

Eating binges

The fewer and fewer calories we give the body, the harder it is to maintain the diet. A return to a normal eating pattern will cause an inevitable increase in weight as body stores of glycogen are replaced. This is extremely depressing if you have made a great effort to shed excess weight. It is common for a person coming off a starvation diet to go on eating binges and find themselves on a treadmill of intermittent starving and bingeing that is extremely damaging to their health and self-image.

Changing body shape

One of the first changes in girls approaching adolescence is the appearance of fat on the hips, breasts, upper arms, and upper thighs. **Throughout fertile life, oestrogen and progesterone are responsible for maintaining the female shape, with its narrow waist and rounded hips.** We now know that these proportions are more than simply an expression of the female gender. They have a much greater significance for both health and longevity.

The narrow waist and rounded hips pattern of fat distribution is closely and unequivocally related to coronary health. The usual ratio of the waist to hip measurement is less than one and this is associated with a low risk of a heart attack. If your waist to hip ratio creeps above 0.8, you are much more at risk.

After the menopause, when levels of oestrogen and progesterone are low or absent, one of the first things that a woman may notice is a thickening of the waist and the appearance of "middle-age spread". She may also notice abdominal swelling because of increased fat on the front of her abdomen. Her shape comes to resemble a more masculine outline, **and her risk of having a heart attack increases in relation to this increased fat distribution.**

The first place a man puts on weight is the abdomen, with an accompanying increase in girth. A similar rule about the ratio of waist to hips applies to women. If it goes up, then the risk of a heart attack goes up too.

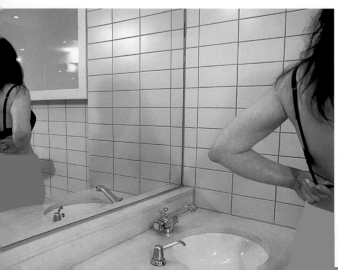

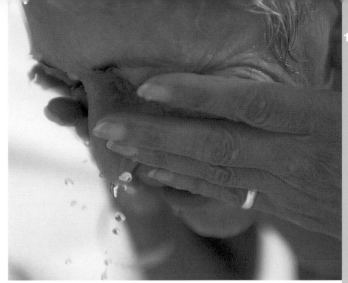

Wrinkling

Wrinkling is traditionally thought to be the most obvious sign of ageing skin. But wrinkling actually begins as early as our 20s and continues at a fairly steady pace for the rest of our lives. We use our facial expressions as a way of communicating with others and recording anger, rage, disappointment, happiness, surprise, consternation and so on. These expressions are captured on our faces by lines which begin to form in the places that move most. Very few of us get to our 40s without any of these telltale signs.

Lessening the effect of wrinkling – both sexes

● Splash water on your face and keep it there with a moisturizer to prevent your skin dehydrating.
● Never go out in the sun without wearing a sunscreen – the higher the number, the greater the protection. Remember, a day on the ski slopes can do as much damage as a day on the beach.
● If you have tiny surface veins on your face, avoid eating hot, spicy food and drinking alcohol; these will aggravate face flushing.
● Stop smoking. Cigarette smoking may hasten crow's feet and causes deep lines. The skin is 10 years older in a smoker than a non-smoker.
● Keep your body well rested by adequate sleep to improve your complexion.
● Facial exercises help to relax the facial muscles, which cause "tension" wrinkles and lines. They can also help keep facial and neck muscles mobile and relieve tension headaches. They cannot, however, stop wrinkles forming. Try a smile all the time instead of a frown as it exercises more muscles.

For women

● If you don't wear make-up, be sure to wear a fairly liberal covering of rich moisturizer that prevents water loss.
● If you do put on some make-up, it will help to reduce water loss from the skin. Avoid astringent toners; switch from cleansing soaps to creams.

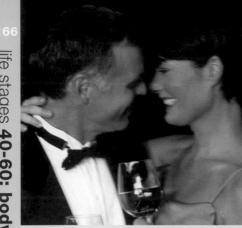

40-60 declining sexuality

High, medium and low sex drives are all normal. All that matters is whether a couple can accommodate each other's needs, however limited or great these may be.

Vaginal dryness

A common myth about the menopause is that it marks the beginning of a woman's sexual decline. Nothing could be further from the truth. **The majority of women can continue to experience sexual pleasure well into old age, indeed as long as their health remains good**. Some women even report that their sexual enjoyment starts to increase after the menopause. This may be due to a higher testosterone to oestrogen ratio than before.

Most menopausal women, however, notice some changes in the way their bodies respond during arousal and sex. This is often due to physical changes in the urogenital tract rather than a decreased psychological desire for sex. Research on sexual pleasure by Alfred Kinsey some decades ago has shown that women who have an enjoyable sex life before the menopause are likely to continue to enjoy sex after it. On the other hand, for women who have not enjoyed sex throughout their lives, the menopause is more likely to be associated with a decrease in all kinds of sexual activity.

One of the most common sexual problems after the menopause is lack of lubrication. In youth, blood flow out of the genitals is slow during

arousal, causing swelling and sensitivity to touch. After the menopause, there is less engorgement of the clitoris, the vagina, and the vulva, leading to subdued arousal.

In a young woman, the vagina expands during sexual arousal to allow easy penetration. After the menopause, the vagina does not expand so much, but it still remains large enough to accommodate an erect penis (as long as you allow time to achieve proper lubrication).

Healthy adrenal glands are also critical to sex drive. Long-term stress, such as bereavement and divorce, can adversely affect glandular activity. Sexual desire can also be diminished by drugs such as tranquillizers and antidepressants. Alcohol, smoking, coffee, overwork, tension and depression have the same effect.

Self-help tips

● Before sex, put some sterile, water-soluble jelly on your vaginal entrance. You may want to put a small amount inside your vagina and on your partner's penis or fingers. Water-based jellies are better than oil-based ones because they are less likely to promote bacterial growth and infections, and they will not cause the rubber of a condom to perish.

● Avoid douches, talcum powder, perfumed toilet papers and any fragranced bath oils and foams, which can irritate the vagina.
● Avoid washing the inside of your labia with soap as it will dry the skin.
● Avoid remedies for genital itchiness containing antihistamine or perfume.
● Spend longer on foreplay to give your body more time to produce its own lubrication. Gentle massage of the breasts, belly, thighs and genitals can help and be extremely erotic.
● Research shows that regular sex or masturbation may help to keep the vagina lubricated. This may be because sexual activity stimulates the adrenal glands that in turn help to keep the vagina lubricated.
● Women who have low histamine levels may find it difficult to reach orgasm, whereas women with high histamine levels achieve orgasm easily. Women who take antihistamines regularly need to be aware of the possibility of decreased sexual desire and delayed orgasm.
● Pelvic floor exercises (see p.169) will make you more aware of your vagina and will increase your sexual enjoyment, as better-toned muscles will enable you to grip your partner's penis more tightly.

Loss of libido

Sex is a highly complex part of our lives and it is influenced by our current moods and emotions outside the bedroom. If we are depressed, tired or ill, we will have little inclination for it. One of the most common and frustrating problems a couple can face is that one partner wants sex much more than the other. It is important to realize that no matter how well matched you are there will be times when your sex drives are out of phase with each other. Like any other appetite, desire for sex waxes and wanes. It is a popular myth that men are always ready and willing for sex, but they are not.

If you find there is a substantial difference in your appetites, you will need to work out some long-term strategy that prevents you feeling continually dissatisfied, rejected and unloved and for your partner not to feel he is continually under pressure to have sex more than he wants.

Remember sex need not involve intercourse. Even if your partner is not aroused himself he can still arouse you using manual or oral stimulation. To awaken desire for sex, the following suggestions may be helpful.

● Make love somewhere other than in bed (on a chair, sofa, etc).
● Take a bath or shower together.
● Create an intimate atmosphere with music and candlelight.
● Give each other a massage with scented body oils.
● Make love at an unusual time.
● Make love in the dark if you usually prefer some light and vice versa.
● Allow enough time for lovemaking. Don't make an issue of masturbation because sometimes a man finds it easier to achieve and sustain an erection this way. It's possible that he's noticed some differences in his performance which are perfectly normal but worrying for him.

Ageing does have an influence on sex. It takes a man longer to become sexually aroused and his erection may not be as strong. He may need much more direct manual or oral stimulation of his penis. His erection will not be quite as hard or its angle as acute as when he was younger. Orgasms themselves may be less intense than before. And because ejaculation generally becomes less powerful with age, semen seeps rather than spurts out.

Many men feel desire should be spontaneous, that they should not need direct stimulation in order to become aroused. This is not the case, even less so as as they grow older. So encourage your partner to let you arouse him.

Viagra

There are many treatments now available for the treatment of waning sexual potency: the best known is Viagra. It was hailed as the answer to a failing man's prayer but it can't be used by everyone to pep up their libido. It has side effects and for it to be effective a man's equipment must be in moderately good working order.

Health requirements

For starters, the blood vessels and nerves in the penis must be intact, otherwise no form of medication could bring about an erection. And the heart and blood pressure must be close to normal. With these provisos, men with the following conditions may experience an improvement in their sexual performance by taking Viagra: diabetes, multiple sclerosis, Parkinson's disease, poliomyelitis, prostate cancer, prostatectomy, radical pelvic surgery, renal failure treated by dialysis or transplant, severe pelvic injury, single gene neurological disease, spinal cord injury and spina bifida.

Does it work?

Viagra isn't a miracle cure. In the original research, almost half of the subjects had better erections than previously, erections sufficient to allow penetrative sex, but not the rigidity of youth. Half did not.

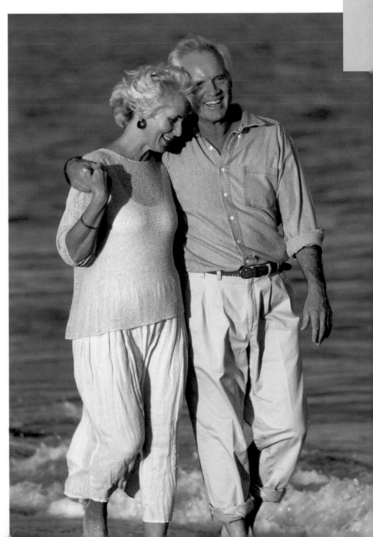

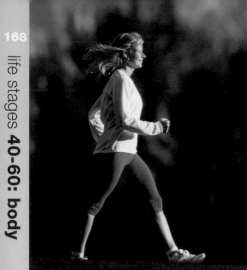

40-60
how to stop your body falling apart

Don't fall into the trap of taking less and less care of yourself, otherwise your muscles will get slacker, and your heart and lungs will be less able to deal with exertion.

Walking

Like other good habits, exercise should be undertaken regularly and be a lifelong habit. Doing a reasonable amount of walking – 20 or 30 minutes or so each day – is a good habit to develop, and you can build this up over a period of months. This kind of routine becomes important after retirement, when most people use up less energy but carry on eating and drinking the same amounts they did before.

Tips for walking

● Do some gentle flexibility exercises before you go out.

● Begin by walking on level ground and progress to hill-walking as you become fitter.

● Walk at a speed that makes you slightly short of breath but don't get too out of breath to talk.

● Never push yourself farther than you feel you can comfortably go.

● Try to increase the distance or the time you spend walking, rather than the speed at which you walk.

● Don't walk into the wind as this requires more effort. If you suffer from heart disease, you should be able to walk quite comfortably in calm weather, but walking into the wind may cause angina pains.

Exercise as a mental tonic

Regular exercise may also have a significant effect on our mental agility by increasing the amount of oxygen supplied to the brain. In a comparison between sedentary older women and older women who took regular exercise, after four months the latter group processed information faster in tests. This effect of exercise is particularly marked in older people.

Apart from increasing the oxygen supply to the brain, exercise may also slow down the loss of dopamine in the brain. Dopamine is a neurotransmitter that helps to prevent the shaking and stiffness that can come with old age. A severe shortage of dopamine results in the exaggerated tremors of Parkinson's disease. Dopamine decreases in the brain by about one percent a year from our mid-20s, and if we lived to be 100, we would all appear to have Parkinson's disease. Since exercise can slow down dopamine loss, it is particularly beneficial as we grow older. Exercise can also prevent our reaction times from slowing down.

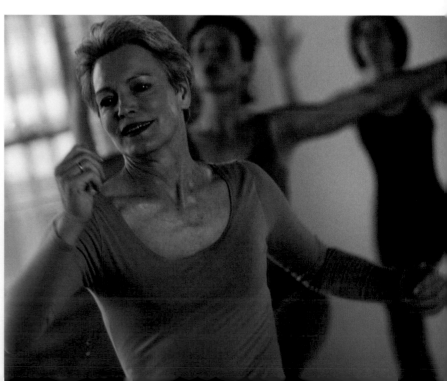

The benefits of regular exercise

Exercise is vital throughout your life, but as you get older these benefits are particularly valuable:

● a reduced risk of heart disease
● a lower chance of developing diabetes
● maintenance of muscle strength
● higher levels of the healthy type of cholesterol in the blood
● better bone health and less chance of developing osteoporosis (if you do weight-bearing exercise)
● a more efficient immune system
● reduced body fat
● better appetite control
● reduced risk of constipation
● increased mental agility
● fewer headaches
● improved sleep quality
● flexible joints.

The type of exercise you take will obviously depend largely on resources, how much time is available and personal preference. To gain the best effects from exercise, try to find a form that you enjoy. There is a wide range of opportunities available in sports centres and fitness classes and, for those who need or prefer to exercise in their own home, there are lots of books, videos and tapes on the market.

You may prefer a sport such as tennis or squash, which offers the added attraction of meeting people. Likewise, joining a class may encourage you to exercise regularly. Less rigorous, more traditional forms of exercise such as brisk walking and swimming offer a viable alternative and keep the body fit and supple.

Recently, there has been a move away from aerobic training towards strength-training and weight-bearing exercise. Research suggests that any form of exercise involving weights can delay loss of bone and muscle tissue, which is a natural consequence of ageing. Weight-bearing exercise also helps to normalize the flow of sugar from the blood into muscle tissue, where it can be properly metabolized. This may lower the risk of diabetes and heart disease.

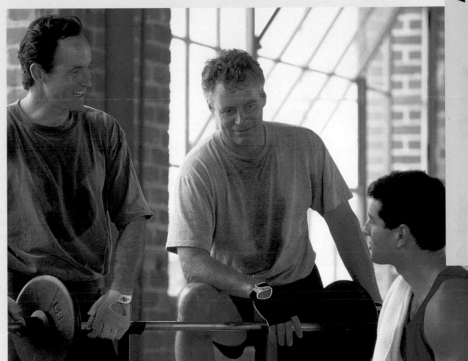

Pelvic floor exercises

Almost all women who've had children notice slight leakage when they cough or lift a heavy weight. But regular pelvic floor exercises will do much to put things right. Here's how to do your pelvic floor exercises.

● The first step is to find the group of muscles that form a figure of eight around the vagina, urethra and anus. You can do this by stopping the flow several times while you're urinating.

● Tighten the muscles for five seconds, relax them for five seconds, then tense them again. Make sure you're not just tightening your buttocks and try not to tighten your tummy muscles at the same time. You may not be able to hold the tension for the full five seconds at first, but you are likely to develop this ability once your pelvic floor muscles grow stronger.

● The next stage is to tighten and relax the muscles 10 times, as quickly as you can so that they seem to "flutter". You will probably need to practise for a while to control the muscles in this way.

● Next, contract the muscles long and steadily as though you were trying to draw an object into your vagina. Hold the contraction for five seconds.

● The final step is to bear down, as if emptying the bowels, but pushing more through the vagina than the anus. Hold the tension for five seconds.

Gradually build up to 10 contractions, 10 times daily or more, spaced over several hours, and check your progress once or twice a week by stopping the flow when you urinate. After about six weeks of these exercises you should find stopping the flow is much easier than it was in the beginning. The beauty of pelvic floor exercises is that, once you've mastered the technique, you can do them anywhere, any time – lying down, watching television, even when you're washing up or waiting for the bus!

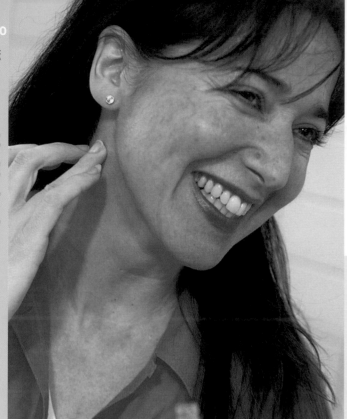

40-60 looking good

Re-thinking hairstyles and make-up and modernizing skin-care routines can take 10 years off your looks. You need a look to suit the woman you are now rather than the woman you were.

Creams

No substance yet known to science can permanently restore the collagen, protein, fat and moisture that we lose from the skin as we grow older. Nor is it possible to repair the fractures that develop in the collagen within the dermis as our faces start to wrinkle. Creams cannot hold lines and wrinkles at bay, no matter what exotic ingredients they contain, but rich cleansing creams and moisturizers may prevent the top layer of our skin from drying out.

Hair

After the menopause, hair growth starts to slow down, the diameter of the hair shaft reduces and grey hairs become more prominent. It is a myth that grey hair is coarser. Grey hair only appears coarser because it starts to appear as the scalp becomes drier. This is due to the oil glands slowing down. Now is the time to switch your shampoo and conditioners to richer, more moisturizing formulations. They aren't sales gimmicks – they really can add moisture to your hair.

Tips on hair care

If you've had the same style for years, ask your hairdresser what style would update your look. Look through magazines and cut out pictures of styles you like. Contrary to popular belief, most hairdressers like to see pictures of the hairstyles you favour because if you simply describe them there is too much room for misinterpretation.

● To cover the first few grey hairs use a semi-permanent hair colour one shade lighter than your natural colour.
● The addition of highlights or lowlights can even out the effect of grey hairs.
● Never be tempted to stay the colour you were when younger. Skin tones change along with hair colour so lighter hair colours become more flattering.
● Soften salt-and-pepper hair colouring with a pale blonde semi-permanent hair colour. It gives the effect of expensive highlights.
● If you wish to grey gracefully but your hair has yellow tones, use pearl or silver shampoos and toners to enhance your hair.

Make-up colours

There are rainbows of shades to choose from, but fortunately nature tells us what colours suit us. Take a magnifying glass and look in a mirror for flecks of different colours in the iris of your eye. All of these, if used as an eyeshadow, will suit you. When selecting colours, take your skin tone into consideration. If you have a warm skin tone, choose warmer colours like golds and bronzes. Cooler skins should opt for cooler colours like silver and lilacs. If your skin is pale, avoid colours that are too dark. If you are olive-skinned, pale colours will be lost so more intense shades are better.

Brunettes

More intense shades suit you better. Try olive green, bronze and terracotta eyeshadows teamed with warm peach or tawny-brown blusher and rust, wine or warm neutral corals on the lips.

Blondes with cool skin tones

Heather, soft greys, lilac and ice blues are good eyeshadow shades to try, along with soft pinks or tea rose blushers. Try lipsticks in dusky rose or raspberry.

Grey hair

Slate blue or steel blue eyeshadows flatter grey hair, along with soft fuchsia blusher. Lips can take raspberry or tea rose shades.

Black skin

Try jewel shades or coppers and bronze for eyeshadows, and rust and fuchsia blushers. Rich gold wine or bronze look good on lips.

Changing your make-up

When you were 17 you wore make-up to look older. If you are stuck in a make-up rut, you could still be making yourself look older. Go through your make-up bag and be ruthless. The colours that suited you a few years ago might not suit you now. As you get older your skin changes tone, so treat yourself to some new, more flattering colours. Look through magazines to see what's popular this year, what new products are around and how you can include them in your lifestyle. If you feel magazines cater only for the young, then book a consultation at a make-up counter and see what the trained beauticians recommend. Don't forget that they are there to sell their own products, so try a few different counters before deciding what you really need to buy.

One of the easiest ways to look younger is to re-think how you use foundation. A thick one won't hide the lines – quite the opposite. Foundation collects in any tiny lines, emphasizing wrinkles. The older you get, the less you should use.

Make-up tips

● Try making up without using any foundation at all. Concealer can be used to hide under-eye shadows or broken veins and you can always use a little skin-toned pressed powder to take away any shine.

● If you feel you need foundation, choose light-reflective formulations or switch to a tinted moisturizer.

● Don't be tempted to add colour with foundation, leave that to blusher. Make sure foundation matches your skin tone exactly then you don't have to apply it all over your face, just where you need it, usually across the cheeks, chin and nose area.

● Plucking the stray hairs from underneath your eyebrows can instantly open up eyes.

● If you have over-plucked your brows in the past, try using brow powder make-up instead of filling in with pencil, which can look too hard. Apply the colour with a small angled brush to create soft, more natural brows.

● Avoid frosted eyeshadows, which draw attention to any lines. Choose shadows with semi-sheen, as matt shadows can look dull.

● A hard line of eyeliner only looks good if you are 18. Use an eyeliner brush and a dark powder eyeshadow and brush a fine line as close to the lashes as possible. The effect is softer and much more flattering.

● Blusher brushes can be too small and so narrow you end up with a stripe of colour across your cheek. Use a powder brush instead as they tend to be fatter. Don't stop at the cheeks, brush on blusher across the chin, temples and forehead for a healthy glow.

● The perfect blusher shade for your skin tone is the colour your cheeks go when you're naturally flushed.

● Build up the colour in gentle layers. Not only will it look more natural but it will last longer too.

● If your skin is naturally dry, switch from powder blusher to cream. Dot along the cheekbone after moisturizing and blend while the skin is still dewy.

● Lips can loose their plumpness and the edges become less defined. Sharpen the outline with a lip pencil.

● Avoid lip liners darker than your lipstick; they look too hard. Choose a shade that matches your natural lip colour. As well as sharpening the outline it also stops lipstick from bleeding.

Skin care

After the menopause, skin becomes drier and thinner. Dead cells aren't shed as quickly, resulting in dull, dry patches. To keep skin as dewy as possible, switch to richer day moisturizers and night creams and exfoliate twice a week to remove sluggish dead cells.

Remember that the basic rule of cleanse, moisturize and protect is more important than ever now.

● **Protect your skin from the sun.** About 80 percent of wrinkles are caused by earlier sun damage. Protect from further damage by using a SPF of at least 15.

● **Don't forget to protect both your neck and hands.** Both are just as much exposed to the sun as your face.

● **Increase your water intake** – water does aid the metabolic rate of the body. So does exercise, even if it is only walking or swimming.

● **Don't use rich moisturizers near your eyes.** You simply end up with puffy eyes in the morning. Use an eye cream for this area, dotting along the bone under your eye, and blend it by gently patting with your ring finger.

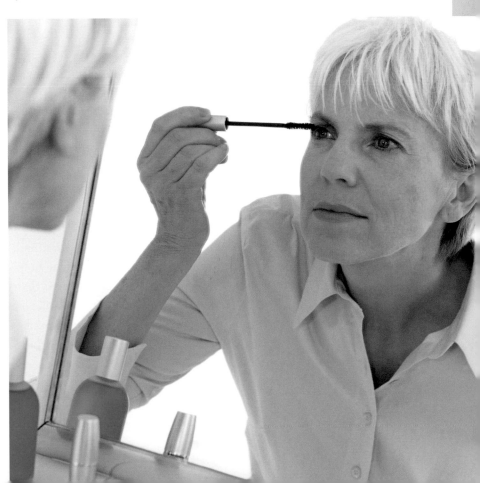

40-60
male menopause

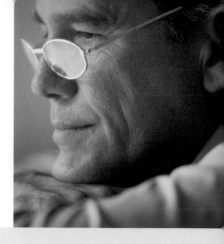

Little is known about the male menopause, or "male climacteric", other than it doesn't exist in the same form as a woman's: hormonally speaking it may not exist at all.

Is there a male menopause?

Do all men experience a menopause or "climacteric"? If there is such a thing, what are the symptoms? Drawing a parallel from the menopausal symptoms in women, should men be the beneficiaries of hormone replacement therapy (HRT)? Once this question is advanced, others follow. What would happen to the male climacteric if HRT were widely used? What would the success rate be? What are the harmful effects? There are very few answers to any of these questions because so little research has been done in this area, though this is sure to change in the near future as more people take an interest in male symptoms.

The male menopause hasn't the same drama as a woman's. It is more gradual, gentle and in a way more insidious than a woman's; nor does it occur during exactly the same years. It is much better thought of as a male climacteric, which envelops all the changes going on in the body and mind as the male genital system begins to wane.

Fear of failure

There is no doubt that "fear of failure" plays a very important part in the ageing man's withdrawal from sexual activities.

Once a man has noticed that his potency is declining, or he experiences one occasion when he is unable to achieve sexual satisfaction through impotence, he may withdraw voluntarily from any kind of sexual activity. This is mainly because most men are unable to face the ego-shattering experience of repeated episodes of sexual inadequacy. Most men are unable to accept the fact that a lessening of sexual drive and a lowering of sexual performance are parts of the normal ageing process, and they make all sorts of excuses and will blame many different kinds of external factors rather than face the truth that their bodies are maturing.

Researchers Masters and Johnson hypothesized in 1970 that a man who finds his potency declining may be showing signs of lowered levels of androgens that may amount to a deficiency. They went on to say that until studies had shown that there was a general requirement by the body for androgen (testosterone) replacement therapy during the male climacteric, cases had to be treated on an individual basis.

There are endocrinologists in many parts of the world who make a special study of the male climacteric, employing hormone replacement therapy for their male patients. The whole area, however, still awaits clear definition and guidelines. **Until then HRT for men will remain a highly specialized field not generally practised.** In this respect women are better off than men. It may be because women are honest and courageous enough to declare that their bodies are deficient, whereas men, particularly in the sensitive area of sexual activities, have yet to come to terms with their bodily changes.

Work/family tensions

Most men between the ages of 40 and 60 are going through the most competitive stages of their careers. The tensions of work are not eased by the financial necessity to look after a growing family with many needs and activities. **On the one hand, men are striving for personal eminence, and on the other they are preoccupied with the security of the "family".** A man in this situation often finds that he spends more time following his professional career than with his family. This leaves a smaller amount of time for loving relationships with his partner, and the stress may lead to gradual lessening in sexual activity.

Both mental and physical fatigue have an ever-increasing influence on sexual activity. **An active sex life in the middle years means being in good condition**, for if a job requires a great deal of physical effort, a man may simply not be fit enough to have stamina left over at the end of a day to enjoy an active sex life. Sometimes, if a man is not fit, a weekend of recreation is more exhausting than the demands of his job, particularly in the age group of 50 and over. Again, this leaves very little energy for sexual activity. If a man is exposed to unaccustomed or excessive physical activity he may feel a loss of sexual responsiveness for a day or so, which will add to his feeling of despondency.

Sexuality in older men

Masters and Johnson, a pioneering research team in human sexuality, made a detailed study of the psychological and physiological factors that might contribute to a decline in a man's sexual prowess as he grows older. From their studies it became obvious that there are factors that affect a man's sexual responsiveness:
- monotony, described as being the result of repetitive sexual relationships
- preoccupation with career and economic pursuits
- mental or physical fatigue
- overindulgence in food and drink
- any physical or mental infirmities in either of the partners
- fear that his performance does not come up to scratch may be greater than at any other time in his life, especially during a time of stressful career decisions.

Monotony is quoted most often and most constantly as the factor that leads to a loss of interest in sex and sexual performance. The end result of this may be one of dutiful indulgence and the need for sexual release. This sometimes arises from a failure of the sexual part of a relationship to grow throughout the marriage. Overfamiliarity with a partner is often blamed; the female partner may no longer be stimulating to her man. She herself may be engrossed in looking after children, or busy with her career. Furthermore, women generally do age more during their 40s and 50s in terms of physical appearance than men. Without attention to her appearance, a woman may become older-looking than her partner.

Sexual problems

As men grow older they eat and drink more, which has a tendency to repress their sex drives. Also, if men feel satisfied from good food this lowers their capacity to achieve in other areas. Overindulgence in alcohol has a particularly negative effect on potency. Impotence developing in a hitherto potent man often makes him drink excessive alcohol and otherwise behave in a way that has not been in his nature.

Most men approaching middle age become concerned about performance. One of the ways of handling any concern is to withdraw from having to perform. This leads to total avoidance of sex within the marriage. If a man is also drinking heavily it only makes matters worse. A problem may arise within the marriage. A man may find that he is impotent with his wife but with another partner, who cannot measure present sexual performance against past, he is perfectly normal.

At any age, physical or mental infirmity can lower or even eliminate sexual drive. After the age of 40 physical or emotional difficulties have a much greater effect, and above the age of 60 a tremendously negative influence. Being physically disabled in the short or long term lowers sexual responsiveness in either sex, but if the illness is acute, such as pneumonia, loss of libido is usually transient and accepted by both partners. With more long-standing disabilities, such as arthritis, interest in sex may decline slowly until it becomes non-existent. Conditions such as long-standing diabetes can lead to impotence in men for medical reasons, and such problems need to be discussed with a partner.

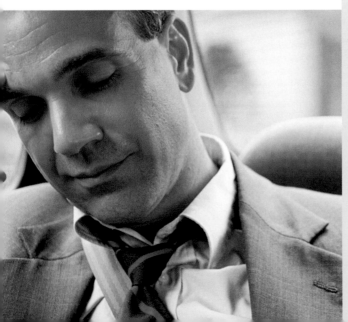

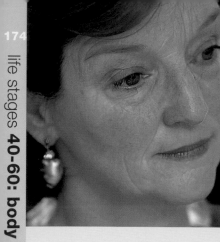

40-60 female menopause

For many women, the menopause can be a psychological, emotional and intellectual turning point as well as a physical one, but it does not have to mean a decline.

Overcoming stereotypes

Referring to the menopause as "the change of life" is misleading and can be counterproductive. The menopause isn't the only change that will occur during your life and it is unlikely to be the most significant change. **Life is a series of gradual changes – we don't suddenly reach a turning point and start growing old when we reach midlife.** Ageing is a continuous process that begins the moment we are born. I believe that a healthy attitude to the menopause is to see it as a time in which to rediscover yourself, to assess your life and its purpose, and to establish new aims and goals.

Many of us have spent much of our lives trying to please other people. We put a great deal of effort into taking care of our children, husbands, parents and friends. We try to be what they would like us to be, and very often we lose sight of who we

are and what we want. By trying to become everything to everyone, we can end up being nothing to ourselves. By the time we reach middle age most of us carry around the received "wisdom" of society, left-overs from old customs and traditions, fears that are often obsolete, and beliefs that may be borrowed. Without clearing out all these redundant feelings, we can lose touch with our inner selves.

It is important to resist negative stereotypes associated with the menopause. These are often culturally created, and do not reflect the reality of our individual experiences. In countries where age is venerated and older women are respected for their experience and wisdom, fewer physical and psychological symptoms of the menopause are reported. Many Asian, Arabic and African women

positively welcome the end of fertility and childbearing, and, perhaps as a result, they seem to encounter fewer difficulties than Western women. In countries that lack a tradition of myths and misconceptions about the menopause, ageing seems to be regarded as a more natural process; women aren't adversely affected by negative images and may feel less confused by what is happening.

If you believe that in order to be beautiful and successful you must be young, then you may not enjoy your middle age to the full. If you are convinced that the quality of life deteriorates from the age of 50 onwards, this can become a self-fulfilling prophecy; because you believe it is going to happen, you may inadvertently make it happen by not taking care of yourself and adopting resigned, negative attitudes.

The menopause

The word "menopause" is usually used to describe the time in a woman's life between the ages of 45 and 55, when her fertility declines and her menstruation stops. The word literally means "cessation of menstruation". The menopause has quite rightly been given a good deal of attention because it is a dramatic event.

There are many changes: hormonal, physical, mental and emotional, which occur during the change, and there is the obvious and inescapable punctuation mark of no more menstrual periods. To feel confident, it is necessary that we know what is taking place in our bodies, so that we can understand that the

mechanism is normal (see p.497).

The menopause is closely involved with gaining new insights, maturing, changing standards, choosing new lifestyles and developing new opinions and priorities. It may be a confused state, or it may be plain sailing. We must draw on our reserves of serenity and maturity.

Developing a positive attitude

The first step in developing a positive attitude towards the menopause is to look back and assess what we have already accomplished. This can reassure us and give us the impetus we need to make decisions about the future. If we forget to acknowledge what we've already done, we can make future goals seem much less attainable.

No matter how active we've been, or what contributions we have made to our work and our family, contemplation of the future can bring mixed emotions. We may find ourselves debating two alternatives: trying to continue living and working as we have always done; or starting to make changes, perhaps reducing our workload. You might justifiably say to yourself that you've been working all your life, so why should you feel guilty for not working now? **It's important as we get older to learn how to enjoy leisure time and to find new and varied diversions.**

Find out what excites and motivates you. Stop spending time on things that don't interest you, household chores for example. You have as much potential as when you were young, but now you are better equipped to harness it. **Make a list of things you "must" do in the rest of your life, things you may never have attempted before.**

Some women break out of their usual lifestyle after many years as wife, mother, and family caretaker to indulge an entrepreneurial spirit and branch out entirely on their own, perhaps setting up a guest house, opening a shop, or running a small business. You may remember your mother in her 50s claiming that she was growing old. If you're still alive at 85, as my mother is, 35 years is a long time to be old, and an intolerable length of time to be inactive.

We have a responsibility to ourselves to make the most of each month, year and decade. Repeat this to yourself every day, and if you feel you lack energy, the best technique is to get angry, particularly if you feel you've stifled your anger and held back in the past. Put yourself in touch with your anger, and use it as fuel. It's absolutely crucial to respect and to trust who you are. You need self-respect before you can respect others and understand them as individuals. Older women are perceptive, experienced and wise about relationships and life. We can benefit even more from joining a group of women of a similar age to us and sharing our experiences.

The strong interaction between your mind and your body means that you can make your menopause more difficult with negative thoughts. If you believe you're sick, you can start to behave like a sick person.

Repeat some of these statements like a mantra each day and you will gradually become convinced of their truth. Positive attitudes will maintain your self-esteem.

● My body is strong and healthy and can become healthier each day.
● My female organs are in good shape.
● My body chemistry is effective and balanced.
● I eat healthy, nourishing food.
● I'm learning to handle stress.
● I'm calm and relaxed.
● I work efficiently and competently.
● I have the freedom and confidence to enjoy life.
● I can be happy and optimistic at this time of my life.
● My life belongs to me and it brings me pleasure.
● I devote time to myself each day.
● My friends and family are more enjoyable than they have ever been.
● I'm going through the menopause more easily and more comfortably with each passing day.

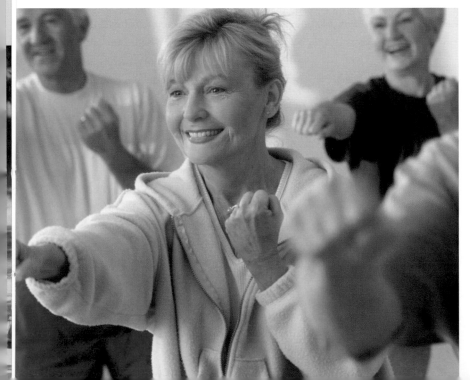

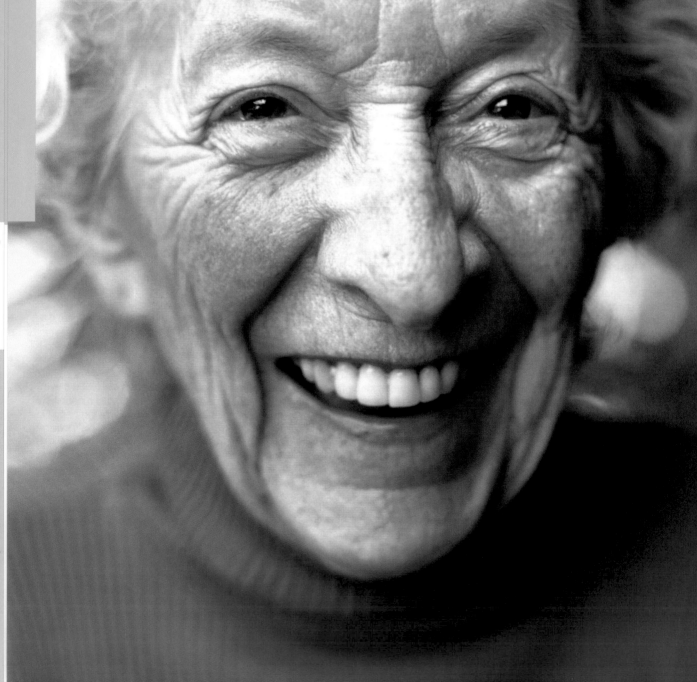

"optimism is the most important personality trait to have if you wish to live a long life"

life stages: 60+ years

The 60-plus age group is the largest and fastest growing in the Western world. Sixty is no longer old, and for the first time ever it's possible to say that ageing isn't inevitable. The reason we age is not because we're programmed to die, but because our tissues accumulate a range of faults that eventually overwhelm us. Now we know this, we can naturally enhance the body's own repair systems and extend life. There's more and more evidence to support this optimism that ageing is controllable.

The two main struts of longevity are, and will always be, eating well and staying active. Of the two, being active is the more important because it keeps the brain alert, with the added bonus that fit muscles burn so many calories that weight gain is controlled. Furthermore, keeping muscles fit acts as a natural appetite suppressant in that active muscles "demand" healthy nutrients. The brain interprets that demand as a command to make healthy choices when you decide what to eat.

Remember – it's never too late to change; it's never too late to start. Alterations to your lifestyle take effect immediately.

Positive attitudes

There are other key factors in controlling ageing. **Positive attitudes**, social networks and a strong spiritual life will increase your lifespan through a sense of wellbeing and life satisfaction. The stress-resistant personality lives longest. People who live to 100 are often strong-willed characters with youthful, can-do attitudes. These same people score high when it comes to self-confidence and resilience, which helps them cope with major stressful events such as war or death in the family.

Strong social networks are important for physical and spiritual wellbeing. Close ties with family and friends can actually strengthen the resilience of the immune system, which affects a person's resistance to disease, including cancer, and can protect against illness and premature death. Nonetheless, a fair

amount of independence may be one of the reasons why the oldest folk can be active and self-supporting in the community until very old age.

Adaptability is another key to long life. Stress accelerates ageing and it may do so by causing shrinkage of the hippocampus in the brain, the main area for memory. It's the negative responses to stress that do the harm in causing premature ageing and there's convincing evidence that adapting to stressful life events through coping is one of the most important factors for successful ageing. It would seem that the key to this talent for adapting is not to perceive events as stressful. So it's important how we react to modern life's stresses – excessive noise, air pollution, traffic jams, rude people and time pressures. People who live to 100 are much better at managing stress than the average person.

Be optimistic

Optimism is the most important personality trait to have if you wish to live a long life. A recent study on men with AIDS showed that those who were optimistic about their future lived nine months longer than those who weren't. In other words, optimism about our health may influence our life expectancy. Optimism has a positive effect on the immune system too. Men undergoing coronary bypass surgery recover more quickly if their outlook is optimistic. The opposite is also true. The belief that we are powerless to influence situations – known as "learned helplessness" – describes a loss of willpower that promotes stress-induced illness. An emotionally stable, flexible personality helps us to stay healthy far into our senior years. Strength of will and assertiveness are an added bonus.

Today we expect to live much longer than our ancestors did. By looking after ourselves well, we can make sure we enjoy those years. In the pages that follow I offer guidelines where appropriate, advice where I feel there may be a need and strategies for dealing with potentially difficult situations.

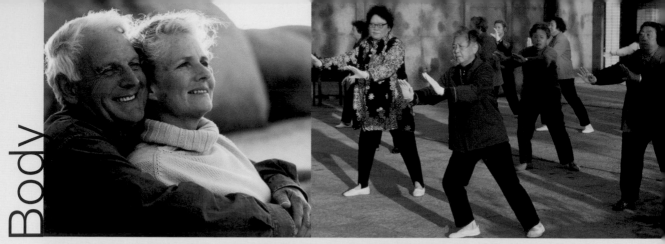

Body

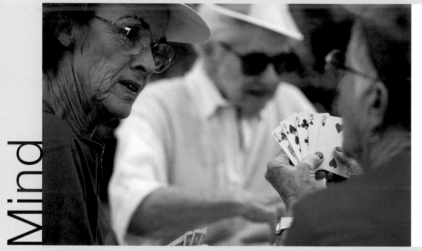

Mind

" long life is determined more by a positive outloo than any other factor "

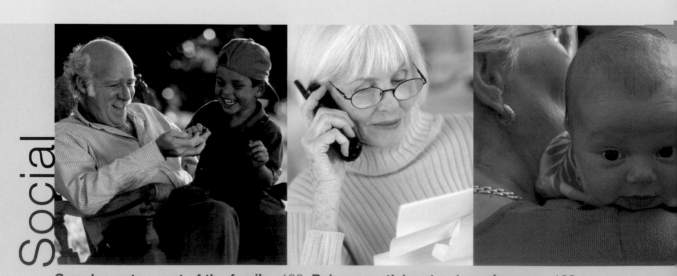

Social

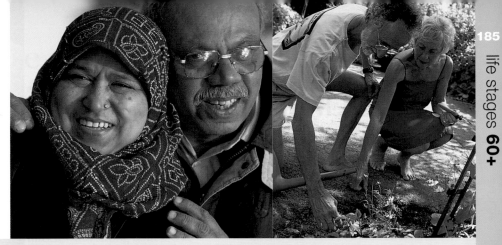

about 80 percent of older people are sexually active

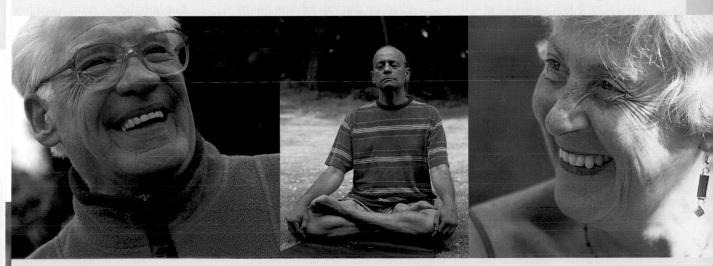

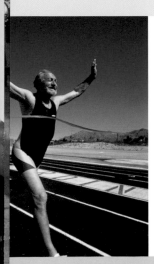

retirement is a time to acquire new skills and new interests

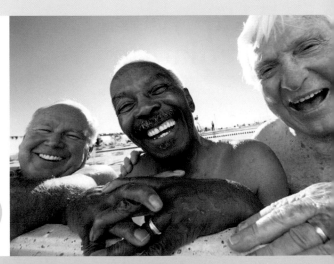

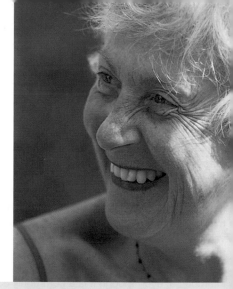

60+ planning for a healthy mind

The latest research suggests that a long life is determined more by a positive outlook and a determination to overcome obstacles than by any other single factor.

Tips for coping with loneliness

One of the best ways of coping with loneliness is to face up to it. You will get great insight into just how lonely you are if you keep a diary. Write down the times when you feel you are at your lowest ebb, when you are the most lonely. For instance, you may realize that the worst times are evenings from about six o'clock, Sundays and holidays. Once you have narrowed those times down, they may be much less frequent than you think.

Planning time

Start splitting up your evenings during the week by allocating them to different activities. You could go to night school on one and take up a new hobby, craft or subject for study. You could make one evening a time for having some friends to your house, and another for visiting someone else. You could make another evening an occasion for going to the cinema, theatre or a concert with a friend. Another could be devoted to keeping fit by going along to a yoga class, having a game of tennis or going to a gym for a workout. One could be for a home hobby like painting, gardening, carpentry or odd jobs around the house. Saturday night could be something special. You could join a local club whose members are interested in the same things as you.

Sundays should be carefully planned. Unless you invite distractions or go out to meet others, it is a long day because it is less easy to shop or do errands. The best and most satisfying way of occupying your Sundays is to invite friends to your home for lunch or brunch. Make it a very relaxed occasion and arrange the food so that people can come and go as they like.

Finding new interests

You are never going to meet people staying alone at home. One of the best ways of getting yourself out of the house is to decide to take up one of your pet passions. Have you always been interested in politics? If so, go along to the next local political meeting. Have you always wanted to paint or sculpt? Enrol at evening classes at the local school. If you have oodles of self-confidence, go along to the local singles club. If you are interested in travel, you could go on a cruise or take up a travel-study programme where you can learn while holidaying in a foreign country.

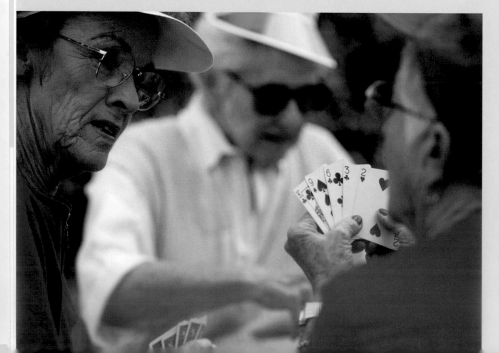

Successful and unsuccessful ageing

Many of us are likely to have evolved ways of making personal adjustments that help us to avoid disturbing situations, but there are still factors that can make adjustment difficult. **Anxiety** increases steadily with age, especially among women. Anxiety arising from what psychologists call "cross pressures", which are typical of adolescence, probably diminishes with age because the older we get the more likely we are to have ironed out the difficulties and contradictions in our circumstances and relationships with others. We all differ as we get older, but many of us become more cautious and less confident.

Rigidity is the inability to modify habits. Naturally habitual ways of thinking and behaving increase with age, partly because the long familiarity with a stable environment has "shaped" behaviour in this direction. Clinging to old ways will ultimately make ageing a difficult transition.

Intelligence, too, is an important determinant of personal adjustment, so that changes in intelligence bring about changes in personality that make ageing more or less difficult.

Personal adjustment is considered to be high if a person can overcome frustrations, resolve conflict and achieve socially acceptable satisfactions and achievements. As you'd expect, good adjustment expresses itself in happiness, confidence, sociability, self-esteem and productive activity.

Personal adjustment is felt to be low if the individual cannot overcome frustrations, resolve conflicts or achieve satisfactory results by means of socially acceptable forms of behaviour. Common signs of poor adjustment are hostility, unhappiness, fear of people, morbid anxiety, dependence, guilt, feelings of inferiority, apathy, withdrawal or incompetence.

Our later years of life need not be static and unchanging. We can continue to learn and grow until the day we die. If we are prepared, personal adjustment should evolve smoothly and logically out of earlier patterns of behaviour. If a sense of continuity and identity can be maintained in spite of physiological, social and psychological changes, the process of re-engagement can proceed successfully. This is essential for adjustment and secures a more effective use of our reduced resources. Normal ageing is gradual, by psychological standards at least, and with foresight, planning and social support, much can be done to ease the problems of adjustment and improve the general level of achievement and happiness.

Adequate adjustment to old age requires certain abilities before we can be happy.

● Our mental state and external circumstances are in balance. There is a degree of continuity between past and present patterns of adjustment.

● We accept old age and death.

● We feel a degree of euphoria arising out of security and relief from responsibilities.

● We have security and adequate financial circumstances to maintain the lifestyle we are used to.

Keeping a tranquil mind

Tranquil young people will probably grow into tranquil old people; **as a general rule, our personalities don't change as we grow older.**

If we are placid and easy-going with a rather philosophical attitude to life, this attitude will almost certainly extend to our middle and later years. If we are excitable, enthusiastic and precipitate, there is a good chance that we will remain this way. If we have been anxious, nervous and inclined to worry, it will be similar later on. If we have had bouts of depression, moodiness and withdrawal from society, the chances are we won't change as we get older.

As we grow older our mental wellbeing is threatened by all kinds of environmental stresses. We may suffer bouts of depression during and after disruptive life events such as retirement, breakdown of marriage or bereavement.

As at any other time of life, we are much better equipped to cope with setbacks, even such serious ones as mentioned, if we are well prepared for them and know where to turn for help. **If you feel strong and supported, mental traumas will be less distressing** and enable you to face the future more calmly and confidently with a greater prospect of happiness.

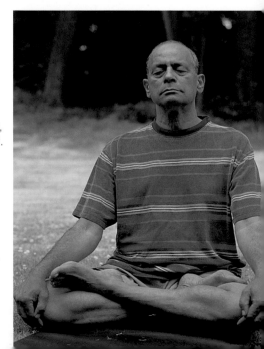

60+ overcoming depression

Depression isn't inevitable as we age, but the problems we may have to face as we get older, such as divorce, bereavement and ill health, can predispose to it.

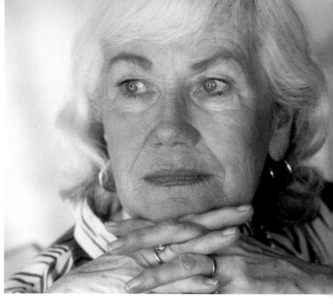

Depression and ageing

At certain stages of our development we may become more vulnerable to external changes and we will show this internal strain by being depressed. Our own individual vulnerability will be based on hereditary factors, our own strengths and weaknesses and our psychological make-up. It is possible to see how depression may express itself as we age and face a life of retirement.

It's lowering to find we can't do the things we used to, nor do we have the status of holding down a job. A woman entering the menopause still cherishes her sexuality and her capacity to bear children. A man cherishes his power, largely represented by his earning capacity. **As we go through middle age we may start to feel that we are lagging behind.** As we reach retirement and get older, we begin

to recognize that we are slower than we once were.

Depression is not inevitable at any critical stage of life, but it is usually those people who have suffered an early loss in infancy, or who have not had their needs met when they were young, who are more likely in later life to become depressed when either internal or external change exposes them to stress.

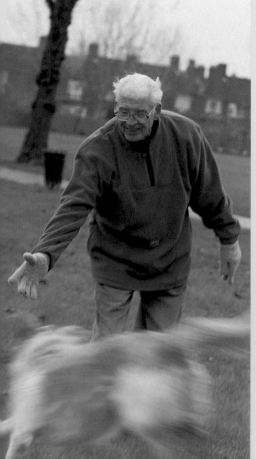

Causes of depression

Depression has physical, psychological and social causes. Some of the physical causes, including infections – particularly viral infections and most commonly influenza, encephalitis and hepatitis – are frequently followed by a period of depression that lasts up to several months. Changes in the brain, such as epilepsy or a stroke, can lead to mood changes, alteration of behaviour and depression. Women undergo certain biochemical changes in their bodies such as those that occur during the menopause, which can lead to depression. Some drugs while dealing with one illness can lead to depression as a side effect in certain susceptible people.

The social causes of depression are nearly always associated with separation and loss. Being poor does not necessarily lead to depression, but if poverty means a loss of status, it may. Bad weather doesn't necessarily lead to depression, but if bad weather means that you have to abandon a treat, then it can. Belonging to a minority

group doesn't cause depression, but if by being so you are cut off from others or persecuted then it wouldn't be surprising if you did get depressed.

Most people believe that there is one social factor – isolation – that seems to be linked very closely with a tendency to depression. Studies have shown that self-destructive acts are more common in people who are cut off from one another. The isolated spinster or bachelor, widow or widower is the one more likely to end up attempting suicide. Marriage, because it avoids social isolation, is less likely to cause suicide, despite the unhappiness it may bring.

As we get older, a wide range of social and psychological stresses may contribute to depression. Bereavement would be the most dramatic for all of us, but other causes of isolation, such as our children getting married or their moving to another part of the country, or our re-housing away from a familiar neighbourhood, are examples that can cause disquiet.

Bereavement

The grief associated with bereavement is not always easy to describe. There may be a good deal of ambivalence at the time – for example, sorrow and disappointment may be mixed with anger, guilt and anxiety. Bereavement is a stress that can precipitate psychiatric disorders, psychosomatic illness or suicide. Many women, for example, experience guilt about their role in the events leading up to the death of their husbands, and widowhood reduces life expectancy.

The reorganization that is called for following the death of a spouse introduces an added source of stress with regard to emotional deprivation and living arrangements, and the increased risk of death of the bereaved person. There are good reasons for supposing that preparation and psychological support help to alleviate the distress that leads to personal conflict. In older people, the awareness of dying has developed slowly. There has been enough time to adapt to the prevailing circumstances and time to learn appropriate strategies of adjustment. Without such adaptation, bereavement and the awareness of dying may evoke feelings of dread associated with a sense of isolation or rejection.

The importance of grief

Bereavement is the loss of someone very precious; grief is the resulting emotional experience of being bereaved. Most people think of grief as a natural response to bereavement. Indeed, they are suspicious of those who deny their grief. Nearly all of us see grief as therapeutic, and we are often told "Get it off your chest and have a good cry".

Grief is more complicated than that. It is dynamic and we live through it. We go through several steps, each of which is hard work. It is not a passive process of the letting out of pent-up feelings but an active process of adjustment. It is a positive "letting go" of something or someone that has been very precious to you for a long time.

Coping with bereavement

● It is important to realize that the feelings you are experiencing are normal. It is normal to feel rage and anger. You wouldn't be human if you didn't feel guilty, so don't spend a lot of emotional energy on self-recrimination.

● Try to find an understanding person to talk to. You can work out quite a lot of your anger, guilt, shame and grief on someone who will just listen, correct you when you over-react and sympathize with what you are going through. At this moment, when you are in the depths of despair, an objective viewpoint that doesn't see life as entirely white or entirely black is one of the best helps you can have.

● It is important to grieve. Grieve in your own time. Don't take any notice of people who encourage you to snap out of it or get back to normal. You will know when your grieving work is done, because you will feel it has worked its way out of your system and you will feel like starting afresh. So if you really want to have a good cry, if you want to have a conversation with your dead partner, go ahead and do so.

● Once the grieving is over, it is important that you start to think about regaining your identity, or even possibly building a new one. Resist the temptation to live in the past. Try to become your own person and to assert your own identity. Start shaping your life as it suits you by doing things that you are really interested in rather than continuing a past way of life.

● Don't make any big decisions quickly, rather let yourself grow into them gradually. Some decisions may be quite hard to take at first. If left for several months or a year, a problem that seemed insoluble will have a very ready solution.

● Whatever you do, try to stay mobile. Don't find yourself chained to the house, unable to get out. Not only see people, but also do essential shopping to give yourself vital changes of routine.

● Don't neglect your finances. This is not a time for them to get out of control and find yourself in debt. So keep an eye on them, budget your expenses and keep a good check on all your sources of income.

● Though it seems unlikely while you are grieving, life does go on and you will live again. Meanwhile you should take good care of yourself. Reward yourself with a holiday. Spend some time in your favourite surroundings or take a course to study a hobby. Go and see members of your family and perhaps stay for a few days.

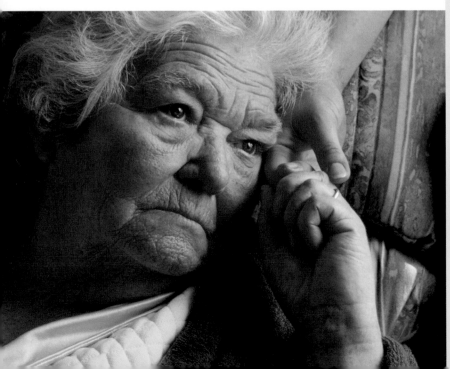

60+ planning for retirement

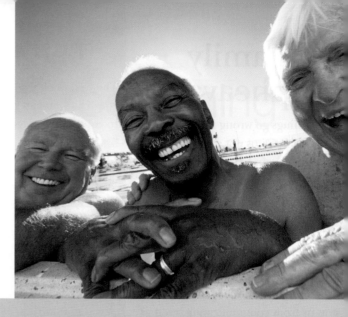

If you are healthy, with reasonable financial resources, and have planned for your retirement, then you will adapt both quickly and completely to your new life.

Preparing to give up work

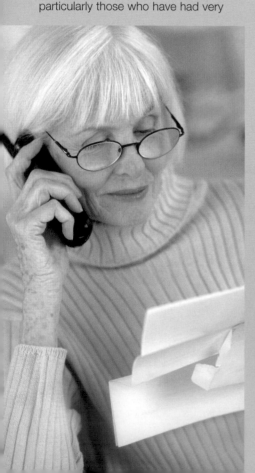

As you near retirement, you may start to reduce your workload, seek financial advice or decide to move to a smaller house. On a personal level, you may start to place more emphasis on your relationships with family and friends.

Whereas some people find retirement a natural transition, others, particularly those who have had very fulfilling careers, may find it harder. You need to prepare for this time because there may be little space for adjustment if you don't.

Retirement preparation is now a widely recognized need. Many firms, voluntary organizations and adult education centres give advice or run courses about financial planning, buying and dispersing personal property and assets, attending to health needs and organizing leisure time.

Financial planning

● Take the best advice you can to make your money work for you during your retirement years. Several years before you retire, think about investments, insurance, mortgages and a will. An accountant or a bank manager will be happy to give you advice. Try to work out a comprehensive budget based on what your income will be after you leave work and what your expenses are likely to be.

● Start living on your projected retirement income about six months before you or your partner retire. If you ease into retirement this way, before you are under the strain of other changes that go with retirement, financial adjustments will be easier to cope with. You will also have saved up the money that you didn't use in the previous six months, which will give you a nest egg and a sense of security. You may get a pleasant surprise and find out that it isn't nearly as difficult as you thought it would be.

Organizing your time

● If your partner retires and you carry on working, or vice versa, you will find that your days are suddenly out of sync. Instead of both getting up early in the morning and going to bed at the same time, one of you will be tired while the other is still raring to go. If this becomes a problem, talk about it and find a solution that works for you both. Make a point of doing things together at weekends when your body clocks become synchronized again.

● If you find yourself at home with time on your hands and you feel at a loss for something to do, you are probably having problems making the emotional transition to retirement. Your partner may be able to help by adapting slightly. Discuss a rota for the chores. Make a list of friends and relatives who are free at certain times during the week (perhaps people whom you haven't seen for several years), and share your interests with these people.

● If you've retired while your partner is still working, take up new projects and revive old hobbies. If you have lots of spare time, spend some of it pampering yourself. Sleep in late, meet a friend for lunch, read in the afternoon and put your feet up whenever you feel like it.

Commit yourself to action

It's never too late to make changes in your life. Once you've made up your mind about what you want to change and how to go about it, take the leap and commit yourself. This doesn't have to mean moving house or filing for divorce, it just means taking a step in the right direction, whether it be looking around at other places you might live or spending more leisure time away from your partner.

Try to avoid thinking of yourself as selfish – others close to you, such as your partner, can also benefit from any changes that you decide to make. For instance, if you have spent most of your life at home bringing up a family, a new part-time job or a course could increase your sense of independence and make you feel more fulfilled, and this can have a positive effect on your relationship. Alternatively, if you've always worked full-time you may be looking forward to a restful retirement.

Remember, you have already made many decisions and experienced many changes in your life and you're well equipped to cope with new experiences. Think of retirement as a period of self-renewal and it shouldn't be the crushing change that people often perceive it to be.

When asked what they miss most about working life, many people mention money and the social environment of work. But there are many advantages to retiring: you can follow your own body clock – eating, sleeping and studying when you feel like it; you no longer have to comply with authority; you have more time to spend on your family, friends and hobbies; and being out of the rat race can dramatically reduce your stress levels.

Pre-retirement

- Other people can dictate your life.
- Your life is structured around work.
- Your leisure time is limited.
- Your tax burdens may be heavy.
- You worry about getting ahead.

Post-retirement

- You can live life as you please.
- You can set your own pace.
- You can choose your own friends.
- You have fewer expectations.
- You have time to be with your family.

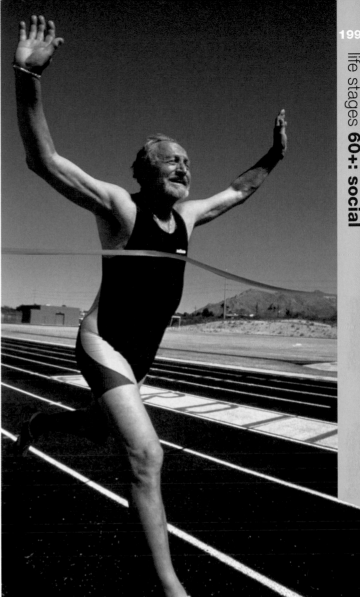

Changing for the better

As you grow older, you may go through a period of major reassessment. You may have a nagging feeling about something in your life you would like to change but, consciously or subconsciously, you have deferred making changes because the time was never right. You may be dissatisfied with where you live. You may feel that you don't spend enough time doing the things that you want to do. Your marriage may feel claustrophobic, and you may want to make some changes in your relationship, or even arrange some time away from your partner.

If any of the above apply to you, confront your feelings and try to be honest with yourself. Talk over your thoughts with your partner, friends or perhaps even with a counsellor. If you let people know what you are looking for, sharing your thoughts may open the door to new opportunities.

60+ dying well

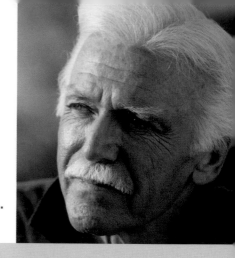

The living will – also known as an advance directive – lets you set out treatments you don't want if you are seriously ill in the future and can't indicate what you want to happen. A living will can help you to die well.

Living will

Through a living will, you can make sure you're not given life-prolonging treatment if, for example you suffer from a massive stroke from which you won't get better. It's your chance to take control over your treatment and make sure that you're not kept alive in a situation that you would find intolerable. You can add to, or amend, the basic living-will form to fit with your personal feelings and beliefs.

Advantages of the living will

The living will makes sure you won't have any treatment you don't want, even if you cannot tell the doctors your decision at the time.
● The living will ensures that your family and friends are not left with difficult decisions because they are not what you would have wanted.
● Knowing what you want will help doctors to make the right decision in difficult situations.
● The living will gives you the chance to discuss your views calmly with doctors treating you and with your close family and friends long before a decision has to be taken.
● When a medical team is faced with a difficult decision about what treatment or care to give you when you aren't able to make a decision, a living will helps the team to understand what you would have wanted if you'd been conscious.
    However, the living will still has to be interpreted to make sure that the situation it describes applies to the patient. Apart from allowing you to control the treatment you receive, the

living will also gives you the opportunity to discuss difficult issues with family and friends without any pressure.

Show your willpower

You never know what's around the corner or what lies in the future for you. By the time you find out, it may be too late to make any decisions for yourself because you're not physically or mentally able to do so. This leaves your friends and family looking after you with difficult decisions to make about your treatment, hampered by not knowing what you would have wanted. You may have a serious or terminal illness, brain damage due to stroke or injury, dementia or Alzheimer's disease, or advanced nervous system disease, such as motor neuron disease.
    You could have severe or lasting brain damage due to an accident. You could be left on a life-support machine or in a deep coma being fed through a tube or intravenously, with all your bodily functions being under the control of a machine to keep you alive. Treatments may offer you little or no chance of recovery and they may have side effects that you would consider worse than the illness itself, or leave you in a condition you would find unbearable.
    You may feel strongly that you don't want to go through this treatment. That is what a living will is for – to ask doctors not to subject you to any medical intervention aimed at sustaining your life beyond a certain point.
    Patients in the UK have called for living wills in our hospitals because they

think the government should adopt American-style living-will consent forms. The British Medical Association, the Patients' Association, the Royal College of Nursing and the government have all confirmed their support for living wills. Any patient entering hospital in the US is asked to register their views on resuscitation, so that action in accordance with their wishes will be taken should an emergency like a cardiac arrest occur.

What does a living will do?

Many people fear that, if they become ill, they could face a situation where they may be given overzealous treatment when there's little or no chance of recovery, or given treatment which would leave them in a condition they couldn't cope with. A living will shows that, in the future, under clearly defined circumstances, you don't want treatment which will help you live longer – treatment such as antibiotics, tube feeding and being kept alive indefinitely on a life-support machine.

Updating your living will

If you have a living will, it's sensible to read it through every few years. Updating a living will isn't a requirement of law. Nonetheless, it makes good sense to review it, reassuring medical staff that it's current and you haven't changed your mind. Every three to five years, simply re-sign and re-date every copy of your living will. Make sure that your GP has the most up-to-date version on file.

Is a living will legally binding?

Although there's no law that governs the use of living wills, in common law, refusing treatment before you need it will have a legal effect as long as it meets the following conditions.

● You were mentally able, not suffering any mental distress and over 18 when you made the request.

● You were fully informed about the nature and consequence of the living will at the time you made it.

● You're clear that the living will should apply to all situations or circumstances that arise later.

● You weren't pressured or influenced by anyone else when you made the decisions set out in your living will.

● The living will hasn't been changed, either verbally or in writing, since it was drawn up.

● You're now mentally incapable of making any decision because you are unconscious or otherwise unfit.

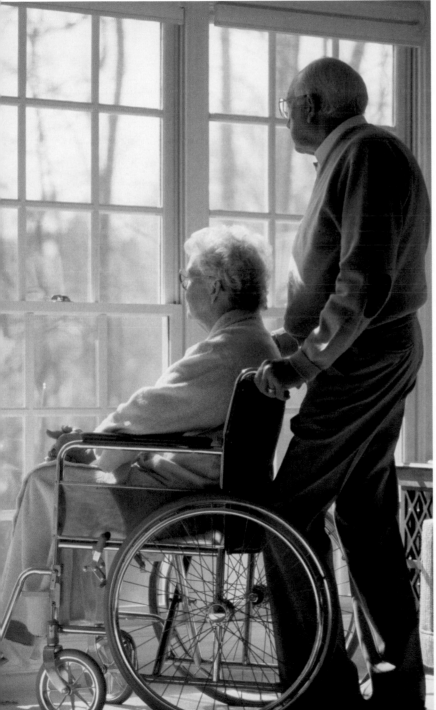

Adjusting to the idea of dying

It's possible to die badly and it's possible to die well. Having been close to two of each kind of death, it became clear to me that what distinguishes dying well from dying badly is the effect on those who are left behind after the death – partners, children, family and friends.

When someone dies well, as my uncle did, we all felt whole, complete, happy for him, unashamed. None of us wished his death had been any different, none of us wished we had done more for him or felt there were things we wanted to say or do for him. This calm and serenity is impossible when someone dies badly. They leave us feeling uneasy, discomforted, guilty, ashamed, angry, cheated, unfulfilled.

Allowing "closure"

I have no ready recipe for how we should die well, but what I've noticed in those who do, and have the time, is that they put the comfort of their family and friends before selfish considerations. So they are open, accepting, generous. They talk intimately to those who surround them, allowing deep, spiritual conversations and contact before the moment of dying. They allow "closure" with all those who love them. They are physically open, too, hugging, kissing and holding others. The flow of love and energy is tangible all around them and it makes for such peace for everyone. To create that peace is our responsibility as we face death.

Symptom Guides

3

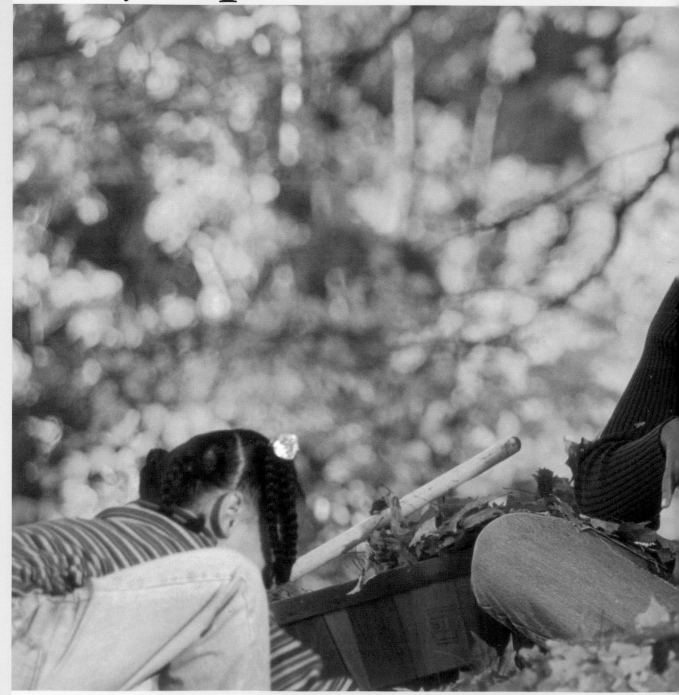

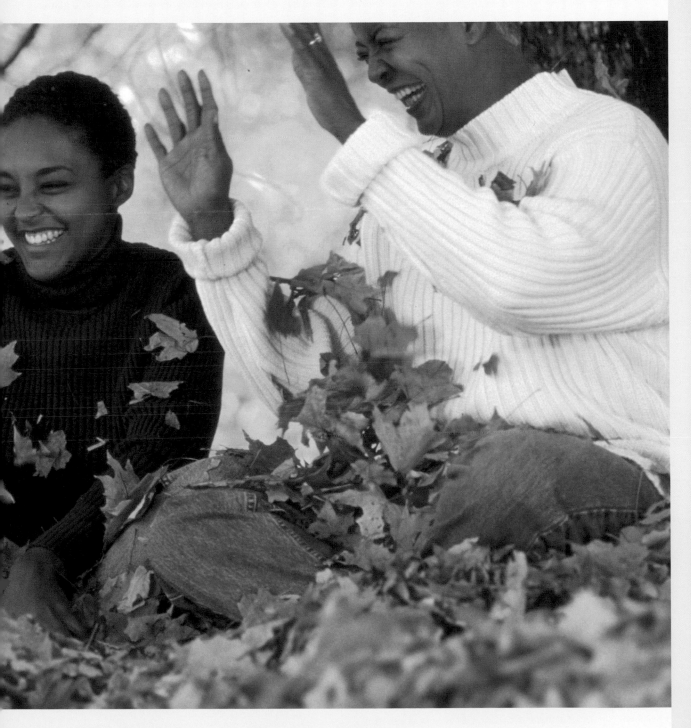

SYMPTOM GUIDES

It can be difficult at times to decide whether you should see the doctor or whether you can treat an illness at home using self-help measures. The symptom guides in this section are designed to help you make that decision. They cover the main symptoms you and your family are likely to experience, and suggest the illnesses that the symptoms could denote. The symptom guides are NOT a substitute for medical advice, and you should always consult a doctor if you are concerned.

HOW TO USE THE SYMPTOM GUIDES
Symptoms are categorized by determining factors such as age, distinguishing features and location. Where a category is not

relevant in diagnosing the problem, it does not appear.

Starting with the age category, you can see at a glance which conditions might be relevant to your symptoms. By proceeding to the distinguishing features category, you can review features of your symptoms that are relevant to diagnosis. Finally, looking at the location map will help you to differentiate symptoms according to where they appear.

"Call" the doctor means just that: speak to him or her, by telephone, to get an opinion about what you should do. "See" the doctor means that you should seek an appointment with your doctor at the earliest opportunity.

RASHES
By location

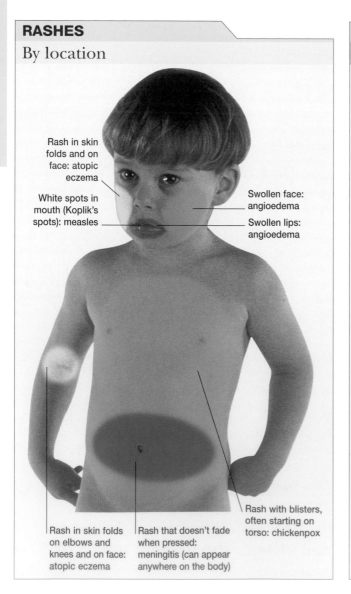

Rash in skin folds and on face: atopic eczema

White spots in mouth (Koplik's spots): measles

Swollen face: angioedema

Swollen lips: angioedema

Rash in skin folds on elbows and knees and on face: atopic eczema

Rash that doesn't fade when pressed: meningitis (can appear anywhere on the body)

Rash with blisters, often starting on torso: chickenpox

ITCHING
By age

In a baby or child
- If on fingers could be scabies (p.452) **see doctor for whole family treatment**
- If rash all over body could be flea bites **see doctor; take cat or dog to veterinarian**
- If face, hands, skin creases affected probably baby eczema **self-help (see Eczema in babies and children, p.313); see doctor and possibly dermatologist**

In an adult
Could be:
- Scabies (p.452) **see doctor**
- Neurodermatitis (a form of atopic eczema, p.312) due to chronic scratching **see doctor**
- Insect bites **self-help (see Bites and stings, p.564)**

In an older person
The skin becomes more prone to itching with age.
- Neurodermatitis (a form of atopic eczema, p.312) **see doctor**
- If persistent can be a sign of a hidden cancer **see doctor for investigation**

CHEST PAIN

By age

In a child
There are few causes of chest pain in children and young people, the main one being a muscle strain or bruise of some kind.

In a young adult
A healthy adult will rarely suffer chest pain, with a few exceptions.

Could be:
- Pneumothorax (p.395), most common in healthy young men **call doctor**
- Bronchitis (p.390), pneumonia (p.392) **call doctor**
- Bornholm disease or intercostal myalgia – a viral inflammation of the muscles between the ribs **see doctor**

In an older person
Could be:
- Angina (p.224), not relieved by rest (could be heart attack) **call ambulance**
- Heartburn (p.350) (could be hiatus hernia, indigestion) **see doctor for endoscopy**
- Peptic ulcer (p.353) **see doctor for endoscopy and biopsy**
- Gallstones (p.357) **see doctor for cholecystography**
- Shingles (p.335) **see doctor**
- Angina (p.224), relieved by rest **call doctor for ECG immediately**
- Pleurisy (inflammation of the covering of the lungs, p.393) causes pain that is worse on breathing and coughing **call doctor**
- Pulmonary embolism (p.395) complicating deep vein thrombosis (p.235) of leg or surgery **call doctor immediately**
- Pericarditis **call doctor**

By location

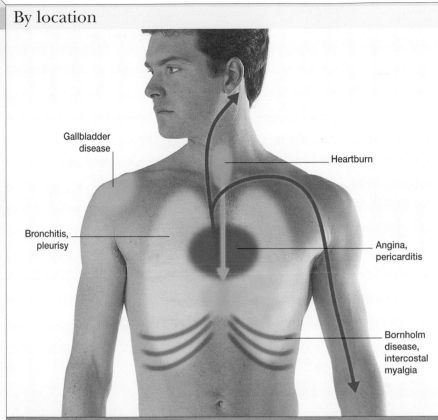

Gallbladder disease

Heartburn

Bronchitis, pleurisy

Angina, pericarditis

Bornholm disease, intercostal myalgia

Distinguishing features

Breathing is difficult
Could be:
- Pulmonary embolism (p.395) **call doctor**
- Pneumothorax (p.395) **call doctor**

Pain worse on breathing or coughing
Could be:
- Bornholm disease (viral inflammation of muscles between ribs) **see doctor**
- Bronchitis (p.390) **call doctor**
- Pleurisy (p.393) **call doctor**

Pain relieved by
- Alkaline food, could be peptic ulcer (p.353) or heartburn (p.350) **see doctor**
- Rest, could be angina (p.224) **see doctor**
- Sitting forward, could be pericarditis (inflammation of the membrane that surrounds the heart) **call doctor**

Pain made worse by food
- Unrelieved by alkaline food Need to exclude stomach cancer (p.354) **see doctor immediately**
- Especially by fatty food Could be gallstones (p.357) **see doctor**

JOINT PAIN

By age

In an infant
Joint pain is always serious **call doctor**

In a young adult
Joint pain could be rheumatoid arthritis (p.429) but most commonly is due to prolonged, unusual activity or body position e.g.:
- Home decorating
- Weeding the garden
- A sports injury **get X-ray**
- Trans-continental flight

In an older person
It's most probably a touch of osteoarthritis (p.428) – the natural ageing process of joints which we all have to some degree or other – but could also be:
- Sudden onset osteoarthritis in a joint which has been injured in the past and possibly over-used **self-help (see Exercises for people with osteoarthritis, p.429)**
- Unusual over-use such as hanging pictures, cleaning windows
- Osteoporosis (p.423) if you're a woman and there's a family history of brittle bones or you're post-menopausal **get bone density scan**
- Osteoporotic fracture if you have osteoporosis and have had a fall or a knock **see doctor**

By location

Peripheral joints of the fingers, hands and wrists, toes, feet and ankle
- **NB** in a child could be a virus or rheumatic fever
- In a young adult nearly always caused by a virus **see doctor**
- In an older adult could be rheumatoid arthritis (p.429) or part of an autoimmune disorder like lupus (p.324)
- **NB** common in last trimester of pregnancy and disappears after the birth spontaneously

Weight-bearing joints, the knees, hips
- Nearly always osteoarthritis (p.428) due to obesity or past injury **see doctor for diagnosis; try self-help (see Exercises for people with osteoarthritis, p.429)**

Joints of the trunk such as the neck, shoulders, spine and lower back
- In a young adult could be part of an autoimmune disease like ankylosing spondylitis (p.430) **see doctor**
- In an older adult probably osteoarthritis of spine (spondylosis; p.432) with or without inflammation (spondylitis; p.430) **see doctor for diagnosis**
- Osteoarthritis (p.428) of vertebrae with osteophyte (bony) formation of vertebrae causing nerve compression and referred pain (pain that originates elsewhere) to shoulder, arm and hand if in neck or sciatica if in lower back **get X-ray**
- Slipped disc (p.437) occurs in the spine where most movement occurs, i.e. back and lower back, giving rise to nerve root pain, numbness and tingling over the distribution of the nerve **get X-ray; try self-help (see Preventing back pain, p.436); try osteopath**

Distinguishing features

Joint is hot
Means that there is some kind of inflammation in the joint and the commonest causes of inflammation are:
- Infection, usually a virus
- Trauma
- An allergic reaction to an external allergen (a drug, say or internal autoimmune reaction) **see doctor**

Joint is swollen
Means that there is fluid in the joint formed to protect the bony surfaces of the joint from injury – it's the body's response to injury to minimize further damage and always denotes pathology in the joint **see doctor**

Joint is red
Means that there is very active inflammation going on inside the joint and it should probably not be moved since rest will ensure that healing can proceed **see doctor**

Joints are stiff/painful to move
- In the early morning nearly always signifies rheumatoid arthritis (p.429) or a related condition
- Later on in the day is classical of an osteoarthritic joint after use **self-help (see Exercises for people with osteoarthritis, p.429)**
- If there is a fracture the joint CAN'T be moved and SHOULDN'T be moved **call doctor**
- If there's a lot of fluid in the joint it's almost impossible to move for mechanical reasons **call doctor**
- Child is limping and won't walk or won't move joint; could signify a greenstick fracture near the joint or a bone condition and is always serious **call doctor**

Fever
Denotes that the joint pain is only a symptom of an illness which is affecting the rest of the body too and it's ALWAYS serious **call doctor**

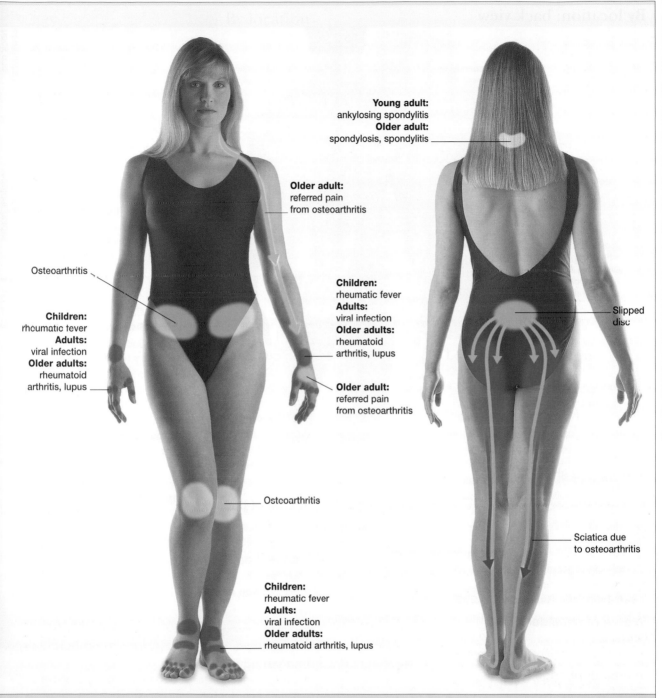

Young adult:
ankylosing spondylitis
Older adult:
spondylosis, spondylitis

Older adult:
referred pain
from osteoarthritis

Osteoarthritis

Children:
rheumatic fever
Adults:
viral infection
Older adults:
rheumatoid
arthritis, lupus

Children:
rheumatic fever
Adults:
viral infection
Older adults:
rheumatoid
arthritis, lupus

Older adult:
referred pain
from osteoarthritis

Osteoarthritis

Children:
rheumatic fever
Adults:
viral infection
Older adults:
rheumatoid arthritis, lupus

Slipped
disc

Sciatica due
to osteoarthritis

Self-help

- Rest the joint.
- If suspected fracture, immobilize the joint
  (see Broken bones and soft tissue injuries, p.560).
- If fever very high, tepid sponge
  (see Fever in children, p.540).
- For joints of ankles and feet, raise the joint when possible to
  prevent further swelling.

- For joint stiffness get them working with heat
  (warm bath, infra-red lamp, warm pad).
- For pain anti-inflammatory analgesic.
- For stiff spinal joints try gentle massage.

DIARRHOEA

By age

In an infant
Could be:
- Travel to a foreign country and new bacteria, not necessarily harmful **call doctor, electrolyte solution for 24 hours to replace lost fluids**
- A viral infection (gastroenteritis) **call doctor**
- Food poisoning **see doctor**
- Coeliac disease **see doctor**
- Lactose intolerance (sometimes following gastroenteritis and temporary) **see doctor**

In an adult
Could be:
- Anxiety (p.287) **self-help (see Relaxation, p.292)**
- Travel (see above) **call doctor, electrolyte solution for 24 hours**
- Food poisoning **call doctor**
- Irritable bowel syndrome **see doctor, self-help (see Irritable bowel syndrome, p.362)**
- Ulcerative colitis (p.367) or Crohn's disease (p.366) **see doctor and specialist**
- Side effect of medication **speak to doctor**

In an older person
Could be:
- Diverticulosis (p.364) **change diet, see doctor**
- Diverticulitis (p.364) **change diet, see doctor**
- Colorectal cancer (p.368) **see doctor soon**

Accompanying symptoms

Vomiting
Could be:
- Food poisoning
- Gastroenteritis
- Food allergy (p.320) **call doctor; 24 hours of electrolyte solution to replace lost fluids**

Fever
Could be:
- Dysentery

NB Diarrhoea and fever can lead to dehydration **get advice from your doctor soon; 24 hours of electrolyte solution to replace lost fluids**

Blood in the stool
In an infant:
Could be:
- Intussusception (p.546) **emergency – go to casualty**

In an adult:
Could be:
- Haemorrhoids (p.370) **see doctor soon**
- Crohn's disease (p.366) **see doctor soon**
- Ulcerative colitis (p.367) **see doctor soon**
- Colorectal cancer (p.368) **see doctor soon**
- Anal fissure (p.370) **see doctor soon**

Distinguishing features

After food
- Up to 6 hours after – Bacterium (probably staphylococcus)
- 6–12 hours after – Bacterium (probably clostridium)
- 12–48 hours after – Bacterium (probably salmonella)

Bowel habit
NB A sudden change in bowel habit at any age requires immediate investigation **see doctor soon**

CONSTIPATION

Distinguishing features/periodicity

Always had it
Could be:
- Too little fibre in diet **change diet**
- Overuse of laxatives leading to inactive bowel **stop laxatives; re-train bowel**
- Ignoring call to stool so it dries out in the rectum **heed call to stool**

Comes and goes
Could be:
- Irritable bowel syndrome (p.362) **change diet, see doctor**
- Diverticulosis, diverticulitis (p.364) **change diet, see doctor**

Recent origin
Could be:
- Hypothyroidism (p.507) (you feel the cold) **see doctor for tests**
- Haemorrhoids (p.370) **see doctor**
- Anal fissure (p.370) (painful) **see doctor**
- Colorectal cancer (p.368) **see doctor for tests**

LOSS OF APPETITE

By age

In a child
Always a serious sign especially if accompanied by any or all:
- Diarrhoea **call doctor**
- Vomiting **call doctor**
- Abdominal pain **call doctor**
- Fever **call doctor**

In a young adult
Could be:
- Anorexia (see Eating disorders, p.300) **see doctor**
- Anxiety disorder (p.287) **see doctor**
- Depression (p.298) **see doctor**
- Drug abuse **get advice from doctor**
- Kidney infection (p.376; with back pain) **call doctor**
- Hangover
- Viral infection
- Food poisoning (with vomiting and diarrhoea) **call doctor if no improvement in 48 hours**

In an older person
Could be:
- Gastric ulcer **see doctor**
- Alcohol abuse **see doctor**
- Liver disease **see doctor**
- Old age **home care**

WEIGHT LOSS

By age

In an infant
Failure to gain weight may be due to:
- Coeliac disease (stools are clay-coloured, bulky, small and float) **see doctor with stool sample**

In a teenager
The commonest causes of weight loss are:
- Dieting **see doctor and counsellor**
- Anorexia (see Eating disorders, p.300) **see doctor and counsellor**

- Bulimia (see Eating disorders, p.300) **see doctor and counsellor**
- Juvenile diabetes (p.504) (hungry, passing lots of urine) **see doctor soon**

In an adult
Could be:
- Dieting
- Malabsorption syndrome (p.365) (stools as for coeliac disease) **see doctor with stool sample**

- Diabetes (p.504) **see doctor soon**
- Cancer **see doctor soon**
- Hyperthyroidism (p.506) (hot, palpitations, clammy palms) **see doctor**

In an older person
Could be:
- Not eating **get advice from doctor**
- Depression (p.298) **get advice from doctor**

FEVER

By age

In an infant
- Always serious if it lasts longer than six hours **call doctor** (Remember, babies can become "feverish" for many reasons, not all of them serious, so if your child isn't listless, vomiting or having diarrhoea try one dose of paracetamol elixir)
- With vomiting and diarrhoea (p.364) **call doctor immediately**

In a child with loss of appetite
Can be the first signs of:
- Appendicitis (p.547) confirmed by abdominal pain **call doctor**
- Any infection (including ear, nose, throat, urinary tract, stomach, bowel) **call doctor if not normal in 24 hours**
- Heat stroke, after sun **get advice from doctor**

In an adult
The commonest cause is a virus infection:
- Flu **self-help (see Influenza, p.334)**
- A bacterial infection, e.g. food poisoning, bronchitis (p.390) **call doctor if not better in 48 hours**

Up to 100°F. (38°C.)
- This is almost within the realm of normality **try paracetamol and monitor**

Up to 102°F. (39°C.)
- Definitely something wrong but not too serious, e.g. cold (p.333), flu (p.334) **try paracetamol, call doctor if not better in 24 hours**

Up to 104°F. (40°C.)
- Could be a serious infection, e.g. kidney infection (p.376) or salmonella **call doctor**

Over 104°F. (40°C. +)
- Could be very serious, such as malaria (p.343) **call doctor or take to casualty**

Distinguishing features/periodicity

Higher at night
- Everyone's temperature is higher at night than in the morning
- Night sweats are a symptom of the menopause (p.497) **see doctor**
- In a man, night sweats can be caused by lymphoma (p.328) **see doctor**

Comes and goes
- Everyone's temperature is higher after exercise
- The fever of tuberculosis classically comes and goes **see doctor**

Long term
- A raised temperature that grumbles on may signify a chronic infection like brucellosis (a rare bacterial infection) **see doctor; keep temperature chart and show to doctor**

Middle of the month
- In women, temperature rises at ovulation and remains up for the rest of the month

Accompanying symptoms

Rash
- With fever in a child could be an infectious disease of childhood, e.g. measles (p.544) or chickenpox (p.335) **call doctor**

IMPORTANT A rash that doesn't fade on pressure (see Thrombocytopaenia, p.239) is a sign of meningitis (p.404) **emergency – take to casualty**

Vomiting
- Always potentially serious if it continues for six hours or more because of risk of dehydration

NB Vomiting can be a sign of brain irritation as in meningitis (p.404), middle ear infection **call doctor**

Diarrhoea
- Always potentially serious if it continues for six hours or more because of risk of dehydration **call doctor**

FATIGUE

By age

In a child
- Listlessness is always serious **see doctor**

In a teenager or young adult
Could be:
- Viral infection, e.g. flu (p.334)
- Post-viral fatigue, e.g. glandular fever, which may take 6–9 months to clear **wait a week or so before seeing a doctor**

In an older person
Could be:
- As for teenager and young adult **wait a week or so before seeing a doctor**
- Anaemia (p.236) or other blood disorder **see doctor for blood test and cause**
- Malabsorption syndrome (p.365) **take stool specimen to doctor**

- Depression (p.298) **examine lifestyle for stress; see doctor for possible treatment with antidepressants; talking therapy with a counsellor; try self-help with yoga, relaxation exercises (see p.292)**
- Hypothyroidism (p.507) (feel cold, hair thinning, skin dry and coarse) **see doctor for thyroid tests and treatment**

Distinguishing features

Worse in early morning
Could be:
- the endogenous form of depression (i.e. not caused by external events) (p.298), especially if it's accompanied by early waking **see doctor**

Worst just before periods
Could be:
- part of PMS (p.302) (other symptoms – lack of concentration, tearfulness,

insomnia) **see doctor; self-help (see Premenstrual syndrome, p.302)**

Worst since periods stopped
Could be:
- menopause (p.497) **see doctor for HRT (p.502); self-help without HRT, including diet, exercise, herbs (see Coping

with menopause the non-hormonal way, p.497)**

Worse at night
Could be:
- stress (p.288), anxiety (p.287), overwork **examine lifestyle for areas to change; self-help (see p.288)**

FAINTNESS/DIZZINESS

By age

In an adult
Could be:
- Pregnancy **test**
- Low blood pressure (p.234) **see doctor (no treatment)**
- Low blood sugar **eat regularly**
- Overbreathing as a reaction to anxiety, a shock **self-help (see Anxiety, p.288)**
- Heatstroke (after sun) **get advice from doctor**

In an older person
Could be:
- High blood pressure (p.226) **get advice from doctor**
- Ménière's disease (p.477) **get advice from doctor**
- Labyrinthitis (p.478) **get advice from doctor**
- Osteoarthritis (p.428) of the neck **get advice from doctor, get X-ray**
- Transient ischaemic attack (TIA; p.402) **get advice from doctor**
- Brain tumour (p.409) **call doctor**

BLURRED VISION

By distinguishing feature

- Followed by headache could be migraine (p.408) **see doctor**
- Lasts only 20–30 minutes could be optical migraine (p.470) **see doctor**
- Gradual onset, getting worse could be shortsightedness (p.469) **see optician**
- Or longsightedness (p.469) **see optician**
- Or astigmatism (p.470) **see optician**
- Accompanied by dry eyes could be Sjögren's syndrome (p.473) **see doctor**
- Loss of part of visual field with attacks of vertigo (p.418), pins and needles or muscle stiffness could be multiple sclerosis (p.412) **see doctor and neurologist**
- Very sudden onset in an older person, like a curtain falling, could be retinal detachment (p.467) **see doctor and ophthalmologist**

HEADACHE
By age

In a child
Could be:
- Migraine (p.408) (is there a family history?) **get advice from doctor**
- Middle ear infection; sinusitis (p.481) **call doctor**
- Meningitis (p.404) (is there a rash?) **call doctor**
- Depression (p.299) (is child a loner?) **get advice from doctor**
- School phobia **get advice from doctor**

In an adult
Could be:
- Side effect of drug you're taking **get advice from doctor**
- Sinusitis (p.481) **see doctor**
- Migraine (p.403) **get advice from doctor**
- High blood pressure (p.226) **check with doctor**
- Very rarely, if severe recurrent headaches start out of the blue, brain tumour (p.409) is a possibility **see doctor**
- Tension due to stress (p.288); anxiety (p.287) **self-help (see Relaxation, p.292)**

In an older person
Could be:
- Temporal arteritis (throbbing pain in temple(s) **see doctor soon**
- Post-herpetic neuralgia (p.408) (after shingles, p.335) **see doctor**
- Trigeminal neuralgia (p.408) **see doctor**

EARACHE
By age

In a baby or a child
- If fever is present could be middle ear infection **call doctor immediately**
- With red spot on cheek and baby pulling her ear could be teething **get advice from doctor**
- If discharge from ear could be otitis externa (infection of outer ear) **see doctor**
- With cough, cold, sore throat could be tonsillitis (p.536) **see doctor**
- If intermittent could be dental problem **see doctor, then dentist**

In an older person
Could be:
- Dental problem **see dentist**
- Temporomandibular joint disorder (p.494) **see doctor**
- Shingles (p.335) **see doctor**
- If persistent and constant (exclude cancer of pharynx) **see doctor**

LUMP IN SCROTUM
By anatomical criteria

Related to testis
Will probably be:
- Spermatocoele (see Why it's important to check your testicles, p.264) **see doctor soon**
- Cystocoele (see Why it's important to check your testicles, p.264) **see doctor soon**
- Hydrocoele (see Why it's important to check your testicles, p.264) **see doctor soon**

None of these is sinister.

- Exclude cancer **see doctor soon**

Unrelated to testis
Could be:
- Varicocoele (see Why it's important to check your testicles, p.264) (feels like a bag of worms) **see doctor**

BREAST PAIN
By distinguishing feature

Cyclical prior to periods
Could be:
- Normal menstrual changes in breasts **keep pain calendar; see doctor; try high dose of evening primrose oil (see Breast pain, p.243)**

Non-cyclical or unrelated to periods
- If stabbing pain around nipple could be duct ectasia (p.246) **see doctor**
- Tender spot in the breast could be a cyst (p.246) **see doctor for ultrasound**
- Could be unrelated to breast such as intercostal myalgia (inflammation of muscles between ribs) **see doctor**
- Tietze's syndrome (arthritis in rib joints) **see doctor**
- Injury or strain to pectoral muscles **see doctor**

Symptoms that may denote cancer if they arise suddenly

- **Headache**
- **Hoarseness**
- **Cough**
- **Blood in sputum**
- **Blood in stool**
- **Blood in urine**
- **Change in bowel habit**
- **Indigestion or heartburn**
- **Loss of weight**
- **Loss of appetite**
- **Breathlessness**

Directory

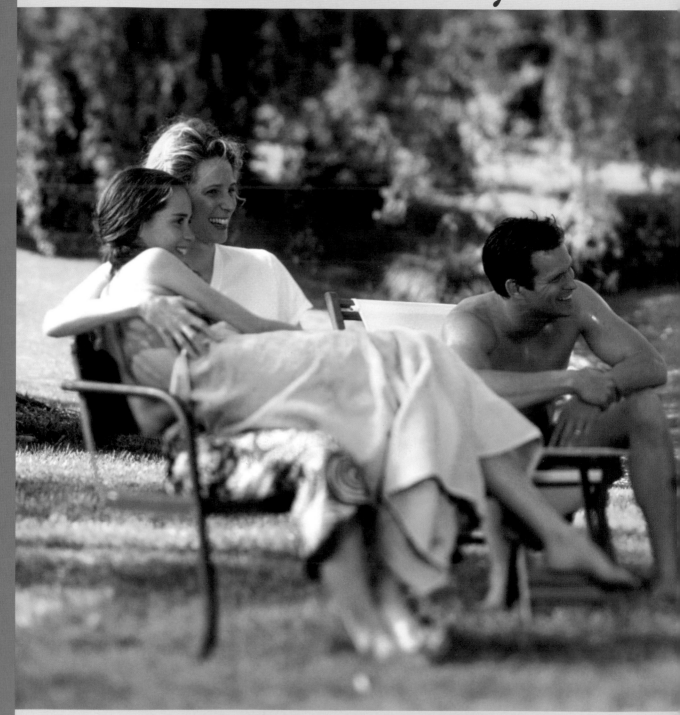

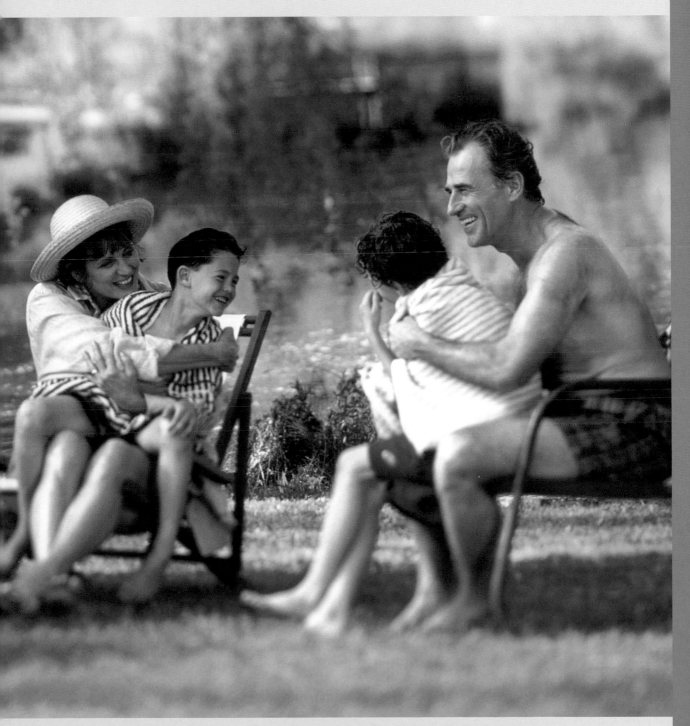

How to use this section

The Directory section covers a wide range of the medical conditions that you and your family may encounter. There are 16 chapters, including one on children's conditions, each devoted to a body system or an area of medical specialization. Each chapter has an introductory essay, which highlights the main conditions and serves as a personal overview of the body system. Conditions listed within each chapter are grouped into related topics, making it easier to find related conditions and to understand shared causes of a group of conditions. Sometimes a chapter will have sections of its own if this is helpful in explaining a group of conditions.

Each condition listed covers the reasons why it might arise (including any relevant risk factors, such as age or gender), how it is diagnosed, how your doctor might treat it, what you can do to help yourself and what the outlook might be. Test and treatment boxes offer up-to-the-minute information on the latest diagnostic procedures and treatments, explaining each procedure in a patient-friendly way. Each chapter also features special "Focus On" topics, where issues of particular interest are discussed in greater depth. Cross-references to related topics appear at the end of entries, so that the flow of information is not interrupted.

How each chapter works

PERSONAL OVERVIEW   **ANATOMY**   **FOCUS ON**

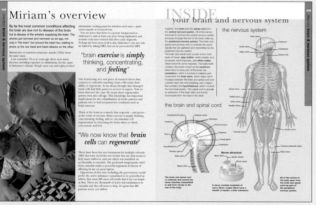

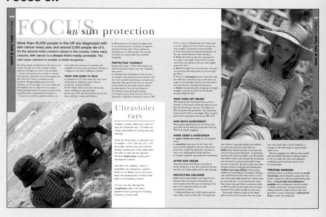

▲ **Dr Stoppard's** unique overview of each body system explains its basic concepts in a friendly way.

▲ **The anatomy** pages show the location of structures discussed in the articles in each section.

▲ **Focus on** articles give Dr. Stoppard's personal view on topics of special interest today.

Find your way around a typical spread

Common conditions are explained in full, with information on causes, symptoms, diagnosis and treatment.

Self-help panels include essential information on what you can do to help yourself.

Warning boxes highlight important advice.

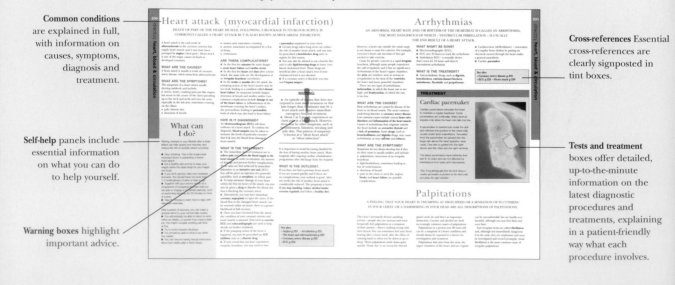

Cross-references Essential cross-references are clearly signposted in tint boxes.

Tests and treatment boxes offer detailed, up-to-the-minute information on the latest diagnostic procedures and treatments, explaining in a patient-friendly way what each procedure involves.

Heart, Blood and Circulation

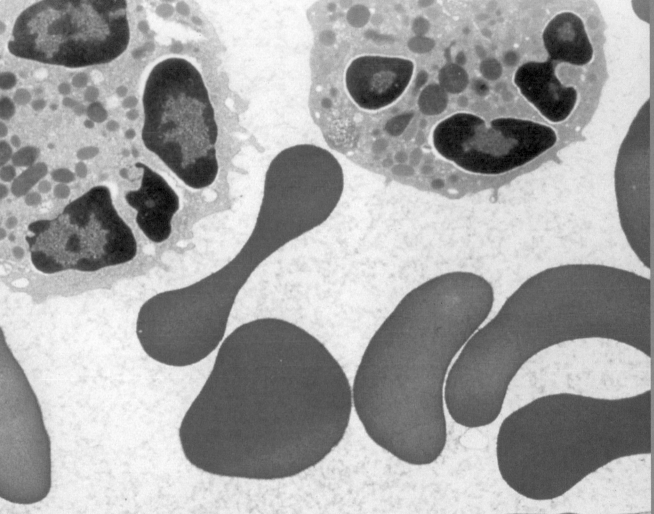

Image shows a coloured transmission electron micrograph of red and white blood cells

Miriam's overview

The headlines in this chapter are heart attacks and high blood pressure. The first can, by and large, be prevented. The second can't but can be successfully treated almost every time.

Your heart health is in your hands once you've excluded a genetic cause for a raised blood cholesterol. All that's required is a heart-healthy lifestyle that encompasses healthy eating – including five fruits a day and if possible two more portions of vegetables.

It also means you won't allow yourself to succumb to a sedentary life. The body is like a muscle – it's better for being exercised. Brisk walking is good enough, fast enough to pant a bit, done for half an hour three times a week.

The heart itself is entirely muscle and like any muscle it requires a workout, once a day if you can but three times a week will keep it in trim.

Without taking that kind of care, your coronary arteries could fur up with fat, giving you coronary artery disease (CAD). It will invariably show up as angina and may then proceed to a heart attack that might, if the CAD is gross, lead to heart failure, or even death.

How will you know if you're a candidate for a heart attack? The best indicator is having a mother or father who had a heart attack. If so, you stand a chance of having inherited a gene that could increase your risk of developing heart disease.

In that case, a healthy lifestyle is a must and if you're a woman you should start taking HRT early in your menopause so that the oestrogen can protect your heart.

A normal blood pressure is essential to lower your chance

> ## "the body is *like a muscle* – it's *better* for being *exercised*"

of ever having a stroke. High blood pressure is the major risk factor for stroke and if yours is raised it's essential that you be assessed by your doctor for treatment.

First-line treatment is very simple and cheap – a diuretic to get rid of any excess fluid. It alone can lower your chances of ever having a stroke.

With the emphasis these days on a balanced diet anaemias of any kind are much less common than they used to be, but particularly those due to deficiencies, such as iron-deficiency anaemia.

It has also meant that inherited anaemias such as sickle-cell anaemia have received the attention they deserve.

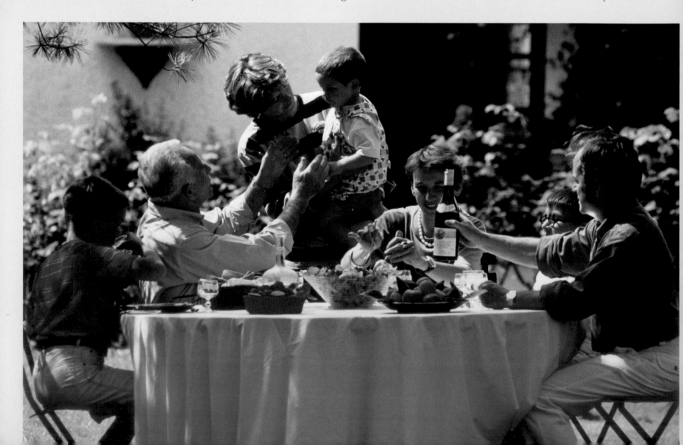

INSIDE
your heart

The **heart** is a hollow muscular organ about the size of your fist whose function is to pump **blood** around the body. The heart itself is divided into four chambers: two upper chambers, called **atria**, and two lower chambers, called **ventricles**. When deoxygenated blood from the body enters the heart it collects in the right atrium, then flows into the right ventricle. From there it is pumped to the lungs. Oxygenated blood from the **lungs** enters the left atrium, then flows into the left ventricle. From there it is pumped around the body.

the structure of the heart

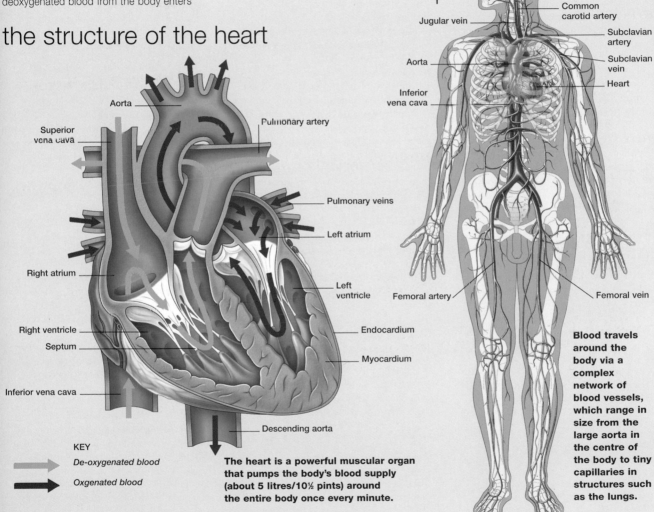

Aorta

Superior vena cava

Pulmonary artery

Pulmonary veins

Left atrium

Right atrium

Left ventricle

Right ventricle

Endocardium

Septum

Myocardium

Inferior vena cava

Descending aorta

KEY

De-oxygenated blood

Oxgenated blood

The heart is a powerful muscular organ that pumps the body's blood supply (about 5 litres/10½ pints) around the entire body once every minute.

the major blood vessels

Jugular vein

Common carotid artery

Subclavian artery

Aorta

Subclavian vein

Heart

Inferior vena cava

Femoral artery

Femoral vein

Blood travels around the body via a complex network of blood vessels, which range in size from the large aorta in the centre of the body to tiny capillaries in structures such as the lungs.

Blood typing

Your blood type is determined by the presence of certain proteins, called antigens, on the surface of your red blood cells. If you are given blood containing antigens that are incompatible with your own, your immune system will attack and destroy them. Blood typing ensures that your are given blood that is compatible with your own.

The major blood types are ABO and Rh (Rhesus). All blood, regardless of ABO type, is classified as either Rh positive or Rh negative. In pregnancy an Rh negative mother's blood may produce antibodies against her baby's blood if it is Rh positive. This problem can be successfully treated if it is identified before the birth.

The heart and atherosclerosis

FURRING UP OF THE WALLS OF THE ARTERIES WITH CHOLESTEROL AND OTHER FATTY SUBSTANCES
THAT CAUSE THEM TO NARROW IS A SERIOUS CONDITION CALLED ATHEROSCLEROSIS.

When the arteries of the heart and brain are affected by atherosclerosis, many common symptoms and diseases develop. **In the case of the heart**, common symptoms are **angina** and **palpitations**, and diseases include **coronary heart disease** and **heart attack**. **In the case of the brain**, symptoms are **dizziness**, **drop attacks** and **memory loss**, and diseases include **stroke** and **dementia**. Seen like this, atherosclerosis is the common denominator of many important conditions and the explanation for many symptoms.

Because of its importance I start with atherosclerosis in this section on the heart and circulation. If you understand atherosclerosis you'll automatically understand a lot about heart (cardiovascular) disease and strokes (cerebrovascular disease).

You'll also become aware of how to lower your chances of getting it and much of the treatment and recommended changes in lifestyle will become obvious and logical.

I also feel a brief discussion of cholesterol is useful for understanding how your heart condition has come about and how you can manage it. Cholesterol has been demonized but not all of it is bad. Indeed, some cholesterol, namely high-density lipoproteins (HDL), is positively good for you and actually protects against heart disease.

Atherosclerosis is a disease that results in the arteries becoming narrowed. The condition can affect arteries in any area of the body and is a major cause of stroke, heart attack and poor circulation in the legs. Platelets (tiny blood cells responsible for clotting) may collect in clumps on the surface of the fatty deposits and form blood clots. A large clot may then completely block the artery.

Atherosclerosis becomes more common with age. However, it rarely causes symptoms until around 45–50 years. The female sex hormone oestrogen helps protect against the development of atherosclerosis. As a result, the incidence of atherosclerosis is much lower in women before they reach the menopause than in men. By the age of 60, however, the risk of women developing atherosclerosis has increased until it is equal to the risk for men. On the other hand, women who take hormone replacement therapy that contains oestrogen will continue to be protected.

WHAT ARE THE CAUSES?

The risk of developing atherosclerosis is determined largely by two things: the level of cholesterol in the bloodstream, which depends on dietary and genetic factors, and whether or not you have the tendency, partly genetic, for cholesterol to collect on the walls of the arteries.

Since cholesterol levels are closely linked with a diet high in fat, atherosclerosis is most common in Western countries where people eat a high-fat diet. In some conditions, such as diabetes mellitus, there is a high blood fat level regardless of diet. Some inherited disorders, such as inherited hyperlipidaemia (see opposite), also cause a high blood fat level.

Factors that make atherosclerosis more likely are smoking, not exercising regularly, having high blood pressure and being overweight, especially if fat accumulates around the waist.

WHAT ARE THE RISK FACTORS?

There are several proven risk factors for atherosclerosis and given that atherosclerosis precedes most heart disease, the risk factors for atherosclerosis apply to heart conditions such as angina, coronary heart disease and heart attacks. These are:

- family history of angina or heart attack
- smoking
- diabetes mellitus
- high blood cholesterol
- not taking exercise or being overweight
- high blood pressure.

WHAT ARE THE SYMPTOMS?

There are usually no symptoms in the early stages of atherosclerosis. If the coronary arteries that supply the heart muscle become blocked, however, symptoms include the chest pain of angina. If atherosclerosis affects the arteries in the legs, the first symptom may be cramping pain when walking caused by poor blood flow to the leg muscles.

HOW IS IT DIAGNOSED?

Since atherosclerosis has no symptoms until blood flow has been restricted, it's important to screen for it, checking on blood cholesterol levels, blood pressure and diabetes mellitus. You should have your cholesterol levels measured at intervals of five years after the age of 20, if you are at risk (see above).

We have sophisticated imaging techniques using X-rays (angiography) and ultrasound (Doppler scanning) that show up the blood flow in the blood vessels of the heart, brain and lungs. An electrocardiogram (ECG) will monitor the electrical activity of the heart. Some of these tests may be done as you exercise to check how your heart functions when it's put under stress.

WHAT IS THE TREATMENT?

■ **Preventive measures** include following a **healthy lifestyle** by eating a low-fat diet, not

Cholesterol

Cholesterol is a fatty substance made in the liver from the saturated fats in food. Too much cholesterol in the blood can increase your risk of getting coronary heart disease.

Cholesterol comes in two main forms:

- low-density lipoproteins (LDL), which carry cholesterol from the liver to the cells in the body, including the arteries
- high-density lipoproteins (HDL), which return excess cholesterol to the liver.

LDLs are the body's natural enemy. High LDLs are a serious risk factor for coronary heart disease, especially with a low HDL. HDLs on the other hand are the good guys and high levels are extremely healthy. The best position to be in therefore is to have a high HDL and a low LDL.

Now we come to the tricky role of diet. A diet high in saturated fat (i.e. animal fat, mainly from full-fat dairy products) raises your LDL and lowers your HDL – the opposite of what

you want. On the other hand, by changing your saturated fats to unsaturated fat (oils) you'll reverse this tendency. The average blood cholesterol level of people living in the UK is 5.8mmol/l (millimoles of cholesterol per 1 litre of blood). This is high compared to other countries. For example, in China the average is 3.2mmol/l. If your measurement is over 5.8mmol/l, your doctor will want you to try to reduce it with changes to your diet and lifestyle, and possibly by prescribing drugs.

Cholesterol is only one risk for getting heart disease. If you have any other risk factors, such as smoking, being overweight or high blood pressure, then these risk factors multiply your chances of having a heart attack.

About 1 in 10 people has a high blood cholesterol as the result of a familial condition called inherited hyperlipidaemia. If this condition is left untreated it can lead to coronary artery disease and heart attack at an exceptionally young age.

TESTS

Blood chemistry and blood cholesterol

Blood chemistry tests

Blood chemistry tests measure the levels of certain chemicals and minerals in the blood and are a simple way of discovering whether particular cells and tissues are functioning normally. They are usually used to check the levels of chemicals produced by the kidneys, the liver or the muscles. The tests can also be used to check levels of bone minerals, such as calcium.

Blood cholesterol tests

Blood cholesterol tests measure levels of certain fatty substances, known as lipids, in the blood. High levels of the lipids cholesterol and triglycerides cause fatty deposits to develop on the walls of the arteries, resulting in atherosclerosis. The fatty deposits interfere with blood flow and can cause coronary artery disease (CAD) and stroke.

As well as measuring the total level of cholesterol in the blood and the levels of other lipids such as triglycerides, the tests also measure the levels of two specific types of cholesterol: high-density lipoprotein (HDL) and low-density lipoprotein (LDL). HDL seems to protect against atherosclerosis, while a high level of LDL is a risk factor for developing atherosclerosis. A result of 5.0 mmol/l (millimoles of cholesterol per 1 litre of blood) or lower is generally considered desirable. The ratio of HDL to LDL is also important; ideally the ratio should be less than 4. Depending on the results of blood cholesterol tests, your doctor may advise you to make diet and lifestyle changes or may prescribe lipid-lowering drugs, or both.

smoking, exercising regularly, and maintaining the recommended weight for your height.

■ If you are in a good state of health but have been found to have a high blood cholesterol level, your doctor will advise a **low-fat diet**.

■ You may also be offered **drugs** that decrease your blood cholesterol level. For people who have had a heart attack, research has shown that there is a benefit in lowering blood cholesterol levels, even if the cholesterol level is within the average range for healthy people.

■ Your doctor may prescribe a drug such as **low-dose aspirin** to reduce the risk of blood

clots forming on the damaged artery lining.

■ If you are thought to be at a high risk of severe complications, your doctor may recommend other treatment, such as **coronary angioplasty**, in which a balloon is inflated inside the artery to widen it and improve blood flow.

■ If blood flow to the heart is seriously obstructed, you may have **coronary bypass surgery** to restore blood flow.

WHAT IS THE OUTLOOK?

A healthy diet and lifestyle can slow the development of atherosclerosis in most

people. If you do have a heart attack or a stroke, you can reduce the risk of having further complications by taking preventive measures.

See also:
• Angina p.224 • Coronary angiography p.224 • ECG p. 224

Inherited hyperlipidaemia

THE CONDITION IN WHICH THE BLOOD CONTAINS ABNORMALLY HIGH LEVELS OF CHOLESTEROL AND/OR TRIGLYCERIDES (ANOTHER TYPE OF FAT) IS KNOWN AS INHERITED HYPERLIPIDAEMIA.

Inherited hyperlipidaemia is present from birth, but usually only becomes apparent in early childhood and is due to an abnormal gene inherited from one or both parents. A high-fat diet and lack of exercise aggravate the condition. Elevated levels of triglycerides, or, especially, cholesterol increase the risk of **atherosclerosis** and **coronary artery disease**.

WHAT ARE THE RISKS?

■ The most common form affects about 1 in 500 people of European descent, who inherit one copy of an abnormal gene. Affected people have a cholesterol level **two or three times** higher than normal.

■ There is a **one in a million** risk that people will inherit the abnormal gene from both parents. If two copies of the gene are inherited, the cholesterol level is **six to eight times** higher than normal.

■ Affected people have a high probability of a **heart attack**, which may occur **even in childhood**.

WHAT ARE THE SYMPTOMS?

Besides the symptoms of atherosclerosis, very high cholesterol levels associated with inherited hyperlipidaemia may cause some of the following symptoms, which develop gradually over a period of several years:

● yellow swellings under the skin (xanthomas) on the back of the hands

● swellings in the tendons around the ankle and wrist joints

● yellow swellings on the skin of the eyelids (xanthelasmas)

● pale yellow ring around the iris (the coloured part of the eye).

Men with these disorders can develop symptoms of coronary artery disease, such as angina, as early as their 20s or 30s. In women,

oestrogen usually gives protection from these problems until after the menopause.

WHAT MIGHT BE DONE?

■ There is no cure for inherited hyperlipidaemia so cholesterol-lowering drugs must be given early.

■ Symptoms can be treated with a combination of exercise, a diet that is low in saturated fats and drugs.

■ The prognosis varies, but early treatment can reduce the risk of a heart attack.

■ Relatives of an affected person should be screened for the disorder.

See also:
• Angina p.224
• The heart and atherosclerosis p.222

Angina

THE TYPICAL CHEST PAIN OF ANGINA IS OFTEN DESCRIBED AS HEAVINESS OR TIGHTNESS IN THE
CENTRE OF THE CHEST SPREADING TO THE ARMS, ELBOWS, NECK, JAW, FACE AND BACK, USUALLY
BROUGHT ON BY EXERTION OR ANXIETY AND RELIEVED BY RESTING FOR ABOUT 10 MINUTES.

TEST

Coronary angiography

Coronary angiography is used to give
a picture of the arteries that supply the
heart muscle with blood. Angiography
can show up narrowed or blocked
coronary arteries, which are not visible
on a normal X-ray. A local anaesthetic
is injected to numb the skin, and a fine
flexible catheter is passed into the femoral
artery, through the aorta, and into a
coronary artery. Contrast dye is injected
through the catheter, and a series of
X-rays is taken. The procedure is
painless, but you may feel a flushing
sensation as the dye is injected.

During the procedure

The catheter is positioned in the heart
so that its tip rests in a coronary artery
and contrast dye is then injected. The
artery and the small vessels leading from
it are visualized by a series of X-rays.
The catheter may be repositioned and
the procedure repeated to check all the
coronary arteries.

Angina affects both sexes but rarely occurs in
women before the age of 60 because oestrogen
protects against it. After the menopause,
however, the protective effect of oestrogen
gradually disappears and angina is as common
in women as in men, as is heart disease.

Angina is the most common symptom
caused by furring up of the coronary arteries
(atherosclerosis). Since atherosclerosis
precedes most heart conditions, angina is a
warning sign for many different heart diseases.

WHAT BRINGS IT ON?

The pain originates in the heart muscle and
is due to an inadequate supply of blood. It is
a sign of coronary artery disease (CAD; see
opposite) and coronary heart disease (CHD).
It may come on when you're walking,
particularly on a cold day or after a meal, but it
can also come on when you're resting and may
even wake you up at night. Some people notice
that getting upset or anxious brings on angina.

WHAT DO I DO IF ANGINA COMES ON?

1. Stop what you're doing.
2. Rest. Don't move until the pain has
completely gone.
3. Take your medication (e.g. a nitrate tablet
under your tongue) to relieve the pain.
4. If the pain lasts longer than 15 minutes
or isn't relieved by a nitrate tablet, call your
doctor – it could be a heart attack. Also inform

your doctor if your angina comes on with less
and less effort.

IS IT REALLY ANGINA?

There are many causes of central chest pain
but they don't all have the significance of
angina. Here are just a few:
- heartburn
- indigestion
- peptic ulcer
- gallstones
- anxiety
- muscle strain or inflammation.

Your doctor can usually distinguish these from
a heart condition by the nature of the pain, but
you may have electrocardiography (ECG), a
radionuclide (thallium) scan, an angiogram or
coronary catheterization. An exercise ECG will
show a heart that's under stress on exertion.

WHAT IS THE TREATMENT?
DRUG TREATMENT

■ Nitrate drugs increase the blood supply to
your heart by widening the coronary arteries.
You can get immediate relief by putting a
glyceryl trinitrate (GTN) tablet under your
tongue. Always keep them with you and never
run out. You can also use them as a preventive
before exertion, such as before sex.

■ Beta-blockers, calcium-channel blockers
or potassium-channel blockers reduce the
amount of work your heart does by slowing
down the heart rate and reducing the heart's

TEST

ECG

Electrocardiography (ECG) is used to
record the electrical activity of the heart,
to investigate the cause of chest pain
and to diagnose abnormal heart rhythms.
Several electrodes are attached to the
skin to transmit the electrical activity of the
heart to an ECG machine. Each trace shows
electrical activity in different areas of the
heart. The test usually takes several minutes
to complete and is safe and painless.

*The trace (paper record) produced by the ECG
machine shows the electrical activity of the heart
as it contracts and relaxes.*

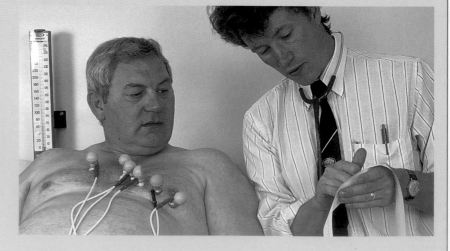

need for oxygen. Side effects are uncommon but include impotence, so report anything untoward to your doctor and your tablet could be changed.

SURGICAL TREATMENT
■ Coronary angioplasty will improve the flow of blood to your heart. This isn't major surgery and you'll be home in two days.
■ Coronary bypass is when the narrowed sections of your coronary arteries are bypassed by an artery or vein grafted from another part of your body, usually your leg. This is major surgery and you'll be in hospital for a week.

LIFESTYLE CHANGES
An angina attack is an early warning sign. You must alter your lifestyle if you want to prevent another attack and stop your heart condition getting worse.
■ Stop smoking.
■ Lose weight and eat a heart-healthy diet with more oily fish and fresh fruit and vegetables.
■ Start exercising gradually.
■ Control your blood pressure, under your doctor's supervision.
■ Keep an eye on your cholesterol (a level under 5mmol/l is best).

With these changes and treatment from your doctor you should be able to get back to normal life, work and sex.

> **See also:**
> • **The heart and atherosclerosis p.222**

Coronary artery disease

IN CORONARY ARTERY DISEASE, THE CORONARY ARTERIES (WHICH SUPPLY BLOOD TO THE HEART MUSCLE) HAVE BECOME SO FURRED UP WITH FATTY MATERIAL THAT THE BLOOD SUPPLY TO THE HEART MUSCLE IS COMPROMISED, LEADING TO HEART DAMAGE.

The underlying condition is atherosclerosis and the most prominent symptom is **angina** (chest pain). I've included a detailed discussion of risks, causes, investigations, treatment and changes to lifestyle under those headings and I suggest you read them in conjunction with this one.

In coronary artery disease (CAD), which can progress to **coronary heart disease**, one or more of the coronary arteries is narrowed. Blood flow through the arteries is restricted, leading to damage to the heart muscle. Impending damage to the heart muscle is signalled by the chest pain angina. Serious heart disorders, including heart attacks, are usually caused by CAD. The condition is therefore a leading cause of death in many Western countries.

WHAT ARE THE CAUSES?
Coronary artery disease is usually due to **atherosclerosis**, in which fatty deposits accumulate on the inside of the artery walls. These deposits narrow the arteries and restrict the blood flow. If a blood clot forms or lodges in the narrowed area of an artery, it can become completely blocked. CAD caused by atherosclerosis is more likely if your blood cholesterol is high and you eat a diet high in animal fat. CAD is also linked to smoking, obesity, lack of exercise, diabetes mellitus and high blood pressure.

In women, the hormone oestrogen reduces the risk of developing CAD.

WHAT ARE THE SYMPTOMS?
■ **Chest pain** (angina).
■ **Palpitations** (awareness of the heartbeat).
■ **Light-headedness** or **loss of consciousness.**
■ **Irregular heartbeats** in some people. These

are a result of an abnormality of the heart rhythm (arrhythmia). Some severe arrhythmias can cause the heart to stop pumping completely – cardiac arrest – which accounts for most of the sudden deaths from CAD.
■ In elderly people, CAD may lead to chronic heart failure, a condition in which the heart gradually becomes too weak to pump an adequate circulation of blood around the body. Chronic heart failure may then lead to the accumulation of **excess fluid in the lungs** and tissues, causing additional symptoms such as **shortness of breath** and **swollen ankles**.

WHAT IS THE TREATMENT?
■ Treatment for CAD falls into three categories: lifestyle changes, drug treatments and surgical procedures.
■ If tests show that you have a high blood cholesterol level, you will be treated with lipid-lowering drugs to slow the progression of CAD and, as a consequence, reduce the risk of a heart attack.
■ Angina may be treated with drugs, such as nitrate drugs and beta-blocker drugs, that improve the blood flow through the arteries and help the heart pump effectively. An abnormal heart rhythm is often treated using anti-arrhythmic drugs.
■ Surgical treatment includes angioplasty and coronary bypass surgery.

> **See also:**
> • Angina p.224 • Arrhythmias p.231
> • The heart and atherosclerosis p.222
> • Chronic heart failure p.233
> • Heart attack p.230
> • High blood pressure p.226

TEST
Exercise testing
Exercise testing is usually done when coronary artery disease is suspected. It is used to assess heart function when the heart is put under stress. The test involves raising your heart rate by exercising, generally using a treadmill with an adjustable slope or an exercise bicycle, and monitoring the heart's function. The exercise is tailored to ensure your heart is tested adequately without putting you at risk. Various methods of monitoring may be used, including radionuclide (thallium) scanning, which can image the heart's function, and electrocardiography (ECG), which monitors the heart's electrical activity.

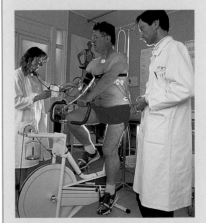

Riding an exercise bicycle tests the heart safely.

FOCUS *on* high blood pressure

Persistently high blood pressure may damage the arteries and the heart. Untreated high blood pressure is the most common cause of a stroke. In the West, at least 1 in 5 people has high blood pressure, also known as hypertension.

High blood pressure is harmful because it puts a strain on the heart and arteries, resulting in damage to delicate tissues. If it's left untreated, high blood pressure may eventually affect the eyes and kidneys. The higher your blood pressure the greater the risk that complications, such as heart attack, coronary artery disease and stroke, will shorten your life. Lowering your blood pressure even a little can cut your risk of having a heart attack by as much as 20 percent.

Your blood pressure varies naturally during the day with activity, rising when you exercise or feel stressed and falling when you rest and sleep. It also varies among people, gradually increasing with age and weight.

High blood pressure per se rarely makes you feel ill. A small number of people get headaches but only if their blood pressure is very high. If your blood pressure is that high, you may have dizziness, blurry vision or nosebleeds. Hypertension is sometimes called the "silent killer" because people may have a fatal stroke or heart attack without warning.

However, if you know you have high blood pressure you're not alone and you're luckier than many because at least you're aware that you have it. Over one-third of people with high blood pressure aren't being treated and their health is at risk.

WHAT ARE THE CAUSES?
Even though high blood pressure is more common among men there is no single cause. All these factors can contribute:
- being overweight
- drinking large amounts of alcohol
- a stressful lifestyle
- excessive salt intake
- physical inactivity
- kidney disease.

In pregnant women, the development of high blood pressure can lead to the potentially life-threatening conditions pre-eclampsia and eclampsia, in which the elevated blood pressure usually returns to normal after the birth.

WHAT MIGHT BE DONE?
- To detect high blood pressure it's important to have your blood pressure measured routinely at least every two years after the age of 30.
- If your blood pressure is more than 140/90mmHg, your doctor will ask you to return in a few weeks so that it can be checked again.
- A diagnosis of hypertension isn't usually made unless you have a raised blood pressure on three separate occasions.

Your doctor may arrange these other tests:
- heart tests including electrocardiography (ECG) or echocardiography
- eye tests to look for damaged blood vessels
- tests to identify the underlying cause. For example, urine and blood tests and ultrasound scanning may be arranged to look for kidney disease or a hormonal disorder.

ARE THERE COMPLICATIONS?
There is risk of damage to the arteries, heart and kidneys with severe hypertension that's left untreated. Arteries that have been damaged are at greater risk of being affected by atherosclerosis, in which fatty deposits build up in blood vessel walls, causing them to narrow and restrict blood flow.

After many years, damage to the arteries in the kidneys may lead to chronic kidney failure. The arteries in the retina of the eye may also be damaged by hypertension.

WILL I NEED TREATMENT STRAIGHT AWAY?
The need for treatment is contingent on the level of blood pressure PLUS other risk factors

Measuring blood pressure

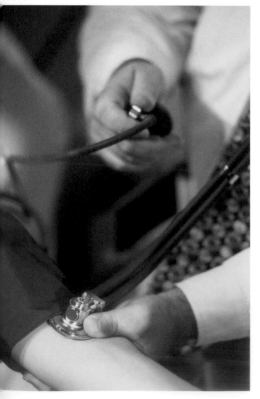

An inflatable cuff is wrapped around your upper arm and inflated using a bulb. The cuff is slowly deflated while the doctor listens to the blood flow through an artery in your arm using a stethoscope.

Blood pressure is expressed as two figures given in millimetres of mercury (mmHg). The blood pressure of a healthy young person who's been sitting down for five minutes shouldn't be more than 120/80mmHg. In general, a person is considered to have high blood pressure when their blood pressure is persistently higher than 140/90mmHg after three readings on separate occasions, even at rest.

140/90 – what it means
140 – Systolic pressure
The pressure when the contraction of the heart forces blood around the body
90 – Diastolic pressure
The lowest pressure occurring between heartbeats

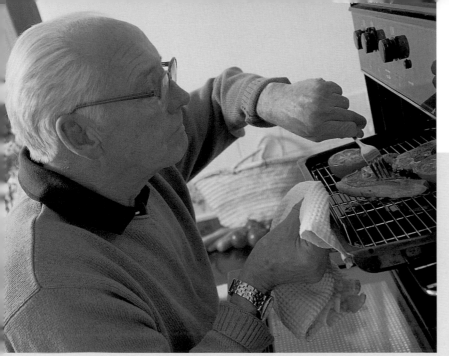

• If self-help measures aren't effective your doctor may prescribe antihypertensive drugs. These drugs work in different ways, and you may be prescribed just one type of drug or a combination of several. There are many drugs for treating blood pressure and they'll lower your blood pressure gradually over several weeks or months.

DO ANY OF THESE DRUGS HAVE SIDE EFFECTS?

Most people will feel well but some will suffer side effects. Fortunately these are few but one of the most distressing is impotence. If you experience impotence ask your doctor if your tablets could be responsible and whether you can change treatments.

WOMEN:

• with high blood pressure can take HRT
• who take the contraceptive pill should have blood pressure checks every six months.

WHAT IS THE OUTLOOK?

In most cases, lifestyle changes and drug treatment can control blood pressure and reduce the risk of complications. You'll probably have to stick to these measures for the rest of your life.

that may damage blood vessels, for example diabetes, continued smoking or being overweight. So, treatment can vary from person to person and isn't always dependent on a certain level of blood pressure.
• Blood pressure that averages 160/100mmHg or higher over many readings is best treated with drugs (see table, below).
• Mild high blood pressure (between 140/90 and 159/99mmHg) may be checked regularly but not treated if the risk of damage to the arteries is low. This is often the case in young people, particularly in young women.
• On the other hand, mild blood pressure

is best treated in older people and those who already have symptoms of blood pressure damage, such as those who suffer from angina.
• You'll probably be checked by your GP for three or six months before starting treatment.
• For mild hypertension the first line of medical treatment is often water tablets (diuretics).

WHAT IS THE TREATMENT?

• High blood pressure can't usually be cured but it can be controlled with treatment. If you have very mild hypertension, changing your lifestyle is often the most effective way of lowering your blood pressure.

Drugs used to treat high blood pressure

Drug type	What they do	Used for	Not used for	Occasional side effects
DIURETICS	Get rid of salt and water	Older people	People with gout or diabetes	Gout Impotence
BETA-BLOCKERS	Slow your heartbeat	Younger people	People with angina People with asthma	Cold fingers and toes Tired legs Vivid dreams, Impotence
ACE INHIBITORS	Relax walls of arteries	People with diabetes or heart failure	Women who are or may be pregnant	Dry cough Throat discomfort, Diarrhoea
CALCIUM-CHANNEL BLOCKERS	Relax walls of arteries	People with angina	People with heart failure	Ankle swelling Skin flushing, Constipation
ALPHA-BLOCKERS	Slow your heartbeat	Men with prostate problems	People with asthma	Headaches, Dizziness Dry mouth
ANGIOTENSIN II ANTAGONISTS	Relax walls of arteries	People with angina	People with heart failure	Ankle swelling Skin flushing

SELF-HELP:
CHANGING YOUR LIFESTYLE

You can help yourself a great deal by changing your lifestyle. There's a strong link between being overweight and having high blood pressure.

If your weight's above normal for your height, you should aim to lose the extra pounds and bring your blood pressure down. You don't need to aim for an ideal weight. Try to be within the healthy range for your height. Losing 10kg (22lbs) can reduce the bottom figure of your blood pressure by 20 points.

If you can't lose weight yourself, your doctor may refer you to a dietician for advice on ways to change how and what you eat. You don't have to give up eating all the food you enjoy. Some people find a slimming group or club very helpful to give moral support.

DO'S

Eat fish, white meat (for example, chicken without the skin), cottage cheese, low-fat yoghurt, semi-skimmed or skimmed milk. Aim for seven items a day of fresh fruit and vegetables (eat seasonal vegetables and fruit when you can); when fresh vegetables are expensive eat frozen ones instead. When possible, grill food instead of frying it.

A diet containing plenty of fruit, vegetables and grains increases potassium intake, and this can help to lower your blood pressure too.

DON'TS

Don't eat butter, cheese and full-fat milk, fried foods and snacks, cakes, biscuits, chocolate and fatty meat.

KEEP YOUR ALCOHOL LEVELS DOWN

High alcohol intake increases your chance of developing high blood pressure.

● Limit your alcohol to no more than 21 units a week if you're a man, 14 units if you're a woman. One unit is equal to a glass of wine OR a half pint of ordinary-strength beer, cider or lager OR a single measure of spirits.

● Try to spread your units evenly over the week and avoid a big drinking session.

● A large amount of alcohol the night before can raise your blood pressure significantly the following day.

● Talk to your doctor if you're drinking more alcohol than you should and finding it difficult to reduce the amount you drink.

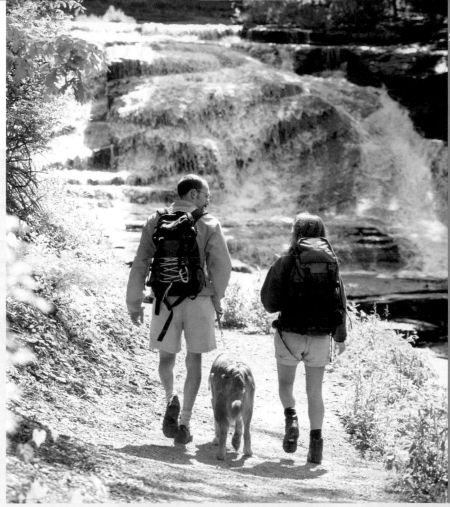

AN ABNORMAL
THE M

However, a heart rate outsi
is not always a cause for col
everyone's heart rate incre:
excited or take exercise.

Cause for greater concer
heartbeat, although many
the odd irregularity and it
Arrhythmias of the heart's
the **atria**, are nowhere nea
irregularities in the beat o
the lower and more powe

There are two types of a
tachycardias, in which the
high, and **bradycardias**, ii
is too low.

WHAT ARE THE CA

Most arrhythmias are cau
heart or its blood vessels.
underlying disorder is co
Less common causes incl
disorders and **inflammati**
Causes of arrhythmias th
the heart include an **ove**
a **lack of potassium**. Sor
bronchodilators and **dig**
arrhythmias, as may **caf**

WHAT ARE THE S

Symptoms do not alway
do their onset is usually
● palpitations (awaren
heartbeat)
● light-headedness, so
loss of consciousness
● shortness of breath
● pain in the chest or
Stroke and **heart fail**
complications.

A FEELIN
IN YOUR

They don't necessaril
serious – people who
frequently feel palpit
of their anxiety – the
their hearts. You can
beating after a heavy
running hard or wh
sleep. These palpita
quickly. Those due t

LIMIT YOUR SALT

A high salt intake raises your blood pressure
about 10 points. Salt can also increase the
amount of fluid that you retain in your body.

Fresh food contains very little salt. Most of
the salt we eat is in processed foods, or in salt
added to food while cooking or at the table.
So to reduce the amount of salt you eat:
● Look at food labels. If it says sodium
chloride (NaCl), sodium benzoate or
monosodium glutamate then you may be
eating extra salt without realizing it.
● Cut down on processed foods. Salt is hidden
in many processed foods, e.g. tinned or packet
soups, breakfast cereals, bread, tinned or
processed fish, crisps, nuts, hamburgers and
prepacked meals.
● Look for low-salt bread.
● Cut down on corned beef, hard cheese, ham,
bacon and sausages, which contain lots of salt.
● Use salt very sparingly in cooking, if at all.
If you feel that you can't do without salt, you
might try a salt substitute (after checking with
your doctor). Rock salt and sea salt are not salt
substitutes.

It's preferable to avoid the taste of salt
altogether. You'll find fairly quickly that your
sense of taste adjusts so that you no longer
like the taste of salt, especially if you add herbs
such as basil, thyme and rosemary to your
cooking, which release the natural salts in food.

EXERCISE

Exercise can help reduce your blood pressure
and keep your weight down. It is also a good
stress reliever. Stress isn't always a cause of
high blood pressure. It will, however, aggravate
raised blood pressure.

If you haven't done any exercise recently,
check with your doctor first.

WHAT TYPE OF EXERCISE SHOULD I DO?

Any vigorous activity such as walking,
swimming, cycling, jogging, dancing or
gardening is good for you. The important
thing is to choose an activity that you enjoy –
if you don't like a particular form of exercise
you'll find it much harder to do it regularly.

Exercise doesn't need to be too strenuous
either. You should start slowly and build up
the amount of exercise that you do. Start by
walking briskly. You don't have to jog unless
you wish to. Walk the dog; use the stairs, not
the lift, and keep active!

Aim to do 20–30 minutes of exercise at least
three times a week.

For some people, it isn't advisable to lift very
heavy weights or to do certain very strenuous
activities such as playing squash. Check with
your doctor first if you're thinking of taking
up a new sport that is very strenuous.

STOP SMOKING

Giving up smoking won't lower your blood
pressure directly, but it lowers your risk factors
for high blood pressure by greatly reducing
the chance of blood vessel damage that can
lead to a heart attack or stroke.

It's so important that you stop smoking that
I suggest you make a plan and prepare yourself
to stop. Have an action plan, prepare well, and
you'll succeed.

Your pharmacist, GP or practice nurse can
advise on stopping smoking and on aids such
as chewing gum and skin patches.

What about a home blood pressure monitor?

It's only worth monitoring your own blood
pressure if you stick to the correct
procedure, like resting for at least five
minutes before each reading and not taking
readings in isolation but averaging out three
consecutive readings.

There are two types of monitor:

● an inflatable cuff that can be pumped
up and the blood pressure is read off a dial
● a digital electronic monitor that provides
a digitally displayed blood pressure reading.

NB Only buy a monitor that's approved
for use in the UK.

Hear...

DEATH ...
COMM...

A heart attack is the...
atherosclerosis in th...
supply heart muscle...
presaged by **angina**...
is one of the major...
developed countrie...

WHAT ARE TH...
A heart attack is us...
artery disease, whic...

WHAT ARE TH...
The symptoms of a...
develop suddenly a...
● severe, heavy, cr...
but worse in the c...
up to the neck and...
especially in the le...
on the elbow
● pale clammy sk...
● shortness of br...

Wh...
I...

Making changes i...
attack can help sp...
reduce the risk of...

■ Stop smoking...
important factor i...
heart attack.
■ Eat a healthy...
weight within the...
and build.
■ If you drink al...
amounts. You sh...
1–2 small glasse...
■ Together with...
programme of i...
are able to enga...
as swimming re...
at a time.
■ Take the trou...
relaxation exerc...

After a period o...
gradual return t...
■ You will prob...
within six week...
job. You might...
at first.
■ Try to avoid...
■ You should...
four weeks.
■ You can res...
about four we...

Low blood pressure (hypotension)

SOME PEOPLE HAVE BLOOD PRESSURE THAT IS PERSISTENTLY BELOW NORMAL LEVELS. IN MOST CIRCUMSTANCES, HOWEVER, SUCH LOW BLOOD PRESSURE OR HYPOTENSION IS HEALTHY AND THE LONGER YOUR BLOOD PRESSURE IS ON THE LOW SIDE THE HEALTHIER YOUR HEART WILL BE.

Except in very old people low blood pressure therefore needn't be treated.

A common type of low blood pressure is **postural hypotension**, in which suddenly standing or sitting up leads to light-headedness or fainting. This can be caused by several drugs, including those for high blood pressure. Shock is a serious form of low blood pressure due to rapid loss of fluids or blood or a heart attack, and requires emergency treatment.

WHAT ARE THE CAUSES?
Dehydration following loss of large amounts of fluid or salts from the body will lower the blood pressure. For example, heavy sweating, loss of blood or profuse diarrhoea may cause varying degrees of low blood pressure.

WHAT ARE THE SYMPTOMS?
You may not have any symptoms unless your blood pressure is very low. Symptoms that do occur may include:
● fatigue
● general weakness
● light-headedness and fainting
● blurry vision
● nausea.

SHOCK
However, if no pulse is present because the blood pressure is too low to provide an adequate blood supply to vital organs, it can be fatal. The low blood pressure that follows a heart attack, acute heart failure and serious cardiac arrhythmias must be treated in an intensive care unit as life is threatened.

SELF-HELP FOR POSTURAL HYPOTENSION
1. Sit up slowly and rest for a few minutes.
2. Slowly lower your legs over the side of the bed and wait a few minutes.
3. Stand slowly holding firmly onto the bedhead or a chair to steady yourself.

These symptoms are usually temporary, and blood pressure rises when the cause is treated.

> **See also:**
> ● **Shock p.560**

CIRCULATION

Into this group of conditions fall disorders of the **peripheral blood vessels – the arteries and veins** of the **arms** and **legs**. Within the remit of this book I feel there's only room for the three most common conditions: one of the arteries, **Raynaud's disease and Raynaud's phenomenon**, and two of the veins, **varicose veins** and **deep vein thrombosis** (DVT).

It's worth just mentioning the word phlebitis, which is used to describe **inflammation** (not a clot) in a vein. It's important to distinguish between phlebitis and DVT. With the former, there's little risk of a clot breaking off and going to the lungs or heart; in the latter, there is. Treatment of the two conditions is therefore quite different.

Raynaud's phenomenon and Raynaud's disease

OFTEN CALLED "DEAD FINGERS", THESE TWO SIMILAR CONDITIONS CAUSE NUMBNESS AND TINGLING IN THE FINGERS OR TOES; THEY ARE MORE COMMON IN WOMEN AND SOMETIMES RUN IN FAMILIES.

The symptoms are due to sudden narrowing of the arteries in the hands or, rarely, the feet because of **hypersensitivity** to cold. **Smoking** and **exposure** to cold may trigger attacks.

In about half of all people with Raynaud's phenomenon, the condition is associated with another disorder such as rheumatoid arthritis. Certain drugs, such as beta-blockers, are known to produce the symptoms of Raynaud's phenomenon as a side effect.

If there is no apparent cause for the condition, it's known as Raynaud's disease, which is most common in women between the ages of 15 and 45 and is usually mild. It can be triggered by smoking, because the nicotine in cigarettes constricts the arteries. Exposure to cold and handling frozen items can also trigger an attack.

Rarely the condition is due to abnormal proteins, **cold agglutinins**, in the blood, which show up when the extremities get cold or the body cools down.

WHAT ARE THE SYMPTOMS?
Both the hands and feet can be affected and an attack can last from a few minutes to a few hours. Symptoms include:
● numbness and tingling in the fingers or toes that may worsen and progress to a painful burning sensation
● progressive change of colour in the fingers or toes, which initially turn white, then blue and finally red again as blood returns to the tissues.

There may be a marked colour difference between the affected area and the surrounding tissues. In severe untreated cases, skin ulcers or gangrene may form on the tips of the fingers or toes.

WHAT MIGHT BE DONE?
■ Your doctor will carry out tests to look for an underlying cause of your symptoms. For

example, blood tests may be performed to look for evidence of **rheumatoid arthritis** or **cold agglutinins**.

■ Your doctor may suggest that you take drugs to dilate the blood vessels during an attack.

■ If you smoke, you should stop immediately.
■ Keeping the body covered up with several layers of warm clothing is helpful.
■ Wearing a thermal hat, gloves and socks in cold weather helps avoid the onset of symptoms.

■ Central heating should keep the ambient temperature on the warm side.
■ If symptoms are very severe, surgery may be considered to cut the nerves that control arterial constriction.

Varicose veins

MANY PEOPLE HAVE VISIBLY SWOLLEN AND DISTORTED VEINS THAT LIE JUST
BENEATH THE SKIN, MAINLY IN THE LOWER LEGS.

These varicose veins may also be found at the **lower end of the oesophagus** as the result of **liver disease** and in the **rectum** as piles **(haemorrhoids)**. Varicose veins tend to run in families and pregnancy, excess weight and prolonged standing are risk factors. Sometimes they are a result of a deep vein thrombosis in the lower leg.

Varicose veins affect about 1 in 5 adults and are more common with increasing age. Although the condition may cause discomfort and appear unsightly, it's not usually harmful to your health. Varicose veins mainly affect the legs. Veins have one-way valves to stop blood from flowing backwards down into the legs. If the valves in the deep veins do not close adequately, the blood flows back into the superficial veins near the skin. The pressure of returning blood causes these veins to become swollen and distorted, and they are then known as varicose veins. If left untreated, the condition often worsens. Sometimes **dermatitis** and even an **ulcer** may develop at the site of a varicose vein, often on the inner side of the ankle.

WHAT ARE THE CAUSES?

■ An inherited weakness of the valves in the veins can cause varicose veins to develop.
■ The female hormone **progesterone** – the pregnancy hormone – causes the veins to dilate and may encourage the formation of varicose veins. The condition is therefore more common during pregnancy. Increased pressure is placed on the veins in the pelvic

region during pregnancy as the uterus gradually grows larger.
■ Being overweight is a factor.
■ Occupations that involve standing still for long periods and little walking can be to blame.
■ A blood clot blocking a deep vein in the lower leg – deep vein thrombosis (DVT) – sometimes known as a "white leg". It may follow major surgery if the patient doesn't wear elastic stockings or remains immobile.

WHAT IS THE TREATMENT?

■ In the majority of cases, varicose veins do not require treatment. Self-help measures such as wearing elastic stockings may be enough.
■ If your varicose veins are small and below the knee, your doctor may recommend that the veins be injected with a solution to make their walls stick together and thus prevent blood from entering them.
■ For varicose veins above the knee, the usual treatment is to tie off the connection with the deep vein so that blood does not enter the varicose vein.
■ For entire varicose veins, surgical removal by "stripping" is an option. However, even after surgery, varicose veins may eventually recur, and treatment may need to be repeated.
■ **Varicose dermatitis** and/or **ulcer** requires special treatment with topical creams and supportive bandaging.
■ Varices at the **lower end of the oesophagus**, usually as the result of alcohol-related liver cirrhosis, can bleed internally and must be treated as a medical emergency.

SELF-HELP

Coping with varicose veins

There are a number of measures you can take if you have troublesome symptoms caused by varicose veins.
■ Avoid prolonged standing.
■ Take regular walks to keep blood flowing in the legs.
■ Keep your legs elevated when sitting, if possible.
■ If your doctor has recommended that you wear elastic stockings, put them on before you get out of bed in the morning while your legs are still elevated.
■ Avoid clothing, such as girdles, that may restrict the flow of blood at the top of the legs.
■ If you are overweight, you should try to lose weight.

■ Varices in the rectum are **haemorrhoids** and they may cause rectal bleeding.

See also:
• **Cirrhosis p.357**
• **Haemorrhoids p.370**

Deep vein thrombosis

THE FORMATION OF A BLOOD CLOT IN A DEEP-LYING VEIN, USUALLY IN THE LEG, IS CALLED DEEP
VEIN THROMBOSIS (DVT). DVT USED TO BE CALLED "WHITE LEG" BECAUSE IF A BLOOD
CLOT FORMS WITHIN A DEEP VEIN IN THE LEG IT SWELLS AND LOOKS WHITE.

DVT is more common over the age of 40 and slightly more common in females. It can run in families and risk factors include prolonged immobility after surgery or childbirth and excess weight. A combination of **age** (being

over 35 years), **cigarette smoking**, **obesity** and the **oral contraceptive pill** increases the risk of DVT too.

The formation of a clot in a deep vein is usually not dangerous in itself. However,

there's a risk that a fragment of the clot may break off and travel to the heart via the circulation. If the fragment lodges in a vessel supplying the lungs, a potentially fatal blockage called a **pulmonary embolism** occurs.

WHAT ARE THE CAUSES?

Deep vein thrombosis is usually caused by a combination of:
- slow blood flow through a vein
- an increase in the natural tendency of the blood to clot, such as after surgery
- damage to the wall of the vein.

Long periods of immobility, such as those experienced during air or road **travel** or while **bedridden**, are a common cause of slow blood flow. Other causes include compression of a vein by the fetus during **pregnancy** or by a tumour. **Leg injury** may also cause a clot to form in the deep veins of the leg.

WHAT ARE THE SYMPTOMS?

A blood clot in a deep vein may produce:
- pain or tenderness in the calf of the leg
- swelling of the lower leg or thigh
- enlarged veins beneath the skin.

WHAT MIGHT BE DONE?

To confirm the diagnosis you may have **Doppler ultrasound scanning** to measure blood flow through the veins and sometimes a **venogram**, in which dye is injected into a vein and then X-rays are taken to reveal blood clots. A sample of your blood may be taken and analyzed to see how easily it clots.

WHAT IS THE TREATMENT?

■ **Thrombolytic drugs** are used to **dissolve** the blood clot in the vein and reduce the risk of a pulmonary embolism.

■ Injections of **anticoagulants** are administered to **prevent** further clots. Although treatment can take place in the hospital, you may be able to self-administer anticoagulant drugs at home.

■ Rarely, the clot is removed surgically.

After you have had the initial treatment, your doctor will prescribe drugs to reduce the risk that the condition will recur.

CAN IT BE PREVENTED?

■ If there is a high risk, low doses of short-acting anticoagulant drugs will probably be given before and after any surgery, to prevent the blood from clotting.

■ Your doctor may also advise you to wear special elastic stockings for a few days after the operation to help maintain blood flow to the veins of the leg.

■ Women who use a **combined oral contraceptive** should stop it two or three months before surgery and will need to switch to an alternative form of contraception.

■ If you are **confined to bed**, you should regularly stretch your legs and flex your ankles. Your doctor may also recommend that you **wear elastic stockings**.

■ **During a flight**, walk around at least once an hour, and, during a long drive, stop regularly to stretch your legs. If you're going to undertake a **long journey** where you'll be sitting most of the time, discuss with your doctor the possibility of **taking a small dose of aspirin** just before, during and after the journey.

ARE THERE COMPLICATIONS?

■ A fragment of the clot may break off and find its way to the lungs. Such a **pulmonary embolism occurs in about 1 in 5 cases of deep vein thrombosis**. The seriousness depends on the size of the fragment. The symptoms associated with pulmonary embolism usually include shortness of breath and chest pain. Rarely, if the clot is large enough to compromise the blood supply to the lungs severely, the condition is life-threatening.

■ In some cases, thrombosis causes permanent damage to the vein and **varicose veins may appear later**.

WHAT IS THE OUTLOOK?

Usually, if deep vein thrombosis is diagnosed in its early stages, treatment with **thrombolytic drugs** and **anticoagulants** is successful. However, if the affected vein is permanently damaged, persistent swelling of the leg or varicose veins may develop and there's a risk that the condition may recur.

See also:
- **Pulmonary embolism p.395**

BLOOD

There are textbooks devoted to this subject but here I only have space for the most common, the **anaemias**, and those that are lodged in the public consciousness, the **leukaemias**. **Haemophilia** is mentioned because it's inherited and **thrombocytopaenia** because it causes the classical rash of **meningitis** and all parents should be on the look out for it should their child be ill with a high temperature. They should know how to recognize the rash of thrombocytopaenia, which is called **purpura**, with tiny haemorrhages in the skin called **petechiae** that remain visible if a glass is pressed onto the skin.

Anaemias

THERE ARE FOUR MAIN TYPES OF ANAEMIA, WHICH IS A DISORDER OF THE BLOOD IN WHICH HAEMOGLOBIN (THE OXYGEN-CARRYING PIGMENT IN RED BLOOD CELLS) IS DEFICIENT OR ABNORMAL.

As the oxygen-carrying power of the blood is reduced, the tissues of the body may not receive sufficient oxygen giving rise to the classical symptoms of anaemia – **paleness**, **tiredness** and **shortness of breath**.

WHAT ARE THE TYPES?

There are four forms of anaemia.

■ By far the most common type is **deficiency anaemia**, one of which results from low levels of **iron** in the body – **iron-deficiency anaemia**. Low levels of other substances, such as vitamin B_{12} and folic acid, can lead to another deficiency anaemia – **megaloblastic anaemia**.

■ **Inherited abnormalities of haemoglobin production**, such as **sickle-cell anaemia** and **thalassaemia**. The haemoglobin is abnormal from shortly after birth, but symptoms of anaemia may not develop until later in childhood.

■ Excessively rapid destruction of red blood cells (haemolysis) is called **haemolytic anaemia**.

■ Failure of the bone marrow to produce enough normal red blood cells and often all the other types of blood cells as well. One form, **aplastic anaemia**, can be congenital or, rarely, can be brought on by exposure to poisons, such as benzene, and certain drugs.

WHAT ARE THE SYMPTOMS?

All anaemias have the same symptoms:
- fatigue and a feeling of faintness
- pale skin
- shortness of breath on mild exertion
- palpitations.

If the anaemia is severe and long term, stress on the heart may result in **chronic heart failure**, with swollen ankles and increasing shortness of breath.

WHAT MIGHT BE DONE?

Tests are aimed at discovering two things.
1. Finding out what kind of anaemia you have.
2. Finding out why you have that particular anaemia, i.e. the cause.

Investigation starts with simple **blood tests** but sometimes more complicated tests, such as taking a specimen of **bone marrow from the hip bone**, may be needed.

WHAT IS THE TREATMENT?

Most anaemias respond well to treatment, although some severe cases may require blood transfusion to ensure immediate improvement. If there is an underlying condition, such as a chronic peptic ulcer, your doctor will treat it too.

IRON-DEFICIENCY ANAEMIA

Iron-deficiency anaemia is the most common form of anaemia. Iron is an essential component of haemoglobin. If insufficient iron is available, the production of haemoglobin and its incorporation into red blood cells in the bone marrow are reduced. As a result, there is less haemoglobin to bind with oxygen in the lungs and carry it to the body tissues. Consequently, the tissues receive insufficient oxygen.

WHAT ARE THE CAUSES?

■ Iron-deficiency anaemia is most commonly caused by the loss of significant amounts of iron through persistent bleeding. Iron-deficiency anaemia occurs mainly in women who experience regular blood loss over a period of time from heavy menstrual bleeding. Persistent loss of blood may also be due to peptic ulcers. The prolonged use of aspirin or long-term use of non-steroidal anti-inflammatory drugs (NSAIDS) are possible causes of bleeding from the stomach lining. In people over the age of 60, a common cause of blood loss is cancer of the bowel. Bleeding in the stomach or upper intestine may go unnoticed, while blood lost from the lower part of the intestine or rectum may be visible in the faeces.
■ The second cause of iron-deficiency anaemia is insufficient iron in the diet. People whose diet contains little or no iron, such as vegans, may be at particular risk of developing this condition.

■ Iron-deficiency anaemia is also more likely to develop when the body needs higher levels of iron than normal and these extra demands are not met by the existing diet. For example, women who are pregnant and children who are growing rapidly, especially adolescents, have an increased risk of developing iron-deficiency anaemia if their diet does not contain plenty of iron.
■ Some other causes of iron-deficiency anaemia include disorders that prevent absorption of iron from the diet. Iron is absorbed from food while it passes through the small intestine and conditions that damage it, such as coeliac disease, may result in iron deficiency.

WHAT ARE THE SYMPTOMS?

You may experience the symptoms of an underlying disorder, along with the general symptoms of anaemia, such as:
- fatigue and a feeling of faintness
- pale skin
- shortness of breath on mild exertion
- palpitations.

You may also have symptoms that are specifically due to a marked deficiency of iron. These include:
- brittle, concave-shaped nails
- painful cracks in the skin at the side of the mouth
- a smooth, reddened tongue.

If your anaemia is severe you may be at risk of chronic heart failure because your heart has to work harder to supply blood to the rest of the body.

WHAT MIGHT BE DONE?

Your doctor will arrange for blood tests to measure the levels of haemoglobin and iron in your blood. If the cause of the iron deficiency is not obvious, other laboratory tests may also be necessary. For example, a sample of faeces may be tested for signs of intestinal bleeding.

Your doctor will treat any underlying disorder such as a stomach ulcer. Iron tablets (syrup for children) or, less commonly, iron injections for several months will replace iron stores. Severe cases of anaemia may require blood transfusion.

MEGALOBLASTIC ANAEMIA

Megaloblastic anaemia is a type of anaemia caused by lack of vitamin B_{12} or folic acid. These two important vitamins play an essential role in the production of healthy red blood cells. Deficiency of either vitamin may lead to megaloblastic anaemia, in which large, abnormal red blood cells (megaloblasts) form in the bone marrow and the production of normal red blood cells is reduced.

WHAT ARE THE CAUSES?

In the West, lack of vitamin B_{12} is rarely due to a dietary deficiency. The problem is usually

TEST

Blood tests

Blood tests are among the most frequently performed medical tests. The chemical composition of the blood can tell a lot about a person's general health and more specific tests can be used to confirm a diagnosis, screen for specific diseases or assess the extent of a disease. Blood samples are easily obtained and are one of the quickest ways for your doctor to confirm a diagnosis or evaluate your health. Some common blood tests are explained below.

Blood cell tests

Blood is composed of three main types of cell: red blood cells, which contain the oxygen-carrying pigment known as haemoglobin; white blood cells, which help defend the body against disease; and platelets, which are cells that help blood clot. Blood cell tests look at the numbers and composition of these cells and can help doctors diagnose diseases of the blood, such as anaemia, or bone marrow, such as leukaemia. Blood tests can also show evidence of infection or inflammation because both cause the number of white blood cells in the blood to rise.

due to an autoimmune disorder, in which antibodies damage the stomach lining and prevent it from forming intrinsic factor, which is vital for absorption of vitamin B_{12} from food in the intestines. The resulting anaemia, called pernicious anaemia, tends to run in families and is more common in women and in people with other autoimmune disorders. Intestinal disorders, such as coeliac disease, or surgery on the stomach can also interfere with vitamin B_{12} absorption.

Folic acid deficiency is often due to a poor diet. People who abuse alcohol are at particular risk because alcohol interferes with the absorption of folic acid. Pregnant women may also be at risk because folic acid requirements are higher in pregnancy. Disorders causing a rapid turnover of cells, including severe psoriasis, may also cause folic acid deficiency. In rare cases, the deficiency is a side effect of certain drugs, such as anticonvulsants and anticancer drugs.

WHAT ARE THE SYMPTOMS?

The initial symptoms of megaloblastic anaemia, which are common to all anaemias, develop slowly and may include:

- fatigue and a feeling of faintness
- pale skin
- shortness of breath on mild exertion
- palpitations.

These symptoms of megaloblastic anaemia may worsen over time. Although lack of folic acid does not produce additional symptoms, lack of vitamin B$_{12}$ may eventually damage the nervous system, possibly leading to:

- tingling of the hands and feet
- weakness and loss of balance
- loss of memory and confusion.

WHAT MIGHT BE DONE?

The diagnosis requires blood tests to look for megaloblasts and to measure the levels of vitamin B$_{12}$ and folic acid. You may also have a bone marrow aspiration and biopsy to obtain tissue samples for further examination.

Megaloblastic anaemia caused by an inability to absorb vitamin B$_{12}$ may be improved by treating the underlying disorder, but some people, such as those with pernicious anaemia and malabsorption caused by surgery, need lifelong monthly injections of vitamin B$_{12}$. Symptoms should begin to subside within days, but existing damage to the nervous system may be irreversible.

If megaloblastic anaemia is caused by an inadequate diet, the condition usually disappears with an improved diet and a short course of folic acid tablets.

SICKLE-CELL ANAEMIA

Sickle-cell anaemia is an inherited condition caused by an abnormal form of haemoglobin in the blood. The inheritance is recessive; that is, both parents carry an abnormal gene but are themselves healthy. The anaemia that results from the blood condition is not present at birth but develops in the first six months. Sickle-cell anaemia is more common in people of African descent.

WHAT ARE THE CAUSES?

Haemoglobin is the protein contained in red cells in the blood. It picks up oxygen from the blood and carries it to various parts of the body. Sickle-cell anaemia occurs when the abnormal haemoglobin causes the red blood cells to become sickle-shaped as a result of low oxygen levels. This may lead to a sickle-cell crisis, involving severe joint and abdominal pain. Immediate medical attention is needed.

WHAT ARE THE SYMPTOMS?

People with sickle-cell anaemia may have the following symptoms:

- anaemia
- fatigue
- mild jaundice – the whites of the eyes may be slightly yellowed
- pain in the limbs and abdomen
- susceptibility to infection leading to frequent colds and illnesses.

WHAT MIGHT BE DONE?

It is essential for people with sickle-cell anaemia to be fully immunized against all infectious diseases and to take any prescribed vitamin supplements. Some people may need to take penicillin regularly to prevent certain bacterial infections. A sickle-cell crisis may be precipitated by strenuous exercise, particularly in the cold and damp, and this should be avoided. If a sickle-cell crisis occurs, it will be treated with painkilling drugs.

As sickle-cell anaemia is inherited, it is important for potential carriers to seek genetic counselling before deciding to have a baby. A blood test will show if the prospective parents are carriers of the disease.

THALASSAEMIA

Thalassaemia is a form of genetically inherited anaemia. It occurs mostly in people from the Mediterranean area but it can also affect people from India and Southeast Asia. Thalassaemia can be passed on to a child if both parents carry the faulty gene.

In thalassaemia, the body cannot make normal haemoglobin, the substance in the blood that makes the cells red and carries oxygen through the body. The problem reveals itself when a baby is about three months old with symptoms of severe anaemia.

WHAT ARE THE SYMPTOMS?

Thalassaemia causes the following symptoms:

- fatigue
- breathlessness
- pallor of the lips, tongue, hands and feet
- loss of appetite accompanied by a swollen abdomen.

WHAT MIGHT BE DONE?

Treatment for thalassaemia requires regular blood transfusions, usually every 6–8 weeks, to prevent severe anaemia from developing. The spleen is also sometimes removed, reducing the need for frequent transfusions. If a person with thalassaemia has too many transfusions, iron can build up in the body and damage the liver, pancreas and heart. There is now a drug available that helps the body get rid of excess iron; the treatment is sometimes carried out overnight by means of a continuous injection into the skin.

If you are from a group particularly susceptible to the disease, you and your partner may wish to seek genetic counselling before trying to conceive to find out if one or both of you might be a carrier of the gene responsible for thalassaemia.

See also:
- **Malabsorption p.365**

Haemophilia

NORMALLY A CUT STOPS BLEEDING WITHIN 10 MINUTES UNLESS IT IS VERY SERIOUS. IN HAEMOPHILIA, AN INHERITED DEFICIENCY OF BLOOD CLOTTING FACTORS DUE TO ABNORMAL GENES, EVEN A SMALL CUT MAY BLEED FOR HOURS OR DAYS, AND THERE MAY BE EPISODES OF SPONTANEOUS BLEEDING.

The much rarer **Christmas disease** has similar features and is named after the person in whom the disease was first diagnosed. Both conditions affect only **males.**

WHAT ARE THE CAUSES?

Haemophilia and Christmas disease are both due to a deficiency of a protein involved in blood clotting. In haemophilia, the deficient protein is **Factor VIII**; in Christmas disease, the protein is **Factor IX**. In both these

conditions, the deficiency is the result of a faulty gene. The particular gene involved is different in the two disorders.

In both disorders, the abnormal gene is located on an X chromosome (X- or sex-linked inheritance). Women do not develop the disease because they have two X chromosomes and the normal gene on the other X chromosome compensates for the abnormal gene. Men with the abnormal gene do develop the disease because they have only

one X chromosome (the other is a Y chromosome) and so do not have a normal copy of the gene to compensate for the abnormal one. Women, however, may pass on the faulty gene to their children. Each child, male or female, has a 1 in 2 chance of inheriting the faulty gene.

In one-third of all cases, the conditions are due to a spontaneous gene abnormality and there is no family history of haemophilia or Christmas disease.

WHAT ARE THE SYMPTOMS?

The symptoms are highly variable, and their severity depends on how much Factor VIII or IX is actually produced. The symptoms usually develop in infancy and include:

● easy bruising, even after minor injury
● sudden, painful swelling of muscles and joints due to internal bleeding
● prolonged bleeding after an injury or a minor surgical operation
● blood in the urine.

Without treatment, prolonged episodes of bleeding into the joints may result in long-term damage and, eventually, may lead to **deformity** of the joints.

WHAT MIGHT BE DONE?

The doctor will arrange for tests to see how long your blood takes to clot and to measure the level of Factor VIII or IX.

The aim of treatment is to maintain the clotting factors at a high enough level to prevent bleeding. If you have a severe form of either condition, you will probably need regular **intravenous injections of Factor VIII or IX** to boost the levels of these factors in the blood. If you have a mild form of either condition, you may need injections only after an injury or before surgery. You may also be prescribed **desmopressin**, which contains **pituitary hormone**, to boost levels of Factor VIII. Some people develop antibodies to Factor VIII supplements, which makes treatment difficult. These people may need to take an immunosuppressant drug to destroy the antibodies.

WHAT IS THE OUTLOOK?

If you have haemophilia or Christmas disease, you can lead an active life but need to avoid sustaining any injuries. Activities such as swimming, running and walking are beneficial, but contact sports, such as wrestling and football, should be avoided. Regular dental care is necessary to avoid the risk of bleeding from inflamed gums.

If you have a family history of either disorder, you should obtain medical advice when planning a pregnancy.

Leukaemia

IN EVERY TYPE OF LEUKAEMIA (BONE MARROW CANCER), ABNORMAL OR VERY IMMATURE WHITE BLOOD CELLS MULTIPLY RAPIDLY AND ACCUMULATE WITHIN THE BONE MARROW, WHERE ALL TYPES OF BLOOD CELL ARE NORMALLY PRODUCED.

The usual production of normal white blood cells, normal red blood cells and platelets within the bone marrow is reduced by the invading cancerous white cells leading to symptoms of **anaemia** and **purpura** (bleeding under the skin that may appear as unprovoked bruising). Leukaemia may therefore show up as anaemia. Other symptoms may include weight loss, fever, night sweats, excessive bleeding and recurrent infections.

In most of the leukaemias, the cancerous white blood cells spread, causing enlargement of the lymph nodes (glands), liver and spleen.

WHAT ARE THE TYPES?

The two main types of leukaemia are **acute leukaemia**, in which the symptoms develop rapidly, and **chronic leukaemia**, in which symptoms may take years to develop.

1. Adults may develop either type but children usually have the acute form. Acute leukaemia can be divided into acute lymphoblastic and acute myeloid leukaemia, depending on which type of white blood cell is involved.
2. Chronic leukaemia is also divided into two types: chronic lymphocytic leukaemia and chronic myeloid leukaemia.

HOW IS IT DIAGNOSED?

Leukaemia may be diagnosed from blood tests and examination of the bone marrow.

WHAT IS THE TREATMENT?

■ Treatment is tailored to each kind of leukaemia and often to each individual case.
■ Chemotherapy is usually given, often as combinations or "cocktails" of several drugs.
■ In some cases, radiotherapy is given.
■ Blood transfusions are sometimes necessary.
■ In some cases, a bone marrow transplant will be done, provided a suitable donor is found.

WHAT IS THE OUTLOOK?

The prognosis varies depending on the type of leukaemia and its severity. For instance, chronic lymphocytic leukaemia may run a long, benign course and need little radical treatment.

Treatment of leukaemia in children is a success story. Due to decades of intensive research into chemotherapeutic regimens, it's fair to say that the majority of children will be successfully treated.

TREATMENT

Bone marrow transplants

To perform a bone marrow transplant, cells in the centre of certain bones are collected from a living donor and are then transfused directly into one of the recipient's veins after his or her existing bone marrow has been destroyed. Alternatively, cells may be collected from the recipient's own bone marrow during a period when his or her underlying disease is in remission and frozen for later use. The stored bone marrow may then be thawed and used to replace abnormal bone marrow in the recipient's body if disease recurs.

Thrombocytopaenia

Thrombocytopaenia is a reduced level of cells called platelets in the blood. Platelets are necessary for blood to clot normally, therefore platelet deficiency causes bleeding into the skin and internal organs. Bleeding into the skin causes bruising and a rash called purpura where there are tiny haemorrhages (petechiae) into the skin. There are many causes of thrombocytopaenia but I wish to mention only one here, meningitis.

Meningitis

■ Thrombocytopaenia may be an early complication of meningitis and shows up in the skin as a purpuric rash.

■ The rash is simple to distinguish from all others: because it's caused by small haemorrhages in the skin, it therefore DOESN'T DISAPPEAR ON APPLYING PRESSURE as nearly all other rashes do.

■ If your child is ill with a high temperature and a rash appears, use a glass to press down on the skin. If the rash remains, take your child immediately to hospital.

■ The thrombocytopaenia of meningitis will correct itself when the infection is treated. It needs no specific treatment.

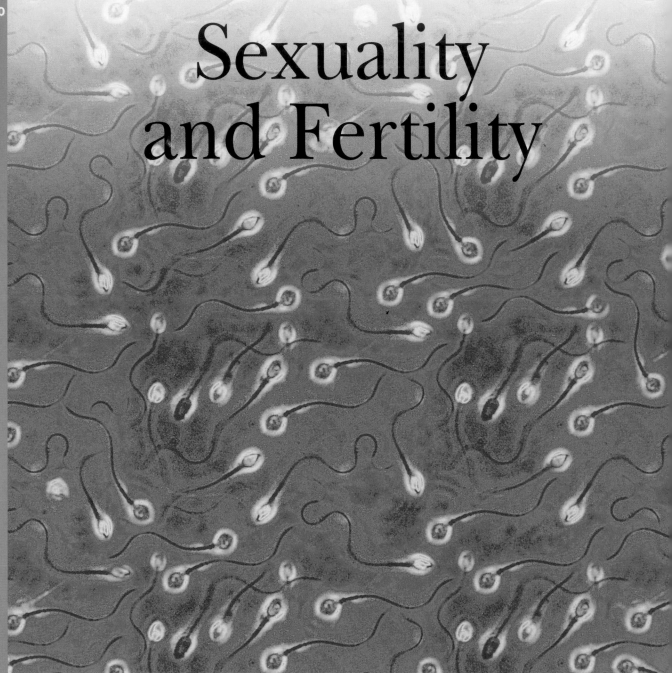

Sexuality and Fertility

Image shows a computer artwork of human sperm

Miriam's overview

This topic is so huge, taking in as it does the whole of gynaecology, I hardly know where to begin. The span is the whole of reproductive life and beyond, starting at perhaps the age of 10 with the appearance of menstruation and stretching to the end of our lives in the case of our sexuality.

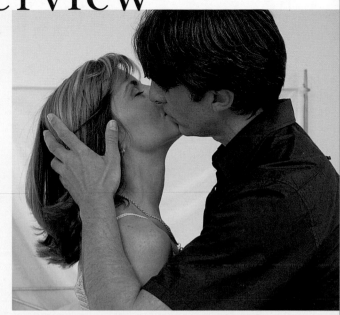

Oh yes, sex may diminish in importance and frequency as we age and performance may slump, but it remains the greatest source of comfort and companionship there is until we die.

Indeed all the news on sex is good. In an American study 80-year-old women confessed to still being very keen on sex. All they lacked was a suitable partner.

As we entered the millennium a very interesting finding emerged from demographic research. It revealed that 1 in 6 girls is menstruating by the age of 8, and 1 in 14 boys of a similar age is producing sperm.

I can remember thinking when the average age of the menarche fell to 11.5 years, it couldn't get any younger, but it has, with implications for society in general, and for teachers and parents in particular.

If your daughter is fertile at the age of 8 when do you start sex education? If your child might be sexually active at 9 or 10 when do you give them advice on contraception? Fertile 8-year-olds raises the spectre of parents aged 10 or even less. This possibility forces us to change our approach to burgeoning sexuality in our children.

"all the *news* on sex *is good*"

Two new vaginal infections have received, rightly in my view, much attention of late. One is usually self-induced, albeit unwittingly – bacterial vaginosis – due to over-zealous personal hygiene with vaginal deodorants, cleansers and putting disinfectants in bath water. They all change the protective bacterial population of the vagina, leading to unhealthy overgrowth of certain bacteria with a characteristic unpleasant odour. Only antibiotics will bring it under control.

The second is chlamydia, often a hidden infection because it's symptomless, especially in men, and used to be difficult to diagnose. Chlamydia can cause pelvic inflammatory disease and subsequent infertility. When this was realized, research focused on devising a reliable diagnostic test so that treatment can be started before any damage is done.

We tend to take for granted that our wishes will be considered when facing mutilating surgery such as mastectomy and hysterectomy but as little as five years ago it wasn't so, and in pockets around the country it still isn't.

In the last 10 years we've seen a revolution in patient power that's been paralleled by a more humane approach by surgeons. In a matter of a few years mastectomy became largely a thing of the past when research showed that the less disfiguring lumpectomy had the same cure rate.

And when it was realized a woman could retain her uterus, women drove surgeons to question hysterectomy as a routine (and often unnecessary) operation in middle age. Suddenly women were directing their surgeons to leave behind their ovaries and cervix – crucial if you wish to remain orgasmic – when hysterectomy was discussed.

For the first time ever, the cure rate for breast cancer is improving and, in the UK, it's rising faster than anywhere else in Europe. Tamoxifen, an anticancer drug, is single-handedly responsible for this turnaround. Given routinely to all women whose cancers are sensitive to oestrogen it will control the cancer and prevent spread and regrowth. There's probably never been as powerful an anticancer drug.

Most women are aware of breast self-examination but few men are aware of testicular self-examination or the importance of doing it to detect testicular cancer early, when the cure rate is over 90 percent.

Nor are many men aware that there is a screening test, PSA, for cancer of the prostate and that it's available on the NHS to men who have prostatic symptoms.

INSIDE
your reproductive system

Male reproductive system

The external parts of the male reproductive system include the **penis**, **scrotum** and the two **testicles**, which hang in the scrotum. Behind each testicle is a coiled tube known as the **epididymis**, which leads to another tube called the **vas deferens**. The top of each vas deferens is joined by a duct that drains from the seminal vesicle. These join the **urethra**, where they are surrounded by the **prostate gland**, and the urethra passes through the penis to the outside.

After puberty, the two testicles manufacture sperm continuously at the rate of about 125 million sperm a day. Sperm mature in the **epididymis**, and travel from there through the vas deferens before ejaculation. On this journey sperm are mixed with secretions from other glands to form semen. Semen contains about 50 million sperm per millilitre.

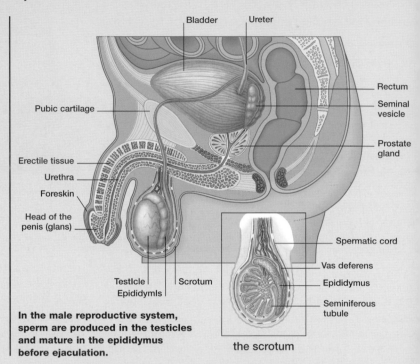

In the male reproductive system, sperm are produced in the testicles and mature in the epididymus before ejaculation.

the scrotum

Female reproductive system

The external organs of the female reproductive system consist of the **clitoris** and the **labia**, which surround it – together they are known as the **vulva**. Inside the labia are the entrances to the **vagina** and the **urethra**. In the lower part of the abdomen are the two **ovaries**. These organs store eggs and, following puberty, release them into the **fallopian tubes**, which in turn lead to the **uterus**. The neck of the uterus, called the **cervix**, projects down into the vagina.

Fertilization of an egg by a sperm usually takes place in one of the fallopian tubes, after which the fertilized egg travels down the tube into the uterus. It implants in the uterine lining and continues development there.

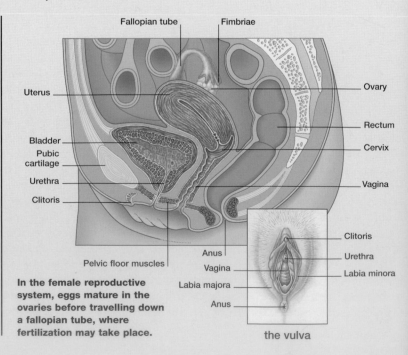

In the female reproductive system, eggs mature in the ovaries before travelling down a fallopian tube, where fertilization may take place.

the vulva

THE BREASTS

I recommend breast awareness (see box, below) for all women, at all stages of their lives. Further checks are advisable for older women, who have a higher risk of breast cancer, and for women in other high-risk groups – those with breast cancer in the family, for instance. There's now clear evidence that early detection by screening cuts down the number of women dying from breast cancer. Studies in Sweden and the US show that screening can reduce deaths from breast cancer by up to one-third in women between the ages of 50 and 65. Early detection automatically means earlier treatment and increases the chances of a full recovery if a lump turns out to be breast cancer. Early detection also means you have greater choice over how your cancer will be treated. It's understandable to feel anxious about having regular mammograms. However, the chances are you'll be one of the 99 women out of every 100 routinely screened who are found not to have cancer.

Breast pain

BREAST PAIN, OR MASTALGIA, IS PAIN OR DISCOMFORT IN ONE OR BOTH BREASTS. SIXTY PERCENT OF WOMEN SUFFER SOME KIND OF BREAST DISCOMFORT. BREAST PAIN CAN BE DIVIDED INTO TWO TYPES: CYCLICAL, WHICH IS ASSOCIATED WITH MENSTRUAL PERIODS, AND NON-CYCLICAL.

Non-cyclical pain may originate in the breast or in the nearby muscles and joints, in which case it is not true breast pain.

CYCLICAL BREAST PAIN

The most common kind of breast pain is associated with the menstrual cycle, and is nearly always related to fluctuations in hormone levels, which every woman experiences as part of the cycle. Pain is probably related to the sensitivity of breast tissue to hormones and this can differ within a breast and between your two breasts. Hormones aren't the whole story, however, because in the majority of women the pain is more severe in one breast than in the other. Most women experience some degree of breast pain when their breasts become sensitive just prior to menstruation. Some women, however, may experience soreness and tenderness starting with ovulation, in the middle of the cycle, and continuing for about two weeks until menstruation takes place. Others find that this premenstrual soreness becomes even worse after the birth of their first child.

WHAT IS THE TREATMENT?

■ **Evening primrose oil**: this natural remedy has to be taken in a large dose (3g daily) to be effective. It also has to be taken over a long period of time since its effects build up slowly; in most cases, it takes as long as four months to see if there are benefits. Notwithstanding the large dose and prolonged usage, evening primrose oil has very few side effects, which is why it should be the first-line treatment of choice.

■ **Danazol**: this drug, which blocks ovulation, has a success rate of nearly 80 percent, making it the ideal second-line treatment. Despite its success, it is not suitable for everyone: some women may experience side effects such as weight gain and irregular periods. Danazol is given in a dose of 200mg daily for two months; if this is effective, the dose will be gradually reduced.

■ **Tamoxifen**: this drug may be prescribed for women with severe breast pain. The usual dose in this case is 10mg, which may cause hot flushes but does not cause more severe side effects that are seen with higher doses. Tamoxifen may be used continuously or may be restricted to the second half of the menstrual cycle.

NON-CYCLICAL BREAST PAIN

There are two types of non-cyclical breast pain: true breast pain, which comes from the

Breast awareness

Women used to be advised to examine their breasts every month at the same point in their menstrual cycle. However, this made some women anxious and others felt guilty if they didn't do it or responsible if there was a problem. Now doctors are advising women that it is more important for them to be familiar with the shape and texture of their breasts than to examine them on a regular basis. This "breast awareness" means that you will be able to spot any unexpected changes in your breasts and can consult your doctor straight away.

In order to be breast aware, you need to know what your breasts look like. Try to get into the habit of looking at your breasts in the mirror from time to time – you can easily do this after a bath or shower or before you get dressed.

Raise your arms over your head and notice how your breasts move, so that you know what is normal for you. Possible changes to watch out for include a difference in the shape of the breast, such as puckering or pulling of the skin, areas of swelling in the breast or changes in the nipple, such as puckering.

You also need to be aware of how your breasts feel. So that you can identify changes, feel your breasts every day for several days until you are aware of their usual texture and how it changes throughout your menstrual cycle. Most women's breasts are a bit lumpy, especially in the days before a period. After your period lumpiness may lessen and disappear altogether.

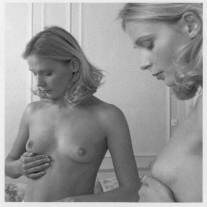

If you do note any unusual changes in your breasts, see your doctor as soon as possible. It's normal to feel anxious, but remember that 9 out of 10 breast lumps turn out not to be cancerous.

breast but is unrelated to the menstrual cycle, and pain that is felt in the region of the breast but is actually coming from somewhere else. This latter kind nearly always involves the muscles, bones or joints and for this reason it is called **musculoskeletal pain**. Two-thirds of non-cyclical mastalgia is pain of musculoskeletal origin. Rarely what appears to be breast pain is due to underlying **lung** or **gallbladder disease**.

TRUE NON-CYCLICAL BREAST PAIN
Some benign breast conditions may be associated with true breast pain. Burning or stabbing pains centred around or under the nipple may be due to dilatation of the ducts (duct ectasia) and tend to run an intermittent, though harmless, course. They may also be due to periductal mastitis, a condition that affects young women, the majority of whom are smokers.

A tender spot with occasional stabbing pain or an ache is common. Its cause is unknown, but it is no reason for anxiety. The pain can be relieved by an injection of local anaesthetic mixed with prednisone to help to reduce any inflammation. A cyst occasionally underlies a tender spot; removal of fluid from the cyst can ease the pain.

PAIN OF NON-BREAST ORIGIN
Pain originating in the chest wall or spine may be felt in the breast area. The most usual cause is a form of **arthritis**, called **costochondritis**, which affects the ends of the ribs where they join the breastbone; this condition is called **Tietze's syndrome**. If your pain is worse when you take a deep breath or press on your breastbone and ribs, it's likely to be costochondritis. Taking a painkiller, such as paracetamol, or a non-steroidal anti-inflammatory drug (NSAID), such as ibuprofen, is often effective.

Breast lumps

BREAST LUMPS ARE ANY MASSES OR SWELLINGS IN THE BREAST TISSUE. WHEN YOU FIND A LUMP IN YOUR BREAST, DOCTORS USE MANY INVESTIGATIVE TECHNIQUES TO ARRIVE AT AS SPECIFIC A DIAGNOSIS AS POSSIBLE.

The initial test sequence varies, depending on whether you have found the lump yourself or it has been detected during routine mammogram screening, in which case it may be too small to feel. In all cases, however, a sample of cells or tissue will have to be examined under a microscope to determine whether the lump is malignant. If it is, further tests will be done to assess the precise origin of the tumour and to see if it has spread.

YOUR BILL OF RIGHTS
When you find any lump in your breast, you're entitled to the best possible treatment. You have the right to expect the following things.
■ A prompt referral by your family doctor to a team specializing in the diagnosis and treatment of breast cancer, including a consultant.
■ A firm diagnosis within one week of being examined.

■ The opportunity to have a confirmed diagnosis before consenting to any form of treatment, including surgery.
■ Full information about types of surgery (including breast reconstruction where appropriate) and the role of additional treatments such as radiotherapy, chemotherapy, hormone therapy and so on.
■ A clear and detailed explanation of the aims and benefits of the proposed treatments and any possible side effects, including long-term ones.

HOW IS IT DIAGNOSED?
Your doctor will start the examination by looking at your breasts while you sit with your hands by your sides and then with your arms raised above your head, so that asymmetry between the breasts, nipple retraction (the nipple will appear drawn in), difference in level between nipples or dimpling of the skin

can easily be seen. You'll then be asked to lie back with your arms above your head while the doctor examines your breasts carefully, feeling each quadrant of both breasts with the flat of the hand.

The aim is to decide whether there's an obvious lump and if the breasts are just generally lumpy – and many are!

FINE-NEEDLE ASPIRATION CYTOLOGY (FNAC)
One of the three procedures in assessing a breast lump is **FNAC**. It's used to sample cells from the lump.

Under mammography or ultrasound guidance, a fine needle is inserted painlessly into your lump. If fluid is withdrawn, the lump is a cyst; the fluid can be drawn off and the cyst will disappear. If your lump is solid, a sample of cells is removed and spread on a glass slide for microscopic examination.

CORE NEEDLE BIOPSY
FNAC yields only a tiny sample of cells from breast tissue, so it's impossible to be specific about where they've come from. A core needle biopsy provides a sample of cells from the lump that can be analyzed to make this distinction.
1. Under a local anaesthetic, a special needle with a sheath is painlessly inserted into your lump in order to withdraw a fine core of tissue from it.
2. The sheath is drawn back and some tissue from your lump falls into the notch.
3. The sheath is closed, trapping a tiny core of tissue from your lump inside the notch and the needle is withdrawn.
4. The skin is left virtually intact; although there may be a little bruising afterwards, there's hardly any discomfort.

Fibroadenomas

Common in teenagers and women in their 20s, fibroadenomas are simply over-developed lobules and are completely benign. You don't always need to have one removed, as long as you agree to a further ultrasound scan and examination in six months' time. The majority of women, when offered excision or observation, opt for the latter.

Fibroadenomas can be very large – they vary from pea size to larger than a lemon. While they can grow anywhere in the breast, quite often they're found near the nipple. They feel smooth and firm and quite distinct, and move freely in your breast. Most doctors can recognize one simply by feeling it, but

the diagnosis should be clinched with mammography or ultrasound and fine-needle aspiration cytology (**FNAC**) or core needle biopsy.

Although they are most common in young women, fibroadenomas can occur at any age up to the menopause (or later if you are on **HRT**). Most women who get a fibroadenoma will never get another one, but a few women will have several over a lifetime. It is possible to have more than one at a time or a single large fibroadenoma involving more than one lobule. In very rare cases there may be a tendency for them to run in families.

Mammograms

A mammogram is a low-dose X-ray of the breast. It's such a refined method of imaging the breast that it can pick up small cancers and other abnormalities that neither you nor your doctor can feel.

Why after 50?

Mammograms are not done with the same frequency in all age groups. Breast cancer is comparatively rare in women under 50, so mammograms are recommended only after the age of 50. Women who fall into high-risk groups may be offered yearly mammograms at an earlier age.

What about younger women?

Mammography is less effective in women under 50, since their breast tissue is more dense and abnormalities don't show up so well, but it's still more sensitive than self-examination.

This is why it can be used as a diagnostic tool, to investigate a lump found in physical examination, for example, or to look for further lumps when one has already been found. **Ultrasound scans** may be used to investigate breast lumps found in women aged 35 and below.

How often?

At present, mammography is offered to women over 50 every three years, although there's a continuing debate about this.

Getting the results

After your screening, the films are developed and examined by a radiologist who specializes in interpreting mammograms.

The results usually take only a few days to come through and most women will be told that they're fine and just need regular screening. A small number will be asked to come back for further tests. This can be worrying, but the chances of getting an all-clear are still high.

Although mammograms are good for detecting small lumps, they cannot determine a lump's precise character, so extra tests may be needed to pin that down.

Microcalcifications are tiny deposits of calcium that show up as very fine specks on

a mammogram. They may be quite normal and many women have them but, because they have been occasionally linked with cancer, the radiologist will always mention their presence and you'll wonder why. They're only worrying if they suddenly appear in a cluster in one breast.

If it's your first mammogram, your doctor may wait a year before doing another one to see if there's any change. If the pattern of microcalcifications is very abnormal, a biopsy will be carried out at once.

If a lump is found

If your mammogram shows any kind of lump, further tests will be necessary.

■ If the lump is large enough to feel easily with your fingers, a fine needle can be inserted to draw off some of the cells. This is called **fine-needle aspiration cytology**, or **FNAC**.

■ If the lump is fluid-filled, it's a cyst, which is nearly always perfectly harmless. Your specialist will draw off the fluid with a needle and will usually discard it. A sample will be sent for laboratory tests only rarely.

■ If the lump is solid, some of the cells that have been drawn off will be smeared on a

slide, stained, and examined in the laboratory.

■ If the lump isn't easy to feel, you'll probably have an ultrasound scan to determine whether it's a solid lump or a cyst. Either way it will be investigated with FNAC or cutting-needle biopsy.

When a lump can't be felt, FNAC and core needle biopsy are done with guidance of ultrasound so that the tumour can be precisely located.

Putting you in the picture

To have a mammogram done:
1. You'll be asked to strip to the waist and remove any deodorant or talc from your breasts. The reason for this is that they may show up as microcalcifications.
2. You will then be asked to stand in front of the machine and the radiologist will compress your breast between two plates. The procedure is not without a degree of discomfort, particularly if the plates are cold. The sensation lasts no more than 10 or 15 seconds, however, so it's easily bearable.
3. Two views of each breast will usually be taken. The radiologist compresses each breast in turn between two plates so that a good image is obtained.

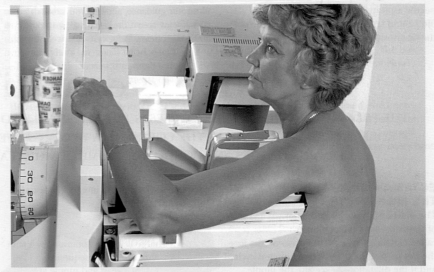

Having a mammogram takes only a few minutes and is not painful, although some women may find the procedure uncomfortable.

OPEN BIOPSY

This kind of biopsy is an alternative to a core needle biopsy. As the name implies, the skin is cut open to reveal the lump, which is then removed with a margin of healthy breast tissue. In practical terms, open biopsy nearly always

means removing the whole lump – **lumpectomy**. It is always carried out in hospital under a general anaesthetic.

Not every woman over age 30 with an obvious breast lump should have it removed. The aim is to diagnose the lump – those

that are benign are in the main left alone and not excised.

Analyzing the biopsy

The biopsy or lump is sent to the pathology laboratory where it's very finely sliced,

VAGINAL INFECTIONS

Vaginal infections are important because some of them have the habit of "ascending", meaning they travel upwards through the uterus and into the fallopian tubes and thence even into the pelvis. Here they can give rise to **pelvic inflammatory disease** (PID), which can result in **chronic pelvic pain** and more alarmingly, infertility.

A vaginal infection due to chlamydia or gonorrhoea therefore must be eradicated by vigorous treatment not just for you but for your partner too. Many women with chronic infections are being reinfected by their largely symptomless partners. Men must accept this and be assessed and treated at the same time.

Chronic pelvic pain

CHRONIC PELVIC PAIN IS LONG-TERM PAIN IN THE LOWER ABDOMEN OR PELVIS. THE PAIN MUST HAVE LASTED FOR AT LEAST SIX MONTHS AND ISN'T LINKED TO MENSTRUATION OR SEXUAL INTERCOURSE. ABOUT 1 IN 6 WOMEN HAS CHRONIC PELVIC PAIN.

Recent studies suggest that chronic pelvic pain may even be more common than low back pain.

It's hard to assess the cost, but in the UK about £160 million a year is spent on medical investigations into chronic pelvic pain, and women with this condition may need several days off work every month.

There's much that can be done to relieve their misery, yet women often feel they have to fight to get anything done.

Most GPs do refer women with undiagnosed chronic pelvic pain to a gynaecologist but, even so, women often feel dismissed and find that their symptoms are not taken seriously.

Armed with some information, it's important for every woman to insist on investigation and treatment because the alternative may be the inability to have children some time in the future.

WHAT ARE THE CAUSES?

Several conditions may give rise to the condition, including **endometriosis**, **irritable bowel syndrome**, **pelvic inflammatory disease** (see opposite) and **musculoskeletal damage**.

Women are often aware that stress increases their pain, and some researchers have shown that deep-rooted psychological trauma, such as sexual abuse, may reveal itself as pelvic pain.

Sometimes several of these factors may be present at the same time, making investigation and diagnosis of chronic pelvic pain quite difficult.

HOW IS IT DIAGNOSED?

You may need a specialist to sort out the cause, so I advise asking for a referral to a gynaecologist early. Don't wait and suffer.

LAPAROSCOPY

Your gynaecologist will probably suggest an investigation called diagnostic laparoscopy (see box, left). It can be done as a day case under a general anaesthetic, using a thin viewing instrument inserted through a small incision just below your navel. This allows the gynaecologist to see your pelvic organs directly.

To see the pelvic organs clearly, carbon dioxide gas is pumped into the abdominal cavity so that the abdominal wall is lifted out of the way.

Don't be surprised if it takes you a week or two to recover fully. Relatively minor complications, such as nausea and pain, occur after about 3 in 100 laparoscopies. More serious complications are rare but bowel perforation or blood vessel damage, requiring further surgery and a longer hospital stay, occur after about 1 in 500 laparoscopies.

ULTRASOUND

Adhesions (scar tissue) and endometriosis don't show up clearly on an ultrasound scan, so ultrasound isn't much use in investigating pelvic pain unless an ovarian cyst is suspected.

MRI

Magnetic resonance imaging (MRI) can help identify endometriosis.

WHAT MIGHT BE DIAGNOSED?
ENDOMETRIOSIS AND ADHESIONS
The purpose of the laparoscopy is to look for endometriosis and adhesions resulting from

TEST

Laparoscopy

Certain conditions can be diagnosed accurately only if the organs are directly seen. Laparoscopy is a procedure that enables a doctor to see the inside of the abdominal cavity and organs such as the gallbladder, liver and uterus through an instrument called a laparoscope. The most common use of laparoscopy is in gynaecology, where it is commonly used for the following:
- tubal surgery, including sterilization
- infertility investigations
- ovarian cysts
- fibroids
- ectopic pregnancy
- laparoscopic hysterectomy
- bladder operations for stress incontinence.

How is it done?
■ The procedure is usually done under a general anaesthetic. A tiny cut is made in the abdomen, usually just below the navel so that no scar is visible afterwards. A needle is inserted into the abdomen and carbon dioxide gas is pumped into the abdominal cavity so that organs can be visualized.

■ The laparoscope is passed in and the doctor can angle it to get a clear view. If other instruments are being used, these are inserted through a second incision above the pubic line.

■ The procedure takes about 30–40 minutes and you will have one or two stitches in the skin. After about two hours, depending on the reason for the laparoscopy, you should be allowed to go home.

You may have a little discomfort from any gas that remains in your pelvic cavity, and the incision site may be sore. However, laparoscopy is very safe and you should have few problems.

pelvic infection, but in over 50 percent of cases no cause for the pain is found. Even when adhesions or endometriosis are detected, gynaecologists disagree about whether either of these conditions is really the cause of the pain.

IRRITABLE BOWEL SYNDROME (IBS)
IBS can be detected reliably using a checklist of symptoms called the Rome Criteria.

This is a set of symptoms that includes pain relieved by defecation, bloating and a change in bowel habit associated with pain.

MUSCULOSKELETAL CAUSES OF PAIN
If the pain is worse on moving and bending, musculoskeletal causes of pain, such as a trapped nerve, may be the cause. A skilled physiotherapist, chiropractor or osteopath can offer the best help if this is the case. Your doctor may offer you an appointment with a psychologist, too.

If your gynaecologist fails to pinpoint the cause of your pain, it is possible that it may not be of gynaecological origin. Unfortunately, gynaecologists aren't always well trained to detect non-gynaecological causes of pelvic pain. In one study of women attending a gynaecology clinic with pain, half had symptoms of IBS, but they were less likely than the other women to receive a diagnosis and more likely to have pain persisting 12 months later.

But you need to get to the bottom of it, so if your gynaecologist can't find the cause of the pain, seek referral to a gastroenterologist.

WHAT IS THE TREATMENT?
It depends on the diagnosis.

■ Endometriosis can be removed surgically, or treated by suppressing the ovaries using drugs such as the **combined oral contraceptive** or a group of drugs called **GnRH analogues**.

■ However, endometriosis is a recurrent disease and some women eventually choose **hysterectomy** with removal of their ovaries. This relieves the symptoms but does not cure the endometriosis.

■ Surgical division of adhesions works for some but not all women. Quite often the adhesions simply grow back again in time.

■ IBS often responds well to dietary changes or **antispasmodic drugs** and **bulking agents**.

■ Musculoskeletal pain is probably best treated with painkilling drugs, particularly non-steroidal anti-inflammatory drugs (NSAIDs), manipulation and a graded exercise programme from a physiotherapist.

■ If psychological factors play a part, they need to be recognized and sympathetically addressed alongside any other treatment.

DRUGS TO COMBAT PAIN
For some women, no clear diagnosis is reached. Nonetheless, much can be done to relieve symptoms.

■ The most effective painkillers are NSAIDs such as ibuprofen. They may be used in combination with other types of painkillers such as paracetamol or dihydrocodeine.

■ Drugs such as **amitriptyline** (an antidepressant) or **carbamazepine** (an anticonvulsant) can be used for chronic pelvic pain; they are also effective in conditions such as acute low back pain. This is because they have an effect on pain in addition to their other effects.

■ Some women find pain management, with careful pacing of activities and fitness training, can help them to live with chronic pelvic pain. And many derive great comfort and support from self-help groups. In many women the pain resolves on its own.

> **See also:**
> • **Endometriosis p.254**
> • **Irritable bowel syndrome p.362**
> • **MRI p.409**
> • **Ultrasound scanning p.277**

Pelvic inflammatory disease

PELVIC INFLAMMATORY DISEASE (PID) IS GRUMBLING INFECTION OR INFLAMMATION OF ANY OF THE PELVIC ORGANS – THE UTERUS, FALLOPIAN TUBES AND OVARIES. PELVIC INFLAMMATORY DISEASE IS A POWERFUL THREAT TO FERTILITY.

Irrevocable scarring of the fallopian tubes and ovaries is the most serious complication because it causes sterility. Other complications include **painful intercourse** (dyspareunia). At one time, the most common cause of PID was tuberculosis. Now it is **chlamydia**. There is a little evidence that the use of **intrauterine contraceptive devices** (IUDs) may be a contributing factor.

WHAT ARE THE SYMPTOMS?
■ Abdominal pain.
■ Back pain.
■ Persistent menstrual-like cramps.
■ Vaginal spotting of blood.
■ Tiredness.
■ Pain during and after intercourse.
■ Foul-smelling vaginal discharge.
■ Flu-like symptoms of fever and chills.
■ Sub-fertility or infertility.

PID must be treated early to prevent long-term problems. The symptoms can be those of an **acute infection** with fever, nausea, discomfort and pain, which should alert you to the fact that there is something wrong. A chronic infection may only cause recurrent mild pain and sometimes backache. But both forms must be investigated. Don't wait for it to go away, see your doctor as soon as possible. If you have an IUD, go to your clinic immediately.

WHAT WILL THE DOCTOR DO?
■ You will be examined and tested to identify the organism causing the infection. Your doctor will probably prescribe antibiotics and bed rest. Eat well and don't have sexual intercourse during the course of treatment. If antibiotics are not suitable for you, you may have to have other treatment.

■ If PID develops into a chronic infection, it can be difficult to eradicate. You may need investigative laparoscopy (see box, opposite) to confirm the diagnosis. In severe cases, for a long-term infection, **hysterectomy** with removal of the fallopian tubes can be the only course of action, although you should go into the alternatives fully before agreeing to this operation.

WHAT CAN I DO?
■ Don't let any vaginal discharge continue for any length of time without full investigation and treatment. Because PID can recur, have a full check-up to confirm that your infection has been completely eradicated.

■ If you suspect that you or your partner may have a sexually transmitted disease, go to an STD clinic straight away.

> **See also:**
> • **Chlamydia p.278**
> • **Hysterectomy p.256**

Endometriosis

ENDOMETRIOSIS IS A VERY COMMON CONDITION, DEFINED
AS THE PRESENCE OF CELLS FROM THE LINING OF
THE UTERUS AT OTHER SITES IN THE PELVIS.

The principal route of spread for these "seedlings" is via the fallopian tubes. Deposits find their way to the ovaries, bowel, bladder and the pelvis, forming very small cysts and localized scarring. The seedlings respond to the cyclical changes of ovarian hormones, so bleeding occurs into the cysts when you are menstruating, but the blood cannot escape. The cysts become swollen and tender, and in the ovary may enlarge to 5–6cm (2–3in) in diameter, causing menstrual pain, painful sexual intercourse and generalized pelvic tenderness. Adhesions may form around the cysts, interfering with ovulation and, possibly, conception.

WHAT ARE THE SYMPTOMS?

■ Heavy or abnormal bleeding.
■ Severe abdominal and pelvic pain, often leading to painful intercourse.
■ Severe cramping pain, starting before the period is due and continuing during menstruation, after which it gradually eases.
■ Urinary or bowel pain, including diarrhoea.
■ Fertility problems.

If you are in your late 20s and have been unable to conceive, or if you suffer very painful periods or pain deep in your pelvis during intercourse, you should see your doctor as soon as possible. If you have never suffered from **dysmenorrhoea** (painful periods) before, it is very unlikely to develop in your late 20s without there being a major reason.

WHAT MIGHT THE DOCTOR DO?

The drugs used to treat endometriosis suppress ovulation and menstruation, thus permitting the disease to regress. The drugs include the continuous use of high-dose oestrogens and/or progestogens or drugs, called **GnRH analogues**, to suppress ovarian-stimulating hormones. All these treatments are contraceptive.

Medical treatment of endometriosis is usually only offered to women who are not trying to conceive; it has not been shown to improve fertility rates.

For women wishing to conceive, surgical treatment, usually laparoscopic, includes **diathermy** or **laser vaporization** of the endometriosis deposits (see box, right) and **adhesiolysis** (removal of adhesions).

Radical surgery with removal of the uterus and ovaries (**hysterectomy**) may be necessary in older patients with advanced disease who don't wish to have more children.

NB In vitro fertilization (IVF) should be offered immediately to women trying to conceive who have dense, widespread adhesions that are not amenable to, or recur after, surgery.

SELF-HELP

Join a self-help group where you can share your experience with other women and discuss the latest treatments and side effects of treatment.

See also:
- Dysmenorrhoea p.247
- Hysterectomy p.256
- Infertility p.274
- Laparoscopy p.250

- Dysmenorrhoea p.247
- Hysterectomy p.256
- Infertility p.274
- Laparoscopy p.250

TREATMENT

Laser treatment

Light from a laser beam can cut or destroy tissue or repair damaged tissue by fusing together torn edges. This allows lasers to be used in a number of surgical procedures in place of scalpels, scissors and stitches. Since laser beams can be focused precisely, small sections of tissue can be treated without causing damage to the surrounding tissues.

Laser treatment is commonly used in gynaecological procedures. A laser beam can be directed into the body through an endoscope to remove scar tissue inside the fallopian tubes, which may be a cause of infertility. Lasers are also used to remove cysts that form in the pelvic area due to endometriosis and to destroy abnormal cells on the cervix which, if untreated, may develop into cancer. Similarly, small tumours or pre-cancerous cells in other internal body areas, such as the larynx or inside the digestive tract, can be destroyed by laser beams directed through an endoscope. The technique can also be used to open arteries that have been narrowed by fatty deposits. In ophthalmic surgery, laser beams can be used to seal small tears in the retina, the light-sensitive layer at the back of the eye.

Laser treatment is often used on the skin, especially on the face, for reducing scar tissue and birthmarks, non-cancerous moles, tattoos or wrinkles. The results depend on the extent of the problem but in most cases scarring is minimal, and the appearance of the skin is much improved. External laser treatment can also be used to treat conditions such as spider veins and to remove warts on the skin and genital warts.

Most forms of laser treatment are done under either local or general anaesthesia, depending on the type of surgery and the area to be treated. However, for minor skin conditions, laser treatment causes little discomfort and may be performed without anaesthesia. There may be some swelling, redness and blistering, which usually disappear within a week. Large areas of skin may have to be treated over several sessions.

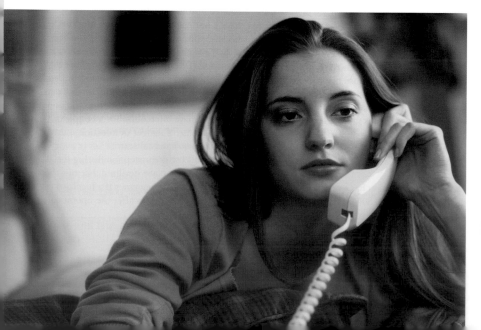

A support group can help women with endometriosis cope with the psychological impact of the condition.

Prolapse of the uterus

PROLAPSE IS WHEN ONE OR SEVERAL PELVIC ORGANS DROP DOWN INTO THE VAGINA.
IF THE PELVIC FLOOR MUSCLES ARE WEAKENED, THE VAGINAL WALLS
BECOME DISPLACED, RESULTING IN A PROLAPSE.

Any of the pelvic organs, including the **uterus**, **bladder**, **rectum**, **bowel** and **urethra**, can prolapse into the vagina, but prolapse of the uterus is the most common.

Depending on the severity, the cervix may drop and actually protrude from the vagina. Prolapse tends to occur in older women, and hardly ever occurs in those who haven't had children.

Pelvic floor muscles can weaken with age, but prolapse is nearly always caused by earlier injury to the pelvic floor muscles **during labour**.

This happens especially if you had a rapid delivery, you were allowed to go on too long in labour or if your babies were on the large side.

To understand what your doctor is talking about these names can be helpful.

■ If the **rectum** bulges into the back of the vaginal wall, it is called a **rectocoele**.
■ When the **urethra** bulges into the front of the vaginal wall, it is called a **urethrocoele**.
■ If the **bladder** drops into the front of the vaginal wall, it is called a **cystocoele**.

WHAT ARE THE SYMPTOMS?
■ Backache.
■ A feeling of something bulging from the vagina; difficulty inserting and removing a tampon.
■ Stress incontinence – leaking urine when you lift a heavy weight, cough or sneeze.
■ With uterine prolapse, a dragging down feeling in the pelvis.
■ With a urethrocoele or a cystocoele, frequent urination and an urgent need to pass urine.
■ With a rectocoele, discomfort on moving the bowels and difficulty in passing a stool.

Don't wait for symptoms to become really troublesome; consult your doctor as soon as possible.

WHAT MIGHT THE DOCTOR DO?
■ Your doctor will give you an internal pelvic examination to confirm a prolapse and to determine which type you have.
■ You'll be asked about the births you've had, whether they were difficult, if your babies were larger than normal, if the second stage of labour lasted a long time and if forceps were used to aid delivery of any of your babies.
■ Being overweight makes a prolapse worse, so you'll be advised to lose weight.
■ If you have a severe prolapse, your doctor will recommend surgery (see box, right). I would always advise going ahead because it will improve your quality of life by controlling incontinence and improving your sexual enjoyment. Surgery works by tightening up all the support structures in your pelvis – a sort of **pelvic face-lift**. Treatment will depend on the type of prolapse and your age.
■ Most prolapse repairs are performed through the vagina and involve a general anaesthetic. Occasionally, the operation may be performed with an epidural anaesthetic, especially if the patient is old and infirm.
■ You will probably stay in hospital for 5–7 days. An outpatient appointment is usually made six weeks later, after which sexual intercourse can be resumed if there are no problems.

SELF-HELP
■ If you suffer from backache, try to avoid standing for long periods at a time. Wear a tight girdle to counteract any dragging feeling you may have in your pelvis.
■ If you are having difficulty with sexual intercourse, you and your partner may need to explore alternative non-penetrative ways of achieving sexual pleasure.
■ Wear panty liners if you are troubled by leakage (stress incontinence). If the leakage becomes worse, see your doctor.
■ The most important preventative treatment is being conscientious about doing pelvic floor exercises regularly during pregnancy and

Retroverted uterus

A mobile retroverted uterus is a harmless variation of normal in which the uterus is tilted backwards. It is often blamed for failure to conceive but in no way implicated.

especially after the birth of your baby, whether or not you have stitches.
■ You should continue pelvic floor exercises until the day you die, each day going through them on five or six separate occasions.
■ If you stop your pelvic floor exercises for a few weeks, do start again.
■ Mild incontinence can be controlled with pelvic floor exercises alone done five times a day for a couple of weeks.

See also:
● **Pelvic floor exercises p.375**

TREATMENT

Surgery for prolapse

To correct prolapse, an operation is performed under general anaesthesia to shorten the supporting ligaments and muscles of the uterus. The surgery can usually be performed through the vagina. After the operation patients usually remain in hospital for 5–7 days.

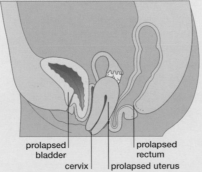

Prolapsed uterus

prolapsed bladder | prolapsed rectum
cervix | prolapsed uterus

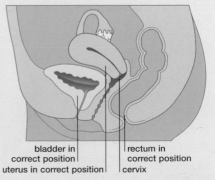

Correctly positioned uterus

bladder in correct position | rectum in correct position
uterus in correct position | cervix

Hysterectomy

HYSTERECTOMY IS THE SURGICAL REMOVAL OF THE UTERUS. IN THE US, A SHOCKING 25 PERCENT OF ALL WOMEN OVER THE AGE OF 50 HAVE HAD A HYSTERECTOMY. THE OPERATION IS OFTEN PERFORMED FOR NO GOOD REASON, SUCH AS THE REMOVAL OF SMALL FIBROIDS.

In the UK, there has been a reluctance by doctors until recently to remove the uterus unless the symptoms warranted it. However, the American attitude is beginning to creep in here. The decision to have a hysterectomy should never be taken lightly and in young women the instant menopause that follows a hysterectomy in which the ovaries are removed must be treated with hormone replacement therapy (HRT); conception is never an option.

WHAT ARE THE TYPES?

■ **Subtotal abdominal hysterectomy**, in which the uterus and sometimes the ovaries and fallopian tubes are removed, but the cervix is left intact.

■ **Total abdominal hysterectomy**, in which the ovaries, fallopian tubes, uterus and cervix are removed.

■ **Radical hysterectomy**, in which the uterus, cervix and pelvic lymph nodes are removed through an abdominal incision.

■ **Vaginal hysterectomy**, in which a hysterectomy is performed through the vagina instead of through an abdominal incision.

If the ovaries are removed, a woman no longer produces the female sex hormones and HRT must be considered.

WHY IS IT DONE?

Hysterectomy can be done for any of the following reasons:

● to remove **cancer** in the pelvic organs

● to treat any severe and uncontrollable **pelvic infection**

● to stop life-threatening **uterine haemorrhage**

● in certain life-threatening **conditions affecting the intestines and bladder**, when it's impossible to deal with the primary problem without removal of the uterus

● to remove multiple **fibroids** that are causing **excessive bleeding** and **pain**

● to treat **prolapse**

● to treat severe **endometriosis**

● in repairing **uterine and vaginal prolapse**.

NB HYSTERECTOMY SHOULD NEVER BE THE FIRST-LINE TREATMENT FOR HEAVY, LONG PERIODS.

HOW IS IT DONE?

■ Under general anaesthesia, an incision is made in the lower abdomen, and the uterus, and if required the ovaries and fallopian tubes, are removed.

■ After the operation you'll have a drip for fluids and perhaps a catheter to drain urine. There'll be some discharge from the vagina for a day or two.

■ If your ovaries were removed, HRT will soon be started. If not, ask about it.

■ Alternatively, you may have a vaginal hysterectomy, in which the abdominal cavity isn't opened but the uterus is removed through the vagina. Recovery is quicker this way and complications are minimized or avoided altogether. This is the ideal operation

to correct uncomplicated uterine prolapse. Vaginal hysterectomy is only performed if the uterus is not too bulky and if the supporting structures aren't too tight.

WHAT ABOUT AFTERWARDS?

■ When you go home after the operation, maintain a moderate level of activity, but stop the minute you feel any discomfort.

■ Gradually build up your strength. Gentle activities can be started by the fourth week after the operation; moderate activity such as light shopping or housework can be undertaken by about the fifth week. By the sixth week, you should start to feel nearly back to normal, although you may still feel tired.

■ By the sixth week, you can resume sexual intercourse as the top of the vagina will have healed. If you've kept your cervix there is no reason why sex should be any different for you.

ARE THERE PSYCHOLOGICAL CHANGES?

■ Most women who are appropriately counselled and have hysterectomies are happy with the operation. The vagina will be the same size as it was before unless it was a radical hysterectomy, when it will be slightly shorter.

■ Dissatisfaction is related to whether the operation was done for a very good reason and after full consideration by the woman and her partner of the options available.

■ Women who wanted more children find it difficult, as do some whose ovaries are removed premenopausally.

■ The women who suffer depression after hysterectomy are usually those who weren't convinced that the operation was necessary, especially if it was done for a condition that was not life-threatening. It's easier to adjust if you know the operation saved your life.

What should I do if hysterectomy is suggested?

■ Question your gynaecologist very carefully about the reasons for your hysterectomy and be satisfied in your mind that it's absolutely necessary.

■ Don't make a decision quickly – complications after a hysterectomy are most common in women who remain unconvinced the operation was necessary.

■ If you are in doubt about the advice or wish to avoid hysterectomy, seek a second opinion from another gynaecologist. Many conditions respond

to much less radical approaches than hysterectomy.

■ Check to see whether your ovaries need to be removed as well as your uterus, and find out about hormone replacement treatments available for premature menopause, which will occur if your ovaries are removed. It's no longer medically accepted that the ovaries should be removed in case cancer should develop, so don't be persuaded by this argument.

FEMALE CANCERS

Cancer of the cervix and breast cancer are two of the most common cancers seen in women. Fortunately, cancer of the cervix can largely be prevented provided that women attend appointments for cervical smears regularly. Breast awareness and screening can also help detect breast cancer while it is still at a curable stage. Cancer of the ovary and cancer of the uterus are two rarer forms of cancer that also affect women.

Cervical pre-cancer and cancer

CANCER OF THE CERVIX IS THE SECOND MOST COMMON FEMALE CANCER (BREAST CANCER IS THE FIRST) AND IT'S BECOMING MORE COMMON, PARTICULARLY AMONG YOUNG WOMEN. UNTREATED, IT MAY SPREAD TO MOST OF THE ORGANS IN THE PELVIS.

The chances of a cure for cervical cancer depend very much on what stage the cancer has reached when first detected.

Cervical cancer has a **pre-cancerous stage**, often called **cervical intraepithelial neoplasia** (**CIN**), during which time abnormal cells grow but are not cancerous. As this pre-cancerous stage may last for several years, any woman who has regular smear tests will be identified early enough for the abnormal cells to be totally removed by simply taking out the tissue from the cervix long before there's any threat of cancer.

Despite the fact that pre-cancerous changes *continued on page 259*

TREATMENT

Chemotherapy

Chemotherapy uses powerful chemicals in the form of pills, injections or a drip into a vein to kill cancer cells. Chemotherapy drugs interrupt cell growth, so they end up killing large numbers of cells, both cancerous ones and healthy ones. Many "normal" body cells (such as the bone marrow and the lining of the intestine and mouth) divide rapidly and are therefore vulnerable to cancer drugs, giving rise to many of the side effects of chemotherapy.

Most chemotherapy is given as outpatient treatment, either as a short injection into a vein or as an intravenous drip over an hour or so. It rarely involves staying in hospital overnight.

Depending on the type of cancer being treated, chemotherapy is usually given once every three or four weeks, but some treatments may be given weekly. You'll probably receive 6–8 courses of treatment, and treatment usually lasts 5–6 months.

Hormonal drugs

For certain types of cancer, special hormonal drugs may be used. One of the best known of these drugs is tamoxifen, which is used to block the effect of oestrogen, implicated in the growth of certain tumours (and especially in breast cancer). In women with a family history of breast cancer, tamoxifen may be given as a preventive measure, but the risks have not yet been fully investigated.

In chemotherapy, cancer cells are killed off faster than normal cells, until no cancer cells are detectable.

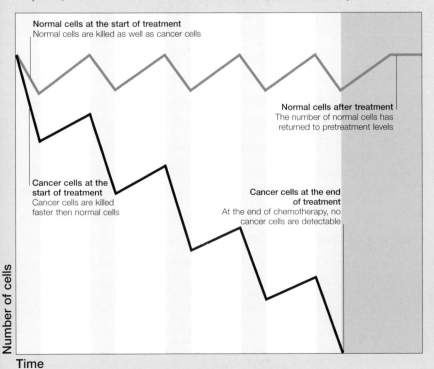

Normal cells at the start of treatment
Normal cells are killed as well as cancer cells

Normal cells after treatment
The number of normal cells has returned to pretreatment levels

Cancer cells at the start of treatment
Cancer cells are killed faster then normal cells

Cancer cells at the end of treatment
At the end of chemotherapy, no cancer cells are detectable

Number of cells

Time

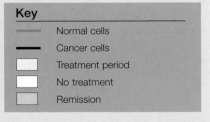

Key

———	Normal cells
———	Cancer cells
	Treatment period
	No treatment
	Remission

FOCUS *on* smear tests

Nearly all of us harbour some trepidation about having a smear test. It's natural to feel vulnerable about exposing ourselves to a stranger, and there's also the added fear the test may show up a worrying result. But it's up to us all to take responsibility for our own health.

A smear taken regularly can detect the earliest pre-cancerous changes, which can be treated promptly so that the cancer never develops.

As cervical cancer is one of the few cancers over which we can exert some positive control, it's madness to allow a few minutes of embarrassment to prevent us having regular checks. It's a very quick procedure and before you know it, it'll be time to go home.

DID YOU KNOW?
● The human papilloma virus (HPV) raises the risk of cervical cancer.

Colposcopy

Colposcopy is a simple, non-invasive procedure and can be used as a treatment as well as a diagnostic tool following an abnormal smear test. It requires no anaesthetic and can be done in your gynaecologist's surgery or outpatient clinic. The colposcope, a kind of microscope, is placed at the entrance to the vagina. The doctor examines the tissue to identify the precise area of abnormal cells. (A smear test doesn't pinpoint this exactly.) He'll then remove the speculum slowly so that he can inspect the vaginal walls.

Abnormal cells inside the cervical canal can't be detected with a colposcope. If these are suspected, a cone biopsy (in which a cone of cervical tissue is removed) will be recommended.

Areas confirmed as abnormal by biopsy are treated by electrocoagulation or laser (both use heat to destroy tissue), by cryosurgery (which uses cold to destroy tissue) or may be removed by diathermy loop excision (DLE). Treatment may be carried out at the same time as colposcopy if the abnormal area is small and well-defined. If a woman is pregnant, treatment is usually delayed.

● 95 percent of women with cervical cancer carry HPV.
● HPV is symptomless in many women.
● Having many sexual partners puts you at risk as it increases your likelihood of being exposed to HPV.
● Cervical cancer won't have time to develop if you have regular smear tests.

A cervical smear, also known as a **Pap smear** after the doctor (Papanicolau) who invented it, is done during a pelvic examination. It's used primarily to detect precancerous and cancerous cells on the cervix – the neck of the uterus.

It detects very early abnormal changes in the cells of the cervix, which can be destroyed thus preventing cervical cancer from developing.

Cancerous change is even more likely if you have several partners. Promiscuous sex also increases the risk of being infected with HPV, the virus that promotes cervical cancer.

The test offers a 95 percent chance of detecting **CIN** (abnormal cell changes which, if not discovered and treated, could become cancerous).

WHAT IS THE CERVIX?
The cervix is small, cylindrical, several centimetres in length and forms the lower part and neck of the uterus. The cervix dips down into the vagina. Running through the centre of the cervix is a canal through which sperm pass from the vagina into the uterus on their way to fertilize an egg and through which blood passes during menstruation.

WHO SHOULD HAVE SMEARS?
Cervical smears should be performed on all women once they begin having intercourse and then every three years up to the age of 65. The test is also important for women who have or have had infection with the human papilloma virus (HPV). A smear may incidentally detect sexually transmitted diseases.

WHEN AND WHERE IS IT DONE?
A woman should have a cervical smear within a year of her 20th birthday. Cervical smears may be performed by GPs or Well Woman or Family Planning Clinics. You shouldn't be menstruating or have had intercourse within 24 hours of having your test as blood and semen make the result unreliable. Ideally you should be at mid-cycle to obtain the best quality smear.

HOW IS IT DONE?
You lie on your back with your knees bent. A warmed speculum is passed into the vagina to separate the walls so the doctor can see your cervix.

A wooden spatula is wiped across the cervix to collect cells, and the smear is transferred to a glass slide and sent to a laboratory. The whole thing takes less than a minute and, although uncomfortable, isn't painful. The results should be available within 6 weeks.

THE RESULTS
Results of a smear test are classified into three categories:
● **Negative** gives you the all-clear.
● **Mild dysplasia** or CIN I means that you have some infection and should be screened more frequently.
● A **positive** smear test, although not always indicating cancer, means there is a detectable change in the cells necessitating further investigation.

The table below gives you a comprehensive run down of the sort of results you're likely to get and what you'll need to do in response.

Result	Action
Negative	No follow-up needed: next smear in three years' time
Mild dysplasia or CIN I	Another smear in no more than 6 months' time
Moderate dysplasia or CIN II	Colposcopy
Severe dysplasia	Colposcopy

See also:
● **Cervical pre-cancer and cancer p.257**

continued from page 257
can be detected by **regular smear tests** and treated, each year about 25 percent of women with cervical cancer die, usually because they have not had a smear test. As the condition has no early warning symptoms it can only be detected by routine cervical smear screening.

STAGES OF CERVICAL PRE-CANCER AND CANCER
PRE-CANCER
- The mildest stage is known as CIN I.
- More severe changes, NOT CANCER, is called CIN II.
- The most severe stage is called CIN III.

CANCER
- Stage 1: cancer confined to the cervix.
- Stage 2: cancer extends beyond the cervix to involve the top of the vagina and/or tissue immediately surrounding the cervix.
- Stage 3: cancer extends to the lower part of the vagina and/or the side wall of the pelvis.
- Stage 4: cancer extends beyond the pelvis and/or involves the bladder or rectum.

TEST

Tissue tests

Some disorders change the number of different types of cell within an organ or make individual cells abnormal. Tissue tests can show up these changes. In a tissue test, a small sample of a particular tissue is removed and examined under a microscope. One of the most frequently performed tissue tests is the cervical or Pap smear, in which a sample of tissue is taken from the cervix to look for pre-cancerous changes in the cells.

Biopsy

The procedure in which a sample of tissue is taken specifically for testing is known as a biopsy. Biopsy may be done to confirm a diagnosis or to investigate a suspicious lump or a tumour. For example, if cirrhosis is suspected, a biopsy of liver tissue may be done and if characteristic changes are found, the diagnosis is confirmed. If it is not known whether a tumour is malignant (cancerous) or benign (non-cancerous), a biopsy can provide tissue that can be tested for cancerous changes. Further tests are sometimes needed if tissue tests do not provide a definitive diagnosis.

WHAT ARE THE SYMPTOMS?
- In its early pre-cancerous stages (CIN I and II), there are no symptoms.
- By Stage 1 or 2, **intermenstrual bleeding** and **spotting after intercourse** can show up as a warning sign that must always be investigated.
- An **offensive vaginal discharge** may be a symptom of cervical cancer and needs medical assessment.

WHAT ARE THE CAUSES?
While the exact cause of cervical cancer is not known, certain risk factors have been identified. These include infection with certain types of the human papilloma virus (HPV), which is linked with 95 percent of all cases of cervical cancer. Other risk factors include having multiple sexual partners, smoking, long-term use of the contraceptive pill, early pregnancy and many pregnancies. Women who have not recently had a smear test are most at risk of developing cervical cancer simply because these women will not receive treatment for any pre-cancerous changes to the cervix. Thus the biggest risk factor for cervical cancer is non-attendance for cervical screening.

WHAT'S THE TREATMENT?
MEDICAL
- All stages of CIN should be treated, although some doctors adopt a "wait and see" approach, involving repeat smear tests for early CIN.
- Treatment of CIN involves performing a **colposcopy** usually in the outpatient department, when the cervix is viewed with a special microscope. Areas with abnormal cells may be identified and, if necessary, a biopsy may be taken to examine the tissue in the laboratory.
- Following a colposcopy a woman will either be reassured, or have a follow-up smear or have further treatment.

SURGICAL
- The simplest surgical treatment of CIN involves removing the pre-cancerous tissue under a local anaesthetic with a **laser**, or **freezing** or **cutting** away the tissue with an electric loop (known as large loop excision of the transformation zones, or LLETZ, or diathermy loop excision, or DLE).
- A **cone biopsy** involves removing a larger piece of tissue and this may require a general anaesthetic. This may be done with a scalpel or a laser beam. A cone of cervical tissue is taken out to remove all abnormal tissue plus a wedge of surrounding normal tissue. After the tissue is examined microscopically, doctors decide if you require any further treatment.

Treatment of full-blown cancer of the cervix depends on the stage that the disease has reached. Treatment may involve either **surgery**

or **radiotherapy**, or both. As a general rule radiotherapy is more often used for older women and surgery for younger, fitter patients, irrespective of the stage of the disease.
- Surgery involves removing all affected tissue and organs. A **radical hysterectomy** is most often performed. This involves removing the uterus, the cervix, the upper vagina and the surrounding tissues, including some lymph nodes.
- If the cancer involves the bladder or bowel, major surgery involving removal of the bladder or bowel, as well as a hysterectomy, may be necessary.

Nearly half of all cases of cervical cancer are treated with radiotherapy. The aim is to give a fatal dose of radiation to the centre of the cancer. Radiation also kills those parts of the growth that were invading other areas. However, surgery alone with conservation of the ovaries is preferred for younger women because of the adverse effect of radiotherapy on bowel and sexual function.

WHAT IS THE OUTLOOK?
- You'll be required to have regular checks over the next five years or so to make sure the cancer spread has been stopped.
- You'll almost certainly not be able to have any or any more children and, if your ovaries are removed, you'll go through a **premature menopause**. You must be aware of this because you'll need HRT from day one after the operation, so do enquire of your surgeons.

Remember

If you maintain regular appointments for **smear tests**, any cancer will be caught at a time when chances of a cure are high. Even if cancerous cells are found, try to take an interest in the disease and co-operate with your medical advisers as much as possible to fight it. Cancer cures do depend to a certain extent on your determination to beat the disease.

See also:
- HRT p.502
- Hysterectomy p.256
- Smear tests p.258

Cancer of the ovary

CANCER OF THE OVARY IS A MALIGNANT TUMOUR THAT CAN DEVELOP IN ONE OR BOTH OVARIES,
USUALLY IN WOMEN AFTER THE MENOPAUSE BUT OCCASIONALLY IN YOUNGER WOMEN.

Unfortunately ovarian cancer does not usually cause any symptoms until it is advanced, by which time it may be very difficult to treat effectively. Ovarian cancer is usually aggressive and can spread quite early in the course of the disease.

WHAT ARE THE CAUSES?

There are many theories about what causes ovarian cancer to develop. It is more common in older women and in women who have not had any children, and less common in women who have used the oral contraceptive pill or HRT for a number of years and in those women who had a late start to their periods and an early menopause.

"Resting" the ovary by suppressing ovulation, for example during pregnancy or while on the pill, may protect a woman against developing ovarian cancer. Genetic factors are important in ovarian cancer: sometimes it runs in families. A triad of cancers – ovary, breast and colon – run through some cancer families where a gene is at work.

WHAT ARE THE SYMPTOMS?
■ Abdominal pain.
■ Swelling of the abdomen.
■ A hard lump in the abdomen.
■ If the tumour is large, pressure on the bladder can cause frequent urination.
■ Occasional breathlessness if the tumour presses upwards on the diaphragm.

WHAT MIGHT BE DONE?
Some families carry a **gene** called BRCA1 that increases the likelihood of both ovarian and breast cancer. Genetic tests for this gene are now available to help identify those women at risk of developing ovarian and breast cancer.

If you have a strong history of ovarian or breast cancer in your family, it is important to tell your doctor.

Treatment of ovarian cancer usually involves several things.
■ Your surgeon will attempt to remove the whole tumour and any local spread. The extent of surgery depends on the type of tumour found.

■ Minimal surgery involves the removal of both ovaries and the fallopian tubes as well as the uterus.
■ If the disease has already spread beyond the reproductive organs, much more extensive surgery may be necessary. This may involve surgery to other organs, such as removing part of the bowel and bladder.
■ Drugs containing platinum are commonly used to treat ovarian cancer, but radiotherapy has been found to have limited effect.
■ Further surgery may well be performed to remove any recurrences.

WHAT IS THE OUTLOOK?
The outlook in the longer term depends on the stage of the disease and the type of malignant cell present in the ovary, but the figures are not reassuring. If the cancer is restricted to the ovary, 60–70 percent of women can expect to live for five years; if the growth has spread, the five-year survival rate is only 10–20 percent.

Cancer of the uterus

CANCER OF THE UTERUS IS A TUMOUR THAT GROWS IN THE LINING OF THE
UTERUS, THE ENDOMETRIUM, AND IS SOMETIMES KNOWN AS ENDOMETRIAL CANCER.
IT HAS A RELATIVELY LOW MALIGNANCY.

WHAT CAUSES IT?
Cancer of the uterus is more common in obese women and those taking the drug tamoxifen, which is used to prevent or treat breast cancer. Hormone replacement therapy (HRT) using oestrogen alone also increases the risk but addition of a progestogen for 14 days at least every three months prevents this, and the continuous "non-bleeding" form of HRT actually reduces the risk of developing this cancer.

There has been a lot of controversy in recent years about the possible association of uterine cancer with taking HRT for menopausal symptoms. If a menstrual period is induced at least every three months by a 14-day course of progestogen, endometrial overgrowth is avoided. Inserting a progesterone IUD that can be left in situ for five years accomplishes the same aim.

WHAT ARE THE SYMPTOMS?
■ Postmenopausal bleeding or brown discharge.
■ Discomfort in the lower abdomen.
■ Bleeding after intercourse.
■ Heavy menstrual periods.

WHAT WILL THE DOCTOR DO?
If you have any post-menopausal vaginal bleeding or any change in your normal menstrual pattern, consult your doctor immediately.
■ If your doctor suspects that you have a growth in your uterus, the only effective way to check whether there is any malignancy is to undergo an investigation. You are likely to have an ultrasound scan; if this shows a thickened endometrium, an endometrial biopsy may done via the cervix, or the inside of the uterus may be examined using hysteroscopy with a biopsy at the same time.

■ If the uterine lining contains cancerous cells, your doctor will recommend a total hysterectomy with removal of the ovaries and fallopian tubes as well as the cervix. Radiotherapy may be advised if the tumour has spread through the wall of the uterus.
■ If the growth is advanced, a radical hysterectomy will be performed to remove some vagina and the lymph nodes of the pelvis too.

WHAT IS THE OUTLOOK?
The news is good. The overall cure rate is as high as 90 percent when the cancer is localized to the lining of the uterus itself. If the spread is beyond the lining and the muscles of the uterus, the figure after five years is reduced to 40 percent.

FOCUS *on* breast cancer

I wish I could wave a magic wand and make women less afraid of breast cancer. I feel you, and every woman, would be less fearful if you knew the good news, and could take the reassuring facts on board. Fear can stop you from doing this.

I want to try to reassure women by starting with this very positive statistic, and then following with a lot more. **Of every 15 women referred to a breast clinic, 14 do not have cancer.**

Understanding breast cancer can greatly improve your chances of avoiding it and defeating it. You can reduce the risk of ever getting breast cancer by knowing how to prevent it. This includes making life choices such as having your first baby before 30. Lifestyle changes, such as keeping your weight down and your consumption of alcohol low, also helps. You should also eat at least five fresh fruits and vegetables every day.

Early detection and diagnosis play an important role in the successful treatment of breast cancer, and in the long-term outlook.

It's important to know that, even when a diagnosis of breast cancer is made, there are different types. Not all cancers have the same degree of invasiveness or potential for spread, so not all, by any means, have a poor outlook.

A positive attitude is a real asset, possibly as vital as some medical treatments.

PUTTING BREAST CANCER INTO PERSPECTIVE

● For every breast lump found to be cancerous, approximately eight others will prove to be benign and therefore harmless.
● If the lump is diagnosed and treated early, you'll have a better chance of a successful outcome.
● Even with cancerous lumps, 6 or 7 out of 10 will be treated without removing the breast.
● In post-menopausal women, deaths from breast cancer pale into insignificance when compared with the number of deaths caused by heart disease – **four** times as many!
● Five times more women suffer from the disease than die from it. In a given year, of 100,000 women with breast cancer, 80,000 **do not die**.
● More than 70 percent of women who have operable disease will be alive and well five years after diagnosis.
● By the age of 50, your chances of dying of

breast cancer, compared to other causes of death such as heart disease, will have dropped dramatically from 1 in 12 to 1 in 70, and the odds get better with every year you live after that without developing it.
● By the time you are in your sixties, your chances of dying from breast cancer are probably less than half what they were when you were 50.

HORMONE REPLACEMENT THERAPY (HRT) AND BREAST CANCER
The risk of breast cancer increases slightly if you take HRT. The increase rises a little depending on the time you are on HRT. Here are the real figures:

Women aged 50 (per 1,000 women)	Breast cancer risk over next 10 years
No HRT (baseline risk we all have)	45
5 years HRT	47
10 years HRT	51
15 years HRT	57

A woman who stops HRT treatment returns to the normal risk rate after five years. However,

the risk of breast cancer should be weighed against the benefits of HRT.

Four times as many women die from coronary artery disease and the consequences of osteoporosis, both of which HRT may help to guard against.

FAMILY HISTORY
About 5 percent of breast cancers may be due to genes inherited from your family. Women are at increased risk if their mother or sister developed breast cancer before the age of 40, if two of these relatives developed it before the age of 60, or if three relatives developed breast cancer at any age.

Any woman who's worried should ask her doctor to refer her to a Cancer Family Clinic for advice.

WHAT IS A TUMOUR?
The word tumour simply means a lump. Most breast tumours aren't cancerous. They're usually benign, i.e. the growth of cells is confined to the area where the tumour starts. Tumours whose cells don't spread to other parts of the body aren't fatal.

In contrast, the cells that make up cancerous tumours are invasive. They spread beyond their original location, not just into adjacent tissues but to other distant parts of the body and as they invade they destroy.

The original tumour is known as the **primary**. Tumours that arise from cancerous cells that have spread elsewhere are called **secondaries** or **metastases**.

continued on page 262

What happens to your sex life if you lose a breast?

It's quite natural for the loss of one of your breasts to radically change your self-image and lower your self-esteem.
You may feel unattractive or embarrassed by it and not surprisingly you may become inhibited and lose your sex drive.
About 1 in 5 women has a loss of sexual interest a few months after mastectomy and at two years the figure rises to 1 in 3. Interest in sex declines in over a quarter of sexually active women, irrespective of the

kind of surgical treatment they have. The psychological impact of knowing you have cancer and coping with its treatment may preoccupy you with thoughts of survival, so that sexual desire is at the bottom of your priority list.
Some couples will, however, find the trauma of breast cancer brings them closer together, especially if you involve your partner in every step from day one.

To determine how aggressive cancer cells are, and how far they have spread, if at all, grading and staging tests are done, which are also a basis for deciding on treatment.

SPREAD

Invasive cancers tend to spread first into the **regional glands** – the axillary lymph nodes in the armpits in the case of the breasts – causing swellings. They may also spread to lymph nodes under the breastbone and above the collarbone.

Spread via the bloodstream, through "seeds", is probably more important in determining the long-term outlook. This is why modern treatments, such as hormonal therapy and chemotherapy, are aimed at eradicating cancer cells from the body as a whole rather than just dealing with the tumour locally.

1 IN 11

You may have heard that 1 in 11 women develops breast cancer. This figure, although true, may be misleading because it doesn't tell the whole story, only the alarming part of it.

1 in 11 represents the lifetime risk. This means 1 in 11 women will develop breast cancer during the course of their whole lives – that means over 70 or 80 years.

Not today, not this week, not this month. As risk increases with age, the risk at any point in time is much lower than 1 in 11; in point of fact, it's closer to 1 in 1,000.

HOPE FOR THE FUTURE

● Women who have treatment for early breast cancer can expect to live a normal life span.
● For women who get local recurrences,

radiotherapy can sometimes cure without the need for other treatment.
● While breast cancer is predominantly a disease of older women, many women live to die from causes other than their breast cancer.

SURGERY

Mastectomy, the removal of a breast, is less common nowadays – or should be. Radical surgery is no longer the norm for breast cancer and there are currently several possible variations of mastectomy.

More than 80 percent of breast cancers are localized and caught early enough to be suitable for lumpectomy – removal of the lump alone leaving the breast virtually intact.

The type of surgery selected to treat cancer depends on the size of the tumour and other factors.

The majority of women qualify for additional treatments after surgery. It's called **adjuvant therapy**.

CHEMOTHERAPY

Several drugs are designed to target rapidly dividing cancer cells anywhere in the body, and the use of these drugs can increase the cure rate by 10 percent.

Side effects, including hair loss and nausea, are unpleasant but usually only temporary.

Other non-cancerous cells that are rapidly dividing, such as those in bone marrow, are susceptible to damage from chemotherapy.

HORMONAL DRUGS

Tamoxifen, a very promising hormonal drug, can block tumour growth in certain patients and is used widely. Tamoxifen may even be given as a preventive measure in women who are at high risk of getting breast cancer. The latest UK figures show that tamoxifen has cut the death rate from breast cancer by nearly 40 percent.

Because it has an anti-oestrogenic effect, tamoxifen has side effects when taken for long periods, including menopausal symptoms. It slightly increases the risk of uterine cancer.

RADIOTHERAPY

Radiation destroys or slows the development of cancerous cells.

It's usually given after surgery, to kill any remaining cancerous cells, but may be used in place of surgery to reduce the size of breast tumours and thus to relieve symptoms.

Lumpectomy

Lumpectomy (also called breast-conserving surgery) is the removal of a breast lump along with some surrounding normal tissue. If the procedure is done to remove a cancerous lump, some of the lymph nodes in the armpit are usually also

removed. The procedure is done in hospital under either a local or, more usually, a general anaesthetic. Lumpectomy to remove a cancerous lump is usually followed by 3–5 weeks of radiotherapy to ensure that the cancer is eradicated.

Sites of incisions

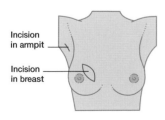

Incision in armpit

Incision in breast

The breast lump, some surrounding normal tissue and some lymph nodes are usually removed during a lumpectomy.

Areas treated in a lumpectomy

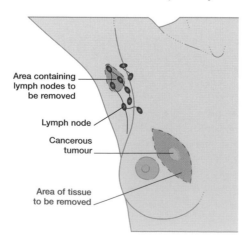

Area containing lymph nodes to be removed

Lymph node

Cancerous tumour

Area of tissue to be removed

A certain percentage of women may be left with discomfort and stiffness in the shoulders and arms following radiotherapy and you may lose some sensation in the treated breast; it may also be slightly swollen and feel different. If your breasts were an important source of sexual stimulation prior to surgery, counselling could help you to find other means of enhancing your enjoyment of lovemaking.

BREAST RECONSTRUCTION

Every woman who has a mastectomy has the right to a new, reconstructed breast. It can be done at the same time as mastectomy or at a later date.

Most breast reconstructions involve a flap of skin, fat and muscle swung round from the back that's folded into a breast shape. An implant may be inserted too.

New nipples can be created by tissue grafting and tattooing. The new breast is often better than the breast that's left!

FALSE BREASTS OR PROSTHESES

Breast prostheses are very sophisticated now and feel like a natural breast. They can be fitted into a bra or swimsuit. Bras containing breast prostheses can also be obtained. Prostheses are designed to simulate the appearance and feel of a natural breast.

WHAT IS THE OUTLOOK?

Remember, modern techniques mean that doctors can tailor treatment to the particular needs of each woman, so you will be given every chance of a cure. Rigorous follow-up will be necessary to pick up any problems and to check for recurrence of cancer. After months of intensive medical attention you may feel alone and fearful, and this is a time when a care network such as a local breast-cancer group can be invaluable.

In conclusion, bear in mind that 1 in 3 women who have treatment for early breast cancer can expect to live a normal life span.

Being aware of the normal appearance and texture of your breasts enables you to bring any changes to your doctor's attention promptly.

MEN'S CONDITIONS

With some famous men going public and owning up to testicular and prostatic disease, men's conditions are much more high-profile than they were, and about time too.

Men need a lot of encouragement to be open about their health problems, particularly intimate ones such as testicular and prostatic cancer.

Men don't easily talk about themselves. They are sometimes loath to consult a doctor because they see confessing to being concerned about health as somehow un-macho.

That's not only a great shame but also dangerous, especially as testicular cancer, caught early, is one of the most curable cancers there is.

Why it's important to check your testicles

WOMEN ARE GETTING THE MESSAGE THAT IT MAKES GOOD HEALTH SENSE TO CHECK THEIR BREASTS REGULARLY FOR LUMPS. BY COMPARISON, ONLY 1 IN 30 MEN EXAMINES HIS TESTICLES.

It's a pity more men don't do testicular self-examination because testicular cancer is **highly curable** when detected at an early stage. And self-examination couldn't be simpler, it only takes a few minutes every month. It's best done after a bath or shower when the scrotum is warm and relaxed as this will increase the chances of detecting any abnormality. Self-examination is really worth doing – the latest treatments mean 9 out of 10 men will make a complete recovery.

Men need to check their bodies for cancer, just as women do. Here's the simple self-examination you can use to test for first signs of testicular cancer.

1. Stand in front of a mirror and look for **any swelling** on the skin of the scrotum. One testicle may appear larger than the other and one may hang lower, which is usually normal.

2. Hold each testicle gently between the thumb and fingertips of both hands and slowly bring the thumb and fingertips of one hand together while relaxing the fingertips of the other.

3. Alternate this several times so the testicle glides smoothly between both sets of fingers. This lets you assess its shape and texture.

4. You mustn't press too hard and you must be careful not to twist the testicle.

5. Each testicle should feel soft and smooth, like a hard-boiled egg without its shell.

WHAT YOU'RE LOOKING FOR

Any lump, swelling, irregularity, abnormal hardness, tenderness or any change within the body of the testicle itself. Testicular cancer almost always occurs in only one testicle.

WHAT YOU MIGHT FIND

There are causes of testicular swellings other than sinister ones; these include a **hydrocoele, epididymal cyst**, **spermatocoele** or **varicocoele**.

■ A **hydrocoele** is a soft painless cyst surrounding the testicle. During development, the lining of the abdomen pouches down into the scrotum as the testicle descends. This closes off to leave an empty remnant in the scrotum.

In middle age, this remnant often fills with fluid and can grow quite large. In most cases there is no underlying cause, but occasionally a hydrocoele forms as a result of inflammation, infection, injury or, rarely, an underlying tumour of the testicle on that side.

A doctor tests for a hydrocoele by holding a **pen torch** next to the scrotal skin. The swelling will light up if it is due to a fluid-filled hydrocoele and you can do this for yourself. Small hydrocoeles are often left alone and larger ones may be drained off under a local anaesthetic, though they may recur, so surgery is the most effective treatment.

■ An **epididymal cyst** is a harmless swelling arising from the epididymis, the coiled collecting tube attached to the back of each testis. Small, pea-sized epididymal cysts are common in men over the age of 40. These cysts are often multiple and may affect both sides. They are filled with a clear, colourless fluid and are usually left in place rather than removed.

■ A **spermatocoele** is similar to an epididymal cyst, but instead of containing clear fluid it is filled with milky semen and sperm. If you shine a torch through it, it doesn't light up like a hydrocoele. The two can only be differentiated if fluid is drained for examination.

Spermatocoeles are harmless and are usually left in place unless they become troublesome.

■ A **varicocoele** is a collection of **varicose veins** surrounding a testicle and is one of the most common reasons for an enlarged testicle.

It feels like a warm tangle of worms in the scrotum and it's a condition that affects about 10–15 percent of men; it is usually harmless although there may be aching discomfort in the scrotum or an abnormally low sperm count. Diagnosis is confirmed by examination of the scrotum while the patient is standing. Any aching may be relieved by wearing an athletic support or tight underpants.

WHAT CAUSES TESTICULAR CANCER?

Testicular cancer is still quite rare, with just over 1,500 new cases a year in the UK. However, it is one of the most curable cancers, with 90 percent making a complete recovery. We don't know what causes it yet, but we do know that men who were born with an **undescended, or partly descended, testicle are between 3 and 14 times** more likely to develop testicular cancer. Other research has suggested that there may be a **hereditary** factor involved. Treatment shouldn't affect your sex life or fertility in the long term.

See also:
• **Testicular cancer p.270**

Younger men are at risk

■ Testicular cancer is the most common form of cancer in young men in the UK and it occurs mostly in those aged between 19 and 44.

■ It's easily treated and, if caught at an early stage, testicular cancer is nearly always curable.

■ The risk of developing it has risen by 70 percent in the past 20 years.

■ Only 3 percent of young men check their testicles; most are unaware of this simple method of early detection of cancer.

■ More than 50 percent of sufferers consult their doctors after the cancer has started to spread. This makes it more difficult to treat successfully and the side effects of treatment become more unpleasant.

Gynaecomastia

GYNAECOMASTIA IS COMMON, NORMAL ENLARGEMENT OF ONE OR BOTH BREASTS IN MALES AND
HAS NO SINISTER SIGNIFICANCE. IT'S MOST OFTEN SEEN IN NEWBORN BABIES AND OLDER MEN.

All men produce small amounts of the female sex hormone oestrogen. If oestrogen levels are higher than normal, breast enlargement – gynaecomastia – occurs. Either one or both breasts may become enlarged. Gynaecomastia is common in newborn boys because of their mother's oestrogen crossing the placenta. It affects a fair number of male adolescents too,

because their own oestrogen levels are swinging about. In babies and adolescent boys it is almost always temporary. Gynaecomastia can also affect older men when they have stopped producing the male hormone testosterone but their adrenal glands and fat are still producing oestrogen. The condition may also be a side effect of certain drugs, for example digoxin.

WHAT MIGHT BE DONE?
In baby boys the swelling settles down after a week or so and in adolescent boys it disappears when their hormones level out. In these cases no treatment is usually needed. In older men, the doctor will ask about lifestyle factors and carry out an examination to exclude breast lumps. If a drug is the cause, it may be changed.

Peyronie's disease

PEYRONIE'S DISEASE IS A CONDITION IN WHICH THE SHAPE OF THE PENIS IS DISTORTED,
CAUSING IT TO BEND TO ONE SIDE OR UP AND DOWN WHEN ERECT. IT'S VERY
RARE UNDER THE AGE OF 40 AND SOMETIMES RUNS IN FAMILIES.

Some penises **always** bend when erect and this is just a variation of normal. In Peyronie's disease, the fibrous tissue of the penis becomes thickened, causing it to bend during erection. The penis may bend so much that sexual intercourse is difficult and painful. Peyronie's disease occurs in about 1 in 100 men.

Often no cause can be identified, but previous damage to the penis may be a risk factor. Peyronie's disease is also associated with **Dupuytren's contracture**, a condition in which the fibrous tissue in the palm of the hand becomes thick and shortened, causing the fingers to bend inwards. Peyronie's disease can run in families, which implies that a genetic factor is involved.

WHAT ARE THE SYMPTOMS?
The symptoms of Peyronie's disease develop gradually and include:
● curvature of the penis to one side during an erection
● pain in the penis on erection
● a thickened area in the penis, usually be felt as a firm nodule when the penis is flaccid.

Eventually, the thickened region of the penis may extend to include parts of the erectile tissue. In this case, Peyronie's disease may lead to impotence if it is not treated.

WHAT IS THE TREATMENT?
In some cases, Peyronie's disease improves without treatment. Some surgeons **excise** the

fibrosed tissue, others **remove a wedge** on the opposite side to encourage a straight erection. A vein patch may be inserted. Poor results are usually due to disease progression or scarring. If the condition is advanced, the best solution may be to implant a **penile prosthesis**.

Prostate cancer

THE PROSTATE GLAND IS ONE OF THE ORGANS THAT CAN DEVELOP CANCEROUS
TUMOURS, AND THIS FORM OF CANCER CAN HIT ANY MAN.

HOW DOES PROSTATE CANCER GROW?
At first, the tumour stays inside the prostate's outer capsule but, as it enlarges, it spreads through the capsule and grows into tissues around the prostate gland.

Cancer cells can also break off from the primary tumour. They are trapped by the lymph glands near the prostate and here they can grow into secondary tumours or **metastases**.

The tumour can also spread via blood vessels, giving rise to **metastases** in the **bones of the back, spine and pelvis**.

HOW IS PROSTATE CANCER DIAGNOSED?
A doctor will suspect a tumour if, when he does a **rectal examination**, he finds a hard, irregular lump in the prostate or if the whole prostate feels hard and uneven. As with breast cancer, very small tumours may be impossible to feel.

HOW COMMON IS PROSTATE CANCER?
It's much more common than we used to think. We now know that almost **three-quarters** of men over the age of 80 have it, but in many of these men the cancer is quiescent and most will die of something else.

Prostate cancer is the second most common cause of male cancer death in England and Wales and men have a 10 percent lifetime risk.

As with breast cancer in women, it's important to catch the disease **early**, especially in men who are at high risk. A **family history** of prostate cancer, or even breast cancer, would put a man in the high-risk group.

Prostate cancer may be preventable. A study published last year from Finland suggests that taking **vitamin E supplements** may reduce the chance of developing the disease by about a third and of dying from it by nearly a half. There's also some evidence that **selenium**
continued on page 268

FOCUS *on* prostate problems

Most men will suffer from an enlarged prostate to some degree. It's part of normal male ageing and Western men suffer from it more than Asian men. What is the prostate anyway? Most people have heard of it, but have little idea what it's for, and many people don't even know where it is.

Indeed doctors and scientists don't fully understand its functions, and there's still a lot to be learned about the prostate and about the diseases affecting it.

The prostate gland lies underneath the bladder. Its main job is to produce a thin, clear fluid that nourishes sperm while they're being stored in the seminal vesicles awaiting release through ejaculation. The prostate needs hormones from the testicles (mainly **testosterone** but also **prostaglandin**) so that it can work properly, and if they're low the prostate shrinks.

Close to the prostate are two important bladder muscles called sphincters, one above and one below the prostate. They control the outlet from the bladder, stopping it from leaking urine. They also help to expel semen at ejaculation.

WHY DOES THE PROSTATE CAUSE TROUBLE?

A man's prostate usually becomes larger after the age of 50. The fact that the prostate grows isn't important in itself, and indeed the trouble it causes doesn't depend on its actual size.

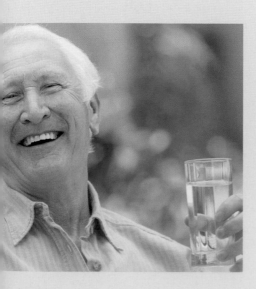

However, the prostate surrounds the tube from the bladder called the **urethra** and as it enlarges it squeezes the urethra and narrows the opening out of the bladder. This is called **obstruction** and it impedes the flow of urine. 25 percent of men aged 50 and over will experience urinary symptoms due to prostate enlargement.

SYMPTOMS OF OBSTRUCTION

As obstruction occurs gradually, many men don't realize it's happening. They may notice that their urine stream doesn't travel as far as it did when they were young and they may be aware that it's less forceful.

Then there may be a delay in getting started (called **hesitancy**), and the urine stream tails off at the end, sometimes causing troublesome dribbling.

There may be a feeling that the bladder isn't quite empty, known as incomplete emptying.

WHY DOES THE PROSTATE GET BIGGER?

The main cause is simply **age**. The benign non-cancerous enlargement is called benign prostatic hyperplasia (BPH).

The exact reason for enlargement is uncertain, but male hormones are required so it doesn't occur in men castrated at an early age.

Most men over the age of 80 have the condition, and about half will have some symptoms from it.

WHAT HAPPENS TO THE PROSTATE?

BPH starts in the inner part of the gland and, as it enlarges, it squashes the rest of the gland into a fairly thin shell, called the capsule. BPH never spreads outside the gland. However big the prostate, it remains covered by the capsule rather like a chestnut in its shell.

A doctor examines a prostate by doing a rectal examination (the prostate lies right up against the back passage). A prostate with BPH has a smooth surface with an even shape and feels rubbery, rather than hard.

PROSTATITIS

Inflammation of the prostate (prostatitis) from infection or other causes is not uncommon and can occur at most ages, affecting approximately 1 man in 10. Sometimes it causes symptoms like **cystitis** – such as **burning pain while passing urine**. In older men it might cause a sudden increase in prostate symptoms. The prostate is very **tender** when the doctor does an internal rectal examination.

DO I HAVE AN ENLARGED PROSTATE?

If you've read this far and you're a man of the right age for prostate problems, you'll probably be wondering whether you need to have your prostate seen to, so ask yourself some questions.
- Do you have difficulty starting to pass urine?
- Does it take longer to pass urine than it did?
- Do you stop and start?
- Do you need to pass urine twice or more during the night?
- Are you sometimes caught short?

If your answer to two or more questions is yes, see your doctor.

TREATMENT OF AN ENLARGED PROSTATE

If you have a prostate problem, your doctor will ask you about your symptoms then do a rectal examination to assess the size of your prostate. Tests will be arranged for confirmation and to help plan your treatment.

You'll be asked to give a sample of your urine and a blood sample is usually taken to check how your kidneys are working and to measure a substance called **prostate-specific antigen (PSA)** (see opposite).

WHAT ARE MY TREATMENT OPTIONS?

Until very recently, virtually the only treatment for benign enlargement of the prostate was an operation. Operations on the prostate are usually very successful if a man has severe symptoms, but are sometimes disappointing if symptoms are only mild.

SURGERY

Transurethral versus open surgery

The earliest operations on the prostate were done as open surgery – removing the enlarged part of the gland through a surgical incision in the front of the abdomen.

Just before the Second World War, urologists

in America started doing an operation called **transurethral resection** (TUR).

It was one of the earliest types of endoscopic or **"keyhole" surgery** and now nearly all prostate operations are done this way.

An instrument called a **resectoscope** is passed into the prostate via the urethra.

The urologist can see the prostate directly and sends a special type of localized electric current through a metal loop to cut the prostate out in pieces, leaving a cavity in the middle of the gland through which urine will pass easily.

A general anaesthetic may be used, but as the operation only takes about half an hour, it's often done with the patient awake but numb from the waist down under an epidural anaesthetic, given through a needle in the back.

It's quite possible for a man to watch his operation being done on a TV screen in front of him if he wants to.

DRUG TREATMENT

Drug treatment of BPH is usually for mild symptoms where the obstruction isn't too bad. Drugs may be tried in more severe cases if there are medical reasons to avoid surgery, or for temporary relief when waiting lists are long.

HORMONE TREATMENT

● The drugs that shrink the prostate interfere with the action of the male hormone testosterone, which is part of the cause of BPH.

Only one, called **finasteride**, is used at present, given as a single tablet once a day. It may take three months or more before the prostate shrinks enough to improve the symptoms, so don't stop taking it after a week or two because it doesn't seem to be working. A small number of men do experience failure of erections and other sexual difficulties. If sex is very important, you might feel that this treatment isn't right for you – although sexual

problems are more common with a TUR and then they aren't reversible.

As soon as the drug is stopped, the prostate grows again very rapidly, so if it is working, keep on taking it.

ALPHA-BLOCKER DRUGS

The other type of drug used for treating BPH is called an alpha-blocker. Alpha-blockers relax the muscle, reduce the obstruction and improve symptoms almost immediately, although they can cause side effects such as faintness, weakness and tiredness.

OTHER TREATMENTS

● **Laser treatment** is more like a TUR and is an alternative way of removing the enlarged part of the prostate or of simply widening the urethra: it can be done as a day case or short stay and is associated with less bleeding.
● Microwave or thermotherapy, where heat treatment is used to destroy prostate tissue, may help some patients with less severe symptoms.

PROSTATE-SPECIFIC ANTIGEN TESTING

Any man with an enlarged prostate will have a fairly new test that measures the level of prostate-specific antigen (PSA) in the blood. The test has been given a lot of publicity as a method of early diagnosis of prostate cancer. Just because your doctor does a PSA test doesn't mean he suspects cancer. He's just being thorough.

Think of the PSA in the blood as if it's "leaking" out of the prostate. More PSA will come from a large prostate than from a small one, so as you get older the PSA can increase quite normally as the prostate enlarges. PSA is **prostate** specific but not **cancer** specific. So if your PSA is higher than normal, it doesn't mean you have cancer.

As older men have larger prostates and also more have non-cancerous diseases of the prostate the average PSA is higher in men of 75 than in men of 55.

After the operation

● Will it be painful?

Postoperative pain is uncommon but the **catheter** can be uncomfortable, and may make the bladder feel full.

Sometimes painful spasms occur.

If they're severe you'll get drugs to control them. You'll be asked to drink a lot of water each day to help flush out your bladder.

● Getting back to normal

It's usual to have some **frequency** for a day or two, and often it's difficult to control the urine at first. A physiotherpist (or a nurse) will teach you some **exercises** to help control the urine flow.

Sometimes it's difficult to start passing urine but persevering for a few hours usually does the trick. If not, the catheter may be re-inserted. Don't despair – usually everything's fine when it's taken out again. Inside, the prostate is raw and needs time to heal. Continue to drink plenty of fluid (but no alcohol). Avoid driving, heavy lifting and sex for two to three weeks.

You'll see some bits of tissue and blood in

the urine from time to time – this is like a scab coming off the skin and, as when a scab comes off, there's sometimes a little bleeding.

Frequency (an abnormally short time between passing urine) may take longer to improve and may not return completely to normal. Needing to pass urine **in the night** may persist after the operation but it's a symptom of getting old as much as of prostate trouble.

Leakage at the end of passing urine may persist, but can usually be controlled by taking a little care.

● Interference with sex

At the end of sex, a man may have a normal climax but no semen is ejaculated. This is called **retrograde ejaculation**. "Having a dry run" describes exactly what happens and it's because semen is leaking back into the bladder rather than coming out normally. A few men do experience difficulty in getting an **erection** after the operation, so ask your surgeon before having the operation for his opinion.

See also:
● **Endoscopic surgery p.358**

lead to fears that she might be abandoned by her partner. It is not surprising therefore that such women may try to avoid sexual contact altogether.

The man frequently becomes frustrated by his inability to penetrate his partner, and often feels she is rejecting him.

WHAT CAN I DO?

The first stage in correcting vaginismus is to reduce the anxiety connected with sexual intercourse. This should be done by using a **relaxation technique**.

1. The woman should lie on the bed, close her eyes, and then relax all the muscles in her body, starting from the toes and working upwards, until all the other muscles in the body are relaxed as well.

2. When she is fully relaxed, **she should first imagine** being in bed with her partner, and then gradually increase the degree of intimacy until she can imagine him penetrating her without this making her anxious. She may then go on to the next stage.

3. This involves gently inserting either **one of her own fingers** or letting her partner insert one of his fingers into her vagina, whichever

produces less anxiety. The finger should remain there quite still until all her feelings of discomfort have subsided. Then the finger should be moved forwards and backwards in the vagina until she can tolerate this without any discomfort.

4. The next stage is the insertion of two fingers, and providing that this is successful, the woman or the couple can then try moving the fingers round and round in her vagina. It is helpful if she can be encouraged to cope with her feelings of discomfort rather than avoiding them.

5. Sexual intercourse must on no account take place until the woman can tolerate her own or her partner's fingers in the vagina without any discomfort whatsoever. It is helpful if she learns to tense and relax her vaginal muscles because this gives her the feeling that she has got some control over her own vagina. **Pelvic floor exercises** show a woman where her vagina is and let her feel it tightening up then loosening.

6. Also, it is helpful **if she "bears down"** when her partner inserts the penis for the first time.

7. It is extremely important that the first attempt at sexual intercourse should be

carried out very gently, with the assistance of a lubricating jelly.

8. The woman should **guide the man's penis into her vagina**, and once inserted, it should be held there without any movement taking place at all. Then he should start slow thrusting movements at her signal, and should withdraw his penis immediately she wants him to do so.

9. All these stages may need **to be repeated several times** before she is sufficiently confident to allow normal sexual intercourse to take place.

10. **Thrusting to orgasm** should not take place on the first occasion and it is far better for the couple to wait until they are less anxious about sexual intercourse before either of them reach orgasm.

If the couple still find that they are having problems with sexual intercourse, then it is recommended that they seek expert advice from an experienced therapist, after discussion with their GP.

> **See also:**
> • Pelvic floor exercises p.375

Impotence

IMPOTENCE IS INABILITY TO ACHIEVE OR MAINTAIN AN ERECTION. DON'T PANIC, IT'S VERY COMMON… DESPITE THE FACT THAT 1 IN 10 MEN OVER THE AGE OF 21 SUFFERS FROM IMPOTENCE, VERY FEW UNDERSTAND HOW IT ARISES.

Impotence can be a side effect of **accidents**, **disease** and most importantly, of **prescription drugs**. This latter cause would fall into the category of medically-induced, or **iatrogenic**, impotence. A quarter of all cases of impotence arise as a side effect of drugs given to treat other conditions. The list of drugs that can interfere with erection (see opposite) is really very long. If you're on any one of them it could be the cause.

Impotence can be a feature of many conditions, including **heart diseases** such as **high blood pressure** and **angina**, **liver disease**, **thyroid disease**, **diabetes**, **chronic bronchitis** and **emphysema**.

HOW ERECTION WORKS

In youth, no man worries about how his erection might work. He takes erections as a matter of course and never expects his penis to fail him. But erection is quite a complicated physiological event and a lot can go wrong.

■ The stiffness of an erection depends on blood being pumped into specially designed spaces (the corpus cavernosum) in the penis, in much the same way as we blow up a balloon with air.

■ To keep the spaces full of blood, and an erection stiff, blood must be prevented from escaping from the spaces by valves snapping shut.

■ Both of these events are controlled by nerves running down the sides of the penis that are in direct connection with the brain. Hence a man can see a sexual image and a split second later feel his erection begin – the **brain–penis connection**.

■ Any interference with that connection, or damage to the penile nerves themselves, can result in too little blood getting into the penis to bring about erection (or only a limp erection). Alternatively, once in the penis, the blood necessary to maintain turgidity can simply seep away through leaky valves.

■ It also has to be said that, if the arteries bringing blood into the penis get furred up, there's insufficient blood to stretch the corpus cavernosum and expand the penis, so erection will be a pretty half-hearted affair. This could happen to any man who has hardening of the arteries.

■ Given the importance of the brain in the complicated circuit of an erection it's not surprising that emotional or psychological disturbance can interfere with a man's potency.

Given this interaction of the brain, the nerves and a healthy blood supply, it isn't difficult to see how the complicated mechanism of erection could go wrong. And go wrong it will, if anything damages either the health of the nerves and arteries of the penis.

WHAT ARE THE CAUSES?
ACCIDENTS

Any accident that involves a **fractured penis** could, theoretically, cause impotence, either by damaging nerves, arteries and veins, or by causing scars to form when injuries heal that distort the normal anatomy.

SURGERY

It's estimated that roughly **half of all men having surgery to or around their prostate gland** will end up with a degree of impotence, in some due to nerve damage, in some due to scarring and in some due to leakage of blood away from the penis in veins that form as the result of surgery.

So, if you're contemplating having surgery for prostate troubles, ask your surgeon about his record of post-operative impotence.

Drugs that can cause impotence

Sleeping pills and tranquillizers
- Phenothiazines: sedatives, anti-sickness pills
- Benzodiazepines: tranquillizers and sleeping pills
- Lithium – antimanic drug

Anti-depressants
- Tricyclic antidepressants, e.g. amitriptyline
- Monoamine oxidase inhibitors (MAOIs)

Almost all antihypertensives for high blood pressure and some heart drugs
- Digoxin ■ Diuretics (water tablets)
- Beta-blockers ■ ACE inhibitors

Endocrine drugs
- Anti-androgens ■ Oestrogens

Cholesterol-lowering drugs
- Statins ■ Fibrates

Any drugs used to treat an enlarged prostate gland

Others
- Cimetidine – antiulcer drug
- Phenytoin – anti-epileptic drug
- Carbamazepine – antithyroid drug

Recreational drugs
- Alcohol ■ Nicotine ■ Marijuana
- Amphetamines ■ Barbiturates

RADIOTHERAPY
Radical radiotherapy treatment for cancer of the prostate, bladder or rectum can lead to impotence. The radiotherapy probably causes damage to the penile nerves.

INFECTIONS
Any virus has the potential to cause nerve damage, anywhere. But some viruses seem to go for the nerves supplying the penis. The commonest ones are the **mumps virus** and the virus of **glandular fever**. Recovery may take 1–2 years but impotence may be permanent.

DYSFUNCTION OF THE PENILE NERVES
■ **Diabetes** causes nerve damage and doesn't spare the penis. Impotence is common in diabetes.
■ **Multiple sclerosis** causes patchy inflammation of the nerves – sometimes in the penis, which can lead to impotence.
■ **Motor-neuron disease** and a stroke can also damage penile nerves.

HARDENING OF THE ARTERIES (ATHEROSCLEROSIS)
If you have **hardening of the arteries** then the arteries supplying your penis are hardened too and you could experience impotence. Warning signs are: **angina**, **high blood pressure**, **kidney disease**.

LIFESTYLE
The mildest impotence is made worse by heavy smoking and heavy drinking.

WHAT IS THE TREATMENT?
Doctors divide impotence into two main categories. First, men who have never been able to produce a satisfactory erection, and second, men who have had a good and active sex life, but who then find that they can no longer produce an adequate erection.

Men in the first category will need to seek professional help as impotence may be the expression of a **deep-seated emotional problem** that is unlikely to respond to simple measures. However, most men who complain of impotence will fall into the second category and are likely to benefit from a straightforward approach. Sometimes a couple have only to make a few lifestyle changes to see a surprising improvement.

LIFESTYLE
Time of day
Choose your moment carefully. The first important step when tackling impotence is to make sure that the man is not over-tired. Tiredness is death to an erection.

Many men find that they are able to produce an erection in the morning, but that it is quite impossible for them to do so at night. Also, it is well to remember that alcohol may well increase sexual desire, but at the same time, it reduces the capacity to produce an erection.

Reduce anxiety
It is extremely important to reduce the amount of anxiety and in the early stages, the couple should not even attempt sexual intercourse and just enjoy each other's bodies again without trying to reach orgasm. In this way, the erection will be strengthened.

Fear of failure
Often the man fears that he will not perform properly and he is over-concerned about what his partner may think of him. It is extremely helpful if the man is allowed just to concentrate all his energies on his own sexual desires instead of being over-concerned with what his partner is feeling. He should just abandon himself to his own sexual feelings, and temporarily think of nothing else at all.

A relaxing bath
It may be helpful for the couple to have a bath before attempting sexual activity, or for him to ask her to put on his favourite perfume, as smell is an extremely important aspect of sexual arousal. Some men will find that the playing of

---

SELF-HELP

What you can do

Sexual positions
I'd like to suggest you take a fresh look at the positions you're using for intercourse. Traditionally, the missionary position has been the most popular with couples. This is where the man lies on top of his partner supporting his weight on his arms.
For the older man, this can be quite tiring and for the woman uncomfortable if her partner is much heavier than she is. **Lying side by side** with the man behind is probably a more suitable position as it is less tiring and also provides the opportunity for maximum manual stimulation.

Kind of lovemaking
All women know that wonderful orgasms can be achieved without penetration. If a man transfers his concern from his penis to his partner's enjoyment, he'll go a long way towards forgetting about his male obsession with erection. Concentrating on non-penetrative sex is one of the best cures for impotence.

What about complementary methods?
There are many herbal remedies that claim to help impotence. I stress the word "claim" because none of them has been really tested; most of the evidence is anecdotal. They claim to "tone up the genital tissues" or "promote healthy testosterone production" or "stimulate the circulation to the penis". This is all pseudo-science aimed at seducing you to buy the products. And they're not cheap. Most of them cost £20 or more. My advice is to save your money.

soft music is helpful, others may prefer to make love in the dark. You should use any measures that are likely to increase sexual desire and remove anything likely to reduce it.

Give it time
No two men will respond to these measures in the same way, and your partner will have to be patient. It may be several weeks before you can get an adequate erection. Take your time.

ERECTION AIDS
There's a wide range of implants available, from relatively simple, rigid supports to sophisticated pumps that can inflate a tube in the penis to make it erect. These implants do not increase a man's desire for sex but they do make sex play and intercourse possible. Again, your GP can help you here.

No matter how tempting, I wouldn't respond to newspaper advertisements if I were you. They promise the earth and deliver very little.

DRUGS
In 1982 it was discovered that some drugs when injected into the penis could provoke an erection and this revolutionized the diagnosis and treatment of impotence. The latest drug,

alprostadil, relaxes the muscles in the erectile tissue of the penis, allowing increased blood flow, which is the basis of a normal erection.

Injectables
The idea of injecting the penis with anything makes me wince, but men do. Injectable alprostadil is available and it comes in a box containing a syringe with the dry, sterile powder form of the drug. The solution must be carefully prepared and the correct dose injected into the side of the penis through a very fine needle. Some discomfort is common but it's seldom troublesome. Overdosage may lead to a prolonged erection. Should the erection last more than six hours, seek medical advice.

Pellets
Developed in the USA, MUSE (medicated urethral system for erection) is a fairly new addition to the treatment of impotence. It's alprostadil in the form of a small pellet. The pellet is pushed directly into the urethra by a urethral stick – so there are no needles.

When this kind of treatment is effective, an erection generally lasts 30 to 60 minutes. Not more than two doses are recommended in 24 hours. It's available only on prescription.

Viagra warning

There's been a lot of hype about Viagra but the reality is quite sobering. For Viagra to work, the penis should have adequately healthy nerves and arteries. So while it may be worth a try if you have diabetes, in trials, only half the diabetic men tested had an improvement in their erections. If your pelvic nerves or pelvic arteries have been damaged by an accident or by surgery, Viagra might not perform miracles for you either; the success rate is only 40–50 percent.

In addition to normal nerves and arteries, you need to have normal sexual desire for Viagra to work. If you don't want sex, Viagra won't give you an erection.

Infertility

AS MANY AS 1 IN 6 COUPLES CONSULT THEIR DOCTOR BECAUSE OF AN INABILITY TO CONCEIVE. MOST DOCTORS WOULD FEEL THAT INVESTIGATION IS CALLED FOR IF NO PREGNANCY OCCURS AFTER A YEAR OF REGULAR, UNPROTECTED SEXUAL INTERCOURSE.

That, of itself, isn't a cause for gloom – most couples who are infertile after trying for a year do eventually conceive a child.

In addition, fertility isn't always a straightforward case of being able, or unable, to conceive.

WHAT ARE THE CAUSES?
Of all the cases of infertility, about 40 percent are due to the man, about 30 percent are due to the woman and about 20 percent are the result of combined factors. Ten percent remain unexplained.

Female infertility has been studied for years by gynaecologists, whereas the study of male fertility, known as andrology, is relatively new.

Given the ready availability of sperm, however, **a semen analysis should always be the first investigation of infertility**. This includes a sperm count and tests the motility and quality of sperm.

Remember, infertility should **always be investigated as a couple – the fertility of a couple is the sum of their individual fertilities**.

MALE INFERTILITY
■ **Hormonal problems.** The brain sex hormones (gonadotrophins) of a man, luteinizing hormone (LH) and follicle-stimulating hormone (FSH), need to be in balance for sperm to be produced.
■ **Anatomical problems** with the penis or testicles, or the man's ability to ejaculate, can affect fertility.
■ **Immunological problems**, when a man's immune system produces antibodies that attack and destroy his sperm, reducing their ability to fertilize an egg.
■ **Decreasing sperm counts.** Studies suggest that sperm counts decreased over the course of the 20th century, owing to environmental factors such as exposure to oestrogens in foodstuffs and indestructible chemicals such as polychlorinated biphenyls (PCBs), used in the plastics industry, that enter the food chain. But, despite lower numbers of sperm, **actual fertility remains unaffected**, presumably because sperm are produced in such excessive numbers. **Smoking**, **alcohol** and **stress** lower the quantity and quality of sperm. **Coffee** and

social drugs may produce abnormal sperm.

FEMALE INFERTILITY
Female infertility has many different causes such as the **inability to ovulate**, **endometriosis**, **blocked fallopian tubes**, **ovarian cysts** or an **abnormal uterus**. A woman's **cervical mucus** may also be hostile to her partner's sperm.

When a woman's fertility is marginal, as when ovulation is irregular, it's known as subfertility. Usually this only becomes a problem if her partner's fertility is also marginal – if a man has a low-to-average sperm count, for instance – because subfertility in one partner can be balanced by strong fertility in the other.

HORMONAL PROBLEMS
About one-third of female infertility is due to a **failure to ovulate**. Ovulation is controlled by the same finely orchestrated release of hormones that controls the menstrual cycle. If the precise reason for a failure to ovulate can be pinpointed, it can be treated using synthetic hormones (fertility drugs).

A hormonal imbalance can result in two faults:

1. The ovary fails to produce properly mature follicles in which the ova can develop fully.

2. A slightly different hormonal imbalance can mean that, although the ovum matures, the ovary isn't triggered to release it.

Deep in the brains of both men and women, the **hypothalamus** is responsible for sending signals to the pituitary gland, which then sends hormonal messages to the ovaries and testicles triggering them to produce ova and sperm. A malfunctioning **hypothalamus**, therefore, may result in infertility of both men and women.

A malfunctioning **pituitary gland** – under-active, over-active, or injured in some way – may not produce the precise amount of follicle-stimulating hormone (FSH) and luteinizing hormone (LH) necessary for normal ovulation and sperm production.

REPRODUCTIVE ORGAN PROBLEMS
Ovaries
In addition to hormonal problems, the ovaries may be affected by **cysts**, **past surgery**, **radiation** or **chemotherapy**, and **lifestyle** factors such as smoking (passive smoking too).

Fallopian tubes
About 50 percent of infertile women have blocked fallopian tubes. Healthy fallopian tubes are essential for conception because they're the pathways that allow the ovum and sperm to meet and fuse, and then enable the resulting fertilized ovum to reach the uterus. The fallopian tubes usually become blocked because of **pelvic inflammation** from an STD infection such as **chlamydia**. They're extremely delicate structures and it's difficult for them to be made fully functional once damaged.

Uterus
Uterine problems account for 10 percent of all cases of female infertility and may be due to fibroids or an abnormally shaped uterus. Other, more rare, uterine problems include polyps and internal adhesions that

Secondary infertility

The term secondary infertility applies if a woman already has a child but is unable to conceive another. The problem may be caused by an infection of the fallopian tubes, which are particularly vulnerable to STDs such as chlamydia, but may also be due to failure to ovulate or may be unexplained.

make the walls of the uterus stick together. The majority of these problems can be treated successfully.

Fibroids
Fibroids, benign muscle tumours of the uterine wall, don't necessarily affect fertility. 1 in 5 women over the age of 30 has them, and 1 in 3 women over 35, but many conceive nonetheless.

Cervix
Cervical mucus that is hostile to sperm may play a part in infertility.

INVESTIGATING THE PROBLEM
The investigation of infertility may try your patience and resolve. It may even humiliate you. Whichever partner is found to have low fertility will feel threatened and guilty. Be prepared to be long-suffering and very generous. And please see the counsellor affiliated to your fertility centre for guidance.

Tracking down the cause of infertility proceeds logically.

PART ONE: YOUR GP
One couple in six consults their doctor about infertility. Your doctor first assesses how healthy you both are and will ask about your sex life.

The woman will be asked for dates of her last six periods to establish she's menstruating regularly.

If further investigation is needed, the couple will be referred to a special fertility clinic and further tests will be done there.

PART TWO: A SPECIAL FERTILITY CLINIC
Women may be asked to keep an ovulation temperature chart and will have a blood test to check that ovulation has occurred. Men will have investigations too. You can expect the following steps to be taken.

■ **Checking on ovulation:** If your doctor suspects there's a problem with ovulation, you'll be tested for the level of **progesterone in your blood on day 21 of a 28-day cycle,** or seven days before an expected period if your cycles are usually shorter or longer than 28 days. This is because progesterone levels rise after ovulation and a high level will indicate that if you're ovulating. You may be asked to keep a record of your basal body temperature (BBT) each morning for several cycles. Ovulation prediction kits can also be useful.

■ **The man is asked to provide a semen sample.**

■ **If a man's sperm are normal,** the woman

Reasons for female infertility

Primary reason	Frequency	Causes	Results
FAILURE TO OVULATE	30 percent	● Underactive pituitary gland ● Polycystic ovary syndrome	● No ova ● Ova not maturing ● Mature ova not able to be released
PROBLEMS WITH TRANSPORT OF OVA	50 percent	● Abnormalities of fallopian tubes, pelvic disease or surgery ● Endometriosis	● Ova cannot reach uterus
UTERINE PROBLEMS	10 percent	● Fibroids ● Abnormally shaped uterus ● Adhesions in uterus	● Fertilized ovum unable to develop properly

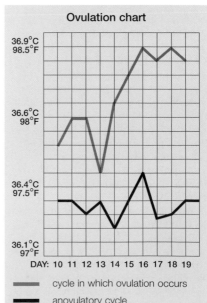

Ovulation chart

36.9°C 98.5°F

36.6°C 98°F

36.4°C 97.5°F

36.1°C 97°F

DAY: 10 11 12 13 14 15 16 17 18 19

——— cycle in which ovulation occurs

——— anovulatory cycle

Basal body temperature (BBT) drops sharply before ovulation occurs and rises sharply afterwards. Keeping a chart helps track ovulation.

will then be offered an **ultrasound scan** and possibly **laparoscopy** if she's ovulating.

Once the cause of infertility is pinpointed a suitable treatment will be suggested.

CHECKING MALE INFERTILITY
SPERM ASSESSMENT
Your doctor will arrange for preliminary tests on your semen before making more detailed investigations of your fertility. The semen samples are examined by a trained technician, using a microscope and a computer-assisted semen motility analyzer.

Sperm tests
Sperm tests are performed to assess whether your sperm appear normal and are capable of swimming to and penetrating your partner's egg.

■ In the **sperm invasion test** the interaction between your sperm and your partner's cervical mucus is examined under a microscope. If sperm are unable to cross into the mucus or cannot move through it properly, the finding doesn't itself indicate whether the problem lies with the sperm or the mucus.

■ The **crossover sperm invasion test** is performed to answer that question. This uses exactly the same procedure as the sperm invasion test – but first, your sperm and normal mucus from a donor female will be used, and second, the normal sperm from a donor male will be combined with your partner's mucus.

These may reveal the problem but, if not, further tests such as the egg penetration test may be necessary.

■ The **egg penetration test** examines the potential of sperm to fertilize an egg. The test involves introducing the sperm to hamster eggs (yes, I know it sounds strange, but read on) and measuring how well the sperm penetrate and fuse with them.

The use of hamster eggs means that your partner doesn't have to go through stressful IVF treatment in order to provide eggs for testing. There's no danger of an embryo resulting from the fusion of sperm and hamster eggs.

CHECKING FEMALE INFERTILITY
LAPAROSCOPY
A slender telescope that's equipped with fibre optics, a laparoscope is about the width of a fountain pen.

It can be inserted through a tiny incision in the navel to view the abdominal cavity directly.

In addition to offering the surgeon a superb view of the organs, high-quality videos can be taken through the laparoscope for later reference.

Laparoscopy allows the condition of the reproductive organs to be assessed under direct vision. The procedure is often timed for

the second half of the cycle to confirm that ovulation has occurred.

HYSTEROSALPINGOGRAPHY
Hysterosalpingography (HSG) is usually reserved for women found to have damaged fallopian tubes via laparoscopy, or if doctors suspect there's something wrong with the uterus – say, a cyst.

HSG is an X-ray picture of the uterus and tubes and can show up problems within the cavity of the womb and within the tubes.

Dye is useful for checking the fallopian tubes as it will only enter and travel through open tubes, thus showing up any damage, distortion or complete blockage. The injected dye is monitored on an X-ray screen. Ultrasound may be used to do a similar test since it does not expose the ovaries to X-rays.

ENDOMETRIAL BIOPSY
In this procedure a tiny amount of the endometrium (uterine lining) is removed and then examined for any changes.

An endometrial biopsy is performed in order to assess whether a woman's hormones are bringing about normal alterations to her endometrium during the second half of her cycle in preparation for conception.

When the hormones are balanced correctly, there's an increase in the production of progesterone, which thickens the endometrium.

If progesterone is being underproduced, the uterine lining won't develop sufficiently for an embryo to implant. If there's little or no alteration, then fertility drugs are an option.

ULTRASOUND SCANNING
Ultrasound scanning is used to check the development of ovarian follicles, so that doctors can track the growth of follicles and the release of the ovum or ova at ovulation.

WHAT IS THE TREATMENT?
Though you're desperate for a baby, if you're a candidate for infertility treatment of any kind, try to be rational and balanced. Get to know the success rate for any treatment from your doctors so that your expectations are reasonable.

Some treatments involve complicated regimes that will test your emotional and physical stamina. As a couple, you're going to have to be strong, so take advantage of the counselling service attached to all fertility centres.

FERTILITY DRUGS
Step one
A woman's ovaries can nearly always be encouraged to produce good-quality eggs using fertility drugs, so when failure to ovulate is the reason for female infertility, fertility drugs are the usual treatment.

■ The most common fertility drug is

clomiphene, which is taken for five days at the beginning of each menstrual cycle.

■ Clomiphene stimulates the release of follicle-stimulating hormone (FSH) by the pituitary gland. This acts on the ovaries and often initiates the ripening of a follicle and then ovulation.

■ Clomiphene's advantages are that it's free from major side effects and has a low multiple pregnancy rate – only 5–10 percent – usually twins and occasionally triplets; quadruplets and quintuplets are now very rare because we know so much more about the correct dosage.

■ Clomiphene is an **anti-oestrogen** (the drug was first developed as a contraceptive), so it may impede conception if prescribed inappropriately.

Step two
If clomiphene fails, it's usual to try daily injections of human menopausal gonadotrophin (hMG), which is similar in action and effect to FSH, followed by an injection of **human chorionic gonadotrophin** (hCG).

This complicated treatment requires close monitoring of the ovaries with blood tests and daily ultrasound scans in order to avoid the risk of multiple pregnancy. Some women require even more complex medical management in order to achieve ovulation.

OTHER METHODS
Artificial insemination
In this procedure, a partner's sperm (artificial insemination by partner, or AIP) or a donor's sperm (donor insemination, or DI) is introduced into the cervix from a syringe. Insemination is done just before or during ovulation.

DI may be considered when a man has a very low sperm count, is sterile or is known to be a carrier of a hereditary abnormality (see Sperm donation, below).

Single women who want a baby also consider DI, although UK infertility doctors are bound by the Human Fertilization and Embryology Act to take into account the need of the child for a father.

Sperm donation
The best sperm donor is your partner, but, if not, sperm donors should be healthy, fertile men who have children of their own.

All sperm is screened for infectious diseases, such as AIDS, and all donors are asked about their genetic family background.

Clinics also try to match the donor's physical characteristics to those of the couple but, because a different donor's sperm is usually used at every attempt, the closest match may not be the one that actually results in pregnancy.

Egg donation
More complicated than sperm donation, this involves the female donor using fertility drugs

so that her ovaries will be stimulated to produce several ova at once.

A couple of trips to the fertility clinic will be necessary and perhaps an overnight stay when the ova are collected. For this reason, many ovum donors are women who are undergoing in vitro fertilization (IVF).

The medical data on each donor is archived and can be accessed by the resulting child once she or he is 18.

In vitro fertilization (IVF)

For IVF to work, two things are necessary.

1. Eggs from the female partner, if necessary harvested after clomiphene or hMG/hCG treatment.

2. Sperm from the male partner, if necessary isolated microscopically from a specimen of semen or the testicles themselves.

Both, of course, can be obtained from donors (see opposite).

Children conceived by IVF used to be known as test-tube babies. IVF was pioneered by British doctors Patrick Steptoe and Robert Edwards in 1978, when the very first IVF baby, Louise Brown, was born.

Since then, about 35,000 IVF babies have been born in the UK. Although this figure sounds high, IVF only has about a 20 percent success rate per cycle of treatment, although it can be as high as 30 percent under the best circumstances. Everyone contemplating IVF should know that it's physically and emotionally very demanding and stressful. You should always have **counselling** before and during IVF and it's available at all IVF clinics.

1. Once her partner's sperm have been tested for viability, the woman is given fertility drugs to stimulate her ovaries into producing ova.

She's then carefully monitored using ultrasound until the follicles are ripe, when the ova will be collected by her gynaecologist using laparoscopy.

2. A long hollow needle will be inserted through the upper vagina or the abdominal wall to reach the ovaries, under constant monitoring with ultrasound.

The ova are gently suctioned out of the follicles into the probe, transferred to a culture medium in a petri dish, and then stored in an incubator, where they continue to grow.

3. Once they have reached full maturity (within 2–24 hours), the sperm are introduced. Fertilization usually occurs within 18 hours.

The fertilized ova are then kept inside the incubator for an additional 48 hours, by which time each will have divided into about four cells.

A maximum of three embryos can then be transferred into the woman's uterus. Further embryos can be stored.

GIFT and ZIFT

Gamete intrafallopian transfer (GIFT) and zygote intrafallopian transfer (ZIFT) are two variations on IVF. In GIFT, the egg and sperm (both medically known as gametes) are transferred to one of the woman's fallopian tubes, where conception may then take place naturally. In ZIFT, the fertilized egg (medically known as a zygote) is transferred to one of the fallopian tubes before it has begun to grow into an embryo. There seems to be a slightly higher chance that an embryo will implant in the uterine wall if it travels down the fallopian tube at the correct time in a woman's cycle as it would if conception had occurred naturally. For both of these procedures, a woman must have at least one open and undamaged fallopian tube. Pregnancy success rates for GIFT and ZIFT are thought to be about 25–30 percent per cycle.

ICSI

Intracytoplasmic sperm injection (ICSI) is a new technique, not available everywhere, allowing a man with a very low sperm count to father a baby.

Sperm are sucked up into a syringe and, under a microscope, are injected into a harvested ovum to fertilize it. After 48 hours of incubation, the resulting embryo is replaced in the woman's body using the procedure for IVF.

TEST

Ultrasound scanning

Ultrasound scanning is a way of producing a photographic picture by using sound waves. The picture is formed by the echoes of sound waves bouncing off different parts of the body. The echoes differ in their waves according to the density of the organ. Ultrasound scanning can give pictures of soft tissue in great detail. If it is done during pregnancy, it will show fetal heartbeat and movement and can be used as a non-invasive means of examining the fetus. An accurate picture of the fetus in utero may be printed out.

Ultrasound is used in many areas of medicine as a diagnostic tool, particularly to detect breast lumps and the cause of abdominal pains, such as gallstones or hiatus hernia. It can also sometimes be used to treat abnormalities. For example, high levels of ultrasound waves can destroy stones in the bladder. Ultrasound scanning is also used widely in fertility treatment and to tell whether a pregnancy is viable or not.

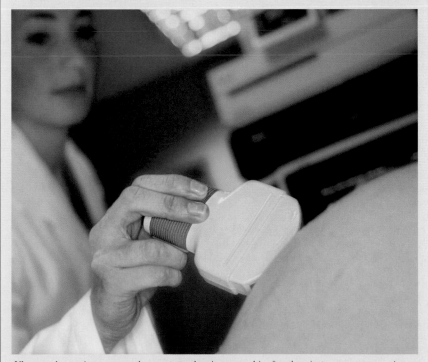

Ultrasound scanning uses sound waves to produce images and is often done in pregnancy to examine the fetus. The procedure is quick and painless and does not involve exposure to radiation.

SEXUAL HEALTH

The group of diseases classed as sexually transmitted are those that are passed on primarily by sexual contact between people. Many people delay seeking treatment for these diseases because of embarrassment, but if you suspect that either you or your partner are suffering from a sexually transmitted disease (STD), it's essential to seek help from your doctor or an STD or genito-urinary medicine (GUM) clinic as soon as you can.

I begin with chlamydia, an STD that's on the increase and is especially dangerous because it can rob a woman of her fertility if not treated promptly. Next I cover thrush, which affects many people and is not necessarily sexually transmitted. Then come genital herpes and genital warts, followed by bacterial vaginosis and trichomoniasis. Syphilis and gonorrhoea are also covered. I also discuss the importance of safe sex in preventing STDs.

Chlamydia

CHLAMYDIA IS THE MOST COMMON BACTERIAL SEXUALLY TRANSMITTED INFECTION
AND IT'S ON THE INCREASE. THE NUMBER OF CASES OF CHLAMYDIA
IN ENGLAND ROSE BY 74 PERCENT BETWEEN 1995 AND 1999.

Rates have been consistently higher in women than men, and particularly in those aged 16–24. Part of this increase is due to new diagnostic methods and publicity, which mean that more people are being screened and seeking care. Up to 70 percent of women and at least 25 percent of men infected with chlamydia have no symptoms, so a substantial number of infections remain undiagnosed and untreated. Where there are symptoms, **women** may have discharge, pain when passing urine, heavy periods or bleeding between periods, low abdominal pain or abdominal pain during vaginal sex. **Men** may notice discharge from the penis and/or burning when passing urine.

New methods of testing for chlamydia are now available that will allow easier and more widespread detection and treatment. Over 56,000 cases of chlamydia infection were treated in STD or genito-urinary medicine (GUM) clinics in England and Wales in 1999 – that's more than three times the number of cases of gonorrhoea reported.

HOW IS CHLAMYDIA PASSED ON?
Chlamydia is almost always transmitted through vaginal or anal sex, and very occasionally through oral-genital contact. Occasionally a pregnant woman can pass the infection to her baby. In this case infection is usually limited to the eyes, but can rarely cause pneumonia.

HOW DOES CHLAMYDIA HARM YOU?
After infection with chlamydia, the fine hairs can be destroyed that waft the fertilized egg down the fallopian tube to the uterus. This sets the scene for tubal or ectopic pregnancy.

In Britain, the **ectopic pregnancy rate** has quadrupled since the early 1960s, in parallel with chlamydia infection. The damage can also set up tubal inflammation, swelling and

---

Who should be tested for chlamydia?

■ All sexually active women under 25 and women over 25 with a new sexual partner.
■ Those with more than two sexual partners a year.
■ All men and women attending STD clinics: nearly 1 in 5 has chlamydia.
■ Women seeking termination of pregnancy: nearly 1 in 10 has chlamydia.

---

complete blockage of the tubes, though why this develops in some women and not others isn't known. **Teenagers** are more vulnerable to this bacterial attack, so threatening the fertility of future generations of mothers.

LONG-TERM EFFECTS
Chlamydia infection in women has serious fall-out. Untreated infections can persist for a long time and up to one-third of inadequately treated women may go on to develop **pelvic inflammatory disease**.

Up to half of all cases of pelvic inflammatory disease can be attributed to chlamydia.

Among women with pelvic inflammatory disease, **one-fifth** may become infertile, and one-tenth will go on to have an ectopic pregnancy once they conceive. So the personal and economic costs of untreated chlamydia infection are considerable.

SCREENING
Given the prevalence of chlamydia and the long-term effects of infection, could women be screened for its presence so cases are caught

and treated early before lasting damage has been done?

The first trial of chlamydia screening in women aged 18–34 in the US showed that pelvic inflammatory disease was 56 percent lower in screened and treated women than in those who were unscreened. All women and men with a discharge should therefore be tested for chlamydia. Since this infection is often without symptoms, those who have frequent partner changes should also be tested.

LATEST TESTS FOR CHLAMYDIA
At one time chlamydia was notoriously elusive to track down but tests are becoming more sophisticated with increasing use of **DNA urine check**; there is even talk of a future test being available over the counter. Anyone can request a test at any STD or GUM clinic.

CHLAMYDIA – THE FERTILITY TIME-BOMB
Often neglected by patients and doctors alike, chlamydia infection may not be life-threatening but it can be life-ruining. It has come to be known as the fertility time-bomb, capable of lurking silently for years before causing irreparable damage.

CARRIERS OF CHLAMYDIA
Because chlamydia is virtually symptomless in men, they can carry the disease without knowing. Male carriers can reinfect women and keep a chronic low-grade infection simmering even after a woman has had antibiotics. This means that if chlamydia is found in a woman, her partner(s) must be treated too.

See also:
• **Pelvic inflammatory disease p.251**

FOCUS *on* vaginal thrush

Vaginal thrush is inflammation of the vagina caused by the candida fungus. Thrush is a very common, not to mention miserable, problem. Three-quarters of all women will get thrush at some stage in their lives. Although the lucky ones only suffer one attack, many get it several times a year.

WHAT EVERY WOMAN SHOULD KNOW

- While thrush isn't life-threatening, it can cause a lot of distress – the more you know the less it will worry you.
- As a woman, you're likely to suffer from some form of **genito-urinary infection** at some point in your life. The most common infections are **thrush, cystitis** and **bacterial vaginosis**.
- Men very often re-infect their partners because usually women seek medical treatment.

HOW CAN I TELL IF I HAVE THRUSH?

Do you have any of the following symptoms?
Women
- Itching and/or soreness in and around the entrance to the vagina.
- A thick, whitish discharge that does not smell unpleasant.
- Swelling of the labia.
- Stinging on passing water.
- Pain during sexual intercourse.

Men
- Irritation, burning or itching under the foreskin or on the tip of the penis.
- Redness or red patches under foreskin or on the tip of the penis.
- A thick, cheesy discharge under the foreskin.
- Difficulty in pulling back the foreskin.
- Slight discharge from the penis.
- Discomfort when passing water.

If you have any of these symptoms, see your GP to confirm that you have a thrush infection.

Once your thrush has been diagnosed by your doctor, on future occasions you may wish to treat yourself with an over-the-counter remedy.

The symptoms listed are experienced by some but not all sufferers. They can also be a sign of another type of infection – for example, cystitis, of which pain on passing urine is a common symptom.

HOW TO AVOID THRUSH

While there's no simple solution to prevent thrush, there are a number of things you can do to prevent getting it so frequently.

- Avoid wearing tights, underwear not made of cotton, leggings, Lycra shorts and tight jeans or trousers.
- Wash and wipe the genital area from front to back. You can wet a couple of clean cotton wool balls in water and use to wipe once and then throw them away.
- If possible, don't scratch because the fungus can be spread by hand. Any constant scratching can cause thickening of the skin and proneness to infection.
- Use sanitary pads rather than tampons during a period.
- Avoid perfumed soaps, genital sprays and deodorants and any other irritants such as disinfectants.
- If prescribed an antibiotic, remind your doctor that you tend to get thrush.
- Thrush can sometimes be passed on through sex. Even though you might be treated, you could be getting it straight back again if your sexual partner isn't having treatment as well. While you're on any treatment for thrush, it's not advisable to have sex until given the all-clear.
- As the fungus likes warm, moist conditions, folds of fat around the groin may be the reason for recurrent infections. If you're overweight it might help to shed some of those extra pounds.
- Although any man can carry thrush, all uncircumcized men should clean under their foreskins as part of their daily routine.

> **See also:**
> • **Bacterial vaginosis p.283** • **Candidiasis p.450** • **Cystitis p.378**

Common myths

THE MYTH: Thrush is a sexually transmitted disease that affects women who have poor personal hygiene or who are promiscuous. The facts: Vaginal thrush is NOT necessarily a sexually-transmitted disease – it results from an imbalance of bacteria and yeasts in the vagina. The imbalance can allow one type of yeast, *Candida albicans,* to breed faster than usual and this can cause thrush. The imbalance that can lead to thrush can be caused by many things, such as hormonal changes experienced during menstruation, in pregnancy and at the menopause. Other common triggers are **antibiotics** and **poorly-controlled diabetes, disinfectant** in the bath and **vaginal deodorants**. Being a thrush sufferer does =not mean you're "dirty" – in fact being over-zealous with douching can upset the natural balance in the vagina and start an attack of thrush. Men can get thrush as well.

THE MYTH: Thrush has to be treated by a doctor and requires an internal examination and questions about your sex life. The facts: If this is your first bout of thrush, you should visit your doctor to confirm that thrush is the problem. Your doctor may take samples from the vagina to check for infection. If you're getting recurrent attacks of thrush, your doctor may ask about your sex life to find out whether your partner may be reinfecting you. If you've had thrush before, had a diagnosis from a doctor and recognize the symptoms, you may find it easier and more convenient to use an over-the-counter treatment.

THE MYTH: All thrush treatments involve either pessaries or creams, which have to be inserted into the vagina. The facts: Treatment can be by insertion of a **pessary** or **cream** into the vagina, but oral treatments have been available from the doctor for more than eight years and this form of treatment is preferred by most women. Home remedies such as **live yoghurt** applied to the vagina are NOT proven cures for thrush. If any treatment causes soreness, stop using it immediately.

Safe sex

- Safe sex helps protect you from STDs and HIV/AIDS.
- Safe sex means being responsible about sex.
- Always practise safe sex; nothing less will do.

Condoms and STDs

In order for sex to be safe from STDs, you should always use a condom for vaginal and anal sex – for oral sex too if you're worried about HIV (but HIV infection from oral sex is rare). Make sure that you know how to use one properly, and never use condoms from out-of-date packets. Practise safe sex; think carefully about your sexual behaviour.

Your rights

Demanding safe sex is your right. If your partner resents this, he or she is not thinking about you, and you should question your relationship. If your partner won't use a condom, refuse to have sex, and consider ending the relationship. By acting irresponsibly he or she puts you in danger.

Preventing pregnancy too

While condoms are great for safe sex, don't rely on them alone to prevent pregnancy. Semen can leak if you haven't managed to use the condom correctly, or if you've used an out-of-date one. It's best for women to either be on the pill or to use a diaphragm as well.

Getting help...

Your doctor, family planning clinic or advice centre will gladly give you information on condoms. A whole variety of condoms is available, and some of them have been designed to make sex a little more interesting! Condoms are available from retail outlets, supermarkets, pharmacies and even public toilets. You can get advice on safe sex practices from AIDS charities, hospitals and gay helplines (see Useful addresses, p.567).

Next time...

Don't drop your guard for a second; always practise safe sex. You want to be able to relax when you have sex; you don't want to have to worry about pregnancy and STDs.

Do's and Don'ts

Carry a condom
Do carry a condom with you at all times, women as well as men.

Practise first
Do make sure you know how to use a condom before you have sex with someone.

Condoms every time
Do use a condom until you're absolutely sure there's no risk to or from your partner.

Be frank
Do be open when you start a relationship. Tell your partner about any chronic infections, such as herpes.

Once only
Don't ever try to use a condom more than once.

No casual sex
Don't have sex with someone at a party, or on holiday, who you hardly know and may never meet again.

How do I protect myself?

Try saying something like this:

1. Talking to a partner:
"My ex has sent me a card...no, not for my birthday – it says he's got something nasty and I might have caught it. So that could include you too. We'd better go to the STD clinic and get this sorted."

But your partner may not know he or she has an STD so...

2. Going for a health check:
"Contraception's sorted – but why don't we both get a health check?"
"Right. Good idea. Let's call the STD clinic."

3. Using a condom for protection:
If he says: "You don't think I'd wear one of those...", tell him:
"You've obviously not looked at some of them recently."

A condom will protect you from infection, and the pill will protect you from pregnancy.

Genital herpes

HERPES SIMPLEX IS THE NAME OF A VIRUS THAT CAN CAUSE COLD SORES OR GENITAL SORES, DEPENDING ON WHICHEVER BIT OF SKIN IS INFECTED.

Herpes is called a cold sore on the face but you can get it on the genitals or anywhere else. Cold sores are often due to a mother passing on the virus to her children through kissing. In genital herpes the virus is transmitted through infected skin coming into contact with a partner's skin – for example, during sex or from mouth to genitals during oral sex. It's more common in women because their genital areas are warmer and moister than men's.

WHAT ARE THE CAUSES?

■ Genital herpes was originally thought to be caused only by the **herpes simplex virus type 2**, while cold sores on the lips were thought more likely to be due to **herpes simplex type 1**. However, with the increase in oral sex this distinction has become blurred.

■ In Europe, genital herpes infection is the commonest cause of genital ulceration and it's increasing among women.

HOW COMMON IS GENITAL HERPES?

Blood tests show that most of us have been exposed to the **herpes simplex** virus by the time we reach middle age. Millions of people are infected with the virus but probably only one-quarter of those infected have symptoms of any kind. Many people have what is called a **sub-clinical attack** – with no visible signs of infection and no ill effects. These people don't know they've been infected.

WHAT HAPPENS TO THE VIRUS?

Once in the body, the virus can retreat to nerve cells near the base of the spine. If the virus is reactivated, it can return to where it entered the body and cause a recurrence. Not all people have recurrences; some have a few and for some the problem recurs from time to time. Usually the initial attack is the most severe.

HOW INFECTIOUS IS IT?

As you'd expect, genital herpes is highly contagious. New research indicates that the

virus can also be transmitted by people who don't have any symptoms. Symptoms appear between three and seven days after sexual contact with an infected partner.

WHAT ARE THE SYMPTOMS?

■ The genital skin feels oversensitive to the touch.

■ Itching and irritation around the genitals.

■ A general feeling of being unwell.

■ Headache.

■ Muscle aches and joint pains.

■ Abdominal pain.

■ Shooting pain in the lower limbs.

■ Enlarged tender glands in the groin.

■ Pain on passing urine.

■ Blisters appear within a few hours, enlarge, burst and become painful ulcers within two or three days.

■ The ulcers form scabs and take 14–21 days to heal completely.

WHAT ARE THE TRIGGERS FOR GENITAL HERPES?

Recurrences don't depend on having intercourse with an infected partner. Attacks can be triggered by:

● physical and mental stress
● excessive cold or heat, including fever
● irritation of delicate genital tissues
● local genital trauma (e.g. rough sexual intercourse, plucking or shaving pubic hair)
● general ill health and other infections such as a cold causing fever.

WHAT IS THE TREATMENT?

■ Genital herpes should always be looked at by a doctor and not treated by yourself at home.

■ See your doctor immediately if you feel numb or sensitive in the genital area or if you've had sexual relations with anyone with the herpes virus.

■ There's no cure for genital herpes but the sooner treatment is given the more likely it will prevent or ameliorate an attack. Antiviral drugs, such as **acyclovir**, taken as tablets make the ulcers less painful and encourage healing if taken early in the attack.

■ Other remedies include bathing the area with salt solution (a heaped teaspoon of salt to a pint of water).

■ Over-the-counter acyclovir cream shouldn't be used to treat genital herpes, though it works better on facial cold sores.

SELF-HELP

■ Always use a condom to protect yourself from genital herpes.

NEVER!

Once you have got herpes it's for life, so here are a few nevers:

NEVER have sex if you have symptoms, except with the person from whom you got it (or who you gave it to). When both partners have the same virus they don't reinfect each other.

NEVER have unprotected sex with a comparative stranger.

NEVER have oral-genital sex if you have a cold sore.

NEVER be dishonest about your herpes. It's best to be open about herpes simplex and tell your partner. And you must avoid skin contact when the virus is active. It may be easier to explain that you sometimes get cold sores on your genitals.

NEVER be shy to tell your doctor about possible contacts.

Genital herpes and pregnancy

If you or your partner has had an attack of genital herpes, it should be recorded on your medical notes, but you should still tell your doctor if you have or have had herpes. Swabs during the last stage of pregnancy are no longer thought necessary as we now know that the delay in getting the results makes it pointless. Caesarean sections are rarely performed except when the mother is experiencing a primary infection. A mother's antibodies protect her baby from becoming infected during birth.

■ Painful blisters can be relieved by a soak in a tepid bath with salt added and cold packs (not ice) applied to the infected area.

■ To prevent genital herpes recurring get plenty of rest and eat a balanced diet with nutritional foodstuffs – fresh fruit and vegetables, wholefoods and plenty of liquids.

■ Manage stress by learning relaxation exercises or taking up yoga.

■ Wear loose underwear so air can circulate and keep your genitals cool. Leave the sores exposed to air as much as possible.

■ Keep a record of when you get recurrent attacks in an attempt to find a pattern. If, for example, recurrences are related to rough sex, try using a lubricant such as KY jelly.

■ You could try taking 200 IU (international units) of vitamin E daily, which may improve your body's immune response.

> **See also:**
> ● **Herpes simplex p.336**

> **WARNING:**
> The herpes virus MAY have a role in the development of cervical cancer, so women who have had genital herpes should have a cervical smear test regularly, preferably every year, though NHS guidelines state every three years.

Threats to mental wellbeing

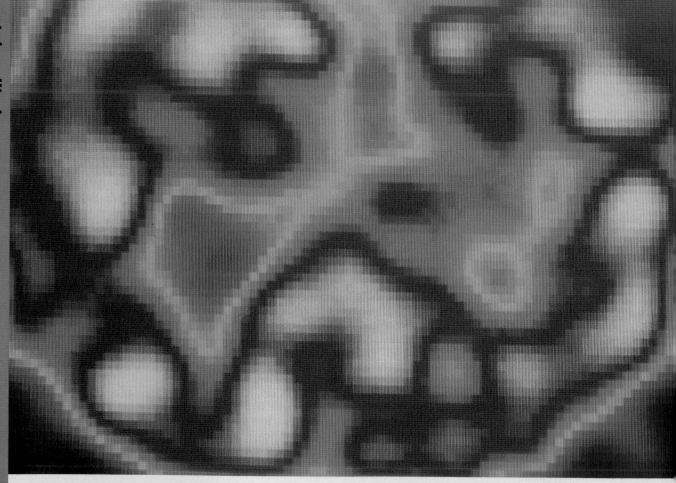

Image shows a positron emission tomography scan of the brain during hallucination

Miriam's overview

Few people hesitate to seek treatment for a physical illness, but many find it hard to accept they have a mental health problem. That's a great pity because depression, anxiety and irrational fears are common, well understood and often treatable.

No one need feel embarrassed about a mental illness or believe that they must deal with it alone. Anxiety disorders, including panic attacks, are among the most common mental health problems in the UK. Feeling worried is a natural reaction to problems and stress. But persistent anxiety, often with no obvious cause, needs treatment to prevent it from becoming a long-term problem.

Anxious personalities may be prey to obsessive-compulsive disorder (OCD) and phobias, irrational fears of anything from spiders to confined spaces – which can dominate a person's life. Other anxiety-related illnesses include post-traumatic stress disorder, a prolonged reaction to events such as serious accidents and natural disasters.

Depression affects as many as 1 in 3 people at some time in their lives but is quite difficult to understand.

"*harness* stress and *manage it*"

Nonetheless it requires prompt treatment to relieve symptoms and prevent long-term feelings of despair, possibly culminating in suicide.

The two eating disorders anorexia nervosa and bulimia are most common in teenage girls, but they're also being diagnosed at a younger age and in boys too. They have been falsely attributed to the desire to be slim but that's to misunderstand what's going on. Anorexia is the expression of profound psychological disturbance and the desire to exert some control over life with the only tool at the anorexic person's disposal – a refusal to eat. Losing weight is a consequence, not a cause, of anorexia.

A new syndrome in men is related to anorexia where there's a similar obsession with shape and weight, but it's to do with muscular development rather than thinness. Men spend hours in the gym "purging" themselves on the treadmill rather than with laxatives.

Stress is ever present and virtually unavoidable in modern life. But that doesn't mean we have to succumb to it. A better strategy, if you can do it, is to harness stress and manage it so that stress leads to greater, not less,

productivity. Learn to do that and you'll be able to defuse stressful situations – you may even find you thrive on a bit of stress every now and then.

A phenomenon of the new millennium seems to be a preoccupation with appearance to the point where feelings of ugliness may become obsessive. This disturbance of the way we see our bodies is called body dysmorphic disorder but it goes way beyond the common belief that our thighs are on the wide side or our faces are asymmetrical.

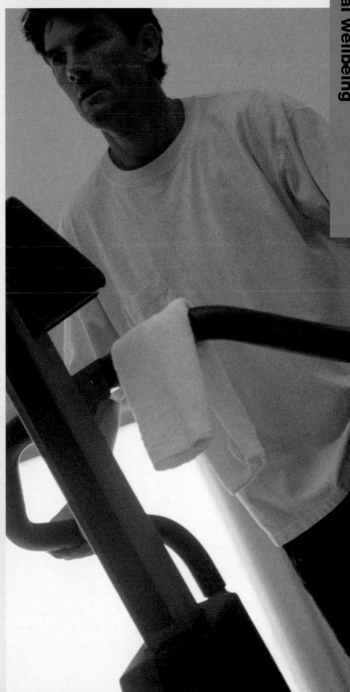

PSYCHOLOGICAL THERAPIES

Counselling

In days gone by, when faced with an emotional crisis we might have gone to a local priest, family doctor or village "wise woman". Nowadays a counsellor can fill that role. Trained to listen while you talk through your personal problems, a counsellor can support you through a bad patch and help you see the overall picture. Friends can be wonderful but they can't give the same kind of concentrated time and objectivity.

Counselling is gentle and supportive, relying on trust. The aim is to help you develop your own insights into what's gone wrong so you can approach the problem in a fresh way. That should mean you feel less like the victim of circumstances and have more control over your life. In the course of counselling you can reassess your coping skills – how you deal with problems, challenges, relationships, work – and learn new ways that would be more effective. It can also help to make you clearer and more direct when communicating with others – saying what you mean and asking for what you want, being assertive without being aggressive.

Short-term counselling for a specific difficulty may only take a few weekly sessions while more complex deep-rooted problems will need longer, perhaps an hour every week for several months.

Some family practices now have a counsellor as a member of their primary care team. Community counselling services exist in many areas and there's almost certainly an individual practitioner within travelling distance of your home. Many counsellors try to offer a sliding scale of fees that takes your ability to pay into account.

Self-help groups have branches in most parts of the country and you should find the address you need in your local telephone directory. There can sometimes be long waiting lists, but talk to the appointments secretary if you feel you need to be seen urgently and most groups will do their best to help. It's sometimes possible to obtain an early appointment if you can attend a day-time session.

If you're between 16 and 25 you might prefer to see a counsellor who specializes in helping young people. Look in the telephone directory to see if there's a youth counselling and advice centre in your area or see Useful addresses (p. 567) for further information.

Counselling is about trust so it's important that you feel comfortable with a counsellor. The more open you can be, the more you gain from the experience. The British Association for Counselling recommends you "shop around" by talking to two or three practitioners before deciding which one is the right counsellor for you.

Cognitive therapy

Cognitive therapy is based on the idea that some psychological problems stem from inappropriate ways of thinking. It helps people to recognize and understand their current thought patterns and shows them ways to consciously change the way they think. Cognitive therapy does not look into past events and is often used in conjunction with behaviour therapy.

Psychoanalysis

Psychoanalysis in its purest form is inevitably lengthy and therefore expensive. It is not uncommon for a course of therapy to demand daily attendance at the analyst's office for several years. An acceptable minimum might still involve two or three visits a week for more than a year.

One of the reasons why psychoanalysis i s so protracted is that the analyst and the patient join in a contract to explore every aspect of the patient's feelings in a close, intimate way in order to understand all facets of the patient's life as far back as the patient can remember. During the therapy, the analyst will attempt to interpret the patient's personality, motivations, inadequacies and symptoms and relate them to family, personal, social and professional

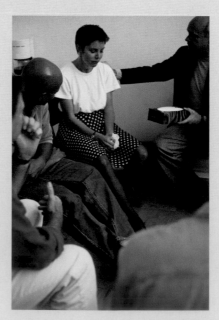

relationships. Such a complex exploration is necessarily long.

The aim of psychoanalysis – and every other form of psychological treatment – is to help people to have insight into themselves. In doing so, it attempts to explain the underlying reasons for psychological disturbance and symptoms. Once explained, the technique then builds in a positive way to provide support while patients face their difficulties and cope with them.

Short-term psychotherapy

Psychotherapy is an important form of treatment because it doesn't require hospital admission and can be fitted into daily life. So a mother can stay at home, and an employed woman needn't be absent from her job.

As with most other forms of psychological treatment, psychotherapy must cover all aspects of the patient's life. It is useless to embark on a course of psychotherapy if you are not prepared to explore your feelings candidly and accept the involvement of your psychotherapist in the intimate details of your problems and in forming a treatment plan.

In the broadest sense, psychotherapy is useful for managing any illness that has a psychological component, the commonest being an inability to adjust to stress. As just being alive in the 21st century is stressful, most of us would probably be better off for having psychotherapy.

Group therapy

There are many forms of group therapy but all rely on one basic premise: they set out to help individuals to take well-defined steps towards being able to deal with their problems alone. There are usually four steps:
1. to discover what the real problems are
2. to rationalize them
3. to adjust to them
4. to cope with them.

Whatever the form of group therapy, this step-by-step progress is facilitated by the presence of others. It may be possible to identify with another group member and share experiences. It may be possible to assess behaviour in others as irrational even though it's difficult to recognize and admit to the same thing in oneself when alone.

In group therapy, members use the group as a crutch, a cathartic and an instrument to work through their own difficulties. With successful group therapy, however, the patient ceases to be dependent on the group and has the confidence to face life alone.

Anxiety

TEMPORARY FEELINGS OF NERVOUSNESS OR WORRY IN STRESSFUL SITUATIONS ARE NATURAL AND APPROPRIATE. HOWEVER, WHEN ANXIETY BECOMES A GENERAL RESPONSE TO MANY ORDINARY SITUATIONS AND CAUSES PROBLEMS IN COPING WITH EVERYDAY LIFE IT IS DIAGNOSED AS ABNORMAL.

Anxiety disorders occur in a number of different forms, the most common being generalized, persistent background anxiety that is difficult to control.

Any type of anxiety can escalate to **panic**, in which there are recurrent attacks of intense anxiety and alarming physical symptoms (see box, above). These attacks occur unpredictably and usually have no obvious cause.

In another type of anxiety disorder known as a **phobia**, severe anxiety is provoked by an irrational fear of a situation, creature or object, such as fear of enclosed spaces (claustrophobia) and fear of spiders (arachnophobia).

Generalized anxiety disorder affects about 1 in 25 people, usually beginning in middle age, with women more commonly affected than men, and often related to the menopause and the withdrawal of the female hormone oestrogen. This kind of anxiety can respond well to oestrogen in the form of hormone replacement therapy (HRT) as it's one of the most powerful natural tranquillizers known.

WHAT ARE THE CAUSES?

An increased susceptibility to anxiety disorders may be inherited or may be due to childhood experiences. For example, poor bonding between a parent and child and abrupt separation of a child from a parent have been shown to play a part in some anxiety disorders. Generalized anxiety disorder may develop after a stressful life event, such as the death of a close relative. However, the anxiety frequently has no particular cause. Similarly, panic attacks often develop for no obvious reason.

WHAT ARE THE SYMPTOMS?

People with generalized anxiety disorder and panic attacks experience both psychological and physical symptoms. However, in someone with generalized anxiety disorder, psychological symptoms tend to persist while physical symptoms are intermittent. In panic attacks, both psychological and physical symptoms come on together suddenly and unpredictably. The psychological symptoms of anxiety include:
- a sense of nameless foreboding with no obvious reason or cause

- being on edge and unable to relax
- impaired concentration
- repetitive worrying thoughts
- disturbed sleep and sometimes nightmares.

In addition, you may have symptoms of depression, such as early waking or a general sense of hopelessness. **Physical symptoms** of the disorder, which occur intermittently, include:
- headache
- abdominal cramps, sometimes with diarrhoea and vomiting
- frequent urination
- sweating, flushing and tremor
- a feeling of something being stuck in the throat.

Psychological and physical symptoms of **panic attacks** include the following:
- shortness of breath
- sweating, trembling and nausea
- palpitations (awareness of an abnormally rapid heartbeat)
- dizziness and fainting
- fear of choking or of imminent death

continued on page 292

Panic attacks

A panic attack is a short burst of overwhelming anxiety. It occurs without warning and quite unpredictably and tends to happen in public places such as a crowded supermarket or a cramped lift. The symptoms begin suddenly with a sense of breathing difficulty, chest pains, palpitations, feeling light-headed and dizzy, sweating, trembling and faintness, fast, shallow breathing and pins and needles. Although very unpleasant and frightening, panic attacks usually last for only a few minutes, cause no physical harm and are rarely associated with a serious physical illness.

How to help yourself:

- **Exercise** can be very helpful by diverting the mind and alleviating mental stress. It also increases blood flow to the brain. Studies have shown that **jogging** for 30 minutes three times a week is as effective as psychotherapy in treating depression and will work just as well for you. So, if you can, establish a **routine of regular exercise** – walking, swimming or whatever appeals. Start gradually, building up to a more energetic pace as you progress.
- **Avoid junk food and sugar** and increase your intake of wholegrain cereal, vegetables, fruit, lean meats, low-fat dairy products and fish. The amino

acid tryptophan has been found to relieve anxiety and natural sources include turkey, chicken, fish, peas, nuts and peanut butter; where possible you should eat them with a carbohydrate such as potatoes, pasta or rice, which facilitates the brain's uptake of tryptophan.
- You might also find it helpful to use **essential oil of clary sage** (available from health food shops and pharmacies). This is both a powerful relaxant and mentally uplifting. It eases mental fatigue and depression and helps bring good sleep. Put two to three drops into a bowl of steaming water and inhale or add a little to your bath water. You could also place four to six drops on a tissue when you're going out and inhale whenever you feel particularly tense.
- **Passion flower** and **valerian root** taken as a tea or tincture have a calming effect. Some people have also found **ginger, cayenne pepper, dandelion root** and **Siberian ginseng** to have helpful, calming properties.
- **Instant help during a panic attack:** You also need to have a way of relaxing **instantly** when you are in public if you feel a panic attack coming on and you'll be able to do that once you have got used to practising relaxation techniques in your own time at home. Try the following exercise

when you are out. (I think it is a particularly good one to try when you are waiting in a queue.)
1. Stand as comfortably and as relaxed as you can.
2. Take a deep breath to the count of five, and then breathe slowly out.
3. Mentally tell all your muscles to relax.
4. Repeat this two or three times until you're feeling relaxed.
5. Imagine yourself in a pleasant situation such as walking along a beach, or sitting in a beautiful garden.

If you find yourself hyperventilating (breathing rapidly and shallowly) cover your mouth and nose with a **small paper bag** and breathe into it for a few minutes. You will soon feel much calmer. During an attack **concentrate as hard as you can** on something you can see, such as the pattern on the carpet or a picture on the wall. Stay calm. Try to continue with what you were doing but take it slowly.
- **Further help:** Panic attacks may be a symptom of a more deep-seated problem that may be helped by **counselling** (see Psychological therapies, opposite). This could be a way of finding your own inner resources – resources you may have forgotten you possess because of your present anxiety.

FOCUS *on* stress

Many people need some stress to optimize their performance and, up to a point, stress can help us to pull out the stops. However, too much stress, particularly if it is continuous, can cause serious health problems.

Although many people still think of stress as wholly negative, it can, in fact, be either positive or negative. Stress is energy that's generated by change and can range from something as minor as getting out of bed in the morning to a major life event such as giving birth or bereavement.

WHAT MAKES US STRESSED?

The short answer is potentially anything. In general the greater the number of events that happen to us in a given time, say a year, and the higher the combined rating (see below), the more likely we are to suffer a physical or emotional stress response.

And, of course, a stress-related illness such as indigestion, heart pain or irritable bowel syndrome will add to the pressure.

PHYSICAL EFFECTS OF STRESS

The stress reaction is a natural response to fear. It prepares the body for **fight** or **flight**.

It follows that if we're in a constant state of fear, we're in a constant state of stress. And that can make us ill. This is called **stress-related illness**.

When faced with a stressful situation, the brain and then the body respond by increasing production of certain hormones such as cortisol and adrenaline. These hormones lead to changes in heart rate, blood pressure, metabolism and physical activity designed to improve overall performance.

We all recognize the physical effects of adrenaline:

● Our hearts begin to pound so that the maximum amount of blood is being pumped round our bodies to make them ready for action.

● The rate at which we breathe increases so that our blood carries the maximum amount of oxygen to our muscles to make them work efficiently.

● Our blood pressure increases so that our essential organs are well supplied with blood.

● Blood vessels in our skin and internal organs constrict, diverting blood to our muscles, making us ready to run.

● Our pupils enlarge so that we can see both what's frightening us and a clear path to get away from it.

● The blood sugar rises steeply, providing the large amount of energy we'll need if we have to fight with, or flee from, an adversary.

A certain amount of stress isn't all bad as it helps us to meet challenges and stay motivated. But when stress levels rocket, our ability to cope is disrupted. Fewer than 20 percent of people are effective in the face of crises such as fires or floods.

WHY STRESS MAKES US ILL

Living in the 21st century means that we feel more stress than any member of the human race has ever felt. We live in a success-oriented society where it's impossible to escape from competitiveness and the desire to succeed.

We suffer from stress because we've evolved a long way from the time when stressful situations could be resolved by fighting or fleeing. Yet adrenaline is being pumped into our bodies and makes us ready to do both. Our bodies are switched on, but our instincts to run or face the enemy are repressed.

The resulting tension and frustration promotes further stress, and a vicious circle is set up that may develop into physical and mental illness.

STRESS-RELATED ILLNESSES

Continued exposure to stress (fear) often leads to stress-related illnesses such as depression, headaches, indigestion, palpitations and muscular aches and pains.

Constriction of the blood vessels due to long-term stress can give you **high blood pressure** too. If blood pressure remains elevated for any length of time, it leads to damage to the arteries and possibly to a heart attack.

Migraine headaches, **skin conditions** such as **eczema** (dermatitis) and **itching** (pruritis), and **digestive problems** such as **IBS, dyspepsia** and **peptic ulcer** may also result.

The high stress league

EVENT	STRESS RATING	EVENT	STRESS RATING
Death of spouse	100	Large mortgage/loan	31
Divorce	73	New responsibilities at work	29
Marital separation	65	Children leaving home	29
Prison term	63	In-law trouble	29
Death in the family	63	Outstanding personal achievement	28
Personal injury or illness	63	Spouse begins or stops work	26
Marriage	50	School or college ends or begins	26
Losing job	47	Living conditions change	25
Marital reconciliation	45	Personal habits change	24
Retirement	45	Trouble with boss	23
Illness of family member	44	Change in working conditions	20
Pregnancy	40	Change in residence	20
Sex problems	39	Change in school or college	20
New baby	39	Change in social activities	18
Business readjustment	39	Change in sleeping habits	16
Change in financial circumstances	38	Change in eating habits	15
Death of a close friend	37	Holiday	13
Change in work	36	Christmas	12
Increased marital argument	35	Minor law violation	11

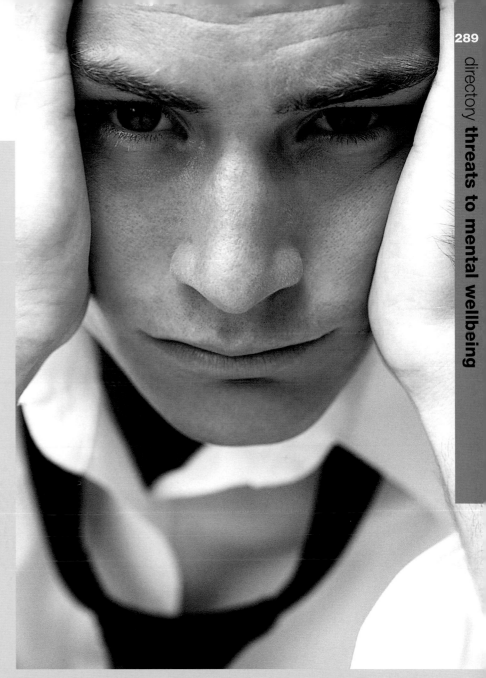

There are other major diseases that may be aggravated by stress, such as **arthritis**, **asthma** and **diabetes**. Research has shown that when we're under stress we're more **susceptible to infection**, particularly from viruses.

Certain stress-related problems specific to women include **menstrual disorders**, **pelvic pain**, **sexual difficulties**, **premenstrual tension**, **unwanted hair growth** and disturbance of **ovarian function** leading to a failure to ovulate.

The stress of modern living isn't going to go away so our only hope is to change our attitude to it.

In other words, we have to manage stress or, even better, harness it and use it as energy.

In order to live with stress, we need to decide what's causing it and if our responses to stress are sensible. If they're not, they'll prevent us from coping and taking control.

Some people are more susceptible to stress than others but with some training and practice most of us can learn to handle it.

LIFESTYLE AND STRESS

To help pinpoint the source of your stress, begin by asking yourself whether there are any social, physical or emotional factors affecting you:

● Are you smoking heavily as a response to stress?

● Is stress making you drink too much?

● Do you exercise or are you a couch potato?

● Could you be ill?

● Is there some new element of challenge in your life?

● Has there been any change in your general circumstances?

● Have long-standing problems recently become worse?

● Is someone close to you facing difficulties that affect you?

OVERCOMING STRESS

Often the hardest thing about stress is recognizing it.

If you're feeling stressed there's every reason to be optimistic that you'll be able to overcome it.

There are several simple and effective things you can try to reduce and overcome stress.

It's a very satisfying feeling to handle stress confidently and once you've done it you'll feel stronger and more confident that you'll be able to do it next time.

TOO MUCH TO DO?

It doesn't have to be this way. Learn to prioritize and make lists.

● What **must** I do?

● What **should** I do?

● What can **"wait"**?

● What **needn't** I do?

Only tackle the first two, let the rest wait.

GAIN CONTROL OF YOUR LIFESTYLE – MANAGING STRESS

● Plan a daily or weekly timetable of things you love doing and include one of them in each day.

● Plan for the future and don't dwell on past mistakes or disappointments.

● Reward your successes and challenge your critics – don't accept criticism at face value.

● Find time every day for rest and relaxation, even if it's just a soak in the bath or 10 minutes with your feet up in a comfy chair reading a magazine.

● Involve your family – especially your kids – and friends in helping you to change your lifestyle. Children will force you to relax or put your feet up.

DIET

How well we handle stress can be helped by how well we eat.

People who eat a diet high in wholegrain breads and cereals, fruit and vegetables, and low in refined carbohydrates, sugar, caffeine and fat, show greater ability to cope with stress.

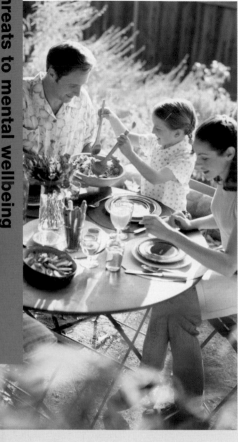

THE ANTI-STRESS DIET
Every day have:
- **An orange**, fresh vegetables and dark green leaves for vitamin C, folic cacid, selenium, antioxidants.
- **Fish**, such as tuna, herring, salmon and salad oil on your salads for vitamins A, D and E, essential fatty acids for your brain, zinc and manganese for your immune system.
- **Half a pint of skimmed milk** or two low-fat yoghurts for calcium.
- **Unrefined carbohydrates**, like wholemeal bread, brown rice, porridge – eat three portions, to keep brain serotonin levels up, provide mood-regulating B vitamins and make you feel optimistic and positive.
- **Onions, broccoli and tomatoes** and **drink tea** for flavonoids – potent antioxidants that may help prevent cell death (ageing) and cancer.

In addition:
- **Don't eat your largest meal** after 8 p.m. – it may interfere with a good night's sleep
- **Drink something hot and sweet** (diet chocolate will do) in bed and go to sleep listening to music or read a book.
- **If you can cuddle up close** to someone – it's the best antidote to stress and anxiety.

LOSS OF APPETITE
Stress often puts you off your food. So:
- Eat small portions of food that you particularly like.
- Take your time eating.
- Temporarily avoid situations that put you under pressure to finish eating.
- Drink plenty of fluids, especially water, fruit juices and skimmed milk.

Weight loss may be an important indicator of the extent of stress, so if you continue to lose weight seek help from your GP.

LOSS OF SEX DRIVE
Waning sexual interest is frequently a feature of stress and a cause of much distress – and as a consequence more stress.

It won't last forever, so stay calm but in the meantime try to enjoy those parts of your sexual relationship that are still a pleasure. Cuddling, caressing and kissing always are.

DEFUSING STRESS
In my book, anything that helps you defuse stress is good for you. Here are a few suggestions.

EXERCISE
Exercise is what the body instinctively wants to do under stress – fight or flight – and it's extremely beneficial in relaxing the mind and body.

Regular running, walking, cycling, swimming or any other aerobic exercise, ideally carried out for at least 20 minutes three times a week, can make a big difference.

Even a walk around the block can help let off steam and ease stress. Choose an exercise that you find pleasurable.
- Warm up for two or three minutes before by stretching before starting exercising vigorously.
- Build up slowly and don't over-extend yourself. Always exercise within the limits of comfort, letting your breathing be your guide. If it hurts, stop.
- If you feel tired, stop and rest.
- When stopping exercise, cool down gradually and slowly to avoid stiffness.
- Exercising at a pace that keeps you moderately "puffed" but not gasping for breath is best for stimulating both your muscles and circulation and for burning calories.
- Keep an eye on your heart rate; if you're a medically fit person (check with your doctor) your heart rate shouldn't exceed 110 beats per minute during warm-up, and during vigorous

Aromatherapy to help stress

- Keep some essential oil of lavender by you – it has been shown in studies to reduce stress.
- Use five or six drops in a bath or on a handkerchief. If you have sensitive skin, it's advisable to test a little of the diluted essential oil on a small area.
- You should avoid contact with the eyes and always close them when inhaling. Smells are interpreted by the inner core of the brain, the area that is concerned with emotions. Scents therefore tend to have powerful effects on mood and health.
- Concentrated essences, such as those used by aromatherapists, are a complex mixture of chemicals. Different essences have specific properties.

Oil	Effect
Bergamot	Antidepressant
Camomile	Tranquillizer
Clary sage	Stimulant
Geranium	Antidepressant
Jasmine	Antidepressant
Lavender	Tranquillizer
Marjoram	Sedative
Neroli	Sedative
Rose	Sedative

Warning: Aromatherapy oils should never be taken internally. Except for bergamot, rose and neroli, the oils in this chart should be avoided in pregnancy, although lavender and camomile need to be avoided only for the first three months.

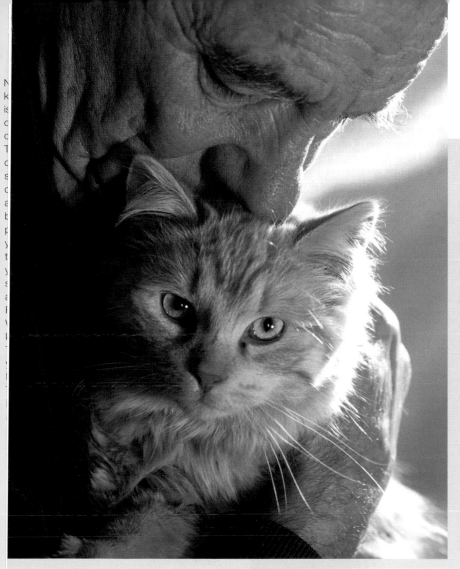

People with pets live longer than people without them and this is thought to be due to the calming effect of stroking.

BE POSITIVE
● Make a list of your three best attributes. Do people describe you, for example, as generous, affectionate and trustworthy? Carry the list with you and read it to yourself whenever you find yourself thinking unpleasant thoughts.
● Keep a daily diary of all the small, unpleasant events that happen and talk about them with your partner or a friend each day. Write down what you did for enjoyment or fun. Look back at your diary every week to see what progress you have made and to make plans for what you intend to achieve next week.
● Recall pleasant occasions in the past and plan pleasant ones for the future.
● Avoid talking about your unpleasant feelings.
● Keep your mind occupied by planning and doing constructive tasks – avoid sitting or lying around day-dreaming or doing nothing.
● Keep a list of affirmations to say to yourself when under stress. It's amazing – chanting simple phrases such as "I really can handle this" can divert the stress response.

WAYS TO COPE
● Be reasonable with yourself.
● Avoid perfectionism.
● Sort out what really matters in your life.
● Think ahead and try to anticipate how to get round problems.
● Share your worries with family or friends.
● Exercise regularly.
● Give yourself treats and rewards for positive actions, attitudes and thoughts.
● Relax every day.
● Make small, regular changes to your lifestyle.
● Learn to delegate.
● Take short rests throughout the day.
● Have proper breaks for meals.
● Make time for yourself every day and every week.
● Know your limits and try to work within them.

TOP TIP
The secret of coping with stress is similar to coping with a child who's having a tantrum – yes, honestly. Take control and use distraction tactics. Then stress is what it should be – a sudden brief reaction to a threatening situation, not a long, drawn-out state of affairs.

exercise it shouldn't exceed 130 beats per minute.
● If you're prepared to exercise for 30 minutes, your own endorphins kick in and they're wonderful. They suppress your appetite, give you an amazing high, cure headaches and make you sleep well.

RELAXATION
Yogic breathing:
Kneel on the floor, place one hand on your stomach and the other on your chest. Inhale for about two seconds, allowing your stomach to bulge out, then slowly exhale for about four to eight seconds, feeling your stomach deflate. Then place your hand on your chest and repeat the procedure, allowing your chest to bulge and deflate. Repeat this pattern for several minutes.

Attending a yoga class and practising yoga and meditation at home will divert your mind from stress, relax muscle tension through stretching, and teach you to breathe more completely. If you'd rather give yoga a miss, the following relaxation routine might help.

1. Lie on a firm surface, close your eyes and become aware of how your body feels.
2. Imagine a calm scene. Blue is a relaxing colour, so try a clear blue sky and calm sea.
3. Focus your attention on each part of your body, starting with the tips of the toes and finishing with your face and eyes.
4. Consciously try to relax every part of your body in turn.
5. The whole procedure should take at least 10 minutes and you should carry it out at least once a day to benefit. If you prefer, buy a relaxation tape or borrow one from the library.

THE IMPORTANCE OF TOUCH
Touch is essential for health. People can become depressed and irritable if they aren't touched enough.

In addition, touch lowers blood pressure. Massage not only relaxes and soothes, it also stimulates the circulatory and lymphatic systems – both are important in preventing swelling of the face, hands and feet from developing.

If necessary, touch, stroke and massage yourself – you'll feel your stress ebbing away.

Depression

DEPRESSION IS THE MOST COMMON SERIOUS PSYCHIATRIC ILLNESS,
AND IT BECOMES MORE COMMON WITH AGE. WOMEN ARE PARTICULARLY
VULNERABLE BECAUSE OF THEIR HORMONES.

Plummeting hormone levels can trigger depression when menstruation stops at the menopause, after the birth of a child and after a miscarriage or termination. About 1 in 6 women seek help for depression at some time in their lives, as opposed to only 1 in 9 men. Most depressed people find they feel slightly better as the day progresses.

RISK FACTORS

■ Depression in the past or a family history of depression.
■ Poor health (such as a stroke or heart attack).
■ Widowhood and widowerhood.
■ Loss of a partner.
■ Personality problems.
■ Isolation.
■ Lack of confidence.
■ With elderly people, alterations in health and circumstances, such as giving up the family home.

WHAT ARE THE CAUSES?

The cause of depression is complex but is probably related to a reduction in the level of certain chemicals in the brain, called **neurotransmitters**, which keep us in a good mood by stimulating brain cells. The best known of these mood elevators is **serotonin**.

WHAT ARE THE SYMPTOMS?

■ Tiredness.
■ Sleep problems.
■ Worry.
■ Weepiness.
■ Sadness, despair, misery, gloom and blackness.
■ Loss of affection towards oneself and others.
■ A sense of failure, unworthiness, even self-loathing.
■ Loss of interest in life.
■ Loss of sex drive.
■ Loss of self-esteem and confidence.
■ Altered appetite (usually a loss of appetite).
■ Lethargy, slovenliness and apathy.
■ Insomnia or sleeping for long periods as a means of escape.
■ Early-morning waking – typically between 2 a.m. and 4 a.m.
■ A conviction that the world is against you, paranoia, recurrent thoughts of death, even suicide.

WHAT IS THE TREATMENT?

Try to see your doctor at once if you feel depressed. Don't wait and hope your mood will pass. In the case of weepiness after the birth of a baby, see your doctor if you're still depressed after two weeks. The longer postnatal depression stays untreated the harder it is to cure.

■ **Psychotherapy**, whether individual or in a group, is most useful for those whose personality and life experiences are the main causes of their illness. The aim of one of the most successful treatments, **cognitive therapy**, is to change the way you think about problems and therefore be able to deal with them.

■ **Drug treatment** is used for people with predominantly **physical** symptoms. There are two main groups of antidepressants: **tricyclics**, introduced in the 1950s with well-known side effects, and **selective serotonin re-uptake inhibitors** (SSRIs), which appeared mainly in the 1990s. The newer antidepressants, such as SSRIs, are costly but have fewer side effects than the older drugs and patients seem to like them. Yet large studies show tricyclics work equally well to cure depression if you can tolerate them. Antidepressant drugs are effective in more than two-thirds of patients, provided the drugs are taken in a sufficient dosage over a long enough period of time. They take between two and three weeks to work. Patient compliance is high – important because halting medication too early is a big factor in depression returning.

■ **Antidepressants and psychotherapy in combination.** Patients who stop drug therapy before six months will relapse. But maintenance therapy with either drugs or psychotherapy will halve the relapse rate. What's more, **cognitive therapy** continues to work after it's stopped, its effectiveness being the same as maintenance drug therapy – something to remember if you don't like taking drugs for long periods.

GETTING HELP

Don't try to cope alone. Lean on people. Join a self-help group and get help dealing with your everyday problems. Avoid being alone and make a point of being with people you like. Don't be afraid to approach organizations such as the Samaritans.

SELF-HELP

For mild depression

WORK: If work distracts you, increase your workload.

KEEPING ACTIVE: Any kind of activity helps reduce sadness and will bring the pleasure of achievement. Completing a task gives you a sense of self-worth, which itself is an antidote to depression.

SEX: Good, wholesome sex makes all aspects of life seem brighter, so if your libido isn't depressed, keep sexually active.

DIET: Avoid junk food and sugar and increase your intake of wholegrain cereals, vegetables, fruit, lean meats, low-fat dairy products and fish.

The amino acid **tryptophan** has been found to relieve depression and natural sources include turkey, chicken, fish, peas, nuts and peanut butter. Where possible eat them with carbohydrates, such as potatoes, pasta and rice, which facilitate the brain's uptake of tryptophan. Cut out or cut down on caffeine and alcohol.

EXERCISE: Exercise alleviates all kinds of mental stress. It also increases blood flow to the brain. Jogging for 30 minutes three times a week can be as effective as psychotherapy in treating depression. So, a regular routine of exercise – walking, swimming or whatever appeals – is good for your mood.

AROMATHERAPY: Essential oil of clary sage is both a powerful relaxant and mentally uplifting. It can ease mental fatigue and promote sound sleep. Put two to three drops into a bowl of steaming water and inhale or inhale four to six drops from a tissue.

RELAXATION: Relaxation techniques to reduce stress, such as massage, yoga, aromatherapy and meditation, are helpful in alleviating the anxiety that is common with depression.

See also:
• **Psychological therapies p.286**

Depression in children and teenagers

GOOD PARENTS ENCOURAGE THEIR CHILDREN TO TALK ABOUT THEIR WORRIES FROM
A VERY EARLY AGE, ALWAYS LISTEN AND OFFER HELP. CHILDREN CAN QUICKLY FEEL ISOLATED,
MISUNDERSTOOD AND IGNORED IF PARENTS ARE PREOCCUPIED WITH THEIR OWN PROBLEMS.

It's difficult to pin down why children become depressed and often it's a combination of factors. But some classical situations seriously affect children and precipitate depression, such as:

- death in the family
- bullying
- exam anxiety
- feeling ugly
- unsympathetic parents
- girls/boys don't like me
- parental illness
- parental discord.

TELL-TALE SIGNS FOR PARENTS

Parents often wonder what's wrong with a child who seems out of sorts a lot of the time. Here's a guide to what to look out for.

BABIES AND TODDLERS

They can't tell us if they're sad, so they express themselves through their behaviour and:

- become unresponsive
- are clingy but can't accept comfort
- refuse to eat
- can't settle down to sleep.

PRE-SCHOOLERS MIGHT:

- be tearful all the time
- stop eating
- wake up during the night
- have frequent nightmares and night terrors
- become very demanding and naughty
- bully, hit and bite other children
- start telling lies
- behave destructively.

A few children can put their sad feelings into words – I well remember one of my sons, normally outgoing and happy, saying "The world doesn't feel right, Mum". Children quickly blame themselves if things go wrong and think they're worthless. Then their behaviour seems to ask for punishment – lying, stealing or playing truant from school. Remember – a naughty, depressed child isn't an innately bad child.

SCHOOL-AGE CHILDREN

If they are depressed they may:

- find it hard to concentrate and lose interest in schoolwork and play
- become loners
- refuse to go to school
- complain of feeling bored all the time
- say they're lonely
- lose confidence
- become difficult to control
- become slovenly.

ADOLESCENTS

Almost without exception, adolescents go through periods of being moody and antisocial and it can be difficult to spot the difference between what's normal and what's depression. Look out for these signs of depression – one or two signs could be a passing phase but three, four or more mean you should see your doctor:

- being much more moody and irritable than normal
- becoming withdrawn, giving up on friends and hobbies
- losing interest in or not doing well at school
- taking no interest in hair, clothes, music
- not eating enough, even anorexia, or eating too much, even bulimia
- having low self-esteem
- not being able to get out of bed until mid-day
- getting into bad habits and bad company
- taking drugs
- getting drunk
- becoming preoccupied with thoughts of death
- harming themselves by cutting their skin.

WHAT IS THE TREATMENT?

Getting professional help early from your GP for any child whose unhappiness is more than a passing phase can often prevent long-term depression. The mainstay of treating childhood depression is what's called talk therapy, sessions with a **psychotherapist**, **clinical psychologist** or **family therapist**, where the child can vent their anger, frustration, fear and hopelessness. Loving, caring attention is very powerful medicine for every depressed child.

HOW CAN ADULTS HELP?

By themselves, children simply can't make sense of feeling depressed; they feel helpless. Depressed children need a caring adult to take a loving interest in them and show understanding. Then they can help them deal with their feelings over time.

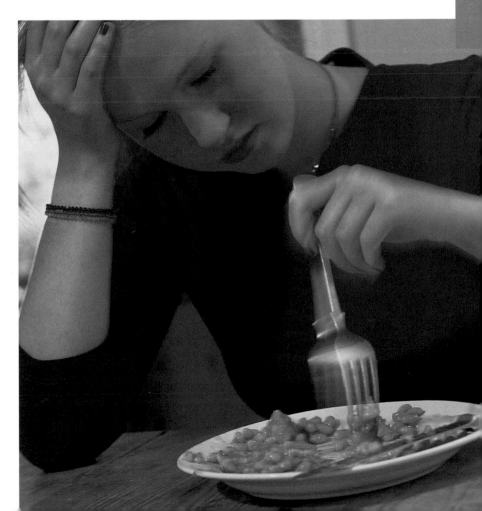

FOCUS *on* eating disorders

Anorexia and bulimia are abnormal ways of controlling weight but neither is what is popularly described as the "slimmer's disease". Both are expressions of deep inner turmoil, of psychological problems that are too difficult for the person to cope with in any other way.

Dieting is easy to be good at – you just have to starve yourself. But it's possible for an ANOREXIC to believe it's the only thing she's good at, so thinness becomes an obsession. Anorexics judge themselves only according to how much they've eaten – the less they eat the more successful they judge themselves to be. All their self-worth becomes bound up in not eating and so starving becomes very difficult to give up.

Anorexics hate food and crave love. They remember the time when they felt secure in being loved and didn't have to take any grown-up responsibilities, so they may subconsciously try to remain a child. As a child they didn't have to perform and they didn't have to excel. By starving they fight against their developing body – they lose or don't develop breasts and they don't menstruate.

BULIMICS go for several days with very little food and then become crazed with an uncontrollable desire to eat so that they gorge on almost anything in sight that is edible. This may mean eating extraordinary mixtures of raw and cooked food, sweet and savoury mixed in huge quantities. Some women have died after a binge because their stomachs have ruptured under the strain. Some women eat normally but then force themselves to vomit immediately afterwards or take huge quantities of laxatives to induce purging. This pattern of starving, bingeing, vomiting and purging is very hard to break. It's also much more common than people think, but treatments can help.

WHAT ARE THE CAUSES?

Desire for control: Dieting can be very satisfying, especially for girls in their teens who feel that weight is the only part of their lives over which they have control. Not eating becomes an end in itself.

Social pressure: In societies that don't value thinness, eating disorders are very rare. In surroundings such as ballet schools, where people value thinness highly, they're common.

Cultural pressure: Generally in Western culture "thin is beautiful". Television, newspapers and magazines are full of pictures of slim, attractive young men and women and there's huge pressure to conform.

Family: Some children and teenagers find saying no to food is the only way they can make their feelings felt and have influence in the family. Eating becomes an important social tool with which to exert pressure on parents.

Not growing up: A girl with anorexia may lose or not develop some of the physical traits of an adult woman, such as pubic hair, breasts and monthly periods. As a result, she may look very young for her age. Not eating can therefore be seen as a way of putting off some of the demands of growing up, particularly the sexual ones.

Depression: Many bulimics are depressed and binges may start off as a way of coping with unhappiness. A third of people with eating disorders are depressed and can be helped with the new generation of antidepressants.

Upsets: For some people, anorexia and bulimia seem to be triggered off by an upsetting event, such as the break-up of a relationship. Sometimes it needn't even be a bad event, just an important one, such as marriage or leaving home.

CONSEQUENCES OF ANOREXIA AND BULIMIA

Starvation leads to broken sleep, constipation, difficulty in concentrating or thinking straight, depression, feeling the cold, brittle bones that break easily (osteoporosis), muscles becoming weaker – it becomes an effort to do anything, menstruation failing to start or stopping, inability to have a baby, death.

Vomiting stomach acid dissolves the enamel on teeth and leads to a puffy face (due to swollen salivary glands), irregular heartbeat, muscle weakness, eventually to kidney damage and even epileptic fits.

Laxative use causes persistent tummy pain, swollen fingers and damage to bowel muscles that may lead to long-term constipation.

Bladder problems become common. New research shows that women with anorexia are far more likely to have bladder problems than other women. Nearly two-thirds of women with anorexia, at least three times more than non-sufferers, had symptoms suggestive of an **unstable bladder**, with a sudden and overwhelming desire to go to the lavatory eight times or more in 24 hours, and sometimes actual incontinence. These symptoms usually start about a year after anorexia began.

Symptoms of anorexia and bulimia

Anorexia symptoms:
● Severe weight loss.
● Distorted ideas about body size and weight.
● Excessive exercising.
● Vomiting or purging.
● Social isolation.
● Emotional and irritable behaviour.
● Difficulty sleeping.
● Loss of menstrual periods.
● Perfectionism.
● Feeling cold, poor circulation.
● Growth of downy body hair.

Bulimia symptoms:
● Normal weight.
● Binge-eating large amounts of food.
● Vomiting or purging after eating.
● Disappearing to the toilet after meals.
● Secretive and ritual behaviour.
● Feeling helpless and lonely.
● Erratic menstrual periods.
● Sore throat and tooth decay caused by vomiting.
● Dehydration and poor skin condition.
● Social isolation.
● Swollen salivary glands.

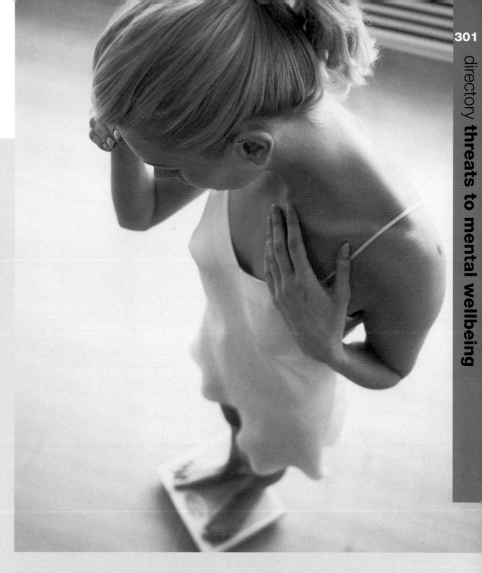

GETTING HELP

As with alcohol or drug dependence, the sooner you admit to having an eating disorder and accept help, the better the chance of a cure. Left untreated, anorexia has one of the highest death rates of all psychiatric illnesses, though deaths can be prevented by proper treatment.

No one form of treatment is 100 percent effective; what's effective for one person may not be effective for you. And despite best efforts, some people only partly recover. But there are lots of avenues to explore.

YOUR GENERAL PRACTITIONER

To help yourself, you have to be open and honest with your family doctor. Don't be ashamed of being anorexic or bulimic or reluctant to admit you have a problem.

Don't be frightened of the consequences of admitting you have an eating disorder. You're entitled to complete confidentiality; this means that your parents and carers needn't know.

It's your right to be referred for assessment by a specialist who has training in eating disorders; you should be seen as soon as possible so that delays and waiting lists can be avoided. You may get worse if you wait too long and then need in-patient rather than day-patient treatment.

SELF-HELP

Self-help groups can be a useful addition to treatment but they aren't an alternative. They're very helpful in getting patients and families to understand they aren't alone with the illness.

GENERAL TREATMENT

Treatment must address the psychological aspects of anorexia and bulimia nervosa as well as the abnormal eating. All these treatments work so don't be afraid to try them.
- Counselling.
- Psychotherapy.
- Cognitive therapy.
- Group therapy.
- Family therapy.
- Day hospital programmes.
- In-patient treatment.
- Dietetic advice.
- Drugs can be of help in the short term, particularly to bulimics who are depressed.
- Re-feeding is a last resort but may be necessary to save life. Alone, however, it's only successful in short-term weight restoration, but usually isn't effective in the long term.

COUNSELLING

For anorexia, counselling is more effective during the early stages (when less than 25 percent of body weight has been lost). Research shows that cognitive behaviour therapy is especially effective for people with bulimia.

SPECIALIST TREATMENT

You should be involved as much as possible in your treatment programme and care plan, so you should be able to see your case notes and be involved in setting target weights. Therapy should not be conditional on weight gain, and vegetarian menus and appropriate food for minority groups should be available.

HOSPITAL TREATMENT

Some severely underweight people with anorexia nervosa can be treated successfully as **day-patients** rather than in-patients. If you need in-patient treatment, you have the right to:
- a quiet and safe environment

- continuity of care from staff with an understanding of eating disorders
- support during and after your meals
- appropriate food
- on-going counselling or psychotherapy
- follow-up and support after in-patient care.

COMPULSORY ADMISSION

Out of people who had been admitted or detained against their wishes, 50 percent said they thought it had been "a good thing" in retrospect.

So, in extreme circumstances and when all other alternatives have failed, people may be detained under the Mental Health Act in order to save life or reduce risk.

TEAMWORK

Good treatment demands selfless teamwork with families, carers and friends all working together. The impact on the family of someone with an eating disorder can be enormous. Families also need support. They need advice on what they should and shouldn't do to help a person's recovery.

WOMEN AND MENTAL HEALTH

In this section, I cover a group of topics that have a direct effect on the mental health of a great many women, as well as an indirect but often considerable effect on women's partners, family members, friends and colleagues. All women are prey to their hormones, variations in which affect them throughout their lives, not least once a month through the menstrual cycle. **Premenstrual syndrome** (PMS) can be a problem throughout a woman's fertile years. After childbirth, changes in female hormone levels may cause the "baby blues" or the more serious condition known as **postnatal depression** (PND). Then, later in life, women may experience depression and other emotional problems due to hormonal adjustments at the **menopause**. I also look at the effects on mental and physical wellbeing that may follow from **sexual assault**.

Premenstrual syndrome

PREMENSTRUAL SYNDROME, OR PMS, IS A COLLECTION OF UNCOMFORTABLE, PAINFUL AND ANNOYING SYMPTOMS THAT AFFECT SOME WOMEN BEFORE THEIR PERIODS. ROUGHLY 50 PERCENT OF WOMEN SUFFER FROM PREMENSTRUAL SYNDROME.

Half of those suffer very badly, quite a number so badly that they have to take time off school or work. But what exactly is premenstrual syndrome?

WHAT ARE THE SYMPTOMS?

The symptoms that we associate with PMS vary but include **tension**, **irritability**, **depression**, **headaches** and an **inability to concentrate**.

They also consist of **breast tenderness, swollen ankles**, **palpitations**, **a change in sexual interest**, **faintness**, **dizziness**, **changes in eating habits**, **an inability to get to sleep at night**, **indigestion** and either **diarrhoea** or **constipation**.

In addition:
■ All stress-related illnesses – such as **migraine**, **asthma** and **eczema** – may get worse before a menstrual period.
■ The effects of alcohol are worse just before a period, so a woman may find herself in a double-bind: she drinks to relieve her symptoms of PMS but the effects of drinking are much worse than usual.
■ The severity of symptoms can also vary each month. In addition to the symptoms already mentioned some women complain of **bloating**, **weight gain**, **skin problems**, **mood swings** and **depression, aggression, fatigue, tearfulness, feeling irrational, difficulty with decision making** and the **feeling of being misunderstood**.
■ No woman experiences all of these symptoms and the most important factor is their timing. The symptoms are present at some time in the second half of the cycle. Then they disappear or significantly improve either on the first day of your period or the day after the flow is heaviest. You should then be symptom-free.

Simple self-help measures, such as a hot bath and time to relax, can help ease premenstrual symptoms.

NOTE: If you have symptoms after these few days, it's unlikely that you're suffering from PMS and you should see your doctor so that a cause can be found and the appropriate treatment given.

Before blaming symptoms on PMS, it's important to confirm that there's a tie-up between symptoms and menstrual cycle. The way to do this is to keep a **diary**. Start filling in a daily chart showing exactly when symptoms appear, when they get worse and when they go away. When symptoms don't disappear or improve after a period, they're unlikely to be anything to do with PMS.

WHAT CAUSES PMS?

Premenstrual syndrome is now widely accepted as a true medical condition that affects women during their fertile years.
■ It's related to menstrual hormones and it can cause **physical** and **psychological** symptoms. There are more than 150 symptoms associated with PMS and the number and type vary from person to person.
■ PMS usually increases in severity when there are **alterations in hormone levels** such as after **pregnancy**, after a **miscarriage** or **termination**, when starting or **stopping the contraceptive pill**, or even occasionally **after a hysterectomy**.

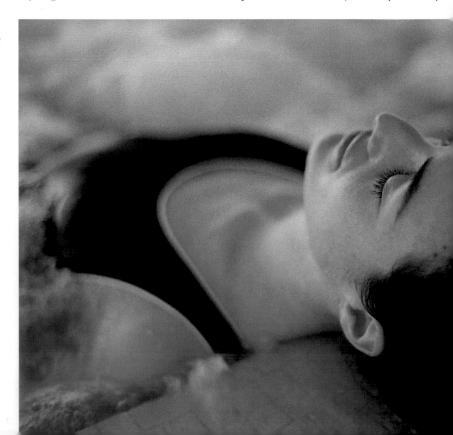

■ If you've suffered from postnatal depression, you are also more likely to suffer from PMS.

■ We used to think that PMS was brought on by the lack of one of our sex hormones, progesterone, in the week prior to menstruation. But, in fact, progesterone levels are quite high until just before a period starts. Our other sex hormone, oestrogen, however, is very low seven days before menstruation and experts agree that it's a **shortage of oestrogen** that causes symptoms of PMS.

■ PMS can get worse as we get older and after each baby. By the time I was in my 40s, PMS felt like a mini-menopause each month and I dreaded having to do a TV show that week.

■ PMS sometimes seems to run in families, but a genetic link has not been established. If you feel able to talk to other family members about PMS, you may find that they also suffer and have found some treatment that has helped them and may help you too.

PMS can wreak havoc in families when a normally lovely wife and mum becomes a shrew. All you have to do is warn your loved ones of your PMS and ask them to understand. Tell your children sooner rather than later.

WHAT CAN I DO?

There are many theories about the best ways to treat PMS but here are several things you can try.

■ Oil of evening primrose may bring relief.

■ If you retain fluid and swell up before a period (fluid sometimes collects in the breasts, sometimes around the waist and sometimes around the ankles, hands, fingers and face), try restricting your salt intake for a week to ten days before your period starts.

■ If your breasts swell and become especially tender try experimenting with different bras until you find one that's comfortable with plenty of support; you may find it a help to wear a bra in bed, too, and you may need one a cup bigger for your premenstrual week.

■ Don't add salt at the table, cook with less salt (use seasonings such as pepper and garlic instead) and limit salt-rich foods such as hard cheese, ready meals, smoked bacon and fish, salted peanuts, crisps, etc. Look at the labels to find out which other foods contain salt. The recommended limit for women is 5g of salt per day.

■ Try cutting down on your consumption of caffeine too (that means going easy on coffee, tea and cola drinks); there is thought to be a link between caffeine and menstrual cramps, breast tenderness and other symptoms. If you find that cutting down on caffeine helps, do so all the time – not just before a period.

■ Keep up your blood sugar levels by eating regular small meals rather than irregular large meals; some experts feel that low blood sugar levels can worsen irritability and aggressiveness.

■ If you suffer from constipation then try a high-fibre diet by simply increasing your intake of green vegetables, fresh fruit and wholemeal bread; or you can try a teaspoon of psyllium husk each morning (you can get it from a health food store).

■ Of the many over-the-counter remedies for PMS, aspirin and paracetamol are still the best painkillers you can buy.

■ Many women find exercise helps PMS, even if it's only taking the dog for a walk. If you go to the gym regularly don't give it up in the PMS week. Exercise such as swimming and walking, deep breathing, and relaxation techniques can all be helpful in bringing relief from tension and insomnia.

■ Help your PMS with diet (see box, right).

■ Herbs such as black cohosh may help.

WHAT IS THE TREATMENT?
DIET

Not all women require medical help with PMS and often your symptoms will be sufficiently controlled by changes to diet and lifestyle.

There's quite a lot of evidence that a healthy diet, particularly one low in fat and high in fruit, vegetables and wholegrains, can go a long way to relieving PMS.

What's really helpful is to eat starchy food every two to three hours to keep your blood-sugar level up. You can do this by having three main meals and three smaller snacks each day. Eating this way is particularly important in the second half of your cycle when your PMS is likely to occur. On the face of it, it seems to be a lot of food, but try to eat small meals so that you can manage the snacks.

WHAT YOUR DOCTOR MIGHT PRESCRIBE
Progestogen

No matter what you read, there's no evidence that taking progestogen in whatever form – not even progesterone cream – will help to relieve symptoms of PMS, and there may also be unpleasant side effects such as breast tenderness, water retention and loss of sex drive.

Oestrogen

■ Oestrogen is known to exert a profound effect on mood and mental state. Rapidly falling levels of oestrogen run parallel with PMS, postnatal depression and postmenopausal depression.

■ Doctors at Chelsea and Westminster Hospital in London have developed a treatment for PMS based on giving natural oestrogen by means of skin patches. This has the effect of suppressing ovulation and eliminating fluctuations in the menstrual cycle. The patches are like sticky clingfilm and women can swim, bathe or shower as usual. Oestrogen skin patches are one of the few treatments proven scientifically to be highly effective for PMS.

Helping PMS with diet

Try to eat LESS:
■ Saturated fat
■ Sugar
■ Salt
■ Caffeine
■ Alcohol

Try to eat MORE:
■ Starchy foods
■ Fibre
■ Vegetables
■ Fruit
■ Nuts and seeds

Snack ideas

■ Bowl of unsweetened cereal (with low-fat milk).
■ Sandwich with low-fat filling.
■ Fruit, low-fat yoghurt or rice pudding.
■ A plain biscuit, for example, digestive or rich tea.
■ Any of the following with a thin layer of spread: crispbread, crackers, rice cakes, oatcakes, bread, crumpets, teacakes, malt loaf, scones or buns.

Antidepressants

Until recently, I was against the use of tranquillizers and antidepressants for PMS, but a new generation of antidepressants has been developed called **selective serotonin re-uptake inhibitors** (SSRIs), which will bring relief to some PMS sufferers. It is worth discussing these with your doctor.

Fortunately, the new antidepressants, which include fluoxetine and paroxetine, are not addictive. They work to increase levels of serotonin in the brain and restore emotional balance. Studies have shown that SSRIs work faster in PMS than in depression (three weeks).

BREATHING TECHNIQUES

The way you breathe is closely related to the way you feel. If you're angry or upset, breathing is fast, shallow and irregular. When you're calm and relaxed, your breathing is slow and deep. You can consciously affect the way you feel by altering your breathing. Here are two ways to make yourself calmer.

■ **Breath awareness:** close your eyes and just be aware of your breathing. You don't have to change your breathing in any way, just notice your breath as it flows in and out.

■ **Alternate nostril breathing:** there's a greater flow of air through one nostril than through the other. You can activate the relaxation response by blocking the right nostril or by lying on your right side. This allows the right side of the brain to be associated with the relaxation response – to become dominant.

Depression after childbirth

CHANGES IN HORMONE LEVELS AFTER CHILDBIRTH CAN PROFOUNDLY AFFECT THE EMOTIONS. IN
MOST WOMEN, EMOTIONAL SWINGS – THE "BABY BLUES" – LAST ONLY A FEW DAYS, BUT IN OTHERS
THEY LEAD TO THE MORE PROLONGED, SERIOUS CONDITION CALLED POSTNATAL DEPRESSION.

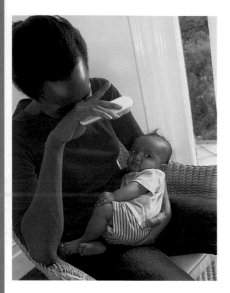

It's certainly true that nothing can prepare
you for caring for a new baby. The physical
and emotional upheaval is bound to have an
impact; quite often when most mothers think
they're going to be happiest, they feel very
low – the "baby blues". In most instances
this only lasts a few days but, sadly, in others,
these feelings can continue for months due
to a condition known as postnatal depression.
It's important for a father to be aware of
the symptoms and recognize the difference
between the normal "blues" and real
depression so that he knows how to help
and when to seek medical advice.

BABY BLUES

The "baby blues" are mood swings caused
by hormonal changes. In all likelihood this
period of feeling low one minute and
euphoric the next won't last beyond the first
week but you'll still need a lot of support to
get you through it. Maybe the "baby blues"
are a natural sign to those around you that
you need time and space to come to terms
with being a mother. That's certainly how a
concerned partner, relative or friend should
deal with it, although you'll find that because
your hormones are all over the place, you'll
also cry when someone's nice to you!

WHY DO YOU GET THE BLUES?

Your hormones, progesterone and oestrogen,
will have been high during pregnancy. After you
have had your baby, these hormone levels drop
and your body may find it difficult to adjust.
This can have a marked effect on your emotions.

With this, and the fact that you're probably
completely exhausted from the labour and
lack of sleep, it's not at all surprising that
you may not be feeling on top of the world.

WHAT CAN YOU DO TO HELP YOURSELF?

■ Give yourself time: accept that you'll feel
like this for a short time and that what you're
going through is incredibly common.
■ Accept offers of help and don't try to do
everything yourself.
■ Try to talk about your feelings and have
a good cry if it helps.
■ Tell your partner you need a lot of love
and affection, but remember this is a time
of upheaval and change for him too.

DO FATHERS GET THE BLUES?

Most fathers feel an anti-climax after the
birth. There are the extra responsibilities
and sudden changes in lifestyle. If your
partner is feeling low, you'll be called on
to be a tower of strength, which can be
a huge strain. Try to think of the first few
months as a period of rapid change that
is testing for both of you; when you come
through it, you'll emerge closer than you
were before. If you get really unhappy,
talk things over with your health visitor, doctor
or a close friend.

POSTNATAL DEPRESSION (PND)

If symptoms that started out as the common
"baby blues" don't go away and, in fact, start
to become worse, you could be suffering from
postnatal depression. This is a temporary and
treatable condition that varies from woman to
woman. It can develop slowly and not become
obvious until several weeks after the baby's
birth, but if it's diagnosed and addressed early
enough, there's a good chance of a fast cure.
Health visitors are trained to recognize the
symptoms, and treatment ranges from
something as simple as talking to a friend,
health visitor or doctor about how you feel,
to taking medication, such as antidepressants,
for more severe cases.

WHY POSTNATAL DEPRESSION HAPPENS

There are many reasons why postnatal
depression occurs. It depends on you as a
person, your personal circumstances and the
way your baby behaves. Research shows that
the following risk factors may make you more
susceptible to postnatal depression.

SELF-HELP

Overcoming postnatal depression

If you are feeling low, there are a number of
things you can do to help yourself.
Believe in recovery Convince yourself that
you will get better, no matter how much
time that takes.
Correct potassium deficiency Severe
exhaustion, another possible problem after
giving birth, may be made worse by a lack
of potassium in your body. **Low potassium**
levels are easily corrected by eating plenty
of potassium-rich foods such as bananas
or tomatoes.
Rest as much as possible Being tired
definitely makes depression worse and
harder to cope with. Catnap during the day
and, if possible, get someone to help with
night feeds.
Maintain a proper diet Eat plenty of fruit
and raw vegetables; don't snack or binge on
chocolate, sweets, and cookies. Eat little and
often. Do not go on a strict diet.

Get gentle exercise Give yourself a rest
from being indoors or taking care of the
baby. A brisk walk in the fresh air can lift
your spirits.
Avoid major upheavals Don't start a new
job, move to a new home or redecorate.
Try not to worry unduly Aches and pains
are common after childbirth, and more so if
you are depressed. Try to take them in stride;
they will almost certainly fade away as soon
as you can relax.
Be kind to yourself Don't force yourself to
do things you don't want to do or that might
upset you. Don't worry about not keeping
the house spotless or letting household
tasks lapse. Concern yourself with small,
undemanding tasks and reward yourself
when you finish them.
Talk about your feelings Don't bottle up
your concerns; this can make matters worse.
Talk to others, particularly your partner.

- If you enjoyed a senior position at work or high-flying career before the birth, it can be difficult to adjust to the status change.
- If you already have difficulties in your relationship, the baby may make them worse; this in itself may lead to disillusionment and low self-esteem.
- If you had an unexpectedly difficult birth experience, you could easily feel demoralized and feel that you've failed in some way.
- If you've had depression in the past, you may be more prone to PND now.
- A very demanding, sleepless baby can trigger postnatal depression from sheer exhaustion.
- If you have particularly difficult living conditions and no support network, this can exacerbate postnatal depression.
- If you've bottled up your emotions and not sought help early on, PND may develop.

SEEKING HELP

Many women are too embarrassed to admit how they feel, fearing that it will appear that they have somehow failed. Talking about how you feel is the most important thing you can do; once you accept that you're not "mad" and that there are things you can do to help yourself, you are one step on the road to recovery. Once you seek help you'll be guided to:
- understand how you feel and learn to express this
- learn to prioritize and go with the flow
- devote more time to yourself and find ways to relax
- visit the health visitor more regularly and seek support
- begin taking medication if your postnatal depression is very extreme.

WHAT FATHERS CAN DO

As a father, you may feel helpless because you don't understand PND. Remember, it's temporary and treatable, so try to be patient. You can be a huge help if you make an effort to understand and do the following:
- Talk and listen to your partner. Never tell her to pull herself together – she can't. Don't assume she'll snap out of it – she won't.
- Mother the mother: encourage her to rest and eat and drink properly.
- Encourage her to be with the baby as much as she wants, so that she can take things slowly and gradually work out how the baby will fit in.
- Make sure she's not alone too much.
- See the doctor first for advice; your partner may refuse to accept she's ill. The doctor may arrange to visit her informally at home.

Menopausal depression

FEELINGS SUCH AS TENSION, ANXIETY, DEPRESSION, LISTLESSNESS, IRRITABILITY, TEARFULNESS AND MOOD SWINGS CAN OCCUR AT ANY AGE, BUT THEY RARELY OCCUR TOGETHER OR AS FREQUENTLY AS THEY DO DURING THE MENOPAUSE.

If you are experiencing several negative feelings simultaneously, it may be helpful to know that the menopause is the reason.

For many women, menopausal mood changes resemble a roller coaster ride. Women describe subtle sensations such as trembling, fluttering, unease and discomfort. More severe feelings of anxiety or panic can arise with little provocation. Tasks that you used to be able to tackle can leave you in total disarray. Mood swings from elation to despondency are common. Your patience is easily exhausted. The future may look hopeless, your loss of self-esteem is precipitous, and you may feel truly depressed.

WHAT ARE THE CAUSES?

- The centres in the brain that control a sense of wellbeing, a positive state of mind, and a feeling of control and tranquillity are affected by the absence of oestrogen. Taking oestrogen supplements as hormone replacement therapy (HRT) can cause a dramatic return to normality.
- For some women, the emotional troubles they experience around the menopause may mainly be due to the fact that their sleep is being interrupted by night sweats. People who are tired are often irritable and anxious. If you're experiencing this problem, try the self-help tips for promoting sleep on p.297.
- A major depression, although rare, can descend upon you during your menopausal years, and this is distinct from other emotional symptoms that you may experience, such as tearfulness and anxiety. These are possible predictors of depression during the menopause:

- a past or recent history of stressful events, such as divorce or bereavement
- a surgically-induced menopause
- having negative expectations of menopause
- severe hot flushes or night sweats
- a family history of depressive illness
- "empty nest" syndrome.

Depression can be a debilitating illness that can last for weeks, months or even years if left untreated. It affects your body, your mood, your thoughts and severely interferes with normal life. As a woman, you're more likely to experience depression than a man is.

Consult your doctor if you have experienced four of these symptoms for at least two weeks:
- any extreme eating patterns, such as bingeing or loss of appetite
- unusual sleeping patterns, such as sleeping all the time or insomnia
- being exceptionally lethargic or restless
- an inability to enjoy a once pleasurable activity, including a loss of sex drive
- debilitating fatigue or loss of energy
- feelings of worthlessness and self-reproach
- difficulty concentrating, remembering and making decisions
- thoughts of death or suicide, or suicide attempts (seek help straight away).

COMPLEMENTARY THERAPIES

Herbs that may have a calming effect are **passion flower** and **valerian root**, taken as a tea or a tincture. Passion flower helps insomnia, and elevates the levels of serotonin in the blood, which creates a feeling of well-being. A herbal bath can also be therapeutic.

SELF-HELP

Managing depression

- Severe mood swings and irritability can distance you from your partner and occasionally can jeopardize a relationship. However, if you share your feelings you may find your partner is very supportive. Several studies show that partners are keen to understand menopausal symptoms and would prefer to have insight into potential problems before the onset of menopause.
- Women who go to self-help groups may be better able to deal with depression. Think about joining such a group or starting one yourself.
- 20–30 minutes of strenuous exercise results in the release of endorphins, which are brain opioids similar to morphine. This can lift mood and produce an "exercise high" that lasts up to eight hours. Exercise can also reduce hot flushes and night sweats, which is helpful if these are the root cause of your depression.
- Yoga, relaxation techniques and meditation all promote tranquillity and combat anxiety and tension.

Some women find that menopausal depression and stress may be alleviated by **ginger**, **cayenne pepper**, **dandelion root** and **Siberian ginseng**. These may work because they contain essential nutrients; for instance:
● dandelion root contains magnesium, potassium and vitamin E
● cayenne pepper contains a high level of magnesium and bioflavonoids
● ginseng contains oestrogenic compounds, and Siberian ginseng and liquorice root, which have been important medicines in the Far East for thousands of years, are said to combat lassitude and depression.

MEDICAL TREATMENT
The mainstay of treatment for emotional symptoms is HRT. Studies from all over the world show that after a short period (between two weeks and two months) HRT can bring about a significant decline in anxiety and depression. Oestrogen even lifts the mood in non-depressed, healthy young women. It acts through several well-known antidepressive mechanisms in the brain, on which other antidepressant drugs also act. The tranquillizing effect of oestrogen is at least the equivalent of that of tranquillizers such as diazepam and chlorodiazepoxide, and oestrogen is a great deal healthier to take.

Sexual assault

THE PHYSICAL AND PSYCHOLOGICAL AFTER EFFECTS OF BEING SEXUALLY ASSAULTED CAN BE DEVASTATING. HERE I INCLUDE ADVICE ON REDUCING THE RISKS OF BEING RAPED AND ON WHAT TO DO BOTH DURING AN ATTACK AND AFTERWARDS.

Rape of women and children (of both sexes) is growing and, although not as prevalent in Britain as in America, it is increasing at an alarming rate. Although it is a fact not often recognized, adult men may also be victims of rape. Most cases of rape occur between people who know each other, making it difficult for the victim to prove that rape has taken place. Moreover, it often occurs in circumstances where the victim is unlikely to tell anyone about it or where she is not likely to be believed as there are no witnesses.

This last situation, which says a lot about prevailing double-standards in society, has further repercussions for rape victims. Even if the ordeal of rape is bad, going to the police and courts can be worse. Most rape victims find insensitivity and callousness, if not downright obstructiveness and disbelief, at all levels of the legal process – from police questioning, to the gynaecological examination, to the questioning of the prosecutor and lawyer. It is a brave woman who follows up a rape charge to the end; most women do not want every detail of their daily lives laid bare in court or to deal with innuendos or implications about their sexual behaviour. The present rape laws are designed to protect men from women, and quite innocent behaviour on the part of women can be misinterpreted in a very sinister way against them.

THE POTENTIAL RAPIST
While it is impossible to generalize about the kind of man who rapes women, certain characteristics occur too frequently to be coincidental. Rapists very often dislike women and find their desire to intimidate and humiliate them difficult to control. Frequently they are described as immature and are often known to be violent. Usually they believe that the only way they can achieve sexual satisfaction is through violence, and many have sexual problems such as impotence or an inability to reach orgasm. Very often rapists have been subjected to humiliation at some time in their lives and they feel they have to get rid of their resentment by attacking other human beings.

Alcohol is frequently connected with rape. One study in America revealed that 50 percent of rapists had taken alcohol before the rape, and 35 percent of them were actually alcoholics.

AVOIDING RAPE
There are certain things that you can do to reduce your risk of being raped.

ON THE STREET
■ Don't venture alone into areas where you know there has been trouble and where there are street gangs.
■ If you suspect that someone is following you, walk out into the middle of the street where there are cars, and run.
■ If you feel that you may be about to be attacked, run into the middle of the street and start screaming. It is quite likely (though not certain) that if a potential attacker is faced with a crowd, he will not attack you.

BY YOUR CAR
■ Never leave your parked car unlocked.
■ Park by a street lamp at night, if possible.
■ Before you get into your parked car, look at the back seat.

AT HOME
■ Have strong locks on your windows and doors.
■ Install and use a peephole.
■ Never open your front door to a man who has come to do a job in your house without checking his identity.

ONCE ATTACKED
■ If you find yourself in a situation where you are being sexually assaulted, scream as loudly as you can and fight as hard as you can. Try to get a finger in the man's eye or pull your knee up sharply into his groin.
■ On the other hand, if your assailant is armed, lack of resistance on your part may be necessary to save your life.

BEING RAPED
Once you determine that resistance is useless or is likely to lead to more violence against yourself, do the following things.
■ Stay calm. Talk quietly and carefully to your attacker to remind him that you are human.
■ Don't excite him further by answering leading questions about your feelings during rape – reply with a calm, factual statement about something else, for example, "You're hurting my back".
■ Concentrate on his features and clothing and on any regional accent or speech patterns, or other identifying factors.
■ Think about something concrete and routine – like what you are going to do about notifying the authorities once you're free.
■ Try not to show any pain or weakness as it will only make him more violent.

INFORMING THE AUTHORITIES
When you have to report the case to the police it is almost certain to be embarrassing, so ask for your interview to be in a private room, and by a female officer if there is one at that police station. If at any time you think that your investigator is becoming offensive, don't be afraid to say so. Always have a second person with you while your statement is being taken.

If your case goes to trial, you will find it at the least embarrassing and, possibly, psychologically traumatic. However, all the questions that you can be asked either for the police report or in court must, by law, be confined to the rape incident, and questions into your private sex life are not permitted. Many women's groups have volunteers on call who will accompany rape victims to court. If you cannot get one of these women to accompany you, take a friend.

The legal definition of rape is contact between a penis and the vagina against the will of the victim. One of the most difficult things to prove is that there was force, particularly if there is no bodily injury. This is why you should contact your doctor as soon as you can after rape, so that he or she can perform a careful medical examination; the testimony may count in your favour in court.

Also by legal definition, fear of bodily injury is considered force, and you will have to prove that in court too. In other words, you must prove you did not willingly engage in sexual activities.

THE MEDICAL EXAMINATION

The presence of sperm or semen in your vagina is considered to be very strong corroborative evidence of rape. However, it is possible that your rapist did not ejaculate – 1 in 3 don't – and therefore the medical examination becomes crucial to see if there is any evidence of injury. It is very important for you to tell the doctor and the police if you think that the man didn't ejaculate.

■ You will first have a general examination of your whole body, so that the doctor can describe bruises, redness, cuts, pain and tenderness.

■ Then you will have an internal pelvic examination, partly to look for evidence of injury and partly to take a sample of the vaginal secretions. Examination of these secretions will show if there are any sperm present. It will also identify a chemical called **acid phosphitase**, which is found in seminal fluid and will be present in your vagina if the man ejaculated but had no sperm.

■ It is possible that your mouth and anus will be examined to see if the attacker has harmed these areas.

■ Blood samples will be taken to check for HIV infection and syphilis. If there is a risk of developing HIV infection, you may be prescribed a course of antiviral drugs to reduce this risk.

■ The doctor will probably prescribe antibiotics to prevent STDs, such as syphilis and gonorrhoea. You will be offered emergency contraception if there is a risk of pregnancy. Doctors are familiar with the use of the morning-after pill to prevent conception. You can discuss this possibility with the doctor, and if you find that your period is delayed, discuss with the doctor the possibility of having a menstrual extraction.

■ Don't let the doctor put you off by saying that the chances of you having caught an STD or being pregnant are very small. Assert yourself and get your rights.

■ Never leave the doctor's surgery without getting a name, address and telephone number, so that you can phone him or her

Checklist for post-rape action

1. If there is no one in the house, telephone a friend or relative who can get to you fairly quickly, so that they can give you support. Try to keep them with you all the time.

2. Report the crime to the police: if you feel you cannot do this, tell your nearest and dearest friend immediately, who may be able to persuade you to report the incident.

3. Contact your doctor and ask to see him or her as soon as possible or go to hospital if your doctor is not immediately available.

4. Do not take a bath. Take off the clothing you were wearing. Do not wash or change it, as doctors and police may want to examine it.

5. Try to remember every detail you can about the man who assaulted you. Keep a notepad by you and write down everything you can remember: not just physical features, but perhaps a regional accent or peculiar words that the rapist used.

6. After you have made your report to the police, don't go home alone. Don't stay at home by yourself. Try always to have a friend with you or if that is not possible, go and stay with friends or relatives.

7. There are rape crisis centres in many areas, or local women's groups that will give you advice. Contact one of them quickly.

back if any problems arise, and say that you will do so.

■ Subsequent visits may be necessary after six weeks to test for syphilis and gonorrohea and at three and six months for repeat HIV and hepatitis B and C testing.

Your state of mind after being raped makes it quite difficult for you to think calmly and coolly about all the things that you should be doing and asking. Indeed, you may be so shocked that you cannot think straight or say anything. This is one of the reasons why it is very important to have a friend with you so that she can act as your advocate to ensure that nothing is forgotten and that everything is done.

COPING WITH RAPE

The after effects of rape are both physical and psychological. You may discover a vaginal discharge and you may have itching of the perineum – this could be due to an infection of candidiasis (thrush) or trichomoniasis. Quite often bruises, swelling and tenderness appear several hours after the rape. If they do, go back to the same doctor who examined you to make sure that they are recorded. It is possible for slight tears to occur in the lining of the rectum if your assailant involved this area. Sometimes they may bleed when you move your bowels. Make sure that you report this also to the doctor who examined you, even if some time has elapsed.

No woman who is raped does not suffer some sort of psychological after effect, though it differs greatly. Some women are completely stunned, and others are quite calm. However, it is quite normal to suffer some anxiety, which may go as far as hysterical behaviour. It is also

perfectly normal to be afraid of being left alone, even for a few minutes; it is normal not to be able to sleep, and it is normal to want to run away and hide yourself. With the help of family and friends, these feelings will pass more quickly than if you stay alone. When choosing a friend that you want to stay with, choose the one that cares most about you and not about the fact that you were raped. This is because many people have conflicting ideas about rape and they may give more attention to the incident than to your particular needs.

One of the best ways to help yourself is through women's groups and through rape crisis centres; this is because they are experienced in dealing with all the various reactions that a woman can feel after being raped. They will counsel you and give you comfort. They will seek legal advice on your behalf and they will help to get you through your serious psychological upsets. One of the most important things is that you get help and support from friends and sympathetic groups as soon as possible. This way you are giving yourself the best chance of coming through your rape experience without long-term psychological trauma.

Women's rape crisis centres say that one of the most helpful emotions for you to express after rape is rage, so get angry if you feel like it. They also point out that the least helpful emotion is guilt. Sympathetic and understanding friends, and qualified counsellors from rape crisis centres, can help you to come to terms with both of these emotions.

Body dysmorphic disorder

PEOPLE WITH BODY DYSMORPHIC DISORDER (BDD) HAVE A DISTORTED PERCEPTION
OF THEIR OWN BODY SHAPE, BECOMING PREOCCUPIED WITH AN IMAGINED DEFECT
OR SHOWING EXCESSIVE CONCERN ABOUT SOME MINOR ANOMALY.

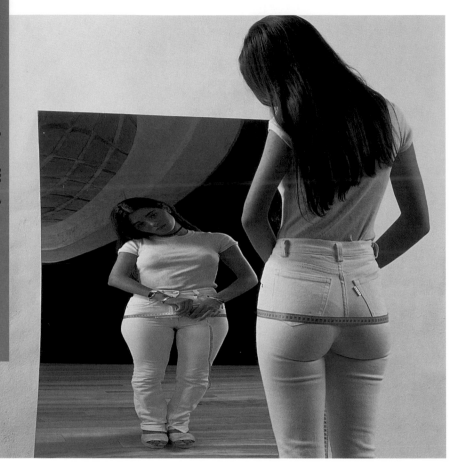

These are normal adolescent anxieties blown up to monstrous proportions, so that eventually you may believe that if anyone even looks at you in the street they're condemning you for living. Like one man with BDD said, "The only place you feel comfortable is in book shops looking at pictures of people with horrible deformities".

Self-loathing can be so intense that you repeatedly mutilate yourself. Life may become one complex ritual. You check your face in the mirror hundreds of times a day and it can take you five hours to get ready to go out.

Just why someone tumbles into the BDD pit of self-loathing no one knows. There's speculation about triggering events in childhood. Researchers at Great Ormond Street Hospital have shown that anorexics have reduced blood flow to the part of their brain that controls vision, which might be linked with the distortion of their body image.

Brain scans have revealed that several areas in the brain malfunction in cases of obsessive-compulsive disorder. Is something similar going on with BDD? No one knows yet. However, about 60 percent of those affected recover with therapy.

What's so fascinating about BDD is that, although it involves a level of obsession and isolation that most of us can barely imagine, we can all dimly empathize with it. We all feel our noses could be smaller or that we could be shorter or taller or fatter or thinner, and we wish we had perfect skin, longer legs or more or less hair.

In our body-beautiful and celebrity-obsessed culture, the BDD sufferer is like the rest of us, only more so.

WHAT IS THE TREATMENT?

The recommended treatment for BDD is cognitive therapy. This involves being exposed to more and more challenging situations until you can begin to function in society again. Selective serotonin re-uptake inhibitor (SSRI) drugs can help too. Also, self-help groups give support and advice.

Body dysmorphic disorder (BDDsufferers typically try to hide their "affliction". We have known for some time that anorexics have a distorted perception of their bodies: no matter how thin they are they still see themselves like the Michelin man. And it's not restricted to women – men are increasingly perceiving themselves as too thin and becoming obsessive about weight training and body building, even to the extent of taking anabolic steroids. In the most severe cases people go to extraordinary lengths to rid themselves of their ugly feature, in some cases amputating an unwanted limb.

WHAT ARE THE CAUSES?
Body dysmorphic disorder shares features with several other psychiatric conditions, including anorexia and obsessive-compulsive disorder (OCD). Like anorexics, BDD sufferers see

their body in a distorted way, but while anorexics flaunt their thinness and are proud of it, people with BDD regard their affliction as a terrible secret.

Preoccupation with an imagined defect in appearance is the basis of this disorder. If a slight physical anomaly is present, the person's concern is markedly excessive.

BDD quite often starts in adolescence when teenagers are plagued with insecurity and shyness. It wouldn't be uncommon to feel that everything about you was wrong, the size of your head, your hands, your height, your thinness, your fatness, your spots. You may resort to all sorts – Charles Atlas to build you up, cream to stop your hair falling out, powerful skin treatments because you're convinced your skin looks like the lunar surface.

See also:
• **Psychological therapies p.286**

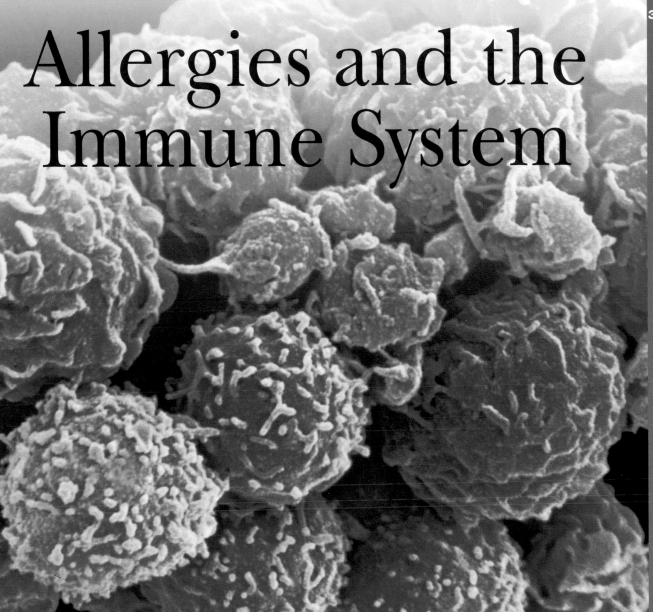

Allergies and the Immune System

Image shows a coloured scanning electron micrograph of white blood cells and platelets

Miriam's overview

The immune system makes us immune – immune to infections, foreign proteins and to cancer. It brings together a complex array of interacting genes, cells, enzymes and chemicals, so complex that much of it still remains a mystery.

We've managed to make sense of a few small corners but are still miles away from making sense of the whole.

I'd be the first to admit that anything I have to say merely scratches the surface. My aim is to throw light on some common conditions involving the immune system so that you'll have a better understanding of what's going on and how to deal with them.

"Boosting your immune system" is a phrase bandied about by manufacturers in the hope that you'll buy their product for which this claim is made. I wish I understood what the phrase means, I'd probably be seduced into buying the product too. But I don't.

I don't know of anything that boosts the immune system, certainly not by a supplement of any vitamin or mineral. The immune system doesn't work like that. The only way that I know of giving the immune system a boost is a dose of an infection. Then the whole defence system swings into action, the T cells get busy and antibodies start pumping.

That's why immunization works so well and why childhood vaccinations are so important. They put our immune systems through their paces. Vaccinations do this so efficiently that they may make us immune for life.

An allergy is simply an expression of an immune system

that has got out of hand – it's become too sensitive – so it tries to protect us from things that most immune systems don't even bother about – pollen, house dust and the like.

Now it's possible to retrain that trigger-happy immune system with desensitizing injections, but most of the time doctors simply have to numb it with anti-allergic medicines, as we do in most cases of asthma.

Sometimes the immune system can get out of hand and start protecting the body against itself. When it does, the resulting condition is called an autoimmune disorder. Rheumatoid arthritis is an example, when the body turns on its own joints.

"it's possible *to retrain* that trigger-happy *immune system* with desensitizing injections"

And if the immune system falls down on its protective job we can be in an awful lot of trouble. AIDS is one instance of that, where the virus, the HIV virus, systematically dismantles the fundamental elements of the immune system, making us prey to opportunistic infections and cancers, often fatally (see p.338).

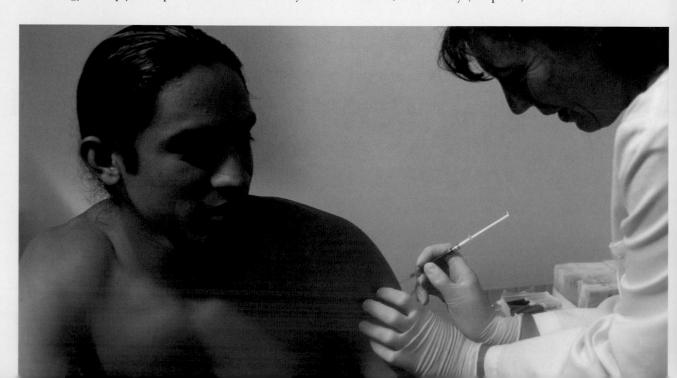

INSIDE
your immune system

The body has many barriers to infection and various types of **immune response** to invading organisms and cancerous cells. For example, **sebum** and **sweat**, excreted by the skin, are mildly antiseptic. **Tears** contain a more powerful antiseptic. **Mucus**, secreted by the lining of the respiratory tract and the stomach, protects the body by trapping harmful organisms. In the **antibody immune response**, white blood cells known as **B lymphocytes** or **B cells** attack and destroy invading bacteria. In the **cellular immune** response, white blood cells known as **T lymphocytes** or T cells attack and destroy viruses, parasites and cancer cells.

In an **allergic reaction**, the immune system becomes sensitized to a substance that is normally harmless, such as pollen. Subsequent exposure to the substance causes **mast cells**, which are located in the skin and nasal lining as well as in other tissues, to be destroyed, releasing **histamine**. Histamine causes an **inflammatory response** and brings on the symptoms of allergy.

the body's defences

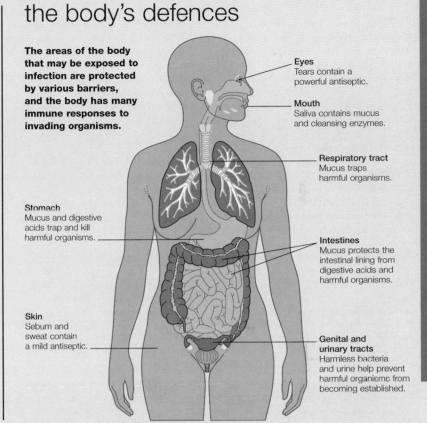

The areas of the body that may be exposed to infection are protected by various barriers, and the body has many immune responses to invading organisms.

Eyes
Tears contain a powerful antiseptic.

Mouth
Saliva contains mucus and cleansing enzymes.

Respiratory tract
Mucus traps harmful organisms.

Stomach
Mucus and digestive acids trap and kill harmful organisms.

Intestines
Mucus protects the intestinal lining from digestive acids and harmful organisms.

Skin
Sebum and sweat contain a mild antiseptic.

Genital and urinary tracts
Harmless bacteria and urine help prevent harmful organisms from becoming established.

THE ATOPIC FAMILY OF CONDITIONS

I'd like to tell you about a particular and common form of allergy. What is atopy? The word "atopic" means that a person is born with an extra sensitivity to certain things, usually invisible proteins called allergens, in the environment. The commonest triggers or allergens in these people are the house dust mite (more accurately the droppings of house dust mite), grass, tree and weed pollen, proteins on cat and dog fur, feathers and occasionally foods, such as egg, milk or nuts.

Atopic people have a hypersensitivity of their immune system and produce too much of the IgE allergy antibody. They have no other problem with their immune system, but this sensitivity leads to ATOPY. A gene is responsible and the gene can be passed down through a family. Family members show up this atopic gene in any or all of several different ways.

So if you belong to an "atopic" family you'll be able to track your "atopic" gene showing up as any of these conditions:

- childhood eczema
- adult dermatitis
- childhood asthma
- hay fever
- allergies
- migraine (I describe this with other headaches, see p.407).

At first glance these conditions don't seem to be closely related, but they're all expressions of the atopic gene so I describe them here as a family of conditions.

Eczema

ECZEMA DESCRIBES AN ITCHY, INFLAMED SKIN RASH. THE TERM ECZEMA COMES FROM A GREEK WORD MEANING TO "BOIL OVER" AND IS USED INTERCHANGEABLY WITH ANOTHER TERM, DERMATITIS. THERE ARE SEVERAL DIFFERENT TYPES, INCLUDING ATOPIC OR ALLERGIC ECZEMA.

The most common type of eczema is atopic eczema, sometimes referred to as "allergic eczema". If someone is atopic they carry a gene that makes their skin react to stress (a virus infection, an irritant in contact with the skin, psychological disturbances) with patches of eczema. Once you have eczema or dermatitis you will **always** have the tendency to develop it, so episodes may return throughout your life.

Atopic eczema sufferers may also develop asthma or hay fever or may have relations who have those conditions. The gene for atopy tends to run in families but may express itself differently in family members, for example migraine in one, hay fever in another, allergies in another, asthma, etc. All these conditions are close relatives of eczema (dermatitis) and all run in my atopic family.

Though the tendency to develop eczema is undoubtedly genetic, certain foods (most commonly dairy products, eggs and wheat) and skin irritants (such as pet fur, wool or washing powders) can act as triggers, especially in children.

WHAT ARE THE SYMPTOMS?

■ Dry, red, scaly rash, which is extremely itchy, occurring on the face, neck and hands, and in the creases of the limbs.
■ The rash usually starts off as minute pearly blisters beneath the skin's surface.
■ When very severe, the rash may weep.
■ Sleeplessness may result if the itchiness is very bad.

AGGRAVATING FACTORS

Symptoms vary from mild to severe and can be made worse by:
● climate changes, especially if exposed to cold winds or excessive heat
● water, especially hard water
● soaps, detergents, cleansers, bubble bath, cosmetics, perfume
● pollen, pet hair, animal dander, dust
● stress and anxiety
● synthetic or wool fibres
● certain chemicals: acids, alkalis, oxidizing or reducing agents, oils, solvents
● colds, flu, infections of any kind.

LIFESTYLE

■ People with eczema should avoid contact with soap, detergents and other irritants. This means wearing rubber gloves for household wet work, or cotton gloves for cleaning.
■ They should avoid jobs or occupations that expose their skin to irritants, such as in hairdressing, catering, mechanical engineering and perhaps nursing, especially if the eczema affects the hands.
■ Reduce the population of house dust mites in the home by regular dusting and vacuuming of carpets. Dust mite bed covers have benefited some eczema patients, and frequent airing and changing of bed linen should reduce the house dust mite population in bedding.
■ Bed clothes should be washed at 50°C (122°F) or more to kill house dust mites.
■ Old mattresses are more likely to harbour large populations of house dust mite, and furry toys are another source of exposure.
■ Shaking soft toys vigorously or placing them into a plastic bag in the freezer for a few hours helps.
■ Some atopic people are sensitive to cat or dog fur and it makes sense to avoid having these animals as pets when a family member suffers from atopic eczema.
■ The use of make-up can irritate facial skin in a person with eczema, and these preparations should be used with care.
■ It is best to keep the central heating turned as low as is comfortable as it has a tendency to dry out the skin.
■ Cotton clothes are less irritating on eczema skin than polyester or wool.
■ Bathing and showering are safe, provided that a soap substitute such as aqueous cream is used, or a bath oil is added.
■ Bubble bath should be avoided, as it is a detergent. The moisturizer that the person uses should be applied after the skin has been patted dry.
■ Holidays in a warm environment are beneficial as the skin's moisture is improved and, of course, the person is more relaxed.
■ Although sunlight is usually helpful, atopic eczema may make the skin more sun-sensitive and covering up with cotton clothes and using a sunblocking cream are advised in hot climates to avoid burning.
■ People with eczema can **go swimming**. Putting an emollient ointment or a barrier cream on the skin before and after swimming reduces irritation.

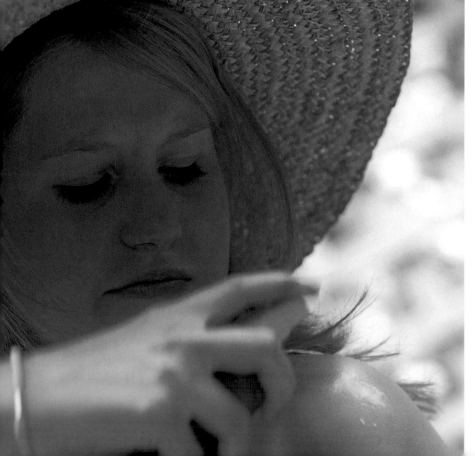

IS DIET IMPORTANT?

■ In very young children, atopic eczema may be worsened by **cow's milk formula** and so infants with eczema are often put on to soya milk, or low-allergy milk feeds. This problem generally settles in the second year of life and cow's milk may then be tolerated in slowly increasing amounts.

■ **Eggs** may worsen eczema, although they may be tolerated in highly processed form, such as in cakes.

■ Families may feel that other food items are important and if several foods are suspected or you decide to put your child on a restricted diet, then it is wise to discuss this with a dietitian to make sure your child is getting enough protein, calcium and calories.

■ Fortunately, most apparent food allergies get better during childhood.

■ One food item that continues to cause problems in a few atopic individuals is **peanuts**.

■ **Tomato sauce** and **citrus fruits** seem to worsen facial eczema because they irritate broken skin and can produce weals around the mouth.

CHINESE HERBAL TREATMENTS

Recent research has shown ancient Chinese herbal remedies can be very helpful. There are tablets to take, infusions to drink and creams to rub on. Most dermatologists recognize the effectiveness of these treatments.

WHAT MIGHT THE DOCTOR DO?

■ Your doctor will question you on your family's medical history, particularly whether anyone has ever suffered from eczema or related conditions such as asthma and hay fever.

■ The doctor will ask you about any changes in diet, whether you have recently changed your washing powders, whether you have just brought a pet into the house and whether natural or synthetic fibres are worn next to the skin.

■ If your baby has eczema and you've just started weaning him from the breast or bottle, your doctor may recommend that you avoid dairy products and continue breast-feeding or use formula milk. If you don't want to do this, your doctor may recommend that you wean your baby on to soya milk instead.

■ Your doctor may prescribe an anti-inflammatory skin cream to reduce redness, scaliness and itchiness. In severe cases, very weak steroid creams may be prescribed. These creams should be used very sparingly, especially on a child's skin.

■ If the itching is causing sleepless nights, your doctor may prescribe antihistamine medicine to improve sleep.

■ If the skin has become infected through scratching, your doctor may prescribe an antiseptic cream or antibiotics.

■ Your doctor will advise you to add bath oil to bath water and to stop using soap. Soap can be an irritant to the already sensitive skin; the oil will help to keep the skin supple and less dry.

WHAT'S THE OUTLOOK?

Many children outgrow eczema (and asthma) around the age of seven. They will, however, retain a life-long tendency to develop transient eczema if the body is put under stress and may pass on this tendency to their children.

In adult life, dermatitis isn't the same as that in a child. The eczema looks different, it's in different places and it may come and go. It may take the form of seborrhoeic, contact or photo-dermatitis (caused by light).

Eczema in babies and children

Baby eczema, also called infantile eczema, is common and usually develops when a baby is about 2–3 months old, or at 4–5 months when solid foods are introduced. Most children grow out of eczema by the age of three or, if not, by seven.

Some important points

■ **Baby** eczema is less common in breast-fed babies than those fed on the bottle.

■ **Baby** eczema isn't caused by an allergy and allergy tests don't help.

■ **Children** with eczema don't benefit from a special diet.

What should I do first?

■ If your baby is scratching, look at his neck and scalp, his face, his hands and the creases of his elbows, knees and groin, classic sites for baby dermatitis.

■ Keep his fingernails short to minimize the possibility of breaking the skin. If the skin becomes broken, put mittens on him to prevent infection.

■ If you've just started weaning your breast-fed child, return to breast-feeds until you've seen your doctor. If you've been using formula milk, return to that.

■ Apply oily calamine lotion to ease irritation and soothe the skin.

■ Soap should be avoided as it de-fats the skin and makes it drier, more scaly and irritable.

■ Avoid woollen or hairy garments; use cotton or linen instead.

What else can I do?

■ Use an emollient cream whenever your child washes. This will keep his skin soft, prevent it from drying out and damp down the itchiness.

■ Underplay the condition in front of your child. Your anxiety can make the condition worse.

■ Keep your child's fingernails short so that scratching doesn't cause the skin to break and give rise to infection.

■ Make sure all your child's clothes, and anything that comes next to his skin, are rinsed thoroughly to remove all traces of powders and conditioners.

■ If the eczema is found to be made worse by pet fur, you may need to consider giving your family pet away.

■ Use an aqueous cream from your chemist as a soap substitute.

■ Use a bath emollient (available from your pharmacist) dissolved in bath water to put a protective layer over your child's skin.

■ Think about installing a domestic water softener.

■ Dress your child with cotton next to his skin at all times.

■ Don't eliminate any foods from your child's diet without your doctor's supervision.

■ Remove as many irritants from your child's environment as possible. For example, feather and down pillows can be a source of irritation.

Vaccinations

It is generally safe to vaccinate children with eczema in the usual way. However, if a child has a proven egg allergy, their MMR (measles, mumps and rubella) vaccination should be given in a hospital setting in case there are problems, although this is very rare in practice.

Contact dermatitis

THE NAME CONTACT DERMATITIS IS USED TO DESCRIBE AN ITCHY, INFLAMED SKIN RASH THAT
DEVELOPS WHEN SOMETHING IN THE OUTSIDE WORLD COMES INTO CONTACT WITH THE SKIN.
OCCUPATIONAL DERMATITIS IS A TYPE OF CONTACT DERMATITIS.

Contact dermatitis may develop if an offending substance is touched directly or sometimes if there is contact with particles of the substance carried in the air. If all further contact with this substance is avoided the dermatitis should get better.

There are two main types of contact dermatitis: **irritant** and **allergic**.

Irritant contact dermatitis is a very common skin problem that affects many people at some stage of their life. It is caused by contact with substances that damage the outer layers of the skin and typically affects the hands. One of the commonest situations giving rise to irritant contact dermatitis is repeated contact with mildly irritant substances such as water and detergents (washing-up liquid, soaps, etc.). Other irritant substances include solvents, for example petrol, cleaning chemicals, oils and metalworking fluids used in industry. The skin problem often starts as chapping, soreness and redness, and if untreated leads to a stubborn dermatitis. Once damaged, the skin is no longer a barrier against the outside world and can easily be irritated further. This sets up a vicious circle that can be difficult to break.

Allergic contact dermatitis is less common than irritant contact dermatitis and you're born with the tendency to get it. It happens because the body's immune system reacts against a specific substance or "allergen", making the skin hypersensitive. The tendency to allergic response, or "atopy", is genetic, and you and your relatives may have other atopic conditions such as eczema, asthma, hay fever and migraine. People are not born with this type of allergy, but develop it later, usually in adulthood.

Allergic contact dermatitis usually affects only a minority of people who come into contact with the allergen. What makes an allergy develop at a certain time is unknown, and why one person gets affected while others don't is also unclear. **The commonest cause of allergic contact dermatitis in women is nickel**, which is found in metallic jewellery. About 1 in 10 women has this type of allergy and typically develops itchy, sore, red patches on the ear lobes after wearing inexpensive earrings. Other things that commonly cause allergic contact dermatitis include perfumes, rubber, additives, leather additives and preservatives in creams and cosmetics. Allergies can also develop to medicated creams and ointments, and sunscreens.

A person can actually suffer from more than one type of dermatitis. For example, someone with atopic eczema (i.e. constitutional eczema) who works as a hairdresser could get skin irritation on their hands from frequent shampooing (i.e. irritant contact dermatitis).

OCCUPATIONAL DERMATITIS
In some cases a person's dermatitis is caused primarily by substances to which they are exposed at work. These may be irritants or allergens depending on the nature of the job. Patch tests should be carried out if the work involves exposure to substances that can cause allergy.

PREVENTING FURTHER DERMATITIS
■ Minimize contact with all irritant substances at work and at home.
■ Avoid skin contact with the substances you are allergic to.
■ Take general skin care measures to keep the skin strong and healthy.

ACTIVE TREATMENT
Treat the dermatitis with frequent application of moisturizers and regular use of steroid creams or ointments once or twice a day. If the dermatitis has become additionally infected, a course of antibiotic cream may be necessary.

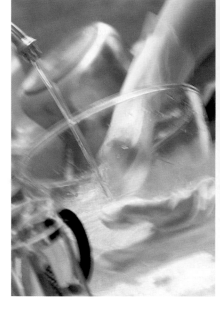

GENERAL HAND CARE
The hands are one of the commonest parts of the body to be affected with dermatitis. Because they are so important for carrying out the tasks of daily life, skin problems here can be especially troublesome. Good general skin care measures can help to look after the skin and are a major part of the treatment of hand dermatitis.
■ Avoid frequent contact with water and use protective gloves where possible.
■ Use gloves and barrier creams if provided at work.
■ Avoid direct contact with other harsh substances such as the juices from fruit and vegetables, detergents and cleaning agents.
■ Use a gentle skin cleanser instead of soap for washing with warm water, and dry the hands thoroughly afterwards to prevent chapping.
■ Use plenty of moisturizers and reapply them frequently (e.g. during tea and coffee breaks, while watching television and before going to sleep at night).

It can take several months for the skin to recover completely from an episode of dermatitis, so even when it looks apparently normal it is still vulnerable. Try to find the time to look after your skin and treat it with respect – it's got to last you a lifetime!

Common causes of allergic contact dermatitis

Substance	Where is it often found
Nickel	Cheap jewellery, studs on jeans, metal objects including coins
Fragrance	Perfumes, toiletries, cosmetics
Chromate	Leather items, wet cement
Preservatives	Cosmetics, especially creams (cleansers, moisturizers, etc.)
Rubber additives	Rubber gloves, shoes

See also:
• **The atopic family of conditions p.311**

Seborrhoeic dermatitis

THE TERM SEBORRHOEIC DERMATITIS DESCRIBES PATCHES OF RED, SCALY, ITCHY
SKIN THAT OCCUR MAINLY ON OILY PARTS OF THE SKIN SUCH AS THE SIDES OF THE NOSE,
SCALP, FACE AND CHEST. STRESS IS OFTEN A TRIGGER.

Some people are born with the tendency
to get seborrhoeic dermatitis and may get
recurrent episodes throughout their life.
Seborrhoeic dermatitis is a skin rash that
commonly occurs in infants and adults. In
infants, either the scalp (cradle cap) or the
nappy area (nappy rash) may be affected.
In adults, the rash tends to occur on the
central part of the face, the eyebrows and
the scalp, where it often leads to flaking of the
skin. Sometimes seborrhoeic dermatitis also
develops in the armpits, the groin or the
middle of the chest and back. In men, the
condition may develop in the beard area.

WHAT IS THE TREATMENT?
- Avoid soap and water.
- Use moisturizing emollient creams.
- Use a weak steroid preparation, such as
1 percent hydrocortisone cream, sparingly
and only under medical supervision.
- Avoid stress as much as possible.

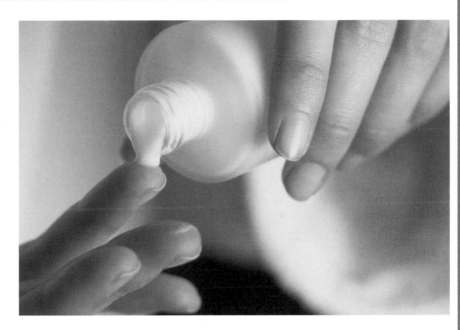

ALLERGIES

Some people become ill when they come into contact
with a substance that may have no effect on other
people. Their illness is due to an allergy – an abnormal
response by the immune system to a foreign invader.
When a person's immune system reacts abnormally to a
substance that has no effect on most people, we say that
the affected person has an "allergy" to the substance and
that they are suffering from an allergic reaction.

An allergic reaction can show itself in different ways,
such as sneezing, an itching or runny nose, breathing
problems, swelling of the face (angioedema) and the
most serious form, anaphylaxis.

The substance that causes such a reaction is known
as an allergen. Common examples of allergens that
affect the lungs include pollens from grass and trees,
house dust mite and animal fur.

Some people – between a quarter and a third of
us – are more likely than others to have allergies
of one kind or another. This tendency runs in
families and is called "atopy". However, not all
the people who have this tendency will actually
get allergy problems.

HOW THE BODY RESPONDS
TO ALLERGENS
Allergens, usually proteins, are seen by the body
as "foreign" and the body's natural response to
anything foreign is to repel it.

The body makes antibodies to neutralize
and repel the allergen. If you make the allergic
type of antibodies (IgE), when allergens and
antibodies meet up inside the body there's
quite an explosion, with the release of many
chemicals that can irritate tissues and even cause
disease and illness. An example would be

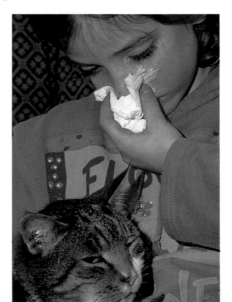

histamine, which narrows the bronchial tubes
and causes wheezing as in asthma.

The symptoms of an allergic disease simply
depend on where this explosion happens. So
if it's in the skin, you'll get a rash; if it's in the
nose, you'll get itching and sneezing; if it's in
the lungs, you'll get wheezing.

Very rarely, and for reasons we don't understand,
the body may see part of itself as the allergen
and attack the thyroid gland or the joints or
the pancreas and we then get thyroid disease,
arthritis and diabetes respectively, which are
called "autoimmune diseases".

THE COMMONEST ALLERGIES
1. Some allergies can cause problems all
through the year; others only affect us at
certain times. The most common cause of year-
round allergy is the **house dust mite**. These tiny

continued on page 318

FOCUS *on* asthma in children

More cases of asthma are being reported than ever before. Is this because we're all more allergic than we were? Is it because, in towns at least, there's more pollution? Or is it because we don't understand what we have to do to prevent asthma? There's quite a lot of evidence that it is the latter.

Studies from Europe show that children raised on farms and in touch with livestock are two-thirds less likely to develop asthma. The same has been shown in Italian soldiers.

The suggestion is that contact with common-or-garden bacteria at a young age gives protection.

One theory for the sharp increase in asthma is that children today are so protected against dirt and everyday infections that their immune systems fail to develop normally and are prone to become hypersensitive and then prey to allergies.

WHAT IS ASTHMA?

In children, asthma is primarily an allergic disease that affects air passages (bronchi) that are extra sensitive to triggers.

When the allergic reaction takes place, the bronchi constrict and become clogged with mucus, making breathing difficult. The muscle around the walls of the airways tightens so that inhaled air can't be forced out. An asthma

attack can be very frightening for a child because the feeling of suffocation can cause panic, making breathing even more laboured.

The initial cause of the allergic reaction, the **allergen**, is usually airborne – pollen or house dust, for example. Once asthma is established, emotional stress or a mild infection such as a cold can also bring on an attack.

Asthma doesn't usually begin until a child is about two years old. The condition tends to run in families and may, unfortunately, be accompanied by other allergic diseases, such as eczema, hay fever and penicillin sensitivity.

However, the good news is that most children get better as they get older.

WHEEZING IN BABIES

Many babies under one year wheeze if they suffer from bronchiolitis, when their small air passages become inflamed. These babies aren't necessarily suffering from asthma; as they grow, their air passages widen and the

wheezing will stop. Infection and not an allergic reaction is the usual cause of this kind of wheezing.

IS IT SERIOUS?

Asthma attacks can be frightening but, with medication and advice from your doctor, your child should suffer no serious complications.

POSSIBLE SYMPTOMS

● Laboured breathing: breathing out become difficult and the abdomen may be drawn inwards with the effort of breathing in.
● Sensation of suffocation.
● Wheezing.
● Persistent cough, particularly at night.
● Getting short of breath – a child doesn't run around as much as usual.
● Blueness around the lips (cyanosis) because of lack of oxygen.

WHAT SHOULD I DO FIRST?

1. Consult your doctor immediately if your child is having any kind of difficulty with breathing.
2. If the attack occurs when your child is in bed, sit him up, propped up with pillows. Otherwise, sit him on a chair with his arms braced against the back to take the weight off his chest; this allows the chest muscles to force air out of the lungs more efficiently.
3. Stay calm; a show of anxiety would only make your child more fearful.
4. While waiting for the doctor, try to take your child's mind off the asthma attack. Sing to him, for example, to try to help him forget about the wheezing.
5. Put a humidifier in the room to ease his sensitive air passages.
6. Give him lots of reassuring cuddles.

CONSULTING YOUR DOCTOR

The mainstays of treatment are **reliever** drugs to relieve an attack of asthma and **preventer** drugs to stop an attack from happening. Preventer drugs must be taken all the time to keep a child free of asthma symptoms.
● Your doctor will treat the attack with a reliever drug, usually a bronchodilator, which opens up the bronchi by relaxing muscles in the lining of the air passages. This drug is inhaled directly into the bronchi and gets right to the site of the obstruction. A severe attack may need treatment in hospital, where bigger doses of bronchodilator drugs may be given by inhalation or by intravenous drip.

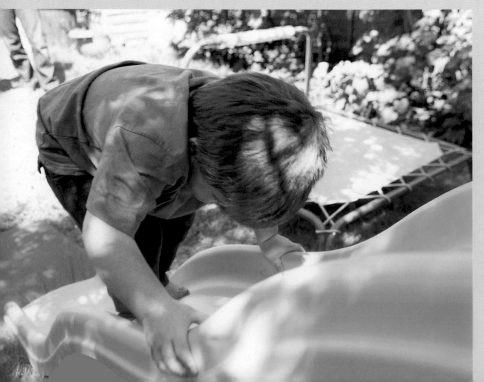

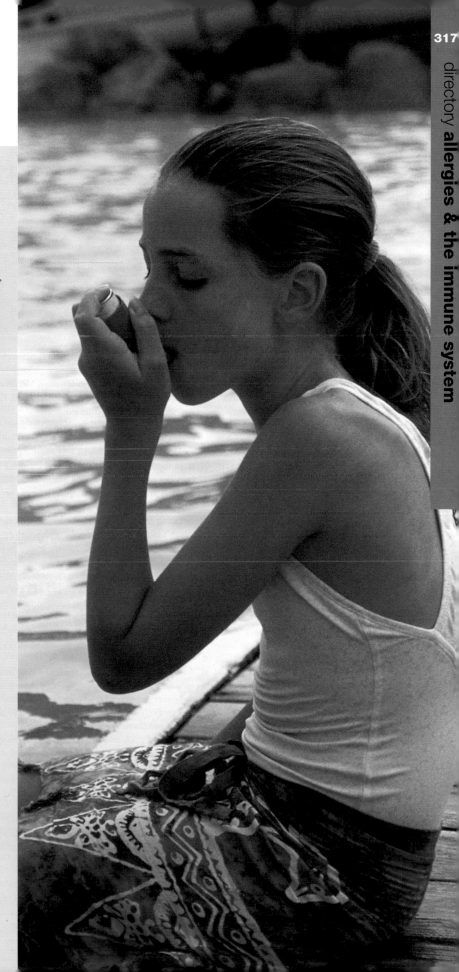

- If there's evidence of a chest infection, your doctor will prescribe antibiotics.
- Your doctor will want to prevent further attacks. He may, for instance, try to determine the allergen, so that your child can avoid it, probably by performing skin tests for the most likely allergens, such as pollen and house dust.
- He'll give you a supply of a bronchodilator drug, usually as an inhaler used with a "spacer" that is easy for children to use, to be taken as soon as an attack begins.
- Your doctor will ask you to inform him if your child has a severe attack, or if an attack doesn't respond to two doses of the bronchodilator.
- Your doctor may prescribe a steroid drug if other simple measures don't stop further attacks. Don't be afraid, steroids for asthma are nearly always inhaled into the deepest parts of the lungs, and are quite safe. A small dose of steroid may be inhaled three or four times a day.

WHAT CAN I DO TO HELP?

- If your doctor has not pinpointed the allergen, try to track it down yourself. Notice when the attacks occur and at what time of the day or year. Avoid obvious allergens such as feather pillows and keep the dust down in your house by damp-dusting and vacuuming floors rather than sweeping them.
- Many asthmatics are allergic to animals – their hair, fur and saliva. If you have a pet, ask a friend to look after it for two weeks and see if your child's attacks reduce in frequency.
- Make sure your child has the prescribed drugs nearby at all times.
- Inform his school about the possibility of attacks occurring.
- It's vital your child takes his preventer medicine continuously and does not stop just because he's feeling fine. Never stop a preventer without consulting your doctor.
- Ask to be referred to a physiotherapist so your child can learn breathing exercises to help him to relax during an attack.
- Encourage your child to stand and sit up straight so that his lungs have more space. Don't let him get overweight, as this will put an extra burden on his lungs.
- Moderate exercise can help his breathing, but too much can bring on an asthma attack. Swimming, however, can be especially helpful for children with asthma.

Food allergy

MANY PEOPLE CONFUSE FOOD ALLERGY AND FOOD INTOLERANCE BUT THE TWO ARE QUITE DIFFERENT. FOOD ALLERGY INVOLVES AN ABNORMAL REACTION BY THE IMMUNE SYSTEM AND CAN BE VERY SERIOUS. FOOD INTOLERANCE NEVER INVOLVES THE IMMUNE SYSTEM.

Let's clear up a common misunderstanding.
■ Food INTOLERANCE is common.
■ Food ALLERGY is relatively rare.
The two must not be confused.
■ An easy way to distinguish them is that an intolerance makes you feel uncomfortable; a food "doesn't suit you" but you can still eat it. You're NOT allergic to it.
■ If you're allergic to a food, you can't eat it at all. The minutest amount, even on a knife, can cause very severe symptoms like angioedema.
■ Food allergy causes serious illness; intolerance NEVER does.

Food allergy is an uncommon condition in which the immune system reacts in an inappropriate or an exaggerated way to a specific food or foods, causing development of various symptoms such as an itchy rash. In contrast, food intolerance, which often causes abdominal discomfort and indigestion, does not involve the immune system in any way.

WHAT ARE THE CAUSES?

■ Food allergy is more common in **atopic** people with other allergy-related conditions such as asthma, eczema or hay fever. There is a greater risk of developing a food allergy if a close relative is allergic to a particular food.
■ Although allergic reactions can occur with any food, nuts (especially peanuts) are probably the most common cause.
■ Other relatively common causes of food allergy include seafood, strawberries and eggs.
■ Though often blamed in the media and by wishful parents, food colourings and preservatives **rarely** cause allergic reactions, but **intolerance** to the food additive monosodium glutamate (MSG) is common.
■ Wheat (gluten) allergy may cause a condition known as **coeliac disease**.
■ An allergic reaction to the protein in cow's milk is especially common in infants and young children.
■ Both of these conditions differ from immediate sensitivity to nuts or other foods in that they are more chronic conditions.

WHAT ARE THE SYMPTOMS?

Symptoms may appear almost immediately after eating the food or develop over a few hours. They may include:
● an itchy, red rash anywhere on the body (urticaria)
● nausea, vomiting and diarrhoea
● difficulty in swallowing (a medical emergency)

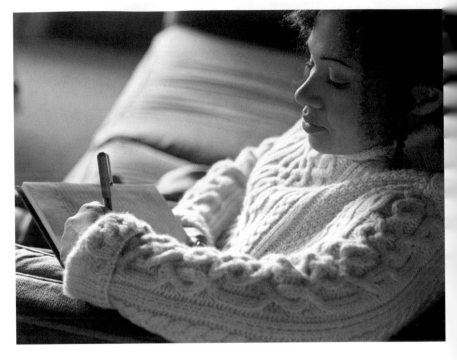

● itching and swelling affecting the face, lips, mouth and throat (angioedema)
● shortness of breath or wheezing – **anaphylaxis**, a **life-threatening** allergic response that causes sudden difficulty in breathing and collapse. If you develop the symptoms of a severe reaction, call an ambulance immediately.

WHAT MIGHT BE DONE?

1. You may be able to diagnose food allergy yourself if the symptoms occur soon after you eat a particular food. However, you should consult your doctor. If he or she is unsure what is responsible for the reaction, you may have a **skin prick test**.
2. Your doctor may also recommend an **exclusion diet** (don't embark on one yourself). By eating a restricted diet for one or two weeks, you may avoid the foods that cause your symptoms. If your symptoms improve substantially while on the diet, you may have one or more food allergies. You can gradually add other foods to your diet, but if symptoms recur when a particular food is eaten, you should avoid it in the future. You should NEVER embark on an exclusion diet without first consulting your doctor. Nor should you follow a nutritionally restricted diet for more than two weeks. Interpreting the results of an exclusion diet is often difficult.

Keeping a food diary can help you identify particular foods to which you may be allergic.

SELF-HELP

■ Keep a food diary and note symptoms. Show it to your doctor.
■ Avoiding the problem food is the only effective treatment.
■ Always ask about ingredients when eating out, and check labels on packaged foods.
■ Consult a diet or nutrition counsellor if you need to exclude a food that is a major part of a normal diet, such as wheat.
■ If a major permanent dietary change is needed, be sure to maintain a balanced diet.

WHAT IS THE OUTLOOK?

Many food allergies, particularly nut allergies, are permanent, and people must avoid the relevant foods throughout their lives. Some food allergies may disappear. Children under age 4 who completely avoid problem foods such as wheat for two years have an excellent chance of outgrowing their allergy.

See also:
● Anaphylaxis p.321 ● Angioedema p.321
● Malabsorption p.365 ● The atopic family of conditions p.311 ● Urticaria p.322

Angioedema

ANGIOEDEMA IS AN ALLERGIC CONDITION THAT TYPICALLY AFFECTS THE LIPS, MOUTH, THROAT, AIR PASSAGES AND EYES, CAUSING SUDDEN AND SOMETIMES SEVERE SWELLING. BECAUSE THE SWELLING CAN INTERFERE WITH BREATHING, IT SHOULD BE TREATED AS AN EMERGENCY.

In angioedema, the mucous membranes and tissues under the skin suddenly become swollen due to an allergic reaction. In some cases, swelling of the mouth, throat and air passages is severe enough to prevent swallowing, even breathing. For this reason, angioedema requires emergency medical treatment.

WARNING:

■ Any severe allergy may develop at some time into an attack of angioedema. The swelling may affect the larynx (voice box) and can be life-threatening if the airway becomes blocked. Angioedema may occur at the same time as ANAPHYLAXIS, a potentially fatal allergic reaction that requires urgent medical attention.

■ If you develop the symptoms of angioedema or experience difficulty breathing, you should call an ambulance immediately.

WHAT ARE THE CAUSES?

■ The most common cause of angioedema is an allergic reaction to a type of **food**, such as seafood, nuts or strawberries.

■ Less commonly, the condition may result from an allergic reaction to **drugs**, most often to **antibiotics**.

■ Angioedema may also develop after an **insect bite or sting**.

■ Rarely, a person may inherit a tendency to develop angioedema that is unrelated to an allergy. In such cases, episodes of unexplained angioedema may begin in childhood and may be triggered by **stressful events**, such as an injury or a dental extraction.

■ It is not unusual for people to have only a single episode of angioedema, for which no cause can be determined.

WHAT ARE THE SYMPTOMS?

Swelling usually develops within a few minutes and is often asymmetrical; for example, only one side of a lip may be affected. The main symptoms are:

● swelling of any part of the body, especially the face, lips, tongue, throat and genitals

● sudden difficulty breathing, speaking or swallowing due to swelling of the tongue, mouth and airways

● in about half of all cases, an itchy rash (urticaria) affecting areas that are not swollen.

WHAT MIGHT BE DONE?

EMERGENCY!

■ Severe angioedema requires an urgent injection with **adrenaline**, followed by observation in hospital. In milder cases, a **corticosteroid** or an **antihistamine** may be prescribed to reduce the swelling; this may take hours or days to subside.

■ Your doctor may carry out tests to determine the cause. If a food allergy is suspected, a **skin prick test** may identify the substances to which you are allergic. If you suffer from severe angioedema, your doctor may teach you how to self-inject adrenaline.

See also:
● **Drug allergy p.322**
● **Food allergy p.320**
● **Urticaria p.322**

Anaphylaxis

ALSO CALLED ANAPHYLACTIC SHOCK, ANAPHYLAXIS IS A RARE BUT POTENTIALLY FATAL CONDITION. IT IS A SEVERE ALLERGIC REACTION THAT SPREADS THROUGHOUT THE BODY, CAUSING SHOCK WITH A SUDDEN DROP IN BLOOD PRESSURE AND NARROWING OF THE AIRWAYS.

Anaphylaxis occurs in people who have developed an extreme sensitivity to a specific substance (allergen). The allergic reaction is so severe that it can be fatal unless immediate treatment is available.

WHAT ARE THE CAUSES?

Anaphylaxis is most commonly triggered by **insect stings** or certain **drugs** such as **penicillin**. Foods such as **nuts** or **strawberries** may also trigger this serious form of allergic reaction.

WHAT ARE THE SYMPTOMS?

If you have an extreme sensitivity to a substance, you may experience some or all of the following symptoms as soon as you are exposed to it:

● sudden feeling of extreme anxiety

● swollen face, lips and tongue

● wheezing and difficulty breathing

● in some cases, an itchy, red rash (urticaria) and flushing of the skin

● lightheadedness or, in some cases, loss of consciousness.

If either you or anyone you are with develops these symptoms, you should call an ambulance immediately.

WHAT IS THE TREATMENT?

EMERGENCY!

■ Emergency treatment for anaphylaxis is an **immediate injection of adrenaline**. Injections of **antihistamines** or **corticosteroids**, together with **intravenous fluids**, are also given.

■ You should avoid any substance to which you are sensitive, especially if you have had a previous anaphylactic reaction. You may be given **adrenaline to self-inject** (an Epi-Pen).

■ You will also be advised to carry an **emergency card** or **bracelet** to alert others to your allergy.

See also:
● **Drug allergy p.322** ● **Food allergy p.320**
● **Urticaria p.322**

Emergency aid for anaphylaxis

If you have previously experienced anaphylaxis or severe angioedema, your doctor may provide you with syringes of injectable adrenaline, often called Epi-Pens

(keep one at home and one at work and carry one with you at all times). In the event of an episode of anaphylaxis, inject adrenaline immediately, then call for an ambulance.

Drug allergy

TREATMENT WITH VARIOUS DRUGS CAN RESULT IN A RANGE OF DIFFERENT SIDE EFFECTS. THE REACTION IS CAUSED BY AN ALLERGIC RESPONSE TO THE DRUG OR TO SUBSTANCES FORMED WHEN THE DRUG IS BROKEN DOWN BY THE BODY.

Rashes are a common side effect of drug treatment. Antibiotics and aspirin, for example, commonly cause urticaria (also called hives or nettle rash; see below). There may be other, more dramatic, effects such as nausea, diarrhoea, wheezing, swelling of the face and tongue (**angioedema**) and collapse. People with severe reactions need hospital treatment. Repeated exposure to a drug that causes a rash or angioedema can precipitate **anaphylaxis**.

The drugs that most often produce rashes are antibiotics, such as **penicillin**, but almost all drug treatments can cause an allergic reaction if a person becomes sensitive to them. Drug-induced rashes usually develop within

the first few days of starting treatment but they can also occur after a course of treatment has finished.

Sensitivity can only develop after at least one previous exposure to a drug. It is usual for people to take a certain drug for the first time without experiencing any allergic reaction and then to develop a rash when the drug is taken in a subsequent course of treatment.

WHAT MIGHT BE DONE?

■ If you develop a rash while you are taking a drug, you should consult your doctor before the next dose is due.
■ Most drug-induced rashes disappear when the drug responsible is stopped.

■ If itching is a problem, your doctor may advise that you apply a topical corticosteroid or take an oral antihistamine, but something simple like calamine lotion can bring relief.
■ Once you know you are allergic to a drug, you should make sure you notify any doctor who treats you in the future.
■ If you have had a severe reaction to a particular drug, you should consider wearing a **medical alert** tag or bracelet.

See also:
• Anaphylaxis p.321
• Angioedema p.321

Urticaria (nettle rash)

URTICARIA, ALSO KNOWN AS NETTLE RASH OR HIVES, IS AN INTENSELY ITCHY RASH THAT MAY AFFECT THE WHOLE BODY OR JUST A SMALL AREA OF SKIN. IT IS AN ALLERGIC REACTION TO VARIOUS SUBSTANCES, INCLUDING FOODS, DRUGS AND STINGS.

The rash consists of raised, red areas and, sometimes, white lumps. The inflamed areas usually vary in size and may merge to involve very large areas of skin. Urticaria comes and goes. Typically it lasts for only a few minutes or hours and there may be only one or two attacks. But sometimes it recurs for several months (chronic urticaria). Sometimes urticaria occurs at the same time as the more serious condition affecting the face called **angioedema**. Urticaria is sometimes an early symptom of **anaphylaxis**, a severe and potentially fatal allergic reaction to something.

WHAT ARE THE CAUSES?

■ The tendency to develop urticaria may run in families – atopic families.
■ Urticaria can occur as a result of an allergic

reaction to a particular food, such as shellfish, fruits and nuts – peanuts having received publicity.
■ The condition may also be due to a **drug allergy** (see above).
■ It may be due to an allergy to plants.
■ It may develop after an insect bite or sting.
■ However, when urticaria occurs for the first time in an adult, it is often difficult to identify the cause.

WHAT MIGHT BE DONE?

A one-off bout of urticaria generally disappears with treatment within a few hours.

The chronic form of the condition may take several weeks or months to clear up. Over-the-counter products such as calamine lotion and oral antihistamines may help relieve itching.

If your symptoms persist or recur and the cause of the problem is not obvious, you should consult your doctor. A skin prick test will identify the substances to which you are allergic (allergens). When the substance causing your urticaria has been identified, you should take all possible steps to avoid coming into contact with it in future in order to prevent a recurrence of the condition.

Never again eat a food to which you've been proven to be allergic. Avoid dishes and cutlery that may have touched the food.

See also:
• Anaphylaxis p.321 • Angioedema p.321
• Food allergy p.320
• The atopic family of conditions p.311

AUTOIMMUNE DISORDERS

If someone has an autoimmune disorder, their immune system mistakenly interprets their body's own tissues as **foreign**. As a result, antibodies are formed that attack the tissues and try to destroy them.

In general terms an autoimmune disease shows up in those tissues that are attacked by a particular antibody; for instance, the kidneys in glomerulonephritis and the joints in rheumatoid arthritis.

WHAT ARE THE TYPES?

1. In some autoimmune disorders, the tissues of a **single organ** are damaged, preventing normal function. Here are some examples of organs that may be affected:
- the **thyroid** gland in Hashimoto's disease
- the **pancreas** in diabetes mellitus
- the **adrenal glands** in Addison's disease.

2. A second group of autoimmune disorders affects **connective tissue**, the "glue" that holds together the structures of the body, e.g. **scleroderma** and **lupus**. In these disorders, the immune system may react against connective tissues **anywhere and everywhere** in the body, resulting in many and varied symptoms.

WHAT MIGHT BE DONE?

If your doctor suspects an autoimmune disorder, you'll have blood tests to assess your immune function and look for evidence of tissue inflammation.

The **treatment** of autoimmune disorders depends on which organs are affected. In Hashimoto's thyroiditis or Addison's disease, damage to the affected organs leads to a deficiency in the hormones they normally produce. However, replacement can often restore health. In other cases the aim of treatment is to block antibody production in the first place with drugs such as **immunosuppressants** and **corticosteroids** or limit the effects of antibodies. **Non-steroidal** anti-inflammatory drugs (NSAIDs) can treat symptoms such as pain and stiffness.

WHAT IS THE OUTLOOK?

The outlook for people who have autoimmune disorders depends on the amount of damage to the body's tissues and organs. Autoimmune disorders are nearly always chronic, but the symptoms can often be controlled with drugs. In some cases, serious complications such as kidney failure may develop. Quite often, though, the disease eventually "burns out" in middle age and symptoms subside.

Acquired immunodeficiency

IMMUNODEFICIENCY IS THE COMPLETE OR PARTIAL FAILURE OF THE IMMUNE SYSTEM, THE BODY'S NATURAL DEFENCE SYSTEM AGAINST DISEASE. IF THE IMMUNE SYSTEM FAILS AT SOME POINT DURING LIFE, THE CONDITION IS KNOWN AS "ACQUIRED" IMMUNODEFICIENCY.

WHAT ARE THE CAUSES?

■ In the most infamous form of this condition, acquired immunodeficiency syndrome (AIDS), the **human immunodeficiency virus** (HIV) destroys a particular type of white blood cell, the T cell, and this causes progressive weakness and vulnerability of the immune system.

■ Infections such as **measles** or **flu** damage the body's ability to fight infection. They do this partly by reducing the number of white blood cells involved in fighting the infection. Usually, this type of immunodeficiency is mild, and the immune system returns to normal once the infection is overcome.

■ A mild form of immunodeficiency may develop in some chronic disorders, including **diabetes mellitus** and **rheumatoid arthritis**. This may occur partly because these diseases put stress on the immune system, reducing its ability to resist other diseases.

■ Certain types of **cancer**, particularly tumours of the lymphatic system (lymphomas), may cause a more severe form of immunodeficiency by damaging the cells of the immune system and by reducing the production of normal white blood cells.

■ The long-term use of **corticosteroids** suppresses the immune system and has the inevitable effect of causing immunodeficiency.

■ **Immunosuppressant drugs**, which may be given to prevent the rejection of an organ following transplant surgery, also produce immunodeficiency and affect the body's ability to fight infections.

■ **Chemotherapy** can damage the bone marrow, where the majority of blood cells are made, and may also lead to the development of acquired immunodeficiency.

■ Immunodeficiency may also develop **after removal of the spleen**, an organ in which some of the white blood cells are produced.

WHAT MIGHT BE DONE?

Your doctor may suggest continual low doses of **antibiotics**, **antiviral drugs** and/or **antifungal drugs** and various **immunizations**, such as the pneumococcus vaccine, to protect against pneumococcal pneumonia.

The effects of immunodeficiency can usually be controlled by treatment, although immunodeficiency due to HIV infection tends to worsen over time.

See also:
- Chemotherapy p.257
- Diabetes mellitus p.504
- HIV infection and AIDS p.338
- Influenza p.334 • Lymphoma p.328
- Measles (chart) p.544
- Rheumatoid arthritis p.429

FOCUS *on* lupus

Lupus (sometimes known as systemic lupus erythematosis or SLE) is an autoimmune disease that can attack many different parts of the body and produces a great variety of different symptoms. Because the effects of lupus are so variable, this disorder can be very difficult to diagnose.

Although few people have heard of lupus, worldwide it's far more common than leukaemia, muscular dystrophy and multiple sclerosis, which, after extensive publicity, have become household names.

Lupus mainly attacks women during their child-bearing years, but sometimes men and even young children are affected. It's estimated that 1 in 750 women suffers from lupus in the UK and, for reasons we don't understand, it is more common in some races than in others. For instance, the frequency in white women is 1 in 1000 compared with that in black women of 1 in 250.

WHAT ARE THE SYMPTOMS?

Because lupus can attack so many parts of the body, it can show up in a bewildering number of ways, even to the extent of mimicking other diseases such as rheumatoid arthritis, multiple sclerosis or chronic fatigue syndrome (ME). So lupus can be difficult to diagnose and it can be overlooked, often for years.

Lupus is a disease that can present many different facets. Rarely do two people have exactly the same symptoms, and they can vary from just one to many:
- joint and muscle aches and pains
- permanent rash, which may be raised and scaly, over the nose and cheeks
- extreme fatigue and weakness
- rashes from sunlight
- recurring flu-like symptoms and/or night sweats
- poor blood circulation causing the tips of the fingers and toes to turn white then blue on exposure to cold – Raynaud's phenomenon
- anaemia
- headaches, migraine
- increased risk of miscarriage
- kidney problems
- oral ulcers
- hair loss
- depression.

Some drugs, such as certain antihypertensive drugs, may cause similar symptoms.

THE TREATMENT OF LUPUS

At present, there's no cure for lupus, but it can be controlled with specialist treatment so that most patients are able to live a normal life span. The majority of lupus patients should be in the ongoing care of their specialist.

If you have a lupus-like condition that has been triggered by a particular drug, your doctor may be able to prescribe an alternative drug. Symptoms should then disappear gradually over a period of weeks or months.

WHAT CAN I EXPECT AT THE LUPUS CLINIC?

- You'll have your urine tested for protein, blood and glucose to check on your kidneys and for diabetes.

Lupus triggers

Lupus can be triggered:
- at puberty
- after childbirth
- through sunlight
- by some medications
- during the menopause
- after a viral infection
- as a result of injury.

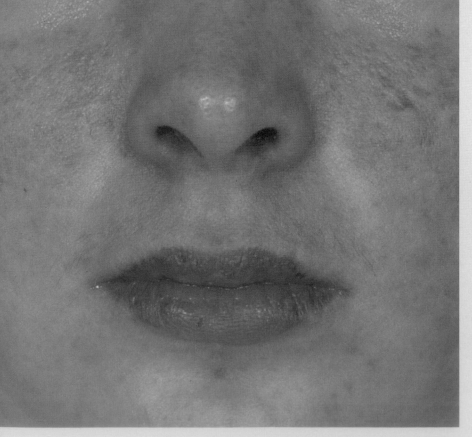

The typical rash of lupus is butterfly-shaped and spreads across the nose and cheeks.

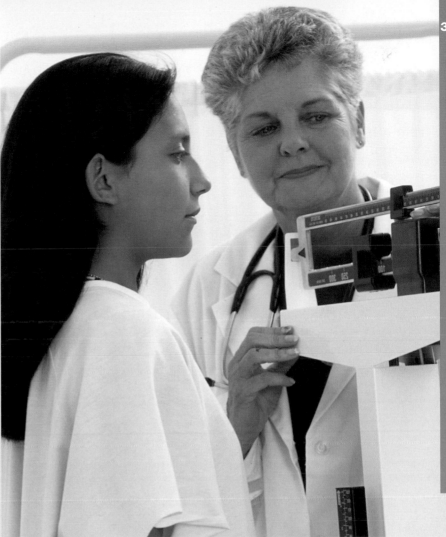

- You'll be weighed at each visit as some treatments, such as steroids, can cause water retention.
- You'll have a blood test to check for anaemia.
- An MRI scan, X-rays and nerve conduction tests may be done.
- Eye checks will be done before starting some treatments.
- When you start new medication, you'll be given booklets so you can understand how your treatment works.
- You may need a lot of support and understanding in coming to terms with lupus. You may have gone undiagnosed for several years, and feel frustrated that no one understands what you're going through. If there's a nurse counsellor attached to the clinic, get her help.

WHAT KIND OF TREATMENT WILL I GET?

Lupus is usually treated with four main groups of drugs, depending on the severity of the disease.

Aspirin and non-steroidals: Non-steroidal anti-inflammatory drugs (NSAIDs) are used for patients with mainly joint and muscle pain. In the case of patients with sticky blood, aspirin in low dosage, 75–150mg daily, is used to thin the blood.

Antimalarials: These drugs are of help in patients with skin and joint disease. They may be sufficient for patients with moderately active lupus to avoid using steroids. Hydroxychloroquine and mepacrine are most commonly used.

Steroids: Drugs such as prednisone have been vital in the improvement in lupus and for some people can be life-saving. They have a profound effect on inflammation and can suppress the disease. Once lupus is under control, you can be weaned off steroids gradually under your doctor's supervision.

Immunosuppressants: These drugs are used in more severe disease. The most commonly used are azathioprine, methotrexate and cyclophosphamide. You'll have regular blood tests to check on your bone marrow and liver.

You may also have physiotherapy to help improve mobility in affected joints. It's important to remain as physically active as the condition will allow, so try to take moderate exercise regularly.

With treatment, most people with lupus are able to lead normal, active lives.

Self-help

- Become well educated on lupus.
- Try to prepare for the up and down nature of the disease. Plan for alternatives. Allow for rest when the disease is active but try to maintain general fitness.
- Reduce fatigue by developing priorities and learning to pace yourself. Break down big, long-term goals into small, manageable steps that can be easily accomplished.
- Be open with family and friends about the unpredictable pattern of lupus, and how the disease affects you.
- By listening to your pain, you can begin to control it.
- Try to accept the things you cannot change, rather than feeling constantly frustrated and upset over situations beyond your control.
- Remember that stress, depression and pain are all closely connected and each affects the other. Reduce one and you reduce them all.
- Approximately one-third of lupus patients are sensitive to light, so avoid direct and prolonged sun exposure and ultraviolet light from artificial sources (such as fluorescent lights). Wear broad-brimmed hats and cover other exposed parts of the body when out in sunlight and use sunblock creams.
- Ask for help. Family, friends and health-care professionals, together with Lupus UK (see Useful addresses, p.567), are all sources of support.

Polymyositis and dermatomyositis

THE NAME POLYMYOSITIS MEANS INFLAMMATION OF MANY MUSCLES. THE DISEASE MAY AFFECT BOTH SKELETAL MUSCLES AND MUSCLES ELSEWHERE IN THE BODY SUCH AS IN THE THROAT OR HEART. IN DERMATOMYOSITIS, THE SYMPTOMS OF POLYMYOSITIS ARE ACCOMPANIED BY A RASH.

WHAT ARE THE SYMPTOMS?

Polymyositis results in the following symptoms:
- weakness of affected muscles, leading to, for example, difficulty raising the arms or getting up from a sitting or squatting position
- painful, swollen joints
- fatigue
- difficulty swallowing if the muscles of the throat are affected
- shortness of breath if the heart or chest muscles are involved.

In cases of dermatomyositis, the symptoms outlined above may be preceded, accompanied or followed by the following additional symptoms:
- a red rash, often on the face, chest or backs of the hands over the knuckles
- swollen, reddish-purple eyelids.

WHAT IS THE TREATMENT?

This condition must always be treated by a specialist. Usually, high-dose steroids are given along with analgesics for symptomatic relief.

Scleroderma

SCLERODERMA IS THICKENING AND HARDENING OF THE CONNECTIVE TISSUES IN THE SKIN, JOINTS, ARTERIES AND INTERNAL ORGANS. IT IS A RARE AUTOIMMUNE CONDITION THAT IS TWICE AS COMMON IN WOMEN AS IN MEN AND USUALLY DEVELOPS BETWEEN THE AGES OF 40 AND 60.

WHAT ARE THE SYMPTOMS?

These include:
- fingers or toes that are sensitive to the cold, becoming white and painful (Raynaud's phenomenon)
- small, hardened areas that appear on the fingers and may go on to ulcerate
- swollen fingers or hands
- pain in the joints, especially the joints in the hands
- thickening and tightening of the skin, which is most severe on the limbs but may affect the trunk and face
- muscle weakness
- difficulty swallowing due to stiffening of the tissues of the oesophagus (the tube that runs from the mouth to the stomach).

If the lungs are affected, shortness of breath may develop. Sometimes it causes high blood pressure and, rarely, eventual kidney failure.

WHAT IS THE TREATMENT?

- Immune-suppressing drugs or drugs that interfere with collagen production may be given.
- Support and education are important.

See also:
- **High blood pressure p.226** • **Acute, chronic and end-stage kidney failure p.380**
- **Raynaud's phenomenon p.232**

LYMPHATIC SYSTEM

The lymphatic system is quite difficult to get your mind around because it's distributed around the body with no real shape. There are some main features, however. Firstly, the lymphatic channels are vague, shapeless spaces between muscles, under the skin and around joints through which the lymph flows, always in a direction towards the heart. At certain points the channels join up in a group of glands – you find them in the groin, neck and armpit. From there they run into one large lymph tube that joins the main vein of the heart. But the lymphatic system extends further than

that. Its main cell is called a lymphocyte and it's made in the liver and the bone marrow. So it's useful to think of the liver and bone marrow as connected with the lymphatic system. Then there's the spleen, lying under the left ribcage, whose job it is to break down old red blood cells. So add the spleen to the lymphatic family. The lymph, the colourless fluid that's slowly flowing around this system, seeps out from cells, from blood vessels and from veins. It then circulates back to the heart. So there is a true lymphatic "circulation", not that different from the circulation of the blood.

Swollen glands

SWOLLEN GLANDS (ENLARGED LYMPH NODES) ARE A COMMON SYMPTOM OF MANY CONDITIONS, MOST OF THEM NO CAUSE FOR CONCERN. HOWEVER, THEY MAY ALSO INDICATE THE SPREAD OF CANCER, SUCH AS FROM THE BREAST TO NODES IN THE ARMPIT.

Swollen glands, known medically as lymphadenopathy, are really enlarged lymph nodes. They usually develop in response to a **bacterial or viral infection**, and are most likely to be noticed in the neck, groin or armpit, because the nodes in these places lie closest to the skin. Infection anywhere can spread to the glands. So, for example, an infection spreading from an ingrown toenail can give you swollen glands in your groin.

Swollen lymph nodes in the neck are usual with a **throat infection** and can be tender. Swollen glands **at the back of the head** usually indicate German measles (rubella). If swollen glands are due to an infection, the swelling subsides when the infection clears up.

A SPECIAL NOTE ON THE SPREAD OF BREAST CANCER

The glands, also called nodes, in the armpit swell up and can be felt when breast cancer spreads.

Treatment for breast cancer involves surgery as a first step then further treatment with radiotherapy, hormones and chemotherapy to contain the tumour and catch any cancer cells that are spreading.

To help doctors decide what will be the best regime for each individual woman, they have to know how far her cancer has spread.

The simplest way to do this is to **sample or remove** the glands in the armpit. The surgeon will hope that he can take a deeper and deeper sample until he reaches a gland that's completely clear. Then he will have a good idea of how far the tumour's spread and be able to come up with a plan for radiotherapy, hormones or chemotherapy tailor-made to give the best chance of recovery.

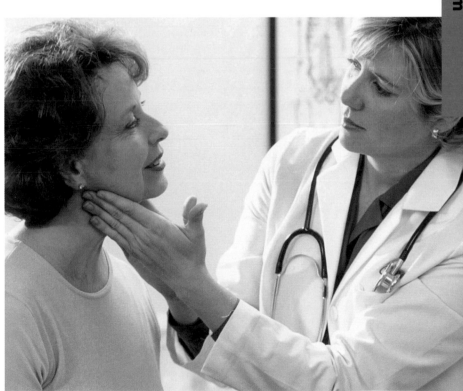

There are several surgical operations to remove a breast tumour, such as lumpectomy (only the lump) and partial and simple mastectomy, but in all of them the surgeon will aim to take away the smallest part of the breast that will get rid of the cancer. At the same time the glands in the armpit will be sampled and may be removed to reduce the risk of cancer spread to other parts of the body.

See also:
- **Breast cancer p.261**
- **Chemotherapy p.257**
- **German measles (chart) p.544**
- **Lumpectomy p.262**

Lymphoedema

LYMPHOEDEMA IS A LOCALIZED ACCUMULATION OF FLUID IN THE LYMPHATIC VESSELS, CAUSING
PAINLESS SWELLING OF A LIMB. IT RESULTS FROM DISRUPTION OF THE NORMAL DRAINAGE OF
LYMPH DUE TO LOCAL BLOCKAGE, DAMAGE OR REMOVAL OF LYMPH VESSELS.

Most commonly, lymphoedema is caused by damage to the lymphatic vessels following **surgery** or **radiotherapy**, for example in **the arm** in the treatment of **breast cancer** and in **the leg** after treatment of **ovarian cancer**.

The skin over the affected limb often becomes rough and thickened. You should contact your doctor immediately if you injure a limb affected by lymphoedema, even if it only seems trivial, because lymphangitis (see box, right) may ensue. However, it is also a condition where often there is no known cause and, for reasons we still do not understand, it affects twice as many women as men.

See also:
- **Breast cancer p.261**
- **Cancer of the ovary p.260**
- **Lumpectomy p.262**
- **Radiotherapy p.395**

WHAT IS THE TREATMENT?

■ In most cases, lymphoedema is a life-long disorder and treatment is aimed at relieving symptoms. You can reduce swelling by keeping the affected limb elevated. Wearing an elastic stocking or sleeve can prevent further swelling.

■ There is no cure as such and treatment consists of taking diuretic drugs, massage, wearing an elastic bandage or compression sleeve, and performing exercises with the affected limb elevated. Surgery is possible in the most severe cases and this involves removing the swollen tissues and some of the overlying skin.

■ **Lymphatic drainage** can bring relief in some cases although, again, this is not a cure and will only bring temporary respite. It's done through massage, which encourages the tissues to expel the excess fluid back into the blood vessels and so out of the body. Qualified practitioners will do this massage for you and most aromatherapists are trained to carry out lymphatic drainage.

Lymphangitis

Lymphangitis develops when bacteria spread into lymphatic vessels close to the site of an infection, possibly as a result of an injury. The condition usually affects lymphatic vessels in an arm or leg. The infected vessels become inflamed and tender, and hot, red streaks may appear on the skin over the inflamed vessels. Lymph nodes near to the affected area sometimes become swollen. If you develop any of these symptoms following an injury, you should consult your doctor immediately. You'll need antibiotic treatment to prevent further spread.

Lymphoma

THE WORD LYMPHOMA STRIKES FEAR INTO MANY PEOPLE BECAUSE IT'S ILL-UNDERSTOOD.
LYMPHOMAS ARE CANCERS OF THE GLANDS (LYMPH GLANDS OR LYMPH NODES) AFFECTING BOTH
ADULTS AND CHILDREN, BUT THE OUTLOOK FOR CANCERS OF THIS TYPE IS BETTER THAN MOST.

Cancers are simply cells whose growth has got out of hand; they invade healthy organs with differing degrees of aggressiveness according to how malignant they are.

There are two types of lymphoma – Hodgkin's disease (HD) and non-Hodgkin's lymphoma (NHL), which differ in their behaviour and treatment.

The first symptom may be a painless lump in the neck, armpits or groin. Tiredness, weight loss, fever, night sweats and itching can be prominent symptoms too.

HOW IS LYMPHOMA DIAGNOSED?

Your doctor will ask you many questions and examine you to see if the glands in your neck, armpits and abdomen are enlarged.

After a small operation (biopsy) to remove one of the glands, the gland will be examined under a microscope.

This enables an accurate diagnosis to be made and with the results of other tests (X-rays, blood tests, scans) helps to decide the best form of treatment.

WHAT IS THE TREATMENT?

Some low-grade (non-aggressive) lymphomas need no treatment but most require treatment with radiotherapy, chemotherapy or a combination of both.

Radiotherapy uses powerful X-rays that kill cancer cells. Chemotherapy uses powerful chemicals in the form of pills, injections or a drip into a vein to do the same thing.

CHEMOTHERAPY

Lymphomas are one of the most sensitive cancers to chemotherapy. The overall aim of chemotherapy is to give drugs that have maximum anti-cancer effect, but with the least possible damage to the body's normal cells.

Chemotherapy drugs interrupt cell growth so they end up killing large numbers of cells.

However, many "normal" body cells (such as the bone marrow and the lining of the intestine and the mouth) divide rapidly and are vulnerable to cancer drugs, giving rise to many of the side effects caused by chemotherapy.

WHICH CHEMOTHERAPY?

The type of chemotherapy you'll get depends on the type of lymphoma, and the extent to which it may have spread.

Although some chemotherapy drugs are given as tablets, most people with lymphoma are treated with intravenous chemotherapy.

Several drugs are usually given in combination to help stop cancer cells becoming resistant to any one drug.

There are several combinations in routine use, and new ones are being tried all the time. If you're asked to take part in a clinical trial, don't be afraid – trials usually compare a standard treatment with one that's judged to be better.

HOW IT IS GIVEN
Method

Most chemotherapy is given as out-patient treatment, either as a short injection into a vein, or as an intravenous drip over an hour or so. It rarely involves staying in hospital overnight.

Timing
■ Chemotherapy is given once every 3–4 weeks.
■ You'll receive 6–8 courses of treatment.
■ Treatment usually lasts around 5–6 months.
■ Some treatments may be given on a weekly basis.

Questions you may want to ask

About your diagnosis
- What kind of lymphoma do I have?
- What is the spread of the lymphoma?
- If it's non-Hodgkin's lymphoma, is it high- or low-grade? What's the difference?
- Where is it? Is there any doubt?
- What do these tests I'm having tell you? What are they for?

At the hospital
- Does the hospital have modern radiotherapy equipment, specialists in radiotherapy and chemotherapy, hormone therapy and surgery?
- Does it have supportive care and counselling?

About the treatment
- What kind of treatment will I have – radiotherapy, chemotherapy or none?
- Is it aimed at curing the disease or relieving the symptoms?
- Are there any other options?
- How will the drugs be given?
- Are there any special instructions about taking the tablets at home?
- How do these tablets help?
- When will the treatment start and how often will it be given?
- Are there things I should or shouldn't do during treatment?
- What are the possible side effects?

- Will the treatment affect the possibility of having children?
- Do I contact the hospital or my GP if I'm unwell at home?
- Can I drive during and after treatment?
- May I drink alcohol and take medicines for other complaints?
- Are there foods I should or shouldn't eat during the treatment?
- When will I know if the treatment has worked?

Coping with chemotherapy

SIDE EFFECTS
You may well have no, or very few, side effects. However, it's preferable to know something about possible consequences so that you can let your medical team know if you get them.

Nausea and vomiting
Chemotherapy drugs can cause nausea and vomiting. However, this can largely be controlled by new anti-sickness medications, given as injections or tablets. You may be given them before chemotherapy to avoid sickness in the first place.

Tiredness
Tiredness is one of the most common side effects of chemotherapy, though we don't know exactly why. If the cause is anaemia then a simple blood transfusion may correct the problem.

Hair loss (alopecia)
Hair loss is an effect of the chemotherapy on the rapidly dividing cells of the hair follicle but many patients have no hair loss at all. If it does occur, it will only be temporary

and your hair will grow back when the chemotherapy is over.

Many people find that a wig is helpful and it is worth organizing one sooner rather than later, so that your hair can be matched. Scalp cooling slows blood flow to the scalp and can stop the chemotherapy reaching hair follicles. Ask your medical team about it.

LONG-TERM SIDE EFFECTS
Sterility
Chemotherapy agents can affect fertility, though it's usually temporary. Women may stop having periods. Rarely, chemotherapy has been known to cause permanent sterility.

Low white-cell blood count
If your white cell count drops (neutropaenia) – a fairly common side effect of chemotherapy – you'll have an increased risk of infection. Look out for signs of infection and let your doctor know if you have any of the following symptoms:
- Fever, with temperature above 38°C (100°F).

- Chills and sweating.
- Mouth sores and ulcers.
- Coughs and sore throat.
- Redness or swelling around sores on the skin.
- Loose stools/diarrhoea.
- Cystitis or burning sensation during urination.
- Unusual vaginal discharge or itching.

Questions to ask
- What are the possible side effects?
- Will the treatment affect my ability to have children?
- Should I contact the hospital or my own GP if I'm unwell?
- Will I be able to drive during and after treatment?
- Can I drink alcohol and take medicines for other complaints during treatment?
- Are there foods I should or shouldn't eat during the treatment?
- When will I know if the treatment has been successful?

Infections

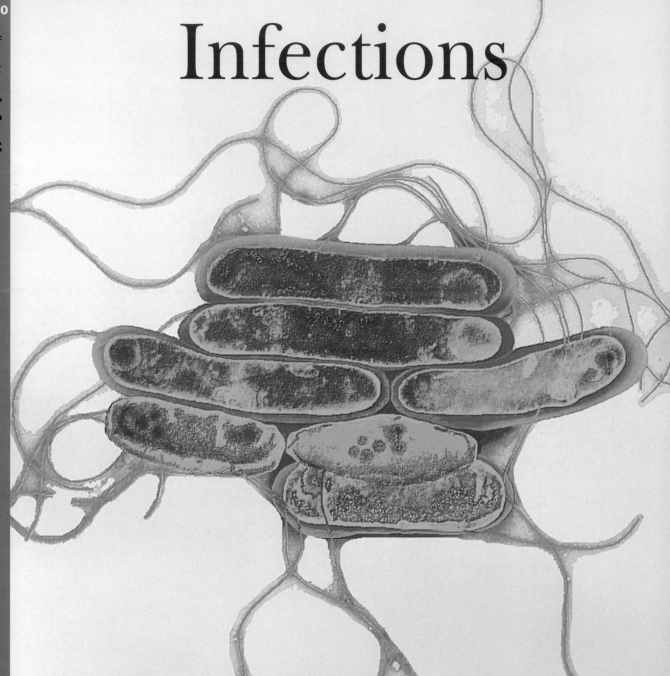

Image shows a coloured transmission electron micrograph of Legionella pneumophilia *bacteria*

Miriam's overview

I'm making the distinction in this book between infections and "infectious diseases", which are historically confined to childhood and usually to the under-fives and school children.

So you'll find diseases such as measles and whooping cough in the chapter on children's conditions.

You won't find sexually transmitted diseases here either. Gonorrhoea, thrush and the like are all together with STDs in the chapter on sexuality, though infection with the HIV virus and AIDS are in this chapter.

By and large, few infections are serious and very few indeed are life-threatening. On these grounds most need not be a cause for concern and don't even require the attentions of a doctor. All that's required is symptomatic relief with over-the-counter medicines you can buy from the pharmacy.

By the same token antibiotics are rarely required since most infections are self-limiting, meaning your healthy body will fight the infection, limit its effect and cure you of it without outside help.

As an extension of such a principle you can see that I'd be an advocate of only the most judicious use of antibiotics. I'd define judicious as meaning strictly when needed, and except in the case of emergencies, when it's known which bacterium is to be treated. The reasons for this caution are compelling, the most persuasive being the increasing numbers of resistant bacteria, a problem caused by abuse of antibiotics in the past. This abuse took the form of unnecessary overuse that actually encouraged bacteria to breed forms that could survive the presence of antibiotics rather than succumbing to them.

As a result we are now left with monster forms of bacteria

> ## "*antibiotics are rarely required* since most infections are *self-limiting*"

and no antibiotics to curb their growth. The most notorious is methicillin-resistant *Staphylococcus aureus* (MRSA), invariably picked up in hospitals, where the use of antibiotics has been traditionally concentrated, and once the organism takes hold there is often little doctors can do.

continued on p.332

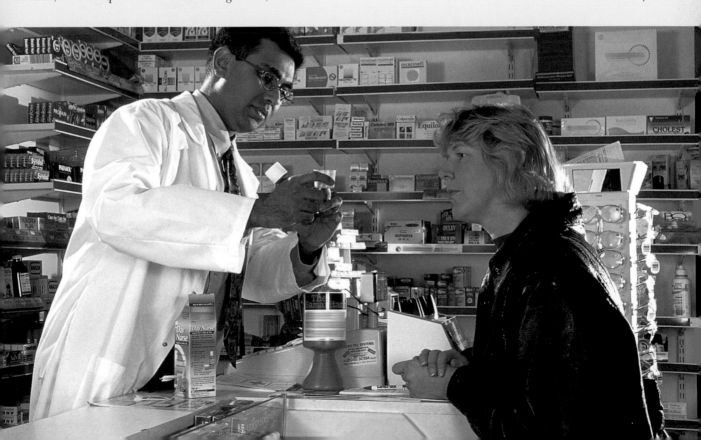

Miriam's overview *continued from p.331*

Because it releases a potent poison – a toxin – the bug can spread through the body very quickly leaving tissue destruction in its path, sometimes with a rapidly fatal outcome. The latest figures in the UK show that 5000 people

"we're infected by *very few* organisms"

die in hospital from opportunistic infections every year.

Researchers are constantly pursuing a new super-antibiotic to cope with this new breed of super-bug, but such is the speed of bacterial mutation there's the chance that our best research efforts will be outstripped by nature's ingenuity.

Besides bacteria, viruses, fungi and parasites we've become aware of a new and potent infecting agent – the PRION – a small, sub-viral particle that enters cells and

destroys DNA, the cell's reproductive code. These prions cause BSE in cattle, scrapie in sheep and new variant CJD in human beings.

At first it was thought that prions were species-specific, meaning they could not escape from one species (cattle, for instance) to another (man). Given the new variant of CJD only recently described it would appear that our assumptions were wrong.

The truth is that we're infected by very few organisms be they bacteria, viruses, fungi or parasites despite there being many millions of potential invaders out there.

In trying to decide what I could possibly cover for you here I've been guided by what's most common, what infections you're likely to meet and what's serious enough to have the potential to make us very ill or kill us. So, for instance, I consider it very important to tell you how to spot the early signs of meningitis, always very serious and becoming more common, so that you can take rapid action to safeguard the wellbeing of your family.

INSIDE
infections and infestations

There are a number of organisms and microorganisms that cause infection and infestation, including lice and mites, worms, fungi, protozoa, bacteria and viruses. **Lice** and **scabies mites** are easily transmitted and infestations are common in children. **Worms** may be microscopic or several feet in length. Two types, **flatworms** and **roundworms**, may infest humans. **Fungi**, broadly divided into the filamentous type (which grow threads) and the single-celled yeasts, are responsible for many infections in humans, such as candida. The single-celled organisms known as **protozoa** are responsible for diseases such as malaria and toxoplasmosis. **Bacteria** form a large group of single-celled organisms, of which relatively few types cause disease. **Viruses** are the smallest infectious agents, much smaller than a single human cell. A virus can only reproduce by invading a host cell and copying its own genetic material using substances from the host cell, which it then usually destroys.

how infections invade the body

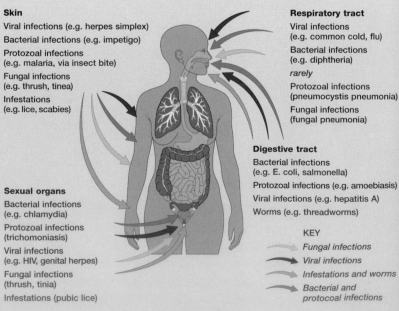

Skin
Viral infections (e.g. herpes simplex)
Bacterial infections (e.g. impetigo)
Protozoal infections
(e.g. malaria, via insect bite)
Fungal infections
(e.g. thrush, tinea)
Infestations
(e.g. lice, scabies)

Respiratory tract
Viral infections
(e.g. common cold, flu)
Bacterial infections
(e.g. diphtheria)
rarely
Protozoal infections
(pneumocystis pneumonia)
Fungal infections
(fungal pneumonia)

Digestive tract
Bacterial infections
(e.g. E. coli, salmonella)
Protozoal infections (e.g. amoebiasis)
Viral infections (e.g. hepatitis A)
Worms (e.g. threadworms)

Sexual organs
Bacterial infections
(e.g. chlamydia)
Protozoal infections
(trichomoniasis)
Viral infections
(e.g. HIV, genital herpes)
Fungal infections
(thrush, tinia)
Infestations (pubic lice)

KEY
Fungal infections
Viral infections
Infestations and worms
Bacterial and protocoal infections

Common cold

A COMMON COLD IS AN INFECTION OF THE NOSE AND THROAT CAUSED BY
ANY OF A GROUP OF VIRUSES. THERE ARE AT LEAST 200 HIGHLY CONTAGIOUS
VIRUSES THAT CAN CAUSE THE COMMON COLD.

The viruses that cause colds are easily transmitted in minute airborne droplets from the coughs or sneezes of infected people. However, the most common route of spread is by hand-to-hand contact with an infected person or by way of things that are contaminated with the virus, such as a cup or towel. Per se, the common cold is not serious, but it can predispose to a chest infection in a vulnerable person with, say, chronic obstructive pulmonary disease, or in a baby.

Colds can occur at any time of the year, although infections are more frequent in the autumn and winter. About half the population of Europe and the US develops at least one cold each year. Children are more susceptible to colds than adults because they have not yet developed immunity to the most common viruses and also because viruses spread very quickly in communities such as nurseries and schools.

WHAT ARE THE SYMPTOMS?
The initial symptoms of a cold develop between 12 hours and 3 days after infection. Symptoms usually intensify over 24–48 hours, unlike those of influenza, which worsen rapidly over a few hours. Symptoms include:

- frequent sneezing
- runny nose with a clear, watery discharge that later becomes thick and green-coloured
- mild fever and headache
- sore throat and sometimes a cough
- aching muscles
- irritability
- catarrh.

In some people, a common cold may be complicated by a bacterial infection of the chest (bronchitis), or of the sinuses (sinusitis). Bacterial ear infections, which may cause earache, are a common complication of colds.

WHAT CAN I DO?
Most people recognize their symptoms as those of a common cold and do not seek medical advice.

Despite a great deal of scientific research there is no cure for the common cold but over-the-counter drugs might help to relieve symptoms.

■ **Painkillers** will relieve a headache and reduce a fever.

■ **Decongestants** will clear a stuffy nose.

■ **Cough remedies** will soothe a tickling throat.

■ It is important to drink plenty of cool fluids, particularly if you have a fever.

Many people mistakenly take large quantities of vitamin C to prevent infection and treat the common cold, but the latest research shows this remedy to be without value, indeed dangerous, because mega-doses of vitamin C predispose to heart disease.

If your symptoms do not improve in a week, or your child is no better in two days, you should consult a doctor.

If you have a bacterial infection, your doctor may prescribe **antibiotics, although they are ineffective against cold viruses**.

The common cold usually clears up with or without treatment within two weeks, but a cough may last longer.

See also:
- **Bronchitis p.390**
- **Fever in children p.540**
- **Sinusitis p.481**

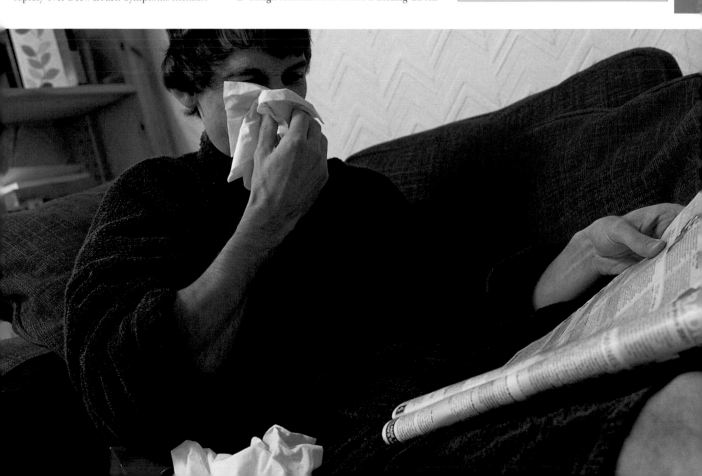

Influenza

INFLUENZA IS A VIRAL INFECTION OF THE UPPER RESPIRATORY TRACT (AIRWAYS),
COMMONLY KNOWN AS FLU. INFLUENZA IS A HIGHLY CONTAGIOUS VIRAL DISEASE
THAT TENDS TO OCCUR IN EPIDEMICS DURING THE WINTER.

Influenza mainly affects the upper airways and can be transmitted easily in airborne droplets from the coughs and sneezes of infected people. However, the influenza virus is usually transmitted from person to person through direct contact.

Many different viral infections can result in mild flu-like symptoms, but true influenza is caused by two principal types of influenza virus, A and B. **The type A virus**, in particular, frequently changes its structure (mutates) and produces new strains to which few people have immunity.

The number of influenza cases varies from year to year, but particularly virulent strains have spread worldwide and caused millions of deaths. Such major outbreaks, called pandemics, occurred in 1918 with Spanish flu, in 1957 with Asian flu, in 1968 with Hong Kong flu and in 1977 with Russian flu.

WHAT ARE THE SYMPTOMS?

The symptoms of influenza develop 24–48 hours after infection. Many people think they have influenza when they have only a common cold, but the symptoms of influenza are far more severe than those of a cold, and develop much faster. The first symptom may be **slight chills**. Other symptoms, which develop later and worsen rapidly in just a few hours, may include the following:

- high fever, sweating and shivering
- aching muscles, especially in the back
- severe exhaustion
- frequent sneezing, stuffy or runny nose, sore throat, and cough.

Following an attack of flu, **fatigue** and **depression** are often experienced after other symptoms have disappeared.

The most common complications are bacterial infections of the **airways** (bronchitis) and **lungs** (pneumonia). Such infections can be life-threatening in babies, elderly people, those with **chronic heart** or **lung disease**, and people with reduced immunity, such as those with AIDS or **diabetes mellitus**.

WHAT MIGHT BE DONE?

■ For most normally healthy people, the best way to relieve the symptoms of influenza is to rest in bed, drink plenty of cool fluids and follow the advice for bringing down a fever.

■ Painkillers, such as **paracetamol**, and other over-the-counter remedies may help ease aching muscles and other symptoms.

■ If self-help measures are ineffective, you may be prescribed **antiviral drugs**, such as **amantadine** or **rimantadine**, which are effective against influenza viruses provided that they are given within 24 hours of the onset of symptoms.

■ You should see your doctor immediately if you have difficulty breathing or if your fever lasts for longer than two days. You may be given a chest X-ray to rule out a chest infection such as pneumonia.

■ If a bacterial infection is found, your doctor will prescribe antibiotics. **However, these drugs have no effect on the influenza virus itself**.

■ Vulnerable people, such as babies, young children, the elderly, those with chronic heart or lung conditions, and people with reduced immunity, are at increased risk of serious complications. A doctor should be consulted immediately when anyone in a vulnerable group gets flu.

WHAT IS THE OUTLOOK?

■ If there are no complications, most of the symptoms of influenza usually disappear after 6–7 days, although a cough may persist over two weeks.

■ Fatigue and depression may last even longer.

■ However, for anyone who is in one of the high-risk groups, the complications of influenza may be life-threatening and in epidemics, deaths from associated pneumonia are very common.

■ **Immunization** is effective protection. It is especially recommended for people in high-risk groups (excluding babies) and people who are particularly likely to be exposed to the virus, such as health workers or carers or elderly people.

Immunization prevents infections in about two-thirds of people who are vaccinated annually. However, the vaccine can never be completely effective because the viruses frequently mutate, and different strains are responsible for outbreaks each year. The World Health Organization recommends the types of vaccines issued each autumn, depending on which strains are expected to be most prevalent in a particular region. However, if a virus mutates substantially, protection from the vaccine will be minimal and epidemics may occur.

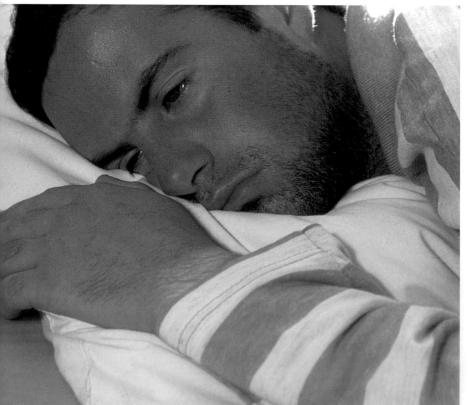

> **See also:**
> • Diabetes mellitus p.504
> • Fever in children p.540
> • HIV infection and AIDS p.338
> • Pneumonia p.392

Chickenpox

CHICKENPOX IS AN INFECTION THAT CAUSES A FEVER AND WIDESPREAD CROPS
OF BLISTERS. THE INFECTION IS CAUSED BY THE VARICELLA ZOSTER VIRUS,
WHICH ALSO CAUSES SHINGLES (HERPES ZOSTER).

The chickenpox virus is transmitted in airborne droplets from the coughs and sneezes of infected people or by direct contact with the blisters.

The illness is usually mild in children, but symptoms are more severe in young babies, older adolescents and adults. Chickenpox can also be more serious in people with reduced immunity, such as those with AIDS.

WHAT ARE THE SYMPTOMS?

The symptoms of chickenpox appear 1–3 weeks after infection. In children, the illness often starts with a mild fever or headache; in adults, there may be more pronounced flu-like symptoms. As infection with the virus progresses, the following symptoms usually become apparent.

■ Rash in the form of crops of tiny red spots that rapidly turn into itchy, fluid-filled blisters; within 24 hours the blisters dry out, forming scabs; successive crops occur for 1–6 days. The rash may be widespread or consist of only a few spots, and it can occur anywhere on the head or body.

■ Sometimes, discomfort during eating

caused by spots in the mouth that have developed into ulcers.

A person is contagious from about two days before the rash first appears until it fully crusts over in about 10–14 days.

The most common complication of chickenpox is bacterial infection of the blisters due to scratching. Other complications include **pneumonia**, which is more common in adults, and, rarely, inflammation of the brain (encephalitis). Newborn babies and people with reduced immunity are at high risk of complications. Very rarely, if a woman gets chickenpox in early pregnancy, the infection may result in fetal abnormalities.

WHAT MIGHT BE DONE?

Chickenpox can usually be diagnosed from the appearance of the rash. Children with mild infections do not need to see a doctor, and rest and simple measures to reduce fever are all that are needed for full recovery. Calamine lotion may help relieve itching. To prevent skin infections, keep fingernails short and avoid scratching.

People at risk of severe attacks, such as

babies, older adolescents, adults and people with reduced immunity, should see their doctor immediately. An antiviral drug may be given to limit the effects of the infection, but it must be taken in the early stages of the illness in order to be effective.

Children who are otherwise healthy usually recover within 10–14 days from the onset of the rash, but they may have permanent scars where blisters have become infected with bacteria. Adolescents, adults and people with reduced immunity take longer to recover.

CAN IT BE PREVENTED?

One attack of chickenpox gives **life-long immunity** to the disease. However, the varicella zoster virus remains dormant within nerve cells and may reactivate years later, causing shingles (see below).

See also:
• **Fever in children p.540**
• **Influenza p.334**
• **Pneumonia p.392**

Shingles

SHINGLES IS AN INFECTION THAT CAUSES A PAINFUL RASH OF BLISTERS FOLLOWING THE PATH
OF A NERVE, SOMETIMES ON THE FACE AND OCCASIONALLY AFFECTING THE EYE, WHEN
TREATMENT MUST BE ONGOING TO PREVENT INFECTION.

Shingles is most common between the ages of 50 and 70. People with reduced immunity, such as those with AIDS or those undergoing chemotherapy, are also especially susceptible to this infection. People with AIDS are particularly likely to have severe outbreaks of shingles.

The shingles rash commonly occurs on only one side of the body and usually affects the skin on the chest, abdomen or face. In older people, discomfort may continue for months after the rash has disappeared. This prolonged pain is called **post-herpetic neuralgia**.

Shingles is caused by the same virus that causes chickenpox, which remains dormant in nerve cells. When it is reactivated later in life, it causes shingles. The reason for reactivation is unknown but shingles often occurs at times of stress or ill health.

The virus is easily spread by direct contact

with a blister and will cause chickenpox in someone who has not already had it.

WHAT ARE THE SYMPTOMS?

Initially, you may experience tingling, itching and a sharp pain in part of your skin. After a few days, the following symptoms may develop:
● painful rash of fluid-filled blisters
● fever
● headache and fatigue.

Within 3–4 days blisters form scabs. The scabs heal in 10 days but may leave scars. If a nerve that supplies the eye is affected, blisters may cause inflammation of the cornea. Rarely, infection of a facial nerve causes paralysis of one side of the face.

WHAT MIGHT BE DONE?

■ Shingles can be difficult to diagnose until the rash appears, and severe pain following the

line of the ribs (where nerves run around the body) can be mistaken for the chest pain of angina.

■ Your doctor may prescribe antiviral drugs to reduce the severity of the symptoms and the risk of post-herpetic neuralgia.

■ Immediate treatment with antiviral drugs is important if your eyes are affected or if you have reduced immunity.

■ Painkillers may help relieve discomfort, and **carbamazepine** may help relieve the prolonged pain of post-herpetic neuralgia.

■ Most people who develop shingles recover within 2–6 weeks, but up to half of people over the age of 50 develop post-herpetic neuralgia.

See also:
• **Post-herpetic neuralgia p.408**
• **Facial palsy p.417**

FOCUS *on* herpes simplex

Herpes simplex is the name given to a virus that can cause cold sores (usually herpes simplex type 1) or genital herpes (usually herpes simplex type 2). The sores appear on whichever part of your skin is infected.

In either type of herpes the virus is transmitted mainly through infected skin coming into contact with another person's skin, for example through kissing, during sex or from mouth to genitals during oral sex. However, the disease can also be spread by contact with other parts of the body, especially the fingers if a sore has been touched, and herpes may be spread to the eyes in this way. A cold sore that develops near the eye is potentially dangerous and should be seen by a doctor as soon as symptoms, such as tingling or itching, begin.

Originally it was thought that cold sores on the lips were only due to herpes simplex type 1 (HSV1) and genital herpes only due to the herpes simplex virus type 2 (HSV2). This distinction has become blurred, however, with the increased practice of oral sex. In Europe, genital herpes infection is the most common cause of genital ulceration and it is increasing among women. Genital herpes infection is more common in women than in men because their genital area is warmer and moister than a man's.

HOW COMMON IS HERPES?

Blood tests show that most people have been exposed to herpes simplex type 1 by the time we reach middle age. This means that millions of people are infected with the virus, but probably only a quarter of those infected have symptoms of any kind.

Many people have what is called a **subclinical** attack, with no visible signs of infection and no ill effects. These people are then naturally immune to further infection but don't know they've been infected.

WHAT HAPPENS TO THE VIRUS?

Once in the body, the virus can retreat to nerve cells in the face in the case of HSV1, or near the base of the spine in the case of HSV2. If the virus is reactivated, it can return to where it entered the body and cause a recurrence. Not all people have recurrences; some have a few and for some herpes recurs regularly. Normally the initial attack is the most severe. Recurrences don't necessarily depend on having contact with an infected person. Irritation of affected skin from other

causes is known to trigger attacks. If you have genital herpes, you mustn't have sex if the virus is active, i.e. if you have genital blisters or any tingling or soreness, and you should always avoid oral sex if a cold sore is present.

As you'd expect, herpes is highly contagious. There is a 90 percent chance of catching it if either partner has an active blister, although new research confirms that **the virus can also be transmitted by people who don't have any symptoms**. Symptoms appear between three and 20 days after contact with an infected person.

WHAT ARE THE SYMPTOMS OF HERPES?

- The **skin** feels oversensitive to touch.
- Itching and irritation around the affected area of skin.
- **Enlarged** tender lymph glands in the neck or groin.
- A general feeling of being unwell.
- Headache.
- Muscle aches and joint pains.
- Blisters that appear within a few hours of the itching and soreness; these enlarge, burst and become painful ulcers after two to three days.
- Ulcers that form scabs and take 14–21 days to heal completely.
- In genital herpes, shooting pain in the lower limbs.
- In genital herpes, pain on passing urine.

WHAT ARE THE TRIGGERS FOR HERPES?

- Physical and mental stress.
- Excessive cold or heat, including fever.
- For herpes infections of the face, exposure to strong sunlight.
- Local trauma to the skin (e.g. in genital herpes, rough sexual intercourse, plucking or shaving pubic hair).
- General ill health and other infections, such as a cold.

WHAT IS THE TREATMENT?

Cold sores caused by HSV1 can be treated at home using **aciclovir cream**, which is available over the counter from chemists. Genital herpes should always be looked at by a doctor and not treated at home. See your doctor immediately if you feel numb or sensitive in the genital area or if you've had sexual relations with anyone with the herpes virus.

There's no cure for genital herpes but the

Family of herpes infections

Type of virus	Condition it causes	Description
Herpes simplex type 1 (HSV1)	Cold sores	Infections of the **lips**, **mouth** and **face**
Herpes simplex type 2 (HSV2)	Genital herpes	Infections of the **genitals**
Herpes zoster	Chickenpox Shingles	Infection causing **blisters** Infection causing **blisters** along the path of a nerve; only occurs in those who have previously had chickenpox

sooner treatment is given the more likely it will prevent or ameliorate an attack. Antiviral drugs, such as **aciclovir**, taken as tablets make the ulcers less painful and encourage healing. Over-the-counter aciclovir cream shouldn't be used to treat genital herpes.

Other remedies for genital herpes include daily douches with **povidone iodine** solution or bathing the area with salt solution (one heaped teaspoon of salt to one pint of water).

SELF-HELP

● Keep separate towels and face cloths for each member of your household. This helps prevent the virus being spread from one person to another.
● To prevent herpes recurring get plenty of rest and eat a balanced diet with nutritional foodstuffs – fresh fruit and vegetables, **wholefoods** and plenty of liquids.

● Manage stress by learning relaxation exercises or taking up yoga.
● For cold sores, wear a high sun-protection factor cream on your lips and any other affected parts of the face when in bright sunlight.
● Keep a record of when your attacks recur in an attempt to find a pattern. If, for example, recurrences of genital herpes are related to rough sex, try using a lubricant jelly.
● Try a cream containing lemon balm, daily or when symptoms start.
● Always use a condom to protect yourself from genital herpes.
● For genital herpes, wear loose underwear so air can circulate and keep your genitals cool. Leave the sores exposed to air as much as possible.
● Painful blisters in the genital area can be relieved by a soak in a tepid bath and cold packs (not ice) applied to the infected area.

WARNING:

The herpes virus may have a role in the development of cervical cancer and women who have had herpes should have a cervical smear test regularly, preferably every year.

See also:
● **Chickenpox p.335** ● **Cold sores p.338**
● **Genital herpes p.281** ● **Shingles p.335**

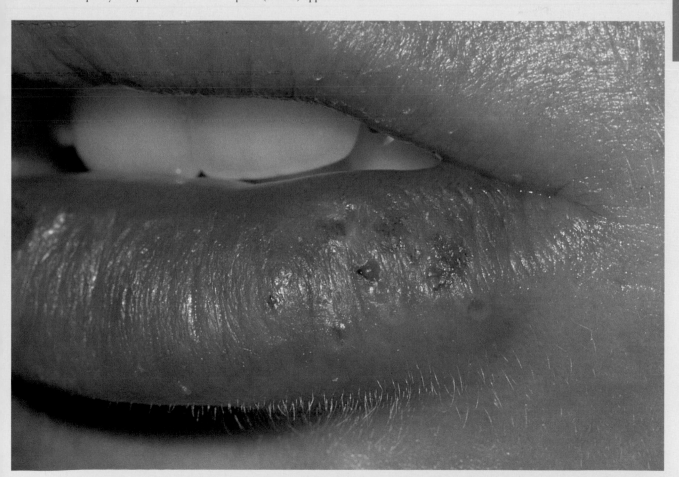

Cold sores

COLD SORES ARE TINY BLISTERS THAT FORM MOSTLY AROUND THE NOSTRILS AND LIPS
BUT SOMETIMES ALSO ELSEWHERE ON THE FACE. THE BLISTERS BREAK OPEN
AND WEEP BEFORE THEY CRUST OVER AND DISAPPEAR.

Cold sores are caused by the herpes simplex virus, of which there are two types: type 1, which causes most cases of facial cold sores, and type 2, which causes about 70–80 percent of cases of genital herpes. A rise in skin temperature – perhaps caused by a cold, or by going out in the sun – activates the virus. The first attack may take the form of painful mouth ulcers. Subsequent attacks take the form of skin blisters. Most cold sores last about 10–14 days.

Cold sores are not serious unless they occur near the eye, where they may rarely cause an ulcer to form on the front of the eyeball.

WHAT ARE THE SYMPTOMS?
■ Raised red area, usually around the nostrils and lips, which tingles and feels itchy. Tiny blisters then form on the spot.
■ Weeping blisters, which then crust over.

WHAT SHOULD I DO FIRST?
■ Once blisters have formed, don't touch them.
■ Surgical spirit dabbed on the cold sores will dry them up (take care, it may sting). I'm more in favour of a soothing cream, such as petroleum jelly, to keep them moist while the virus runs its course.

SHOULD I CONSULT THE DOCTOR?
Consult your doctor as soon as possible if the cold sores become redder and develop pus-filled centres, as they may be infected with bacteria. Also, consult your doctor as soon as possible if a cold sore is near your eye. Ask your doctor's advice if you suffer from recurrent cold sores.

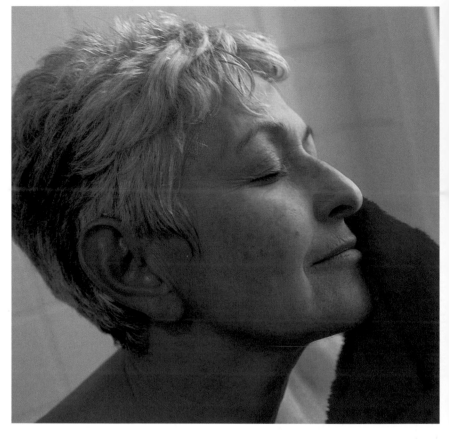

WHAT MIGHT THE DOCTOR DO?
■ If the cold sores are infected, your doctor may prescribe an antibiotic ointment that lubricates the area and treats the infection.
■ Your doctor may prescribe an antiviral cream to spread over the affected area regularly to contain the attack. He may also give you antiviral tablets if attacks are frequent.

WHAT CAN I DO TO HELP?
■ Make sure that you have a personal towel and face cloth.
■ Don't kiss anyone. The virus can be transmitted this way.
■ If you tend to develop cold sores after exposure to sunlight, smear a sunblock on your lips or nose when you go out in the sun.

HIV infection and AIDS

HIV IS A CHRONIC VIRAL INFECTION THAT, LEFT UNTREATED, RESULTS IN REDUCED
IMMUNITY TO OTHER INFECTIONS AND CANCERS (PARTICULARLY KAPOSI'S SARCOMA),
WHICH MAY RESULT IN DEATH.

Infection with the **human immunodeficiency virus** (HIV), which in many cases leads to acquired immunodeficiency syndrome (AIDS), has been the most written about, most researched and most feared infection of the past two decades. Despite the development of highly effective drugs to limit the disease there is still

no vaccine against the virus, and the number of people with HIV infection continues to rise, especially in developing countries.

HIV is believed to have originated in Africa, where a similar virus is carried by some species of primates. The virus is thought to have spread from monkeys to humans through saliva in

bites, then around the world from person to person in body fluids. The first recognized cases of AIDS in the US occurred in 1981, when there was an outbreak of unusual cases of pneumonia and skin cancer in young homosexual men in Los Angeles. Two years later, the virus was isolated and identified as HIV.

HIV infects and gradually destroys cells in the immune system, weakening the body's response to infections and cancers. People infected with HIV may have no symptoms for many years, or they may experience frequent or prolonged mild infections, but they **all** develop **antibodies** to the virus, which can be detected by a **blood test**; they're said to be **HIV positive**. When the immune system becomes severely weakened, an infected person is said to have AIDS. A person with AIDS develops serious infections caused by organisms that are normally harmless to healthy people and is also susceptible to certain cancers.

WHO IS AFFECTED?

By the end of 1998, there were about 22,000 people in the UK who had HIV infection, with 2,000 new cases a year. Worldwide, over 33 million people are thought to be infected, 9 out of 10 of whom are unaware that they have the condition; the number is rising. As a result of developments in drug treatment, deaths due to AIDS have fallen dramatically in the developed world since 1995. The problem of AIDS is much greater in developing countries, where most people with HIV infection live and where the new drugs are unavailable or unaffordable.

HOW IS HIV TRANSMITTED?

The HIV virus is not the common cold – it's not contagious. HIV is carried in body fluids including blood, semen, vaginal secretions, saliva and breast milk, although not to the same degree. All body fluids do not therefore have the same potential for infection. Saliva from an infected person contains the HIV virus but in such a small quantity that it would be exceedingly difficult to be infected by saliva. HIV is most commonly transmitted sexually – by vaginal, anal and, more rarely, oral intercourse. **You are more susceptible to HIV infection and more likely to pass on the virus if you have another sexually transmitted disease.**

You are also at increased risk of HIV infection if you use **intravenous drugs and share or reuse needles** contaminated with the virus. Medical workers are also at risk from contaminated needles or from contact with infected body fluids, but the risk is very low.

HIV infection can be passed from an infected woman to the fetus or to the baby at birth or by breast-feeding. The virus can also be transmitted through organ transplants or blood transfusions. However, in developed countries screening of blood, organs and tissues for HIV is now routine, making the risk of infection extremely low.

HIV infection cannot be transmitted by everyday human contact, such as shaking hands or by coughs or sneezes, and there is no risk to your health from working or living with someone who is infected with the virus.

WHAT IS THE CAUSE?

HIV enters the bloodstream and infects cells that have a special structure, known as the **CD4 receptor**, on their surfaces. The infected cells include a type of **white blood cell**, known as a **CD4 lymphocyte**, which is responsible for fighting infection. The virus reproduces rapidly within the cells and destroys them in the process.

At first, the immune system is able to function normally despite the infection, and symptoms may not develop for years. However, especially if the infection is untreated, the number of CD4 lymphocytes eventually begins to fall, causing increased susceptibility to other infections and some types of cancer.

WHAT ARE THE SYMPTOMS?

The first symptoms of HIV infection usually appear within 6 weeks of infection. Some people experience a flu-like illness that may include some or all of the following symptoms:
- swollen lymph glands
- fever
- fatigue
- rash
- aching muscles
- sore throat.

These symptoms usually clear up after a few weeks, and many people with HIV infection feel completely healthy. However, in some people, any of the following minor disorders may develop:
- persistent, swollen lymph glands
- mouth infections, such as thrush
- gum disease
- severe, persistent herpes simplex infections, such as cold sores
- extensive genital warts
- itchy, flaky skin (seborrhoeic dermatitis)
- weight loss
- neurological symptoms similar to dementia.

The time between infection with HIV and the onset of AIDS varies from person to person, but it can be anywhere between 1 and 14 years. Often people are totally unaware for years that they are infected with HIV until they develop one or more serious infections or cancers, known as "**AIDS-defining illnesses**".

ARE THERE COMPLICATIONS?

The single most dramatic complication of HIV infection is the development of AIDS. A person infected with HIV is said to have developed AIDS if the CD4 lymphocyte count falls below a certain level or if he or she develops a particular AIDS-defining illness. These illnesses include opportunistic infections (infections that occur only in people who have reduced immunity), certain cancers and problems with the nervous system that may result in **dementia**, confusion, behaviour changes and memory loss.

OPPORTUNISTIC INFECTIONS

These infections may be caused by protozoa, fungi, viruses or bacteria, and they can often be life-threatening.
- One of the most common illnesses in people with AIDS is a severe infection of the lungs (pneumonia) by the parasite *Pneumocystis carinii*.
- Other common diseases are protozoal, such as **toxoplasmosis**, which can affect the brain.
- *Candida albicans* is a fungus that causes mild superficial infections in healthy people but may produce much more serious infections in people who have AIDS.
- The cryptococcus fungus may cause fever, headaches and lung infections.
- People with AIDS suffer from severe bacterial and viral infections. Bacterial infections include **tuberculosis** and **listeriosis**, which may lead to **blood poisoning** (septicaemia). Viral infections include those caused by the **herpes viruses**. Herpes simplex infections can affect the brain, causing meningitis and viral encephalitis.
- **Cytomegalovirus** infection may cause a number of severe conditions, including pneumonia, viral encephalitis and a type of

Diagnosing HIV and AIDS

If you suspect that you may have been exposed to HIV infection, you should have a blood test to check for antibodies against the virus. The blood test may also be performed if you have symptoms that suggest HIV infection. Consent is always obtained before the test, and counselling is given both before and afterwards to discuss the implications of a positive result.

If your HIV test result is negative, you may be advised to have another test in three months because antibodies can take time to develop. HIV infection can also be difficult to diagnose in the baby of an infected woman because the mother's antibodies may remain in the baby's blood for up to 18 months.

AIDS is diagnosed when an AIDS-defining illness, such as pneumocystis infection or Kaposi's sarcoma, develops or when a blood test shows that the CD4 lymphocyte count has dropped below a certain level.

Myths about HIV infection

Because HIV/AIDS is a very frightening subject, many myths and half-truths have grown up about how the infection can be transmitted. It should be stressed that HIV is quite difficult to catch. In an infected person, there are large numbers of the virus in blood and semen, but small numbers in saliva and vaginal fluid.

Knowing the truth about HIV helps you to act responsibly.

You won't get HIV

- from swimming in the same pool as an HIV-positive person
- if you kiss an infected person on the mouth, although there is a slight risk if the person has inflamed or bleeding gums
- from drinking from a glass or eating from a plate that's been used by an HIV-positive person
- by going to school or college with an HIV-positive person
- by visiting someone with HIV at their home or in hospital
- by hugging, shaking hands or dancing with someone who's HIV positive
- by sitting on a toilet seat that's been used by an infected person
- by standing next to an infected person who is sneezing; the virus doesn't travel through the air
- if you're bitten by an insect
- if you give blood at a blood transfusion unit.

can take to avoid sexual transmission are to **use a condom during sexual intercourse** and to **avoid sex with multiple partners**. No matter how much you like someone, never give in to the temptation to have sex with a partner you barely know. Talk to him or her before you do anything you might regret. Talk about the risk; if he or she gets angry or resentful, you should ask yourself whether this person is really worth knowing. Men are just as worried about AIDS as women so they're usually grateful if a woman raises the subject as long as it's done in a tactful way.

■ Both partners might think about having an **HIV test before** having unprotected sex in a new relationship.

■ Specific groups also need to take special precautions. For example, if you inject drugs intravenously, you must use a clean needle every time.

■ People who are HIV positive need to take special care to prevent others from coming into contact with their blood or body fluids and should always inform dental or medical staff that they are HIV positive.

■ If you are HIV positive and pregnant, antiviral drugs may be given to reduce the risk of transmission to the fetus. You may also be advised to have a caesarean section.

■ Avoid breast-feeding if you are HIV positive to reduce the risk of transmitting the virus to your baby.

Medical professionals take many steps to prevent transmission of HIV, including screening all blood products and tissues for transplant and using disposable or carefully sterilized equipment.

Extensive research is being carried out either to develop a **vaccine** against HIV or to prevent the development of AIDS. However, although researchers are optimistic they will succeed, there will inevitably be millions more deaths worldwide before an affordable cure is found and made available to everyone.

---

eye inflammation that can result in blindness.

However, people with AIDS are no more susceptible to common infections such as colds.

CANCERS

The most common cancer that affects people with AIDS is **Kaposi's sarcoma**, a type of skin cancer that can also affect the inside of the mouth and internal organs. Other cancers that commonly develop in people with AIDS include **lymphomas,** such as non-Hodgkin's lymphoma. **Cancer of the cervix** is an AIDS-defining illness in women infected with HIV.

WHAT IS THE TREATMENT?

If your HIV test result is positive, you will probably be referred to a special centre where you will receive monitoring, treatment and advice from a team of health-care professionals.

Drug treatment may be started when you are diagnosed with HIV infection or when CD4 lymphocyte levels start to fall. Advances in the use of combinations of specific antiviral drugs, called antiretroviral drugs, that prevent HIV from replicating have made it possible to prevent progression of HIV infection to AIDS and to suppress the viral infection to undetectable levels in some people.

There are two main groups of antiretroviral drugs used in the treatment of HIV infection and AIDS: reverse transcriptase inhibitors and protease inhibitors. The drugs work by blocking the processes necessary for viral replication without significantly damaging the body cells that the virus has invaded. Reverse transcriptase inhibitors, such as zidovudine

(AZT), alter the genetic material of the infected cell (which is needed by the virus to replicate) or the genetic material of the virus itself. Protease inhibitors, such as ritonavir, prevent the production of viral proteins necessary for replication.

Once AIDS has developed, opportunistic infections are dealt with as they occur, usually by treatment with antibiotic drugs, and in some cases, there may also be long-term preventive treatment against the most common infections.

Emotional support and practical advice can be obtained from the many groups and charitable organizations that help people with HIV infection and AIDS.

WHAT IS THE OUTLOOK?

There is no cure for HIV infection, but the drug treatments available in the developed world have made it possible to regard the condition as a chronic illness rather than as a rapidly fatal one. In the two years following the introduction of antiviral drug combination therapies in 1995, deaths from AIDS in the developed world fell dramatically. However, for most of the people with HIV who live in the developing world, the prognosis is bleak. Few have access to up-to-date treatment, and left untreated, half of all people infected with the virus develop AIDS within 10 years and die.

CAN IT BE PREVENTED?

HIV infection can be prevented by teaching everyone about the risks of infection from an early age.

■ The two main precautions that everyone

See also:
- Blood poisoning p.345
- Cold sores p.338
- Genital warts p.282
- Herpes simplex p.336
- Pneumocystis infection p.396
- Safe sex p.280
- Seborrhoeic dermatitis p.315
- Toxoplasmosis p.344

Hepatitis

HEPATITIS IS A USUALLY SUDDEN, SHORT-TERM INFLAMMATION OF THE LIVER
DUE TO A VARIETY OF CAUSES, THE MOST COMMON BEING THE HEPATITIS
VIRUSES A, B AND C; C IS THE MOST SERIOUS.

About 1 in 1000 people in the UK carry the virus for hepatitis at any one time, although not all of them will necessarily go on to develop the disease. The condition has various causes and has a sudden onset. Most people with acute hepatitis recover within a month or two. However, in some cases inflammation of the liver persists for many months or may even persist for years (**chronic hepatitis**) and may progress to liver failure.

WHAT ARE THE CAUSES?

Worldwide, the most common cause of acute hepatitis is infection with any one of the several types of **hepatitis viruses**. Until the late 1980s, there were only two known hepatitis viruses, **hepatitis A and B**. Additional hepatitis viruses have now been identified, including **hepatitis C, D and E**. Other hepatitis viruses are almost certainly yet to be discovered. The known viruses can all cause acute hepatitis, and they have many features in common, although the way in which they are transmitted and their long-term effects may differ.

Infections with some types of bacteria, other non-hepatitis viruses and some parasites can also lead to acute hepatitis. In addition, the condition may be caused by non-infectious agents, such as some **drugs** and **toxins**, including **alcohol**.

OTHER INFECTIOUS CAUSES

Acute hepatitis may also be caused by other viral infections, such as cytomegalovirus and the Epstein–Barr virus (the cause of glandular fever). Some bacterial infections, such as Legionnaires' disease, can cause hepatitis. Parasitic infections that may also result in acute hepatitis include infection with plasmodium, the cause of malaria.

NON-INFECTIOUS CAUSES

In developed countries, **excessive alcohol consumption** is one of the most common causes of acute hepatitis. The condition can also be caused by other toxins, such as those found in poisonous fungi. Acute hepatitis can also be caused by certain drugs, such as some **anticonvulsants**, the **anaesthetic gas halothane** and an overdose of paracetamol.

WHAT ARE THE SYMPTOMS?

Some people infected with a hepatitis virus have no symptoms, or symptoms that are so mild they are not noticed. In other cases, the disorder may be life-threatening. If hepatitis is due to a viral infection, the time from infection to appearance of symptoms can vary from up to six weeks for hepatitis A to six months for hepatitis B. Some people who have no symptoms may become carriers of the virus. If symptoms do develop, they may initially include:

- fatigue and a feeling of ill health
- poor appetite
- nausea and vomiting
- fever
- discomfort in the upper right side of the abdomen.

Several days after the initial symptoms develop, the whites of the eyes and the skin may take on a yellow tinge (**jaundice**). Often, the initial symptoms improve once jaundice appears. At this time, the faeces may become paler than usual, and **widespread itching** may be present. Acute hepatitis caused by the hepatitis B virus may also cause **joint pains**.

Severe acute hepatitis may result in **liver failure**, causing mental confusion, seizures and sometimes coma. Liver failure is relatively common following an overdose with the painkiller **paracetamol**, but it is less common with some types of hepatitis, such as those due to the hepatitis A virus.

HOW IS IT DIAGNOSED?

If your doctor suspects that you have hepatitis, he or she may arrange for you to have blood tests to evaluate your liver function and to look for possible causes of the hepatitis. Blood tests will probably be repeated in order to help monitor your recovery. If the diagnosis is unclear, you may also have an ultrasound scan and in some cases a liver biopsy, in which a small piece of liver is removed and examined under a microscope.

WHAT IS THE TREATMENT?

There is no specific treatment for most cases of acute hepatitis, and people are usually advised to rest.

- **Consult your doctor before taking any medicines**, such as painkillers, because there is a risk of side effects.
- If you have viral hepatitis, you will need to take precautions to prevent the spread of the disease, including **practising safe sex**.
- You should **avoid drinking alcohol** during the illness and for a minimum of three months after you have recovered. However, if the cause was alcohol-related, you will be advised to give up drinking alcohol permanently.

WHAT IS THE OUTLOOK?

- Most people with acute hepatitis feel better after 4–6 weeks and recover after three months.
- However, for some people with **hepatitis C**,

Hepatitis viruses

Hepatitis A virus

The hepatitis A virus is the most common cause of acute viral hepatitis in the West. Often, the virus does not produce symptoms, or symptoms are so mild that the infection passes unrecognized. The hepatitis A virus can be detected in the urine and faeces of infected people, and it can be transmitted to other people in **contaminated food or water**.

Hepatitis B virus

It is estimated that each year about one million people in Europe become infected with the hepatitis B virus. The virus is spread by contact with an infected person's body fluids. For example, the virus can be spread by **sexual intercourse** or by sharing contaminated needles used for taking drugs intravenously. In developing countries, the infection is most commonly transmitted from mother to baby at birth. Before blood banks routinely screened blood for the virus, blood transfusions used to be a source of hepatitis B infection, and many

people with haemophilia contracted hepatitis. All blood used for transfusions is now screened for the hepatitis B virus.

Hepatitis C virus

About 3 percent of people worldwide are infected with the hepatitis C virus each year. The virus is most commonly transmitted by blood, often by sharing contaminated needles used for taking drugs intravenously. All blood used for transfusions in the UK is now screened for the hepatitis C virus. It is also spread by **sexual intercourse**.

Hepatitis D and E viruses

Infection with hepatitis D occurs only in people who already have hepatitis B infection. It is spread by contact with infected body fluids. The hepatitis E virus is a rare cause of hepatitis in the developed world. The virus is excreted in the faeces of infected people and is spread in much the same way as the hepatitis A virus.

recovery is followed by a **series of relapses** over several months.

■ About 3 out of 4 people with hepatitis C, and 1 out of 20 with hepatitis B and D **develop chronic hepatitis.**

■ People with acute hepatitis caused by an infection other than the hepatitis viruses usually recover completely once the infection clears up.

■ Recovery from acute hepatitis due to excessive alcohol consumption, drugs or other toxins depends on the extent of the liver damage. The substances causing the acute hepatitis must be avoided in the future.

■ In the rare cases in which hepatitis progresses to liver failure, a liver transplant may be necessary.

CAN IT BE PREVENTED?

■ Infection with hepatitis A and E may be prevented by good personal hygiene.

■ The risk of infection with hepatitis B, C and D can be reduced by practising safe sex and by not sharing needles or other objects that might be contaminated with infected body fluids.

■ Immunizations to protect against hepatitis A are given to travellers to certain countries, and others at risk of contracting the infection.

■ Hepatitis B vaccination is recommended for high-risk groups, such as health-care workers.

■ To avoid the transmission of hepatitis through blood transfusion, blood banks routinely screen all blood for the hepatitis B and hepatitis C viruses.

See also:
• **Alcohol-related liver disease p.356**
• **Jaundice p.355**
• **Malaria p.343**
• **Safe sex p.280**

Glandular fever

GLANDULAR FEVER, ALSO KNOWN AS INFECTIOUS MONONUCLEOSIS, IS A VIRAL INFECTION CAUSING SWOLLEN LYMPH NODES AND A SORE THROAT THAT IS COMMON IN ADOLESCENCE AND EARLY ADULTHOOD.

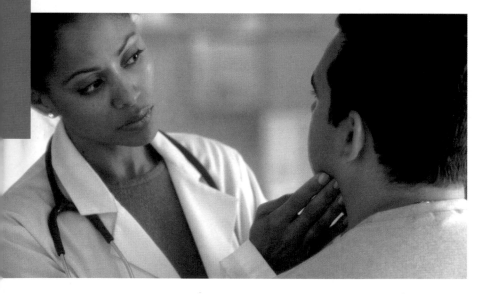

Glandular fever is known as the "kissing disease" of adolescence and early adulthood because it is mainly transmitted in **saliva**. Its name comes from the symptoms, which include widespread swollen lymph glands and a high temperature. Initially, the illness may be **mistaken for tonsillitis**, but it is more severe and lasts longer.

WHAT IS THE CAUSE?

Infectious mononucleosis is caused by the **Epstein–Barr virus** (EBV), which attacks lymphocytes, the white blood cells that are responsible for fighting infection. EBV infection is very common, and about 9 in 10 people have been infected by the age of 50. More than half of infected people do not develop symptoms and, consequently, are unaware that they have been infected.

WHAT ARE THE SYMPTOMS?

If symptoms of infectious mononucleosis develop, they usually do so 4–6 weeks after infection and appear over several days. Symptoms may include:

● high fever and sweating

● extremely sore throat, causing difficulty swallowing

● swollen tonsils, often covered with a thick greyish-white coating

● enlarged, tender lymph glands in the neck, armpits and groin

● tender abdomen as the result of an enlarged spleen

● rash.

These distinctive symptoms are often accompanied by poor appetite, weight loss, headache and fatigue. In some people, the sore throat and fever clear up quickly, and

the other symptoms last less than a month. Other people may be ill longer and may feel lethargic and depressed for months after the infection. Glandular fever was one of the first virus infections recognized as leaving behind post-viral fatigue syndrome.

WHAT MIGHT BE DONE?

Your doctor will probably diagnose the infection from your enlarged lymph nodes, sore throat and fever. A blood test may be carried out to look for antibodies against EBV in order to confirm the diagnosis. A throat swab may also be taken to exclude bacterial infection, which would need to be treated with antibiotics.

There is no specific treatment for infectious mononucleosis, but simple measures may help relieve symptoms.

Drinking plenty of cool fluids, and taking over-the-counter painkillers, such as paracetamol, may help control the high fever and pain. Contact sports should be avoided while the spleen is enlarged because of the risk of rupture, which causes severe internal bleeding and can be life-threatening.

WHAT IS THE OUTLOOK?

Almost everyone who has infectious mononucleosis makes a full recovery eventually. However, in some people, recovery may be slow, and fatigue and depression may last for weeks or even months after the symptoms first appear. One attack of the disease, with or without symptoms, provides life-long protection.

Typhoid and paratyphoid

TYPHOID AND PARATYPHOID ARE INFECTIONS CAUSED BY SALMONELLA BACTERIA
THAT RESULT IN HIGH FEVER FOLLOWED BY A RASH.

Visiting or living in areas where the disease occurs is a risk factor. Typhoid and paratyphoid are almost identical diseases that are caused by the bacteria *Salmonella typhi* and *Salmonella paratyphi*, respectively. The bacteria multiply in the intestines and spread to the blood and to other organs, such as the spleen, gallbladder and liver. The diseases are transmitted through infected faeces and most commonly occur in areas where hygiene and sanitation are poor. Infection is commonly due to food or water contaminated by unwashed hands.

WHAT ARE THE SYMPTOMS?

Symptoms of both diseases appear 7–14 days after infection and may include:

- headache and high fever
- dry cough
- abdominal pain and constipation, usually followed by diarrhoea
- rash of rose-coloured spots appearing on the chest, abdomen and back.

If left untreated, both infections can sometimes lead to serious complications, such as intestinal bleeding and, rarely, perforation of the intestines.

WHAT MIGHT BE DONE?

Typhoid and paratyphoid can be diagnosed by testing blood or faeces samples for the bacteria. The diseases are usually treated with antibiotics in hospital. Symptoms usually subside 2–3 days after treatment has begun, and most people recover fully in a month.

Even with treatment the bacteria are excreted for about three months after the symptoms have disappeared. Some people who do not undergo treatment may become life-long **carriers** of the bacteria and transmit the infection to others, although they appear to be healthy.

Good hygiene is the best protection against infection. Several vaccines are available, and if you intend to travel to a developing country, immunization may be advisable. Consult your doctor before travelling as recommendations change.

Malaria

MORE THAN 1 IN EVERY 3 PEOPLE WORLDWIDE IS AFFECTED BY MALARIA, A PARASITIC
INFECTION THAT LEADS TO THE DESTRUCTION OF RED BLOOD CELLS. MALARIA IS SPREAD BY
INFECTED MOSQUITOES, WHICH PASS THE PARASITE ON THROUGH THEIR BITES.

In tropical countries, about 10 million new cases of malaria and 2 million deaths occur every year. Most of those who die from malaria are children.

WHAT ARE THE SYMPTOMS?

The symptoms of malaria usually begin between 10 days and 6 weeks after being bitten by an infected mosquito. However, in some cases, symptoms may not develop for months or years, especially if preventive drugs were being taken at the time of infection.

If not treated, malaria due to the **plasmodium** parasites – *P. vivax, P. ovale* and *P. malariae* – causes recurrent attacks of symptoms each time the parasites multiply inside red blood cells and destroy them. Each attack usually lasts for 4–8 hours and may occur at intervals of 2–3 days, depending on the species of parasite. Symptoms of an attack include:

- high fever
- shivering and chills
- heavy sweating
- confusion
- fatigue, headaches and muscle pain
- dark brown urine.

Between each attack, extreme fatigue due to anaemia may be the only symptom.

Falciparum malaria (caused by *Plasmodium falciparum*) causes a continuous fever that may be mistaken for influenza. It is more severe than the other types, and attacks may lead to

SELF-HELP

Preventing malaria

If you plan to visit an area where malaria occurs, your doctor will be able to give you up-to-date advice about **antimalarial drugs** for that area. You may need to start taking the drugs several days before you leave and continue taking them during and after your visit. To protect yourself against mosquito bites, you should:

- Keep your body well covered.
- Sleep under a mosquito net that is impregnated with insect repellent.
- Use insect repellent on clothes and exposed skin.

These measures against mosquito bites are especially important between dusk and dawn, when mosquitoes bite.

loss of consciousness, cerebral malaria and kidney failure and may be fatal within 48 hours of symptoms appearing if left untreated.

WHAT MIGHT BE DONE?

Your doctor may suspect malaria if you have an unexplained fever within a year of a trip to a region where the infection occurs. Diagnosis is confirmed by identifying the malarial parasite in a blood smear under a microscope.

If you are diagnosed with malaria, you should be given **antimalarial drugs** as early as possible to avoid complications. Treatment depends on the type of malaria, how resistant the parasite is to drugs and the severity of the symptoms. If you have falciparum malaria,

you may be treated **in hospital** with **oral or intravenous antimalarial drugs**. Treatment may also involve a **blood transfusion** to replace destroyed red blood cells or **kidney dialysis** if kidney function is impaired. Other types of malaria are usually treated on an outpatient basis with oral antimalarial drugs.

If treated early, the prognosis is usually good, and most people make a full recovery. Malaria caused by *P. vivax* and *P. ovale* may recur after treatment.

NB Preventive measures, including taking antimalarial drugs, should always be followed when visiting an area where malaria is known to occur.

Toxoplasmosis

TOXOPLASMOSIS IS A PROTOZOAL INFECTION THAT CAUSES SERIOUS ILLNESS IN THE UNBORN BABY AND IN PEOPLE WHO HAVE REDUCED IMMUNITY, SUCH AS AIDS SUFFERERS, WHO MAY DEVELOP ENCEPHALITIS AS A RESULT OF THIS INFECTION.

Cysts of the parasite are excreted in the faeces of cats and can be passed to people **by direct contact with cats** or by **handling cat litter**. Another source of infection is **raw or undercooked meat** of animals that have eaten cysts from the faeces of infected cats.

In most people, the infection does not cause symptoms because the protozoal cysts are dormant. **If a woman develops toxoplasmosis while she is pregnant, the parasites may infect the fetus and cause blindness.**

WHAT MIGHT BE DONE?

Usually, no treatment is necessary, although **pyrimethamine** and antibiotics may be prescribed for people with reduced immunity or pregnant women. People with reduced immunity may need to take the drugs for life to prevent reactivation of cysts.

Infection can be prevented by avoiding contact with cats, wearing gloves to handle cat litter and for gardening and by not eating undercooked or raw meat.

Lyme disease

LYME DISEASE IS AN INFECTION TRANSMITTED BY TICKS THAT CAUSES A RASH AND FLU-LIKE SYMPTOMS. NAMED AFTER OLD LYME, THE TOWN IN CONNECTICUT, USA, WHERE THE DISEASE WAS FIRST RECOGNIZED, LYME DISEASE IS CAUSED BY A BACTERIUM CALLED *BORRELIA BURGDORFERI.*

If a person is bitten by an infected tick that remains embedded in the skin, bacteria can enter the bloodstream and may then spread throughout the body.

Most reports of Lyme disease have been documented in the northeastern coastal states of the US, but it can be picked up wherever ticks thrive and is prevalent in southwestern France. The disease also occurs in northern and western US states, in Europe and in Central Asia. People who go camping or walking in wooded areas during the summer months are most at risk of being bitten by a tick carrying Lyme disease bacteria.

WHAT ARE THE SYMPTOMS?

A bite from an infected tick usually produces a red lump with a scab on the skin, although some people who have been bitten may not notice this initial sign. Within two days to four weeks after the bite, the following symptoms may develop:
- spreading circular rash at the site of the bite that may clear in the centre
- fatigue
- flu-like chills and fever
- headache and joint pains.

If the infection is left untreated, these symptoms may persist for several weeks. In some people who have Lyme disease dangerous complications may develop up to two years later that may affect the heart, nervous system and joints.

WHAT MIGHT BE DONE?

■ Your doctor may suspect from your symptoms that you have Lyme disease and may also arrange for a blood test to confirm the diagnosis.

■ You will be given prompt treatment with **antibiotics** – most people make a complete recovery.

■ **Non-steroidal anti-inflammatory drugs (NSAIDS)** can help relieve joint pain.

■ **Vaccines** are now available that offer 70 percent protection against Lyme disease. For continued protection, vaccination needs to be repeated every two years.

■ In regions known to be tick-infested, you should cover your arms and legs to reduce the risk of bites and promptly remove any ticks that you find on your skin.

Complications are extremely rare.

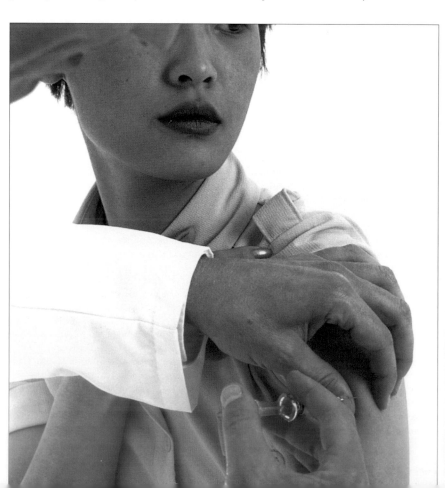

Blood poisoning (septicaemia)

BLOOD POISONING, OR SEPTICAEMIA, IS A RARE INFECTION IN WHICH BACTERIA
MULTIPLY IN THE BLOODSTREAM. QUITE OFTEN WE HAVE BACTERIA
IN THE BLOOD (BACTERAEMIA), BUT THEY DON'T MULTIPLY.

Septicaemia nearly always occurs when bacteria escape from a localized infection, such as peritonitis, meningitis or an abscess, and is more likely to occur in people with a compromised immune system. It is a complication of bacterial meningitis.

WHAT ARE THE SYMPTOMS?
The symptoms of septicaemia develop suddenly and include:
- high fever
- chills and violent shivering.

If septicaemia is left untreated, the bacteria may produce toxins that damage blood vessels, causing a drop in blood pressure and widespread tissue damage. In this dangerous condition, called **septic shock**, which is potentially life-threatening, symptoms include:
- faintness
- cold, pale hands and feet
- restlessness and irritability
- rapid, shallow breathing
- rash
- jaundice
- in many cases, delirium and eventual loss of consciousness.

In some people, bacteria may lodge on the **heart valves**, especially if the heart has previously been damaged by disease. This serious condition is called **infective endocarditis**. Rarely, septicaemia may result in a lack of the blood cells involved in blood clotting (thrombocytopaenia), which increases the risk of bleeding and produces a characteristic **purpuric rash** that doesn't blanch when a glass is pressed on the skin.

WHAT MIGHT BE DONE?
If your doctor suspects that you have septicaemia, you will be admitted to hospital for immediate treatment. **Intravenous antibiotics** are given without delay and blood tests are done to identify the bacterium causing the infection. Once the bacterium has been identified, specific antibiotics are given. With prompt treatment before the onset of septic shock, most people are able to make a complete recovery.

Toxic shock syndrome

TOXIC SHOCK SYNDROME IS A SEPTIC FORM OF BACTERIAL SHOCK, PRODUCED NOT BY BACTERIA
MULTIPLYING IN THE BLOOD BUT BY A TOXIN PRODUCED BY THE COMMON BACTERIUM
STAPHYLOCOCCUS AUREUS AND CERTAIN STREPTOCOCCAL BACTERIA.

When the bacteria multiply, large amounts of the toxin enter the blood and lead to the symptoms of shock.

First described in the 1980s, 7 out of 10 cases were in women using highly absorbent tampons (now taken off the market), but toxic shock syndrome (TSS) can also arise from skin wounds or infections caused by *S. aureus* elsewhere in the body.

In addition to the symptoms of septicaemia, a characteristic reddening of the palms and soles develops, with peeling two weeks later.

Treatment is with antibiotics, sometimes by intravenous infusion.

There seems to be an **individual tendency** to TSS, as it can return to women who've had it. These women, therefore, should avoid using tampons, caps, diaphragms and so forth.

Tetanus

TETANUS IS A WOUND INFECTION CAUSED BY A POTENT TOXIN THAT IS
PRODUCED BY THE BACTERIUM *CLOSTRIDIUM TETANI*.
THE TOXIN INDUCES SEVERE MUSCLE SPASMS.

Tetanus bacteria live in soil and in the intestines of human beings and other animals. If the bacteria enter a wound, they multiply and release their toxin, which affects the nerves controlling muscle contraction. The condition, also known as lockjaw, is rare in developed countries because most people have been immunized.

The symptoms of tetanus usually appear 5–10 days after infection. Fever, headache and muscle stiffness in the jaw, arms, neck and back are typical. As the condition progresses, painful muscle spasms may develop. In some people the muscles of the throat or chest wall are affected, leading to breathing difficulties and possible suffocation.

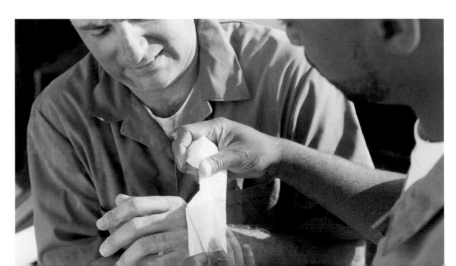

WHAT MIGHT BE DONE?

The disease needs immediate treatment in hospital with **antitoxin** injections, **antibiotics** and **sedatives** to relieve muscle spasm. **Mechanical ventilation** may be necessary to aid breathing. If given prompt treatment, most people make a complete recovery. If treatment is delayed, tetanus is usually fatal.

CAN IT BE PREVENTED?

Essential precautions against tetanus include the following things.
■ Vaccination against tetanus. This is usually given as part of early childhood immunization; it is highly effective.
■ Booster vaccinations every 10 years.
■ Cleaning wounds thoroughly, especially those contaminated with soil, and treating them with antiseptic. Deep puncture wounds,

which are especially likely to become infected, should be seen by your doctor, who may give you antibiotics to prevent infection.
■ A booster vaccination after any deep wound if your booster vaccinations aren't up to date.

See also:
• **Immunization timetable p.519**

Listeriosis

LISTERIOSIS IS A RARE INFECTION TRANSMITTED THROUGH CONTAMINATED FOOD. IT MAINLY AFFECTS VULNERABLE PEOPLE SUCH AS INFANTS, THE AGED, PREGNANT WOMEN (IN WHOM IT CAN CAUSE MISCARRIAGE) AND PEOPLE WITH A COMPROMISED IMMUNE SYSTEM.

The bacterium that causes listeriosis, *Listeria monocytogenes*, is widespread in the soil and is present in most animal species. **It can pass to humans through food products, particularly soft cheeses, milk, meat pastes and pre-packaged salads**. Storing food incorrectly increases the risk. The bacteria multiply in the intestines and may spread in the blood and affect other organs.

The symptoms of listeriosis vary from one person to another. The infection often goes unnoticed in healthy adults, although some

people may develop flu-like symptoms such as fever, sore throat, headache and aching muscles.

WHO IS AT RISK?

In elderly people and people with reduced immunity, such as those with HIV or those taking immunosuppressant drugs, listeriosis can lead to meningitis, a potentially fatal inflammation of the membranes covering the brain. In pregnant women, infection can pass to the fetus, causing miscarriage or stillbirth.

WHAT MIGHT BE DONE?

Listeriosis is usually diagnosed by a blood test. In otherwise healthy people, mild listeriosis clears up with treatment in a few days. People with serious infection, especially during pregnancy, need urgent treatment in hospital with **intravenous antibiotics**.

Hygienic handling and storage of food reduces the risk of listeriosis.

Rabies

RABIES IS A RARE BUT SERIOUS INFECTION OF THE NERVOUS SYSTEM, USUALLY TRANSMITTED IN SALIVA FROM A BITE BY AN INFECTED, RABID ANIMAL, USUALLY A DOG.

Rabies can be prevented by a vaccine, which is recommended for people working with animals in high-risk areas. All travellers in these areas should avoid contact with stray animals.

WHAT ARE THE SYMPTOMS?

An infected person may develop symptoms within 10 days to 2 months of a bite, although rarely the virus can lie dormant for several years. Rabies usually starts with flu-like symptoms that last for about 2–7 days, followed by:

● paralysis of the face and throat muscles
● extreme thirst
● painful throat spasms leading to an inability to drink and a fear of water
● disorientation and agitation
● loss of consciousness
● paralysis of the limbs.
Once symptoms have developed the condition is usually fatal.

WHAT MIGHT BE DONE?

There is no cure once the symptoms have developed. Diagnosis may not be obvious from the symptoms, and blood and saliva tests are usually done to confirm the presence of the virus.

Digestion

Image shows a coloured scanning electron micrograph of a section through the duodenum, with microvilli

Miriam's overview

It can be helpful to think of the digestive system as a tube running through the body with an opening at each end, the mouth at the top and the anus at the bottom.

The tube isn't a neat, constant shape throughout its course. It swells into a muscular storage organ at the stomach where the food you swallow is thoroughly mixed with digestive enzymes that start breaking it up into a form that the body can use.

At the exit from the stomach more essential digestive juices are added from the gallbladder and pancreas. Food particles get smaller and smaller until, in the exquisitely adapted small intestine (small only in diameter, not length) the tiniest fragments of nutrients can pass easily though the intestine wall straight into the bloodstream.

We hear a lot about the large intestine (large in diameter) or colon, or more familiar still, the bowel, because it seems to be the focus of many common complaints. Its function in the body is really very simple, it's there to ensure that precious nutrients and water aren't lost. Its main job is to absorb water from its fluid contents. When the stream of digested food leaves the small intestine it's liquid, very runny. When we pass it as a stool it's solid. Its passage through the large intestine has brought about this change, purely through the absorption of water.

The rectum too can absorb water from faeces, in fact, it will wring faeces dry if they stay in the rectum too long. So if the "call to stool" is ignored for any length of time faeces can become stony hard and difficult, even painful, to pass. This form of constipation is often thought of as a fault of the bowel or diet, but it isn't. It's simply due to not emptying the rectum soon enough. And it can be cured by heeding the call to stool as soon as you're aware of it, even though the pressure to ignore it and do something else is strong.

Laxatives aren't necessary to cure this type of constipation, only retraining yourself to heed what your bowel is telling you to do. If you don't, your bowel won't bother to send you the signal and your "constipation" will worsen.

If I were to try to pull out the headlines of what we've discovered over the last decade two topics would immediately spring to mind, both of them cancer, oesophageal cancer and bowel cancer.

The first is referable to heartburn. For decades heartburn has been thought of as nothing more than a mild irritation, a troublesome form of indigestion. In the last five or so years, however, we've come to realize that recurrent heartburn, especially if it's left untreated, can eventually result in malignant change of the lower end of the gullet where it enters the stomach.

It's caused by the chronic irritation from acid gastric contents, which regurgitate into the lower part of the oesophagus. Here, the lining has no protection from the burning effect of stomach acid. By contrast the stomach lining is covered with a thick protective layer of mucus, so acid never reaches the delicate walls of the stomach lining.

Rigorous treatment of heartburn can prevent cancerous change, so you must seek advice from your doctor if you have a long-term problem.

> "*we can help* the next generation by making *sure our children* eat the magic number of *five fruits a day*"

We know more and more about bowel cancer. In the UK it kills approximately 18,000 people every year and it's almost certainly due to the fact that our Western diet now contains too little fibre (mainly fruit and vegetables). We can help the next generation by making sure our children eat the magic number of five fruits a day.

There are two cardinal signs of bowel cancer. The first is seeing blood in your stool, though that's a rather late sign. Before that you'll probably have noticed a change in your bowel habits, going more or less often than you used to, a touch of constipation or diarrhoea where previously you had none. Or a sudden change in the shape of the stool – narrow where previously it had been round. This change in the bowel habit, in middle age or later, is a sign you must heed and discuss with your doctor.

Peptic ulcer now has a new cause. We used to think it was due to too much stomach acid. We now know it's due to an infection, a new infection, with *Helicobacter pylori*. Treatment has been revolutionized in the last 10 years. Now antibiotics are the lynchpin and, as the bacterium is difficult to eradicate, the course lasts a minimum of two weeks, along with other medicines to increase the effectiveness of the antibiotic. One course of treatment and nearly everyone is cured!

Now, that's an advance on the old days.

INSIDE
your digestive system

The digestive tract can be thought of as a single, long, irregular tube and consists of the **mouth** and **throat** (pharynx), **oesophagus**, **stomach**, **small** and **large intestines** (bowels) and the **anus**. Other organs that are not part of the digestive tract but are important to digestion are the **salivary glands**, the **liver**, the **pancreas** and the **gallbladder**.

Food enters the digestive tract at the mouth, where it is mashed by the **teeth** and mixed with **saliva**. It passes down the oesophagus to the stomach, where it is mixed with **digestive enzymes** and broken down further into a semi-liquid mixture. This mixture passes into the small intestine, where it is broken down into molecules that are absorbed into the blood via the liver. Indigestible material then passes into the large intestine, where some water is reabsorbed before it is excreted as faeces. The liver produces the digestive juice **bile**, which is stored in the gallbladder until it is released into the small intestine.

The pancreas also secretes a digestive juice and produces the hormone **insulin**.

the digestive system

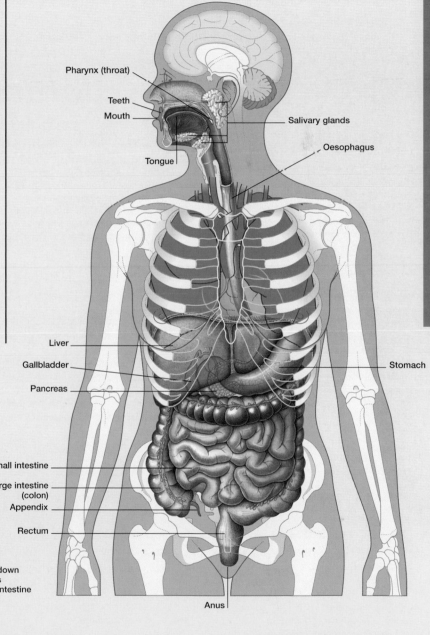

Pharynx (throat)
Teeth
Mouth
Tongue
Salivary glands
Oesophagus
Liver
Gallbladder
Pancreas
Stomach
Small intestine
Large intestine (colon)
Appendix
Rectum
Anus

the digestive process

Mouth
Gallbladder
Liver
Pancreas
Salivary glands
Oesophagus
Ingested food
Stomach
Duodenum
Nutrient breakdown as food passes through small intestine
Jejunum
Ileum
Rectum
Anus
Large intestine (colon)

KEY

Pancreatic fluids and bile

Food

Nutrient transfer to liver

As food passes through the digestive tract it is broken down into nutrients, which are absorbed by the small intestine, and water, which is absorbed by the large intestine. Nutrients pass to the liver in the bloodstream. Faeces form in the large intestine and collect in the rectum before excretion.

DISORDERS OF THE MOUTH, TONGUE AND OESOPHAGUS

It's difficult to know where to start discussing the digestive tract, which runs from mouth to anus. Should the most common conditions come first, in which case flatulence, indigestion, constipation and irritable bowel syndrome (IBS) would head the list? Or do we simply start at the top and work down? That's what I've chosen to do. Nonetheless, inclusion of topics is based on their importance, which itself relies heavily on commonness.

Digestion begins in the mouth, where food is crushed, minced by the teeth and the tongue, and mixed with saliva secreted by the salivary glands. Swallowing forces the food into the oesophagus and thence to the stomach by ripples of muscle contractions.

Causes of mouth ulcers

- The cause of mouth ulcers is not known, but they tend to occur in people who are run down or ill.
- They appear before menstruation in women.
- Mouth ulcers are often stress-related.
- Injuries to the lining of the mouth caused by ill-fitting dentures, a roughened tooth or by careless tooth brushing can also result in mouth ulcers.
- **Rarely**, recurrent mouth ulcers may be due to **anaemia**, a **deficiency** of either vitamin B_{12} or folic acid, an intestinal disorder such as **Crohn's disease** or **coeliac disease**, or **Behçet syndrome**, a rare autoimmune disorder.
- Ulcers may also occur as a result of specific infections, such as **herpes simplex infections**.
- Very rarely, an ulcer that **enlarges** slowly and does not heal may be **mouth** cancer.

Mouth ulcers

PAINFUL SORES IN THE LINING OF THE MOUTH, KNOWN AS MOUTH ULCERS OR APHTHOUS ULCERS, CAN BE EXCRUCIATINGLY PAINFUL.

Mouth ulcers are extremely common, especially in young people and during times of stress or illness. They are slightly more common in girls and women and sometimes run in families, suggesting that a genetic factor may be involved.

Mouth ulcers appear as shallow, grey-white pits with a red border and may occur singly or in clusters anywhere in the mouth. They can cause pain, often excruciating for the first few days and particularly when you are chewing spicy, hot or acidic food.

If they are very painful, mouth ulcers may deter eating and chewing, which in a child can look like loss of appetite. They may recur several times a year but they usually **disappear with or without treatment** within two weeks.

WHAT IS THE TREATMENT?

Mouth ulcers usually heal without treatment. Over-the-counter preparations containing a corticosteroid to reduce the inflammation combined with a local anaesthetic are available in lozenge, gel and paste form, which sticks to most surfaces.

NB If you have an ulcer that does not heal within three weeks, you should consult a doctor.

See also:
- **Anaemia p.236**
- **Crohn's disease p.366**
- **Herpes infections p.336**
- **Malabsorption p.365**

Gastroesophageal reflux, hiatus hernia, heartburn

IN GASTROESOPHAGEAL REFLUX, ACIDIC JUICES ARE REGURGITATED INTO THE OESOPHAGUS FROM THE STOMACH. THIS REGURGITATION CAUSES A PAIN OR DISCOMFORT IN THE UPPER ABDOMEN AND CHEST, KNOWN AS HEARTBURN. ONE CAUSE IS A HIATUS HERNIA.

Gastroesophageal reflux (GOR), commonly known as heartburn or acid reflux, is probably the most common cause of **indigestion**. The discomfort is due to acidic juices from the stomach flowing back up into the oesophagus (the gullet, the tube leading from the throat to the stomach). The lining of the oesophagus does not have adequate defence against the harmful effects of stomach acid, which causes inflammation,

sometimes even ulceration, and a burning pain known as **heartburn.**

Obesity, a high-fat diet, drinking too much coffee or alcohol and smoking are risk factors.

WHAT ARE THE CAUSES?

The stomach contents are prevented from entering the oesophagus by a double-action valve mechanism: the lower end of the oesophagus has a muscular ring, known as the

ower oesophageal sphincter**, which forms one part of the valve mechanism, and the other part consists of the **hiatus**, a narrow opening in the diaphragm muscle. The combination of these two muscular gateways provides an effective one-way valve.

GOR may develop as a result of several factors acting together to make the valve leak. These factors include:

- poor muscle tone in the sphincter

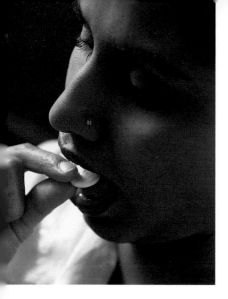

Dangerous heartburn

If heartburn (gastroesophageal reflux) is a daily occurrence it can develop into something far more serious. The irritating acid causes changes in the cells lining the lower end of the oesophagus, leading to a serious form of cancer.

The chances of getting cancer of the oesophagus is eight times higher in people who have chronic heartburn and it's increasing faster than almost any other cancer. So take your heartburn seriously and talk to your doctor about it. Simply taking antacids doesn't reduce the danger.

Gastroesophageal reflux

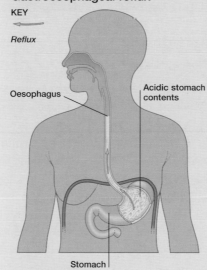

KEY

Reflux

Oesophagus

Acidic stomach contents

Stomach

In gastroesophageal reflux (GOR), the acidic contents of the stomach are regurgitated up into the oesophagus, which lacks the mucus lining of the stomach and becomes irritated.

The oesophagus isn't lined like the stomach and so stomach acid irritates the lower oesophagus and over time triggers pre-cancerous changes that can progress to cancer.

What's the connection between heartburn and cancer?

Researchers reported recently that having frequent, inadequately treated heartburn increased the risk of oesophageal cancer nearly eight-fold. Among those in the study who had particularly severe and long-standing heartburn the risk of cancer rose more than 40 times. The relationship was so strong, researchers concluded that chronic heartburn was likely to be the cause of this cancer.

Pre-cancerous changes in the oesophagus develop in 10–15 percent of patients with chronic heartburn, and these patients face a risk of cancer that is 30–40 times greater than the risk in the general population.

Heartburn is obviously a disease that demands more respect than it gets. It's estimated that at least half the people who suffer from chronic heartburn are not getting the kind of medical care that may protect them from the serious consequences found in the study. The overall risk of developing oesophageal cancer is very low, but only 5–10 patients out of 100 survive more than five years after getting the disease.

● increased abdominal pressure due to pregnancy or obesity

● a weakness in the hiatus that allows part of the stomach to slide into the chest (a **hiatus hernia**).

Many people develop mild attacks of GOR after eating rapidly or eating certain foods, especially pickles, fried or fatty meals, or drinks, especially carbonated soft drinks, alcohol or coffee. Smoking worsens symptoms too.

WHAT ARE THE SYMPTOMS?

The main symptoms of GOR are usually most noticeable immediately after eating a large meal or when bending over. They include:

● a burning pain or discomfort in the centre of the chest behind the breastbone, known as heartburn

● an acidic taste in the mouth due to regurgitation of acidic fluid into the throat or mouth

● erosion of the teeth due to acid

● persistent cough and sometimes asthma at night and sore throat

● hoarseness of the voice

● belching

● streaks of blood in the vomit or faeces.

GOR that persists over many years can cause scarring in the oesophagus, which may eventually be severe enough to cause stricture (narrowing). A stricture can make swallowing very difficult and may lead to weight loss. Chronic GOR may lead to the oesophageal lining replacing the stomach lining, increasing the risk of developing oesophageal cancer.

WHAT IS THE TREATMENT?

The good news is that many products and treatments are now available to alleviate chronic heartburn and prevent stomach acid from damaging cells of the oesophagus, which have no protection against a frequent bath of acid.

■ Acid reflux may also be aggravated by drugs you can take for other conditions, so consult your doctor about the effects of both over-the-counter and prescription medications you take

and ask whether substitutions may be helpful.

■ More severe cases that do not respond to diet and lifestyle changes alone require medication, starting with over-the-counter antacids. Histamine blockers such as Tagamet (cimetidine) and Zantac (ranitidine) help, but may not be strong enough to control acid reflux fully. If not, your doctor can prescribe more potent acid suppressors called proton-pump inhibitors, such as Losec. Other potentially useful drugs protect the lining of the oesophagus and speed stomach emptying.

■ If acid reflux cannot be controlled through diet, habits and drugs, surgery may be required.

■ One of the newest procedures, done through a laparoscope, involves wrapping a defective oesophageal sphincter to strengthen it against reflux.

Experts agree that it's not enough merely to calm all the symptoms of heartburn. Rather, acid reflux must be prevented and any cellular damage that has occurred must be healed.

It isn't enough to treat chronic heartburn sporadically, stopping treatment when symptoms subside. It has to be long-term. To protect the oesophagus adequately, treatment must be aggressive, continuous and indefinite and so involves some major changes to your life.

■ If you have heartburn two or more times in a week, see your doctor and perhaps request a consultation with a gastroenterologist.

■ If the problem has been long-standing, an examination and biopsy of the oesophagus through an endoscope is the only good way to assess what damage has been done, if any. If there are abnormal cell changes, endoscopic examinations should be done every year or two to check for possible progression towards cancer.

■ Should a pre-cancerous condition develop, the oesophagus can be removed and replaced with a piece of intestine or stomach. There are also experimental treatments that use laser or other forms of heat to obliterate the abnormal cells and allow healthy cells to replace them.

See also:
• Endoscopy p.353
• Indigestion p.353

Easing chronic heartburn

If you have chronic heartburn:

■ Chew food well, and eat slowly.
■ Watch what you eat. Stay away from or limit spicy or fatty foods, as well as chocolate, citrus juice, coffee, tea and alcohol.
■ Eat five or six small meals rather than two large meals a day.
■ Immediately after a meal, avoid exercising, bending over or lying down.
■ Lose weight if you need to.
■ You will feel better if there is some food in your stomach, so eat little and often.
■ Raise the head of your bed by about four inches or sleep on at least four pillows.

■ Antacid tablets will help to neutralize the acids and protect the oesophagus.
■ Give up smoking.
■ Consult your doctor if the problem occurs two or more times a week.

If you have recently developed pain in the centre of your chest that seems to be unrelated to mealtimes, you should seek immediate medical help because the heart condition angina may sometimes be mistaken for the pain of severe heartburn.

THE STOMACH AND DUODENUM

When you think about it, the stomach and the duodenum (the short first part of the small intestine) are exposed to quite a few potentially irritating substances, including acid produced by the stomach to help digest food, alcohol and hot foods such as spices. The stomach and duodenum have a natural defence mechanism that protects against damage, but sometimes the mechanism fails, leading to disease.

The two most common conditions that affect the stomach and duodenum are **indigestion** and **peptic ulcer**. We now know that peptic ulcers (ulcers of the duodenum and the stomach) are caused by a **bacterium** and symptoms are made worse by excess stomach acid. The importance of the *Helicobacter pylori* bacterium was only recognized in the early 1980s and it is now estimated that about half the world's population is infected with *H. pylori*. In most people there are no symptoms but others can develop **gastritis**, which is inflammation of the lining of the stomach, **peptic ulcer** and **stomach cancer**, a cancer with a rather poor outlook. *H. pylori* infection can usually be treated successfully with drugs.

Indigestion (dyspepsia)

PAIN OR DISCOMFORT IN THE UPPER ABDOMEN BROUGHT ON BY EATING IS COMMONLY KNOWN AS INDIGESTION. THE MEDICAL NAME IS DYSPEPSIA. THERE ARE VARIOUS CAUSES, AND STRESS, BEING OVERWEIGHT, SMOKING AND CERTAIN DIETARY HABITS ARE RISK FACTORS.

WHAT ARE THE SYMPTOMS?
Indigestion is a rag-bag word covering many upper abdominal symptoms related to eating food, including heartburn, fullness, discomfort, pain, nausea, flatulence and belching.

For most people it's a feeling of discomfort induced by eating too much, too quickly or by eating very rich, spicy or fatty food.

"Nervous" indigestion can be a reaction to stress and it can be a symptom of peptic ulcer, gallstones or heartburn.

WHAT IS THE TREATMENT?
■ Eat small meals often or at least regularly three times a day.
■ Avoid foods and situations that bring on indigestion.
■ Take an antacid when symptoms start.
■ See your doctor if you need to take antacids often or if your pain lasts longer than a few hours.
■ Indigestion starting suddenly in middle age must always be investigated to exclude stomach cancer.

See also:
• Gallstones p.357
• GOR, hiatus hernia, heartburn p.360
• Peptic ulcer p.353

Preventing indigestion

Some measures can be taken to prevent or reduce the frequency of episodes of indigestion. You may find some of the following helpful.

■ Eat small portions of food at regular intervals without rushing or overfilling your stomach.

■ Avoid eating in the three hours before going to bed to allow your body enough time to digest food.

■ Reduce or eliminate your intake of alcohol, coffee and tea.

■ Avoid rich, fatty foods such as butter and fried foods.

■ Keep a food diary to help identify foods that cause indigestion.

■ Learn to overcome stress, which can often trigger episodes of indigestion (see Relaxation, p.292).

■ Try to lose excess weight and avoid tight-fitting clothing.

■ If possible, avoid medicines that irritate the digestive tract, such as aspirin and non-steroidal anti-inflammatory drugs (NSAIDs).

Peptic ulcer

A PEPTIC ULCER OCCURS WHEN THE TISSUE LINING THE STOMACH OR DUODENUM IS ERODED BY ACIDIC DIGESTIVE JUICES. PEPTIC ULCERS ARE ALSO CALLED STOMACH (OR GASTRIC) ULCERS OR DUODENAL ULCERS, DEPENDING ON THEIR LOCATION.

The lining of the stomach and duodenum (the first part of the small intestine) is normally protected from the effects of acidic digestive juices by a barrier of mucus. If this barrier is damaged, acid may cause inflammation and erosion of the lining. The resulting eroded areas are known as peptic ulcers, and there are two different types: duodenal ulcers and stomach (gastric) ulcers.

Stomach ulcers are more common over age 50 but **duodenal** ulcers are more common in men between the ages of 20 and 45. Duodenal ulcers sometimes run in families, and stress, excess alcohol and smoking are risk factors. About 1 in 10 people in the UK develops an ulcer at some time.

WHAT ARE THE CAUSES?

■ Peptic ulcers are most commonly associated with *Helicobacter pylori* infection. This bacterium releases chemicals that increase gastric acid secretion. Acidic digestive juices are then more likely to erode the lining of the stomach or the duodenum, which allows peptic ulcers to develop.

■ Peptic ulcers may sometimes result from the long-term use of aspirin or non-steroidal anti-inflammatory drugs (NSAIDs), such as **ibuprofen**, that damage the lining of the stomach.

■ Other factors that may lead to peptic ulcers include smoking and alcohol.

In some people, there is a strong family history of peptic ulcers, suggesting that a gene may be at work.

NB It is currently thought that psychological stress is probably not one of the primary causes of peptic ulcers; however, it may make an existing ulcer worse.

WHAT ARE THE SYMPTOMS?

Many people with a peptic ulcer do not experience symptoms or dismiss their discomfort as indigestion or heartburn. Those with persistent symptoms may notice:

● pain or discomfort that is felt in the centre of the upper abdomen, often just under the tip of the breastbone

● pain going through to the back

● loss of appetite and weight loss

● a feeling of fullness in the abdomen

● nausea and sometimes vomiting.

Pain comes in attacks and is often present for several weeks and then disappears for months or even years. The pain from a duodenal ulcer can be worse **before** meals

Contrast X-rays

In a contrast X-ray, a substance known as a contrast medium is introduced into the body to help an organ show up better on X-ray film. Contrast media, such as barium, are harmless and are expelled or absorbed by the body after the X-ray has been taken. They are usually given as a drink but may sometimes be given as an injection. A few people may experience a flushing sensation when a contrast medium is injected.

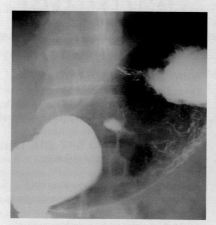

Mass of barium in the digestive tract

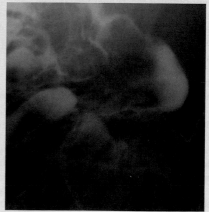

Barium solution coating the intestinal lining

increasing pain. Acute pancreatitis may also lead to shock, a potentially fatal condition in which the blood pressure falls dangerously low.

Blood tests, a computerized tomography (CT) scan or endoscopy of the pancreas (ERCP; see box, right) may be used to confirm a diagnosis of acute pancreatitis.

WHAT IS THE TREATMENT?

■ Your stomach will be kept empty to prevent the pancreas from being stimulated to produce more enzymes. A tube will be passed through your nose into your stomach to remove its contents by suction.

■ You will be given fluids intravenously. If tests have detected a gallstone, ERCP may locate the stone more precisely and remove it.

■ Rarely, if damaged pancreatic tissue becomes infected, surgical drainage may be needed.

■ If the pancreatitis was caused by gallstones, it may be advisable to have your gallbladder removed once you have recovered.

WHAT IS THE OUTLOOK?

About 9 in 10 people survive an attack of acute pancreatitis, but the gland may be damaged so that it is unable to produce adequate amounts of enzymes and you develop **malabsorption syndrome**. You may then need to take enzyme supplements for the rest of your life.

> **See also:**
> • **CT scanning p.401** • **Gallstones p.357**
> • **Inherited hyperlipidaemia p.223**
> • **Shock p.560**

TEST

ERCP

Endoscopic retrograde cholangio-pancreatography (ERCP) is used to look for problems in the bile ducts and pancreatic duct. A contrast dye is injected into the ducts via an endoscope passed through the mouth and the path of the dye is then tracked on X-ray images. Doctors can also look directly down the endoscope. The procedure is done in hospital under a general anaesthetic and takes about an hour.

Pancreatic cancer

PANCREATIC CANCER IS A MALIGNANT TUMOUR OF THE MAIN TISSUE OF THE PANCREAS. SMOKING, A HIGH-FAT DIET AND ALCOHOL ABUSE ARE RISK FACTORS.

Pancreatic cancer is more common over age 50 and almost twice as common in men. Cancer of the pancreas is a relatively uncommon cancer, with about 7000 new cases diagnosed in the UK each year. The tumour may be symptomless in its early stages.

WHAT ARE THE SYMPTOMS?

Symptoms often develop gradually over a few months and may include:

• pain in the upper abdomen that radiates to the back

• loss of weight

• reduced appetite.

Many pancreatic tumours cause obstruction of the bile ducts through which the digestive liquid bile leaves the liver. Such blockage leads to **jaundice**, in which the skin and whites of

the eyes turn yellow. Jaundice may be accompanied by itching, dark-coloured urine and lighter than normal faeces.

WHAT IS THE TREATMENT?

Surgery to remove part, or all, of the pancreas offers the only chance of cure. However, the cancer has usually spread by the time it is diagnosed. In such cases, surgery to relieve symptoms may be possible. For example, if the bile duct is obstructed by a tumour, a rigid tube known as a stent may be inserted to keep the duct open. This procedure is usually done during endoscopic examination of the pancreas (ERCP; see box, above) and helps to reduce jaundice. Treatment such as chemotherapy and radiotherapy may be used to slow the progress of the disease.

Pain can often be relieved with analgesics. Severe pain may be treated by a nerve block, a procedure using an injection of a chemical to inactivate the nerves supplying the pancreas.

WHAT IS THE OUTLOOK?

In many cases, pancreatic cancer is not diagnosed until it is far advanced, at which time the outlook is poor. Fewer than 1 in 50 people survives more than five years. Even with surgery, only 1 in 10 people survives more than five years. Most people survive for less than a year.

> **See also:**
> • **Chemotherapy p.257** • **Jaundice p.355**
> • **Radiotherapy p.395**

DISORDERS OF THE INTESTINES, RECTUM AND ANUS

Irritable bowel syndrome (IBS) is probably the most common bowel condition in the West along with its symptoms of **flatulence** and **bloating**. **Constipation** and **diarrhoea** are almost as common, and then **diverticulosis** and **diverticulitis**, which arise as a consequence of ageing. Malabsorption, such as occurs with **lactose intolerance** and **coeliac disease**, can leave the body short of important nutrients. When the bowel becomes inflamed, **Crohn's disease** and **ulcerative colitis** may result. Finally, **colorectal cancer**, a common cause of death in the West, and disorders of the rectum and anus, such as **haemorrhoids** and **anal fissure**, are covered.

Flatulence and bloating

MOST OF US OCCASIONALLY EXPERIENCE THE EMBARRASSMENT OF BREAKING WIND (FLATULENCE), BUT FOR SOME IT CAN BE A RECURRING AND DISTRESSING PROBLEM. SWELLING OF THE ABDOMEN DUE TO A BUILD UP OF GAS (BLOATING) MAY ACCOMPANY THE MENOPAUSE.

FLATULENCE

This is a feature of many gastrointestinal conditions, in particular **indigestion** and **irritable bowel syndrome (IBS)**, which is said to affect at least a fifth of the population. However, there are other symptoms with IBS, including pain, constipation or diarrhoea or a mixture of both, and as these symptoms also occur in more serious bowel conditions it is important to have them checked out by a doctor. Self-diagnosis is not a good idea. Flatulence is also a feature of **diverticulosis** and **diverticulitis** and can be a problem in pregnancy. Menopausal women are also prone to flatulence due to lack of oestrogen.

WHAT CAN BE DONE TO BRING RELIEF?

Thankfully there is quite a lot we can do to help ourselves. The most common cause of wind is what we eat. So you should look very carefully at your diet. Keep fry-ups to a minimum as these are not only unhealthy in themselves, they are also a frequent cause of wind. Baked beans and peas are notorious for causing wind but there are other foods and drinks that should also be taken in moderation.

■ Eat more fish and skinless white meat instead of red meat.

■ Allow enough time to sit down and have a meal rather than snacking on the hoof, as gulping food and drink is often responsible for a bad bout of wind.

■ For those who are lactose intolerant, milk can cause excessive gas and replacing cow's milk with calcium-fortified soya drinks often helps.

■ As we age, small pockets of tissue may balloon out from the bowel, giving rise to the conditions known as diverticulosis and diverticulitis. Within these small pockets bacteria may accumulate, ferment carbohydrates and produce large amounts of gas.

■ Try to eat foods that can affect fermentation, such as those containing yeast and sugar, only in the early part of the day. A yeast-free alternative to regular bread would be crackers, rice cakes or soda bread.

■ Charcoal tablets available from chemists can provide immediate relief by absorbing gas.

■ Natural herbs and spices contain substances that calm the bowels and prevent a build-up of wind. These include aniseed, camomile, lemon balm, fennel, dill, cloves, black pepper, marjoram, parsley, peppermint, rosemary and spearmint. Use them as a garnish on food or as a soothing, herbal tea.

■ Gulping mouthfuls of air can cause or aggravate wind. If you are inclined to do this, try and break yourself of the habit and you may find the flatulence gradually becomes less frequent. Gum chewing, for example, causes us to take in air.

■ Stress is another important factor in flatulence and if you are feeling stressed you need to identify the reason so you can find effective ways of reducing anxiety. However, as a short-term solution studies have shown essential oil of lavender can reduce stress. Use five or six drops in a bath or on a tissue.

■ Exercise can help reduce wind as it tones up our stomach muscles and prevents our intestine being able to swell up so much that it holds large pockets of wind. Exercise is also very good for relieving stress and even a walk round the block is beneficial, although it isn't sensible to exercise within two hours of eating.

■ For some, an upset in bowel bacteria is a problem. Reducing sugar and yeast, for example in bread, wine and beer, may help, along with a supply of beneficial lactobacillus bacteria from a daily pot of "live" yoghurt.

BLOATING

Bloating with abdominal swelling may be a problem during the menopausal years. It is usually due to **gas** in the large intestine, produced by fermentation in the bowel. As we age, small pockets of tissue may balloon out from the bowel, giving rise to the condition called **diverticulosis**. Within these small pockets bacteria may accumulate, ferment carbohydrates and produce large amounts of gas. The intestine may end up coated with food remnants that form small centres of fermentation.

It is quite common to wake in the morning with a flat stomach and for the abdomen to swell as the day progresses so that by bedtime the swelling resembles a six-month pregnancy! During the night lack of food and sugar in the intestine allows fermentation to abate. After a breakfast that contains sugars and yeasts, fermentation in the bowel flares up again.

WHAT CAN YOU DO TO EASE THE PROBLEM?

■ Try to eat foods with yeast and sugar in the early part of the day only to see if that helps.

■ A high-fibre diet, plenty of fluids and frequent exercise will keep the bowels normal.

■ Try to eat a pot of "live" yoghurt each day.

See also:
• **Diverticulosis and diverticulitis p.364**
• **Indigestion p.352**
• **Irritable bowel syndrome p.362**
• **The menopause p.497**

■ If the ulcerative colitis has spread further up the colon, you will be given the drugs to take orally.

■ If you have severe, sudden attacks of the disorder, your doctor will probably prescribe corticosteroids to be taken orally or as an enema. Long-term use of corticosteroids may cause side effects, such as weight gain and a moon-shaped face. For this reason, the doctor will reduce the dose once your symptoms start to subside and stop the treatment as soon as possible.

SURGERY

■ Surgical treatment is usually necessary for people who experience persistent symptoms despite treatment with drugs.

■ Surgery may be recommended for people who have a sudden, severe attack that does not respond to medical treatment.

■ Surgery may be advisable for people with an increased risk of colorectal cancer. Surgery usually involves the removal of the diseased colon and rectum and creation of a stoma, which is an artificial opening in the abdominal wall through which the small intestine can expel faeces. This procedure is called ileostomy.

■ A newer procedure called a pouch operation is suitable for some people. In this procedure, part of the small intestine is used to create a pouch that connects the small intestine to the anus. This procedure avoids the need for a stoma, but the pouch may become inflamed and the frequency of bowel movements often increases.

WHAT IS THE OUTLOOK?

Some people have only one attack of ulcerative colitis, but most have recurring episodes. About 1 in 5 people needs to have surgery. Colorectal cancer (see below) is the greatest long-term risk, and it eventually develops in about 1 in 6 people whose entire rectum and colon have been affected for 25 years or more. If you have long-standing, extensive ulcerative colitis but have not had surgery, you will need a yearly colonoscopy to detect possible early warning signs of colorectal cancer.

See also:
• **Ankylosing spondylitis p.430**
• **Arthritis p.427**
• **Colostomy and ileostomy p.367**

Colorectal cancer

COLORECTAL CANCER, SOMETIMES CALLED BOWEL CANCER, IS THE GENERAL TERM FOR CANCEROUS TUMOURS OF THE LINING OF THE COLON OR THE RECTUM.

Cancer of the colon (bowel) occurs more often in women but cancer of the rectum is more common in men. Colorectal cancer is a disease of middle and late age. A high-fat, low-fibre diet, alcohol abuse and obesity are risk factors. Taking regular exercise may help to prevent colon cancer.

Colorectal cancer is the **second most common cause of cancer deaths** in the West. It is also one of the few cancers that can be detected at an early stage by screening people thought to be at risk. When it is detected early enough, the disease can often be successfully treated by surgery.

Colorectal cancer is rare under age 40 and most cases occur in people over age 60. Cancer can occur anywhere in the colon or rectum, but about 3 in 5 tumours develop in the part of the colon **nearest the rectum**.

WHAT ARE THE CAUSES?

In less affluent countries, where people traditionally live on a high-fibre diet consisting mainly of cereals and fruit and vegetables, colorectal cancer is rare. However, a typical Western diet, which tends to be high in meat and animal fats and low in fibre, seems to increase the risk of developing colorectal cancer. It is not known how fibre in the diet reduces the risk of the disorder. A possible explanation is that dietary fibre shortens the time that it takes for waste matter to pass through the intestines. As a result, potentially cancer-causing substances (known as carcinogens) in food are expelled from the body at a faster rate. Other lifestyle factors, such as **excessive consumption of alcohol**, **obesity** and **lack of exercise** may also contribute to the risk of developing colorecteral cancer. Inflammatory disorders affecting the large intestine, such as **ulcerative colitis** or **Crohn's disease**, can also increase the risk of developing colorectal cancer if they are long-standing.

GENETICS

About 1 in 8 cases of colorectal cancer is hereditary. Most of these cases are caused by inheritance of an abnormal gene. People who have this gene are at increased risk of developing a form of cancer known as **hereditary non-polyposis colorectal cancer** (HNPCC). Rarely, colorectal cancer may be caused by the inherited disorder **familial adenomatous polyposis** (FAP), in which polyps form inside the large intestine. In FAP, there is a 9 in 10 chance that some of the polyps will become cancerous over time. Another gene may cause a **triad of cancers** of **breast, ovary** and **colon** when it runs through a family.

All members of such a family should have regular screening for all three cancers.

WHAT ARE THE SYMPTOMS?

The symptoms of colorectal cancer vary depending on the site of the tumour. They include the following:

• changes in the frequency of bowel movements or in the general consistency of the faeces; **any change over the age of 50 should be reported to your doctor**

• abdominal pain

• blood in the faeces – always report this to your doctor

• rectal discomfort or a sensation of incomplete emptying of the rectum

• loss of appetite.

The symptoms of colorectal cancer may be mistaken for the symptoms of a less serious disorder, such as **haemorrhoids**. If there is heavy loss of blood from the rectum, iron-deficiency anaemia may result. As the tumour grows bigger, it may eventually cause intestinal obstruction.

You should consult your doctor without delay if you notice an obvious change in your bowel habits or blood in your faeces. Left untreated, colorectal cancer will eventually spread via the bloodstream to the lymph nodes, liver and other organs in the body.

HOW IS IT DIAGNOSED?

■ Colorectal cancer is often diagnosed during screening before symptoms have developed.

■ If you do have symptoms, your doctor may first feel your abdomen to detect swelling.

■ A rectal examination, in which a gloved

WARNING:

■ People with a family history of colorectal cancer should be screened from age 40.

■ An annual faecal occult blood test is advised for people over age 50 who have a family history of the disease, in addition to sigmoidoscopy (a form of colonoscopy) every 3–5 years.

Faecal tests

The faeces may be examined for small amounts of blood that can't be seen by the naked eye. This blood, known as occult blood because it isn't immediately visible, can indicate a disorder that causes bleeding from the digestive tract, such as a peptic ulcer, polyps in the colon or bowel cancer. The test is usually repeated several times over a period of several days because blood may not appear in every sample. If blood is found in the faeces, other tests may be done to look for the cause, including endoscopy of the digestive tract and contrast X-rays to look for ulcers or tumours.

finger is inserted into the rectum, may also be done to see if a tumour can be felt.
■ A stool sample is tested for the presence of blood.
■ A blood sample may be tested for anaemia.
■ The rectum may be examined visually with a viewing instrument inserted through the anus.
■ Your doctor may also arrange for a colonoscopy, in which a flexible viewing instrument is used to examine the entire colon.
■ A biopsy may be taken (in which a small sample of tissue is removed for microscopic examination) during the procedure.
■ You may also have a contrast X-ray in which a barium enema is used to detect an abnormality of the rectum or colon.

If a cancerous tumour is detected, you will probably need to have computerized tomography (CT) scanning to see if the cancer has spread to the lymph nodes in the abdomen or to the liver.

SCREENING
The aim of all screening is to detect disease before symptoms appear. So it's an early warning system.

There are several ways of screening for bowel cancer that are currently being investigated.

Scientists at the Imperial Cancer Research Fund are testing a technique to detect small growths that can be removed before they develop into cancer.

WHAT IS THE TREATMENT?
Treatment for colorectal cancer may involve surgery and/or chemotherapy.

SURGERY
Surgery is the primary treatment for colorectal cancer. If the cancer hasn't spread beyond the wall of the bowel, no further therapy is needed and you'll generally make a full recovery. Unfortunately, cancer is hard to control once it has spread. The search is always going on for more effective ways of treating advanced disease and preventing cancer from spreading in the first place.

CHEMOTHERAPY
A new technique of giving the anticancer drug **5-fluorouracil** (5-FU) directly to the liver after surgery may improve survival in bowel cancer that's spread, and the results of a nationwide trial are due to be released soon.

Another drug, **irinotecan**, has been found to control the spread of colorectal cancer in over 50 percent of patients who had not responded to, or who had relapsed after, conventional treatment with 5-FU.

Trials in America have already shown that the drug **oxaliplatin** could be used as a first-line treatment in cases of advanced colorectal cancer.

Other results suggest that patients may respond better to the traditional treatment with 5-FU if it's given with oxaliplatin. It may be that these drugs given in combination are more effective than either of them given alone.

Studies are underway to identify the best dose and the most effective timing for giving the combination.

See also:
• Anaemias p.236 • CT scanning p.401
• Crohn's disease p.366
• Haemorrhoids p.370
• Ulcerative colitis p.367

Anal itching (pruritus ani)

ANAL ITCHING, KNOWN MEDICALLY AS PRURITUS ANI, IS A FAIRLY COMMON CONDITION THAT MAY OCCUR EITHER IN OR MORE OFTEN AROUND THE ANUS.

Anal itching is rarely serious, although it may be embarrassing and difficult to treat. It may be either localized around the anus or be part of generalized itching. In postmenopausal women, pruritus ani is often associated with itching around the vagina (pruritus vulvae). The condition may be worse in older people because their skin is drier, less elastic and more easily irritated.

WHAT ARE THE CAUSES?
The most common cause of anal itching is **candida** (moniliasis, thrush) with redness and scaling of the adjacent skin. Localized itching may also be caused by poor personal hygiene, **haemorrhoids** or **threadworm infestation**. Generalized itching around the anal area may be a symptom of a skin disease such as psoriasis or eczema or be due to an **allergic reaction** to a substance such as laundry detergent or washing soap. Once the skin has been thickened by chronic scratching (neurodermatitis) it's very difficult to break the itch-scratch-itch cycle.

SELF-HELP
There are several measures you can take to relieve anal itching.
■ It is important to keep the anal area clean by washing and drying carefully (but not excessively) after a bowel movement.
■ Avoid using **soaps** that irritate the skin, and try **not to scratch** because it will worsen the itching.
■ A warm bath or shower before bed may soothe night-time itching.
■ **Loose underclothes** made of **natural fibres** are less likely than synthetic materials to cause irritation.
■ An over-the-counter cream containing a mild **topical corticosteroid** may give relief.
■ Itching that lasts for longer than three days should be assessed by a doctor.

Your doctor may examine your anus and arrange for tests to look for causes that need treatment. For example, severe haemorrhoids may need to be removed.

See also:
• Candidiasis p.450 • Eczema p.312
• Haemorrhoids p.370 • Psoriasis p.448
• Worms p.458

Haemorrhoids

SWOLLEN VEINS INSIDE THE RECTUM AND AROUND THE ANUS ARE KNOWN AS HAEMORRHOIDS
OR PILES. THEY ARE MORE COMMON DURING PREGNANCY AND AFTER CHILDBIRTH.
BEING OVERWEIGHT AND EATING A LOW-FIBRE DIET ARE RISK FACTORS.

Haemorrhoids are a common problem, affecting up to half of all people at some time in their lives. In this disorder, veins in the soft tissues around the anus and inside the lower part of the rectum become swollen. Swellings around the anus are called **external haemorrhoids**, and those within the rectum are called **internal haemorrhoids**. Internal haemorrhoids that protrude outside the anus are known as **prolapsing haemorrhoids** and can be especially painful.

Haemorrhoids often cause bleeding, itching and discomfort. These symptoms are usually intermittent, and the condition is not in itself serious. However, a single so-called "sentinal" haemorrhoid may be a sign of colorectal cancer.

WHAT ARE THE CAUSES?

■ Haemorrhoids most commonly occur as a result of **constipation** when a person strains to pass stools. Straining in this way increases the pressure inside the abdomen, which in turn causes blood vessels around the rectum to swell.
■ Being overweight also **exerts pressure on blood vessels** and increases the risk of haemorrhoids.
■ During **pregnancy** the growing fetus has the same effect, frequently causing haemorrhoids.

WHAT ARE THE SYMPTOMS?

The symptoms of haemorrhoids commonly develop following constipation. They include:
● fresh blood on toilet paper or in the toilet after a bowel movement
● increasing discomfort on defecation
● discharge of mucus from the anus, sometimes leading to itching
● visible swellings around the anus
● feeling that the bowels have not been fully emptied.

A prolapsing haemorrhoid may protrude through the anus after a bowel movement and may then retract or can be pushed back inside with a finger. In some cases, a blood clot (thrombus) may form within a prolapsing haemorrhoid, causing severe pain and a visible, tender, blue, grape-sized swelling.

If you have bleeding from the anus consult your doctor without delay, especially if you are over 40, since it may indicate a more serious disorder, such as **colorectal cancer**.

WHAT MIGHT BE DONE?

■ Your doctor will probably examine your rectum by inserting a gloved finger.
■ If there has been bleeding that suggests a serious underlying disease, your doctor may arrange for colonoscopy.
■ Small haemorrhoids usually do not need treatment.
■ Haemorrhoids due to pregnancy usually disappear soon after the birth.
■ A high-fibre diet helps prevent constipation, and laxatives may help ease defecation.
■ Over-the-counter topical corticosteroids and corticosteroid suppositories can reduce swelling and itching, and anaesthetic sprays may relieve pain. If these measures are not effective within a few days, you should consult your doctor, who may consider surgery.
■ Small internal haemorrhoids may be treated by **sclerotherapy**, in which the affected area is injected with a solution that causes the veins to shrink.
■ Alternatively, the doctor may place a band around the base of an internal haemorrhoid, causing it to shrink and fall off.
■ Persistent, painful bleeding haemorrhoids can be destroyed by electrical, laser or infrared heat treatment. They can also be removed surgically.

Haemorrhoids may recur, although treatment is usually successful.

> See also:
> ● Colorectal cancer p.368
> ● Constipation p.363

Anal fissure

AN ANAL FISSURE IS A SMALL TEAR IN THE ANUS THAT IS
PREVENTED FROM HEALING BECAUSE THE SPHINCTER
(ANAL MUSCLE RING) GOES INTO SPASM AND HOLDS IT OPEN. THE
PROBLEM IS USUALLY CAUSED BY PASSING A LARGE, DRY STOOL.

I'm including this condition because it causes pain disproportionate to its significance. Anal fissure may be so excruciatingly painful that sufferers suspect the worst and fear they may have colorectal cancer. A visit to the doctor can be entirely reassuring so seek advice and put your mind at rest.

SELF-HELP

■ Use bulk-forming agents to soften the stool.
■ Eat a high-fibre diet to overcome constipation.
■ Use a local anaesthetic cream to ease pain and promote healing.

Hernias

A HERNIA, COMMONLY CALLED A RUPTURE, IS USUALLY THE PROTRUSION OF A BIT OF THE INTESTINE THROUGH A WEAKENED MUSCLE. OBESITY AND LIFTING HEAVY WEIGHTS MAY BE RISK FACTORS. DIFFERENT TYPES ARE NAMED ACCORDING TO WHERE THEY OCCUR.

Hernias most often occur at sites in the abdomen where there is a weakness in the muscles. If pressure in the abdomen is increased due to causes such as lifting heavy weights, persistent coughing or straining at defecation, the muscles of the abdomen become stretched at the weak point. A visible bulge can then develop, which may contain fatty tissue or part of the intestine. Abdominal hernias are frequently found in men who have heavy manual jobs.

WHAT ARE THE TYPES?

Hernias are classified according to the site where they occur in the body. Some types occur more often in men; others are more frequently found in women.

INGUINAL HERNIA

This type of hernia occurs when a portion of the intestine pushes through into the inguinal canal, which is a weak spot in the abdominal muscle wall. The hernia causes a visible bulge in the **groin** or **scrotum**. These hernias usually affect men, but sometimes occur in women.

FEMORAL HERNIA

This type of hernia occurs in the part of the groin where the femoral vein and artery pass from the lower abdomen to the thigh. Women who are overweight or who have had several pregnancies are at increased risk of these hernias because their abdominal muscles are weakened.

UMBILICAL HERNIA

Babies may be born with an umbilical hernia, which develops behind the navel due to a weakness in the abdominal wall. Hernias that develop near the navel are known as para-umbilical hernias and are most common in women who are overweight or who have had several pregnancies.

OTHER TYPES OF HERNIA

Epigastric hernias develop in the midline between the navel and the breastbone and are three times more common in men.

Incisional hernias may develop after **abdominal** surgery if there is weakness around the scar. Risk factors include being overweight and having several operations through the same incision.

WHAT MIGHT BE DONE?

Your doctor may be able to feel a hernia by examining the abdomen or groin. Even small hernias eventually need to be repaired because if they are left untreated, they may become strangulated. The type of operation depends largely on the size of the hernia and on your age and general health. Some procedures are done under local anaesthesia as day surgery. Umbilical hernias in babies can usually be left untreated since they tend to disappear naturally by the age of five.

Surgery is usually effective. However, a hernia may recur in the same place or elsewhere. After surgery, you may be advised to avoid strenuous activity for a few weeks. You can help prevent a recurrence by losing excess weight, doing gentle exercise and avoiding constipation.

See also:
• **Constipation** p.363

Types of hernia

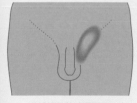
INGUINAL HERNIA

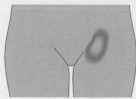
FEMORAL HERNIA

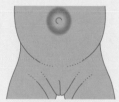
UMBILICAL HERNIA

Kidneys and Bladder

Image shows a coloured X-ray urogram of urine in a healthy human bladder

Miriam's overview

One of the most dramatic scenarios of the whole of modern medicine involves the kidneys – kidney failure, renal dialysis and organ transplant. Patients who would once have died can now miraculously be pulled back from the brink.

A triumph of modern medicine, yes, but on a much wider scale, more minor conditions bring untold discomfort and social embarrassment. I'm referring to cystitis and incontinence.

More than three million women in the UK suffer from incontinence largely as the result of childbirth, including women as young as 30.

I get hundreds of letters from young women embarrassed by incontinence and distressed that they could be looking at another 40 years with this upsetting condition. Few women know that simple pelvic floor exercises can remedy incontinence, especially if they're done frequently each day. This applies to women of all ages. Research shows that pelvic floor exercises can make a huge difference even in women as old as 80 years.

Few women are aware that the bladder needs oestrogen to keep it healthy and so bladder symptoms arising at the menopause are due in great measure to oestrogen deficiency. Furthermore they will respond to oestrogen

> "*pelvic floor exercises* can make a *huge difference* even in women as old as *80 years*"

used locally (creams and pessaries inserted into the vagina). A woman doesn't have to take HRT by mouth if she doesn't want to in order to clear her symptoms.

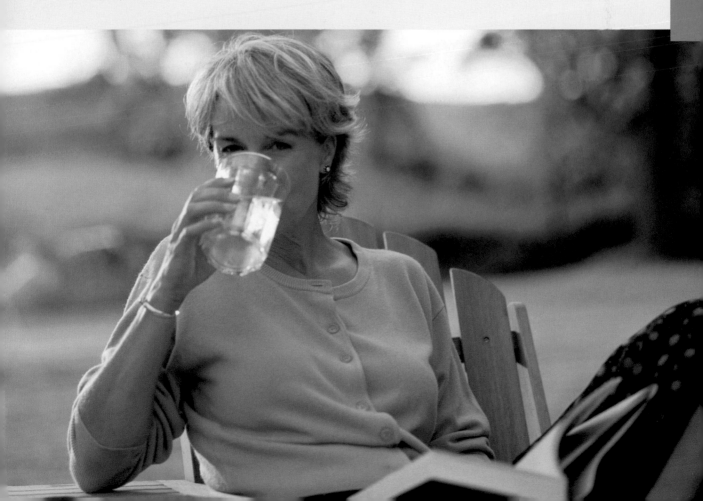

INSIDE
your kidneys and bladder

The kidneys and bladder are the major elements in the **urinary system**, which acts as a **filter** for the blood by removing and excreting waste products and excess water. The urinary system also regulates levels of water in the body and **maintains body fluids** in balance. The kidneys also produce **hormones**, including renin, which is important in the control of blood pressure. The kidneys receive blood from the **aorta**, the main artery connected directly to the heart. Blood passes through filtering units in each kidney, known as **nephrons**, where harmful wastes are removed and the amount of water to remain in the body is regulated. Filtered blood from the kidneys is returned to the heart through the body's largest vein, the **inferior vena cava**. Urine, containing water and waste products, passes through tubes called **ureters** to the **bladder**, where it is temporarily stored until it is emptied through the **urethra** during urination.

the kidney

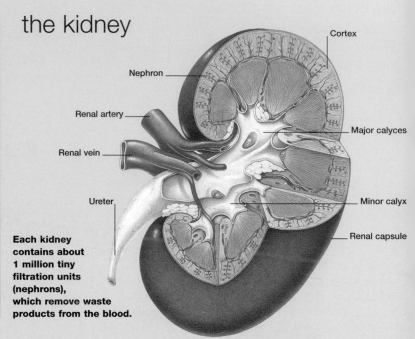

Cortex
Nephron
Renal artery
Renal vein
Ureter
Major calyces
Minor calyx
Renal capsule

Each kidney contains about 1 million tiny filtration units (nephrons), which remove waste products from the blood.

the urinary tract

Waste products and excess water pass from the kidneys via the ureters to the bladder, where they are stored as urine before being excreted through the urethra.

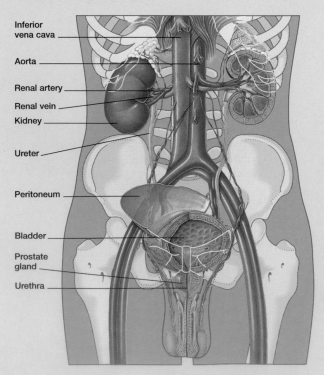

Inferior vena cava
Aorta
Renal artery
Renal vein
Kidney
Ureter
Peritoneum
Bladder
Prostate gland
Urethra

sexual differences

The male urethra passes through the prostate gland and is about 8in (20cm) long. The female urethra is only about 1½in (4cm) long.

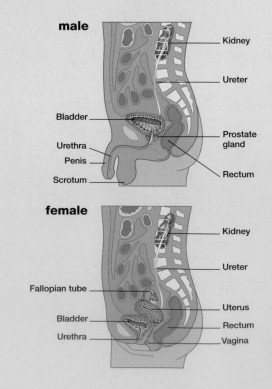

male

Kidney
Ureter
Bladder
Urethra
Penis
Scrotum
Prostate gland
Rectum

female

Kidney
Ureter
Fallopian tube
Uterus
Bladder
Rectum
Urethra
Vagina

Urinary incontinence, including stress incontinence and irritable bladder

ALTHOUGH THERE ARE AN ESTIMATED SIX MILLION SUFFERERS IN THE UK, MOSTLY WOMEN, INCONTINENCE IS A TABOO SUBJECT – NO ONE TALKS ABOUT IT, BUT IT'S IMPORTANT TO BE WELL INFORMED, BECAUSE IT COULD AFFECT ANY ONE OF US.

There are different types of incontinence, all of which are forms of uncontrollable leakage of urine. Although most older women suffer from it occasionally, incontinence can start surprisingly early in life – many women have occasional bouts of incontinence from their mid-20s onwards, particularly if they've had children.

WHAT CAUSES IT?

There are four major causes of incontinence.
■ After pregnancy the pelvic tissues can become so stretched that a slight prolapse of the vaginal wall forms. If even a very small part of the urethra or bladder is trapped in the prolapse, urinary symptoms such as urgency, frequency and pain nearly always follow.
■ After the menopause, lack of oestrogen weakens the exit valve from the bladder, which may then leak.
■ Urine may also leak when pressure inside the abdomen is increased when we sneeze, cough, strain to open our bowels or lift a heavy weight. This is called **stress incontinence**.
■ Post-menopausally the muscles of the bladder become over-sensitive to the presence of **any** urine in the bladder, so they contract spontaneously and try to empty the bladder even when there's only a small amount of urine there. This is sometimes called **irritable bladder**.

WHAT ARE THE SYMPTOMS?

■ Inability to prevent your bladder from leaking urine.
■ The urge to pass urine frequently (frequency) even when your bladder isn't full.
■ Urgency (you can't hold on), even when your bladder isn't full.

SHOULD I SEE THE DOCTOR?

Seek help as soon as symptoms appear. The earlier incontinence is treated, the less likely it is that it will become chronic. Both stress incontinence and irritable bladder can be treated successfully.

WHAT WILL THE DOCTOR DO?

■ Your doctor will want to check a mid-stream urine sample for infection, so take one along when you see her. She may also refer you for a special X-ray of your bladder (cystogram).

■ She will advise you to strengthen your pelvic floor muscles by doing a series of special exercises (see box, below).
■ Since obesity weakens the pelvic floor, you may be advised to reduce your weight.
■ HRT has an almost instant rejuvenating effect on the bladder and urethra. There's no need to take tablets; oestrogen cream inserted in the vagina each night can be enough.
■ A prolapse can be helped by wearing a special support ring internally during the day, so ask if one is appropriate.
■ If you have a prolapse your doctor may advise you to have a surgical operation to tighten up your pelvic floor muscles – a kind of **pelvic facelift** – called a colporrhaphy.
■ If you are suffering from an irritable bladder, she may suggest a muscle-relaxant drug to relax your bladder muscles.
■ If this doesn't work, she may advise a surgical procedure to "desensitize" your bladder by stretching the urethra.

WHAT CAN I DO?

■ Pelvic floor exercises are most important. All women, whether they have bladder symptoms or not, should do pelvic floor exercises every time they pass urine.
■ Research has shown that even women as old as 80 years can benefit from a regime of these exercises carried out regularly. Over as short a time as three months, they can regain bladder control and vastly reduce any leaking.
■ As the pelvic floor muscles contract at orgasm, toning them up can dramatically increase a woman's awareness of vaginal sensation during intercourse, making sex a much more pleasurable experience for her and her partner.
■ Try to avoid smoking, caffeine and alcohol.

Pelvic floor exercises

■ The first step is to find the group of muscles that form a figure of 8 around the vagina, urethra and anus. You can do this by stopping the flow several times while you're urinating.
■ Tighten the muscles for five seconds, relax them for five seconds, then tense them again. Make sure you're not just tightening your buttocks and try not to tighten your tummy muscles at the same time. You may not be able to hold the tension for the full five seconds at first, but you are likely to develop this ability as your pelvic muscles grow stronger.
■ The next stage is to tighten and relax the muscles 10 times, as quickly as you can so that they seem to "flutter". You will probably need to practise for a while to control the muscles in this way.
■ Next, contract the muscles long and steadily as though you were trying to draw an object into your vagina. Hold the contraction for five seconds.
■ The final step is to bear down, as if emptying the bowels, but pushing more through the vagina than the anus. Hold the tension for five seconds.

Gradually build up to 10 contractions, 10 times daily or more, spaced over several hours, and check your progress once or twice a week by stopping the flow when you urinate. After about six weeks of these exercises you should find stopping the flow is much easier than it was in the beginning.

The beauty of pelvic floor exercises is that, once you've mastered the technique, you can do them anywhere, any time – lying down, standing, watching television, even when you're washing up or vacuuming!

Infection of the kidneys (pyelonephritis)

ONE OF THE MOST COMMON KIDNEY DISORDERS, WHICH PARTICULARLY AFFECTS YOUNG AND MIDDLE-AGED ADULTS, PYELONEPHRITIS IS INFLAMMATION OF ONE OR BOTH KIDNEYS, USUALLY AS A RESULT OF A BACTERIAL INFECTION.

Pyelonephritis is much more common in women and it may be related to sexual activity. In adults, the condition causes intense pain around the kidneys in the back. For this reason it can usually be promptly diagnosed and treated, so it rarely leads to long-term kidney damage. However, in children the symptoms of pyelonephritis may not be so obvious. All they may have are vague symptoms such as a headache and feeling sick. As a result,it may go unnoticed and lead to serious kidney problems, possibly resulting in kidney failure in later life.

WHAT ARE THE CAUSES?

There may be a minor **anatomical abnormality** that predisposes to infection and this should always be excluded with special X-rays of the kidneys. Pyelonephritis may be caused by bacteria that enter the urinary tract from the outside through the urethra (the passage from the bladder to the outside of the body). Often, the bacteria migrate upwards from an infection in the bladder. Urinary infections, and therefore pyelonephritis, are much more common in women since the female urethra is shorter than that of the male and its opening is nearer the anus so there's little distance for the bacteria to travel to reach the kidneys. Bacteria from the anal area may enter the urethra during sex or if the area is wiped from back to front after a bowel movement. People with **diabetes mellitus** are more likely to have urinary infections, partly because glucose in the urine may encourage bacterial growth.

In both sexes, pyelonephritis is more likely to develop if there is a **physical obstruction** anywhere in the urinary tract that restricts the normal outflow of urine. Bacteria that have already contaminated the urine are not flushed out as would normally happen, and they multiply in the stagnant urine. An obstruction may be the result of pressure on parts of the urinary tract, such as the **expanding uterus in pregnant women** or an **enlarged prostate gland** in men. Normal urine flow may also be obstructed by **bladder tumours** or **kidney stones**. Kidney stones may harbour bacteria and therefore predispose to urinary tract infection. All of these conditions are likely to lead to recurrent episodes of pyelonephritis.

Bacteria may also enter the bladder during bladder **catheterization**, a procedure in which a tube is passed up the urethra into the bladder to drain urine if the bladder can't empty itself. Sometimes bacteria are carried to the kidneys in the bloodstream from infections elsewhere in the body.

WHAT ARE THE SYMPTOMS?

The symptoms of pyelonephritis may appear suddenly, often over a period of a few hours, and include:
- intense pain that begins in the back just above the waist and then moves to the side and groin
- fever over 38°C (100.4°F), resulting in shivering and headache
- painful and frequent urination
- cloudy, blood-stained urine
- foul-smelling urine
- nausea and vomiting.

If you develop any of these symptoms, consult your doctor immediately.

HOW IS IT DIAGNOSED?

■ If your doctor suspects pyelonephritis, she will probably examine a sample of your urine (see box, left) to find out whether it contains bacteria. If there is evidence of infection, the urine sample will be sent for laboratory analysis to establish which bacterium is responsible.

■ Further investigations may include a blood test so that the function of the kidneys can be assessed. Imaging tests, such as **ultrasound scanning**, **CT scanning** or a type of contrast X-ray known as **intravenous urography** may also be carried out to check for a blockage and signs of kidney damage or kidney stones.

WHAT IS THE TREATMENT?

■ Pyelonephritis is usually treated with a course of **oral antibiotics** and symptoms often improve within two days of treatment, but the full course MUST be taken to prevent bacterial resistance.

■ When the course of antibiotics is finished, further urine tests may be performed to confirm that the infection has cleared up completely. However, if you are vomiting or in pain, or if you are seriously ill, you may be admitted to hospital and given **intravenous fluids** and **antibiotics**.

■ If you experience repeated episodes of pyelonephritis, you may be advised to take low-dose antibiotics over a period of six months to two years to reduce the frequency of the attacks. If you have an underlying disorder, such as kidney stones, this may also need to be treated.

WHAT IS THE OUTLOOK?

In most cases, prompt treatment of pyelonephritis is effective, and the condition causes no permanent damage to the kidneys. However, in rare cases, frequent episodes of pyelonephritis may lead to scarring of the kidneys and may result in irreversible damage.

TEST

Urine test

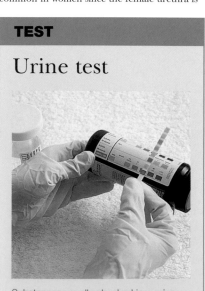

Substances usually checked in a urine analysis include glucose, proteins, calcium, creatinine and certain hormones. A urine sample may also reveal blood cells, bacteria or other substances that indicate an underlying problem.

See also:
- **Bladder tumours p.380**
- **CT scanning p.401**
- **Diabetes mellitus p.504**
- **Kidney stones p.377**
- **Prostate problems p.266**
- **Ultrasound scanning p.277**

Glomerulonephritis

THE KIDNEY CONTAINS MANY TINY FILTERING UNITS, THE GLOMERULI, WHICH VERY RARELY BECOME INFLAMED; THE RESULTING DISORDER, GLOMERULONEPHRITIS, CAN COME ON SUDDENLY (ACUTE) OR DEVELOP PROGRESSIVELY OVER A LONG TIME (CHRONIC).

An acute episode of glomerulonephritis is usually followed by complete recovery; however, in severe cases damage to the glomeruli may be permanent. Glomerulonephritis is a serious condition and must be treated in hospital under the supervision of a renal (kidney) specialist.

WHAT ARE THE CAUSES?
Acute glomerulonephritis may occur as a complication of certain infectious diseases. The antibodies produced by the immune system to fight the infection may attack the glomeruli in the kidneys, causing inflammation and damage. The most common cause, especially in children, is a throat infection due to the streptococcus bacterium. Chronic glomerulonephritis may occur as part of an **autoimmune disorder** such as lupus.

WHAT ARE THE SYMPTOMS?
- Sore throat.
- Fever and shortness of breath.
- Back pain and headache.
- Passing little or no urine.
- Frothy or cloudy urine.
- Blood in the urine.
- Puffiness in the face, with swelling around the eyes in the morning.
- Swollen feet and legs in the evening.
- Loss of appetite.
- Nausea and vomiting.

WHAT IS THE TREATMENT?
- Following a bacterial infection, antibiotics and sometimes corticosteroid drugs may be prescribed.
- If glomerulonephritis is due to an autoimmune disorder it can usually be treated with immunosuppressants and corticosteroids.
- If the blood pressure rises it will be treated at the same time with antihypertensive drugs.
- For chronic glomerulonephritis, a low-salt diet with reduced fluid intake may be recommended to prevent fluid retention in body tissues.

WHAT IS THE OUTLOOK?
In most cases the symptoms of acute glomerulonephritis disappear after 6–8 weeks. In some people, kidney function is impaired but does not deteriorate further. However, other people may develop chronic kidney failure along with irreversible loss of kidney function that may be fatal if not treated promptly.

Kidney stones

NORMALLY, THE WASTE PRODUCTS OF THE BODY'S CHEMICAL PROCESSES PASS OUT OF THE KIDNEYS IN THE URINE. OCCASIONALLY, HOWEVER, THE URINE BECOMES SATURATED WITH WASTE PRODUCTS.

These waste products are able to crystallize into stone-like structures of varying sizes within the kidney – kidney stones. A shortage of chemicals that normally stop crystals forming can lead to kidney stones, which usually start off as fine gravel and take years to reach a size that causes problems.

WHAT ARE THE CAUSES?
- The most common cause of kidney stones is prolonged **inadequate fluid intake**. People who live in hot climates may be susceptible to kidney stones if they do not drink enough to replace fluid lost in sweat.
- Different types of kidney stones can form, depending on the waste products that crystallize out of the urine; most are made of **calcium salts**.
- Kidney stones may also result from a **long-standing urinary tract infection**. In such cases, the stones can grow into a **staghorn** shape, filling the central cavity of the kidney.
- Rare **disorders of metabolism** may be complicated by kidney stones.

WHAT ARE THE SYMPTOMS?
Very small kidney stones may pass unnoticed in the urine. Larger stones, or small fragments of stones that pass down the **ureter** (the tube from the kidney to the bladder), may cause extremely painful spasms of the ureter wall called **renal colic**. The symptoms usually appear suddenly and include:
- excruciating pain that starts in the back, spreads to the abdomen and groin and may be felt in the genitals
- frequent, painful urination
- nausea and vomiting
- blood in the urine.
If a kidney stone is passed in the urine the pain will subside rapidly.

WHAT IS THE TREATMENT?
- If the stones are small and remain in the kidney, you may simply be advised to rest, take painkillers to relieve discomfort and drink plenty of fluids to help flush the stones into the urine.
- In some instances, kidney stones that have become lodged in the lower part of the ureter can be removed via the bladder. In this procedure, a viewing tube is passed into the bladder and ureter. Instruments are then passed through the tube to crush or remove the stone.
- The most frequently used treatment for kidney stones is **lithotripsy**, in which shock waves are used to break the stones into powder that can be passed easily in the urine.
- The underlying cause needs to be treated to prevent a recurrence of kidney stones.

SELF-HELP

Preventing kidney stones

If you have kidney stones, these dietary precautions may help prevent their recurrence:
- drink at least 3 litres (6 pints) of fluids daily to avoid dehydration
- drink fluids before you sleep to ensure that urine production continues overnight
- drink more fluids in hot weather, after strenuous exercise or if you have a fever
- to prevent calcium stones, eat fewer dairy products and avoid calcium-based antacids. If you live in a hard-water area, use a water softener in drinking water
- to prevent oxalate stones (made up of calcium oxalate), avoid rhubarb, spinach and asparagus, which contain oxalic acid.

See also:
- Cystoscopy p.380

FOCUS *on* cystitis

A very common, annoying and inconvenient condition, cystitis causes frequent, painful urination as a result of inflammation of the bladder. It hardly ever occurs in men and in women is most often the result of an infection or bruising after athletic or prolonged sex.

Most women have a bout of cystitis at some time in their lives but it doesn't usually endanger health.

WHAT CAUSES IT?

● The most common bacterium to cause cystitis is *E. coli*, which lives without causing problems in the bowel and on the skin around the anus. It only causes infection when it spreads up the urethra into the bladder. Women are more prone to cystitis than men because the female urethra is shorter than the male one and it's therefore a shorter distance for bacteria to travel from the skin.

● Other organisms that cause **sexually transmitted diseases**, such as **herpes** or **trichomonas**, can cause cystitis too.

● The cystitis known as **honeymoon cystitis** is not restricted to honeymooners. It is caused at any time by unusual amounts of frequent, strenuous sexual intercourse, which can cause bruising of the urethra, especially with the man on top position.

● Occasionally, cystitis can be caused by the use of **antiseptics** in bath water or by over-zealous use of **vaginal deodorants** or **douches** when the normal protective flora in and around the vagina is disturbed.

● As women get older and reach the menopause, a shortage of oestrogen leads to thinning of all the genital organs, including the bladder and urethra, and this can contribute to **menopausal cystitis**.

● Cystitis can sometimes be a side effect of some cancer treatment. Radiotherapy, particularly if cancer of the cervix or prostate cancer are being treated, may lead to cystitis and chemotherapy has the same effect as the powerful drugs are flushed out with the urine.

● Diabetics often suffer from cystitis because the high sugar content of the urine favours multiplication of bacteria, and people with reduced immunity, for example those with an **autoimmune** disease or HIV infection, are also at greater risk of developing the condition.

WHAT ARE THE SYMPTOMS?

● The frequent and urgent need to urinate, although only a small amount of urine may be passed each time.

● A burning or stinging sensation while urinating.

● A severe knife-like pain when you finish urinating.

● The appearance of blood in the urine, which may be pink, red or simply streaks.

● A severe dragging-down pain, usually in

Cystitis triggers

● In a sensitive woman not drinking enough water can be enough to cause cystitis.

● Sex, at any time (although not every time) and for the same reason, that is mechanical trauma, horseriding or riding a bicycle for long periods can induce an attack of cystitis.

● Perfumed soaps, bath foams or oils, talc and vaginal deodorants can irritate the delicate skin around the vagina and urethra and act as triggers.

● Certain foods and drinks like strong tea, coffee, alcohol, fruit juice or highly spiced dishes can cause cystitis attacks or make them worse.

● Holding on too long before going to the lavatory, or wearing tight-fitting trousers, tights or underwear in man-made fibres – creating the warm, moist atmosphere germs love – are also triggers.

the front of the abdomen but quite often radiating up the flanks and to the back, or down the front of the thighs.

● Pain and the urge to get up several times in the night to empty your bladder, even though there may be very little urine present.

● Fever and shivering attacks.

WHAT CAN I DO?

If the self-help measures listed below don't bring relief, seek help from your doctor as soon as possible:

● Drink large volumes of fluid at the first sign. It's important to get urine flowing fast to flush out the bladder, so try to drink the equivalent of at least a glass of water every **half hour**.

● Drink cranberry juice, which is a urinary antiseptic.

● Make your urine alkaline by drinking milk and adding a little bicarbonate of soda to your drinks. You'll find that making your urine alkaline eases bladder pain quite considerably.

● Drink as much bland, non-acidic liquid, such as water, milk or weak tea, as you can. Try to drink around five pints a day during the 48-hour treatment.

● Try to avoid alcohol, coffee, strong tea or fruit juices; they may make matters worse.

● Urinate as often as you feel the need. In this way, you'll produce a flushing-through effect that helps your natural defences.

● For pain relief, take paracetamol every four hours. Don't take anything containing aspirin, it makes urine acidic.

● Keep warm. A warm pad or wrapped hot water bottle placed across the tummy can be very comforting.

● Avoid perfumed soaps, deodorants and bubble baths as these may cause further irritation.

WHAT WILL THE DOCTOR DO?

● Your doctor may take a urine specimen to confirm an infection.

● As soon as the specimen has been taken, he can start you on a course of antibiotics, usually a penicillin derivative. It's essential that you take the full course of treatment, even if your symptoms subside completely within 24 hours, otherwise organisms may become resistant to antibiotics and your cystitis can become chronic.

● If your cystitis doesn't respond to

treatment, your doctor may recommend a full hospital investigation to see whether there's any predisposing internal cause.
● If investigation shows no trace of bacteria or any other cause, you may be suffering from an "irritable bladder", in which emotional factors play a part.

CYSTITIS AND PREGNANCY

● Cystitis is fairly common during pregnancy, particularly in the first few months when the urethra relaxes under the influence of the hormone progesterone and infections spread more easily.
● Later on, pressure from the enlarging uterus may cause a small amount of urine to remain in the bladder and become stagnant, encouraging bacteria to multiply, leading to cystitis.

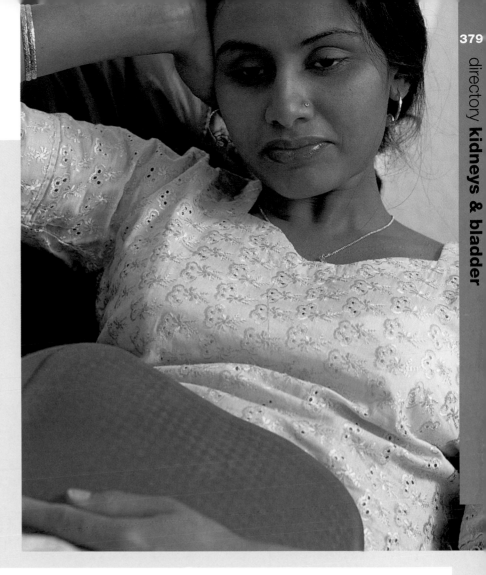

Drinking plenty of fluids, taking paracetamol and applying heat to the abdomen can all help ease the symptoms of cystitis.

How to stay clear

● Drink plenty of water at all times.
● Keep cranberry juice in the fridge at all times and start drinking it at the first sign of cystitis.
● At the first symptom, increase your water intake and make your urine alkaline by adding a little bicarbonate of soda to your drinks. (Don't continue this for too long; you could have unpleasant side effects such as wind.)
● **Never** allow yourself to get dehydrated, carry water with you at all times.
● If you're having sex frequently, drink a lot of fluid to keep the urine flowing. Pass urine before and after sexual intercourse. Drink cranberry juice before and after.

● If you suspect that wearing a diaphragm is a contributory cause, ask your doctor about another form of contraception.
● Use tampons instead of sanitary towels as they're less likely to allow the bacteria to thrive; some women, however, find that tampons irritate the bladder further.
● Remember to wipe from the front towards the back after bowel motions to avoid spreading bacteria to the urethra.
● **Don't** be obsessive about genital hygiene. However, using a bidet after moving your bowels is a good idea to avoid contamination of the vagina and

urethra from the rectum.
● **Don't** use antiseptics in the bath water, and don't use vaginal douches or deodorants.
● Wear cotton panties or cotton liners.
● Avoid tight clothing, especially if made from synthetic material. Stockings and cotton knickers are better than tights.
● Keep a diary so that you can spot anything such as alcohol or spicy food that appears to bring on attacks, and avoid it whenever possible.

If you're susceptible to cystitis it's going to be part of your life so you have to learn to "manage" it.

Bladder tumours

GROWTHS THAT OCCUR IN THE BLADDER MAY BE NON-CANCEROUS (BENIGN) OR CANCEROUS (MALIGNANT), BUT BOTH TYPES CAUSE BLOOD IN YOUR URINE, WHICH MUST ALWAYS BE REPORTED TO YOUR DOCTOR.

From blood in the urine alone it is impossible for your doctor to tell if the cause is relatively minor or something more serious. A tumour is what your doctor will want to exclude. Tests, including ultrasound and intravenous urography (IVU) may be arranged and your specialist may want to perform a **cystoscopy** (see box, below) to take a look directly inside your bladder.

Treatment for shallow tumours can often be done during cystoscopy, although surgery, chemotherapy and radiotherapy may be used for more serious growths. Shallow cancerous tumours diagnosed early have a high cure rate.

TEST

Cystoscopy

During cystoscopy, a thin, hollow viewing tube, known as a cystoscope, is inserted into the urethra and then into the bladder to look for tumours and other abnormalities.

The cystoscope may be rigid or flexible. Instruments to take tissue samples and destroy or remove tumours and stones can be inserted through the cystoscope as required. Cystoscopy may be carried out under either a local or general anaesthetic.

> See also:
> • Chemotherapy p.257 • Radiotherapy p.395 • Ultrasound scanning p.277

Acute, chronic and end-stage kidney failure

WHEN BOTH KIDNEYS STOP WORKING NORMALLY, THE CONDITION IS KNOWN AS KIDNEY FAILURE. IT MAY BE SUDDEN (ACUTE) OR GRADUAL AND PROGRESSIVE (CHRONIC).

Chronic kidney failure may lead to irreversible loss of kidney function (end-stage kidney failure), which is life-threatening if not treated.

ACUTE KIDNEY FAILURE

■ The kidneys will stop working properly if their blood supply is suddenly and greatly reduced. This can happen in **surgical shock,** such as after severe bleeding, serious infection or a heart attack, when there is a profound fall in blood pressure.

■ Kidney failure may result from damage as a result of **glomerulonephritis**, **pyelonephritis**, **toxic chemicals** or **drugs**.

WHAT ARE THE SYMPTOMS?

The symptoms of acute kidney failure may appear rapidly, sometimes over a period of

TREATMENT

Transplant surgery

Many organs and tissues can now be transplanted. Kidney transplants have become common, and liver, heart, lung, cornea and bone marrow transplants are performed routinely. Transplants of the intestines and pancreas are done less often. More than one organ may be transplanted at the same time, as in the case of heart and lung transplants.

Transplants are usually performed only when the tissue types and blood groups of the donor and recipient are similar. This is necessary because the recipient's immune system will attack any organ it identifies as "foreign", a process called rejection. Most transplant organs are taken from donors who have very recently been declared dead and who are unrelated to the recipient. However, bone marrow and single kidneys can be taken from living donors without damaging their health. Bone marrow is always taken from a living donor. When bone marrow or kidneys are donated by a close, living genetic relative, often a brother or sister, the transplants are far less likely to be rejected by the recipient because the tissue types are likely to match more closely.

Most transplant surgery requires general anaesthesia. In an organ transplant, the organ to be transplanted is removed from the donor and chilled in a salt-containing solution until it reaches the operating room. This prolongs the time the organ can safely be deprived of its normal blood supply by a few hours. In most cases, the diseased organ is replaced by the donor organ. However, in kidney transplants the defective organ may be left in place and the new kidney placed in the pelvis, where it is connected to the relevant blood vessels.

After a transplant, you will probably spend several days in a critical care unit. With all transplants except the cornea, you will need immunosuppressants indefinitely in order to prevent your immune system from rejecting the new organ or tissue. You should be able to leave the hospital after a few weeks if the transplant has been successful. Recovery time for a corneal graft is shorter, and it is usually possible to go home after a few days.

hours only, and may include the following things:

- greatly reduced urine volume
- nausea and vomiting
- drowsiness and headache
- back pain.

If you develop these symptoms, you should call your doctor immediately. Without treatment, acute kidney failure may be fatal within a few days.

WHAT IS THE TREATMENT?

If you have acute kidney failure, you will need immediate hospitalization. You will probably be treated in an intensive care unit.

■ You may have to undergo **dialysis** for a short time so that the excess fluid and waste products can be removed from your bloodstream while the doctors investigate the cause of the kidney failure.

■ If you have lost a large amount of blood, you will need to have a **blood transfusion** to restore your normal blood volume.

■ Any underlying cause will be treated.

■ Finally, if there is a blockage anywhere in your urinary tract, you may need to undergo surgery to have the obstruction removed.

WHAT IS THE OUTLOOK?

If your kidneys have not been damaged irreversibly, there is a good chance that you will make a complete recovery, which may take up to 6 weeks. However, in some cases, the damage resulting from acute kidney failure may not be completely reversible, and in this situation **chronic kidney failure** may develop.

CHRONIC KIDNEY FAILURE

Chronic kidney failure is gradual and progressive loss of function in both kidneys so that eventually the kidneys cannot remove excess water and waste from the blood for excretion as urine. As a result, waste substances start to build up in the body and cause problems. In many cases, kidney function is reduced by over 60 percent before the build-up begins. By this time, often after months or perhaps years, the kidneys may be irreversibly damaged. Dialysis or a kidney transplant may therefore become necessary.

WHAT ARE THE SYMPTOMS?

The initial symptoms of chronic kidney failure appear gradually over several weeks or months and are often vague, such as weakness and loss of appetite. The first obvious symptoms of the condition to appear include:

- frequent urination, particularly during the night
- pale, itchy and easily bruised skin
- shortness of breath
- persistent hiccups

Dialysis

Dialysis is used to treat kidney failure by replacing the functions of the kidneys in filtering out waste and excess water from the blood. It can be temporary, as for acute kidney failure, or long-term, as for end-stage kidney failure. There are two forms: **peritoneal dialysis**, in which the peritoneal membrane is used as a filter, and **haemodialysis**, in which a kidney machine filters the blood.

Peritoneal dialysis

In peritoneal dialysis, the peritoneum, the membrane that surrounds the abdominal organs, is used instead of the kidneys to filter the blood. A procedure called an **exchange** is carried out four times a day at home. During an exchange, dialysis fluid that was flowed into the abdomen 4–6 hours earlier is drained out of the peritoneum through a catheter in the abdominal wall. The fluid is replaced with fresh solution, then the equipment is disconnected, and you can carry out normal activities.

Haemodialysis

In haemodialysis, blood is pumped by a kidney machine from your body through a filter attached to the side of the machine. Inside the filter, blood flows on one side of a membrane and dialysate fluid flows on the other. Waste products and water pass from the blood across the membrane and into the fluid; the filtered blood returns to the body.

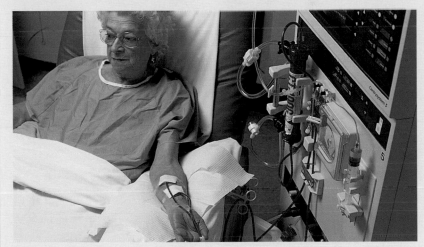

In haemodialysis, a kidney machine filters the blood in place of the kidneys. The procedure takes 3–4 hours and needs to be repeated about three times a week.

- nausea and vomiting
- muscular twitching
- pins and needles
- cramps in the legs.

Chronic kidney failure can lead to a number of complications, such as **high blood pressure** (which may also be a cause of kidney failure), **thinning and weakening of the bones** (osteoporosis) and **anaemia**, in which the oxygen-carrying capacity of the blood is reduced.

If chronic kidney failure progresses to **end-stage kidney failure**, with permanent and almost total loss of kidney function, you will need treatment involving **long-term dialysis** (see box, above) or a **kidney transplant** (see box, opposite).

END-STAGE KIDNEY FAILURE

End-stage kidney failure is the irreversible loss of the function of both kidneys, which is often life-threatening.

WHAT ARE THE SYMPTOMS?

The main symptoms of end-stage kidney failure usually include:

- greatly reduced volume of urine
- swelling of the face, limbs and abdomen
- severe lethargy
- weight loss
- headache and vomiting
- furry tongue
- very itchy skin.

Many people who have end-stage kidney failure also have breath that smells of ammonia.

WHAT IS THE TREATMENT?

Long-term renal dialysis or a kidney transplant will be needed.

See also:
- **Glomerulonephritis p.377**
- **Infection of the kidneys p.376**

Chest and Air Passages

Image shows a coloured angiograph of a normal human lung

Miriam's overview

The most dramatic development in this area is the increase in asthma, which some alarmist commentators liken to an epidemic. I, personally don't think the picture is that bleak but certainly there are growing numbers of people developing asthma and at both ends of the age scale.

Each is for a different reason. In children asthma is becoming more common because we're too clean. Yes, our modern obsession with all things "anti-bacterial" is the primary cause of the increase in childhood asthma. There's much excellent research to support this conclusion. We know, for instance, that children who live on farms and are exposed to countless millions of germs every day hardly ever get asthma. Whereas children brought up in homes where every surface is cleaned with a household cleaner containing anti-bacterial chemicals are prone to asthma.

"without exposure to an array of *household germs* the immune system is *feeble and weak*"

The reason is that a child's developing immune system needs contact with bacteria to become strong and capable. Without exposure to an array of household germs the immune system is feeble and weak and succumbs to asthma.

We've also recently found out that asthma is not caused by air pollution. Pollution may make asthma worse but it isn't the root of the problem. Asthma is increasing most quickly in the least polluted areas.

At the other end of our lives asthma is largely the consequence of smoking. A lifetime of smoking leaves most people with lung damage. Years of smoking leads to chronic bronchitis which can end up as COPD – chronic obstructive pulmonary disease – a component of which may be asthma.

The treatment of asthma has been revolutionized with the concept of "preventers" and "relievers". These two different kinds of asthma medicines are used in different ways. Preventers are taken every day, even in tip-top health, to prevent an asthma attack from happening and by and large they allow a child to live a normal life, playing sports and swimming.

Relievers are always close at hand, usually in the form of an inhaler for use in an asthma attack should it happen. Between these two regimes most children become unafraid of their asthma and take it in their stride – an essential part of successfully controlling asthma.

Because of the importance of asthma you'll find an article on it in this chapter, as well as a special "Focus on" asthma in the chapter on allergies and the immune system.

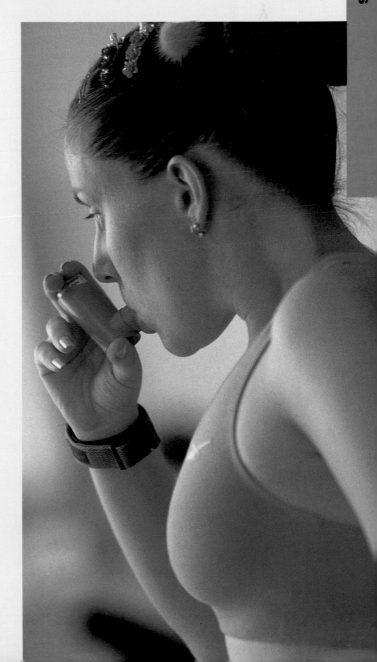

INSIDE
your chest and air passages

The function of the lungs is to supply oxygen to the blood and to remove the waste product carbon dioxide from it. This vital exchange of oxygen and carbon dioxide between the air and the blood is known as **respiration**. Air enters the body and leaves it via the respiratory system, which consists of the **mouth, nose, throat** (pharynx), **voice box** (larynx), **windpipe** (trachea), **branching air passages** (bronchi) and the **lungs** themselves. It is the job of the circulatory system, consisting of the heart and blood vessels, to carry oxygenated blood to body tissues and bring de-oxygenated blood back to the lungs.

Inhaled air is warmed and moistened by the nose before passing into the lungs, where oxygen from the air passes into the blood via blood vessels. Here, oxygen binds to haemoglobin in red blood cells and travels in the blood back to the heart, which pumps the oxygenated blood around the body. At the same time, the lungs remove carbon dioxide from the fluid part of the blood, known as plasma, and exhale it.

the respiratory system

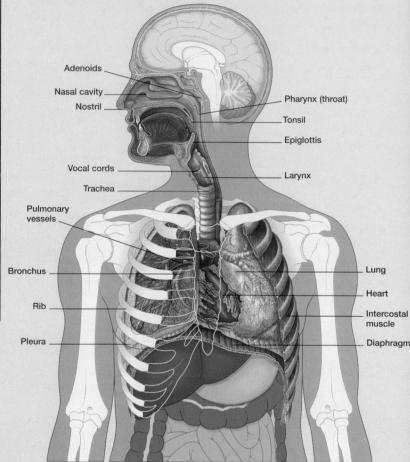

The lungs receive de-oxygenated blood from the body via the heart. The blood is oxygenated through the process of breathing before it is returned to the heart to be pumped around the body.

how breathing works

Decreasing air pressure in the lungs during inhalation causes air to be drawn into the lungs. Air pressure increases in the lungs during exhalation, forcing air out.

Inhaling

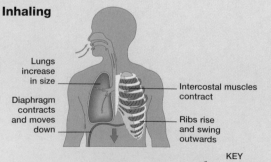

Exhaling

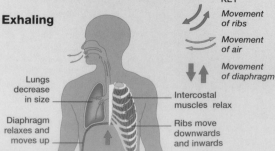

Cross-section of alveoli

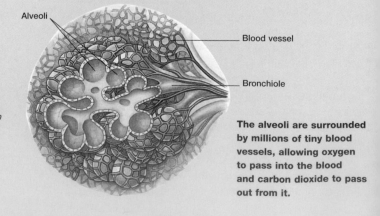

The alveoli are surrounded by millions of tiny blood vessels, allowing oxygen to pass into the blood and carbon dioxide to pass out from it.

Asthma

TO UNDERSTAND ASTHMA, AND INDEED ANY PROBLEMS RELATING TO THE CHEST
AND AIR PASSAGES, IT IS NECESSARY TO KNOW WHAT THE LUNGS DO.

When we breathe air in, the lungs remove oxygen from it and pass the oxygen into the blood. The blood then circulates around the body and delivers the oxygen to the tissues. At the same time the blood collects the waste product carbon dioxide, and takes it back to the lungs. The lungs get rid of the carbon dioxide by mixing it with the air that we breathe out. Air gets in and out of the lungs by a series of branching pipes, often called the "bronchial tubes", which get progressively smaller as they penetrate deeper into the lungs.

WHAT IS ASTHMA?

Asthma is a condition that affects the bronchi (large airways) and bronchioles (small airways) that carry air in and out of the lungs. People with asthma have particularly sensitive airways.

These airways can constrict when you have a cold or other viral infection or when you come into contact with an asthma trigger, making breathing much more of an effort.

Asthma is a common condition that affects about 1 in 7 children and 1 in 20 adults. Many people think of asthma as something that starts in childhood, but it can occur for the first time at any age. Asthma may get better or disappear completely during the teenage years, but about half the children with asthma will still have some problems as adults. There is a tendency for asthma to run in families but many sufferers have no relatives with asthma. Asthma cannot, as yet, be cured but it can be kept under control so that asthma attacks are prevented. With proper treatment taken regularly, most people with asthma can lead entirely normal lives, with no time lost from school or work, and enjoy full involvement in sport and other recreations.

WHAT ARE THE SYMPTOMS?

As it is more difficult to get air in and out of narrowed airways, people with asthma get the following symptoms:
- coughing
- wheezing, or a whistling noise in the chest
- getting short of breath
- a tight feeling in the chest
- coughing up phlegm.

Not everybody will get all of these symptoms. Some people experience them from time to time, perhaps if they get a cold or come into contact with one of their asthma triggers. Others experience the worst symptoms at night, first thing in the morning or after exercise. A few people may experience symptoms all the time.

HOW DO I AVOID TRIGGERS?
COLDS

Colds are very common triggers of asthma attacks. They are also almost impossible to avoid!
- Regular use of a preventer inhaler reduces the risk of asthma attacks due to colds and infections.
- Flu injections each autumn are recommended for people with severe asthma
- A healthy diet with lots of fruit and vegetables containing vitamin C may help to fight viruses.

PETS

Pets can be great fun and a wonderful source of companionship. Unfortunately, furry animals are also a common allergic trigger of asthma symptoms. The allergens are found in the pet's fur, saliva, dander (minute flakes of dead skin) and urine.
- If someone in your family has asthma, or if there is a family history of asthma, don't buy a furry or feathered pet.
- Up to 50 percent of children with asthma have their symptoms triggered by an allergy to cats and/or dogs.
- The urine from guinea pigs, rabbits and gerbils can cause problems too.
- Rarely, even fish can cause problems! Some people have an allergic reaction to the ants' eggs on which tropical fish feed.
- Bathing cats and dogs once a week can help. Ask your vet for advice on how to do this properly.
- Always keep pets out of areas such as the lounge and bedroom.

POLLEN

There are many different types of pollen grains (from grasses, trees and plants) that can trigger asthma symptoms in some people.
- On hot, dry days avoid spending too much time outdoors.
- Avoid long grass.
- Keep car windows closed.

SMOKING
- Give up smoking! Within a few weeks you should start to notice huge benefits to your health – you should feel fitter and your risk of smoking-induced illness will rapidly decline. Your airways will start to recover in 3–6 months.
- If you are planning to have a child, it is very important that neither parent smokes. Studies have shown that children of mothers who smoke are more likely to develop asthma.
- Inhaling other people's smoke is hazardous for people with asthma too. A National Asthma Campaign survey showed that cigarette smoke caused an increase in asthma symptoms in 80 percent of respondents.
- Avoid smoky places. If you are going to be in a smoky room (e.g. at a party or in a pub), remember to take your inhaler with you. Go outside for some fresh air if you start to wheeze.
- Don't be afraid to tell people how you feel. Ask them to stop smoking if you start to feel wheezy.
- If you are concerned about smoke in the workplace, speak to your health and safety representative or your manager.

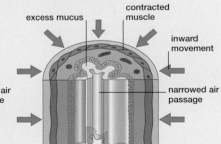

The effect of asthma on the airways

NORMAL AIRWAY

thin layer of mucus — relaxed muscle — normal air passage

CONSTRICTED AIRWAY

excess mucus — contracted muscle — inward movement — narrowed air passage

In a normal airway, the muscle is relaxed and only a thin layer of mucus is present, allowing air to flow freely to the lungs.

During an asthma attack, the muscle in the airway contracts and excess mucus is produced, restricting air flow to the lungs.

HOUSE DUST MITE

Little or no cost measures.

■ Hot wash (at 60°C or 140°F) sheets, duvet covers and pillow cases at least once a week.

■ Children with asthma who sleep in bunk beds should sleep in the top bunk.

■ Put soft toys in the freezer for 24 hours once every two weeks to kill mites. Then wash at 60°C (140°F) to remove dead mites and their droppings.

■ Vacuum frequently, using a high-efficiency vacuum cleaner.

■ Damp dust all surfaces regularly or use the vacuum attachment.

■ Use cotton or synthetic blankets instead of wool.

■ There is no conclusive evidence that feather pillows are better than synthetic ones (in fact, the opposite may be true). Whichever pillows you choose, use a barrier cover and wipe over with a damp cloth once a week.

If the above steps seem to work, you might also like to consider the following measures.

■ Choose short-pile synthetic carpet. It may be better than pure wool carpets, although there is no conclusive proof for this.

■ Replace carpets with lino, tiled or wood flooring.

■ Plain wooden bed frames are better than upholstered beds or headboards, which tend to collect dust.

■ Wash curtains every 2–3 months. Vertical blinds are often a better choice.

House dust mites love warm, humid environments – the following tips will reduce humidity levels in your home:

■ Keep rooms well aired.

■ Open windows during and after cooking, when you are doing the washing or using the bathroom.

■ Keep kitchen and bathroom doors closed to prevent dampness spreading to other parts of the house.

■ Remove damp and mould in the house quickly and avoid condensation.

■ Don't hang wet clothes indoors. It is best to use a tumble dryer that is vented outdoors.

■ A dehumidifier that reduces indoor humidity may be helpful, but the evidence is inconclusive and they can be expensive.

■ Consider using barrier covers for your mattress, duvet and pillow. Make sure all the beds in the room are covered. Covers that completely enclose the mattress are better than ones that just cover the top. Barrier covers need not be expensive, so shop around for ones that suit your budget.

WEATHER

Sudden changes in temperature, cold air, windy days, and poor air quality on dry, still days can all affect your asthma. Thunderstorms can also activate allergens – asthma emergencies rocketed during the summer thunderstorms of 1994, which caused a massive release of pollen into the air.

■ Take a puff of reliever just before going out.

■ Wear a scarf over your face if it's cold and windy. It will help warm the air up before you breathe it in.

■ Try to avoid going out in the middle of the day on hot, smoggy days.

EMOTION

Although it is not true that asthma is "all in the mind", we do know that psychological factors including excitement, stress or even a long fit of laughing can trigger asthma symptoms. Regular monitoring of your condition and taking your medication regularly should help to minimize these problems.

FOOD

Most people with asthma do not have to follow a special diet. In some cases, however, certain foods can make symptoms worse. Dairy products (including eggs), shellfish, fish, yeast products and nuts are some of the offenders. Some people can have a severe allergic, or anaphylactic, reaction to these foods. For more information, see Useful addresses (p.567).

■ If you think you have a food allergy, consult your doctor.

■ Your doctor may ask you to keep a diary of your diet and your symptoms to see if there is a consistent relationship between the two.

■ Your doctor may refer you to a specialist clinic for further tests.

DRUGS

In a few people, certain medications can lead

SELF-HELP

Know your triggers

A trigger is anything that irritates the airways and brings on the symptoms of asthma. There are many different asthma triggers and they vary from person to person. These are some of the common triggers.

Colds, flu and other viral infections:
A recent survey put viral chest infections as the top trigger of asthma symptoms for both adults and children.

House dust mites:
Many people with asthma are allergic to the droppings of the microscopic house dust mites found in our beds and other soft furnishings.

Cigarette smoking (active and passive):
This significantly increases breathlessness and coughing for people with asthma.

Furry or feathery animals:
Fur, feathers and dander (shed flakes of dead skin) are common allergic triggers of asthma symptoms.

Exercise:
Exercise can make some people's asthma worse, especially when outside on cold, dry days or after a change of weather.

Pollen:
Pollen can trigger asthma attacks in some people.

Air pollutants:
These can include cigarette smoke, car fumes, paint fumes, perfumes and certain chemicals.

Weather:
A sudden change in temperature, cold air, windy days, poor air quality (often on hot, humid days), thundery weather.

Mould:
Mould spores in wet weather, damp housing or piles of autumn leaves.

Emotion:
Emotional upset, stress, excitement or even a long fit of laughing.

Drugs:
Some drugs, including aspirin, non-steroidal anti-inflammatory tablets (e.g. ibuprofen) and beta-blockers (tablets and drops) used for heart disease and glaucoma, can lead to asthma attacks in a small number of people. Always tell your pharmacist that you have asthma.

Hormones:
Some women's asthma varies before a period, during pregnancy or during the menopause.

Food:
Although rare, some people have an allergy to specific foods (e.g. dairy products, fish, nuts or yeast) that can bring on an asthma attack.

Work:
Occupational asthma mainly occurs in people who develop a sensitivity to a chemical in the workplace.

REMEMBER Just avoiding your triggers alone is unlikely to control your asthma. You need to take regular asthma medication as well.

TREATMENT

Relievers and preventers

Relievers

■ Relievers are bronchodilators; they work by relaxing the muscles in the walls of the airways, which allows the airways to open.
■ Relievers usually come in blue inhalers.
■ Relievers are medicines that you can take immediately when asthma symptoms appear. They quickly relax the muscles surrounding the narrowed airways. This allows the airways to open wider, making it easier to breathe again. However, relievers do not reduce the swelling in the airways.
■ They are essential in treating asthma attacks.
■ If taken before exercise they reduce your chances of getting asthma symptoms.
■ Salbutamol and terbutaline are two examples of relievers. They work almost immediately to relieve the symptoms of asthma. That is why they are sometimes called rescue relievers.
■ Ipratropium bromide is a different type of reliever, most commonly used by children under age 2 or older people. This drug takes around 45 minutes to work. It is often used to treat chronic obstructive pulmonary disease.

Preventers

■ Most preventers are corticosteroids; they reduce the inflammation in the airways and calm their irritability.
■ Sodium cromoglycate and nedocromil sodium are non-steroid preventers and must be taken regularly, usually three or four times a day. They are not usually as effective as corticosteroids and are rarely used nowadays.
■ Preventers usually come in brown, white, red or orange inhalers.
■ Preventers protect the lining of the airways. They calm down the inflammation in our airways and stop them from being so sensitive. This means that the airways are less likely to react badly when they come across an asthma trigger.
■ They reduce the risk of severe attacks.
■ Their protective effect builds up over a period of time so they need to be taken every day, usually morning and evening, even if you are feeling well.
■ When you first start using them, it may take up to 14 days before you notice any improvement in your symptoms.

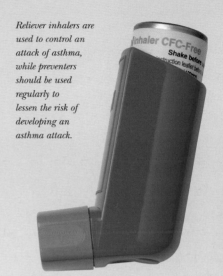

Reliever inhalers are used to control an attack of asthma, while preventers should be used regularly to lessen the risk of developing an asthma attack.

■ There are several kinds of inhaled corticosteroids but they all work in the same way. Sometimes a steroid and bronchodilator are combined in the same dose.

---

to asthma attacks. This occurs most often with medicines containing aspirin, non-steroidal anti-inflammatory tablets (e.g. ibuprofen) and beta-blockers used for heart disease (as tablets) and glaucoma (as eyedrops). Always tell your pharmacist or doctor that you have asthma.

HOW DO I LOOK AFTER MY ASTHMA?

The best way to take control of your asthma is to follow these golden rules:
● get the best treatment you can and take it regularly
● try to avoid things that trigger your asthma.
   Ask your doctor to give you an asthma self-management plan showing you how to alter your own medicine to keep yourself well.

WHAT ARE THE TREATMENTS?

■ Relievers help to relieve breathing difficulties when they happen.
■ Preventers help protect the airways and reduce the chance of getting asthma symptoms.
   Both can be inhaled so that the medication reaches the inflamed airways instantly.

WHAT IS A SPACER?

A spacer is a large plastic container, usually in two halves that click together. At one end there is a mouthpiece and at the other a hole for the inhaler to fit into.

There are several different brands of spacer that fit the different inhalers and which are available on prescription. Spacers are very important.
■ They make inhalers easier to use and more effective.
■ You get more medicine into your lungs than you could using just the inhaler on its own.
■ The medicine is trapped inside the spacer so you don't have to worry about pressing the inhaler and breathing in at the same time; this makes spacers particularly useful for children, for whom co-ordinating breathing and inhaling is almost impossible. For babies and very young children, a mask can be attached so that by breathing normally the drug is inhaled.
■ They are a convenient and compact alternative to a nebulizer. Spacers work just as well as nebulizers in acute attacks of asthma.
■ They help reduce the possibility of side effects from higher doses of inhaled steroids by reducing the concentration of medicine that is swallowed and absorbed into the body.
■ Spacers do need to be used and cleaned correctly and regularly. Ask your doctor or pharmacist for advice on how to do this.

HOW DO I KNOW IF MY ASTHMA'S GETTING WORSE?

A peak flow meter is a simple instrument that determines the maximum rate at which you are able to blow out. If you take peak flow

Worries about steroids

Many people are anxious about the side effects of steroids used in preventer treatment. Here are some points to remember.
■ The steroids used to treat asthma are called corticosteroids and are completely different from the anabolic steroids used by body builders and athletes.
■ Corticosteroids are a copy of chemicals produced naturally in our bodies.
■ Most people use inhaled steroids, which go straight down to the airways, so very little is absorbed into the body.
■ Your doctor will prescribe the lowest possible dose to get your asthma under control.
■ There is a small risk of a mouth infection called thrush and hoarseness of the voice. You can avoid this by using your inhaler before brushing your teeth, and by rinsing out your mouth well afterwards. Using a spacer will also help reduce the possibility of thrush.

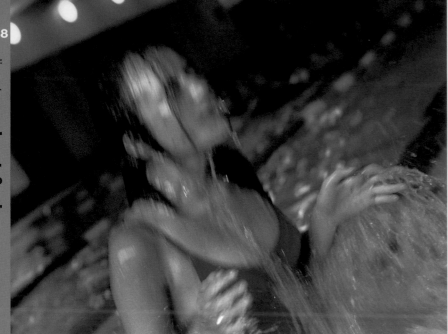

Swimming is ideal exercise for people with asthma.

Asthma self-management

An asthma self-management plan allows you to adjust your own medication according to guidelines you develop and agree in advance with your doctor.

Self-management involves taking a peak flow reading twice a day and keeping track of the results on a chart. You also use other indicators, such as whether your asthma has disturbed your sleep, to determine how well controlled your asthma is each day. You can then adjust your medication accordingly, using the guidelines set out in your plan.

measurements yourself every day to monitor your asthma you will get an early warning sign – a reduced reading – if your condition is worsening.

If you notice any of the following, then you should see your doctor, who can help to bring your asthma back under control.

■ Waking at night with coughing, wheezing, shortness of breath or a tight chest.

■ Increased shortness of breath on waking up in the morning.

■ Needing more and more reliever treatment or reliever doesn't seem to be working as well as it was.

■ Can't keep up with your usual level of activity or exercise.

ASTHMA AND EXERCISE

Exercise is the best way to keep your body in tip-top condition. It is fun and leaves you feeling good about yourself. However, exercise is also a common asthma trigger. But that doesn't mean you should stop! Exercise is good for everyone, including people with asthma.

● Take a couple of puffs of your reliever inhaler (usually blue) about 15 minutes before you start and keep it close at hand at all times.

● Warm up for 5–10 minutes or so with a few short 30-second sprints.

● If you still get wheezy, it's a sign your asthma might not be properly under control. Go and see your doctor, who will be able to adjust your treatment to help get you fighting fit again.

If your asthma is under control, you should be able to do any sport or exercise that you enjoy. However, you might like to try the following.

■ Swimming is a great form of exercise for people with asthma. This is because the air in the pool is warm and moist – a combination that doesn't seem to irritate sensitive airways so much.

■ Yoga can be extremely good for some people with asthma. It helps relax the body and may improve your breathing.

■ Team games are a good idea too – you can always play in a position that doesn't require so much running around.

■ Long spells of exercise are more likely to bring on asthma symptoms than short bursts. So long-distance running is more likely to be a problem than, say, a fitness class involving short periods of aerobic exercise.

There are some sports and activities you should be careful of. These include scuba diving and sports done at high altitudes such as climbing, hiking and skiing. Speak to your doctor if you're thinking about doing any of these activities.

CAN COMPLEMENTARY MEDICINE HELP?

Although some people find that complementary therapies, particularly yoga, acupuncture and homeopathy, seem to improve their asthma symptoms, it is dangerous for a person with asthma to think they can rely on complementary medicines. There is no scientific evidence that complementary treatments used on their own are effective. That is why it is better to regard them as "complementary" rather than "alternative". If you want to try one of the many complementary treatments available, tell your doctor and do not stop taking your normal asthma medication.

What to do in an attack

Sometimes, no matter how careful you are taking medicine and avoiding triggers, you may have an asthma attack. Quite often, a couple of puffs of reliever are all that is needed to get your asthma under control again. At other times, symptoms are more severe and more urgent action is needed. Don't be afraid of causing a fuss, even at night.

1. Take two puffs of your reliever straight away, preferably using a spacer.

2. Keep calm and try to relax as much as your breathing will let you. Sit down, don't lie down. Rest your hands on your knees to help support yourself. Try to slow your breathing down as this will make you less exhausted.

3. Wait 5–10 minutes.

4. If the symptoms disappear, you should be able to go back to whatever you were doing.

5. If the reliever has no effect, call for the doctor or an ambulance.

6. Keep taking your reliever inhaler; use it every few minutes until the ambulance arrives.

7. Take your steroid tablets, if your doctor has written them into your self-management plan.

What if my child has asthma?

Is it easy to be sure?

Diagnosing asthma in very young children can be difficult.

■ If your child is under the age of two, it is even more difficult to tell if they have asthma. There are a number of different wheezing illnesses, including acute bronchiolitis and wheezy bronchitis as well as asthma, that can make your baby wheezy.

■ At least 1 child in 7 will have wheezing at some point during their first five years. Many of these children will not go on to have asthma in later childhood, so your doctor may not want to use the term "asthma" at this stage.

■ It is not easy to measure how well a young child's lungs are working. A peak flow meter is used for older children, but is unsuitable for children under the age of six. The pattern of symptoms that develops **over time** shows whether a child has asthma or not. Your doctor may ask you to keep a record of your child's symptoms and when they happen. This will help the doctor get to the bottom of your child's breathing problems.

The typical symptoms of asthma in young children are:

● coughing, particularly at night and after exercise

● wheezing, or a whistling noise in the chest

● getting short of breath – perhaps your child is not running around as much as usual, or needs to be carried a lot.

Can I prevent it?

If you or your partner have asthma, there are steps you can take that could help reduce the chances of your child developing asthma.

■ Breast-feed for at least four months.

■ Don't keep furry or feathery pets. Avoid allergens such as house-dust mite and pollen during pregnancy and keep your child away from them in the first few months of life.

■ Neither you or your partner should smoke. We know that this increases the likelihood of a child developing asthma. Outdoor air pollution has not been proven to cause asthma although it can make the symptoms of asthma worse.

How will my child cope at school?

Any inhalers that your child needs to take during the school day should be labelled with their name. It is very important that your child can get to their reliever inhaler as soon as they need it. Ideally, children should carry their own reliever inhaler with them at all times. For younger children, their reliever should be kept in a central and accessible place throughout the school day. Make sure that the school knows about your child's asthma.

What about sport?

Exercise is good for everyone, including children with asthma. Nearly all children with asthma become wheezy during exercise. However, if your child takes a few simple precautions, she/he should be able to participate fully in sport at school.

■ Taking a couple of puffs of reliever inhaler 15 minutes before exercise will usually help prevent symptoms.

■ A few short sprints over 5–10 minutes before vigorous games may protect the lungs for an hour or so.

■ If your child takes their reliever inhaler but still gets wheezy after exercising, it's a sign that their asthma might not be properly under control. Go and see your doctor or nurse. They will be able to adjust the treatment to help them get fit and healthy again.

■ And remember – your child should always have their reliever close at hand during exercise.

How do I help?

■ Make sure you tell the school your child has asthma.

■ Tell them about the medication your child requires. Contact the National Asthma Campaign who can provide a free school asthma card to help you do this.

■ Keep the school informed of any changes in your child's medication.

■ Discuss with your teacher any worries you have about your child's asthma.

■ Make sure your child's reliever medication and/or spacer is labelled with his/her name. Make sure the school has a spare inhaler that is also labelled.

■ Make sure your child's medication and the spare are both within their expiry dates.

■ Keep your child at home if he/she is not well enough to attend school.

■ Visit the doctor or nurse regularly to make sure your child's asthma is under good control.

What should the school do?

■ Keep records of children with asthma and the medication they take.

■ Allow children immediate access to their reliever inhaler throughout the school day. That includes during PE, at break time and on school trips.

■ Make sure the school environment is asthma-friendly. For example, do not keep feathery or furry pets in school and adopt a no-smoking policy on school premises.

■ Make sure that pupils take part fully in school life, including PE.

■ Liaise with parents, the school nurse and special educational needs co-ordinator or the Learning Support and Special Educational Needs Department in Scotland if a child is falling behind with their work because of their asthma.

■ Encourage other children to understand asthma. Schools can be associated to the National Asthma Campaign's Junior Asthma Club. Contact the National Asthma Campaign's youth team to find out more (see Useful addresses, p.567).

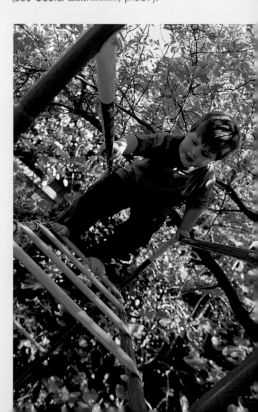

Bronchitis

WHEN THE LARGE AIRWAYS (BRONCHI) BECOME INFLAMED, MOST OFTEN DUE TO A VIRAL
INFECTION, THE BODY'S RESPONSE IS A PRODUCTIVE COUGH, OFTEN WITH YELLOW OR GREENISH
PHLEGM – THESE ARE THE TYPICAL SYMPTOMS OF BRONCHITIS.

There are two forms of bronchitis: **acute**, which starts suddenly and clears quickly, and **chronic**, which is long term and recurs each year with winter cough and phlegm for several months. Chronic bronchitis is one part of chronic obstructive pulmonary disease (COPD; see below) with wheezing, shortness of breath, and eventually serious impairment of lung function due to emphysema. Smoking is undoubtedly the causative factor in COPD.

ACUTE BRONCHITIS

This type of bronchitis is usually a complication of a viral infection such as a cold or flu, when secondary infection by a bacterium supersedes. Attacks usually occur in winter and affect vulnerable people such as smokers, babies, the elderly and people who already have lung disease.

WHAT ARE THE SYMPTOMS?

Inflammation of the lining of the bronchi causes swelling and congestion leading to a feeling of shortness of breath, with or without wheezing, cough and green/yellow phlegm. There may be a temperature and a feeling of soreness behind the breastbone.

WHAT IS THE TREATMENT?

■ Humidify the room or sit in the bathroom with the hot tap filling the bath.
■ Inhalations of steam.
■ Painkillers to bring down a fever.
■ Antibiotics if there is a bacterial infection but they are of no use if the cause is viral. However, antibiotics may be given to protect vulnerable people from a secondary bacterial infection.

ARE THERE COMPLICATIONS?

Rarely, acute bronchitis may develop into the following:
● pneumonia, when the lung tissue becomes inflamed and infected
● pleurisy, when the covering of the lungs is inflamed, usually over a patch of pneumonia.

You should call the doctor if:
● breathlessness is severe
● there is no improvement after three days
● fever exceeds 38.3°C (101°F)
● there is pre-existing lung disease or you belong to a vulnerable group.

WHAT IS THE OUTLOOK?

If smoking continues, or with pre-existing lung disease, there is always the possibility of progression to COPD.

Once you have continuous production of phlegm for three consecutive months during two consecutive years, you have COPD.

Vulnerable people should have a flu vaccination each autumn.

> See also:
> • Pleurisy p.393
> • Pneumonia p.392

Chronic obstructive pulmonary disease

NOWADAYS, PROGRESSIVE DAMAGE TO THE LUNGS – CHRONIC OBSTRUCTIVE PULMONARY DISEASE
(COPD) – IS NEARLY ALWAYS CAUSED BY SMOKING. THE AIRWAYS AND TISSUES OF THE LUNGS BECOME
DAMAGED, EVEN DESTROYED, CAUSING WHEEZING AND INCREASING SHORTNESS OF BREATH.

Some people with COPD eventually become so short of breath that they are seriously disabled and are unable to carry out even simple daily living activities. COPD is rare before age 40 and is twice as common in men, but as more women smoke the prevalence in women is increasing.

People with COPD usually have separate lung conditions, **chronic bronchitis, airway narrowing and emphysema**, and any of these conditions may be dominant.
■ In chronic bronchitis, the airways (bronchi) become inflamed, congested and narrowed, and a cough that produces phlegm is common; in airway narrowing, the flow of air is obstructed.
■ In emphysema, the air sacs (alveoli) within the lungs become enlarged and damaged, making them less efficient in transferring oxygen from the lungs to the bloodstream. The damage to the lungs that is caused by both chronic bronchitis and emphysema is usually irreversible. COPD

is extremely common, affecting about 1 in 6 people in the UK, and is a leading cause of death.

WHAT ARE THE CAUSES?

The main cause of both chronic bronchitis and emphysema, and hence of COPD, is smoking. Occupational exposure to dust, noxious gases or other lung irritants can worsen existing COPD. If you work in a dusty environment, you should wear protective clothing and ask your employer to install air purification systems as appropriate.

In chronic bronchitis, the linings of the airways of the lungs respond to smoke irritation by becoming thickened, narrowing the passages that carry air into and out of the lungs. Mucus glands in the bronchial linings multiply so that great quantities of mucus are produced and the normal mechanism for clearing the airways and coughing up excess

mucus as phlegm is impaired. As the disease progresses, retained mucus in the airways easily becomes infected, which may lead to further damage and bouts of **pneumonia** and **pleurisy**. Repeated infections may eventually cause the linings of the airways to become permanently thickened and scarred, destroying the normal anatomy of the lungs even further.

In emphysema, the air sacs eventually lose their elasticity, and the lungs become distended and can't be properly emptied during exhalation. Eventually, the air sacs tear and merge together, reducing their total surface area, and air becomes trapped in the dilated sacs. As a result, the amount of oxygen that enters the blood with each breath is severely reduced.

People with COPD have restricted lung function, which is evident from lung function tests (see box, opposite).

WHAT ARE THE SYMPTOMS?

Symptoms of COPD may take many years to develop. When they appear, symptoms often include the following:

- shortness of breath on mild exertion, becoming progressively worse so that eventually shortness of breath occurs even when at rest
- coughing in the morning that produces phlegm
- coughing throughout the day
- increasing production of phlegm
- frequent chest infections, especially in winter, producing yellow or green phlegm
- wheezing, especially after coughing.

ARE THERE COMPLICATIONS?

Cold weather and infections, such as flu, cause symptoms to worsen.

■ Some people with emphysema develop a barrel-shaped chest as the lungs become distended.

■ Respiratory failure may develop, in which lack of oxygen causes the lips, tongue, fingers and toes to turn blue.

■ In addition, swelling of the ankles caused by chronic heart failure may occur.

■ Some people who have COPD unconsciously compensate for their lung problems by breathing rapidly to get more oxygen into their blood, and, as a result, they have a **rosy flush** to their skin, the so-called "pink puffers".

■ Other people are unable to compensate in this manner and tend to have a **blue complexion** instead, which is caused by lack of oxygen. These people often have tissue swelling in the feet and legs, which is due to heart failure, the so-called "blue bloaters". These patients may experience drowsiness and headaches.

If you are a smoker and notice symptoms that indicate you may have COPD, consult your doctor as soon as possible and consider stopping smoking immediately.

WHAT CAN I DO?

If you develop COPD and you smoke, giving up permanently is the only action that can delay the progress of COPD. Cutting down on the number of cigarettes you smoke will have little or no effect on the progress of your deterioration.

HOW MIGHT THE DOCTOR TREAT IT?

The damage caused by COPD is largely irreversible, but there are treatments that may ease the symptoms.

■ Your doctor may prescribe an **inhaler** containing a bronchodilator drug.

■ Shortness of breath may also be relieved by continuous **home oxygen therapy**, which also reduces strain on the heart. This therapy concentrates the oxygen available in room air and is used for at least 15 hours a day. It reduces breathlessness, strain on the heart and the risk of heart failure and increases life expectancy.

TEST

Lung function

Two tests are used to detect air flow problems in the lungs: **spirometry**, which measures how quickly the lungs fill and empty, and the **lung volume test**, which can show how much air the lungs can hold. Other tests not shown here include **gas transfer tests**, which use a small amount of inhaled carbon monoxide to determine how fast a gas is absorbed from the lungs into the blood. Tests to measure blood gases show the blood level of oxygen and other gases.

Spirometry

A spirometer is used to measure the volume of air (in litres) that you can inhale and exhale over a period of time. The results show whether the airways are narrowed as a result of lung disorders such as asthma. Spirometry can also be used to monitor the effectiveness of certain treatments for lung disorders, such as bronchodilator drugs, which widen the airways.

Using the spirometer

You will be asked to inhale and exhale fully through a mouthpiece several times. The volume of air inhaled and exhaled is displayed on the monitor.

Lung volume test

This test measures the volume of air (in litres) that can be taken in with a full breath and the volume of air that remains in the lungs when the breath is fully exhaled. The lung volume test is used to help diagnose disorders such as chronic obstructive pulmonary disease that affect the volume of air retained by the lungs after breathing out.

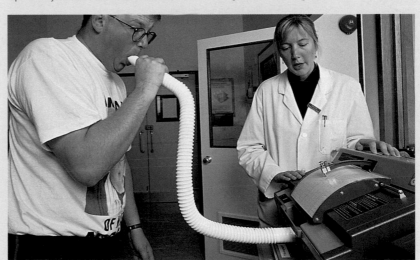

A spirometer is used to measure the volume of air inhaled and exhaled.

■ If you have swollen ankles, your doctor may prescribe **diuretics** to reduce build-up of fluid.

- **Antibiotics** may be prescribed if a chest infection develops.
- You should be **vaccinated against flu** each autumn and you may also be given a further vaccine to protect against infection with the bacterium *Streptococcus pneumoniae*.
- If the lungs are very distended, part of the lung tissue may be removed by **lung volume reduction surgery**. This allows the lungs to inflate and deflate more easily, increasing the amount of oxygen in the blood.
- Pulmonary rehabilitation programmes are run by many hospitals. These last 4–6 weeks and teach patients how to breathe most efficiently and how to exercise within their limits.

WHAT IS THE OUTLOOK?

If your COPD is mild and has been diagnosed at an early stage, you may be able to avoid severe, progressive lung damage if you stop smoking at once. However, most people with COPD do not realize they have the condition until it is well advanced. For these people, the outlook is poor. They often need to retire from work early and may become inactive and housebound through shortness of breath. Although about 3 in 4 people with COPD survive for one year after diagnosis, fewer than 1 in 20 survives longer than 10 years.

See also:
- **Chronic heart failure p.233**
- **Pleurisy p.393** • **Pneumonia p.392**

Pneumonia

IN PNEUMONIA, SOME OF THE TINY AIR SACS (ALVEOLI) IN THE LUNGS BECOME INFLAMED AND FILLED WITH PUS (WHITE BLOOD CELLS) AND FLUID.

When pneumonia develops it is harder for oxygen to pass across the walls of the alveoli into the bloodstream. Usually, only a proportion of one lung is affected, but, in some severe cases, pneumonia affects both lungs ("double" pneumonia) and can be life-threatening. Pneumonia is a result of infection but can occur beyond a blockage due to chronic obstructive pulmonary disease or lung cancer, and as a complication of childhood infections such as whooping cough and measles.

WHO IS AT RISK?

■ Infants, elderly people and people who are already seriously ill or have a chronic disease, such as diabetes mellitus or heart disease, are at greatest risk of developing pneumonia.
■ Other people more likely to develop pneumonia are those who have lowered immunity as a result of a serious disease, such as AIDS. Impaired immunity can also occur during treatment with immunosuppressant drugs or chemotherapy.
■ People who smoke, drink excessive amounts of alcohol or are malnourished are more likely to develop pneumonia.

WHAT ARE THE CAUSES?

■ Most cases of pneumonia in adults are caused by infection with a **bacterium**, most commonly *Streptococcus pneumoniae*. This type of pneumonia may develop as a **complication** of a viral infection in the upper respiratory tract, such as a cold. Other common causes of bacterial pneumonia in healthy adults include infection with the bacteria *Haemophilus influenzae* and *Mycoplasma pneumoniae*. Viral pneumonia can be caused by the organism that is responsible for **influenza** and **chickenpox**.
■ Pneumonia caused by the bacterium *Staphylococcus aureus* usually affects people who are already in hospital with another illness, especially very young children and the elderly.
■ The bacterium known as *Legionella pneumophila* causes a form of pneumonia called **Legionnaires' disease**, which can be spread through air-conditioning systems.
■ A rare type of pneumonia, known as **aspiration pneumonia**, may be caused by accidental inhalation of vomit or a food particle as a result of choking.

WHAT ARE THE SYMPTOMS?

Bacterial pneumonia usually has a rapid onset, and severe symptoms generally develop within a few hours. You may experience the following symptoms:
● cough that may produce rust-coloured or bloody phlegm
● chest pain that becomes worse on inhaling
● shortness of breath at rest
● high fever, delirium or confusion.

In infants, children and elderly people, the symptoms associated with all types of pneumonia are often less obvious. Infants may initially vomit and can develop a high fever that may cause a convulsion. Elderly people may not experience respiratory symptoms but often become progressively confused.

ARE THERE COMPLICATIONS?

■ Inflammation may spread from the alveoli in the lungs to the **pleura** (the membrane that separates the lungs from the chest wall) causing **pleurisy**. Fluid may accumulate between the two layers of the pleura, causing a pleural effusion, compressing the underlying lung and making breathing difficult. If pus

---

TEST

Chest X-ray

A chest X-ray is often one of the first tests used to investigate lung and heart conditions because it is painless, quick and safe. To create the image, X-rays are passed through your chest onto photographic film. Dense tissues, such as the bones, absorb X-rays and appear white; soft tissues appear grey; air appears black. Damaged or abnormal lung tissue or excess fluid in the chest shows up as a white area because it does not contain air as it should. Chest X-rays are usually taken from behind, but in some cases side views may also be required.

Having a chest X-ray

You will be asked to raise your arms to move your shoulderblades away from your lungs and to take a deep breath. While the X-ray is being taken, you must remain still to prevent the image from blurring.

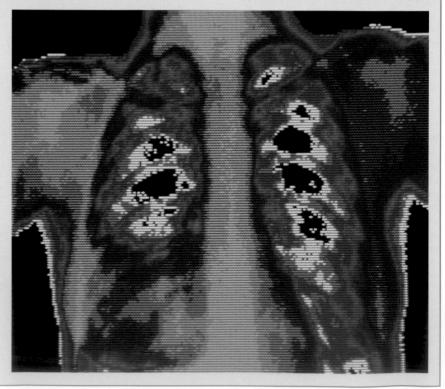

The shadows in this X-ray of the lungs show areas of infection due to pneumonia.

collects between the layers of the pleura, it is known as an **empyema.** This is a serious complication of pneumonia.

■ In severe cases of pneumonia, the microorganism that initially caused the infection may enter the bloodstream, leading to **blood poisoning** (septicaemia).

■ In some vulnerable people, such as young children, elderly people or those with a weakened immune system, the inflammation may spread and result in **respiratory failure**, which is a life-threatening condition. Mechanical ventilation may then be necessary.

WHAT MIGHT BE DONE?

■ Pneumonia can be diagnosed by your doctor examining your chest and listening with a stethoscope.

■ The diagnosis may be confirmed by a chest X-ray (see box, opposite), which will show the extent of infection in the lung.

■ A sample of phlegm may be collected and tested to identify the organism that has caused the infection.

WHAT IS THE TREATMENT?

If you are otherwise healthy and have a mild form of pneumonia, you can probably be treated at home.

■ Painkillers should help reduce your fever and chest pain.

■ If a bacterial infection is the cause of the pneumonia, your doctor will give you antibiotics.

■ Hospital treatment will probably be needed in severe cases of bacterial pneumonia and for infants, children, elderly people and people whose immune systems are suppressed. Drug treatment is essentially the same as it is for people treated at home.

■ If oxygen levels in your blood are low, you will be given oxygen through a face mask. Less commonly, you may require mechanical ventilation in an intensive care unit.

WHAT IS THE OUTLOOK?

Young people who are in good health are generally able to recover from pneumonia within 2–3 weeks, and there is no permanent damage to the lung tissue. Recovery from bacterial pneumonia usually begins within a few hours of starting treatment with antibiotics. However, some severe types of pneumonia, such as Legionnaires' disease, may be fatal, especially in people whose immune systems are weakened.

See also:
• **Blood poisoning (septicaemia) p.345**
• **Chronic obstructive pulmonary disease p.390** • **Lung cancer p.394** • **Pleurisy p.393**

Pleurisy

THIS IS INFLAMMATION OF THE TWO-LAYERED MEMBRANE (PLEURA) THAT SEPARATES THE LUNGS FROM THE CHEST WALL, OFTEN AS A COMPLICATION OF PNEUMONIA.

Normally, when people breathe, the two layers of the pleura slide over each other, allowing the lungs to inflate and deflate smoothly. In pleurisy, inflammation of the pleura prevents the layers from moving over each other easily; they grate as they rub against each other, causing sharp, severe chest pain when inhaling.

WHAT ARE THE CAUSES?

Pleurisy may be caused by a virus, such as **flu**, which affects the pleura itself. However, it's often a reaction to damage to the lung just beneath the pleura. The lung damage may be due to **pneumonia** or **pulmonary embolism**, in which the blood supply to part of the lung is blocked by a blood clot. The pleura can also be affected by primary or secondary **lung cancer**.

Occasionally, an autoimmune disorder such as **rheumatoid arthritis** or **lupus**, in which the immune system attacks healthy tissues, affects the pleura and leads to pleurisy.

WHAT ARE THE SYMPTOMS?

If an infection or a pulmonary embolism is the cause of the inflammation, the symptoms usually develop rapidly over 24 hours. In other cases, the symptoms occur gradually. They include:

• sharp chest pain that causes you to catch your breath on inhaling
• feeling that it is difficult to breathe.

The pain is often restricted to the side of the chest affected by the underlying inflamed pleura. In some cases fluid accumulates between the layers of the pleura (**pleural effusion**). This condition may actually lessen the pain because it eases the movements of the pleural layers over each other.

WHAT MIGHT BE DONE?

If you have chest pain when you breathe consult your doctor immediately. The layers of the pleura rubbing can be heard against each other when your doctor listens to your chest with a stethoscope. You may need a chest X-ray to check for a problem in the underlying lung or for the presence of a pleural effusion.

WHAT IS THE TREATMENT?

■ Non-steroidal anti-inflammatory drugs (NSAIDs) will relieve the pain and inflammation.

■ Holding the affected side while coughing helps relieve the discomfort.

■ If a lung infection is the cause, you will be prescribed a course of antibiotics. If you have a pulmonary embolism, you will probably be given anticoagulant drugs.

In the majority of people the condition clears up within 7–10 days of the start of treatment.

See also:
• **Lung cancer p.394** • **Lupus p.324**
• **Pneumonia p.392** • **Pulmonary embolism p.395** • **Rheumatoid arthritis p.429**

Bronchiectasis

ABNORMAL WIDENING OF THE LARGE AIRWAYS (BRONCHI) IN THE LUNGS THAT CAUSES A PERSISTENT COUGH WITH LARGE AMOUNTS OF PHLEGM IS CALLED BRONCHIECTASIS.

Before mass immunization for childhood infectious diseases, such as **whooping cough** and **measles**, bronchiectasis used to be a common disease. Nowadays, it may still be a complication of pneumonia or occur as part of **cystic fibrosis**. Although bronchiectasis often begins in childhood, the symptoms may not be apparent until after the age of 40.

WHAT ARE THE CAUSES?

■ Childhood infections, such as whooping cough and measles.

■ Repeated lung infections in people with the inherited condition **cystic fibrosis**, in which the mucus produced by the lining of the airways is thicker than normal, blocking the bronchial tubes and collecting in the lungs.

WHAT ARE THE SYMPTOMS?

The symptoms of bronchiectasis gradually worsen over a period of several months or years and include:

• a persistent cough that produces very large quantities of dark green or yellow phlegm and is often worse when lying down
• coughing up blood

- bad breath
- wheezing and shortness of breath
- enlarged fingertips with abnormal fingernails, known as **clubbing**.

Eventually, the effects of long-term infection such as **weight loss** and **anaemia** will show. Bronchiectasis may cause extensive damage to a large area of the lung tissue, and may finally lead to **respiratory failure**.

WHAT MIGHT BE DONE?

- You should not smoke and you should avoid smoke and dust.
- A family member or friend may be taught how to give you chest physiotherapy, which ideally should be carried out on a daily basis.
- Inhaled bronchodilator drugs may be given.
- Any infection will be treated with antibiotics.
- Surgery to remove a single affected area of

the lung may cure the condition, but is very rarely appropriate.

- A small percentage of sufferers may be considered for a lung transplant.

See also:
• Cystic fibrosis p.521 • Measles (chart) p.544 • Whooping cough (chart) p.544

Lung cancer

PRIMARY LUNG CANCER IS NOW THE MOST COMMON TYPE OF CANCER AFTER SKIN CANCER. IT IS THE MOST FREQUENT CAUSE OF CANCER DEATH IN BOTH MEN AND WOMEN. VERY FEW PEOPLE DIAGNOSED WITH PRIMARY LUNG CANCER LIVE LONGER THAN FIVE YEARS.

Lung cancer is a cancerous tumour that develops in the tissue of the lungs; it is most common in men between the ages of 50 and 70, but is rapidly increasing in young women because more people in this group are now smoking.

Smoking is the main cause of lung cancer. The more cigarettes you smoke, the sooner you may develop cancer. For example, if you smoke 20 cigarettes a day you may develop lung cancer 20 years later, if you smoke 40 a day you develop the disease after only 10 years.

WHAT ARE THE TYPES?

Most of these cancers begin in the cells that line the main airways (bronchi) that lead to the lungs. It's important to have an idea about the most common types of lung cancer because each type behaves differently and has a different outlook:

- squamous cell carcinoma and small cell carcinoma are the most common types
- adenocarcinoma and large cell carcinoma make up the rest.

Each type of cancer has a different growth pattern and response to treatment. **Small cell carcinoma** is the most highly malignant type. This type of cancer grows rapidly and spreads very quickly throughout the body. On the other hand, **squamous cell carcinoma** grows more slowly than other types of lung cancer but also spreads to other parts of the body. **Adenocarcinoma** and **large cell carcinoma** both develop at a rate somewhere between small and squamous cell carcinomas.

WHAT ARE THE CAUSES?

About 1 in 7 smokers is likely to develop the disease by the age of 70. The risk is greater for people who have smoked more than 20 cigarettes a day since early adulthood. For people who have never smoked, the risk of lung cancer is small, but it increases slightly for anyone who may be exposed to **other people's cigarette smoke** on a regular basis.

WHAT ARE THE SYMPTOMS?

The symptoms of lung cancer depend on how far advanced the tumour is, but early symptoms include:

- a new persistent cough or change in a long-standing cough, sometimes with blood-streaked phlegm
- chest pain, which may be felt as a dull ache, or as a sharp pain that is worse on inhaling, and usually a symptom of pleurisy that may overlie the tumour
- shortness of breath
- wheezing, if the tumour is positioned so that it blocks an airway
- abnormal curvature of the fingernails, known as clubbing
- sometimes, hoarseness of the voice can signal lung cancer.

Some lung cancers produce no symptoms until they are advanced, when they may cause shortness of breath.

WHAT MIGHT BE DONE?

- A chest X–ray may be done.
- Samples of phlegm may be taken to look for cancerous cells.
- A bronchoscopy may be performed to examine your airways (see box, right). If a tumour is found, a sample will be removed and examined under the microscope.
- Blood tests, CT (computerized tomography) scanning and MRI (magnetic resonance imaging) of the brain, chest, abdomen and bones may be arranged to see if the cancer has spread.

WHAT IS THE TREATMENT?

Treatment of lung cancer depends on the type of cancer and if it has spread to other parts of the body. **Surgery** to remove a tumour in the lung is an option only if the cancer has not spread. Surgery normally involves removal of the whole lung or a major part of it. However, in over 4 out of 5 cases, the cancer has spread to other organs, and surgery is not an option. Small cell carcinoma is usually treated with

chemotherapy, and **radiotherapy** is used to treat cancer that cannot be removed surgically, or to reduce symptoms of cancer that has spread from the lungs. Radiotherapy does not destroy all the cancerous cells but slows tumour growth.

WHAT IS THE OUTLOOK?

About 3 in 4 people who have surgery to remove a tumour survive for two years.

TEST

Bronchoscopy

Bronchoscopy is a type of endoscopy that can be used to diagnose or treat various lung disorders, such as lung cancer and tuberculosis. A rigid or flexible instrument called a bronchoscope is used to view the bronchi (airways) directly and take a specimen of the tumour for analysis – a biopsy. The rigid type is passed through the mouth into the lungs under general anaesthetic. The flexible type is passed through the nose or mouth into the lungs under local anaesthetic. Special instruments can be used to remove tissue samples and if necessary to carry out laser surgery.

Before the procedure, you will be asked not to eat or drink anything for at least six hours. You may be given a sedative, and a local anaesthetic spray will be used to numb your nose and throat. The length of the procedure depends on what your doctor needs to see and whether or not a biopsy is done.

After a bronchoscopy you may have a sore throat and hoarse voice for the next 48 hours. Over-the-counter throat lozenges may help to relieve discomfort.

People with small cell carcinoma usually **survive only 2–10 months after diagnosis**. Although surgery, chemotherapy and radiotherapy may not always prolong life, they can alleviate symptoms and improve quality of life.

ARE THERE COMPLICATIONS?
■ In some cases, **pneumonia** may develop in an area of the lung if an airway is blocked by a tumour.
■ A tumour may also cause **pleural effusion** and **pleurisy**.
■ As the disease progresses, loss of appetite followed by **weight loss** and weakness may develop.
■ There may also be symptoms from tumours that have spread from the lungs to other parts of the body. For example, **headaches** may result from cancer that has spread to the **brain**.

SECONDARY LUNG CANCER (LUNG METASTASES)
Cancerous tumours in the lungs that have spread from another part of the body are called secondary lung cancer or lung metastases. These tumours are most common in people between the ages of 50 and 70 and are more common in women than men because breast cancer may spread to the lungs.

TREATMENT

Radiotherapy

Radiotherapy (exposure of tissue to radiation) destroys or slows the development of cancerous cells. Radiotherapy is usually given after surgery to kill any remaining cancerous cells, but may be used in place of surgery to destroy or reduce the size of certain tumours. Radiotherapy may be external or internal (when radioactive materials are placed in the body).

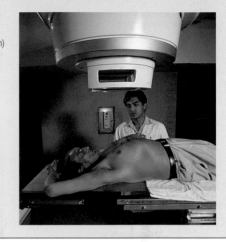

In external radiotherapy, X-rays, gamma rays or electron beams are used to target cancerous tumours. The area to be treated is usually outlined with ink.

Metastases spread to the lungs from other parts of the body via "seedlings" in the bloodstream. The primary cancers that spread most often to the lungs include cancers of the **breast, colon** and **prostate gland**. By the time lung metastases have been detected, there are usually several tumours present and treatment of both the primary and secondary cancers is difficult. Relief of symptoms is the best outcome that can usually be achieved.

See also:
• **CT scanning p.401** • **MRI p.409**
• **Pleurisy p.393** • **Pneumonia p.392**

Pneumothorax

PNEUMOTHORAX, THE PRESENCE OF AIR BETWEEN THE PLEURA (THE TWO-LAYERED MEMBRANE THAT SEPARATES THE LUNGS FROM THE CHEST WALL), MAY OCCUR SPONTANEOUSLY IN HEALTHY YOUNG PEOPLE.

Pneumothorax is thought to be due to the rupture of a congenital blister at the top of the lungs and is rarely serious if treated promptly. It may also result from an injury such as a chest wound or fractured rib or a lung biopsy, or may be a complication of asthma, chronic obstructive pulmonary disease or chest surgery.

WHAT ARE THE SYMPTOMS?
■ Chest pain, which may be sudden and sharp or cause only slight discomfort.
■ Shortness of breath.
■ Chest tightness.
■ With underlying lung disease, pressure may build up and compress the heart, necessitating emergency relief.

■ The windpipe is moved away from the affected side; this can be felt in the neck.

WHAT MIGHT BE DONE?
■ X-rays clearly show air in the pleural cavity.
■ Air may be removed from the pleural cavity by aspiration with a needle or by insertion of a tube.
■ Surgery may be needed to seal the leak.

Pulmonary embolism

IN PULMONARY EMBOLISM, A PIECE OF A BLOOD CLOT (EMBOLUS) BECOMES LODGED IN AN ARTERY IN THE LUNGS AND PARTIALLY OR COMPLETELY BLOCKS BLOOD FLOW IN THE AFFECTED AREA.

Usually, the clot has broken off from a larger clot (thrombus) in the veins of the legs or the pelvic region (**deep vein thrombosis**) and travelled to the lungs in the bloodstream. Rarely, blockage of a major artery may cause sudden severe symptoms and can be fatal. Pulmonary embolism is more common in women over 35 who are overweight, smoke and use oral contraceptives. Being immobile for a long period of time is a risk factor, because blood flow tends to slow down, especially during **pregnancy** and after any **surgery**, when the blood tends to thicken to prevent bleeding.

Pulmonary embolism is most likely to occur in people who have developed deep vein thrombosis as a result of a period of immobility, such as that following childbirth or surgery (especially surgery to repair fractures or pelvic surgery) or, rarely, during a long trip.

A tendency to develop blood clots increases the risk of deep vein thrombosis, as does smoking and taking oral contraceptives.

WHAT ARE THE SYMPTOMS?
A very large embolus that blocks the main pulmonary artery may be fatal. Small clots may cause the following symptoms:
- shortness of breath
- rapid pulse
- low blood pressure and dizziness
- sharp chest pain
- coughing up blood.

WHAT IS THE TREATMENT?
- Anticoagulants to thin the blood and prevent further clots forming.
- Thrombolytic drugs to dissolve the clot.
- Possibly prophylactic daily low-dose aspirin to prevent clots forming in vulnerable people.
- Emergency surgery to remove a large clot.

See also:
- **Deep vein thrombosis p.235**

Hiccups

THE UNMISTAKABLE SOUND PRODUCED BY HICCUPS IS DUE TO A SPONTANEOUS CONTRACTION OF THE DIAPHRAGM FOLLOWED BY INVOLUNTARY CLOSURE OF THE THROAT.

Hiccups occur even before birth; babies hiccup inside the uterus, possibly in preparation for breathing. Most cases settle after a few minutes.

SELF-HELP
There are a vast number of popular home remedies for hiccups, such as holding your breath or drinking a glass of water rapidly. If your hiccups are persistent and exhausting, your doctor may prescribe a drug, such as **chlorpromazine**, that relaxes your diaphragm. In very rare cases, it may be necessary to paralyze the diaphragm by injecting a drug around the nerves that supply it, or by cutting them.

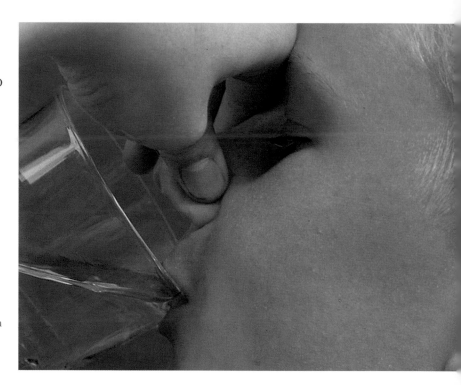

Pneumocystis infection

ALTHOUGH RARE IN HEALTHY PEOPLE, PNEUMOCYSTIS INFECTION IS A COMMON CAUSE OF PNEUMONIA IN PEOPLE WITH REDUCED IMMUNITY, SUCH AS THOSE WITH AIDS. THIS CONDITION IS CAUSED BY INHALATION OF THE PARASITE *PNEUMOCYSTIS CARINII*.

The symptoms, which are the same as other types of pneumonia, are often more striking because of the inability of the immune system to fight back. In severely debilitated patients, pneumocystis pneumonia may be fatal.

See also:
- **HIV infection and AIDS p.338**

Brain and Nervous System

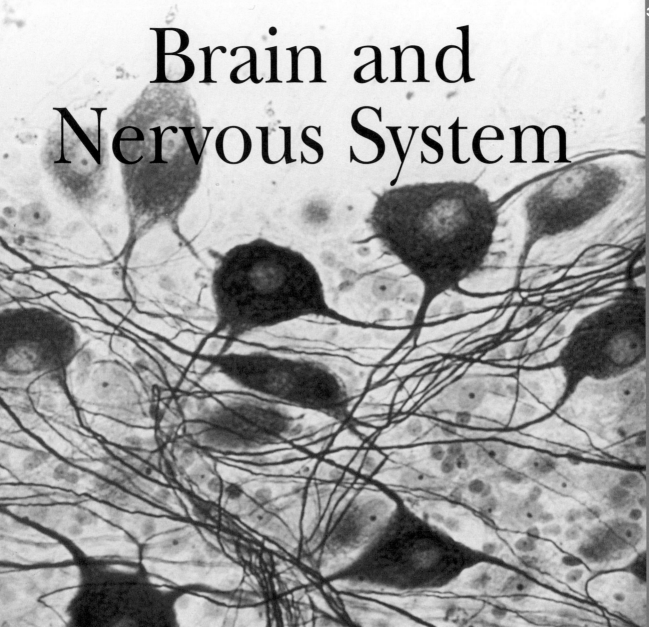

Image shows a light micrograph of neurons in the human brain

Miriam's overview

By far the most common conditions affecting the brain are due not to disease of the brain but to disease of the arteries supplying the brain. The arteries get narrower and narrower as we age, not only in "the brain" but around the heart too, leading to stroke on the one hand and heart attacks on the other.

Mini-strokes or transient ischaemic attacks (TIAs) share the same cause.

I can remember 10 or so years ago there were many theories, including exposure to aluminium, for the cause of Alzheimer's disease. People went out and replaced their aluminium cooking pans for stainless steel ones – quite unnecessarily as it turned out.

Now we know that there is a genetic background to Alzheimer's, with at least one gene being implicated, and sensitive tests have evolved that allow early diagnosis. Perhaps the best news of all is that Alzheimer's can not only be halted by taking HRT, but can be prevented by HRT.

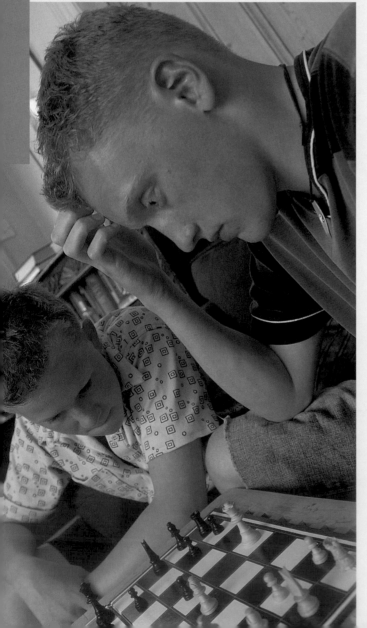

"brain *exercise* is *simply* thinking, concentrating, and

One heartening very new piece of research shows that, contrary to orthodox teaching, brain cells retain their ability to regenerate. It was always thought that damaged brain cells had little power to recover or regrow. Now we know that isn't the case. We retain these regenerative powers even into old age. This knowledge has important implications for the rehabilitation of stroke patients and patients who've had treatment for conditions such as brain tumours.

Think of the brain as a muscle that responds – and grows – as the result of exercise. Brain exercise is simply thinking, concentrating, feeling, and we can stimulate cell regeneration by exercising the brain when we think, concentrate and feel.

"We now know that *brain cells* can *regenerate*"

There have been few new treatments for multiple sclerosis (MS) that have stood the test of time but one that seems to help many sufferers, and one which was stumbled on accidentally, is cannabis. The profound symptomatic relief from cannabis makes a powerful argument in favour of allowing its use on prescription.

Opponents of this view, including the government, would prefer the active substance cannabinol to be prescribed as tablets. But many MS users will testify that it isn't as simple as that. There are thousands of active microsubstances in cannabis and they all seem to help. It's grass that MS patients need, not tablets.

INSIDE
your brain and nervous system

Together, the **brain** and the **spinal cord** form the **central nervous system**. All of the nerves that branch out from the central nervous system and pass through the rest of the body make up the **peripheral nervous system**. The brain and spinal cord process and co-ordinate the nerve signals that are gathered and transmitted by the peripheral nervous system.

The brain and spinal cord consist of two main types of tissue: **grey matter**, which creates and processes nerve impulses, and **white matter**, which transmits nerve impulses. The brain itself contains structures known as the **cerebrum**, which links to every part of the body; the **cerebellum**, which is involved in balance and movement; the **brain stem**, which relays nerve impulses between the brain and spinal cord and controls heart rate and breathing; and a region that contains the **hypothalamus**, which controls the hormonal system. The spinal cord is actually an extension of the brain stem and travels downwards from the base of the skull.

the nervous system

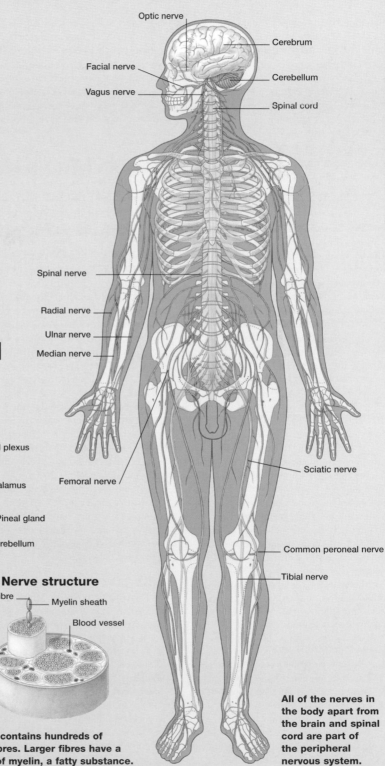

Optic nerve
Cerebrum
Facial nerve
Cerebellum
Vagus nerve
Spinal cord
Spinal nerve
Radial nerve
Ulnar nerve
Median nerve
Femoral nerve
Sciatic nerve
Common peroneal nerve
Tibial nerve

All of the nerves in the body apart from the brain and spinal cord are part of the peripheral nervous system.

the brain and spinal cord

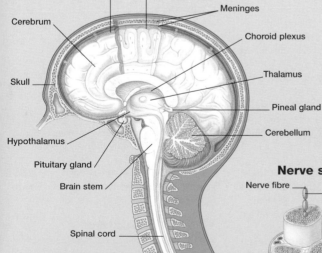

Subarachnoid space
Cerebral cortex
Meninges
Choroid plexus
Cerebrum
Thalamus
Skull
Pineal gland
Cerebellum
Hypothalamus
Pituitary gland
Brain stem
Spinal cord

The brain and spinal cord co-ordinate and control the nerve impulses transmitted to and from nerves in the rest of the body.

Nerve structure

Nerve fibre
Myelin sheath
Blood vessel

A nerve contains hundreds of nerve fibres. Larger fibres have a sheath of myelin, a fatty substance.

ARTERY DISEASE AND THE BRAIN

For most people some degree of "furring up" of the arteries is inevitable as we grow older. Atheroma, as this furring up is called, can affect all of our arteries, but the symptoms are most dramatic if the arteries supplying the heart (see Angina, p.224) and the brain (see Transient ischaemic attacks, p.402 and Stroke, below) are affected, causing the arteries to harden and narrow.

Hardening of the arteries in the brain is exactly the same as hardening of the arteries of the heart and one rarely occurs without the other. Atheroma in any artery interferes with blood supply and predisposes to blood clots forming. When atheroma affects the arteries supplying the brain, the outcome may be a transient ischaemic attack or stroke.

For a doctor, looking at the back of your eyes is like looking through a window at the inside of your body because it's possible to look directly at your arteries on the back of your eye and see if they're becoming furred up. So when your optician or doctor looks at the back of your eyes they aren't simply looking to see if your eyes are healthy, they are looking to see if your arteries are healthy too. Your doctor then has a general idea of the condition of all your arteries, including those supplying the heart and the brain.

So a simple eye examination can alert your doctor to the fact that you could be a candidate for a heart attack or stroke in the future, creating the opportunity to advise you appropriately.

Stroke

A STROKE, SOMETIMES CALLED A CEREBROVASCULAR ACCIDENT (CVA), RESULTS FROM DAMAGE TO PART OF THE BRAIN BECAUSE ITS BLOOD SUPPLY IS CUT OFF.

The blood supply to the brain can be compromised by a blockage (thrombosis or embolism) or a leak (haemorrhage) from one of the arteries in the brain. A CVA is more common in people with high blood pressure, diabetes and high cholesterol levels. People with an irregular heartbeat (atrial fibrillation) are also more susceptible to strokes. After a stroke, part of the brain no longer functions and urgent medical attention is needed.

WHAT HAPPENS?
There is usually little or no warning of a stroke. Immediate admission to hospital for assessment and treatment is essential if there is to be a chance of preventing permanent brain damage. The after effects of a stroke vary depending on the location and extent of the damage. They range from mild, temporary symptoms, such as loss of vision, to life-long disability or, in some people, if the stroke causes extensive brain damage, to coma and death.

If the symptoms disappear within a 24-hour period, the condition is known as a **transient ischaemic attack** or **TIA**, which is a warning sign of a possible future stroke.

HOW COMMON IS IT?
Each year about 100,000 people in the UK have a stroke and the risk increases with age. A 70-year-old living in the UK is about 100 times more likely to have a stroke than a 40-year-old. Although the number of deaths from stroke has fallen over the last 50 years, stroke is still the **third most common cause of death** after heart attacks and cancer in the UK.

WHAT ARE THE CAUSES?
■ About half of all strokes occur when a **blood clot** forms in an artery in the brain, a process called **cerebral thrombosis**.
■ **Cerebral embolism** occurs when a fragment of a blood clot that has formed elsewhere in the body, such as in the heart or the main arteries of the neck, travels in the blood and lodges in an artery supplying the brain. Just under one-third of all strokes are caused by cerebral embolism.
■ **Cerebral haemorrhage** (bleeding), which causes about one-fifth of all strokes, occurs when an artery supplying the brain ruptures and blood seeps out into the brain itself.

Blood clots that lead to cerebral thrombosis and cerebral embolism are more likely to form in an artery that has been damaged by **atherosclerosis**, a condition in which fatty deposits (atheroma) build up in artery walls. Factors that increase the risk of atherosclerosis are a high-fat diet, smoking, diabetes mellitus and raised blood cholesterol levels.

WHAT ARE THE RISKS?
■ The risk of cerebral embolism, thrombosis or haemorrhage is increased by **high blood pressure**, which should always be assessed and treated promptly.
■ Cerebral embolism may be a complication of some heart conditions such as **heart rhythm disorders**, **heart valve disorders** and a **recent heart attack**, all of which can cause blood clots to form in the heart.
■ Sickle-cell anaemia, an abnormality of the red blood cells, also increases the risk of cerebral thrombosis because abnormal blood cells tend to clump together and block blood vessels.

■ Less commonly, thrombosis is caused by narrowing of the arteries supplying the brain due to the inflammation of an autoimmune disorder, such as **polyarteritis nodosa**, in which the immune system attacks the body's own healthy tissues.

WHAT ARE THE SYMPTOMS?
In most people, the symptoms develop rapidly over a matter of seconds or minutes. The exact symptoms depend on the area of the brain affected. The symptoms may include:
● weakness or inability to move on one side of the body
● numbness on one side of the body
● tremor, clumsiness or loss of control of fine movements
● visual disturbances, such as loss of vision in one eye
● slurred speech
● difficulty in finding words and understanding what others are saying
● vomiting, vertigo and difficulty in maintaining balance.

With a severe stroke, the affected person may become unconscious and may decline into coma and die.

HOW IS IT DIAGNOSED?
■ If you suspect that a person has had a stroke, take them to the hospital immediately to find the cause and start treatment.
■ Imaging of the brain, such as computerized tomography (CT) scanning or magnetic resonance imaging (MRI), may be done to find out whether the stroke was due to bleeding or a blockage in a vessel.
■ Antihypertensive drugs, which help control

TEST

CT scanning

Computerized tomography (CT) scanning uses X-rays in conjunction with a computer. A series of X-rays is passed through the body at slightly different angles to produce highly detailed cross-sectional images (slices) of the body, called tomograms. CT scanning makes it possible to gather detailed information about organs painlessly and so that your exposure to radiation is kept to a minimum.

A CT scanner consists of an X-ray source and an X-ray detector, both of which rotate during the procedure so that they remain opposite each other. CT scanning uses X-rays in a different way from an ordinary X-ray machine to give a higher quality image. A CT scan is able to show details that are impossible to see using ordinary X-rays, including fibrous tissue in solid organs such as the liver.

The information from the X-ray detector is sent to the computer, which builds up cross-sectional images of the body and displays them on a monitor. These resulting images can be stored either as computer files or on conventional X-ray film. More sophisticated computers can produce three-dimensional images from standard CT data. Newer CT scanners use the spiral (or helical) technique, in which the scanner rotates around you as

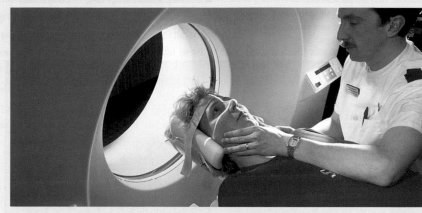

A CT scan is a painless procedure that may take less than one minute to one hour to perform, depending on the condition being investigated.

the bed moves forwards slowly so the X-ray beams follow a spiral course. This type of CT scanning produces three-dimensional images and reduces the time taken for the scans to be completed.

During a CT scan you will lie on a motorized bed that will move you into the scanner. The radiographer will ask you to lie very still and hold your breath while each scan is taken. The bed moves forwards a little more after each scan. If you are very anxious about the procedure you may be given a mild sedative beforehand; you may also be invited to bring a relative or friend with you if you feel you would like moral support. The time it takes

to have a CT scan depends on the nature of the scan and may range from a few seconds to an hour.

CT scans are most often performed on the head and abdomen. However, they can also be used to guide biopsy procedures, in which cells or tissue are taken from internal organs for examination. Like conventional X-rays, CT scanning also produces clear images of bone. Blood vessels and areas of high blood flow, such as the lungs, can also be imaged. These images may be enhanced by using a contrast medium (a substance that makes a hollow or fluid-filled structure visible on the image).

TEST

Carotid Doppler scanning

Carotid Doppler scanning uses ultrasound to look at the flow of blood through blood vessels in the neck. It is generally used to investigate disorders such as transient ischaemic attack or stroke. Ultrasound waves from a transducer produce a picture of the blood flow, which can reveal narrowing of the carotid blood vessels in the neck. Scanning takes about 20 minutes and is painless and safe.

In a carotid Doppler scan, the technician places the ultrasound transducer on one of the carotid arteries to look at the flow of blood through it.

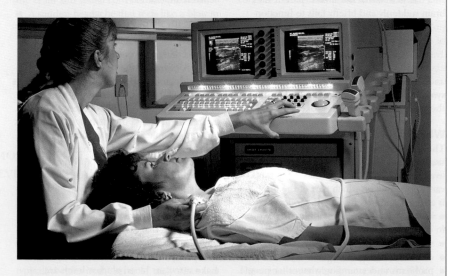

THE MENINGITIS C VACCINE

This is a vaccine against group C **meningococcal** meningitis and **septicaemia** which gives long-lasting protection to babies as young as two months old.

HOW EFFECTIVE IS IT?

Scientists say that the new vaccine is at least 95 percent effective against group C meningococcal meningitis and septicaemia, but it gives absolutely no protection against group B. About 40 percent of cases in the UK are caused by group C, but group B causes most of the rest. **There is no vaccine to prevent group B disease, so it is still very important to be aware of the signs and symptoms of meningitis and septicaemia.**

WHEN SHOULD I BE ON THE LOOK OUT FOR MENINGITIS?

Cases of meningitis and septicaemia increase enormously every winter. The aim of the vaccination programme is to prevent deaths from the disease by protecting as many of those people who are most at risk as possible before winter comes.

WHO IS AT RISK OF MENINGITIS?

Babies and teenagers in the age groups have the highest risk.

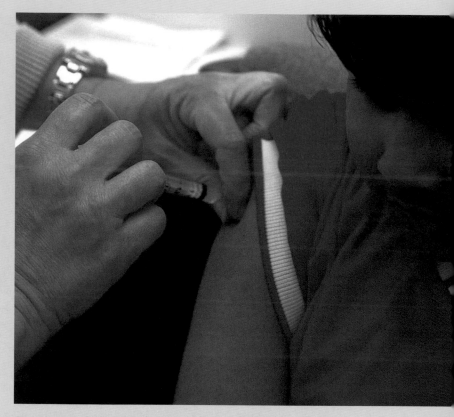

HOW DO PEOPLE GET THE MENINGITIS C VACCINE?

● Babies and toddlers receive the vaccine along with their other routine immunizations. Anyone who hasn't had the vaccine and feels that they should have it should contact their GP.

IS THE MENINGITIS C VACCINE SAFE?

● The meningitis C vaccine has been tested on over 6,000 people in the UK and 21,000 people abroad and has been shown to be safe and to give long-term immunity.
● No serious side effects occurred during safety testing. Some babies and children have had a slight temperature, an unsettled night, or redness and swelling of the skin where they were injected, but the chance of having these mild reactions is no greater than with other childhood vaccines. Older children and teenagers sometimes complain of headache. Vomiting has been reported in some babies, but this is more likely due to other vaccines

that have been given at the same time.
● The vaccine is not "live" and cannot cause even a mild form of meningitis or septicaemia.
● There are no new ingredients in the vaccine. All the ingredients of the new vaccine have already been given to millions of children over many years as components of other vaccines, without causing any harm.

ARE THERE ANY PEOPLE WHO SHOULDN'T HAVE THE VACCINE?

● People who have had a severe reaction to the plain **meningococcal** vaccine or **Hib** or **diphtheria** vaccines should not have the vaccine.
● Vaccination should be postponed in anyone who is ill with a high fever.
● It has not been tested in pregnant women, and although there is no reason to suggest it is not safe during pregnancy, women who think they might be pregnant should speak to their doctor or nurse about it.

IS THERE A PROBLEM WITH "MULTIPLE" VACCINES?

Some parents might be worried that having

DTP, Hib, polio and the new vaccine together will overload babies' immature immune systems.
● There is no danger in having these vaccines at the same time. During trials of the new vaccine, scientists showed that the vaccines could not interact in any way that could harm babies and children.
● These vaccines do not "overload" the immune system. **Vaccines work by arousing a response from the immune system, but getting all the routine vaccinations and the new C-strain vaccine at the same time is less of a challenge to the immune system than everyday events like a baby getting a throat infection or a toddler falling and scraping a knee.**
● Routine vaccinations are timed to protect babies when they need it most.

See also:
● **Chemotherapy p.257**
● **HIV infection and AIDS p.338**
● **Mumps (chart) p.544**
● **Immunization timetable p.519**
● **Thrombocytopaenia p.239**

Preventing a migraine and avoiding the triggers

You should try to be aware of your migraine triggers and avoid them as far as possible. You'll be able to spot warning signs and therefore control the migraine attack better. You can quite often abort a migraine attack if you take some form of treatment as soon as you sense the aura, then the headache may never appear. If an attack starts, try to treat it as quickly as possible with a painkiller such as paracetamol, the soluble form if possible.

Many factors are known to trigger a migraine. You need to identify the ones that affect you. Avoiding these factors may help reduce the frequency and severity of attacks.

■ Keep a diary for a few weeks to help pinpoint trigger factors.
■ Avoid any food you find brings on an attack. Common dietary triggers of migraine include red wine, cheese (especially matured cheese) and chocolate.

■ Eat regularly, because missing a meal may trigger an attack.
■ Follow a regular sleep pattern if possible, because changing it may trigger an attack.
■ If stress is a trigger, you may find it helpful to try relaxation exercises.

continued from page 403

change in brain hormones, resulting first in constriction of blood vessels (causing the flashing lights) then dilatation (causing the thumping headache). There are many well-known triggers that change these brain hormones, the best known of which is **serotonin**.

HOW LONG DO MIGRAINE ATTACKS LAST?
Migraine can vary in severity from being a throbbing headache, usually on one side, which lasts an hour or so, to one that's so excruciating you have to lie immobile in a darkened room for two or more days.

WHAT ARE THE SYMPTOMS?
Migraine symptoms can take a variety of forms.

VISION PROBLEMS
About half an hour prior to the start of the headache you may notice flashing lights or that lights have a halo around them. Part of your visual field may go dark. These symptoms can occur on their own **without a headache**, in which case it's called an **optical migraine**.

HEADACHE
Migraine is a headache plus. The throbbing or knife-like headache, usually above one eye, is followed by nausea (feeling sick), vomiting (being sick) and an aversion to light, sound and movement of any kind. More than one of these symptoms has to be present to be considered a migraine, but not all.

PARALYSIS
Sometimes sensation and movement on one side of the body are affected – like a mini-stroke – and return to normal when the headache goes. This is called **hemiplegic migraine**.

ABDOMINAL PROBLEMS
Migraine where there are mainly abdominal symptoms, such as vomiting and stomach pain, is called **abdominal migraine** and is common in children.

WHAT'S AN AURA?
An aura precedes the headache and can be anything from distorted vision to "pins and needles", or simply an odd feeling.

MIGRAINE IN WOMEN
Many women find that migraine forms a part of the **premenstrual syndrome (PMS)** due to the hormonal changes that take place each month.

Women's hormone levels change constantly throughout their reproductive lives, and this could be why more women suffer from migraine than men. There's also **menopausal migraine** that occurs when hormonal levels sink as menstruation stops.

MIGRAINE IN CHILDREN
Between the ages of 5 and 15, **1 child in 9** suffers from attacks of migraine. Until puberty, boys and girls suffer equally.

Childhood migraine can differ quite dramatically from the adult form. Attacks tend to be shorter (sometimes only an hour) with the emphasis on abdominal pain, nausea and vomiting; the headache can be mild, even absent.

Young children are very often unable to describe the symptoms of migraine and may describe the way they feel as a "sick headache" or "a headache in my tummy". As children get older, abdominal symptoms usually subside and the headache becomes prominent.

The differentiation from **appendicitis** can be difficult and children have been opened up unnecessarily.

CAN CERTAIN FOODS BE A TRIGGER?
Certain foods such as chocolate, cheese, fortified wine like sherry and port, and caffeine may trigger an attack. Missing meals, causing a **drop in blood sugar**, can precipitate a migraine attack.

CAN STRESS CAUSE MIGRAINE?
A period of stress is often followed by a migraine – usually when you're beginning to unwind. If you have a stressful job or very busy lifestyle, you can often have a **weekend or holiday migraine**.

CAN LACK OF SLEEP BE A TRIGGER?
An irregular sleep pattern is a common cause of migraine. Lie-ins or lots of sleep at the weekend are often perceived as a good thing, but in reality are as much a trigger for migraine attacks as lack of sleep.

WHAT OTHER FACTORS CAUSE MIGRAINE?
Travel, weather changes, hormonal factors (in women), loud noises, bright or flickering lights, TV, cinema or VDUs, shopping and strong smells have all been known to trigger attacks.

WHAT IS THE TREATMENT?
Everyone who suffers has their favourite recipe for migraine, arrived at by trial and error over the years. For instance, mine was **Stemetil** suppositories (prescription only) and a darkened room; my stepdaughter's is Solpadeine extra strength, two capsules every four hours.

A hard and fast rule is that any headache can develop into a migraine, so never ignore one.

Your pharmacist will advise you about over-the-counter remedies and medicines for children. However, these are largely for the treatment of symptoms – they don't get at the cause.

From your doctor there are many prescription medicines to try, the latest one being a selective serotonin re-uptake inhibitor (SSRI), which treats the cause. Some of these medicines are injectable, while others can be inhaled or ingested as wafers. Also, if migraine headaches occur frequently (more than about four times a month) there are medications that you take daily to prevent migraines from coming on.

Your emergency kit: When my migraine was worst I never went anywhere without my migraine remedies. Carry yours with you always so that you can take action fast.

See also:
• **The atopic family of conditions p.311**

FOCUS
on chronic fatigue syndrome

The terminology applied to fatigue is confusing for everyone, including doctors. As anyone knows who has got chronically tired, there's a spectrum of fatigue which, at one end, may demand nothing more than a few early nights to catch up but at the other end of the scale may require time off work resting in bed.

So it's important to separate ordinary tiredness from chronic fatigue syndrome (CFS), also known as **myalgic encephalopathy** or ME.

WHAT IS CFS?

Chronic fatigue syndrome is a complex illness with extreme fatigue over a long time. Extreme exhaustion is nearly always a prominent part of CFS, plus muscle pain and a flu-like malaise.

Other symptoms can include problems with concentration and memory, loss of balance, digestive problems, sleep disturbances and mood swings.

CFS affects around 15,000 people in the UK but we know of no exact cause, there's no specific test for it and treatment is purely symptomatic. Many cases arise after a persistent viral infection that has **weakened** the immune system. The association of a viral infection followed by tiredness isn't new of course. We've known for years that the glandular fever virus, for instance, can leave behind it lassitude and depression that can take 9–12 months to get better.

HOW DO WE GET OVERTIRED?

Our fight-and-flight system, the release of adrenaline to prepare us to fight an enemy or run from him, was perfect millennia ago, when stress would consist of the occasional sighting of hostile neighbouring tribesmen.

But today it's constantly on red alert because of the pressured environment we live in. It simply cannot cope with modern-day stresses.

Our bodies are never given the chance to

How can I help myself?

Along with experts in the field, I'm very concerned that supplements are promoted heavily to a vulnerable group of people whose expectations may be falsely raised. I personally would always recommend good eating combined with exercise to relieve chronic tiredness. Exercise is the only way I know of increasing the amount of energy I have. The cornerstone of fitness, exercise is also the antidote to tiredness and ensures refreshing sleep. Run through the benefits of exercise on p. 21. But here are tables of the **foods that contain carbohydrates** and minerals that can also help boost your energy levels.

Minerals

I personally would always recommend good eating combined with exercise to relieve chronic tiredness. But first – here are foods containing minerals that will help to bump up your energy levels.

Best food source	Nutrient	Quantity	Maximum
Broccoli, canned salmon, cheese, fortified orange juice, milk, soy products and yoghurt	Calcium	1,000mg	1,500mg
Barley, legumes, lobster, nuts, organ meats and prunes	Copper	1.5 to 3mg	9mg
Beans, fortified breads and cereals, green leafy vegetables, nuts, oysters and scallops	Magnesium	310mg	700mg
Avocados, beef, dried apricots, fortified breads and cereals, legumes and shellfish	Iron	15mg	65mg
Chicken, mushrooms, nuts, onions, seafood, seeds, garlic, wheatgerm and wholegrain bread	Selenium	55mcg	200mcg
Beef, fortified cereals, legumes, liver, shellfish, wheatgerm and yoghurt	Zinc	12mg	30mg

Carbohydrates

The best source of energy is carbohydrate, so start loading your diet with it.

Food	Grams of carbohydrates
230g serving cooked pasta	50
60g serving cornflakes	50
150g serving rice	45
2 slices of wholemeal bread	30
Toasted bun	30
54g milk chocolate	30
2 scoops of mashed potato	25
1 medium banana, apple or pear	20
160ml serving orange juice	15

And here's how to eat carbohydrates.
Try to eat 5g of carbohydrate per kilogram of body weight each day. For a 70kg man this means having at least 350g of carbohydrate a day and for a 55kg woman, 275g.
To reach these figures have some carbohydrate foods at each meal. Try bread and bread products, pasta, breakfast cereals, rice, potatoes, beans, root vegetables, fruits and **crispbreads**. Ideally eat a meal containing carbohydrate 2–4 hours prior to exercise and a small snack such as a banana about an hour before.
Try to eat around 50g of carbohydrate within 2 hours of finishing exercise. This helps refuel the muscles and should include some quickly absorbed foods such as fruit bars, bananas, **cornflakes** with skimmed milk, sultanas, raisins or a glass of high-energy drink.

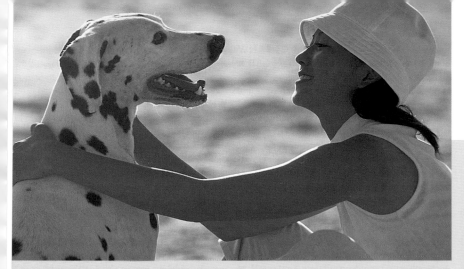

recover from an acute (sudden) stress reaction and soon end up in a state of chronic (long-term) stress, which may compromise the immune system.

When the immune system can't fight off infection we're into a vicious downward spiral to exhaustion.

WHAT ARE THE SYMPTOMS OF CFS?

Although the number and severity of symptoms may vary, the major symptoms of chronic fatigue syndrome are:

- **prolonged** severe fatigue lasting at least six months
- **impairment** of short-term memory or concentration
- **sore** throat
- **tender** lymph nodes
- **muscle** and joint pain without swelling or redness
- **unrefreshing** sleep
- **headaches**
- **prolonged** fatigue and feeling ill after even mild exertion.

Many people who have chronic fatigue syndrome also develop symptoms of depression, such as loss of interest in their work and leisure activities, or of anxiety. This in turn can lead to prolonged inactivity, resulting in "deconditioning" of the whole body that affects the muscles particularly. Conditions involving an allergic reaction, such as eczema and asthma, may become worse in people who have chronic fatigue syndrome.

HOW IS CFS DIAGNOSED?

There are specific criteria which must be present before a diagnosis can be made. Just being plain tired doesn't mean you've got CFS. Your doctor may suspect chronic fatigue syndrome if you have had prolonged fatigue for more than six months with no obvious cause, and you also have at least four of the other symptoms listed. Even

if no underlying cause is identified, the diagnosis of chronic fatigue syndrome will only be made if your symptoms meet the diagnostic criteria.

COPING WITH CFS

If you develop chronic fatigue syndrome, you are likely to have fluctuating energy levels. You may find that you need to be flexible and adjust your lifestyle to help you live with the condition. The following actions may be helpful.

- Try to divide the day into sessions of rest and work.
- Graded exercise may be useful. Try to set yourself a progressive increase in activity week by week.
- Set realistic goals for yourself.
- Make dietary changes, in particular by drinking less alcohol and cutting out drinks containing caffeine.
- Try to reduce stress.
- Join a support group so that you do not feel isolated.

WHAT IS THE TREATMENT FOR CFS?

Although there is no specific treatment for chronic fatigue syndrome, there are a number of measures that may help you cope with the condition.

- Your doctor may give you drugs to help relieve some of your symptoms. For example, headaches and joint pain may be relieved by analgesics, such as aspirin, or **non-steroidal anti-inflammatory drugs**.
- **Antidepressant drugs** may produce an improvement in your condition even if you have not developed the symptoms of depression.
- Your doctor may advise you to have **counselling** to help you cope with your illness and to provide support.
- You may also find **cognitive therapy** and **behaviour therapy** beneficial.

WHAT IS THE OUTLOOK?

Chronic fatigue syndrome is a long-term condition. Many people find that symptoms are at their worst in the first 1–2 years. In more than half of all cases, the condition clears up completely after several years. In some people, the symptoms of chronic fatigue syndrome come and go over a number of years.

See also:
- **Insomnia p.296** • **Depression p.298**
- **The menopause p.497**

TATT syndrome

If you're one of the 38 percent of the UK population who feels exhausted most of the time and wakes up **unrefreshed**, you're in good company.

You have a **recognized** syndrome – TATT – "tired all the time" syndrome. There's no cure, but you could feel a whole lot better if you eat **well**, get eight hours' sleep and set aside time for yourself each day. The simple explanation for present-day long-term tiredness is that we all do too much. We're in overload, even **burn-out**.

A special problem for women Women are often struggling to look after children,

working in the day, doing household chores in the evening and being a wife at night. And women feel under pressure to perform well in all their roles, so it's hardly surprising that many end up chronically tired.

People with chronic tiredness often work too hard. If, on top of everything, you sleep badly you may never recharge your batteries at the end of the day. The key is to have a balance between work and leisure. It's no bad thing to take an inventory of your lifestyle, the time you go to bed, the quality of sleep you get and whether you take time out to relax and enjoy yourself.

Creutzfeldt–Jakob disease

CREUTZFELDT–JAKOB DISEASE (CJD) IS AN EXTREMELY RARE CONDITION IN WHICH
BRAIN TISSUE IS PROGRESSIVELY DESTROYED BY AN UNUSUAL INFECTIOUS AGENT.

A general decline in all areas of mental and physical ability leads ultimately to death. CJD affects about one person in a million each year worldwide.

WHAT IS THE CAUSE?

CJD is caused by an infectious agent known as a **prion**, which replicates in the brain and causes brain damage.

■ One type of CJD, accounting for 15 in 100 cases, has been found to run in families. Most people who develop this form of CJD are over age 50. Usually, the source of the infection is unknown. In about 1 in 20 affected people it can be traced to previous treatment with products derived from human tissue. Before the use of artificial growth hormone to treat growth disorders, one source of infection was human growth hormone injections.

■ In the mid-1990s, a new rare variant of CJD that affects younger people was discovered in the UK. This form of the disease is believed to be linked with eating contaminated meat from cattle with a disease called **bovine spongiform encephalopathy** (**BSE**). It is possible that this form of the disease might be passed from a pregnant mother to her unborn child.

WHAT ARE THE SYMPTOMS?

It is thought that CJD is present for between two and 15 years before symptoms start to appear. Early symptoms develop gradually and may include:

● depression
● poor memory
● unsteadiness and poor coordination.

Other symptoms develop as the condition progresses and include:

● sudden muscle contractions
● seizures
● weakness or paralysis on one side of the body
● progressive dementia
● impaired vision.

Eventually, an affected person may become unable to move and talk. People with late-stage CJD who are confined to bed are also prone to serious lung infections.

WHAT MIGHT BE DONE?

CJD is usually diagnosed from the symptoms. Tests performed on the tonsils and appendix may confirm the presence of the prions associated with the new variant form of CJD. Other tests are:

● magnetic resonance imaging (MRI) to exclude other treatable causes
● brain biopsy, during which a small piece of tissue is surgically removed for microscopic examination.

CJD cannot be cured, but drugs can relieve some of the symptoms.

■ Symptoms of depression may be treated with antidepressant drugs.

■ Muscle contractions may be controlled by muscle relaxants.

The disorder is usually fatal within three years.

Motor neuron disease

IN MOTOR NEURON DISEASE THERE IS PROGRESSIVE DEGENERATION OF THE NERVES IN THE
BRAIN AND SPINAL CORD THAT CONTROL MUSCLE ACTIVITY, LEADING TO WEAKNESS AND WASTING
OF THE MUSCLES. SOME TYPES OF MOTOR NEURON DISEASE ARE INHERITED.

WHAT ARE THE SYMPTOMS?

In the initial stage of the disease, there is weakness and wasting, developing over a few months and usually affecting muscles of the hands, arms or legs.

Other early symptoms may include:
● twitching movements in the muscles
● stiffness and muscle cramps
● difficulty performing twisting movements, such as unscrewing bottle tops and turning keys.

As the disease progresses, other symptoms may include:
● dragging one foot or a tendency to stumble when walking
● difficulty climbing stairs or getting up from low chairs

● less commonly, slurred speech, hoarseness and difficulty swallowing if the muscles of the mouth and throat are involved
● mood swings, anxiety and depression
● recurrent chest infections and possibly pneumonia, if the muscles involved in breathing and swallowing are affected and small particles of food enter the lungs
● the head falling forward because the muscles in the neck are too weak to support it
● eventually, difficulty in breathing due to weakness of the muscles that control respiration.

WHAT IS THE TREATMENT?

At present, no treatment can significantly slow down the progression of motor neuron disease, although a new drug called riluzole may have a small effect. Treatment for symptoms may include antidepressants to relieve depression and antibiotics to treat chest infections. A gastrostomy may be done to treat difficulty swallowing. This is a surgically created opening through which a permanent feeding tube is inserted directly into the stomach or the small intestine.

Usually, a team of specialists will be available to provide support and care for an affected person and members of his or her family. Counselling may be offered to both, and the affected person may be given physiotherapy to help keep joints and muscles supple.

Facial palsy

IN FACIAL PALSY, ALSO CALLED BELL'S PALSY, THERE IS WEAKNESS OR PARALYSIS
OF THE FACIAL MUSCLES ON ONE SIDE OF THE FACE DUE TO DAMAGE TO THE FACIAL
NERVE. THE PROBLEM USUALLY CLEARS UP WITHOUT TREATMENT.

WHAT ARE THE CAUSES?
■ The viral infection **shingles (herpes zoster)** is
a known cause of damage to the facial nerve, and
many other viruses, especially herpes simplex,
also have the potential to cause facial palsy.
■ The bacterial infection **Lyme disease**, carried
by ticks, is also a known cause.
■ Inflammation of the facial nerve is
sometimes due to a middle ear infection.
■ Rarely, the facial nerve may be compressed
by a tumour called an **acoustic neuroma**.

WHAT ARE THE SYMPTOMS?
In some cases, the symptoms of facial palsy
appear suddenly over about 24 hours. In
other cases, including facial palsy caused by
an acoustic neuroma, symptoms may develop
slowly. The symptoms include:
● partial or complete paralysis of the muscles
on one side of the face
● pain behind the ear on the affected side
● drooping of the corner of the mouth,
sometimes associated with drooling
● inability to close the eyelid on the affected
side, and watering of the eye
● impairment of taste.
If facial palsy is very severe, you may have
difficulty speaking and eating. In a few cases,
sounds seem unnaturally loud in the ear on
the affected side. If the eyelid cannot be
closed, the eye may become infected, possibly
leading to ulceration of the cornea, the
transparent front part of the eye. In facial

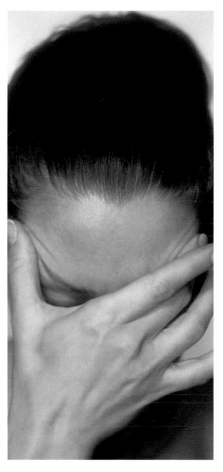

palsy due to shingles, there is also a rash of
crusting blisters on the face.

WHAT MIGHT BE DONE?
■ If your symptoms have appeared in the last
48 hours, your doctor may prescribe
corticosteroids for up to two weeks to reduce
inflammation of the nerve.
■ Analgesics will relieve pain.
■ To prevent damage to the cornea, you
may be given artificial tears and you will
probably be advised to tape the affected eye
shut when you go to sleep.

WHAT IS THE OUTLOOK?
Bell's palsy usually clears up without further
treatment. If facial palsy has an underlying
cause, it will be treated too. For example, if
facial palsy is due to shingles, antiviral drugs
such as **acyclovir** will be prescribed. To be
effective, treatment with acyclovir should begin
as soon as the rash appears. If there is an
acoustic neuroma, it will be removed surgically
to relieve compression of the facial nerve.

If muscle paralysis persists, **plastic surgery**
may be used to re-route another nerve to the
face. Facial exercises and massage may help
maintain tone and facial symmetry.

With appropriate treatment, facial palsy
usually improves in about two weeks. However,
a full recovery may take up to three months.
Some people are left with weakness in the
affected area, and facial palsy may recur.

Persistent vegetative state

PERSISTENT VEGETATIVE STATE IS A LONG-TERM STATE OF UNCONSCIOUSNESS CAUSED BY DAMAGE
TO THE BRAIN. SUFFERERS ARE PHYSICALLY AND MENTALLY UNRESPONSIVE TO EXTERNAL STIMULI,
BUT REQUIRE NO HELP WITH VITAL FUNCTIONS SUCH AS BREATHING AND HEART RATE.

Coma may result from extensive brain damage
as may occur in head injuries or after a heart
attack when the brain has been starved of
oxygen for too long. The most common cause
is a severe head injury. Persistent vegetative
state can also be caused by infection of the
brain, such as **viral encephalitis**, or by oxygen
deprivation of the brain as a result of **near-
drowning**.

In persistent vegetative state, the parts of the
brain that control the higher mental functions
such as thought are damaged, leaving the areas
that control the vital functions such as
breathing and heart rate intact. So although

someone is physically and mentally unresponsive
to noise, light and other stimuli, they can
breathe without assistance. They may also move
the head or limbs.

People in a persistent vegetative state appear
to have normal sleep patterns, with their eyes
closing and opening as if sleeping and waking.
However, they do not appear to feel physical
sensations such as pain or experience emotional
distress. Since areas of the brain that control
breathing and other functions are intact, a
person in a persistent vegetative state can
remain alive for months or even years provided
appropriate medical treatment is given.

WHAT MIGHT BE DONE?
The diagnosis of persistent vegetative state is
made if a person who is unconscious fails to
respond to stimulation or to communicate but
vital functions such as breathing are
maintained. It's generally agreed that the mind
of the person is not functioning consciously.

There is no effective treatment for a person
who is in a persistent vegetative state. However,
general supportive measures and nursing care
will ensure that an affected person is kept
as comfortable as possible. A person in a
persistent vegetative state can live for several
years but recovery is unlikely.

Vertigo

VERTIGO IS AN UNPLEASANT SENSATION OF MOVING OR SPINNING, OFTEN COMBINED WITH NAUSEA AND VOMITING. AN ATTACK OF VERTIGO CAN BE VERY DISTRESSING AND IN SEVERE CASES MAY MAKE IT IMPOSSIBLE TO WALK OR EVEN TO STAND.

Vertigo is a symptom of many different disorders, for example:

- a disorder of the organs of balance in the inner ear (the vestibular apparatus)
- a disorder of the nerve that connects the inner ear to the brain
- problems in the areas of the brain concerned with balance
- a condition such as multiple sclerosis (MS) that requires urgent medical attention.

WHAT ARE THE CAUSES?

There are a number of possible causes.

■ **Infection of the vestibular apparatus**: labyrinthitis usually begins as a viral infection of the respiratory tract, such as a common cold or flu or, less frequently, a bacterial infection of the middle ear. This type of vertigo usually **starts suddenly and lasts for 1–2 weeks**.

■ **Ménière's disease**: recurrent vertigo combined with deafness and **tinnitus** is a conditional sign of Ménière's disease.

■ **Antibiotics**: vertigo is a side effect of certain antibiotics.

■ **Acoustic neuroma**: this type of tumour, affecting the nerve that connects the inner ear to the brain, is a rare cause of vertigo.

■ **Strokes and head injuries** are other rare causes of vertigo.

SELF-HELP

You'll relieve vertigo by lying still, closing your eyes and avoiding sudden movement. If you've been vomiting, take small sips of water every 10 minutes to avoid dehydration until your symptoms go. If the vertigo persists for more than a few minutes, or if it becomes recurrent, you should consult your doctor.

WHAT TESTS MIGHT BE DONE?

■ Your doctor may examine your ears, eye movements and nervous system to look for a cause.

■ Tests may include a caloric test, in which water at different temperatures is poured into the ear to check the function of the vestibular apparatus of the inner ear.

■ A neck X-ray may be done to look for cervical spondylitis.

■ If you also have tinnitus, you may have computerized tomography (CT) scanning or magnetic resonance imaging (MRI) to rule out a tumour pressing on the brain.

WHAT IS THE TREATMENT?

Antisickness drugs and antihistamines will relieve vertigo. If vertigo is a side effect of an antibiotic, you can be given an alternative.

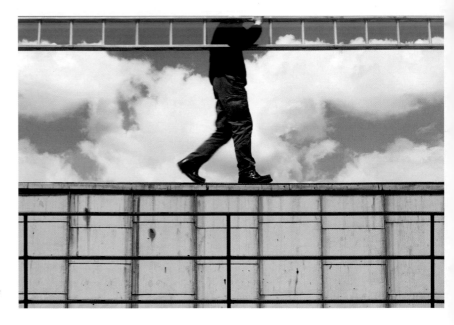

Bones, joints & muscles

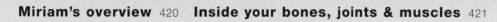

Image shows a coloured scanning electron micrograph of normal spongy bone

Miriam's overview

We take the efficient, comfortable working of the skeleton very much for granted until something goes wrong. It can be a rude awakening when bone, joint and muscle disorders become extremely painful and disabling.

With arthritis in a knee, going about your everyday activities is curtailed, but with a frozen shoulder, you can't even get out of the door as it stops you from putting your clothes on.

Within the body our bony skeleton, our joints and our muscles work in harmony together to make us uniquely mobile and dexterous. The efficiency of our muscles to move joints and leverage bone is quite astonishing, but all components need servicing.

Muscles can't work efficiently if they're unfit. Joints don't remain frictionless if they're damaged or abused and bones can become thin if not properly nourished and exercised.

So it's our responsibility to keep this whole system in good working order by resisting a sedentary lifestyle and taking regular weight-bearing exercise. If we don't, we, and especially women, pay a heavy price.

Peak bone mass – the intrinsic strength of our bones – reaches a maximum before the age of 35. If we've been a dieter or not taken much exercise, or worst of all been anorexic, our peak bone mass is low.

When the menopause arrives and bones suddenly thin – they can lose one-third of their mass in three years due to lack of oestrogen – they are at much greater risk of osteoporosis. And brittle bones are painful, they fracture,

they collapse and can land a woman in hospital from which she may never come out. 1 in 4 women with a fractured hip bone dies in hospital.

Great strides have been taken with the biotechnology of joint replacement. Nowadays almost any joint can be renewed for sufferers of both osteoarthritis and rheumatoid arthritis. The latter is always the most difficult to treat with its acutely tender and swollen joints, so inflamed that some destruction is inevitable, leaving behind ugly deformities. Newer drugs and newer ways of giving them present much hope that the course of rheumatoid arthritis can be arrested.

"it's our *responsibility* to keep this whole system in *good working order*"

Repetitive strain injury (RSI) is an almost entirely modern phenomenon. Never before have jobs called for repetitive fine movements performed for long periods of time. The main trouble is in the brain, not in the fingers, wrist or elbows where we feel the pain. The brain apparently gets confused in RSI and calls on our joints and muscles to perform opposing movements at the same time. Retraining your brain therefore is just as essential a part of treatment for RSI as hand rests and careful positioning of keyboards.

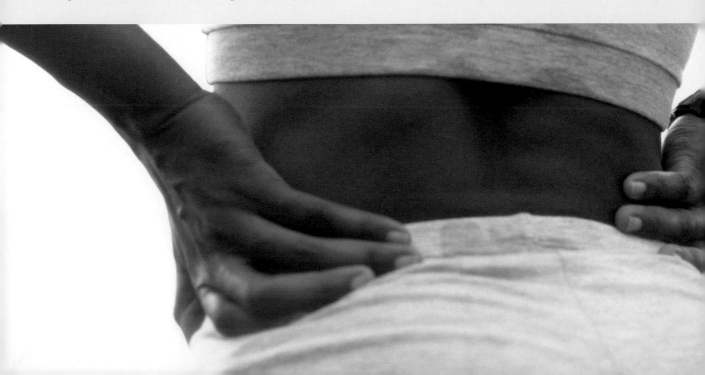

INSIDE
your bones, joints and muscles

The human **skeleton** is made up of 206 **bones** and provides the framework of the body. It protects the internal organs and provides anchor points for the muscles. Bone itself is living tissue, which is constantly being renewed. Inside bone, the soft, fatty substance known as **bone marrow** is responsible for making most of the body's blood cells. A type of connective tissue called **cartilage**, which is not as hard as bone, is also an important component of many parts of the body.

Where two or more bones meet there is a **joint**. Joints that move freely, such as the elbow or the knee, are called **synovial joints** and are lubricated by **synovial fluid** that is secreted by the joint lining. **Semimovable joints**, such as those in the pelvis, do not move freely but are more stable. Certain joints, such as those in the skull, are **fixed** and do not move.

Moving the body is the job of the **muscles**. The skeletal muscles are attached to bones by flexible, fibrous cords of tissue called **tendons**. Muscles normally cross two bones and their joint.

the skeleton

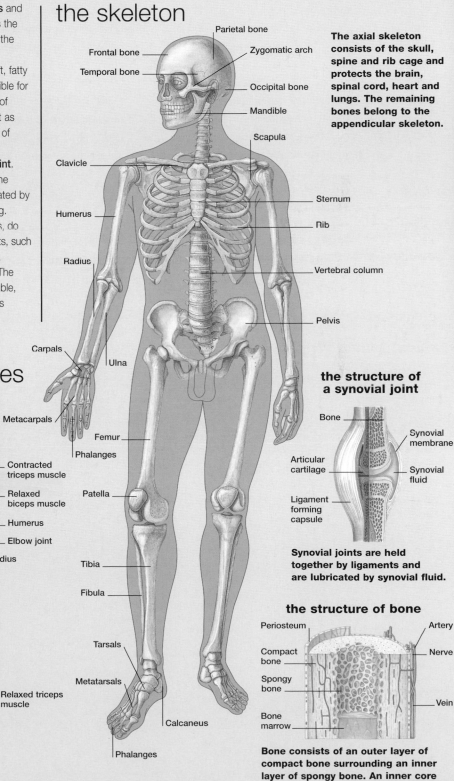

Parietal bone
Frontal bone
Zygomatic arch
Temporal bone
Occipital bone
Mandible
Scapula
Clavicle
Sternum
Humerus
Rib
Radius
Vertebral column
Carpals
Ulna
Metacarpals
Femur
Phalanges
Patella
Tibia
Fibula
Tarsals
Metatarsals
Calcaneus
Phalanges
Pelvis

The axial skeleton consists of the skull, spine and rib cage and protects the brain, spinal cord, heart and lungs. The remaining bones belong to the appendicular skeleton.

how the body moves

Muscles can only contract, not expand. For this reason, muscles work in opposing pairs.

To move the forearm down, the triceps contracts while the biceps relaxes.

KEY
Blue arrows show movement of the forearm

Contracted triceps muscle
Relaxed biceps muscle
Humerus
Elbow joint
Radius
Ulna

Contracted biceps muscle

Relaxed triceps muscle

To move the forearm up, the biceps contracts while the triceps relaxes.

the structure of a synovial joint

Bone
Synovial membrane
Articular cartilage
Synovial fluid
Ligament forming capsule

Synovial joints are held together by ligaments and are lubricated by synovial fluid.

the structure of bone

Periosteum
Artery
Compact bone
Nerve
Spongy bone
Vein
Bone marrow

Bone consists of an outer layer of compact bone surrounding an inner layer of spongy bone. An inner core of bone marrow produces blood cells.

BONES

Bone consists of an elastic protein framework stiffened by calcium and phosphate. Bone isn't lifeless and unchanging, it's very much a living tissue that is continually being broken down and rebuilt. Bone is also the source of blood and most of our blood cells are manufactured in the marrow. Disorders of bone, therefore, can lead to **anaemias**, and abnormal cell growth in the bone marrow to **leukaemia**. Bone can be weakened by nutritional deficiencies, especially of calcium and vitamin D. Hormones guarantee the integrity of bone and with the oestrogen deficiency that occurs with the **menopause** and after, bone becomes weak and brittle (**osteoporosis**) unless we take precautions.

Osteoporosis, which affects 1 in 3 women after the menopause, is the most common bone disorder. Oestrogen normally keeps the natural processes of bone breakdown and replacement in balance. Without oestrogen, replacement can't keep pace with breakdown and so bones become fragile and fracture more easily.

Fractures are common and various and so I've explained them in some detail to give you a clear understanding of them. Primary bone cancers are extremely rare, but secondary bone cancers (**metastases**) are relatively common and are mentioned here.

Fractures

A BREAK OR CRACK IN ANY BONE IN THE BODY IS KNOWN AS A FRACTURE.
FRACTURES ARE USUALLY DUE TO INJURY FROM A FALL BUT THEY CAN BE CAUSED BY BOUTS
OF COUGHING OR EVEN A HUG IF THE BONES ARE SERIOUSLY OSTEOPOROTIC.

Types of fracture

Transverse fracture
In a transverse fracture, there is a straight break across a bone. Transverse fractures, often in the arm or leg, are usually due to a powerful blow, such as that sustained in a collision during a road traffic accident.

Spiral fracture
Spiral fractures, or oblique fractures, are usually caused by sudden, violent, rotating movements, such as twisting the leg during a fall, especially if there's a ski on the end of it.

Greenstick fracture
If a long bone in the arm or leg bends, it may crack on one side only, producing an incomplete break called a "greenstick" fracture. This type of fracture occurs in children, whose bones are still growing and bendy.

Stress fracture
Fractures are caused by repeated jarring of a bone are called stress fractures. They may occur in the foot bones or shin bones of long-distance runners. In the elderly, fractures may result from minor stress such as a chronic cough, which can break a rib.

Comminuted fracture
The bone is broken into small fragments, which increases the likelihood of damage to the soft tissues surrounding the broken bone. These fractures are usually caused by severe, direct forces.

Avulsion fracture
A piece of bone is pulled away from the main bone by a tendon that attaches a muscle to a bone. It usually results from a sudden violent contraction of the muscle.

Compression fracture
A compression fracture occurs if spongy bone, like that in the vertebrae of the spine, is crushed; this type of fracture is often due to osteoporosis.

Fractures due to a bone being twisted or bent occur in athletic sports such as skiing or rugby. Susceptibility to fractures increases with the bone disorder **osteoporosis**, which mainly affects women after the menopause and results in brittle bones. Fractures that occur in bones affected by tumours are known as **pathological fractures** and may occur after minimal injury or even spontaneously. **Greenstick fractures** occur when a long bone bends and cracks on one side only; these fractures are especially common in children.

WHAT ARE THE TYPES?
There are two main types of fracture: **closed** (simple), in which the broken bone does not break through the overlying skin, and **open** (compound), in which the bone pierces the skin and is exposed. Open fractures are more serious because of the risk of infection and damage to nerves and blood vessels.

WHAT ARE THE SYMPTOMS?
The symptoms of a fracture depend on its type and include:
- deformity in the affected area
- pain and tenderness, which limits movement
- swelling and bruising
- crackling noise caused by grating of the ends of the bones on movement or pressure
- in an open fracture, damage to skin, bleeding and visible bone.

All fractures cause a certain amount of **internal bleeding** because of damage to blood

continued on page 426

FOCUS *on* osteoporosis

The painful, crippling and, sometimes, life-threatening bone condition known as osteoporosis is the single most important health hazard for women who have reached the menopause – it is more common than heart disease, stroke, diabetes or breast cancer.

The word "osteoporosis" is derived from the Greek and means "bone that has many holes". A special X-ray of affected bones will show they have a "low bone density", which means there may be an increased risk of fracture. Some bones can be so brittle as to fracture with coughing, even a hug. 1 in 4 elderly women who fracture the neck of the thighbone (femur) after a fall die in hospital. So osteoporosis must be taken seriously and prevented if at all possible. Black women, because they have greater bone density, have a lower risk of osteoporosis than white women. Osteoporosis also occurs in elderly men, although much more rarely than in women.

WHAT HAPPENS?

As oestrogen and progesterone levels fall after the menopause, bones begin to lose mass by up to 3 percent a year. By the time a woman is 80, she can easily have lost **half of her bone mass**.

Healthy bone has blood vessels and nerves and a very efficient repair and maintenance system. There are special cells, called osteoblasts, that renew, repair and lay down new bone, and others, called osteoclasts, that cause bone breakdown. **The activity of osteoblasts is controlled mainly by hormones, including oestrogen, which is thought to increase the repair and renewal rate of bone.** If oestrogen levels fall, bone is not replaced as efficiently.

AM I AT RISK?

• If you're menopausal, yes. **Menopause** is the main cause of osteoporosis.
• If you have **impaired peak bone density**, yes. Bone density normally peaks at around age 25–27. If your peak bone density is low, less bone loss will be required to develop osteoporosis when you reach the menopause. **Anorexia** and **repeated dieting** lower your peak bone density, making you a candidate for osteoporosis later on.
• If your **mother** has osteoporosis your risk is higher than average.
• Osteoporosis occurs in some women with

premenopausal lack of menstrual periods (**amenorrhoea**), because of low oestrogen levels.
• Women such as **ballet dancers,** who exercise excessively while living on restricted diets, are at risk.
• Women who have an **overactive thyroid gland** are at risk of developing osteoporosis.
• The **earlier the age of the menopause**, with its depletion of oestrogen, the greater the risk of osteoporosis.

• The menopause may start up to five years early in heavy smokers, so **smoking** is a risk factor for osteoporosis.
• **Hysterectomy** and **removal of the ovaries** lead to loss of bone mass. Most women show early signs of osteoporosis within four years of removal of the ovaries if HRT is not given.
• If you've taken **corticosteroids**, such as **cortisone** or **prednisone**, for longer than six months you're a candidate for osteoporosis so ask for a bone scan when the treatment is over.
• Malignant disease, a chronic liver disorder or rheumatoid arthritis all increase the risk.

WHAT ARE THE SYMPTOMS?

• If you are 50 or over, any **curvature of the spine (kyphosis)** and **loss of height** deserve particular attention.

Bone density tests

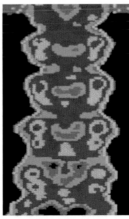

Normal bone mass
Normal bone has a T score above -1 SD units.

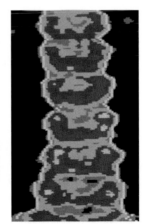

Below-normal bone mass
A T score between -1 and -2.5 SD units is below normal.

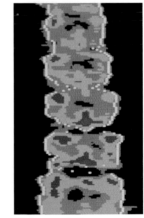

Osteoporotic bone
A T score below -2.5 SD units indicates osteoporosis.

This technique uses low-dose X-rays to measure the density of bone. The test is carried out to screen for and diagnose osteoporosis, a condition that is particularly common in postmenopausal women. The varying absorption of X-rays as they pass through the body is interpreted by a computer and displayed as an image. The computer calculates the average density of the bone and compares it with the normal range for the person's age and sex. The procedure takes about 10–20 minutes and is painless. You will be asked to lie still with your legs raised and your back flat. The X-ray generator and detector move along the length of your spine and transmit information to a computer.

- Symptoms that may signal osteoporosis include upper and low back pain, aches and pains in the joints and limbs, swollen joints at the ends of your fingers.
- Fractures are a very common symptom of osteoporosis, often the first sign that a person has the condition.

- If you are over 40 and you fracture your wrist or hip after a minor fall, you are likely to have osteoporosis. (The working rule is if you sustain a fracture after minor trauma, osteoporosis is present.)
- Fractures of the wrist, **Colles' fractures**, in menopausal women are sustained when they

fall and reach out to save themselves.
- **Hip fractures** are one of the most serious types of fracture because they render an elderly person immobile.
- **Compression fractures of the vertebrae** are also common leading to a reduction in height and an outward curvature of the spine, known as **Dowager's Hump**.

DOWAGER'S HUMP

As the bones of the spine gradually lose density, the vertebrae collapse, causing the ribcage to tilt downwards towards the hips. A curvature in the upper spine creates a second curve in the lower spinal column, pushing the internal organs forwards. Because of the compressed spinal column, up to 20cm (8in) in height can be lost in severe cases. Constipation can be a problem, breathing may become laboured, indigestion and acid reflux are common, and pain in the lower back and limbs results from pressure on the nerves by the collapsed vertebrae. Finding clothes that fit isn't easy and day-to-day life can become increasingly difficult.

HOW IS IT DIAGNOSED?

- At the first sign of the menopause, usually long, heavy periods, ask your doctor to arrange **bone density tests**.
- If you **suddenly** begin to suffer upper or low back pain, you should ask your doctor to do an X-ray of your spine.

There are several ways of assessing bone density, and a scan is considered the best predictor of fractures.

WHAT IS THE TREATMENT?

The aim of prescription drugs, such as HRT, is to halt bone loss, prevent further fractures, and replace or repair bone whenever possible. **Once fractures occur, at least one-third of bone mass** has already been lost; in some cases as much as 60 percent is gone.

NON-HORMONAL TREATMENT

- Ask your doctor about calcium supplements. To **maximize** its benefits, calcium should be taken with other treatments, such as HRT and vitamin D. In parallel you should increase calcium intake through your diet. Eat plenty of calcium-rich foods, including dairy products, canned fish with bones, such as sardines, and vegetables such as broccoli.
- A drug called **etidronate** has been shown to treat effectively established spinal osteoporosis.

The structure of bone

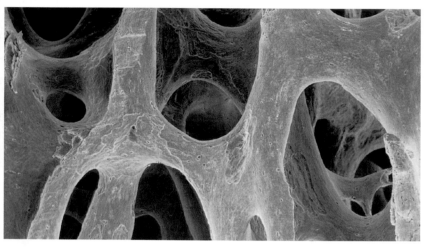

Healthy bone
Bone is living tissue that is constantly being broken down and renewed by the body. Bone is made up of a framework of protein fibres with deposits of calcium and phosphate among them.

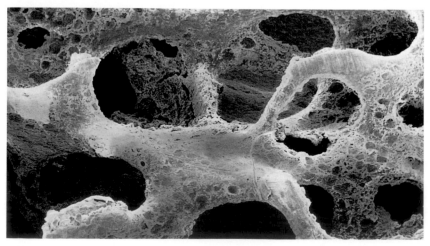

Osteoporotic bone
If the mineral content of bone is not adequately maintained, osteoporosis may result, in which the bones become weak and brittle and more prone to fractures.

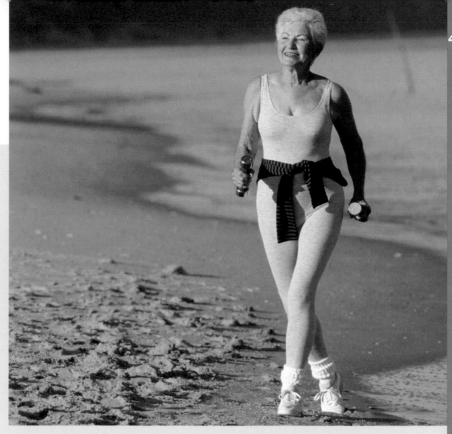

- A new class of drugs called SERMS for menopausal women treats osteoporosis. It also prevents heart disease but is ineffective against menopausal symptoms such as hot flushes and dry vagina.
- Vitamin D supplements will increase the efficiency of your calcium supplements.

PAIN RELIEF

- Women with vertebral osteoporosis can suffer intense back pain, especially after a new fracture, and may need strong prescription painkillers.
- Curvature of the spine produces ongoing muscular and ligament pain, but this can be treated with non-prescription **painkillers**, such as **paracetamol** or codeine.
- Physiotherapists use various forms of **electrotherapy** or **ultrasound** to help relieve pain.
- TENS (**Transcutaneous Electrical Nerve Stimulation**) machines for pain relief are available in most treatment centres and pharmacies.
- **Complementary** techniques such as acupuncture, and the use of heat pads, hot-water bottles or ice packs at home, are sometimes helpful for pain but they don't correct osteoporosis.
- An occupational therapist can advise you on how to **organize your home and work environment** to **minimize pain**. You should sit in a chair with a high back that gives support to the whole spine, and your bed should be firm, but not so hard that it cannot accommodate the altered shape of your spine.

HOW DO I PREVENT OSTEOPOROSIS?

Since all women are at risk of developing osteoporosis, it is important that we adopt self-help measures early in order to build up our resistance to it.

- **Take regular exercise at least from the age of 35**
Exercise is crucial at the menopause. Increased muscle strength, improved spinal power and posture, maintenance of bone strength, relief of pain, and toning of pelvic floor muscles to cope with stress incontinence are all benefits of exercise. Join a keep-fit class. Women who take regular weight-bearing exercise – walking will do – twice a week have denser bones than those who take exercise once a week, who, in turn, have denser bones than those who never

take exercise at all. It is never too late to strengthen your bones.
- **Eat a calcium-rich diet**
From an early age always take the opportunity to eat calcium-rich foods, such as dairy products, fish with bones (such as sardines) and dark green vegetables. Seek them out, keep them in the fridge, choose them from restaurant menus.
- **Consider HRT**
I would suggest that a sensible way of **preventing osteoporosis**, once you are menopausal, is to take enough oestrogen to maintain bone mass. HRT in the form of oestrogen taken continuously in combination with progestogen for 10–13 days per month seems to **optimize** bone health, and prevent fractures. Ideally, you should have a bone density test to assess your bone health before HRT is prescribed but it isn't mandatory. You should discuss the possibility of taking HRT, orally or through the skin via gel or a skin patch, with your doctor. There are over 50 forms on the market so one should suit you. Be sure to give yourself a four-month trial. You need to take HRT for five years for your bones to benefit and the benefit is lost when you stop.

Natural types of HRT, including progesterone cream, have NEVER been shown to have any effect on osteoporosis.

PREVENTING FRACTURES

As the greatest danger of osteoporosis is a fracture, it is vital that you help yourself prevent it happening.

- Regular exercise, a balanced diet and mental alertness can help to maintain overall fitness, which lowers your chance of falling heavily.
- Maintain good vision by having your eyes tested regularly, particularly for a condition known as glaucoma.
- Avoid sedatives and other drugs that might reduce your alertness, such as antihistamines, and try to limit your alcohol intake.
- Reduce the hazards in your home by removing any trailing electrical flexes and loose carpets.
- Make sure that there is always a firm handrail on stairs and be particularly on guard when walking on slippery or uneven surfaces.
- Some women avoid going out and, as a result, may suffer from lack of exercise and vitamin D (through lack of exposure to the sun). This may make their osteoporosis worse.
- Counselling, emotional support and talking to other menopausal women with similar problems can do much to give a woman a more positive attitude to life and help her become more outgoing and confident.
- Have regular health checks with your doctor.
- Ask your doctor to check your heart and blood pressure annually.

continued from page 422

vessels in the bone. The broken bone ends may cause further bleeding by damaging tissues and blood vessels in the injured area. In some fractures, particularly a break in the thighbone (femur), blood loss may be severe and lead to shock.

Various complications may be associated with a fracture. For example, if you fracture a rib, there is a risk that the broken rib may puncture a lung, causing **pneumothorax**.

Delay in treating a fracture properly may result in failure of the bone to heal, causing permanent deformity or disability. Consult a doctor immediately if you think you have a fracture.

HOW IS IT DIAGNOSED?

Your doctor will arrange for you to have X-rays to reveal the type and extent of the fracture. CT scanning or MRI may be needed to investigate complex fractures. If a fracture wasn't due to injury, your doctor may check for a possible underlying disorder that may have weakened your bones.

WHAT IS THE TREATMENT?

If the broken ends of the bone have been displaced, they will be brought into line to restore normal shape by manipulation. This process is known as reduction. Each type of fracture has its own manipulation manoeuvre, which may be carried out under local or general anaesthetic.

TEST

X-rays

X-ray photography is one of the oldest methods of imaging the body. In this technique high-intensity radiation (in the form of X-rays) passes through the body to form an image on film placed on the other side of the body. Hard structures within the body, such as bones, block the radiation and so show up on the X-ray film as white areas. X-rays are therefore useful for imaging hard structures but are not very useful for imaging soft tissues, such as the liver, since they do not block the radiation. However, a special type of X-ray, known as a contrast X-ray, may be used to image certain soft tissues.

During an X-ray, the source of the X-rays is usually positioned directly above the area to be examined. You will be asked to keep completely still during the procedure to ensure that the X-ray picture is clear. You will be exposed to X-ray radiation for less than one second, and the procedure usually takes only a few minutes.

See also:
• **CT scanning p.401** • **MRI p.409**
• **Osteoporosis p.423** • **Pneumothorax p.395** • **Shock p.560**

Bone cancers

THERE ARE TWO TYPES OF CANCEROUS GROWTH THAT OCCUR IN BONE: PRIMARY BONE CANCER, WHICH ORIGINATES IN THE BONE ITSELF AND IS VERY RARE, AND SECONDARY BONE CANCER, WHICH ARISES FROM CANCER ELSEWHERE IN THE BODY AND HAS SPREAD TO THE BONE VIA THE BLOOD.

Secondary cancers, called **metastases**, are much more common than primary bone cancers.

PRIMARY BONE CANCER

Primary bone cancer is a cancerous tumour that originates in bone and is extremely rare. Primary bone cancers are more common in childhood and adolescence and sometimes run in families.

WHAT MIGHT BE DONE?

In most cases the tumour is removed **surgically**. **Radiotherapy** may help reduce the size of the tumour. Post-operative **chemotherapy** helps destroy any remaining cancerous cells. Removed bone is replaced by metal replacements (prostheses) or by bone taken from elsewhere in the body or from a donor.

Most people treated for primary bone cancer have a very small chance of recurrence in the first five years. Thereafter, recurrence is unlikely.

SECONDARY BONE CANCER (BONE METASTASES)

Secondary bone cancer is a cancerous tumour in bone that has spread from a cancer elsewhere in the body. Cancers that typically metastasize to bone include **breast**, **lung** and **prostate cancer** and **cancer of the ovary**, and are often called "secondaries".

Metastases most often develop in the ribs, pelvis, skull or spine. The condition is much more common than primary bone cancer, especially in older people, who are more likely to have cancer elsewhere.

WHAT ARE THE SYMPTOMS?

Bone metastases may cause the following symptoms, in addition to those of the main cancer:
• gnawing bone pain that may become worse at night
• swelling of the affected area
• tenderness over the affected area
• proneness of affected bones to fracture easily, often after minor injury.

WHAT MIGHT BE DONE?

If you already have a cancer somewhere else in your body, you may have X-rays or radionuclide scanning to check whether the cancer has spread to the bones. If the site of the primary cancer is unknown, you may need further tests to find out where the metastasis came from. For example, women may be given **mammography** to look for evidence of breast cancer.

Your doctor will probably direct treatment at your original cancer. He or she may also arrange for you to have **chemotherapy**, **radiotherapy**, or **hormonal therapy** to relieve bone pain.

The prognosis for people with bone metastases usually depends on the site of the original cancer and how successfully it can be treated. However, the best that can usually be achieved for bone metastases is a period of remission and relief from pain.

See also:
• **Breast cancer p.261**
• **Cancer of the ovary p.260**
• **Chemotherapy p.257** • **Lung cancer p.394**
• **Mammograms p.245**
• **Prostate cancer p.265**
• **Radiotherapy p.395**

JOINTS

Joints allow our bodies to be flexible. Their perfect engineering is mainly due to an enveloping capsule and a lining, the **synovium**, which produces lubrication in the form of synovial fluid. Within joints, cartilage lines the ends of bones and prevents friction during movement. Fibrous ligaments surround the joints, giving strength, support and stability. Joints may be damaged by injury, inflammation and the degeneration of bone, cartilage and ligaments that comes with ageing or disease.

Joint disorders are a major cause of disability and immobility, but the treatment of chronic joint disease has improved enormously in the past 20 years due to the availability of new drugs and safe, reliable artificial joints.

The word **arthritis** means inflammation of one or more joints, although there is little evidence of actual inflammation in the most common form, **osteoarthritis**, which comes to affect most joints as they age and especially if they've been injured. **Spondylosis** is a natural deterioration in the spinal joints affecting the parts of the spine where there's most movement – the neck and lower back – and affects all of us from middle age onwards. **Rheumatoid arthritis** is a true inflammatory arthritis and may be the most dramatic feature of a condition in which there is inflammation in many organs of the body other than simply the joints. This kind of disorder is called a **connective tissue disorder** or **autoimmune disease** and rheumatoid arthritis is the most common example. And gout, although comparatively rare, is extremely painful and deserves attention.

Last but not least the common **bunion** gets a mention as it's an inflammation of the tissues around a joint, the bursa of the big toe, affecting many people.

Arthritis

THE TERM ARTHRITIS COVERS A LARGE GROUP OF INFLAMMATORY AND DEGENERATIVE CONDITIONS THAT CAUSE STIFFNESS, SWELLING AND PAIN IN THE JOINTS.

Arthritis may be linked with skin diseases such as **psoriasis**, intestinal disorders such as **Crohn's disease** and autoimmune disease such as **lupus**.

WHAT ARE THE TYPES?
There are several different types of arthritis, each having its own characteristics.
■ The most common form is a degenerative type, **osteoarthritis**, usually affecting middle-aged and older people in the weight-bearing joints – the knees and hips – and after the menopause, the ends of the fingers. **Spondylosis** is a common form of osteoarthritis that affects the joints in the spine, mainly the neck (cervical) and lower back (lumbar) regions.
■ **Rheumatoid arthritis** results from inflammation in the joints and other body tissues, such as the **heart, lungs** and **eyes**.

■ Another chronic disorder is **ankylosing spondylitis**, which affects the spine and joints between the base of the spine and the pelvis. As with rheumatoid arthritis other body tissues, the eyes for example, may be affected. The condition eventually causes the vertebrae (the bones of the spine) to fuse together, making walking extremely difficult.

Living with arthritis

If you have long-term arthritis, you may be able to manage your symptoms so that you can maintain an active lifestyle. Consult your doctor about pain relief and keeping joints mobile. Organizations concerned with arthritis (see Useful addresses, p.567) can also provide valuable information.

Self-help
• If you are overweight, probably the most important single thing you can do is lose weight.
• In addition, exercises to increase muscle power will help stabilize the affected joint and reduce your symptoms.

Mobility
Gentle, regular exercise helps relieve stiffness and improve mobility. Physical activity also helps strengthen the muscles that support the joints. However, if exercise causes swelling or pain, stop the activity and consult your doctor.

Pain relief
Severe joint pain can be improved by applying heat or cold to the area. Heat increases blood flow; cold helps reduce swelling. Both decrease sensitivity to pain.

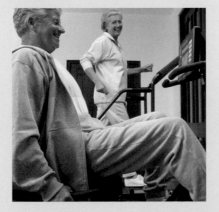

Specialized equipment
Your doctor or a physiotherapist may be able to suggest specially adapted pieces of equipment to help you with household tasks. The equipment may have particular features, such as handles that are easy to grip or extending arms to help you reach objects without bending down.
• If arthritis restricts the movement in your hands, use cutlery with thick handles and glasses with wide stems that will be easier to grip. A plate with a rim may keep the food from spilling, and a nonslip mat will help hold your plate still during a meal.
• Tongs enable you to pick up objects that are out of your reach without bending or stretching. Some types of tongs have a trigger mechanism that operates pincers at the end of the arm.
• A fixed seat in the shower allows you to sit down while you wash. Handrails and a nonslip floor surface reduce the risk of falls.

Joint replacement

Joints that have been severely damaged by arthritis or injury may be surgically replaced with artificial joints made of metal, ceramic or plastic. Most joints in the body can be replaced, but the common ones are the hips, knees and shoulders. During the operation, the ends of damaged bones are removed and the artificial components are fixed in place. The operation usually relieves pain and increases the range of motion in the joint.

Hip replacement

The most commonly replaced joint is the hip. During the operation, both the pelvic socket and the head of the thighbone (femur) are replaced. A general anaesthetic is used and it involves a short stay in hospital. In the first two weeks following the operation the new joint is unstable and patients must be careful not to dislocate it during this time.

Other joints

Many different types of joints in the body can be replaced, from tiny finger joints to large joints such as the knees.

Knee joint replacement

Most artificial knee joints consist of metal and plastic implants that cover worn cartilage in the knee; as much of the original joint as possible is preserved. The operation is performed under a general anaesthetic. A cast fitted during the operation is removed after about five days and the patient can put some weight on the leg after two or three weeks.

Finger joint replacement

Artificial finger joints are made of metal, plastic or silicone rubber and are used to replace damaged joints in the fingers. The operation is done under a local or general anaesthetic and stitches are usually removed after about 10 days.

■ **Reactive arthritis** typically develops in susceptible people after they've had an infection, most often of the **genital tract**, such as **non-specific urethritis**, or of the **intestines**, such as **ulcerative colitis**. This kind of arthritis most commonly causes inflammation in an **ankle** or a **knee**.
■ In **gout**, crystals of **uric acid** are deposited in a joint, leading to swelling and pain. **Treatment** of arthritis depends on the type. **Analgesics** and **non-steroidal anti-inflammatory drugs (NSAIDs)** may help relieve symptoms. **Physiotherapy** helps keep joints mobile. Severely damaged joints may need to be surgically replaced with artificial joints.

> **See also:**
> • **Ankylosing spondylitis p.430**
> • **Crohn's disease p.366**
> • **Gout p.433**
> • **Lupus p.324** • **Psoriasis p.448**
> • **Rheumatoid arthritis p.429**

Osteoarthritis

THE GRADUAL DEGENERATION OF THE CARTILAGE COVERING THE ENDS OF BONE INSIDE JOINTS, DUE TO WEAR AND TEAR OVER MANY YEARS, CAUSES THE PAIN, SWELLING AND STIFFNESS OF OSTEOARTHRITIS.

The condition rarely appears before middle age and primarily affects the weight-bearing joints – the hips and knees. Around the age of the menopause, the terminal joints of the fingers show osteoarthritic change with the appearance of bony outgrowths on the sides of the joints – **Heberden's nodes**. Any joint that is injured could become osteoarthritic at a later date. The greater the wear and tear in early life the greater the chance of osteoarthritis (OA) setting in. OA is almost always asymmetrical.

HOW DOES IT DEVELOP?

OA develops as a result of excessive wear and tear on the joints and it's usually part of the natural ageing process. For example, in OA of the knee, where the thigh bone and shin bone meet, the cartilage preventing them from grinding together has worn away and pain is the result.

OA is common in weight-bearing joints that have been subject to injury in youth or that have been used extensively in certain sports or strained due to obesity. Most people over the age of 60 have some degree of OA and three times as many women are affected as men. The areas most commonly affected are the large spinal joints of the lower back, hips, knees, ankles and feet. A thickening of the bone ends causes bony spurs to appear at the edge of joints.

Exactly the same process occurs at the edges of the neck (cervical) vertebrae, often causing a stiff neck that makes movement painful. This condition is known as **cervical spondylosis**.

WHAT ARE THE SYMPTOMS?

■ As well as pain, OA also causes swelling, creaking and stiffness of the affected joints.
■ Weakness and shrinkage of surrounding muscles may occur if pain prevents the joint being used regularly.
■ Pressure from a bony spur on a nerve in the neck (cervical spondylosis) may cause pain in the shoulder, elbow and fingers.
■ When bony growths occur in the lower back (lumbar spondylosis), pressure on the sciatic nerve will cause pain in the buttock and the back of the legs down to the sole of the foot, pain known as **sciatica**.

WHAT IS THE TREATMENT?

■ Unfortunately, there is no cure although the symptoms can be relieved by painkillers

Formation of osteophytes on bone

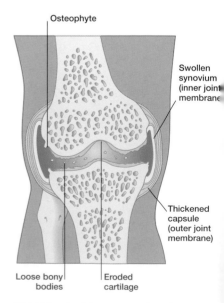

Osteophyte

Swollen synovium (inner joint membrane)

Thickened capsule (outer joint membrane)

Loose bony bodies

Eroded cartilage

Weight-bearing joints may erode and osteophytes (bony outgrowths) may form.

Exercises for people with osteoarthritis

1. Hold your arms straight down but across your body, then lift them upwards and outwards, uncrossing them as you go. With your arms in this position, clasp your hands behind your head.
2. Push your toes and feet down and then pull them up towards you. Move your toes and ankles round in a large circle.
3. Lie down, preferably on the floor, bend each leg in turn up onto your chest towards the opposite shoulder.
4. Rest your arms on a table or arm of a chair without supporting your hand. Bend your hand down towards the floor and then lift it up. Next, move your hand to the left and then to the right. When you are doing this make sure your hand rests in the mid-position and is in line with your forearm and doesn't fall downwards.

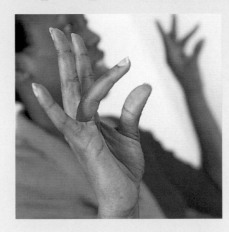

5. Bend your fingers and grip tightly, then stretch and spread your fingers. Touch the tip of each finger in turn with your thumb.

If sitting in a cramped seat becomes painful after half an hour or so, stand up and walk around or massage your knees. **Don't** sit with your legs crossed – it isn't good for the knees.

Swimming is an excellent way to strengthen muscles and maintain joint mobility. As the water supports your body, muscles can be exercised without straining your joints. If you have a heated pool nearby, do use it at least once a week as it increases muscle power without putting undue strain on joints.

---

and non-steroidal anti-inflammatory drugs (NSAIDs).
■ Physiotherapy, heat treatment and exercise are helpful for pain relief and mobility.

■ Corticosteroid injections can sometimes bring instant, if temporary, relief but must be used sparingly.

See also:
• NSAIDS p.431
• Spondylosis p.432

Rheumatoid arthritis

THIS FORM OF ARTHRITIS CAUSES CHRONIC INFLAMMATION OF THE CONNECTIVE TISSUES THROUGHOUT THE BODY, BUT PARTICULARLY AROUND THE JOINTS WHERE THE MAIN SIGN IS OFTEN PAINFUL, SWOLLEN, STIFF JOINTS THAT MAY EVENTUALLY BECOME DEFORMED.

Rheumatoid arthritis (RA) affects about 1 in 100 people, is most common between the ages of 40 and 60, and affects three times more women than men. It sometimes runs in families, suggesting a genetic factor is at play. RA almost always affects the same joints on both sides of the body.

WHAT HAPPENS?
In rheumatoid arthritis, the joints become stiff and swollen as a result of inflammation of the synovial membrane, which lines each joint. Gradually, the cartilage covering the ends of the bones is eroded, together with the bone underlying the cartilage. The tendons and ligaments, which give the joints support, become worn and slack, and the joints may become deformed.

HOW DOES RA AFFECT THE BODY AS A WHOLE?
In most cases rheumatoid arthritis affects several joints. It usually starts first in the small joints of the hands and feet but may develop in any joint. RA usually tends to be symmetrical, appearing in similar joints on both sides of the body. It is classified as one of the **autoimmune disorders**, in which the body produces antibodies that attack its own tissues.

Tissues, mainly connective tissue made out of **collagen**, in other parts of the body, such as the **eyes, lungs, heart** and **blood vessels**, may be affected by inflammation and RA is therefore also described as a **connective tissue disorder**.

RA runs a chronic course and usually recurs in episodes lasting for several weeks or months with relatively symptom-free periods in between. After many years it usually "burns itself out" and becomes quiescent like an extinct volcano.

WHAT ARE THE SYMPTOMS?
Rheumatoid arthritis usually develops slowly, although very occasionally the onset may be sudden and dramatic. General symptoms include **fatigue, pale skin, shortness of breath** on exertion and **poor appetite**. **Specific symptoms** may include:
● stiff, painful and swollen joints, often of the hands, and classically affecting the middle joint of the fingers so that they become spindle-shaped
● classically, the pain and stiffness is worst on waking and improves as the day goes on.
● painless, small bumps (nodules) on areas of pressure such as the elbows.

ARE THERE COMPLICATIONS?
■ In time, the bones around the affected joint may lose density and strength as a result of reduced mobility, becoming increasingly brittle and more susceptible to fracture.
■ The more **general symptoms** of RA are partly due to **anaemia**, caused by a failure of the bone marrow to manufacture enough new red blood cells.
■ **Bursitis** may develop, in which one or more of the fluid-filled sacs around a joint become inflamed.
■ Swelling that compresses the **median nerve in the wrist** may lead to tingling and pain in the fingers. This is called **carpal tunnel syndrome**.
As part of the generalized autoimmune disorder affecting connective tissue throughout the body, complications may include:
● inflammation of the walls of the **arteries** supplying the fingers and toes may result in **Raynaud's phenomenon**, a condition in which the fingers and toes become pale and painful on exposure to cold
● less commonly, the spleen and the lymph nodes may become enlarged
● the membranous sac that surrounds the heart – the pericardium – may also become inflamed (pericarditis)

- some people may also experience inflammation of the eye – iridocyclitis or uveitis.

Symptoms may improve during pregnancy but sometimes flare up again after the birth.

HOW IS IT DIAGNOSED?

■ Joint changes in the hands are so classical as to confirm the diagnosis. However, your doctor may arrange for a blood test to check for the presence of an antibody known as **rheumatoid factor** (RF), which is often associated with RA.

■ Blood tests may also be done to measure the severity of the inflammation.

■ X-rays of the affected joints may be taken to assess the level of bone and joint damage.

WHAT IS THE TREATMENT?

The aim of treatment is twofold: firstly, to relieve your symptoms and, secondly, to reduce further joint damage by arresting inflammation and slowing the progress of the disease. Different drugs are available, and your doctor's recommendation will depend on the severity and progress of your disease, your age and your general health.

■ **If your symptoms are only mild**, your doctor may simply prescribe a non-steroidal anti-inflammatory drug (NSAID).

■ **If your symptoms are severe**, drugs that slow the disease process may be suggested, such as **sulphasalazine** or **chloroquine**. Such drugs should limit permanent damage to the joints but may have to be taken over a few months before their full benefits are felt.

■ **If the symptoms persist**, your doctor may prescribe a drug such as **cyclosporin, penicillamine, methotrexate** or **gold**. As these drugs can have serious side effects, your condition will be monitored closely by your doctor.

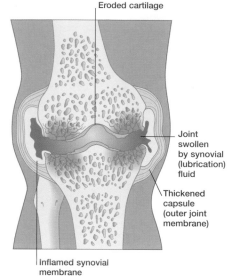

Rheumatoid arthritis

Eroded cartilage

Joint swollen by synovial (lubrication) fluid

Thickened capsule (outer joint membrane)

Inflamed synovial membrane

Characteristic changes in rheumatoid arthritis damage the joint.

■ The **anaemia** that is commonly associated with RA may be improved by treatment with the hormone **erythropoietin**.

■ Your doctor may recommend that you use a **splint or brace**, particularly at night, to support a particularly painful joint and slow the development of deformities.

■ Gentle, regular **exercise** may help keep your joints mobile and prevent muscle weakness.

■ **Physiotherapy** may be given to improve joint mobility and help increase muscle strength.

■ **Hydrotherapy** and **heat or ice treatments** may help relieve pain.

■ If a joint is intensely painful, it may need an **injection** of a corticosteroid.

■ If the joint becomes severely damaged, your doctor may suggest that you have surgery to replace the damaged joint with an **artificial** one.

WHAT IS THE OUTLOOK?

Many people with rheumatoid arthritis are able to lead a normal life, although lifelong drug treatment may be necessary to control the symptoms. About 1 in 10 people have some degree of disability, as repeated attacks gradually destroy the joints.

There are many household items that will help you to lead a normal life so ask your doctor about them.

Regular blood tests will be needed to monitor the progress of the disease and your response to treatment. In some cases, the attacks gradually stop, and the disease is said to **have burned itself out**. After the age of 50, RA quite frequently does so. However, some permanent disability may remain.

> **See also:**
> - Autoimmune disorders p.323
> - Carpal tunnel syndrome p.434
> - Joint replacement p.428
> - Living with arthritis p.427
> - NSAIDS p.431
> - Raynaud's phenomenon p.234

Ankylosing spondylitis

THE CHRONIC, PROGRESSIVE JOINT INFLAMMATION AND STIFFENING (USUALLY OF THE SPINE AND PELVIS) THAT ARE THE MAIN SYMPTOMS OF ANKYLOSING SPONDYLITIS CLASSICALLY AFFECT YOUNG MEN. THE CONDITION TENDS TO RUN IN FAMILIES.

Although the main symptoms are in the joints, ankylosing spondylitis is a connective tissue disorder and also affects other organs in the body. The disorder particularly affects the **sacroiliac joints** that join the back of the pelvis to the bones of the spine (vertebrae). If the spine is severely diseased, new bone starts to grow between the vertebrae and eventually fuses them together so that the spine becomes fixed and immobile.

A variant of ankylosing spondylitis is preceded by the skin disorder **psoriasis** and by inflammatory bowel disease such as **Crohn's disease**.

WHAT ARE THE CAUSES?

The cause of ankylosing spondylitis is unknown, but about 9 out of 10 people with the condition have a particular substance that is capable of stimulating an immune response in the body (**antigen**), called HLA–B27, on the surface of most cells. This antigen is inherited, which helps explain why anklosing spondylitis runs in families. Nonetheless, most people with HLA–B27 don't develop ankylosing spondylitis so there must be other factors at work.

A bacterial infection is thought to trigger ankylosing spondylitis in those who are predisposed.

WHAT ARE THE SYMPTOMS?

The symptoms of ankylosing spondylitis usually appear in late adolescence or early adulthood and develop gradually over a period of months or even years. The main symptoms include:

- low back pain, which may spread down into the buttocks and thighs
- low back stiffness that may be worse in the morning and improves with exercise
- pain in other joints, such as the hips, knees, and shoulders
- pain and tenderness in the heels
- fatigue, weight loss and mild fever.

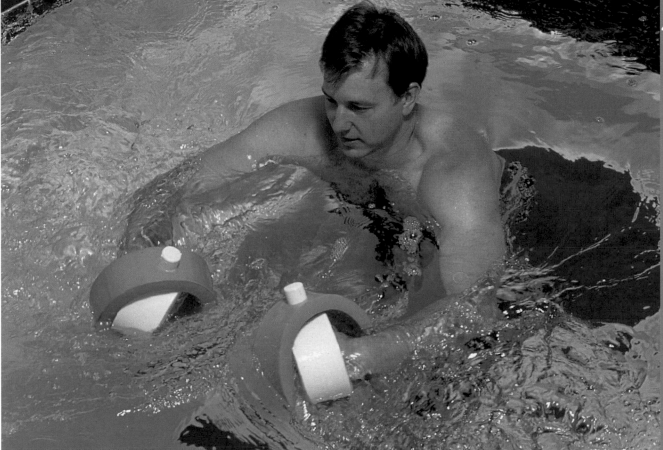

Gentle, regular exercise can help maintain flexibility and relieve the symptoms of ankylosing spondylitis.

WHAT ARE THE COMPLICATIONS?

■ If left untreated, ankylosing spondylitis can cause the spine to become distorted, forming a convex curvature called **kyphosis** that results in a stooped posture.

■ If the joints between the spine and the ribs are affected, **chest expansion** is restricted.

■ In some people, ankylosing spondylitis causes inflammation or damage to the tissues in areas other than the joints, such as the **eyes**.

HOW IS IT DIAGNOSED?

■ Your doctor may suspect ankylosing spondylitis from the pattern of your symptoms.

■ An X-ray will show up evidence of fusion in the joints of the pelvis and the spine.

■ Blood tests will be done to measure the level of inflammation and look for the HLA–B27 antigen.

WHAT IS THE TREATMENT?

The treatment of ankylosing spondylitis is aimed at relieving the symptoms and preventing the development of deformity.

■ Your doctor may prescribe a **non-steroidal anti-inflammatory drug** (NSAID) to control pain and inflammation.

■ You will have physiotherapy, probably including breathing **exercises** and daily exercises to improve posture, strengthen the back muscles and prevent deformities of the spine.

■ You may also benefit from gentle regular physical activity, such as **swimming**, which helps relieve pain and stiffness.

■ If a joint such as the hip is affected, you may eventually need to have it **replaced** surgically.

■ If your mobility becomes severely reduced, you may need **occupational therapy**.

■ Your therapist may suggest that you use **specially designed equipment** and furniture to help make your life easier.

WHAT IS THE OUTLOOK?

Most people with ankylosing spondylitis are only mildly affected, causing minimum disruption to their everyday lives. Even in those people with more severe symptoms, the condition tends to become less severe with age. In many cases, early treatment and regular exercise help relieve pain and stiffness of the back and prevent deformity of the spine. However, about 1 in 20 people with ankylosing spondylitis eventually becomes disabled.

> **See also:**
> • **Crohn's disease p.366**
> • **Joint replacement p.428** • **Psoriasis p.448**

NSAIDs

Non-steroidal anti-inflammatory drugs (NSAIDs) are a group of non-addictive drugs used to relieve pain and inflammation, particularly in muscles, ligaments and joints. They work by limiting the release of prostaglandins, chemicals produced by the body that cause pain and trigger inflammation. One of the best-known NSAIDS is ibuprofen, which is available over the counter.

NSAIDs can cause side effects. One of the most common is irritation of the stomach lining, which may lead to peptic ulcers if NSAIDs are taken for a long period of time. If you are prescribed NSAIDs for a chronic condition, you will probably be prescribed an anti-ulcer drug as well to counter this effect. Another side effect of NSAIDs is allergic reaction, which may appear as a rash or swelling. People with asthma or kidney problems should not take NSAIDs because they can make these conditions worse.

Spondylosis

THE BONES AND CARTILAGE IN THE NECK AND LOWER BACK GRADUALLY DEGENERATE
WITH AGE, LEADING TO THE PAIN AND STIFFNESS OF SPONDYLOSIS.

There are two types of spondylosis: if the symptoms are in the neck it is called **cervical** spondylosis, and if they are in the lower back, it is **lumbar** spondylosis. As everyone over the age of 45 has some degree of cervical and/or lumbar spondylosis, it is considered part of the normal ageing process.

Spondylosis is **osteoarthritis** affecting the spine where the vertebrae and the discs of cartilage between them begin to degenerate. Where movement is greatest, that is in the neck and the lower back, the bones become thickened, and bony spurs called **osteophytes** develop on the edges of the vertebrae. Osteophytes may press on spinal nerves, giving

rise to **root pain** radiating down the arms and legs.

WHAT ARE THE SYMPTOMS?

Many people don't have symptoms. When they become apparent, they include:
● restricted movement of the neck and lower back that may be painful
● pain at the back of the head and in the lower back
● aching or shooting pain that travels from the shoulders to the hands and from the lower back to the buttocks, down the back of the legs to the soles of the feet
● numbness, tingling and muscle weakness in the hands, arms and legs.

Sometimes, if the head is moved too quickly, the bony spurs may temporarily compress blood vessels that supply the brain, resulting in dizziness, unsteadiness and double vision (drop attacks).

HOW IS IT DIAGNOSED?

As spondylosis may be symptomless, the condition is often only diagnosed when an X-ray is taken for another reason.
■ If you experience neck pain or dizziness, you should consult your doctor, who may arrange X-rays to look for signs of cervical spondylosis.
■ If your doctor doubts that your symptoms are due solely to cervical spondylosis, he or she may arrange for further tests to look for other causes, such as a prolapsed or herniated (slipped) disc.

■ You may also have **nerve conduction studies** and electromyography (EMG) to assess the function of nerves in your arms and hands.
■ CT (computerized tomography) scanning or MRI (magnetic resonance imaging) may also be carried out to see whether there have been any changes in the bones of the spine, the discs or cartilage between them, or the tissues around them.

WHAT IS THE TREATMENT?

Degeneration of the spine cannot be halted, but its effects can be reduced with treatment.
■ To relieve pain in mild cases of cervical spondylosis, your doctor may recommend **painkillers**, such as paracetamol, or prescribe non-steroidal anti-inflammatory drugs (NSAIDs).
■ Once the initial pain has been relieved, he or she may suggest **neck exercises** to help maintain mobility and increase muscle strength in your neck.
■ If cervical spondylosis has damaged a nerve, **surgery** may be recommended to prevent the symptoms from getting worse. This involves widening the natural opening between the vertebrae through which the nerve passes when it branches off the spinal cord. In some cases, surgery may also be carried out to stabilize the spine by **fusing together** the affected vertebrae.

See also:
● **Osteoarthritis p.428** ● **Slipped disc p.437**

Complications

Spondylitis
Occasionally spondylosis goes on to become **inflamed** when the condition is called spondylitis. This may require treatment with anti-inflammatory drugs.

Spondylolisthesis
One spinal bone may slide out of position forwards onto another bone, causing pain because the adjacent muscles and ligaments are kept under stretch. This occurs in the lower lumbar region and may be symptomless.

Bunion

A BUNION IS A THICKENED SWELLING AT THE BASE OF THE BIG TOE. IT IS USUALLY CAUSED BY A
MINOR BONE DEFORMITY (HALLUX VALGUS) WHEN THE JOINT AT THE BASE OF THE BIG TOE
PROJECTS OUTWARDS, FORCING THE TIP OF THE TOE TO TURN INWARDS TOWARDS THE OTHER TOES.

This causes a thickening of the soft tissue (bursitis) and a bony overgrowth at the base of the big toe, which often becomes inflamed and painful, making walking difficult. The cause of hallux valgus is multifactorial, that is, due to a number of causes. As a result of pressure on the deformity, the surrounding tissues thicken. The lump caused by a combination of the bony deformity and the thickened soft tissue is called a bunion.

WHAT CAUSES IT?

■ The condition is common in young women as a result of wearing shoes that are too tight or pointed, especially those with high heels. When the big toe joint is overstrained it produces a

cushion of fluid that is held in a sac (a bursa) that surrounds the joint of the big toe.
■ In rare cases, the constant rubbing of tight shoes on the skin over a bunion may cause an abrasion and lead to a bacterial infection.
■ People who have **diabetes mellitus** are particularly susceptible to problems involving bunions because of impaired sensation in their feet and skin that tends to heal more slowly.

WHAT IS THE TREATMENT?

Without attention, a bunion may gradually worsen. Pain may be alleviated by wearing comfortable shoes with good cushioning and a special toe pad or corrective sock that straightens the big toe. However, if a bunion

is causing severe discomfort, your doctor may suggest surgery to correct the underlying deformity by realigning the bone.

If the bunion becomes infected with bacteria, your doctor will prescribe antibiotics.

SELF-HELP

Rest the feet whenever possible. Do not wear high-heeled shoes or ill-fitting shoes; go for wide shoes with low heels.

SURGERY

If the bunion is extremely severe and the feet become very deformed, it is possible to have surgical treatment from an orthopaedic surgeon. The treatment involves completely excising the inflamed bursa and the joint. In doing so, the orthopaedic surgeon fixes the joint, so while it will be entirely painless it will be stiff and immovable. This does not mean that you cannot walk properly, you will, but you will not be able to stand on your toes.

HOW CAN IT BE PREVENTED?
A bunion only forms when the joint of the big toe is overstrained. Prevention is therefore not to overstrain the big toe by not wearing high-heeled shoes for long periods of time and by not wearing ill-fitting shoes, socks or tights.

> See also:
> • **Diabetes mellitus p.504**
> • **Osteoarthritis p.428**

See also:
• **Diabetes mellitus p.504**
• **Osteoarthritis p.428**

TREATMENT

Bunion surgery

Surgery to treat a bunion is aimed at correcting the underlying deformity of the bone, known as hallux valgus. One common type of surgical procedure used to treat a bunion involves reshaping and realigning the deformed bone (the first metatarsal bone) at the base of the big toe.

During the operation the protruding part of the bone is cut away and a V-shaped cut is made in the lower part of the bone. This allows the bone to slide sideways and become realigned. In some cases a temporary wire or a permanent screw may be inserted into the bone. To support the toe, the foot is put in a bandage or plaster that must remain in place for about six weeks.

The operation is performed under general anaesthetic and may require a brief stay in hospital. Crutches or a stick are required for the period during which the foot is bandaged, but normal walking can usually be resumed about six weeks after surgery.

Gout

A TYPE OF ARTHRITIS, IN WHICH CRYSTALLINE DEPOSITS OF URIC ACID FORM WITHIN JOINTS, GOUT IS 20 TIMES MORE COMMON IN MEN, ESPECIALLY THOSE WHO ARE OVERWEIGHT AND INDULGE IN RICH FOODS AND FORTIFIED WINES, CLASSICALLY PORT.

The base of the big toe is the most common site of gout, but any joint may be affected. Gout causes sudden pain and inflammation, usually in a single joint. In women, it rarely appears before the menopause.

WHAT ARE THE CAUSES?
Gout is usually caused by high levels of the waste product uric acid in the blood. Excess uric acid is caused by the over-production and decreased excretion of uric acid and may lead to uric acid **crystals** being deposited in a joint. Why this happens no one knows, but the condition is often

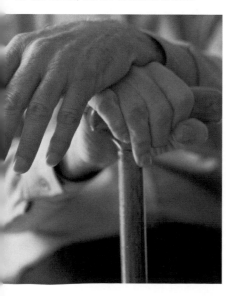

inherited. A few people with gout also develop **kidney stones** formed from excess uric acid crystals.

Gout may occur spontaneously or be brought on by surgery, being overweight, drinking alcohol or excessive cell destruction associated with **chemotherapy**.

WHAT ARE THE SYMPTOMS?
The symptoms of gout usually flare up suddenly. They may include:
• fiery redness, tenderness, warmth, and swelling around the affected area, as in infection
• pain, which may be excruciating, in the affected joint or joints
• mild fever.
    In long-standing gout, deposits of uric acid crystals may collect in the earlobes and the soft tissues of the hands, forming small, creamy lumps called **tophi**.

WHAT MIGHT BE DONE?
■ Your doctor will arrange for blood tests to measure your uric acid levels. Severely raised uric acid levels are diagnostic of gout.
■ To confirm the diagnosis, a joint aspiration, in which fluid is withdrawn from the affected joint, is examined for uric acid crystals. For obvious reasons this procedure is only done when the joint is pain-free.

WHAT IS THE TREATMENT?
Gout may subside by itself after a few days without treatment. If it persists the following treatments may be offered.

■ To reduce severe pain and inflammation, you may be treated with a non-steroidal anti-inflammatory drug (NSAID), the anti-gout drug **colchicine** or with **oral corticosteroids**.
■ If you have recurring gout, you may need **life-long treatment** with preventative drugs such as **allopurinol** to reduce the production of uric acid, or **probenecid** to increase the excretion of uric acid.
■ Your doctor may recommend that you make lifestyle changes and reduce the amount of alcohol you drink and the richness of your diet; in particular you should try to avoid liver, other offal, poultry and pulses.
■ Losing excess weight may help reduce the frequency and severity of attacks of gout.

WHAT IS THE OUTLOOK?
Gout can be very painful and disrupt normal physical activities, but attacks tend to become less frequent and less severe with age. Repeated attacks may cause permanent damage to the affected joint and occasionally to the kidneys.

See also:
• **Chemotherapy p.257**
• **Kidney stones p.377**

MUSCULOSKELETAL DISORDERS

The musculoskeletal system consists of the bones and joints of the skeleton and the hundreds of muscles, tendons and ligaments attached to them. When one of the components of the system is damaged or strained, the whole system is thrown out of kilter, resulting in pain. For instance, most cases of low back pain involve a degree of spondylosis – osteoarthritis – of the spine with some painful **muscle spasm** around the spondylotic vertebra. Similarly there is nearly always **muscle weakness** adjacent to a prolapsed disc.

Carpal tunnel syndrome

COMMONLY AFFLICTING PEOPLE BETWEEN THE AGES OF 40 AND 60, PARTICULARLY WOMEN, CARPAL TUNNEL SYNDROME CAUSES TINGLING AND PAIN IN THE HAND AND FOREARM DUE TO SOFT TISSUE SWELLING AND COMPRESSION OF A NERVE AT THE WRIST.

The carpal tunnel is the narrow space formed by the bones of the wrist (carpal bones) and the strong ligament that lies over them. Nerves and tendons run through this tunnel. In carpal tunnel syndrome, **the median nerve**, which controls some hand muscles and sensation in the thumb, index and middle fingers, is compressed where it passes through the tunnel. This causes painful tingling in the hand, wrist and forearm and often affects both hands. In women the menopause undoubtedly plays a part. Work involving repetitive hand movements is a risk factor.

WHAT ARE THE CAUSES?
Carpal tunnel syndrome occurs because the soft tissues within the carpal tunnel swell and press on the median nerve at the wrist. Such swelling may occur during **pregnancy**, as part of **rheumatoid arthritis** and after a **wrist fracture**. It may be a feature of **RSI**. In most cases there is no clear-cut cause.

WHAT ARE THE SYMPTOMS?
Symptoms mainly affect the areas of the hand supplied by the median nerve, that is the thumb, the index and middle fingers, the inner side of the ring finger, and the palm of the hand. Symptoms initially include:
- burning and tingling in the hand
- pain in the wrist and up the forearm.

As the condition worsens, other symptoms may gradually appear including:
- numbness of the hand
- weakened grip
- wasting of some hand muscles, particularly at the base of the thumb.

Symptoms are usually more severe at night, and pain may interrupt sleep. Shaking the affected arm may temporarily relieve symptoms, but the numbness may become persistent if left untreated.

WHAT MIGHT BE DONE?
The symptoms of carpal tunnel syndrome may be relieved temporarily by **non-steroidal anti-inflammatory drugs** (NSAIDs), or by wearing a **wrist splint**. Resting the hand and arm on a **pillow** often brings relief. In some cases a **corticosteroid injection** under the ligament may reduce swelling. If symptoms persist or recur, **surgery** may be recommended to cut

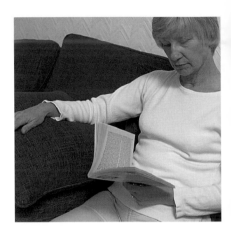

the ligament under local anaesthetic and release pressure on the nerve. After surgery, most people have no further symptoms.

> **See also:**
> - Diabetes mellitus p.504
> - **NSAIDs p.431** • **RSI p.439**

Low back pain

MORE WORKING DAYS ARE LOST DUE TO LOW BACK PAIN THAN TO ANY OTHER MEDICAL CONDITION – IT AFFECTS ABOUT 3 IN 5 ADULTS.

Low back pain occurs in the back below the waist and it may be sudden and sharp or persistent and dull; it may radiate down to the buttock and then down the back of the leg to the sole of the foot.

In most cases low back pain lasts for only a week or so, but many people find that the problem recurs unless they alter their lifestyle and the way in which they perform daily activities. In a minority of people, persistent low back pain causes chronic disability.

Low back pain is usually caused by minor damage to the ligaments and muscles in the back secondary to minor injury (e.g. a twist), overexertion (e.g. digging the garden) or lumbar spondylosis (the natural ageing process of the spine). The lower back is vulnerable to these problems because it supports much of the body's weight and is under continual stress from movement such as bending and twisting. Less commonly, low back pain may be due to an underlying

disorder such as a prolapsed or herniated (slipped) disc in the spine.

WHAT ARE THE CAUSES?
Low back pain may come on suddenly (acute) or develop gradually over a period of weeks. If the pain persists it's described as chronic.

ACUTE
Sudden back pain is often caused by **lifting** or **moving** heavy objects, such as furniture, and is

due to a strained muscle or tendon. The injury may be aggravated by subsequent activity. In most cases, symptoms subside within 2–14 days.

CHRONIC

■ Back pain that tends to be more persistent is often caused by **poor posture**, such as while sitting at a desk or driving a car, or by excessive muscle tension due to emotional stress.

■ In back pain in **pregnancy** there are two factors at work – changes in posture because of the extra weight of the baby and softening of the ligaments supporting the spine due to high levels of pregnancy hormones.

■ In people over age 45, persistent low back pain is caused by **osteoarthritis** of the spine, while in younger people the joints of the spine may be affected by **ankylosing spondylitis**.

■ **Pain** from compression of the nerve root is due to a prolapsed disc or spondylosis exerting pressure on a spinal nerve. Back pain of this type may have a gradual or sudden onset and is often accompanied by **sciatica**, a disorder where severe pain shoots down the back of one or, rarely, both legs.

■ Back pain may rarely come from the **bone** itself, for instance, where cancer has spread to bone from a tumour elsewhere in the body.

■ Conditions affecting the **pelvic organs** can cause pain in the lower back. Examples are **pelvic inflammatory disease** and **kidney infection**. **Peptic ulcers** and gallbladder disease can cause "referred" pain that is felt in the back.

WHAT ARE THE SYMPTOMS?

Low back pain can take various forms. You may experience:
● a sharp pain localized to a small area of the back
● a more general aching pain in the back and buttocks, made worse by sitting and relieved by standing
● back stiffness and pain on bending
● pain in the back that radiates to the buttock, leg and foot, sometimes accompanied by numbness or tingling.

WHAT CAN I DO?

In most cases, you should be able to treat low back pain yourself.

■ An over-the-counter **non-steroidal anti-inflammatory drug** (NSAID) should reduce the pain, and a heating pad or wrapped hot water bottle or sometimes ice placed against your back may provide additional relief.

■ If the pain is severe, you may be more comfortable resting in bed, but you should not stay in bed for more than two days. Start moving around as soon as possible and gradually return to normal activities.

■ If the pain worsens or is still too severe to allow you to move around after a few days, you should consult your doctor.

Back-strengthening exercises

The key is to strengthen your **abdominal** muscles so they will "splint" and support your back from the front. You can help prevent back pain by gently exercising the muscles in your back and abdomen. Consult a doctor or ask for a referral to a physiotherapist before starting an exercise programme. You should not continue any exercise that causes you pain. The movements shown below should make your back muscles stronger and your spine more flexible. Repeat each one 10 times if you can, and try to exercise daily. Do the exercises on a comfortable but firm, flat surface, such as a mat laid on the floor.

Lower back stretch

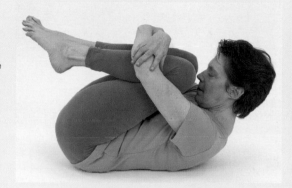

This stretch may relieve aching joints and muscles in the lower back. Lie on your back with your feet flat on the floor and your knees bent. Lift your knees towards your body. With your hands, pull your knees into your chest. Hold for seven seconds and breathe deeply. Keeping your knees bent, lower your feet to the floor one at a time.

Hump and sag

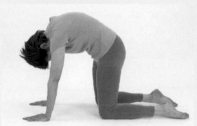 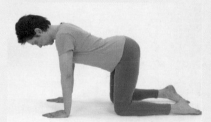

The movements in this exercise should increase suppleness in the joints and muscles of the back. Support yourself on your hands and knees, your knees slightly apart.

Tuck your chin into your chest, then gently arch your back. Hold for about five seconds. Look up, allowing your back to sag, and hold again for about another five seconds.

Pelvic tilt

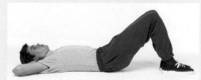 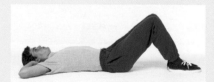

This movement helps to stretch the muscles and ligaments of the lower back. Lie on your back with your knees bent and your feet flat on the floor. Press the small of your back into the floor.

Tighten your buttock and abdominal muscles so that your buttocks rise slightly off the floor and your pelvis tilts upwards. Hold for six seconds, then relax. Once you've learned this exercise you can do it standing at any time.

■ Once the pain has subsided, you can help prevent any recurrences by paying attention to your posture, learning to lift correctly and doing **regular exercises** to strengthen the muscles of your back and make your spine more flexible (see box, above).

WHAT MIGHT THE DOCTOR DO?

■ Your doctor will do a full physical examination to assess your posture, the range of movement in your spine, and any areas of local tenderness.

■ Your reflexes, the strength of different leg muscles, and the sensation in your legs will be

TREATMENT

Self-help: Preventing back pain

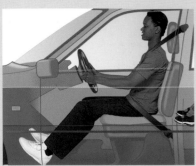

Driving position: Angle your seat backwards a little so it supports your spine, and position the seat so that you can reach the hand and foot controls easily.

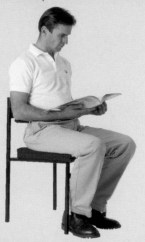

Sitting position: Sit with your back straight and both feet on the floor. Use a chair that supports the small of your back. When using a computer, position the monitor so you can look straight at it.

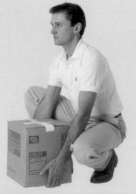

Lifting position: Keep your back straight and hold the object to be lifted as close to your body as possible. Use the muscles of your legs, not your back, to lift the object.

Most people have experienced back pain at some time in their lives, but in many cases the problem could have been avoided. Back pain is often due to poor posture, weak abdominal or back muscles, or sudden muscle strain. You can improve your posture by wearing comfortable shoes, by standing or sitting with your spine properly aligned, and by choosing a supportive mattress for your bed. Gentle, regular exercises may strengthen abdominal and back muscles, and losing excess weight may relieve stress on joints and muscles. Learning how to perform physical tasks safely, such as lifting and carrying objects, can prevent back strain. Ask your doctor or physical therapist for advice on posture, exercises and diet.

Correct body posture

To break bad postural habits, you should be constantly aware of the way in which you stand, sit, move and even sleep. The pictures on the left show how to carry out everyday activities comfortably, with minimal strain on your spine and back muscles.

Lifting an object

When lifting, pushing or pulling a heavy object, keep the object close to you so you can use your full strength to move it. To lift an object, hold the bottom edge so that you support the full weight of the object, and keep your body balanced as you lift to avoid straining your spine.

1. Squat close to the object with your weight evenly on both feet and the object between your legs. Grasp the base of the object.

2. Keep your back straight and lean forwards slightly. Stand up in a single, smooth movement, pushing yourself up with your leg muscles and keeping the object close to you.

3. Once you are upright, keep the weight close to your body. Keep your back straight and head up, so that your body is balanced over its centre of gravity.

tested to look for evidence of pressure on spinal nerves or the spinal cord.

■ A **pelvic or rectal examination** may also be performed to rule out disorders of the internal organs.

■ You may have various **blood tests and X-rays** to look for underlying causes of the pain, such as joint inflammation or bone cancer.

■ If there is evidence of pressure on the spinal cord or spinal nerves, MRI (magnetic resonance imaging) or CT (computerized tomography) scanning may be done to detect abnormalities requiring special treatment, such as a prolapsed or herniated disc.

WHAT IS THE TREATMENT?

■ Unless the physical examination and other tests indicate that there is a serious underlying cause for your back pain, your doctor will probably advise you to continue taking a non-steroidal anti-inflammatory drug (NSAID).

■ You may be given **physiotherapy** to mobilize stiff and painful joints between the vertebrae.

■ A local anaesthetic combined with a corticosteroid may be injected into the tender areas.

■ **Osteopathy** may be effective for treating low back pain and an osteopath is worth consulting. However, chiropractic is less effective.

WHAT IS THE OUTLOOK?

You may think your low back pain will never get better but even the worst attacks do, given time. Most clear up without any specific treatment, but the problem recurs in many people unless factors such as poor posture or ways of lifting are improved.

In a small number of people, low back pain may be a long-standing condition, severely disrupting their work and social life and sometimes leading to depression. Effective pain control is essential in these situations, and many people find that taking the newer **antidepressants**, SSRIs, helps them cope and allows tense muscles to relax.

Once you have "a back" you'll always have a back. As we get older, episodes of pain may get more severe and take longer to resolve but with heat, back-strengthening exercises, painkillers and physiotherapy most resolve after several months. Taking care with posture, sitting and moving or lifting heavy weights should be part of our lives.

See also:
• **Ankylosing spondylitis p.430**
• **Back-strengthening exercises p.435**
• **CT scanning p.401**
• **Infection of the kidneys p.376**
• **MRI p.409** • **Osteoarthritis p.428**
• **Peptic ulcer p.353** • **Slipped disc p.437**
• **X-rays p.426**

Slipped disc

WHEN ONE OF THE SHOCK-ABSORBING PADS THAT LIE BETWEEN THE VERTEBRAE OF
THE SPINE BECOMES DISPLACED AND PROTRUDES, IT IS KNOWN AS A SLIPPED DISC.
DOCTORS REFER TO THE CONDITION AS A PROLAPSED OR HERNIATED DISC.

A slipped disc is most common between the ages of 25 and 45 and is slightly more common in men. Being overweight and lifting objects incorrectly are risk factors.

The shock-absorbing discs between the vertebrae consist of a strong, fibrous outer coat and a soft, gelatinous core. A prolapsed disc occurs when the core pushes outwards, distorting the shape of the disc. If the outer coat ruptures, the condition is termed a **herniated disc**. When a disc prolapses or herniates, the surrounding tissues become inflamed and swollen. Together with the disc, the tissues may press on a spinal nerve, causing pain down the length of that nerve, the most common being the **sciatic nerve**, giving rise to **sciatica**.

WHAT ARE THE CAUSES?

After about the age of 25, the discs begin to **dry out**, being driest on waking, so strenuous activity involving the back shouldn't be undertaken without a good warm-up routine. Discs also become more vulnerable to prolapse or herniation as a result of the normal stress of daily life and minor injury. Sometimes damage to a disc is caused by a sharp bending or twisting movement or by lifting a heavy object incorrectly. From about the age of 45, fibrous tissue forms around the discs, eventually stabilizing them and making them less likely to be damaged.

WHAT ARE THE SYMPTOMS?

Symptoms of a prolapsed or herniated disc may develop progressively over a period of weeks or may appear suddenly. They include:
- dull pain in the affected area
- muscle spasm and stiffness around the affected area that makes movement difficult and pain much worse.

If the disc presses on a spinal nerve, you may also have the following symptoms:
- severe pain, tingling, or numbness in your leg or, if the neck is affected, in your arm
- weakness or restricted movement in your leg or arm.

The pain is usually relieved by rest but can be made worse by walking upstairs, sitting, coughing, sneezing or bending. Bowel movements can also aggravate the pain. Impaired bladder or bowel function may indicate pressure on the spinal cord, and you should consult a doctor immediately.

WHAT MIGHT BE DONE?

■ X-rays will rule out other causes of back pain, such as spondylosis.
■ MRI (magnetic resonance imaging) or CT (computerized tomography) scanning will locate the position of the prolapsed or herniated disc accurately.
■ Even if the disc is permanently damaged, the pain usually improves over 6–8 weeks as the swelling subsides. Your doctor will suggest bed rest and pain medication. If you are free of pain, physiotherapy and exercises may help reduce muscle spasms and hasten recovery. For persistent pain, you will require referral to a hospital.
■ Rarely, pain may be relieved with **traction**,

TREATMENT

Microdiscectomy

Microdiscectomy is a surgical procedure used to treat a prolapsed or herniated disc pressing on a spinal nerve or the spinal cord. The protruding part of the disc is removed through an incision in the fibrous outer coat of the disc using an operating microscope. The operation is performed under general anaesthetic and requires a brief stay in hospital.

in which the spine is gently stretched with weights to create more space around the nerves, reducing pressure on and around them.
■ Some people may benefit from a selective **nerve root block**, in which a local anaesthetic, sometimes combined with a corticosteroid drug, is injected around the compressed nerve to decrease swelling. Occasionally surgery is needed to decompress the affected nerve root.

See also:
- **CT scanning p.401** ● **Low back pain p.434**
- **MRI p.409**
- **Spondylosis p.432**

Restless legs (Ekbom syndrome)

EKBOM SYNDROM CAUSES A BURNING SENSATION IN THE LEGS AND FEET THAT
MAY BE RELIEVED BY MOVING THEM, SOMETIMES CONTINUOUSLY.

We still have a lot to learn about this distressing condition but around 5 percent of the population can expect to experience some or all of the symptoms during their lives.

WHAT CAUSES IT?

Mainly associated with elderly women, restless legs can also affect men and children and there is evidence to suggest that it runs in families. The first symptoms may occur mildly or infrequently in the teenage years, occur again in pregnancy to fade away after the birth, only to reappear later in life.

Some studies have suggested an association with **anxiety, depression** and **stress**. It is known that about one-third of all patients with **rheumatoid arthritis** also suffer from this condition.

WHAT ARE THE SYMPTOMS?

Unpleasant creeping, prickling or burning sensations in one or both calves that can sometimes be felt in the feet, thighs, trunk and arms. The sensations can begin soon after sitting or lying down but usually come on in the evening and at night time, causing severe disruption to sleep.

Although symptoms can vary widely, the one consistent factor is that short-lived relief can be achieved by movement.

If you, or someone you know, suffers frequently from this kind of distressing discomfort, it is important to consult your doctor so a diagnosis can be made. Other disorders – for example, iron deficiency anaemia, circulatory or disc problems – can give rise to similar symptoms.

A similar painful condition, common in the elderly, is **meralgia paraesthetica**, or pain in the outer leg. Unlike restless legs, it can be easily treated by conservative treatment so you can see the importance of an accurate diagnosis.

WHAT CAN I DO?
As yet there is no cure for restless legs, but some sufferers have found regular gentle exercise, swimming, cool showers, yoga and relaxation exercises and vitamin B$_{12}$ helpful.

It is wise to avoid standing or sitting for long periods, cat-naps during the day, heavy meals before bedtime, coffee, restrictive clothing and clothing made from synthetic materials.

Treatment with certain drugs has proved effective, in particular **ropinirole**. No clinical trials have been carried out on ropinirole as a therapy for restless legs (although trials are about to start soon) but there is considerable anecdotal evidence indicating that it has brought relief to many sufferers. It was developed to control leg tremor in people with Parkinson's disease and it has been discovered to have a wider application.

As it is not licensed as a therapy for restless legs, a doctor may need to prescribe it

privately on a "named patient" basis. This is where a doctor notifies the health authorities that he is administering an unlicensed drug to his patient and that you both accept responsibility for the decision.

The support group for sufferers (see Useful addresses p.567) can provide a wealth of information and practical advice on remedies that other people have found effective. Through its quarterly newsletters it shares information about current medical research and investigations.

MUSCLES AND TENDONS

When skeletal muscles contract and relax they move the body by making joints bend and straighten. Muscles are connected to bones by fibrous tissue known as tendons. Both muscles and tendons can be temporarily or permanently damaged by injury and overuse, leading to pain, weakness, restricted movement and fatigue.

Although our muscles account for half the weight of the body they are only rarely affected by disease. Overexertion of a muscle or tendon, through very strenuous exercise, unusual activity or as a result of repetitive movements or immobilization, will cause many of the disorders described in this section, including **muscle cramps**, **frozen shoulder**, **repetitive strain injury**

and **tennis elbow**. Inflammation of a tendon (tendinitis) or tendon sheath (tenosynovitis) is really quite common and quite painful so I've included some personal observations. Probably the most common cause of muscle pain is **fibromyalgia**, a condition whose precise origin remains a mystery but there is nearly always a psychological component.

Some disorders that affect the muscles are covered in other parts of the book. So you'll find **immune system** disorders such as **polymyositis and dermatomyositis** on page 326 and the inherited disease **muscular dystrophy** on page 523. Musculoskeletal conditions are on page 434.

Muscle cramp
PAINFUL SPASM IN A MUSCLE OR GROUP OF MUSCLES, USUALLY IN THE LOWER LEG, IS COMMONLY KNOWN AS CRAMP; THIS UNPLEASANT BUT TEMPORARY CONDITION AFFECTS ALMOST EVERYONE FROM TIME TO TIME.

WHAT CAUSES IT?
Painful spasms of cramp, often lasting only a few minutes, make the muscle become hard and tender; this is usually due to overuse. Protracted pain from muscle spasm is normally because a muscle is protecting an injured part underneath it, as in spondylosis and spondylitis, and won't go until the injured part improves. Muscle cramp may occur in any muscle in the body but it is most common in the large groups of leg muscles, such as the quadriceps on the front of the thighs, the hamstrings at the back of the thighs and the calf muscles. When abdominal muscles are affected, the condition is also known as a "stitch".
■ Muscle cramp often develops during **exercise**, because the working muscle outstrips its oxygen supply or builds up lactic acid during anaerobic exercise.
■ Another possible cause is the loss of salt

and water due to heavy sweating during hot weather or strenuous exercise.
■ Muscle cramp may also develop if you have been sitting or lying in an awkward position for a long time.
■ Cramp is not the only cause of attacks of muscle pain. If you develop recurrent muscle pain in the calves when you are walking, you should consult your doctor; the cause may be poor blood flow when the arteries that supply blood to the leg muscles become furred up by atherosclerosis.

WHAT MIGHT HELP?
■ The immediate self-help treatment for muscle cramp is to stretch and rub the affected area and to apply a heating pad.
■ You should drink plenty of fluids and eat something salty.
■ If you regularly have muscle cramp at night,

your doctor may prescribe a low dose of **quinine**, an antimalarial drug that effectively relieves the symptoms.
■ Muscle-relaxant drugs are sometimes helpful.
■ Flunitrazepam, a sedative with muscle-relaxing effects, may give you a pain-free night's sleep.

See also:
• The heart and atherosclerosis p.222
• Spondylosis p.432

FOCUS *on* RSI

Any person whose work or hobby involves repeated physical movements, particularly of the hands and arms, is at risk of causing damage to tendons, nerves, muscles and other soft body tissues. This type of injury is commonly known as repetitive strain injury (RSI).

Workers ranging from packers to musicians can develop RSI as a result of the tasks they perform. The computer with the flat, light-touch keyboard that permits high-speed typing has produced an epidemic of injuries to the hands, arms and shoulders.

WHAT ARE THE SYMPTOMS?
- **Tightness**, discomfort, stiffness, soreness and burning in the hands, wrists, fingers and forearms or elbows.
- **Tingling**, coldness or numbness in the hands.
- **Clumsiness** or loss of strength and **coordination** in the hands.
- **Pain** that wakes you up at night.
- **Need to massage** your hands, wrists and arms.

RSI CONDITIONS
Specific conditions include **nerve compression, tendonitis** or inflammation of the tendons, **carpal tunnel syndrome** – which causes numbness and pain in the hand – and involuntary movements and spasms of the hand and fingers.

All have different symptoms, from pain and stiffness to jerky movements and cramping.

WHAT IS THE CAUSE?
Researchers around the world have been searching for explanations for RSI. Some doctors aren't so sure that RSI has a single cause and believe that a variety of factors, including genes and personality, could play a part.

One theory says it's psychological and another says it's physical. A third theory says it's an interaction between physical and mental. There isn't just one cause – some people get RSI, others don't while performing an identical task. It may even stem from the brain becoming confused by the repetitive task.

SELF-HELP
Wrist splints, arm rests, split keyboards and spinal adjustment won't get you back to work quickly. Your RSI will relapse unless you make long-term changes in technique and work habits.

If, as some experts think, RSI turns out to be a problem of the brain rather than the hands and arms, re-educating the brain could be more useful. So exercises such as using **Braille cards** or **playing dominoes with the eyes closed** – what the experts call **sensory retraining** – may be the answer for some people (see box, below).

WHAT IS THE TREATMENT?
Treatments range from anti-inflammatory drugs to surgery, but for some people the only cure is a change of job. And compensation can be hard to come by.

HOW DO I AVOID RSI?
- Eliminate unnecessary computer usage. No **amount of ergonomic changes, fancy keyboards or exercises** are going to help if you are simply typing too much.
- **Don't** use computer/video games that often involve long, unbroken sessions of very intense keyboard usage.
- Increase your font sizes. Small fonts encourage you to hunch forwards into the monitor to read, putting pressure on nerves and blood vessels in the neck and shoulders.
- Don't pound on the keys. Use a light touch.
- Use two hands to perform double-key operations instead of twisting one hand to do it. Move your whole hand to hit function keys instead of stretching.
- Take lots of breaks to stretch and relax. This means both momentary breaks every few minutes and longer breaks every hour or so.
- Hold the mouse lightly, don't grip it hard or squeeze it. Place the pointing device close to the keyboard. Pace and plan your computer work.
- **Don't** tuck the telephone between your shoulder and ear so you can type and talk on the phone at the same time, because it's a great strain on your neck, shoulders and arms.
- Keep your arms and hands warm. Cold muscles and tendons are at much greater risk from overuse injuries.
- Take care of your eyes.
- Look at other things you're doing. Problems may be caused or aggravated by other things you do frequently. Sports, carrying children, hobbies requiring intense small work like knitting and excess effort/tension in other daily things may have enormous impact too.
- Pay attention to your body. Pain's a symptom that your body's in trouble, but learning what's comfortable or awkward for your body before you're in pain may prevent injury.
- Kids are at risk, too, with increasing hours in front of the computer at home and school, using equipment that rarely is set up correctly for people of their size.

Handy hints

- Exercise to teach your fingers how to discriminate again.
- Play dominoes with your eyes shut.
- Match a shape to an opening with eyes closed.
- Put together puzzles that have a raised surface with eyes closed.
- Play cards using a Braille deck.
- Ask someone to draw letters and numbers on your fingers and, with eyes closed, try to guess what they are writing.
- Get someone to rub different objects on your hand and try to identify them.
- Carry pairs of different-shaped objects in your pocket and try to match them.
- Make a grab bag of different shaped items and try to identify them.
- Play games requiring orientation, such as pinning the tail on the donkey, blindfolded.

Fibromyalgia

THIS IS A MUSCLE DISORDER THAT CAUSES WIDESPREAD MUSCLE PAIN, ACHING, STIFFNESS AND FATIGUE ASSOCIATED WITH MUSCLE TENDERNESS.

Although the condition has no obvious cause, and no visible abnormality has ever been identified in the muscle itself, fibromyalgia is more common in females, and often develops during periods of stress.

WHAT ARE THE SYMPTOMS?
The symptoms of fibromyalgia develop slowly over weeks and occur in a distinct pattern around the body. They may include the following:
- muscle pain in the upper back, head, thighs, abdomen and hips
- particularly tender areas of muscle, typically at the base of the skull, the neck and near the shoulder blades.

Fibromyalgia is commonly associated with headaches, fatigue, depression, anxiety disorders and disturbed sleep patterns. Some people have irregular bowel movements (irritable bowel syndrome). All of these symptoms usually become worse when levels of stress increase.

WHAT MIGHT BE DONE?
■ The diagnosis of fibromyalgia is often based on the symptoms and a physical examination, but your doctor may arrange for blood tests to rule out other disorders, such as rheumatoid arthritis.
■ Although there is no specific treatment, the pain may be relieved by deep tissue massage and locally applied moist heat, ultrasound treatment,

or an injection with a local anaesthetic.
■ Your doctor may also prescribe a low dose of amitriptyline, which is effective in relieving pain in this condition.
■ Regular exercise is also important to maintain muscle tone and flexibility.

Most people make a full recovery, but in some cases the symptoms recur.

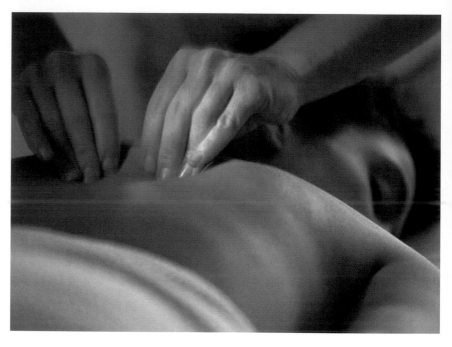

Deep tissue massage can help relieve the pain of fibromyalgia.

See also:
- **Irritable bowel syndrome p.362**
- **Rheumatoid arthritis p.429**

Polymyalgia rheumatica

THE PROMINENT COMPLAINT IN POLYMYALGIA RHEUMATICA IS PAIN AND STIFFNESS IN THE SHOULDERS AND HIPS, ASSOCIATED WITH A LOSS OF ENERGY AND A GENERAL SENSE OF NOT FEELING WELL.

The condition, which may run in families, is rare under the age of 60 and is twice as common in females. Polymyalgia rheumatica is an **autoimmune disorder** in which antibodies attack the body's own tissues, in this case the muscles. It may occur in association with another autoimmune disorder, **temporal arteritis**.

WHAT ARE THE SYMPTOMS?
The symptoms usually appear over a few weeks but sometimes develop suddenly. They include:
- painful, stiff muscles, often causing difficulty getting out of bed and moving around and usually affecting the neck and shoulders

- profound fatigue
- persistent or intermittent fever; night sweats
- weight loss
- depression.

If temporal arteritis is also present, there could be severe headaches on one or both sides of the head and tenderness of the scalp.

WHAT MIGHT BE DONE?
It is important to get advice because treatment is simple and effective.
■ Your doctor will probably be able to make a diagnosis simply on a physical examination and the results of blood tests to look for inflammation.

■ Additional blood tests will be performed to exclude other disorders, such as rheumatoid arthritis.
■ **Oral corticosteroids** reduce the inflammation and pain dramatically. If you also have temporal arteritis, the initial doses may be high. In either case, the dose will be reduced to a maintenance level once the symptoms subside.

Take heart! Symptoms are usually relieved soon after starting corticosteroid treatment. However, polymyalgia rheumatica may persist, in which case you will need to continue taking low doses of a coricosteroid, such as prednisone.

Tennis elbow and golfer's elbow

**THIS IS INFLAMMATION OF A TENDON AT ITS ATTACHMENT TO THE BONE
AT THE ELBOW DUE TO UNACCUSTOMED REPETITIVE MOVEMENT.**

The disorder is rare among professionals but common among recreational tennis players and golfers and among people carrying out repetitive unaccustomed activities like cleaning windows and hanging wallpaper. Music conductors get tennis elbow too!

Tennis elbow and golfer's elbow both occur when the tendon attachment of the muscle to the bone at the elbow becomes damaged. In tennis elbow, the tendon on the outer side of the elbow is injured; in golfer's elbow, the tendon on the inner side of the elbow is affected. It depends if the movement is mainly **backhanded** using the extensor tendon (tennis elbow) or **forehanded** using the flexor tendon (golfer's elbow).

Both conditions are caused by vigorous and repeated use of the forearm against resistance, which can occur when playing certain sports, such as tennis, using a screwdriver or using secateurs for pruning. The tendon is repeatedly pulled at the point at which it is attached to the bone, which may cause small tears to develop. The resulting damage leads to tenderness and pain in the affected arm.

WHAT IS THE TREATMENT?

■ You should rest the affected painful arm as much as possible.
■ Physiotherapy, ice packs and simple exercises to stretch and strengthen the muscles may help.
■ Ultrasound treatment may help relieve symptoms.

■ You may also find that a non-steroidal anti-inflammatory drug (NSAID) helps.
■ If the condition does not improve within 2–6 weeks, your doctor may inject a corticosteroid drug into the tender area.

■ Once the symptoms have subsided, you should seek advice from a physiotherapist on ways to change your technique before resuming the sport or activity that gave rise to the condition.

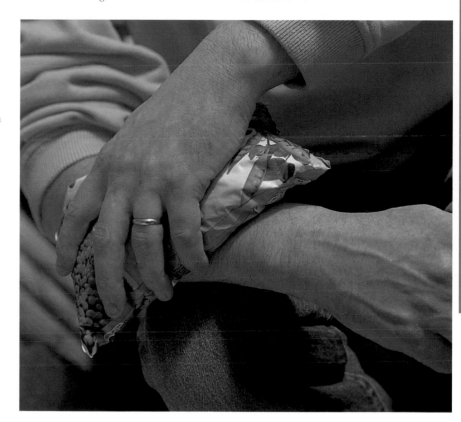

Frozen shoulder

**PAIN AND RESTRICTION OF MOVEMENT IN THE SHOULDER JOINT, COMMONLY FOLLOWING
A MINOR INJURY, IS CALLED FROZEN SHOULDER. THE CONDITION IS MORE COMMON IN WOMEN
THAN MEN. ANY INJURY TO THE SHOULDER CAN END UP AS FROZEN SHOULDER.**

WHAT CAUSES IT?

Frozen shoulder may be caused by inflammation as a result of an injury to the shoulder region. The condition may also occur if the shoulder is kept immobilized for a period of time, for example after a minor injury or stroke. However, in many cases, frozen shoulder develops for no apparent reason. People with **diabetes mellitus** are more susceptible to the condition. The pain probably originates in the muscles around the joint when they go into spasm to protect an injured part underneath them.

WHAT ARE THE SYMPTOMS?

The symptoms of frozen shoulder often begin gradually over a period of weeks or months. They include:
● pain in the shoulder, which can be very severe in the early stage of the condition and often worse at night
● with time, decreasing pain but increasing stiffness and restricted joint movement
● in severe cases, pain travelling down the arm to the elbow and up into the neck.

If you have pain in the shoulder that lasts for more than a few days, consult your doctor

without delay. The longer a frozen shoulder is left, the harder it is to treat. It's quite common for a frozen shoulder to last a year or longer, but it does always get better. It is a matter of retraining the muscles in spasm to relax – and that takes time.

WHAT MIGHT BE DONE?

■ A painkiller or a non-steroidal anti-inflammatory drug (NSAID) will relieve pain and reduce inflammation.
■ If the pain persists or is severe, you may be given a corticosteroid drug by a **direct**

injection around the shoulder joint.

■ You may also be referred for physiotherapy, hydrotherapy, massage and heat treatment. The muscle-relaxant sedative **flunitrazepam** is helpful at night.

■ Despite these measures, your shoulder may remain stiff for up to a year or longer.

■ In very severe, persistent cases you may have to have your shoulder stretched to its limits under a general anaesthetic.

Whatever the severity of the condition, recovery is usually slow and may take up to a further six months after the disappearance of stiffness to be back to normal.

> **See also:**
> • **Diabetes mellitus p.504** • **NSAIDS p.431**

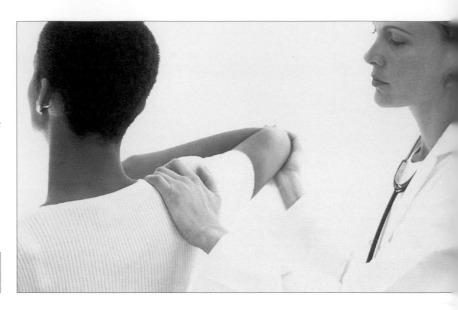

Dupuytren's contracture

IN DUPUYTREN'S CONTRACTURE, THE FIBROUS TISSUE IN THE PALM OF THE HAND
BECOMES THICKENED AND SHORTENED, RESULTING IN DEFORMITY.

One or more of the fingers, often the ring and little fingers, are pulled towards the palm into a bent position and, sometimes, painful lumps develop on the palm and the overlying skin becomes puckered. In about half of all cases, both hands are involved. Rarely, the disorder affects the soles of the feet. Dupuytren's contracture is much more common in men over age 50; alcohol abuse is a risk factor. The disorder may run in families.

The tissue changes in Dupuytren's contracture develop slowly over months or years. The cause is unknown, but it occurs more commonly in people with **diabetes mellitus** or **epilepsy**, and in people who **drink to excess**. About 1 in 10 people with Dupuytren's contracture has a relative with the disorder, so there may be a **gene** at work.

WHAT MIGHT BE DONE?

■ In mild cases no treatment may be needed.

■ If your fingers are slightly bent you may benefit from stretching exercises or short-term splinting.

■ For lumps in your palm, a corticosteroid drug may be injected into the affected area.

■ In severe cases, surgery is the most effective treatment, especially if performed early. Under general or local anaesthetic, the thickened tissue in the palm is removed to allow the fingers to straighten.

■ Further treatment may be needed if the disorder recurs.

> **See also:**
> • **Diabetes mellitus p.504**
> • **Epilepsy p.538**

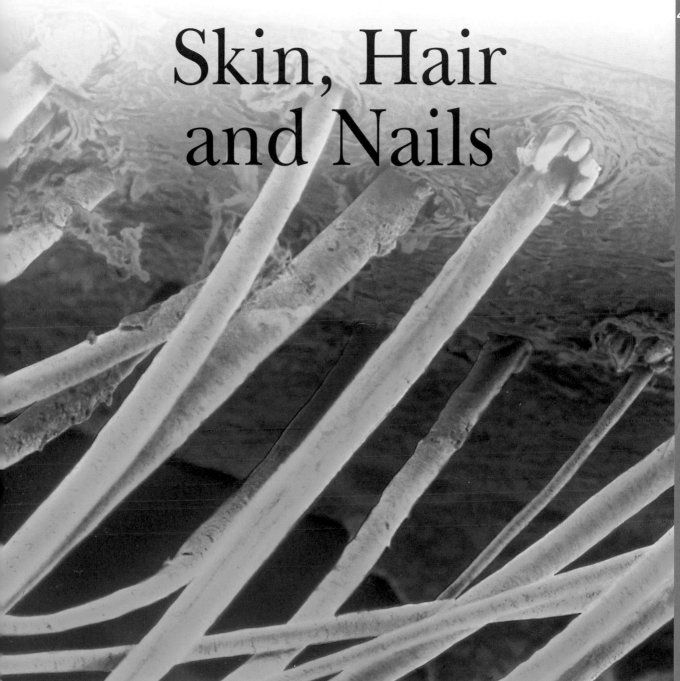

Skin, Hair and Nails

Image shows a coloured scanning electron micrograph of eyelashes

Miriam's overview

The skin is the largest organ in the body. When it gets hot and pink it siphons off half our blood, which is why we can feel faint when we get hot and bothered – there's not enough blood left over to nourish the brain.

The skin is the body's first defence, it's a protective layer that stops harmful things getting in and useful things getting out.

Among other vital jobs it keeps our core temperature constant by conserving heat when we cool down and throwing off calories when we get too hot.

These two main functions of the skin may go awry with dire consequences.

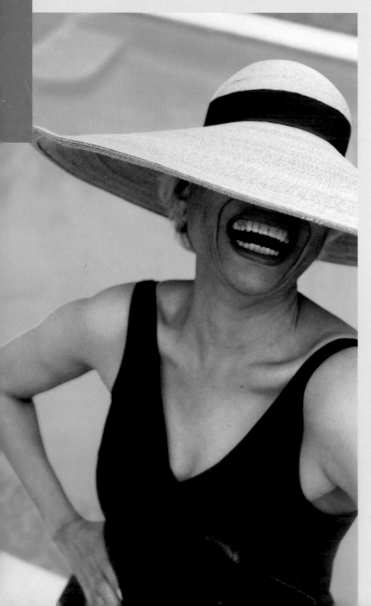

- When more than half the skin is damaged as in severe burns the body loses its ability to keep the temperature steady and we may become dangerously super-heated.
- With most of its covering gone the body can't hang onto vitpal components, they seep away. An example of this is protein which may be lost from burned skin so quickly that life is threatened.

The main message of the millennium about the skin is to stay out of the sun. Wear a sun-block on exposed parts every day, yes, every day. Exposure to sunlight causes skin cancers and the sunshine on a bleak winter's day in England still counts as part of your TOTAL LIFE DOSE. It's this cumulative dose that causes cancer. You will get your total life dose quickly if you live in Australia or slowly if you live in the UK. That means in Australia you'll still be quite young when your skin has soaked up its total life dose of sunshine. Once that's happened you're vulnerable to skin cancer. As the ozone layer gets thinner you get the total life dose earlier and earlier. So the watchword is sun protection at all times, starting as a baby.

"*wear a sun-block* on exposed parts every day, yes, *every day*"

That's crucially important because we've learned that severe sunburn as a child can damage your immune system so that you have an increased tendency to develop skin cancer later in life. I've never understood the obsession with getting a tan. Every day in the sun means a wrinkle later. The sun ages the skin like nothing else. And it can't be undone.

The skin has accessories in the form of hair and nails, both of which are dead. It follows that you can only affect their basic quality while they're growing in the hair follicle and nail-bed respectively. That's about six months before their condition becomes visible to the naked eye so it's a retrospective judgement. Put another way, if you want healthy hair and nails for your summer holidays you lay your plans and take action (mainly what you eat) at Christmas.

Inflammation of the skin, such as eczema (dermatitis), is generally part of genetically programmed reaction to stress called atopy found on p.312.

INSIDE
your skin, hair and nails

The skin is the largest organ of the body and provides our first line of defense against injury and infection. Hair and nails, which grow from the skin, provide the body with further protection.

Skin consists of two layers of tissue: the outer **epidermis**, which is quite thin, and the thicker **inner dermis**. The upper layer of the epidermis consists mostly of dead cells, while the dermis is made of strong, elastic tissue and contains **blood vessels**, **glands** and **nerve endings**. Hair, which is composed mainly of a protein called **keratin**, grows from **follicles** in the skin. Nails are also composed mainly of keratin and grow from an area beneath the nail's **cuticle** called the **matrix**.

the parts of a nail

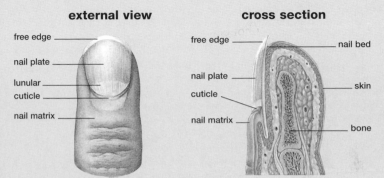

external view

free edge
nail plate
lunular
cuticle
nail matrix

cross section

free edge
nail plate
cuticle
nail matrix
nail bed
skin
bone

The nail itself is dead tissue made up of keratin, the same protein as hair. Nails provide the sensitive ends of the fingers with a protective covering.

the structure of the skin and hair

The skin is the body's largest organ. Skin has two layers, the outer epidermis, and the thicker dermis that lies beneath it.

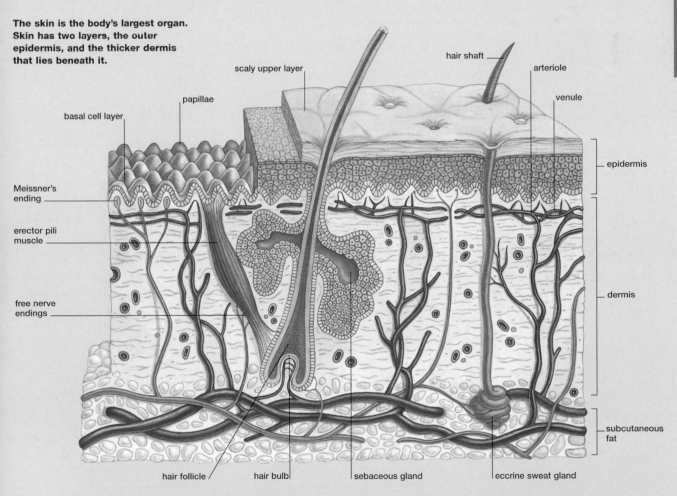

basal cell layer
papillae
scaly upper layer
hair shaft
arteriole
venule
Meissner's ending
erector pili muscle
free nerve endings
epidermis
dermis
subcutaneous fat
hair follicle
hair bulb
sebaceous gland
eccrine sweat gland

Teenage acne

THE GREASY SKIN WITH BLACKHEADS, PUS-FILLED SPOTS, PURPLISH-RED LUMPS AND
POSSIBLY SCARRING THAT CHARACTERIZES ACNE IS MOST COMMON IN ADOLESCENTS,
MORE COMMON IN BOYS AND MAY RUN IN FAMILIES.

Acne mainly affects the face, chest and back and is caused by blockage and inflammation of the grease glands in the skin. There is a persistent adult form of acne.

Our skin contains grease (sebaceous) glands that secrete an oily substance (sebum) to keep the skin supple and moist. If the exits from these glands become blocked, sebum bursts into the deeper layers of skin. Here it's highly irritant and causes inflammation, which can become infected. The result is pus-filled spots and the classical tender, purplish lumps of acne. When the lumps heal, scars and pitting may be left behind.

WHAT ARE THE CAUSES?

■ **Male hormones** are the cause of acne, and this goes for adolescent girls as well as boys. Under the influence of these male hormones (androgens), the best known of which is **testosterone**, cells at the exit from the sebaceous gland overgrow and block the outlet. At puberty, androgens pour into the blood and reach their highest levels in both sexes. In girls, they're even higher than oestrogens. So at **adolescence**, with all those androgens rushing about, sebaceous glands get blocked very easily. To make matters worse, androgens cause overproduction of sebum so sebaceous glands are stretched to bursting and some do.
■ Many women have acne in a mild form just prior to **menstruation,** when oestrogen levels are low.
■ People who take **steroids** may get acne spots.
■ Skin **bacteria** are important too in the formation of the red and yellow spots. After puberty, the skin of the face and upper trunk, with or without acne, contains many bacteria. The most important bacteria in acne are called *Propionibacterium acnes*. They get into the

ducts of the grease glands where they make chemicals that eventually escape into the deeper parts of the skin and cause more inflammation. This does not mean that acne is infective: it isn't. It's not a question of hygiene either. Washing, or the lack of it, does not cause acne.

Sometimes acne persists into the late teens and 20s and, rarely, into the 30s. It's no joke if it does because **adult acne** is more difficult to treat.

FACTORS THAT AFFECT ACNE

■ No matter what you're told or have read, acne **isn't** caused by eating rich or fatty foods, not washing thoroughly or by drinking too much alcohol.
■ There seems to be a tendency for acne to run in families.
■ In girls, a flare of acne is common just before the **monthly period**.
■ Pregnancy does not usually influence acne.
■ **Sunshine** may help acne, but sunbeds give little benefit.
■ **Diet** probably has no role in acne.
■ **Poor personal hygiene** does not worsen it.
■ **Squeezing spots** usually aggravates the problem.
■ **Stress** may make acne worse.
■ Overcleansing, too much rubbing or using products that contain abrasives worsen acne because they liberate bacteria from the grease glands onto the skin and promote more spots.

If acne starts after adolescence, for example in women over the age of 25, the factors above also apply.

SHOULD I SEE A DOCTOR AND WHAT HE CAN DO?

Yes, do, acne can be totally cured these days. But effective treatments are only available on prescription, **not over the counter**. The basis of treatment is four-fold:
1. To reduce the number of bacteria on the skin
2. To stop the multiplication of cells in the sebaceous glands, which results in blockage
3. To unblock pores
4. To lower sebum production.

GENERAL PRINCIPLES OF TREATMENT

With prescription treatment – not over-the-counter remedies – spots can usually be kept under excellent control and scarring prevented. **90 percent of patients show**

a **50 percent improvement in three months** and an 80 percent improvement within six months, but **continuous treatment** is necessary **for many years**.

There are three types of oral therapy: **antibiotics**, **hormones** and **retinoids**. All are available only on prescription and, with the exception of retinoids, should be combined with topical therapy. People who respond to oral antibiotics may need repeat courses, each lasting at least six months.
■ Gels and creams containing **peroxide** are often recommended to help unblock pores.
■ Long-term therapy with **oral antibiotics** often helps. The antibiotics are prescribed regularly for up to six months at a time. They have an effect not only on the bacteria in the skin but may also have a direct effect on inflammatory cells in acne spots, as well as on sebum production. A daily dose of the antibiotic **tetracycline** (750mg once a day) has been shown to help acne sufferers a great deal. There are usually no side effects and the dose is reduced according to the progress of the treatment.
■ Creams based on **vitamin A** reduce sebum production but may have side effects such as reddening of the skin, and should only be used under medical supervision.
■ The treatment of severe acne has greatly improved with the use of oral **retinoid drugs**, such as **isotretinoin** (related to vitamin A), which are prescribed only when antibiotics and other measures haven't helped. Oral

---

Stages of acne

Acne is graded in stages of severity:

Stage 1: An oily skin with blackheads

Stage 2: Stage 1 with pus-filled spots

Stage 3: Stage 2 with deep, tender, hard purplish lumps

Stage 4: Stage 3 with pitted and scarred skin.

WARNING:

SIDE EFFECTS OF ISOTRETINOIN

All patients develop considerable drying of the lips and skin (especially of the face); some have mild aches and pains of their joints, and headaches. However, all these side effects can be easily and well controlled, for example by using a moisturizing cream or a simple painkiller, such as paracetamol. It is very rare to have to stop treatment. BUT the **drug will harm an unborn baby** and **contraception must be used** for two months before, during, and three months after treatment. Oral isotretinoin can also cause liver damage and your doctor will monitor you for this.

isotretinoin is very effective but it can only be prescribed by a dermatologist, whose instructions must be strictly followed. A four-month course is usually needed, **after which most acne will be virtually clear**. These drugs must be used cautiously because they may cause liver damage and will cause malformations in an unborn baby. Depression has also been reported as a possible side effect.

■ Acne cysts can often be treated by **intralesional therapy** (direct injection of a drug into the acne spots), which also helps to reduce scarring.

■ In some cases of severe and extensive scarring, **dermabrasion** (that's the removal of the top layer of skin under a general anaesthetic) may help get rid of pits and scars.

■ A special form of the **oral contraceptive pill** may be prescribed for women because it's often successful in settling acne down. Ordinary contraceptive pills have little or no effect on acne. However, your doctor can prescribe one particular pill (Dianette) that is often helpful. The rationale is that the oestrogen in the pill reduces the production of sebum. It also opposes the effect of male hormones in blocking sebaceous glands and frees them up. It is usually taken for 12–36 months. The side effects of Dianette are the same as those of an ordinary contraceptive pill; ask your doctor to explain these to you if you want further information. A doctor is unlikely to prescribe the pill before the age of 17, unless it's for contraception, because the hormones may interfere with growth.

ESCAPE ROUTE

If you're unhappy with the results of treatment, ask your GP if you can see a **consultant dermatologist** who'll tell you about the very latest advances in acne treatment and special procedures that are available only in hospitals.

Acne is a condition that can be virtually cured in expert hands and if it's really bothering you, insist that you see a dermatologist.

TREATMENT OF SCARS

Carefully selected patients with bad scarring may be considered for dermabrasion. This operation is usually performed by plastic surgeons, under a local or general anaesthetic. The success rate is between 25 and 70 percent. Only patients who are strongly motivated to have the operation should be recommended for it. If in doubt, surgery should be avoided.

HOW SUCCESSFUL IS TREATMENT FOR ACNE?

Acne is usually one of the easiest of the persistent skin conditions to treat, but it must be treated sooner rather than later. Early treatment minimizes the risk of scarring.

Don't give up your treatment. Doctors can now offer therapies that can guarantee a satisfactory result in virtually everyone.

Rosacea

Rosacea is a long-term, possibly permanent skin condition and is most common in women between the ages of 30 and 55 and after the menopause. The features of rosacea include redness and pimples on the cheeks and forehead. The condition often runs in families. Alcohol, coffee and spicy foods may trigger attacks so it's best to avoid them, as well as temperature extremes in winter.

Special treatment will be prescribed by a dermatologist (a skin specialist).

WHAT ABOUT ALTERNATIVE METHODS?

Herbalists will almost certainly recommend special diets and special creams and possibly certain natural or herbal medicines to take by mouth, none of which are proven to work. Sage, plantain, verbascum and ground ivy are said to have useful astringent properties. Shepherd's purse has cleansing properties. Aromatherapists advocate the use of bergamot, camphor, cedarwood, juniper and lavender.

SELF-HELP

Coping with acne

■ **Cleanse** your skin meticulously. Use an **antiseptic soap** or soap solution, brought up to a lather in the palm of your hand, and gently massage it into your skin for at least two minutes, then rinse off. The aim is to de-fat the skin. Wash this way at least three times a day.

■ **Don't** use proprietary acne cleansers as they scrape the skin, break down the pustules and spread germs all over the skin, thereby encouraging acne lesions elsewhere.

■ You can treat blackheads by **steaming** your face. Hold your face about 30cm (12in) above a bowl of hot water from the tap and cover your head with a towel. The steam will cause the pores to open. You can then very gently nudge out the blackhead with a clean fingertip.

■ You should never squeeze anything but a blackhead. Try to keep your fingers away from the acne pimples – touching and rubbing simply spreads germs into the surrounding skin. Much worse, squeezing forces sebum out of the gland and into the skin, causing those hard, tender, purple lumps.

■ Don't put anything greasy on your skin. It'll make your acne worse.

■ If you're female, wear heavy-textured oil-free make-up to cover the spots. Many people mistakenly believe that make-up blocks the pores. That's completely wrong. Nothing put on the skin (except paint) can block pores. Make-up won't make acne worse and it does improve morale, which in turn makes acne better.

■ Moderate exposure to sunlight is helpful as it dries out the skin. Doctors advocate a **mild peel** from mild sunburn to unblock the pores.

■ Don't let acne affect your diet. Research has shown that foods such as chocolate don't have the slightest effect on acne. So eat a good balanced diet to improve your general health.

Mild acne can often be successfully controlled using simple self-help measures.

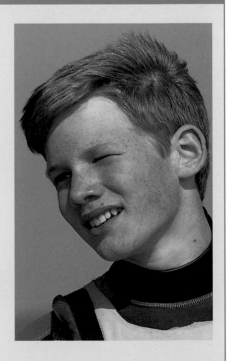

Psoriasis

ABOUT 1 IN 50 PEOPLE SUFFERS FROM PSORIASIS. THE RED, THICKENED, SCALY RASH THAT
CHARACTERIZES THIS CONDITION TENDS TO FLARE UP AT DIFFERENT TIMES THROUGHOUT LIFE.

If psoriasis affects many parts of the body, commonly the fronts of the knees, the backs of the elbows, trunk, scalp and back, it may cause physical discomfort as well as embarrassment in public due to shedding skin scales. The nails can be involved as can the joints. Psoriasis often runs in families and infections and stress can trigger an attack.

In a psoriasis plaque, new skin cells are produced about ten times faster than normal and at a much faster rate than dead cells are shed. The skin cells pile up to form thick, creamy coloured scales. The cause is not known, but psoriasis often has a genetic component. A flare-up of psoriasis may be triggered by infection, injury or stress. Certain drugs, such as **antidepressants**, especially lithium, **antihypertensives**, **beta-blockers** and **antimalarial drugs**, can trigger psoriasis in some people. Drinking alcohol can worsen existing psoriasis.

WHAT ARE THE TYPES?

There are **four** main types of psoriasis, each of which has a distinctive appearance. Some people may be affected by more than one type. Here are the characteristics of each type.

1. PLAQUE PSORIASIS

■ Areas called plaques, consisting of thickened, red skin with cream-coloured scaly surfaces, usually occur on the knees, elbows, lower back and scalp, behind the ears and at the hairline.
■ There is intermittent itching.
■ Nails become discoloured and covered with small pits. In severe cases, the nails thicken and lift away from the nail beds.
■ Plaques tend to last for weeks or months and may recur intermittently.

2. GUTTATE PSORIASIS

This form most commonly affects **children** and **adolescents**, often occurring after a bacterial **throat infection**.
■ Numerous coin-shaped, pink patches of scaly skin, each about 1cm (⅜in) across, appear mainly on the back and chest.
■ There is usually intermittent itching.

These symptoms usually disappear in 4–6 months and do not recur, but more than half of those affected later develop another form of psoriasis.

3. PUSTULAR PSORIASIS

■ Small blisters filled with pus may appear abruptly on the palms of the hands and the soles of the feet.
■ There may be widespread areas of red, inflamed and acutely tender skin.
■ There may be some thickening and scaling of the inflamed areas.

4. INVERSE PSORIASIS

Elderly people are commonly affected by this type of psoriasis in which large, moist, red areas develop in **skin folds**, rather than widespread body areas. The rash often affects the groin, the skin under the breasts and sometimes the armpits. Inverse psoriasis usually clears up with treatment but may recur.

ARE THERE COMPLICATIONS?

About 1 in 10 people with psoriasis of any type develops a form of **arthritis** that usually affects the **fingers** or **knee joints**. In **pustular** and **exfoliative** psoriasis, a massive loss of cells from the surface of the skin may lead to loss of protein, infections and high fever; if it is left untreated, the condition can be life-threatening.

WHAT MIGHT BE DONE?
TOPICAL TREATMENT

■ Psoriasis is commonly treated with **emollients** to soften the skin. Other common treatments are preparations containing **coal tar** or a substance called **anthralin.** These reduce inflammation and scaling. Coal tar and anthralin are effective but have an unpleasant smell and can stain clothing and bed linen. Anthralin should be applied to affected areas only because it can irritate healthy skin.
■ Alternatively, your doctor may prescribe a topical preparation containing the vitamin D derivative **calcipotriol** to be applied twice a day. It has no smell, does not stain skin or clothes, and is normally effective within about four weeks. You should follow the advice of your doctor or dermatologist because this treatment should not be used on the face or in the creases of the skin.

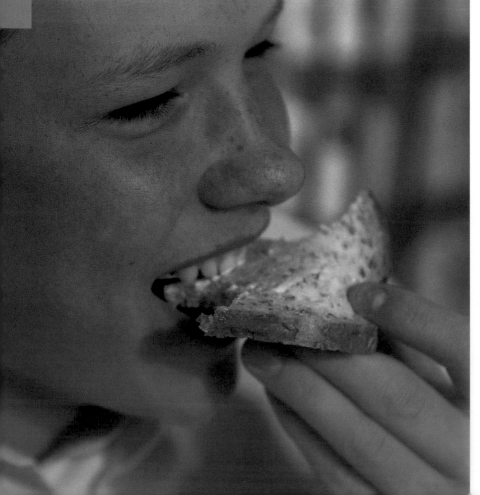

A diet high in wholegrain cereals and low in saturated fats and sugar may help in the treatment of psoriasis.

- Topical corticosteroids may also be used, sparingly.

SPECIAL TREATMENTS

- For widespread psoriasis that does not respond to topical treatments, therapeutic exposure to **ultraviolet (UV) light** is often effective. PUVA therapy involves using UV therapy together with **psoralen**, an oral drug that is taken before the ultraviolet light treatment and helps make the skin more sensitive to the effects of light.
- Regular, short doses of **sunlight** often help clear up psoriasis. Moderate exposure of affected areas to sunlight can be beneficial during the summer months.
- In very severe cases of **pustular psoriasis**, for which topical preparations may not be effective, treatment with oral or intravenous drugs may be recommended. The drugs used for this treatment include **retinoids**, the anticancer drug **methotrexate** and the immunosuppressant drug **cyclosporin**. However, both retinoids and methotrexate can cause abnormalities in a developing fetus. For this reason, you should not take either of these drugs if you are pregnant or you are planning to have a child.
- Chinese herbs in tablet, infusion and cream form can be very successful and are always worth trying.
- The Dead Sea treatment claims a three-year remission. No one knows how it works but it's not solely due to immersion in the Dead Sea. Fellow patients lend support akin to group therapy. But then you have to travel to the Dead Sea for the treatment.

WHAT IS THE OUTLOOK?

Although there is no cure for psoriasis, treatment normally relieves the symptoms and helps many people with the condition lead a normal life. If psoriasis is a long-term problem, you may want to join a self-help group or the Psoriasis Association (see Useful addresses, p.567).

SELF-HELP

It may help to reduce your intake of meat, animal fats, sugar and alcohol and increase intake of fibre – that is, wholegrain cereals, fruit, vegetables, cooked dried beans and peas, and nuts and seeds. Eat more oily fish, particularly mackerel, sardines, herring and salmon. An oatmeal bath can help to soothe irritated skin. Put 1kg (2lb) of oatmeal in cheesecloth bags in a hot bath and soak for 15 minutes. Apply your treatment afterwards.

Photosensitivity

ABNORMAL SENSITIVITY OF THE SKIN TO ULTRAVIOLET LIGHT, RESULTING IN REDNESS AND DISCOMFORT, IS CALLED PHOTOSENSITIVITY.

Various substances may cause photosensitivity, including **drugs** such as **tetracyclines**, **diuretics** and **oral contraceptives**, as well as **chemicals** used in the manufacture of cosmetics. The rare metabolic disorder porphyria can also cause photosensitivity.

WHAT ARE THE SYMPTOMS?

The reaction occurs in areas of skin frequently exposed to sunlight, such as the face and hands. Not much exposure is needed. The effects usually develop shortly after exposure, but may be delayed for 24–48 hours. The symptoms include:
- red, often painful, rash
- small, itchy blisters
- scaly skin.

WHAT IS THE TREATMENT?

- To relieve symptoms, the doctor may prescribe topical corticosteroids.
- Oral **antihistamines** may be prescribed.
- Severe cases are treated with controlled exposure to ultraviolet light, sometimes combined with drugs, to desensitize the skin.
- If a particular drug is causing photosensitivity, your doctor may be able to prescribe a different drug.

SELF-HELP

You can help control the reaction by avoiding sunlight as much as possible. When outdoors, cover your skin, wear a hat and use a total sunblock.

Purpura

THE CHARACTERISTIC RASH OF PURPURA CAUSES REDDISH-PURPLE SPOTS THAT DON'T DISAPPEAR WHEN PRESSED BY A GLASS.

The spots are small areas of bleeding under the skin, and may be caused by damaged blood vessels or by an abnormality in the blood, such as **thrombocytopaenia**, that affects clotting. They can range from the size of a pinhead to about 2.5cm (1in) in diameter. Purpura is a classic sign of one kind of bacterial meningitis. The most common of all types of purpura – senile purpura – mainly affects middle-aged and elderly women.

Purpura is sometimes a sign of a potentially serious disorder so you should always consult your doctor as a matter of urgency if you note a purpuric rash.

See also:
- **Meningitis p.404**
- **Thrombocytopaenia p.239**

Chilblains

WHEN THE SKIN OF A COLD-SENSITIVE PERSON IS EXPOSED TO COLD AND DAMP, THE BLOOD VESSELS CLOSE UP TO CONSERVE HEAT, CAUSING THE SKIN TO BECOME NUMB AND PALE OR PIMPLY.

When the blood vessels dilate again with warmth, the skin becomes red and itchy. The resulting chilblains, due to hypersensitivity to cold, are irritating, but they are not serious. They usually appear on the extremities and other parts of the body where circulation is poor, such as the ankles, hands and feet, and on the back of the legs.

Consult your doctor if chilblains cause a great deal of discomfort. He may prescribe a vasodilator cream to improve circulation.

SELF-HELP

- Keep all the susceptible parts of your body covered up and warm in damp and cold weather.
- Put thermal insoles in your shoes if you suffer from chilblains on your feet.
- If you have been out in the cold without warm clothing and develop chilblains, dust the skin with talcum powder or cornflour to ease the irritation.

SKIN INFECTIONS

Although the skin's surface provides protection from the environment, infectious organisms can enter the skin in various ways. Natural openings, such as a hair follicle or sweat gland, or broken skin at the site of an insect bite or a cut may provide a gateway for bacteria. Warm and moist areas, such as the skin between the toes, are susceptible to fungal infection. Some viral skin infections can easily be spread from the skin on one part of the body to another or passed between people.

Boil

ONE OF THE MOST COMMON TYPES OF SKIN INFECTION IS A BOIL. THIS IS A TENDER LUMP SURROUNDING A HAIR FOLLICLE THAT HAS BECOME INFECTED WITH BACTERIA, USUALLY STAPHYLOCOCCI. BOILS MAY BE LARGE OR SMALL.

The pus-filled lump gradually comes to a head and bursts after about two or three days. It may also heal on its own without bursting and slowly disappear. As the hair follicles are so close together, the bacteria can infect a wide area, causing more boils to occur. This is most likely to happen on the face, especially the shaving area and the back of the neck near the hairline where the hairs may grow back into the skin. Boils usually appear on areas where there are pressure points, such as where a collar rubs or on the buttocks.

Although unsightly, a boil is not serious. However, it can be extremely painful, especially if it develops over a bony area such as the jaw or forehead where the skin is stretched tight. Consult your doctor as soon as possible if a boil does not come to a head within five days, if the boil is causing a lot of pain or if you notice red streaks spreading out from the centre of the boil, which may mean that the infection is spreading.

WHAT IS THE TREATMENT?

■ Your doctor will examine the boil and the surrounding area. If he can feel pus under the skin, your doctor will probably lance the boil with a small scalpel and drain the pus, thus reducing the pain immediately.

■ If there is a spreading infection, or if you have had a number of boils over the previous months, your doctor may prescribe an **anti-infective cream** to treat the skin's surface, or **antibiotic tablets** to prevent the internal spread of the infection lower down into the skin.

■ If there are crops of boils, your doctor may prescribe a special **antiseptic** to put in the bath water.

■ If the boils are recurrent, you will be referred to a **dermatologist** to find out if there is an underlying cause, such as diabetes mellitus.

SELF-HELP

■ Don't scratch or touch the area around the boil. Wash the skin with surgical sprit or a solution of one teaspoonful of salt in a glass of warm water to prevent infection from spreading.

■ **Do not squeeze** the boil, even when it comes to a head. Squeezing will spread the infection to the surrounding area and make the problem much worse.

■ Once the boil has burst, keep the area clean

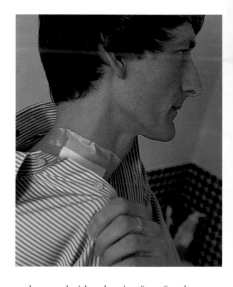

and covered with a dressing for a few days.

■ Keep your towel and face cloth **separate** from those of the family.

■ If the boil is in a place where clothing might rub it, put a **thick pad** over the dressing to prevent any friction.

Candidiasis

CANDIDIASIS IS A YEAST INFECTION THAT USUALLY AFFECTS ONLY ONE PART OF THE BODY BUT CAN BE SERIOUS IF IT SPREADS AROUND THE BODY.

In healthy people, the yeast *Candida albicans* normally exists on the surface of certain areas of the body, including the mouth, throat and vagina. Sometimes, the yeast overgrows in localized areas, causing minor forms of candidiasis such as oral thrush. In people with reduced immunity, such as those with acquired immunodeficiency syndrome (AIDS) or diabetes mellitus, the yeast may spread into the blood and other tissues. Infection that spreads throughout the body may also affect people who have long-term urinary catheters or intravenous catheters, or people who have had prolonged courses of antibiotics or use intravenous drugs.

Widespread candidiasis may be diagnosed by culturing the yeast from a sample of blood or other body fluids or tissue specimens. A chest X-ray may also be done to look for signs of infection in the lungs. Antifungal drugs may be given either orally or intravenously, depending on the severity of the infection.

Untreated, the infection can spread through the body and may eventually be fatal. The prognosis depends on the extent of infection and on the person's general health.

See also:
• **Diabetes mellitus p.504**
• **HIV infection and AIDS p.338**
• **Vaginal thrush p.279**

Impetigo

IMPETIGO IS A BACTERIAL SKIN INFECTION THAT IS MOST OFTEN
SEEN AROUND THE LIPS, NOSE AND EARS.

Impetigo is caused by common bacterial organisms (staphylococcus and streptococcus), which are carried in the nose. The rash starts as small blisters, which break and crust over to become yellow-brown scabs. Impetigo is most often seen in school children and is highly contagious. It should be treated immediately for this reason, although the condition rarely has serious effects.

WHAT IS THE TREATMENT?

■ Your doctor will prescribe an **antibiotic cream** that should clear up the impetigo within five days.
■ Your doctor might also prescribe a course of **antibiotics** to be taken by mouth to eradicate the infection from your body, or a nasal cream to prevent the infection being spread from the nose.

SELF-HELP

■ Before applying the ointment, **wash away** any yellow crusts and pat dry with a paper towel.
■ Be meticulous about hygiene. **Wash your hands** before and after treatment.
■ When the infection has cleared, keep the area soft with emollient cream.

Athlete's foot

A CONTAGIOUS FUNGAL INFECTION, ATHLETE'S FOOT IS USUALLY PICKED UP BY WALKING BAREFOOT
IN COMMUNAL AREAS, SUCH AS SHOWER ROOMS, GYMNASIA AND SWIMMING POOLS.

Athlete's foot affects the soft area between and underneath the toes and seems to have a preference for sweaty feet. The infection is aggravated by **sweaty feet** because the fungus, **tinea**, which also causes ringworm elsewhere in the body, thrives in warm, moist conditions. Athlete's foot may also affect the toenails. Not everyone exposed to the fungus gets the infection.

WHAT ARE THE SYMPTOMS?

■ White, blistered skin between and underneath the toes. The area is itchy and, when scratched, splits and leaves raw, red skin underneath.
■ Dry, peeling skin.

■ Thick, yellow toenails.
  Athlete's foot is a common condition requiring simple treatment and good hygiene to cure it. However, as it is contagious, you should act quickly so that the infection is not spread. Consult your doctor as soon as possible if the underside of the foot is already affected, or if the nails are distorted or yellowing. Consult your doctor if self-help measures (see box, below) fail to improve the condition within two or three weeks.

WHAT MIGHT BE DONE?

If the fungus has affected the toenails, they turn whitish, thicken and sometimes detach from the nail bed. Usually, debris from the

infected nail collects under its free edge. The diagnosis is confirmed by examining a sample of the nail debris under a microscope, where the fungus can be seen growing, and culturing it to determine which fungus is causing the infection.
■ If you have consulted your doctor because self-help measures failed, your doctor will prescribe another **antifungal powder** or cream and will advise you on the correct procedure for good foot hygiene.
■ If your toenails are affected, your doctor will prescribe an antifungal medication that may need to be taken for **three months**. The infected nails will eventually grow out completely.

SELF-HELP

Treating athlete's foot

■ Check the area between and underneath the toes for blisters, redness and cracking.
■ Check the condition of the toenails.
■ Buy an **antifungal powder** or cream from your chemist, and, after washing and drying the feet thoroughly, apply the treatment, following the manufacturer's instructions.
■ Keep your towel and bathmat **separate** from those of the rest of the family and wash them every day.
■ **Don't go barefoot** until the condition has cleared up.
■ Make sure you wear **clean socks every day**, preferably made from natural fibres such as cotton or wool.
■ Rotate your shoes, especially trainers, so they dry out between wearings.

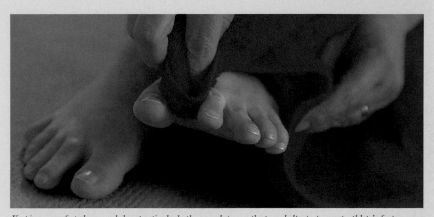

Keeping your feet clean and dry, particularly the area between the toes, helps to prevent athlete's foot.

Warts and verrucae

WARTS ARE SMALL BENIGN LUMPS CAUSED BY THE WART VIRUS.
A VERRUCA IS A PAINFUL WART ON THE SOLE OF THE FOOT THAT HAS BEEN
PUSHED DEEP INTO THE FOOT BY THE PRESSURE OF WALKING.

Warts are made up of an excess of dead cells that protrude above the surface of the skin. They can appear singly or in alarming numbers over all parts of the body, including the face and genitals.

It takes about two years for the body to build up a resistance to the wart virus, and after that time warts usually disappear spontaneously. Warts are spread by direct contact with an infected person.

WHAT ARE THE SYMPTOMS?

■ Hard lumps of dried skin that appear spontaneously and grow singly or in clusters anywhere on the body. Warts are usually round and have a raised surface; verrucae are flat with a thickened surface.
■ Both warts and verrucae may have small black dots within the lumps (these are blood vessels and not dirt).

Warts in the skin are neither serious nor painful, but consult your doctor if the warts continue to multiply or appear on the face and you want them removed. Verrucae can cause pain and discomfort, depending on where they appear on the sole of the foot.

WHAT IS THE TREATMENT?

■ Your doctor may advise you to ignore the warts, or refer you to a hospital dermatologist.
■ Methods of removal include freezing, cauterization and surgical removal.

See also:
• **Genital warts p.282**

SELF-HELP

Wart cures

You can try patent wart cures from the chemist. These work by the application of a weak acid solution to the wart and the daily removal of the resulting burnt skin. You should follow the manufacturer's instructions carefully and avoid applying the solution to healthy skin. Don't use patent wart cures on warts that appear on the face or genitals; you may cause scarring.

SKIN INFESTATIONS

Like other parts of the body, skin can become infested with minute creatures that feed off human blood. The creatures lay eggs and multiply and, when sufficient numbers are reached, irritating symptoms arise, most notably rash and itching.

The most common skin infestations are scabies and lice (head, body and pubic). While none of these causes harmful effects, they are all highly contagious and the itching and scratching they lead to may be embarrassing and a nuisance.

Scabies

SCABIES IS AN IRRITATING, ITCHY RASH CAUSED BY A TINY MITE. THE BURROWING AND EGG-LAYING
OF THESE MITES PRODUCE A RASH THAT NEARLY ALWAYS AFFECTS THE HANDS AND FINGERS,
PARTICULARLY THE CLEFTS BETWEEN THE FINGERS.

Scabies is visible as a fine grey line where the mite has burrowed into the skin, ending in a black dot – the mite. Scabies may also affect the ankles, feet, toes, elbows and the area around the genitals. When the eggs hatch, they are easily passed to another person by direct contact. They can also be picked up from bedding or linen that is infested with the mites.

WHAT ARE THE SYMPTOMS?

■ Intense itching.
■ Burrows – fine, short lines on the backs of the hands and the sides of the fingers that end in a black spot the size of a pinhead.
■ Scabs on the itchy areas.

Scabies is not serious but it is contagious and could run through a family if not treated promptly. Consult your doctor as soon as possible if you suspect scabies or if you are scratching a lot.

WHAT IS THE TREATMENT?

Your doctor will prescribe an **antiparasitic lotion** in sufficient quantity for the whole family to be treated. All the skin must be treated for the lotion to be effective.

SELF-HELP

■ Try **not to scratch** affected areas. This may hinder the doctor's diagnosis and cause sores to form that could become infected.

■ After thorough washing, you should paint the **whole body** below the neck with the lotion and leave to dry. Do not wash it off for 24 hours. To ensure disinfestation, repeat the procedure a further 24 hours in a day or two.
■ Carry out the treatment for **other members of the family** simultaneously.
■ **Launder or air all bedding and clothing** to eradicate the mite. The mite does not live for longer than five or six days after it is removed from human skin.

Lice

LICE ARE WINGLESS INSECTS THAT FEED ON HUMAN BLOOD. THERE ARE THREE KINDS OF HUMAN LICE – PUBIC LICE (ALSO CALLED CRABS), BODY LICE AND HEAD LICE.

PUBIC LICE

Pubic lice need the bodily heat of a person to keep them alive – hence they don't live very long on a lavatory seat, although they may survive on warm bed clothes or garments for a short time.

Medical text books state that crabs are nearly always passed from one person to another during **sexual contact** because they actually live on pubic hair, and sometimes body hair, where they feed on blood and lay eggs called nits. About 10,000 cases of infestation with pubic lice are treated in the UK each year.

With crabs, the most common symptom is itching in the pubic area and around the anus, especially at night. Some people have no symptoms and only realize that they are infested when they see the nits (eggs) or the tiny insects. Normal washing does not remove the nits since they are firmly stuck to the pubic hair.

If you think that you or your partner has pubic lice, you should consult your doctor or go to a clinic specializing in sexually transmitted diseases (STDs).

BODY LICE

Body lice, on the other hand, live on clothing and bed linen and are easily picked up by someone sharing a bed or garments. Body lice do, of course, occasionally stray to the pubic area. Many people confuse the two.

WHAT IS THE TREATMENT?

Your doctor will probably prescribe a preparation containing **lindane** or **permethrin** to apply to affected areas. A second application is needed about **10 days after** the first to destroy freshly hatched lice.

To prevent the spread of lice, **sexual partners** should be checked and treated if necessary. **The clothing and sheets** used by an infested person should be machine washed in hot water.

HEAD LICE

Head lice affect all social classes and have absolutely nothing to do with personal hygiene. They like clean heads as much as they do dirty ones and there is nothing shameful about being infected. If you have a child there is a good chance you will come into contact with head lice at some stage.

Head lice live and suck blood from the scalp, leaving tiny red spots that cause intense itching. Adult lice can live for several weeks and the females lay a daily batch of tiny pale eggs (nits) close to the scalp. These hatch out after several days. Lice are spread through direct contact, but it doesn't necessarily have to be head-to-head.

WHAT IS THE TREATMENT?

The traditional treatment for an outbreak of head lice is the application of powerful lotions containing pesticides. The main advantage is that such lotions can penetrate the hard casing of the lice eggs and kill the nits inside.

However, scientists and parents are beginning to think again, for the following reasons.

■ It seems that with repeated use these pesticides are losing their effectiveness. There are reports from some areas that live nits are not being destroyed and it is suggested that some adult lice may also be resistant.

■ There is concern about using powerful chemicals on young children.

■ They are expensive and unpleasant to use.

However, there are effective alternatives.

ALTERNATIVE TREATMENTS

■ The first and most important weapon against head lice is the **small fine-toothed comb** (often called a nit comb because the teeth are so close together it can remove the lice eggs). Plastic combs are recommended rather than metal because they are more flexible and therefore can get nearer to the scalp. They are also easier to clean and less likely to pull or snag hair.

Use the nit comb every time you wash your own and your children's hair. But do use plenty of **conditioner** after shampooing. Using conditioner makes the procedure simple and painless (no tangles) and makes it possible to dislodge lice from the slippery strands. Pay special attention to anyone with curly hair as it's harder to see the lice or pull the comb through and so they may be more vulnerable.

■ The use of Quassia chips is an alternative remedy that is becoming popular with parents. Quassia chips look like pieces of dried wood. They are cheap, natural and don't smell or leave a greasy residue. To use Quassia chips:

1. Place 25g (1oz) of Quassia chips in a saucepan and pour 560ml (1 pint) of boiling water over them. This loosens the oil in the chips. Leave overnight and the next day bring to the boil and simmer for 10–15 minutes. Let it cool and transfer to a spray bottle.

2. Shampoo hair, rinse and apply conditioner. Comb through with the nit comb. Rinse off the conditioner and towel dry. Spray the Quassia solution all over the hair. Leave to dry naturally. Spray again when dry.

3. Spray again the following morning after brushing and repeat over the next couple of days. You can also use the Quassia solution as a preventive because it creates a bitter, hostile environment that lice do not like.

■ Biz Niz is a blend of five essential oils (citronella, geranium, eucalyptus, lavender and rosemary). It claims to get rid of lice and act as a repellent.

ABNORMALITIES OF PIGMENTATION

The pigmentation of the skin is due to a substance known as melanin. Melanin filters out ultraviolet rays and so helps to protect the skin from damage by the sun (a suntan is caused by the extra melanin the body produces in response to exposure to sunlight). Some conditions, such as vitiligo and chloasma, are caused by changes in the amount of melanin in the skin in localized areas.

Vitiligo

THE CONDITION KNOWN AS VITILIGO IS CHARACTERIZED BY PATCHES OF WHITE SKIN DUE TO LOSS OF NORMAL PIGMENT (MELANIN) FROM PATCHES OF SKIN, MOST COMMONLY OCCURRING ON THE FACE AND HANDS. VITILIGO IS MORE OBVIOUS IN PEOPLE WITH DARK SKIN.

WHAT IS THE CAUSE?

Vitiligo is thought to be an **autoimmune disorder**, in which the body produces antibodies that react against its own tissues. The antibodies destroy the cells in the skin that produce melanin. About 1 in 3 people with vitiligo has a **family history** of the condition. About the same proportion also have **another type** of autoimmune disorder, such as **pernicious anaemia**.

SELF-HELP

■ In mild vitiligo, the discoloured areas can be hidden with concealing cosmetics. No other treatment is needed.

■ The affected areas cannot tan. To prevent sunburn, you should avoid exposure to the sun and use a sunblock in direct sunlight.

■ Phototherapy using ultraviolet (UV) light can help but it takes several months to work.

■ Before UV treatment, you may be given a drug called **psoralen** to increase the sensitivity of the skin to light. This treatment, usually used for psoriasis, is called PUVA (psoralen and ultraviolet light).

WHAT IS THE OUTLOOK?

There is no cure for vitiligo and often the depigmented patches continue to enlarge slowly. However, about 3 in 10 affected people regain their natural skin colour spontaneously.

Chloasma

ALSO CALLED THE MASK OF PREGNANCY, CHLOASMA IS A SPECIAL FORM OF PIGMENTATION THAT CAUSES BROWN PATCHES TO APPEAR ON THE BRIDGE OF THE NOSE, CHEEKS AND NECK.

The only way to handle chloasma is to camouflage it with a blemish stick or the cover-up cosmetics that are used for birthmarks.

Never try to bleach out the pigment; the patches will begin to fade within three months of childbirth. In black women, patches of paler skin develop on their faces and necks. These will probably disappear after delivery and can be camouflaged during pregnancy.

SKIN CANCERS

There are several types of skin cancer, most of which are associated with prolonged exposure to sunlight. Fair-skinned people are most at risk. Exposure to the sun is a risk factor and should be avoided from babyhood; the use of sunbeds is also a risk factor and should likewise be avoided.

Skin cancer is now the **most common** form of cancer in the world. In recent years, the incidence around the world has escalated, and the condition now affects millions of people worldwide. The good news is that skin cancer can usually be cured if it is diagnosed early, though preventive measures are always preferable.

WHAT ARE THE RISKS?

The usual cause of skin cancer is prolonged exposure to the harmful ultraviolet radiation in sunlight. The risk is higher if you are fair-skinned and if you live or take holidays in areas with intense sun; the closer you are to the equator, the greater the risk. It's the **cumulative** hours of sunshine that count so if you live in a very sunny place you'll reach your "**cancer-inducing dose**" earlier than somewhere like the UK where there isn't so much sun. The recent depletion of the ozone layer is thought to have played a part in increasing the incidence of skin cancer because the ozone layer acts as a shield against harmful ultraviolet (UV) light. Sunbeds, which give out ultraviolet light, may also cause skin cancer. You should also bear in mind that the more times you have been sunburned, the greater your chance of developing malignant melanoma, the most dangerous form of skin cancer.

If you work outside or have been sunburned (particularly in childhood), you could be vulnerable to skin cancer. People who have fair skin are especially susceptible because they have low levels of melanin, the pigment that give the skin its colour and helps protect it from the sun's harmful ultraviolet rays.

To reduce the risk of developing skin cancer, try to avoid exposure to the sun and protect your skin when outside. Examine your skin regularly, and ask someone else to check your back and scalp. Wear UV-resistant clothing in areas of intense sunshine and where there's a lot of reflection, for example on snow or water.

WHAT ARE THE TYPES?

There are three main types of skin cancer all linked to over-exposure to the sun.
1. The most common type is **basal cell carcinoma**, which can be easily treated. It rarely spreads.
2. **Squamous cell carcinoma** is a form of skin cancer that may spread and is occasionally fatal, but can be cured completely if detected early.
3. **Malignant melanoma** is still rare but getting more common all the time. It can spread rapidly to other parts of the body and causes more deaths than other skin cancers.

An uncommon skin cancer, known as Kaposi's sarcoma, usually occurs only in people with acquired immunodeficiency syndrome (AIDS).

WHAT MIGHT BE DONE?

Skin cancer can usually be cured if it is diagnosed early. You should consult your doctor promptly if you notice any changes in your skin, such as enlarging lumps or sores that do not heal. You may need to have a skin biopsy. During this procedure, a small area of skin is removed and examined under a microscope for abnormal cells.

The type of skin cancer and spread of the disease determines the treatment and prognosis. Sometimes, only the affected area of skin needs to be treated.

It is possible to remove most types of skin cancers **surgically**. However, **skin grafting** may be necessary if a cancer has invaded large areas of surrounding skin tissue. If the cancer has spread to other parts of the body, **radiotherapy** or **chemotherapy** may also be needed.

Malignant melanoma

OF ALL THE TYPES OF SKIN CANCER, MALIGNANT MELANOMA IS THE MOST SERIOUS. MALIGNANT MELANOMA HAS BECOME MORE COMMON WITH OUR OBSESSION WITH GETTING AND KEEPING A TAN.

A melanoma may begin as a new growth on normal skin or may develop from an existing mole. Left untreated, the cancer can spread rapidly to other parts of the body and may be fatal. As with most other skin cancers, exposure to the sun and the use of sunbeds are risk factors, and fair-skinned people are most at risk. Malignant melanoma is most common between the ages of 40 and 60, increasingly common in young adults and more common in women.

Worldwide, the number of cases of malignant melanoma, particularly in young adults, has increased dramatically over the past 10 years. This rise is probably due to the growing popularity of outdoor activities. However, the condition is still most common in people aged 40–60. In the UK, there are about 4,000 new cases each year, out of a total of 40,000 new cases for all types of skin cancer.

WHAT IS THE CAUSE?

Malignant melanoma is thought to result from damage to **melanocytes** (the skin cells that produce the pigment melanin) by sunlight. The cancer occurs more frequently in people with **fair skin** than in those with dark skin.

People who continually expose themselves to intense sunlight or who live in sunny climates are at greater risk of developing the cancer.

Severe sunburn in childhood has been shown to double the chance of developing malignant melanoma in later life. Reducing exposure to the sun can help decrease the risk of developing any type of skin cancer.

WHAT ARE THE RISKS?

If caught early, most cases of skin cancer can be treated successfully through surgery,

Wearing a high sun protection factor sunscreen and a hat helps reduce sun damage to the skin.

although some can prove fatal.

Skin cancers have increased by 7 percent in fair-skinned people worldwide over the last 10 years. A person's risk of developing skin cancer is increased by several factors, including:
- having fair skin
- having skin that has a tendency towards freckling
- having many moles
- a family history of malignant melanoma
- having had one or more attacks of severe sunburn during childhood
- being aged over 30 years
- many years of exposure to strong sunlight.

WHAT ARE THE SYMPTOMS?

Malignant melanomas can develop on any part of the body but appear most commonly on sun-exposed areas. Some melanomas spread across the skin in irregular flat patches, others appear as fast-growing lumps. In older people, they may occur on the face as freckle-like spots, known as **lentigo maligna**, that grow slowly over many years. If they are not removed, all of these types of melanoma will grow down into the underlying layers of the skin.

continued on page 458

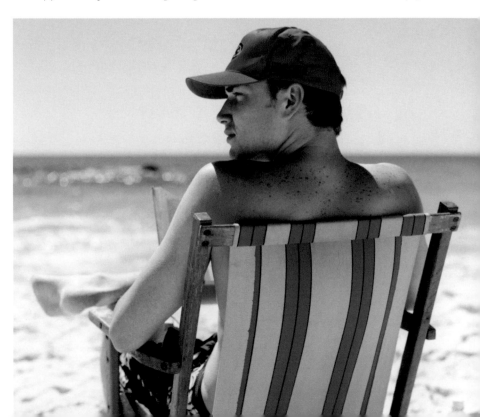

FOCUS *on* sun protection

More than 40,000 people in the UK are diagnosed with skin cancer every year, and around 2,000 people die of it. It's the second most common cancer in the country. Unlike many cancers, skin cancer is a disease that's mostly avoidable. The main cause, exposure to sunlight, is widely recognized.

By taking simple precautions in the sun we can ensure that the rise in the number of skin cancers is brought to a halt, if not reversed.

As you soak up the sun at home or abroad this summer, remember you're damaging your skin. You don't have to sunbathe to get sunburnt. Simply walking around in the sunshine can be enough. A tan may make you feel healthy, but it's a sign that your skin is being damaged and it is trying to protect itself, regardless of how gradually you acquire it.

A burnt face and hot, painful sunburn on your body isn't attractive, it's painful and unsightly and can cause permanent damage to collagen in your skin, leading to wrinkles.

WHAT SUN DOES TO SKIN

● Exposure to UV rays causes the outer layer of the skin to thicken as more cells are produced, causing wrinkles.
● The elastic tissue of the skin also breaks down, resulting in sags and bags.
● On top of this, the sun tends to dry out the skin, making it coarse and leathery.

● Dark patches or liver spots can appear, due to an overproduction of melanin (a pigment produced by skin cells). These patches are normally seen in older people, but can also be found in young people who sunbathe frequently.

PROTECTING YOURSELF

Staying safe is easy – follow these simple tips and you'll greatly reduce your risk of getting skin cancer.

● Clothing is the ideal barrier from the sun – it's cheaper than sunscreens and it doesn't rub off. Cover up with loose-fitting, cool garments and a hat. Take special care of your ears and neck as these are the most common places for skin cancers. You can buy clothes in UV-resistant materials at sports shops.
● On parts of your body you can't cover up, always use a high-factor sunscreen, with an SPF

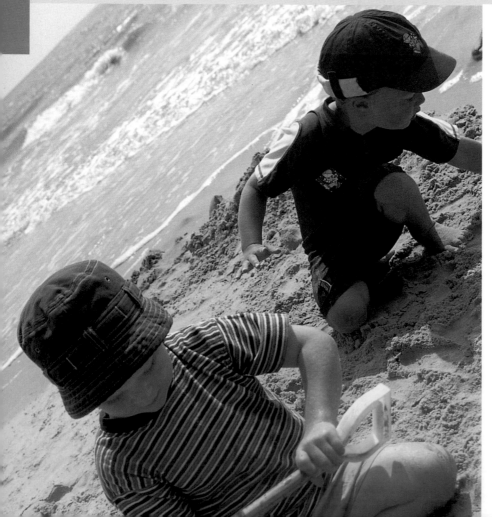

Ultraviolet rays

Sunlight contains visible rays, infra-red rays and ultraviolet rays. The latter are mainly responsible for tanning and skin damage.

There are three types of ultraviolet rays in sunlight – UVA, UVB and UVC. UVA are longer, tanning rays and UVB are shorter, burning rays. Both easily injure the DNA of cells and the pigment-forming **melanocytes** causing skin damage and cancer.

Very little UVC radiation, which is potentially very dangerous, reaches Earth as it is filtered out by the ozone layer; the development of holes in this layer is of increasing concern.

UV rays can also damage the **Langerhans** cells in the skin's epidermis that scavenge for invading bacteria or cancer cells.

of 15 or above. It should also have three stars or more. Apply it an hour before you go out, and re-apply it frequently and generously.

● Find some shade during the hottest part of the day, usually between 11am and 3pm.

● **Never** fall asleep in the sun unprotected – even after a late night. Keep an eye on how much time you spend in the sun and reapply sunscreen often.

● **Don't** be fooled by an overcast day – the sun can penetrate through cloud, so you can still get burnt.

● If you're a **watersport** fanatic, remember that the reflection of the sun's rays on the water can make it even stronger. Protect your skin with a surf suit and use a waterproof sunscreen.

● **Always** wear good-quality sunglasses in bright sunlight. Look on the label for the British Standard BS2724:1987.

WHAT DOES SPF MEAN?

SPF stands for Sun Protection Factor and is a measure of how much a sunscreen protects your skin from burning in the sun. The higher the SPF, the greater the protection. The rating may range from 2 to 30 or even higher. You can get a great surfer's sunscreen that has an SPF of 45.

HOW MUCH SUNSCREEN?

Most people apply sunscreen too thinly and generally end up with less protection than the SPF on the bottle suggests.

WHEN USING A SUNSCREEN

● apply it thickly and evenly over all exposed areas

● remember, those parts of the body that aren't usually exposed to the sun will tend to burn more easily. Pay particular attention to ears, neck, bald patches, hands and feet.

● re-apply regularly, especially after swimming.

AFTER-SUN CREAM

After-sun creams and lotions may help to soothe sunburnt or dry skin caused by the sun, but they can't help repair serious skin damage.

PROTECTING CHILDREN

Babies and young children need special care because they can't protect themselves and aren't aware of how the sun can damage their skin. So it's important that you take precautions for them.

Getting sunburnt as a child leads to greater risk of skin cancer in later life. It's important

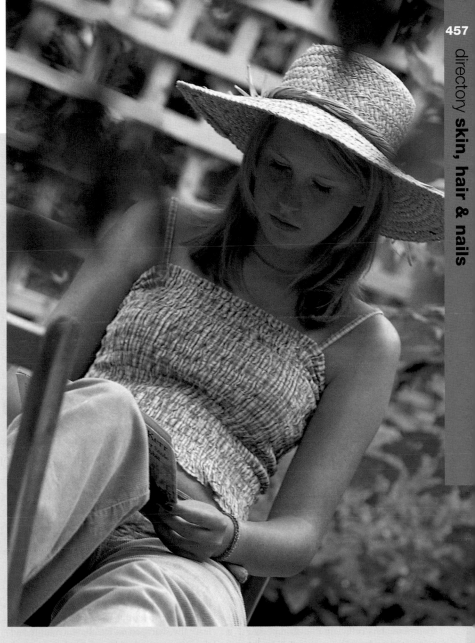

that children, especially babies and toddlers, are given the protection they deserve.

Babies: Keep babies less than 12 months old out of the sun and in the shade. Loose-fitting clothing will help keep babies cool. Remember that babies cannot move around by themselves and may get hot and uncomfortable if they become overheated. Be sure to give your baby frequent drinks to help prevent dehydration.

Toddlers and young children: Dress young children in loose-fitting, UV-resistant clothing and a wide-brimmed hat when they're in the sun. Generously apply sunscreen – before they go out in the sun – to the parts of the body that remain exposed. Select a sunscreen with an SPF of at least 15 and make sure it's water-resistant if they will be going into the water.

Encourage children to play in the shade when the sun is at its hottest. You can create

your own shade with a beach umbrella or canopy, or take advantage of natural shade under trees.

Choose sunglasses for children that comply with the British Standard. If taking children in the car, make sure they have adequate ventilation and never leave them in the car unattended.

TREATING SUNBURN

Calamine lotion or sunburn cream can **soothe burned skin**, which should be protected from further exposure to the sun until healing takes place. A **non-steroidal anti-inflammatory painkiller** such as ibuprofen may be needed to relieve tenderness. A person with severe sunburn should consult a doctor, who may prescribe a cream containing a **corticosteroid drug** to relieve the symptoms.

up to 18 months or two years. Although very disturbing, it is no cause for alarm because it is self-limiting and reversible – although hair may take a long time to grow back, and straight hair may become curly and vice versa.

■ **Chronic scratching of the scalp**, particularly at the back near the nape of the neck, is quite a common symptom of anxiety and can give rise to hair loss. However, this is rarely complete and always recovers when scratching stops.

■ **Hair pulling**, or **trichotillomania**, can occasionally cause bald patches but it can always be diagnosed because hair loss is never complete and there are often broken hairs of different lengths present in the bald patches. Like chronic scratching, trichotillomania nearly always has a **psychological** cause.

> See also:
> • Hypothyroidism p.507

Excessive hair

HAIR GROWTH THAT OCCURS IN AREAS THAT WOULD NOT NORMALLY HAVE HAIR, OR EXCESSIVE HAIR GROWTH, IS MORE COMMON IN WOMEN AND OCCURS ONLY AFTER PUBERTY. IT IS MORE FREQUENT WITH INCREASING AGE AND SOMETIMES RUNS IN FAMILIES.

There are two types of excessive hair growth: **hirsutism** and **hypertrichosis**. **Hirsutism** affects women only. In this condition, excessive hair develops particularly on the face, trunk and limbs. This type of excessive growth is more common in women over the age of 60, due to oestrogen deficiency, especially those who are of Mediterranean, Asian, Hispanic or Arab descent. **Hypertrichosis** can affect both males and females. In this condition, the hair grows all over the body, even in areas that do not normally have hair.

WHAT ARE THE CAUSES?

■ Mild hirsutism in women is often considered normal, especially following the menopause when there is a relative excess of male hormones (androgens) as oestrogen levels fall.

■ Hirsutism may be the result of an increase in normally occurring androgens in women with disorders such as **polycystic ovarian syndrome** (PCOS).

Hypertrichosis may occur with **anorexia nervosa** or may occur as a side effect of **immunosuppressant** or **antihypertensive drugs**.

WHAT MIGHT BE DONE?

■ If you are a young woman with hirsutism, you doctor may arrange for a blood test to measure your male hormone levels and exclude PCOS.

■ If androgens are high, you may be given a drug to block the hormone's effects and be treated for an underlying disorder such as polycystic ovarian syndrome.

■ If hypertrichosis occurs as a side effect of a drug, a change of treatment usually reverses the condition.

TREATMENT

Hair removal

You can deal with excessive hair yourself by bleaching it or by shaving, plucking, waxing or using depilatory creams. The only way to remove hair permanently is by electrolysis and laser treatment but they are slow and can be uncomfortable.

Unlike other body hair, facial hair can actually be made worse by some methods of removal, so it is always wise for a doctor to identify the cause of facial hirsutism before any attempt at treatment is made.

Sugaring and waxing
Sugaring involves painting the skin with a mixture of lemon, sugar, water and herbs, waiting for it to dry and then pulling it off, with the hairs attached. It works on the same principle as waxing, in which warm melted wax is applied to the skin and allowed to dry before removing along with excess hair, but because the mixture is cold it is less likely to cause a reaction on sensitive skin. It doesn't usually cost as much as waxing and lasts for 4–5 weeks.

There are home kits available for both sugaring and waxing but play safe and have it done at a reputable beauty salon. Sugaring and waxing, as well as depilatory cream, can be used to remove hair in the bikini-line area.

Bleaching
This won't remove the hair but it will disguise it. It is most suitable for women with light-coloured hair. Coarse hair is likely to show after bleaching but is not likely to be quite as noticeable because it will be a lighter shade.

Depilatory creams
Hair removal creams specifically designed for the face should be the only ones used on this sensitive part of the body. Normal creams are likely to be too strong and will cause irritation. Regrowth usually occurs between two and three weeks. Hair lighteners and removal creams vary in price and are available from most chemists.

Lasers
Extensive research has recently been carried out into the use of a laser system that can safely slow down or stop hair growth without damaging the surrounding skin. A ruby laser is used that produces a red light. This is highly absorbed by hair and only minimally absorbed by skin. The light is applied for less than a thousandth of a second – enough time to destroy the hair but not to heat the skin. Any part of the body can be treated and it has proved particularly popular with women who have a problem with facial hair.

Electrolysis
This is a very effective and relatively cheap method for removing facial hair. It involves passing an electrical current through the hair, cutting it off at the root. It can take some time to remove all the hair and must be carried out by a qualified operator.

Epilight
The latest concept in permanent hair removal works on the principle of intense pulsed light (IPL) technology. Using camera-flash bursts of multiple light wavelengths pulsed through a quartz crystal, the result is super-fast, long-term removal of all types of hair anywhere on the body. A slight reddening of the skin may be apparent after treatment, but this usually subsides within 24 hours.

Hormone replacement therapy (HRT)
Excessive hair can be counteracted by oestrogen in the form of HRT. A woman who takes female hormones should have few problems with unwanted hair.

NAILS

The nails, like the hair, are dead, except for the growing root, and are made up of compacted **keratin**, the same protein as in hair. It takes a nail nine months to grow out so the nail plate is, in fact, a week-by-week photograph of what's going on inside the body. Consequently, internal events can be "read" in the nails. The chart on the right describes some of them.

Internal disorders that show up in the nails

Nail feature	Significance
Horizontal ridge	Illness, psychological trauma, surgery
Pits like the surface of a thimble	Psoriasis
Pale nail beds	Liver disease
Spoon-shaped nails	Iron deficiency
Brown longitudinal marks (splinter haemorrhages)	Bleeding disorder, septicaemia
Highly curved nails ("clubbing")	Lung, heart or liver disease

Ingrowing toenail

MOST COMMON IN MEN, AN INGROWING TOENAIL IS PAINFUL GROWTH OF THE INNER EDGES OF A TOENAIL INTO THE SURROUNDING SKIN. TIGHT OR BADLY FITTING SHOES INCREASE THE RISK.

WHAT CAUSES IT?

An ingrowing toenail curves under on one or both sides and cuts into the surrounding skin, causing pain, inflammation and sometimes infection. A small toenail with a very fleshy toe predisposes to it. The big toe is particularly vulnerable to ill-fitting shoes pressing on an incorrectly cut nail. In some cases, injury can cause the skin around the nail to overgrow and engulf part of the nail. Poor foot hygiene can also increase the risk of infection, leading to inflammation.

WHAT ARE THE SYMPTOMS?

The symptoms of an ingrowing toenail may include the following:
- pain, redness and swelling around the toenail
- broken skin at the nail edge, which oozes clear fluid, pus or blood.

You should consult your doctor as soon as you notice a toenail has become ingrowing because it is possible that your toe will get infected.

WHAT IS THE TREATMENT?

■ You can relieve the pain of an ingrowing toenail by **bathing** your foot **in warm salt water daily** and by taking **painkillers**.
■ You should protect the affected toe by keeping it covered with **clean, dry gauze**.
■ If your toenail is infected, **oral antibiotics** or **topical antibiotics** will be prescribed.

A couple of simple measures can help prevent an ingrowing toenail from recurring.
■ Keep your feet clean and wear **correctly fitting shoes.**

■ **Cut straight across** your toenails, rather than along a curve, to prevent them growing into the skin.

If the problem recurs, a section or all of the toenail will be removed to prevent the toenail from growing into the flesh of the toe again.

SELF-HELP

■ Examine the skin around the nail to see if the nail has penetrated the skin.
■ Cut a tiny V-shape in the top edge of the nail to relieve pressure on the sides of the nail.
■ Apply an antiseptic cream to the sides of the nail to prevent infection.
■ If there is any sign of redness or pus, lie down with your foot propped up. Apply a sterile dressing to the toe.
■ Cut your toenails straight across and not too short. Cut them regularly; don't let them get too long.
■ Make sure that your shoes and socks are not too tight – you should have enough space to wriggle your toes.
■ If your toenail has become infected, don't wear socks; cut the toe out of an old shoe or wear sandals while the infection clears up.

TREATMENT
CHIROPODY

A chiropodist will cut your toenail to prevent further problems. It's important not to leave splinters of nails at the side but they're best removed by an expert.

Good foot hygiene keeps the feet healthy and reduces the chance of developing ingrowing toenails.

REMOVAL OF THE INGROWING EDGES

Under a local anaesthetic your doctor or chiropodist can lift up the ingrowing edges at the sides of the nail and cut them away so that none is left growing into the skin. This allows the infection to subside and the nail bed to heal. If you adhere to self-help measures the nail should not grow inwards again.

REMOVAL OF AN INGROWING TOENAIL

Minor surgery may be needed for an ingrowing toenail. Your toe will be anaesthetized and cleaned with antiseptic. The nail, or part of it, will be removed, and phenol will be applied to the exposed nail bed to seal the blood vessels. You should be comfortable enough to walk within 24 hours of surgery, and the wound should heal completely within a week.

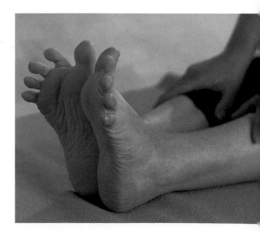

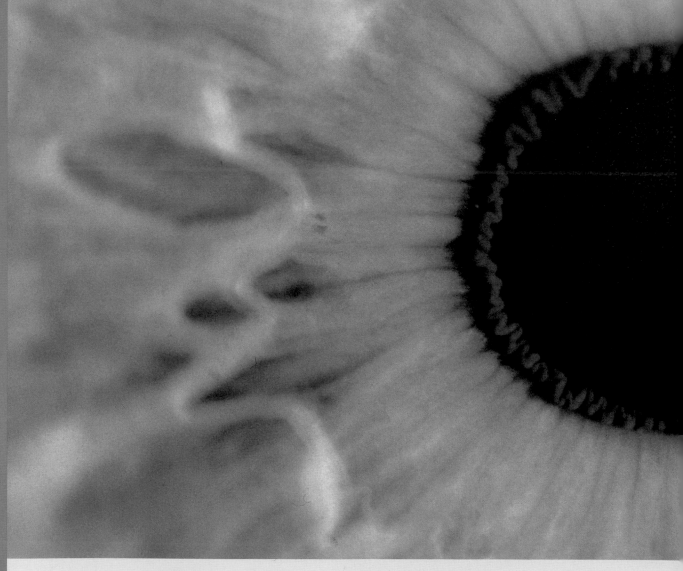

Eyes and Vision

Image shows a macrophotograph of a human iris and pupil

Miriam's overview

The eyes are equipped with one of the most potent antiseptics known to science – the tears. Not only do tears bathe the eyeball continually so that blinking is comfortable, they keep the eye free of infections. The powerful natural antiseptic in tears is called lysozyme – if only we could bottle it.

We think of diminishing sight as a sign of getting old but it isn't. It's a sign that the eyeball is changing shape. The images of objects then fall in front of or behind the retina at the back of the eye and appear blurry.

If the eyeball elongates in the horizontal plane, the image falls in front of the retina and when the eyeball elongates vertically, the reverse happens.

Glasses and contact lenses pull the image back into the right place and laser surgery can alter the shape of the eyeball by shaving off thin slivers of the conjunctiva.

The treatment of cataracts has leapt forward recently so that modern cataract surgery is quick, simple and highly effective. No one these days should have compromised vision because of cataracts.

"modern *cataract surgery* is quick, simple and *highly effective*"

Glaucoma is a treatable condition caught early enough so it's important to have regular tonometry tests done by your optician to measure the pressure inside your eyes. Any "red eye" should take you to your doctor immediately because it could be the first sign of glaucoma.

INSIDE your eyesight

The sensory cells of the eye are an extension of the brain, budding out from the brain during fetal development. The eye shows less growth than any other organ between birth and adulthood.

The eye is sensitive to light, which is focused through the **cornea** and the **lens** onto the **retina** at the back of the eye. The retina contains 137 million **cells**, of which 130 million are **rod-shaped** and used for black and white vision, sensing movement and seeing in poor light, while seven million are **cone-shaped** and used to sense colour and pattern in bright light. Cones are concentrated in the parts of the retina called the **fovea centralis** (central depression) and the **macula**. A network of nerve cells on the surface of the retina changes the light signals into electrical nerve impulses and then relays them to the brain via the **optic nerve**. The eye contains 70 percent of the body's sensors and can deal with one and a half million simultaneous messages. The **pupils** automatically dilate or contract to control the amount of light that falls on the retina.

the parts of the eye

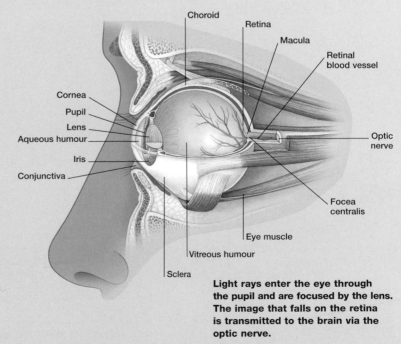

Choroid
Retina
Macula
Retinal blood vessel
Cornea
Pupil
Lens
Aqueous humour
Iris
Conjunctiva
Optic nerve
Focea centralis
Eye muscle
Vitreous humour
Sclera

Light rays enter the eye through the pupil and are focused by the lens. The image that falls on the retina is transmitted to the brain via the optic nerve.

Focusing and sight

The human eye is more efficient at accommodation (ability to resolve fine detail) than the eyes of most mammals. Light enters the eye through the pupil, which dilates or constricts according to lighting conditions, lens adjustment and emotions. The lens then focuses the light on the retina by changing shape. When focusing over long distances (over 7m/20ft), the lens is at its flattest and thinnest. When focusing on near objects, the lens becomes rounder and thicker.

The closest point at which the eye can focus varies with age – from about 7cm (3in) in infancy to only 40cm (16in) in old age. The lens focuses an image upside down on the retina; the conscious mind interprets the image and "sees" it in its true position.

The eye's strength of accommodation is determined by the number of light receptors (rods and cones) present in the retina, and how closely they are packed together. We have 200,000 receptors/mm^2, giving excellent resolution as long as vision during infancy has not been impeded in any way. Some creatures have an even higher resolution – the buzzard's retina, for example, contains one million receptors/mm^2.

how we see

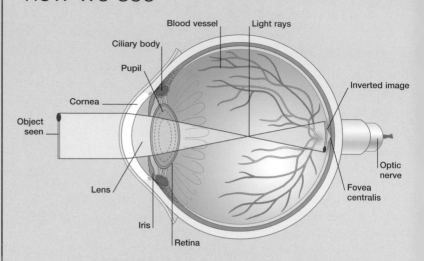

Light rays reflected from an object are partly focused by the cornea before entering the eye through the pupil. The image is focused further by the lens onto the retina, where it appears upside down. Electrical signals from the retina transmit the image to the brain, which interprets it as upright.

Field of vision

Since our eyes are placed on the front of the head we have binocular (three dimensional, or 3D) vision. Binocular vision means that we can see through 180° without moving the head, with an overlap of 90° between the right and left visual fields. This enables us to judge distances and pick out detail, and improves the sensitivity of vision when light is poor.

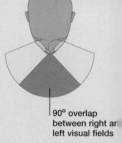

90° overlap between right and left visual fields

Colour vision

Detail of the retina

Connecting nerve cells

Connecting nerve cells

Light entering the eye

Pigment cells

Cones   Rods

In response to light, the rods and cones in the retina produce electrical signals that trigger impulses in the nerve cells to which they connect. These impulses travel along the optic nerve to the brain. Pigment cells behind the rods and the cones prevent reflection of light within the eye.

In common with other primates, we see only part of the colour spectrum since some wavelengths, such as infrared and ultraviolet, are invisible to us. The colour pigments we perceive are blue, green and red. Colour is registered by the **cones** in the retina; the cones are concentrated in the **fovea centralis** and the **macula**, which surrounds it. Each cone has a particular sensitivity for blue, green or red, and intermediate sensitivity to the rest of the colour spectrum. These sensitivities overlap so that wavelengths other than blue, green or red also trigger colour perceptions; for example, where light hits an overlapping curve of red and blue, the colour purple is "seen". We can only see colour in bright light. **Rods** in the retina cannot distinguish colours and are responsible mainly for night vision.

DISORDERS OF THE EYE ITSELF

The eye is a complex organ made up of several highly specialized components. Many eye disorders do not threaten sight, but a few serious conditions such as glaucoma may damage the eye and lead to loss of vision. A few eye disorders, such as conjunctivitis, are very common and early diagnosis usually leads to successful treatment.

I've chosen to start with the condition that is most common, **floaters**, because virtually all of us will get them and they are nothing to worry about. Other common problems, such as **styes** and **squint**, mainly affect children and you will find them in the childhood section. Several conditions, including glaucoma, can cause "**red eye**", the most common being **conjunctivitis** due to an infection, which is easily remedied with local antibiotics. **Glaucoma**, both acute and chronic, is an eminently treatable condition but left undiagnosed and untreated can cause serious loss of vision, so I give both forms prominence in this section.

Floaters

IT'S QUITE COMMON TO SEE SMALL SPECKS THAT APPEAR TO FLOAT IN THE FIELD OF VISION. ALTHOUGH FLOATERS SEEM TO LIE IN FRONT OF THE EYES, THEY ARE IN FACT FRAGMENTS OF TISSUE IN THE JELLY-LIKE FLUID THAT FILLS THE BACK OF THE EYE.

Floaters move rapidly with any eye movement but when the eyes are still, they drift slowly. No treatment is usually necessary.

The reason for most floaters isn't known. They rarely affect vision, but you should consult your doctor immediately if floaters suddenly appear in large numbers or interfere with vision. In an older person or in someone with pre-existing eye problems a sudden increase in the number of floaters, which may be combined with the sensation of flashing lights, could indicate a serious eye disorder that requires urgent treatment, such as the separation of the retina from the back of the eye (retinal detachment).

See also:
- **Retinal detachment p.467**

Conjunctivitis

ALSO CALLED PINK OR RED EYE, CONJUNCTIVITIS IS A COMMON CONDITION. THE CONJUNCTIVA, THE MEMBRANE COVERING THE WHITE OF THE EYE AND THE INSIDE OF THE EYELIDS, BECOMES INFLAMED CAUSING THE EYE TO BECOME RED AND SORE.

Conjunctivitis may look alarming but it is rarely serious. One or both eyes may be affected, and in some cases it begins in one eye and then spreads to the other. Wearing contact lenses and using cosmetics or eye drops are risk factors.

WHAT ARE THE CAUSES?
- Conjunctivitis may be caused by a **bacterial** or **viral** infection. **Bacterial conjunctivitis**, which is common, may be caused by any of several types of bacteria. **Viral conjunctivitis** can occur in epidemics and may be caused by one of the viruses responsible for the common cold. It may also be due to the **herpes simplex virus** that causes cold sores. Conjunctivitis due to a bacterial or viral infection can be spread by hand-to-eye contact and is usually highly contagious.
- Conjunctivitis may result from an allergic reaction or irritation of the conjunctiva, for example by smoke, pollution or ultraviolet light. **Allergic conjunctivitis** is a common feature of hay fever and of allergy to dust,

pollen and other airborne substances. The condition may also be triggered by chemicals found in eye drops, cosmetics or contact lens solutions. Allergic conjunctivitis often runs in families.
- Newborn babies sometimes develop conjunctivitis. This occasionally happens if an infection is transmitted to the baby's eyes from the mother's vagina during birth.

WHAT ARE THE SYMPTOMS?
The symptoms of conjunctivitis usually develop over a few hours and are often first experienced on waking. The symptoms generally include:
- redness of the white of the eye
- gritty and uncomfortable sensation in the eye
- swelling and itching of the eyelids
- discharge that may be yellowish and thick or clear and watery
- crusts on the eyelashes and eyelid margins due to discharge that has dried out during sleep. As a result, the eyelids sometimes stick together on waking.

WARNING:
If an eye becomes painful and red, you should consult your doctor as soon as possible to rule out the possibility of a more serious condition.

WHAT CAN I DO?
The symptoms of conjunctivitis can be relieved by bathing the eye with artificial tears, "comfort" drops, from the pharmacy. To avoid spreading infection, wash your hands after touching the eye and do not share towels or flannels. Once the conjunctivitis has cleared up, vision is rarely affected.

If you are susceptible to allergic conjunctivitis, avoid exposure to triggering substances. Anti-allergy eye drops can be used to ease the symptoms.

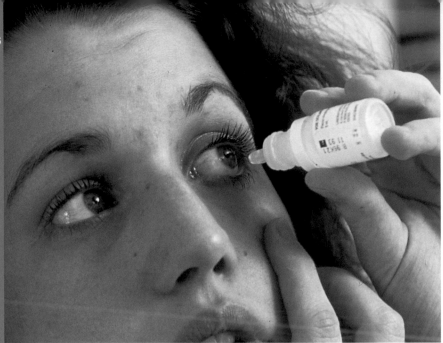

Conjunctivitis caused by a bacterial infection can be easily treated using antibiotic eyedrops, which your doctor may prescribe. Symptoms usually clear up within 48 hours of starting treatment.

WHAT MIGHT THE DOCTOR DO?

■ If infection is suspected, a sample of the discharge may be taken to identify the cause.
■ Bacterial conjunctivitis is treated by applying antibiotic drops or ointment. In such cases, the symptoms usually clear up within 48 hours. However, the treatment should be continued for 2–10 days, even if the symptoms improve, to ensure the infection is eradicated.
■ Viral conjunctivitis that occurs because of a herpes infection may be treated with eye drops containing an antiviral drug. Although other types of viral conjunctivitis cannot be treated, their symptoms usually clear up within 2–3 weeks.
■ Your doctor may prescribe eye drops or oral anti-allergy drugs for allergic conjunctivitis.

See also:
• Allergies p.315
• Hay fever p.319
• Herpes simplex infection p.336

Acute glaucoma

NORMALLY, THE FLUID THAT IS SECRETED INTO THE FRONT OF THE EYE TO MAINTAIN
THE EYE'S SHAPE AND NOURISH THE TISSUES DRAINS AWAY CONTINUOUSLY.

However, in acute glaucoma, the drainage system suddenly develops a blockage, and the fluid pressure inside the eye rises rapidly, causing pain and a "red eye". Acute glaucoma is a medical emergency. Without prompt treatment, the eye can swiftly become damaged and a permanent reduction in vision can result. Acute glaucoma is rare under the age of 40 and most common over the age of 60. The tendency to develop it sometimes runs in families.

WHAT ARE THE CAUSES?
The fluid in the front part of the eye is produced continuously by a ring of tissue called the **ciliary body**, behind the eye's coloured iris. Normally the fluid flows out through the pupil and drains away through the sieve-like meshwork behind the drainage angle at the outer rim of the iris. In acute glaucoma, the iris bulges forwards and closes the drainage angle, so that fluid is trapped within the eye. The pressure inside the eye rises as more fluid is secreted and as the pressure rises, it may damage the optic nerve, which carries nerve signals to the brain, causing reduced vision.

WHAT ARE THE RISKS?
■ Having an eyeball that is smaller than normal is a common cause of farsightedness and increases the risk of developing acute glaucoma.

■ The disorder is more common in older people because the lens of the eye thickens throughout life and may eventually press against the iris. Fluid then builds up behind the iris, which bulges forwards and blocks the drainage angle.
■ Occasionally, acute glaucoma may be triggered when dim light causes the pupil to widen. The iris then thickens and the drainage angle can close.
■ Acute glaucoma sometimes runs in families.

WHAT ARE THE SYMPTOMS?
Mild attacks of acute glaucoma tend to occur in the evening when you are tired, and symptoms include pain in the eyes and haloes appearing around lights. Sleeping usually relieves these symptoms. Full-blown attacks develop suddenly and include these symptoms:
• rapid deterioration of vision
• intense pain in the eye
• redness and watering of the eye
• sensitivity to bright light
• haloes appearing around lights
• nausea and vomiting.

WHAT IS THE TREATMENT?
Applanation tonometry, which measures the pressure inside the eye, is used to detect acute glaucoma. Laser iridotomy (see box, right) is usually performed to correct the condition.

TREATMENT

Laser iridotomy

This technique is used to treat acute glaucoma, in which pressure in the eye rises suddenly due to blockage in the outflow of fluid. First, the pressure is reduced using eye drops, intravenous drugs and, possibly, oral drugs. Anaesthetic eye drops are then put into the eye, and a thick contact lens is placed in front of it to focus a laser beam onto the bulging iris. The laser cuts a small hole in the iris, releasing the fluid behind it. The iris flattens, opening the drainage angle and letting trapped fluid flow out. The hole remains in the iris, harmlessly.

See also:
• Eye tests p.468 • Shortsightedness and longsightedness p.469

Chronic glaucoma

CHRONIC GLAUCOMA IS A GRADUAL, PAINLESS INCREASE IN THE FLUID PRESSURE INSIDE
THE EYE, USUALLY STARTING AFTER THE AGE OF 40 AND SOMETIMES RUNNING IN FAMILIES.
IT IS MORE COMMON IN PEOPLE OF AFRICAN DESCENT.

Chronic glaucoma is also known as **open-angle glaucoma**. The condition causes a gradual deterioration of sight due to a progressive build-up of fluid pressure inside the eye over a period of several years. There are often no symptoms until late in the disease, and loss of vision is permanent. Although the condition can lead to total blindness, early treatment can prevent severe damage. In most cases, both eyes are affected, although symptoms may only occur in one eye initially.

WHAT ARE THE SYMPTOMS?
By the time symptoms appear, it is probable that your vision has been permanently affected. At this late stage, symptoms may include:

● bumping into objects because of loss of the outer edges of vision (peripheral vision)
● blurring of objects that are straight ahead of you.

WHAT MIGHT BE DONE?
Your optician will probably perform a test called applanation tonometry to measure the pressure inside your eye. Various other tests may be done, including a visual field test to check for loss of peripheral vision.

WHAT IS THE TREATMENT?
■ If chronic glaucoma is diagnosed early, eye drops to reduce the pressure in the eye will probably be prescribed. You will probably have

to continue using these eye drops for the rest of your life.
■ If the condition is advanced, or if eye drops do not lower the pressure sufficiently, surgery may be needed to make a drainage channel in the white of the eye.
■ In another surgical technique, called **laser trabeculoplasty**, a laser beam is used to increase the flow through the trabecular meshwork, allowing fluid to drain away.

See also:
• Eye tests p.468

Retinal detachment

THE LIGHT-SENSITIVE RETINA OF THE EYE IS NORMALLY ATTACHED TO THE UNDERLYING TISSUE,
BUT IN RETINAL DETACHMENT PART OF THE RETINA PEELS AWAY FROM THIS TISSUE.

Retinal detachment usually affects one eye only but, without rapid treatment, can cause partial or total blindness in the affected eye. Retinal detachment is more common in people over the age of 50 and sometimes runs in families. Participating in sports that may lead to a blow to the eye, such as boxing, is a risk factor. Severe shortsightedness is also a risk factor.

Retinal detachment usually begins with a small tear in the retina. Fluid is then able to pass through the hole and separates the retina from the supporting tissues underneath.

WHAT ARE THE SYMPTOMS?
■ Flashing lights in the corner of the eye.
■ Sudden appearance of a large number of dark spots (floaters) in the field of vision.
■ Shadow affecting vision.

WHAT MIGHT BE DONE?
Your doctor can diagnose retinal detachment using an ophthalmoscope, an instrument used to examine the back of the eye. If only a small area of retina has detached, the tear may be sealed by laser surgery, which requires only local anaesthetic. However, if a large area has become detached, microsurgery (see box, right) under a general anaesthetic will be necessary. If treated early, normal vision may be restored, but delayed treatment is less effective.

TREATMENT

Microsurgery

Microsurgery is a technique that enables surgeons to operate on extremely small and delicate tissues in the body. In microsurgery a binocular microscope is used to view the operating site and surgeons operate with specially adapted small operating instruments.

Microsurgery is often used to operate on tissue such as nerves and blood vessels and on small structures in the eye, middle ear and reproductive system. For example, microsurgery is regularly used in the repair of detached retinas. It is also used routinely to remove the diseased eye lens of someone with a cataract and replace it with an artificially made lens. In an operation to reattach a severed limb or digit, microsurgery is used to repair severed nerves and blood vessels. Microsurgery may also be used to try to reverse sterilization operations: tubal ligation in females and vasectomy in males.

Microsurgery is usually performed under general anaesthesia, but for some minor

procedures, such as cataract operations, regional or local anaesthesia may be used instead. Since some microsurgical operations take longer than other similar surgical procedures, the time under anaesthesia is longer and this may extend the recovery time from anaesthesia. The risk of infection may also be higher with microsurgery because the operation site is exposed for a relatively long time compared with other procedures.

Microsurgery is usually highly successful for routine procedures such as cataract removal and repairing a detached retina. In other procedures, the success of microsurgery often depends on the extent to which tissues were damaged initially.

IMPERFECT VISION

Most people have a visual problem at some time in their lives so it's important to have regular eye checks with your optometrist throughout your life. The most common disorders of vision are **shortsightedness** (myopia) and **longsightedness** (hypermetropia), which are **focusing** (refractive) errors. If you have a refractive error it means that the image of an object cannot be focused clearly on the retina at the back of the eye and so the object appears fuzzy. Either the eye can't bend the light accurately enough or the eye is the wrong shape and refracted light misses the retina. Another refractive error, **presbyopia**, may develop as you get older for this precise reason – the shape of the eyeball may change as it ages so that images no longer fall on the retina. Most refractive errors can be corrected by glasses or contact lenses, or cured by surgical techniques.

In this section, I include **colour blindness**, which affects far more men than women, and serious visual problems including double vision.

TESTS

Eye tests

Regular eye tests are important, not just to check on your sight but also because a routine check will include tonometry to pick up signs of glaucoma and an examination of the optic nerve at the back of the eye to make sure the retina is healthy.

Vision tests

You should have your vision tested once every two years, especially if you are over 40 years old. The most common vision tests assess the sharpness (acuity) of your distance vision and how well your eyes focus on near objects. The tests also show which corrective lenses you may need. An additional test for glaucoma (see Applanation tonometry, below) may be performed, depending on your age and medical history.
Phoroptor This device holds different lenses in front of each eye, allowing the optician to test each eye separately.
Snellen chart The sharpness of your distance vision is tested separately for each eye. The test involves reading letters of decreasing sizes on a Snellen chart.
Near-vision test Wearing your glasses or contact lenses, if you use them, you will be asked to read very small print on a chart held at normal reading distance. This tests how well you can focus on near objects.
Having a vision test Lenses in the phoroptor are changed until you can read letters near the bottom of the Snellen chart, enabling the optician to make the appropriate prescription for your corrective lenses.
Applanation tonometry The condition glaucoma, in which the pressure inside the eye is raised, can be detected using an instrument called an applanation tonometer. Anaesthetic drops may be put into your eye

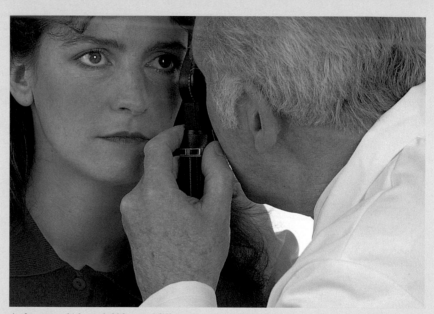

A phoroptor, which can hold lenses of different strengths in front of the eyes, is used with a Snellen chart to test distance vision. Each eye can be tested separately.

and the tonometer is then gently pressed against the cornea (the transparent front part of the eye) to measure the force needed to flatten the cornea. The test lasts only a few seconds and is painless.

Vision tests for children

Vision tests in children are designed according to their age and ability and are performed on a regular basis to look for defects that may delay normal development and learning. Vision can be assessed in infants using special tests, while older children can match shapes or letters. Once a child can read, adult vision tests can be used (see Snellen chart, above).
Retinoscopy This test may be performed on infants. About 30 minutes before the test,

eye drops are given to dilate the pupils and prevent focusing, and a beam of light is shone into each eye in turn from an instrument called a retinoscope. The effect of different lenses on the beam of light tells whether the child needs glasses. The test is performed in a darkened room.
Letter-matching test This test is usually used for children from about the age of three who are able to recognize letters. A child is given a card with letters printed on it. The optometrist then holds up cards with letters of decreasing size at a distance of 3m (10ft) and asks the child to identify the same letters on the card he is holding. Each of the eyes can be tested separately using an eyepatch.

Shortsightedness and longsightedness

SHORTSIGHTEDNESS (MYOPIA) IS THE INABILITY TO SEE DISTANT OBJECTS CLEARLY DUE TO A MISMATCH BETWEEN THE SIZE OR SHAPE OF THE EYEBALL AND THE FOCUSING POWER OF THE EYE.

In shortsightedness, the eyeball is too long and the image forms in front of the retina. Shortsightedness can be corrected with glasses using **concave** lenses or contact lenses (see box, below).

Longsightedness (hypermetropia) is the inability to see close objects clearly because the image cannot be focused precisely on the retina. In longsightedness, the eyeball is too short and the image falls behind the retina. Longsightedness can be corrected with glasses using **convex** lenses or contact lenses (see box, below). Longsightedness in children may interfere with reading and early learning and must be corrected when very young.

WHAT MIGHT BE DONE?

SHORTSIGHTEDNESS

■ Your optician will check your visual acuity and the level of detail you can see and then assess the severity of any visual defect.

■ Shortsightedness can be corrected by wearing contact lenses or glasses that have concave lenses. The focusing power of your own lenses decreases gradually with age, and your prescription may need to be updated regularly.

It's very important to treat shortsightedness in children, particularly once they are in school. Shortsightedness can prevent a child from following lessons written on the blackboard or from participating fully in sports that involve catching a ball.

LONGSIGHTEDNESS

■ Your optician will check your visual acuity and the level of detail you can see, and then assess the severity of any visual defect.

■ Longsightedness can be corrected by wearing contact lenses or glasses that have convex lenses. The focusing power of your own lenses decreases gradually with age, and your prescription may need to be updated regularly.

■ Some people who have longsightedness may be helped by laser treatment, which reshapes the surface of the cornea with a laser beam to increase its focusing power.

■ Longsightedness doesn't cause complications, but people who have it are more prone to **acute glaucoma**, a serious condition that must be treated promptly. You should, therefore, see an optometrist regularly, so that any problems can be spotted early and dealt with.

It's crucial to treat longsightedness in children. Although it may be detected during routine vision tests at school, children with a family history of longsightedness should have a vision test before the age of 3 because early treatment is important for early learning.

Presbyopia

Many of us find that the normal reading distance becomes longer and longer as we get older; this is known as **presbyopia**. As our eyes age they lose the power to focus; deterioration starts around the age of 45 years and by the age of 65 little focusing power remains. Presbyopia can be corrected by simple reading glasses with convex lenses or by contact lenses (see Glasses and contact lenses, below). Lenses may need to be changed four or five times over 20 or 30 years until eventually all focusing is done by lenses.

Focusing errors

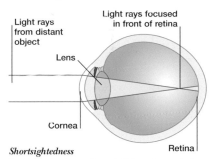

Shortsightedness

In shortsightedness, the eyeball is too long relative to the focusing power of the cornea and lens. Light from distant objects is focused in front of the retina and the image is blurry.

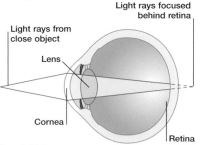

Longsightedness

In a person with longsightedness, the eye is too short relative to the focusing power of the cornea and lens. Light rays are focused behind the retina and the image is blurry.

TREATMENT

Glasses and contact lenses

Most focusing (refractive) errors can be corrected by glasses or, for older children and adults, contact lenses. Glasses can correct most refractive errors and do not cause complications. Contact lenses are most effective for shortsightedness and longsightedness. They require careful cleaning to reduce the chance of an infection of the cornea, over which they are placed.

How corrective lenses work

Glasses and contact lenses correct refractive errors by altering the angle of light rays before the rays reach the surface of the cornea, the transparent front layer of the eye, allowing the lens to focus the rays correctly on the retina.

■ Shortsightedness is corrected by concave lenses, which make light rays diverge, so that they are focused on the retina and not in front of it.

■ Longsightedness requires a convex lens to make light rays converge, focusing them on the retina and not behind it.

Contact lenses

Three types of contact lenses are available: rigid (hard), gas-permeable and soft. Soft lenses are the most widely used and the least rigid. Disposable soft lenses are worn only once or for a few days, then thrown away. Non-disposable lenses should be disinfected and cleaned daily, unless worn for an extended period of time (not usually recommended). If an eye becomes red or painful, stop wearing your lenses and consult your optometrist immediately.

See also:
• **Acute glaucoma p.466** • **Chronic glaucoma p.467** • **Surgery for refractive errors p.470**

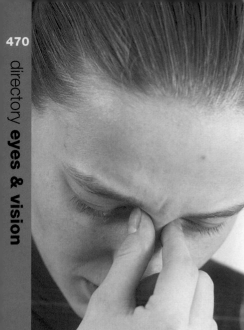

Eyestrain

MOST PEOPLE SUFFER FROM TEMPORARY DISCOMFORT OR ACHING IN OR AROUND THE EYES EVERY SO OFTEN.

Eyestrain is neither a medical term nor a diagnosis. In contrast to widespread belief, you cannot damage or strain your eyes by using them under difficult conditions, such as reading small print in poor light or wearing glasses of the wrong strength. Although aching and discomfort are commonly attributed to eyestrain, more often the cause is a headache due to tension or fatigue of the muscles around the eye as a result of frowning or squinting.

The symptoms normally attributed to eyestrain don't require treatment and normally disappear on their own, but if the problem worsens or persists, you should consult your doctor.

Tips for tired eyes

■ When you're doing close work, rest your eyes by glancing up now and then.
■ If your eyes become sore and dry after close work (as a consequence of forgetting to blink often enough), simply blink a few times to sluice out the eyeball with tears and cure the dryness.
■ "Palming" – the practice of cupping the hands over the eyes to rest them – will do no harm, but shutting the eyes to rest them every so often is just as effective a method of refreshing and relieving them.
■ After a long bout of crying, cold water compresses on the eyelids should help to relieve the discomfort of swollen eyes.
■ It does no harm to rub the eyes, provided that there is no foreign body in either of them and that rubbing them does not cause any pain.

Optical migraine

THE CLASSICAL SYMPTOMS OF MIGRAINE INCLUDE VISUAL DISTURBANCES, HEADACHE AND, POSSIBLY, NAUSEA WITH VOMITING.

Sometimes symptoms are confined to the eyes with **blurred vision**, **flashing lights**, **haloes** around light sources and **sensitivity** to light lasting 30–40 minutes. Neither the headache or nausea develop. When the visual symptoms disappear, the migraine attack resolves too.

Astigmatism

AN UNEVEN CURVATURE OF THE TRANSPARENT CORNEA AT THE FRONT OF THE EYE CAUSES ASTIGMATISM, WHICH IS DISTORTED VISION THAT CAN RESULT IN BLURRING OF SMALL PRINT.

You may notice difficulty in reading and sometimes trouble with both near and distant vision and should seek an eye test from your optician. Most astigmatism is present from birth.

WHAT IS THE TREATMENT?
■ Vision can usually be corrected by glasses that have specially curved lenses to compensate for the unevenly shaped cornea.
■ Rigid contact lenses are also effective for astigmatism because they smooth out the surface of the cornea.
■ Conventional soft contact lenses mould to the shape of the cornea and can normally only correct for mild astigmatism. However, soft contact lenses that are specially designed to correct the condition (known as **toric lenses**) are also available.
■ Astigmatism may be corrected by surgical treatment that reshapes the cornea (see box, right). One of the most widely used and least intrusive forms of surgical treatment for this condition is laser surgery, which causes only minimal scarring.

See also:
• **Glasses and contact lenses p.469**

TREATMENT

Surgery for refractive errors

Surgery can be used to correct some refractive errors permanently. The three main surgical techniques are:
● laser-assisted in-situ keratomileusis (LASIK), in which the cornea is reshaped by a laser
● radial keratotomy (RK), in which the cornea is flattened by scalpel cuts
● photorefractive keratectomy (PRK), in which areas of the cornea are shaved away by laser.

Warning:
Radial keratotomy (RK) can **weaken** the cornea. Photorefractive keratectomy may cause mild corneal scarring. LASIK causes the least scarring and is the most widely used method.

Double vision

IF YOU HAVE DOUBLE VISION, THAT IS, SEEING TWO IMAGES OF ONE OBJECT, YOU MAY
FIND THE DEFECT DISAPPEARS WHEN YOU CLOSE ONE OF YOUR EYES.

However, you should consult your doctor immediately if you suddenly start to experience double vision because it may indicate that you have a serious underlying disorder.

WHAT ARE THE CAUSES?
■ The most common cause of double vision is weakness or paralysis of one or more of the muscles that control the movements of one eye.
■ Many serious conditions that affect the brain and nervous system may cause impaired eye movements leading to double vision. Potential causes include **multiple sclerosis**, **head injuries**, **brain tumours** and bulging of an artery inside the head due to a weakness in the vessel wall (**aneurysm**).
■ In older people, impaired eye movement

resulting in double vision may be linked to **diabetes mellitus**, and, rarely, to **atherosclerosis** and **high blood pressure**.
■ Double vision can also occur as a result of a **tumour** or **blood clot** behind one of the eyes, causing the movement of that eye to be affected.

HOW IS IT DIAGNOSED?
■ Your doctor may ask you to shut one eye at a time to see whether the double vision disappears.
■ Your doctor will probably observe the movements of your eyes closely in order to establish whether any of the eye muscles are weak or paralyzed and do special vision tests to identify weak eye movement.

■ If double vision has come on suddenly, or if no obvious cause can be found, urgent computerized tomography (CT) scanning or magnetic resonance imaging (MRI) may be done to check for any abnormality in the eye sockets or brain that might be affecting the alignment of the eyes. You may also have a neurological examination.

> See also:
> • CT scanning p.401
> • MRI p.409

YOUR EYELIDS AND TEARS

Eyelids and tears work together to protect the eye against damage. The eyelids act as shutters, closing to stop material from entering the eyes. Tears contain one of the most potent antiseptic substances known, called **lysozyme**. It keeps the surface of the eyes moist and helps prevent infection. Disorders of the eyelids or tear system can damage the eyes, but most are easily treated if detected early.

The upper and lower eyelids provide essential protection for the eyes. If anything approaches the eye or face rapidly, the eyelids close together almost instantaneously as a reflex action. Furthermore, each

eyelid has two or three rows of eyelashes, which help prevent small particles from entering the eye.
Tears are another important part of the eye's defences. They are made up of salty fluid produced by the lacrimal (tear) glands, which are located above the upper eyelids. Tears lubricate the exposed surface of the eye and wash away potentially harmful materials, such as dust and chemicals. The production of tears can lessen with age, which is why wearing contact lenses can become increasingly uncomfortable as we age. However, dry eyes per se can be part of a syndrome called Sjögren's syndrome, with arthritis and a dry mouth as well as dry eyes.

Blepharitis

BLEPHARITIS IS INFLAMMATION, REDNESS AND SCALING OF THE MARGIN OF THE UPPER OR LOWER
EYELID OR BOTH, OFTEN ASSOCIATED WITH THE SEBACEOUS GLANDS OF THE EYELASHES AND
WITH THE COMMON SKIN DISORDER SEBORRHOEIC DERMATITIS.

Blepharitis may also occur because of a bacterial infection or may be due to an allergy to cosmetics.

If you have blepharitis, your eyelids will be swollen, red and itchy. The margins of the eyelids may be covered with soft, greasy scales that dry into crusts, sticking the eyelashes together. In some cases, the roots of the eyelashes become infected, causing styes to form.

WHAT IS THE TREATMENT?
■ You can relieve the symptoms by holding a clean, warm, damp cloth against the eyelid.
■ The healing process may be helped by cleaning the eyelids twice a day with baby shampoo diluted half and half with water, or you could use an over-the-counter eyelid wash.
■ If you have seborrhoeic dermatitis, treating it should also help the blepharitis.
■ If the blepharitis recurs repeatedly, see your

doctor, who may prescribe topical antibiotics. The condition often clears up after 2 weeks of treatment but it may recur.
■ Allergic blepharitis usually improves on its own, but you should try to avoid contact with the substance that triggered the condition.

> See also:
> • Seborrhoeic dermatitis p.315 • Stye p.543

FOCUS *on* cataracts

As we get older, cataracts (loss of transparency of the lenses in the eyes) are the most common cause of impaired vision. Cataracts form due to changes in the delicate protein fibres within the lens, in the way that an egg white goes solid when we cook it.

With increasing loss of transparency, the clarity and detail of what we see gets progressively less. Cataracts usually occur in both eyes, but one eye is nearly always more severely affected than the other.

Almost everyone over the age of 65 has cataracts to some degree, but they're usually minor and often confined to the edge of the lens where they don't interfere with sight. Most people over the age of 75 experience some visual impairment due to cataracts.

WHAT ARE THE CAUSES?

You needn't be fearful of getting cataracts – they are so common that they could almost be considered part of the normal ageing process.

● Exposure to the **ultraviolet radiation in strong sunshine** increases the risk, and cataracts are more common in tropical countries than in Europe or North America. They occur more often in those who spend most of their lives outdoors, especially if the eyes are unprotected.

● Exposure to other types of radiation, including **infrared** radiation and **X-rays**, may cause cataracts to form.

● Cataracts may be caused by **direct injury** to the eye, and are almost inevitable if a foreign particle, such as a shard of metal or glass, gets into the lens.

● Cataracts are common in people with **diabetes** and may develop early if the diabetes isn't well controlled and blood-sugar levels get very high.

● The formation of cataracts is promoted by long-term treatment with **corticosteroid drugs**, poisoning by substances such as **naphthalene** (found in mothballs) or **ergot** (formed in stored grain contaminated by a certain type of fungus).

● Mixing **sunshine** and the herbal antidepressant **St John's wort** may lead to cataracts. **Hypericin**, the active ingredient in St John's wort, reacts with visible and ultraviolet light to produce free radicals that damage the lens. Once proteins are damaged they produce cloudiness in the lens, forming a cataract. Hypericin does not cause any protein damage when kept in the dark, so at the very least, those taking St John's wort should wear hats and wraparound sunglasses.

WHAT ARE THE SYMPTOMS?

● Cataracts are entirely painless.

● The onset of visual symptoms is almost imperceptible, and progress is nearly always very slow.

● The main symptom is blurring of vision and **shortsightedness,** which gradually becomes worse. So a person who was previously longsighted may be able to read without using their reading glasses.

● Colours become distorted, with dulling of blues and accentuation of reds, yellow and oranges; the full perception of colour is dramatically restored after surgery.

● Beware! Night driving can be impaired. Often the lens opacity causes scattering of light rays and, even at a fairly early stage, may seriously affect night driving.

WHAT IS THE TREATMENT?

Once a cataract has developed, changes to the lens are irreversible. Nowadays, the need to have thick glasses can be avoided by replacing the removed lens with a tiny plastic implant that is fixed permanently in the eye during surgery. Cataract surgery gives excellent results in most cases.

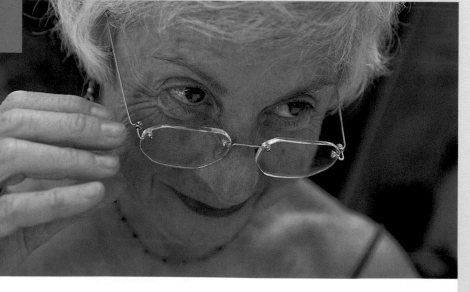

Cataract surgery

A cataract is an opaque region in the lens of the eye causing loss of vision. During cataract surgery, the affected lens is removed and replaced with an artificial lens using microsurgical techniques. The operation is usually performed under local anaesthetic, and you will probably be able to go home the same day. **The lens is first softened by an ultrasound probe** and then the softened tissue is extracted. The back of the natural lens capsule is left in place, and an artificial lens is placed inside it. The incision in the cornea is either closed with surgical **stitches** or will gradually heal on its own.

Dry eye (keratoconjunctivitis sicca)

PERSISTENT DRYNESS OF THE EYE DUE TO INSUFFICIENT PRODUCTION OF TEARS
IS KNOWN MEDICALLY AS KERATOCONJUNCTIVITIS SICCA; THE CONDITION BECOMES
INCREASINGLY COMMON IN WOMEN OVER AGE 35.

WHAT ARE THE CAUSES?

Dry eye can be a feature of certain autoimmune disorders in which the tear glands can be damaged, such as:
- rheumatoid arthritis
- Sjögren's syndrome (see below)
- lupus.

If you notice that your eyes are becoming dry frequently, you should consult your doctor so that he can exclude any possible related condition.

WHAT ARE THE SYMPTOMS?

Symptoms of dry eye include:
- blurred vision
- burning and itching
- grittiness.

If left untreated, corneal ulcers and eventually scarring of the cornea may occur.

WHAT IS THE TREATMENT?

■ Your doctor will prescribe artificial tears to restore moisture to the eye.

■ Investigations should be done to find any underlying cause of the dry eyes and appropriate treatment given.

■ In some cases, surgery may be performed to plug the channel through which the tears normally drain away from the eyes.

See also:
- **Lupus p.324**
- **Rheumatoid arthritis p.429**

Sjögren's syndrome

DRY EYES ARE A MAJOR SYMPTOM OF THE AUTOIMMUNE CONDITION
SJÖGREN'S SYNDROME.

Other normally moist parts of the body – the nose, mouth, throat and vagina – also tend to be dry, causing a range of problems. Arthritis, resembling rheumatoid arthritis, occurs as the autoimmune process begins to destroy glands that produce protective lubricating fluids. 9 out of 10 sufferers are postmenopausal women.

WHAT IS THE TREATMENT?

■ Artificial tears are essential to treat dry eyes.

■ Frequent dental checks will avoid tooth decay due to lack of saliva.

■ Dry vagina responds to vaginal moisturizers, HRT and oestrogen cream or pessaries used vaginally.

■ Arthritis should be treated in the same way as rheumatoid arthritis.

Colour blindness

Some people have a defect in the cones, the specialized cells in the retina at the back of the eye, that reduces their ability to tell certain colours apart. An inability to distinguish between red and green is the most common type of colour blindness, and this is a gender-linked genetic disorder. It is much rarer in women than it is in men.

Non-inherited causes of colour blindness include certain eye conditions, such as macular degeneration. It may also be a side effect of certain drugs, for example some antimalarial drugs.

Colour blindness rarely causes serious problems but it can exclude people from certain jobs where being able to distinguish between colours is essential, such as flying an aeroplane.

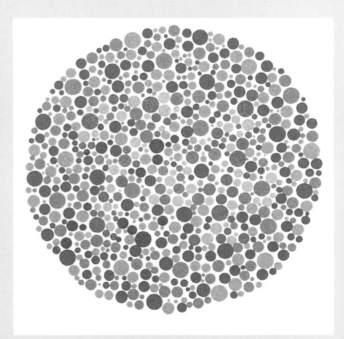

People who are colour blind cannot discern the number in the circle.

Ears, Nose and Throat

Image shows a CT (computerized tomography) section through a human head showing the brain and ear canal

Miriam's overview

When I was a child Ears, Nose and Throat (ENT) or otolaryngology was a major speciality, even though it spans a comparatively small anatomical area.

The popularity of ENT as a medical speciality was mainly due to tonsillectomy – taking out the tonsils – a procedure that enjoyed a great vogue until about 30 years go.

It was felt that infected tonsils were a "bad thing" and every child would be better off without them. That approach seemed logical at the time. But then we realized that the tonsils were, so to speak, the guardians of the throat and chest and by becoming infected they were only doing their job preventing the infection from going any further.

I remember when this approach was first adopted, one ENT surgeon regretting the "tons of tonsils" he had removed unnecessarily.

More medical knowledge means practices change. In the 1990s the ENT operation in vogue was the insertion of grommets. This followed on the realization that much middle ear disease, otitis media, was referable to glue ear, a new description coined to describe the thick gluey mucus that filled the middle ear in small children, causing deafness and difficulty at school later on.

A new operation was devised to drain away this mucus allowing the ear to work normally and hearing to be restored. This was the insertion of grommets, tiny tubes in the eardrum that ventilate the middle ear and keep the tube between the ear and the throat open.

But this fashion too, it would seem, has had its day. Grommets aren't that easy to maintain and they drop out. So they're being inserted less and less.

> ## "*we realized that the tonsils* were, so to speak, the guardians of the *throat and chest*"

Snoring is the butt of jokes and the cause of sleepless nights for wakeful partners. But recently we've realized that some snorers could be in danger of heart attacks. These are people, mainly men, who have periods of "sleep apnoea", spells when they stop breathing. The amount of oxygen in their blood drops, putting heart health in jeopardy.

Snoring needs urgent attention from your doctor, not teasing or jibes.

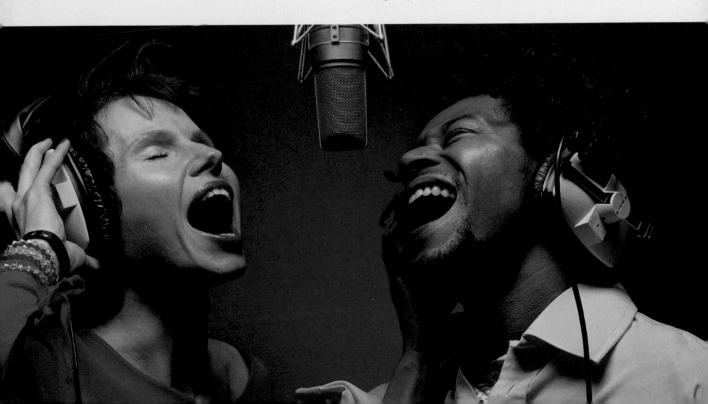

INSIDE
your ears, nose and throat

The ears are responsible for two different senses: hearing and balance. The ear consists of the outer, middle and inner ear. The visible outer part of the ear is called the **pinna**, and the opening into the middle ear is called the **ear canal**. At the end of the ear canal is the **eardrum**, which vibrates in response to sound waves. Beyond the eardrum is the **middle ear**, which contains the **ossicles**, three tiny bones that transmit vibration from the eardrum to a membrane known as the **oval window**. Beyond this membrane lies the **inner ear**. This contains the **cochlea**, which transforms vibration into electrical impulses that are then relayed along nerves to the brain. The inner ear also contains structures responsible for detecting movement and balance.

The **eustachian tube** connects the middle ear to the back of the nose and throat and allows equal air pressure to be maintained on both sides of the eardrum. The nose consists of the visible outer structure, the **nostrils** and the **inner nasal cavity**, which warms and moistens air that is breathed in. Within the skull bones around the nose and eyes are the **sinuses**, cavities that have little use in humans. The back of the nasal cavity connects to the **throat**, or pharynx. At the top of the throat are the **tonsils**, which help protect the body against infection. At the bottom of the throat is the **voice box** (larynx), the structure that contains the **vocal cords** and allows speech to be produced.

how the ear works

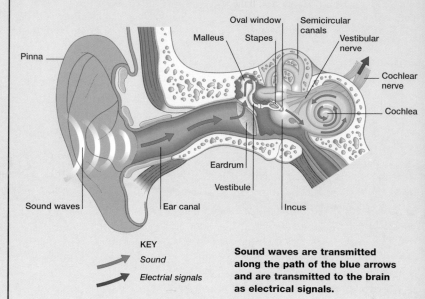

Sound waves are transmitted along the path of the blue arrows and are transmitted to the brain as electrical signals.

KEY
Sound
Electrial signals

the nose and throat

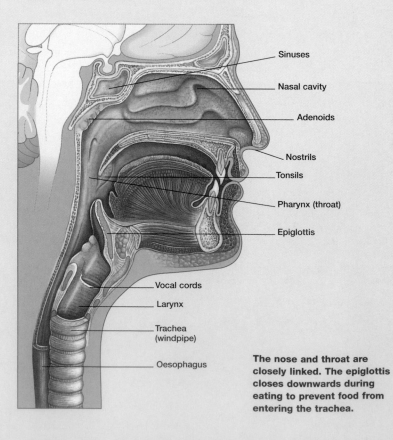

The nose and throat are closely linked. The epiglottis closes downwards during eating to prevent food from entering the trachea.

connecting passageways

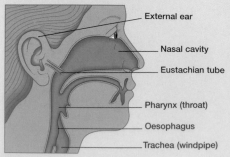

The ears, nose and throat are interconnected. The eustachian tube maintains equal air pressure on both sides of the eardrum.

Wax blockage

EARWAX IS PRODUCED BY GLANDS IN THE EAR CANAL AND ITS JOB IS TO CLEAN,
MOISTEN AND PROTECT THE CANAL. IF WAX IS PRODUCED IN LARGER THAN NORMAL
QUANTITIES, IT MAY CAUSE A BLOCKAGE AND INTERFERE WITH HEARING.

Usually, earwax is produced in small quantities and emerges naturally from the ear. If the canal becomes blocked with wax, it causes a feeling of blockage, itchiness and sometimes hearing loss.

WARNING:

Under normal circumstances the ear canal is a self-cleansing organ and needs no special attention. Never use a cotton swab, hair grip or finger to remove wax from your ears – that simply compacts the wax, making it hard.

WHAT IS THE TREATMENT?

■ Wax blockage can be treated with over-the-counter eardrops, and following the maker's instructions will usually dissolve the earwax in about 4–10 days.
■ If the ear remains blocked, you should consult your doctor.
■ Your doctor will probably use a viewing instrument (an otoscope) to inspect the ear canal.
■ You may have the wax removed with a probe or suction device.
■ The ear may be gently flushed out with warm water from a syringe.
■ Wax blockage sometimes recurs after treatment because some ear canals just produce more wax than others.

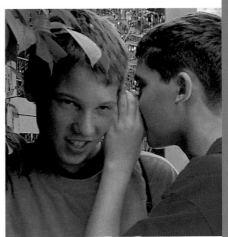

Ménière's disease

IN MÉNIÈRE'S DISEASE, THE FLUID IN THE INNER EAR INCREASES FROM TIME TO TIME.
THE RAISED PRESSURE IN THE INNER EAR DISTURBS THE ORGANS OF HEARING AND BALANCE,
CAUSING SUDDEN ATTACKS OF RINGING IN THE EARS AND SEVERE DIZZINESS.

Attacks of Ménière's disease occur suddenly and may last from a few minutes to several days before gradually subsiding.

WHAT ARE THE SYMPTOMS?
The symptoms may include:
● sudden, severe dizziness and loss of balance (vertigo)
● nausea and vomiting
● abnormal, jerky eye movements
● ringing or buzzing noises in the affected ear (tinnitus)
● loss of hearing, particularly of low-pitched sounds
● feeling of pressure in the affected ear.
The time between attacks of Ménière's disease ranges from a few days to years. Tinnitus may be constant or occur only during an attack. Between attacks, vertigo and nausea cease and hearing may improve. With repeated attacks, hearing can deteriorate progressively.

HOW IS IT DIAGNOSED?
■ Your doctor may arrange for hearing tests to assess your hearing loss.

■ Tests such as CT (computerized tomography) scanning or MRI (magnetic resonance imaging) are also done.

WHAT IS THE TREATMENT?
■ You may be prescribed drugs to relieve nausea (anti-emetic drugs).
■ An antihistamine may give further relief from nausea and vertigo and reduce the frequency of the episodes.
■ Sedative drugs such as diazepam may be prescribed to relieve vertigo, and diuretic drugs may be used to help prevent further attacks.

SELF-HELP
■ During an attack, lie still with your eyes closed and avoid noise, perhaps by wearing ear plugs.
■ Between attacks, try to avoid stress.
■ Relaxation techniques may be helpful.
■ A low-salt diet may help – don't add salt to cooking or use with food, and avoid very salty foods such as smoked fish and sausage.

For people with disabling vertigo, an operation to sever the nerve between part of the inner ear and the brain is the last resort. The operation cures the vertigo and may prevent loss of hearing.

WHAT IS THE OUTLOOK?
■ The symptoms of Ménière's disease are usually improved with medication.
■ The frequency and severity of the episodes tend to decrease over a period of years.
■ However, hearing usually worsens progressively with each successive attack, and permanent hearing loss may be the end result.
■ By the time hearing loss becomes severe, the other symptoms have usually disappeared.

See also:
● CT scanning p.401 ● MRI p.409
● Relaxation p.292
● Tinnitus p.478 ● Vertigo p.418

Otosclerosis

IN OTOSCLEROSIS, BONE OVERGROWS AROUND ONE OF THE THREE TINY BONES (OSSICLES) IN THE MIDDLE EAR, PREVENTING TRANSMISSION OF SOUND VIBRATIONS TO THE INNER EAR AND CAUSING DEAFNESS. USUALLY BOTH EARS ARE AFFECTED, THOUGH NOT ALWAYS EQUALLY.

Abnormal growth of bone in the middle ear, or otosclerosis, affects about 1 in 12 people, sometimes leading to hearing loss, but often symptomless. When symptoms develop it's usually between the ages of 20 and 30. We do not understand why otosclerosis develops but the condition is twice as common in females, and in 3 out of 5 cases someone in the family also has it.

WHAT ARE THE SYMPTOMS?
The symptoms of otosclerosis develop gradually and may include:

- hearing loss in which sounds are muffled but are sometimes clearer if there's background noise
- ringing or buzzing noises in the ears (tinnitus, see below)
- in severe cases, dizziness and imbalance (vertigo).

WHAT MIGHT BE DONE?
Your doctor will probably be able to diagnose otosclerosis from the results of hearing tests and from your family history. The disease can't be halted but a hearing aid may be helpful.

If not, consult your doctor about possible surgery to free up the ossicles.

> **See also:**
> - **Vertigo p.418**

Tinnitus

PEOPLE WITH TINNITUS HEAR SOUNDS THAT ORIGINATE IN THE EAR ITSELF. THESE SOUNDS MAY INCLUDE RINGING, BUZZING, WHISTLING, ROARING OR HISSING NOISES. THEY MAY PULSE IN TIME WITH THE HEARTBEAT OR, MORE COMMONLY, OCCUR CONTINUOUSLY AND PERMANENTLY.

WHAT ARE THE CAUSES?
Tinnitus may have no apparent cause, but it's commonly part of **Ménière's disease**. People with anaemia, an overactive thyroid gland or head injuries may have tinnitus, and treatment with various drugs, such as aspirin and antibiotics, can also cause it.

If you develop tinnitus, particularly if it affects one ear only, you should consult your doctor straight away. When tinnitus is continuous and permanent it may lead to depression and anxiety disorders.

WHAT MIGHT BE DONE?
TESTS
After looking at your eardrum with an otoscope, your doctor may arrange for hearing

tests and a blood test for anaemia as well as CT (computerized tomography) scanning or MRI (magnetic resonance imaging).

TREATMENT
- If an underlying cause, such as thyroid disease, is found and successfully treated, the tinnitus may improve.
- If tinnitus persists, your doctor may recommend a device called a **masker**. This device, worn in or behind the ear like a hearing aid, produces sounds that distract you from the tinnitus.
- If tinnitus accompanies hearing loss, a hearing aid may provide relief by increasing your awareness of background noise while masking the internal sounds.

- Many people with tinnitus find that background noise, such as playing music, reduces their awareness of the sounds in their ears.
- If tinnitus is very distressing or leads to depression or anxiety, counselling, self-help groups or relaxation exercises may help.

> **See also:**
> - **CT scanning p.401**
> - **Ménière's disease p.477**
> - **MRI p.409**

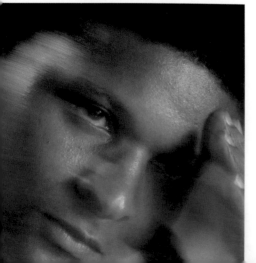

Labyrinthitis

IN LABYRINTHITIS, THE PART OF THE INNER EAR KNOWN AS THE LABYRINTH IS INFLAMED.

Because the labyrinth contains the organs of balance and hearing, inflammation in this part of the ear leads to dizziness, nausea, vomiting and tinnitus.

WHAT IS THE TREATMENT?
Labyrinthitis can often be diagnosed from

your symptoms. Your doctor may suggest:
- antibiotics, for bacterial labyrinthitis
- you lie in a darkened room with your eyes closed
- an anti-emetic drug to ease the nausea.
  It may take several weeks to recover completely from labyrinthitis, so go slowly.

Travel sickness

TRAVEL SICKNESS OCCURS WHEN THE BALANCE ORGANS IN THE EAR ARE UPSET BY MOVEMENT,
CAUSING SYMPTOMS RANGING FROM SLIGHT QUEASINESS TO VOMITING AND FAINTING.

Travel sickness is very common in some families. When the sensation of movement doesn't correspond with what the eyes see, it causes confusion in the brain and may lead to travel sickness. The problem may occur, for example, if you ride a rollercoaster or travel in a car, boat or plane. Children tend to suffer from travel sickness more than adults, though why is not known; most outgrow it by adolescence.

IS IT SERIOUS?
Travel sickness is not serious, but it is inconvenient. With a young child there is a risk that prolonged vomiting could cause dehydration.

WHAT SHOULD I DO FIRST?
1. Lie down flat.
2. Close your eyes to minimize the confusing signals being received by the brain.

POSSIBLE SYMPTOMS
- Nausea.
- Vomiting.
- Pale, clammy forehead.
- Weakness or dizziness.
- Fainting.

SHOULD I CONSULT THE DOCTOR?
Consult your doctor if you suffer from travel sickness even on short journeys, or if proprietary brands of travel-sickness medicine do not help.

WHAT MIGHT THE DOCTOR DO?
After questioning you about the symptoms and their frequency, your doctor may prescribe a drug such as an **antihistamine**, though some antihistamines can have side effects such as drowsiness.

SELF-HELP
- Prevent travel sickness by taking a travel-sickness medicine before you start the journey. There are several good over-the-counter medications available from the chemist.
- Have a small snack before setting out. Don't travel on a full stomach.
- Take plenty of drinks with you, or check that they will be available en route, to prevent the possibility of dehydration through vomiting. Fresh drinks can also reduce the feeling of nausea.
- Carry suitable "sick bags" (strong paper bags are best) in case of vomiting.
- Some people find copper bands worn on the wrist can help.

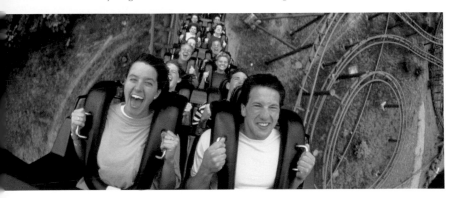

Nosebleed

BLEEDING FROM THE NOSE MAY OCCUR FOR VARIOUS REASONS, INCLUDING INJURY,
NOSE-PICKING, FORCEFUL NOSE-BLOWING, A FOREIGN BODY AND AS A SYMPTOM OF SOME
ILLNESSES. NOSEBLEEDS OCCUR MOST COMMONLY IN CHILDREN AND IN PEOPLE OVER 50.

Bleeding from the nose, usually from one nostril only, is most common in children, but the bleeding usually stops by itself and is minor. It comes from a patch of blood vessels just inside the nostril and just under the nasal lining. Nosebleeds are also common, and sometimes very serious, in people over age 50, when bleeding may come from the back of the nose and be hard to stop, especially when accompanied by high blood pressure.

WHAT ARE THE CAUSES?
Nosebleeds may occur from injury to the nose or from nose-picking or forceful nose-blowing. In children, nosebleeds often occur as a result of rough play. A foreign body in the nose or an infection in the upper respiratory tract may also result in a nosebleed.

continued on page 481

Nasal polyps

Benign fleshy growths of the mucus-secreting lining of the nose, known as nasal polyps, have no known cause. They can block the nose and cause a nasal voice, runny nose and diminished sense of smell.

What might be done?
- A small sample of a single polyp may be removed and examined under a microscope in order to exclude anything sinister.
- Small nasal polyps may be treated by using a corticosteroid spray, which shrinks the polyps over a few weeks.
- Larger polyps may be removed during an endoscopic procedure. A corticosteroid spray may also be necessary for several months after surgery to prevent the polyps from recurring.
- In more severe cases, a course of oral corticosteroids may also be prescribed.

FOCUS *on* snoring

Snoring is a noise caused when floppy tissue at the back of the throat, such as the uvula, blocks the upper air passages during sleep. It may be a symptom of the more serious disorder sleep apnoea, more common in men.

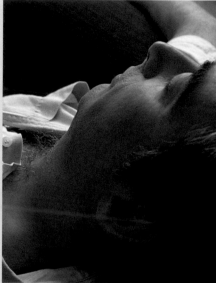

Turbulent airflow creates quite violent vibrations of the soft palate or other structures in the **mouth**, **nose** and **throat**. Depending on how flappable these structures are, vibrations can produce snoring sounds of such resonance that the decibels can be heard throughout the house and curtail the sleep of anyone who's in it.

Most causes of snoring are easily remedied, and there's a good chance that simple treatment or a change in lifestyle will significantly improve things. But other causes are more complex and need specialist investigation and treatment.

WHAT ARE THE CAUSES?

Some factors make us more likely to snore. Smoking, being overweight, consumption of alcohol, use of sleeping pills, poor sleeping position and reaction to house dust and dust mites are all implicated. Avoiding these factors may reduce the likelihood of snoring.

Several things make us more likely to snore:
● obstruction by the tongue if it drops back
● small or collapsing nostrils
● deviated nasal septum, say from a sports injury
● overnight catarrhal congestion
● large, floppy soft palate or uvula
● enlarged nasal bones in the nostrils
● nasal polyps
● in children, enlarged adenoids and mouth breathing.

IS SNORING DANGEROUS?

Snoring in itself isn't serious but it can be a symptom of a more serious disorder, sleep apnoea, in which the snorer stops breathing several times an hour during sleep. The point is that people with sleep apnoea are prone to irregular heartbeats, even possibly heart attacks.

The most vulnerable person is a man over the age of 45 or a woman who's gone through the menopause and isn't taking hormone replacement therapy. So if you're a middle-aged **snorer**, ask your doctor to check you over.

WHAT IS SLEEP APNOEA?

Apnoea literally means a temporary inability to breathe. Sleep apnoea is when a sufferer stops breathing during sleep. The cessation of breathing causes a drop in the blood oxygen level, which arouses the body to start breathing again.

The sleep/arousal cycle is repeated during the night and sufferers get up feeling **unrefreshed** and continually tired. More often than not, they're unaware of their condition.

WHAT ARE THE SYMPTOMS OF SLEEP APNOEA?

Common symptoms are:
● loud snoring
● feelings of choking and shortness of breath at night
● restless, unrefreshing sleep
● excessive daytime sleepiness
● personality changes
● morning headaches.

WHAT CAN BE DONE TO HELP?

Several hospitals have **sleep apnoea and snoring clinics** that can investigate the cause of snoring and diagnose sleep apnoea. Your GP can refer you for special tests to diagnose the cause of your snoring and recommend treatment.

LIFESTYLE CHANGES

Some overweight patients are described as **"weight-sensitive" snorers**. You'll be given a weight-loss programme, and weight reduction alone may provide a complete cure.

HOW DOES LOSING WEIGHT HELP?

Snoring problems are often made worse if you're slightly overweight. Significant relief can often be obtained by some degree of weight reduction, so a sensible eating plan may be of help.

Treating snoring

Surgery

There are a number of new surgical operations for snorers who are found to have obstructions or deformities of the mouth, nose and throat. Such operations are not always guaranteed to work, however.

If snoring is accompanied by sleep apnoea, which is detrimental to your health, treatment may be available on the NHS from an ear, nose and throat surgeon or a respiratory physician. Ask your GP about the possibility.

Somnoplasty

A revolutionary new treatment using low-power, low-temperature, radio-frequency energy will reduce the size of the soft palate.

Laser-assisted uvuloplasty – LAUP

Carbon dioxide laser treatment that will reduce the length and floppiness of the palate and uvula. The technique reshapes your soft palate and is an effective treatment for palatal snorers.

Corrective nasal airway surgery – septoplasty/nasal polypectomy

Minor surgery that opens up the nasal passage by removing a polyp or correcting a deformity that is responsible for reducing the size of the nasal passage.

Tonsillectomy

Where the tonsils and the walls of the pharynx (throat) are causing an obstruction, this operation will be of benefit in a small number of snorers and mild sleep apnoea sufferers.

continued from page 479

WHAT CAN I DO?

■ Put direct pressure on the soft part of your nose by pressing both sides together for at least 15 minutes while breathing through your mouth.
■ Avoid sniffing and/or blowing your nose afterwards because you may dislodge the blood clot that has formed and cause another nosebleed.

■ If bleeding persists for half an hour or more, you should seek medical attention.
■ If membranes in the nose are dry and cracked, rubbing water-based ointment in your nose a few times a day or using a saline spray may help prevent recurrent nosebleeds.

WHAT MIGHT THE DOCTOR DO?

A persistent nosebleed will probably require hospital treatment.
■ The doctor may pack your nose with nasal sponges, which are left in place for about two days.
■ Alternatively, a flexible tube with a small balloon at the tip may be inserted into the back of your nose and inflated to stop the bleeding by applying pressure to leaking vessels.
■ Bleeding vessels may also be cauterized (sealed using heat or a chemical) under local anaesthesia.
■ Blood tests may be done to check how well your blood clots.

Sinusitis

SINUSITIS MEANS INFLAMMATION OF THE SINUSES – THE AIR-FILLED CAVITIES IN THE SKULL SITUATED BEHIND THE NOSE AND EYES AND IN THE CHEEKS AND FOREHEAD. THE PROBLEM USUALLY RESULTS FROM A SECONDARY BACTERIAL INFECTION IN BLOCKED SINUSES.

The sinuses are lined with a mucus-secreting membrane and are connected to the nasal cavity by a number of narrow channels. They have little function in humans.

WHAT ARE THE CAUSES?

The most common primary cause of sinusitis is a viral infection, such as the common cold. If the channels connecting the nose to the sinuses become blocked due to the viral infection, mucus collects in the sinuses. When mucus can't drain away it can become infected with bacteria.

Blockage of the channels is more likely in people with an abnormality in the nose, such as nasal polyps or a deviated nasal septum (twisting of the cartilage that divides the nose internally into two). People with hay fever or cystic fibrosis are also more likely to develop sinusitis.

WHAT ARE THE SYMPTOMS?

In adults, symptoms depend on which sinuses are affected and may include:
● headache
● pain and tenderness in the face that tends to worsen when bending down
● toothache, if the sinuses behind the cheeks are affected
● thick, yellow nasal discharge
● nasal congestion or obstruction.

SELF-HELP

Steam inhalation

Inhaling steam from a bowl of hot water can help relieve the symptoms of colds, sore throats, sinusitis and laryngitis. The moisture in the steam loosens secretions in congested upper airways, making them easier to clear. You can also run hot water while you are in the bathroom and inhale the steam. Children shouldn't carry out steam inhalation unless they are under adult supervision.

Preparation

Fill a bowl about one-third full with hot water. Lean forwards, pull a towel over your head as well as the bowl, and inhale steam for several minutes.

My mum used to put Friar's Balsam into the water and you can use mentholated over-the-counter products to suit your taste. Some people prefer herbal aromatic oils dissolved in the hot water.

Inhaling steam is a good way to clear a blocked nose or sinuses and soothe a sore throat.

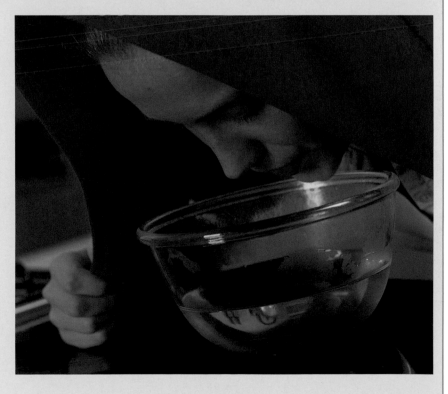

In a few cases, the infection spreads and may cause redness and swelling of the skin around an eye.

SELF-HELP

In many cases, sinusitis clears up without treatment.
■ Painkillers and a decongestant, both available over the counter, may alleviate symptoms.
■ Steam inhalation, which usually helps clear the nose, may also relieve symptoms.
■ If symptoms become worse or do not improve within three days, you should consult a doctor.

WHAT MIGHT THE DOCTOR DO?

Treatments and tests might include:
● antibiotics prescribed to clear up a secondary bacterial infection
● if sinusitis recurs or doesn't clear up completely, X-rays to look for thickening of the lining of the sinuses and excess mucus
● endoscopy of the nose
● CT (computerized tomography) scanning to look for a specific cause, such as nasal polyps
● surgery may be necessary to enlarge drainage channels from the sinuses to the nose or create new ones.

Acute sinusitis usually clears up in a few weeks, but the symptoms of chronic sinusitis may last for a couple of months and need a prolonged course of antibiotics.

> See also:
> • **Hay fever p.319**
> • **CT scanning p.401**
> • **Cystic fibrosis p.521**

Laryngitis

INFLAMMATION OF THE LARYNX (VOICE BOX) IS KNOWN AS LARYNGITIS OR A "SORE THROAT".

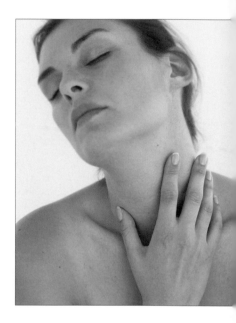

Laryngitis is usually caused by infection, often a viral infection, and results in hoarseness. It's more common in smokers and drinkers.

WHAT ARE THE SYMPTOMS?

The symptoms of laryngitis usually develop over 12–24 hours and vary depending on the underlying cause. Symptoms may include:
● hoarseness
● gradual loss of the voice
● pain in the throat, especially when using the voice.
    Sometimes laryngitis is associated with vocal cord nodules due to overuse or misuse.

WHAT CAN I DO?

When vocal cords are inflamed they need rest. For both forms of laryngitis, resting your voice can help relieve pain and avoid further damage to the vocal cords. Acute laryngitis that's caused by a viral infection usually clears up without treatment. There's no specific treatment for chronic laryngitis.
    Sudden hoarseness in middle or older age must always be investigated by your doctor as it may indicate cancer or an underlying lung disease.

Cancer of the larynx

CANCER OF THE LARYNX (VOICE BOX) OFTEN CAUSES PERSISTENT HOARSENESS. IT'S MOST COMMON BETWEEN THE AGES OF 55 AND 65, AND IS FIVE TIMES MORE COMMON IN MEN, ESPECIALLY IF THEY SMOKE AND DRINK.

In about 3 out of 5 cases, the cancer develops on the vocal cords.

WHAT IS THE TREATMENT?

■ You may be offered surgery to remove part or all of the larynx and/or radiotherapy.
■ If the larynx has to be removed, I'm afraid ordinary speech will no longer be possible.
    However, several techniques have been developed to allow you to speak without a larynx. Speech therapy may enable you to

speak using your oesophagus, or you may be able to learn to speak with the help of a handheld electromechanical device that generates sounds. Alternatively, a small device known as a tracheoesophageal implant may be fitted to help you speak.

GOOD NEWS!

In more than 9 of out 10 cases, treatment is successful if the tumour develops on the vocal cords and is detected and treated early.

WARNING:
Any hoarseness starting for no reason in middle age or older must be checked out by your doctor.

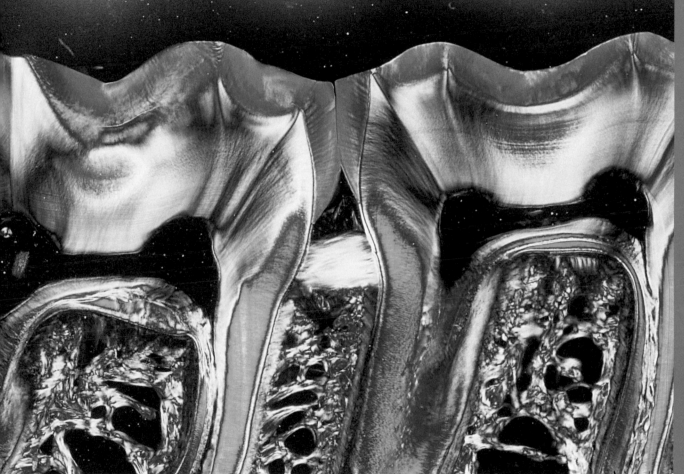

Teeth and Gums

Image shows a polarized light micrograph of molar teeth in the lower jaw

Miriam's overview

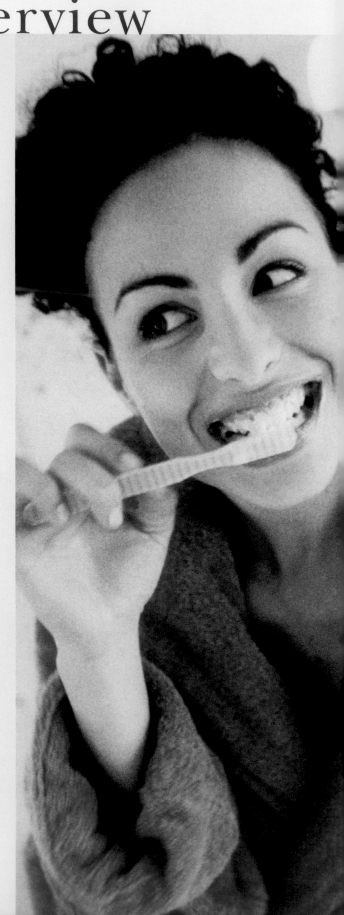

The old joke goes, "Dentist looking into patient's mouth, 'Your teeth are all right but your gums will have to come out'". And there's more than a grain of truth in that.

Without healthy gums the teeth cannot stay healthy. Infections in pockets around the gum margin, caused by the bacteria in plaque, eventually loosen the sealing of the tooth in the jawbone, leading to infections, "sensitive" teeth, pain, difficulty in chewing and eventually loss of teeth – they simply fall out.

"without *healthy gums* the teeth cannot stay healthy"

There are two main ways to maintain gum health – preventing the accumulation of plaque around our children's teeth by cutting down on sugary foods and making sure all youngsters grow up with good dental hygiene habits and continue them through life.

As we get older this requires more than brushing. Spaces open up between the teeth where fermenting food can lodge, creating the conditions where gum-destroying bacteria can thrive. Each meal therefore requires the ritual of tooth brushing and flossing (or the use of dental sticks or micro-brushes) to get rid of all food fragments.

Cosmetic dentistry caught on 20 years ago and is now the prerogative of everyone. It goes a lot further than teenage braces to straighten uneven front teeth. Discoloured teeth can be whitened with a veneer, teeth can be filed down, built-up, replaced, capped, crowned, implanted both to conserve and enhance.

Teeth are seen as accessories whose appearance is important not just for personal morale but also for professional reasons. An attractive smile is just as important to someone whose looks are their fortune as any other part of their body.

"*each meal* requires the ritual of *tooth brushing* and *flossing*"

INSIDE your teeth and gums

A child's first set of 20 teeth, called **primary** or **milk teeth**, erupt from the gums between the ages of about six months and three years. These start to be replaced by 32 **secondary teeth** at about the age of 6, with most secondary teeth in place by the age of 21.

All teeth have the same structure. Each tooth has a hard shell that surrounds a cavity filled with soft tissue, known as **pulp**. The exposed part of the tooth, or the **crown**, is covered by a layer of tough **enamel**, and underneath the enamel is a substance called **dentin**, which is similar to ivory. Long, pointed **roots** extend from the dentin and pulp into the jaw and are sealed by a layer of firm, fleshy tissue called the **gums**.

the structure of a tooth

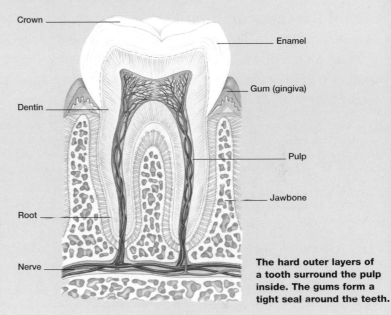

Crown

Enamel

Gum (gingiva)

Dentin

Pulp

Jawbone

Root

Nerve

The hard outer layers of a tooth surround the pulp inside. The gums form a tight seal around the teeth.

Caring for your teeth and gums

THE HEALTH OF THE TEETH IS AT LEAST 50 PERCENT DEPENDENT ON THE HEALTH OF THE GUMS; IN THE WESTERN WORLD, MORE TEETH ARE LOST THROUGH GUM DISEASE THAN THROUGH TOOTH DECAY.

Brushing the teeth regularly and frequently (at least twice a day) is the best possible way to maintain and protect the health of the teeth and gums.

Most dentists would agree that the single most important thing is to use a method that is suitable for you and that is efficient. At one time, a rolling action was propagated, with a downwards motion for the upper teeth and an upwards motion for the lower teeth. This, however, was shown to be only about 50 percent as effective as the technique that is now generally recommended – a gentle, rapid, short, to-and-fro action in the horizontal plane using the **side and edge** of the brush. Don't press too hard or see-saw the toothbrush backwards and forwards – this may damage the delicate gum margin. If you cannot brush between meals, chewing sugar-free gum may help. Avoid sugary foods and drinks. If your water does not contain fluoride, ask your dentist about using fluoride tablets or drops.

DENTAL FLOSS

Using dental floss is an excellent adjunct to tooth brushing. It has to be used carefully so as not to damage the delicate margins of the gum. Use it as follows:
1. Wind a 10–15cm (4–6in) length of floss around the first two fingers of each hand.
2. Slide it gently down between two teeth, pressing it against the side of the tooth (but do not see-saw it against the gum). Then swing it upwards, pressing against the side of the other tooth and removing any debris with it.

DENTAL CARE

■ Your hygienist will descale the teeth and remove any deposits of calculus from the gum margins. Visits should preferably be at six-monthly intervals.
■ Children, whose teeth and bones are still forming, need to have an adequate intake of calcium and vitamin D in their diets.

continued on page 488

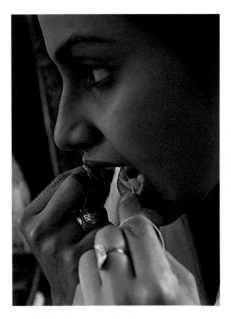

FOCUS *on* fear of dentists

One of the most common phobias is fear of dentists. At the thought of walking into a dentist's waiting room many of us break out into a cold sweat. It's very important to keep our teeth and gums in good shape and that requires regular dental check-ups. But overcoming our fear of dentists can be an uphill struggle.

These days dentistry is a pretty painless exercise. Indeed some dentists go to extraordinary lengths to make sure the procedure is as comfortable as possible. I've come across one dentist, for example, who provides his patients with a headphone so they cannot hear the sound of the drill – so-called "white noise" – and another who sits and chats till the anaesthetic works.

● Another possibility is to ask the dentist to smear a **local anaesthetic gel** on your gums before he injects them. Ask for just half the injection of anaesthetic to begin with, wait for five minutes, then have the rest and you shouldn't feel a thing.

● There is also the **needleless syrijet** or **electrical dental analgesia**, which delivers a mild electrical pulse that the patient controls and that stops their senses sending pain messages to the brain.

● Some dentists now use a technique called **inhalation sedation** when taking out teeth. The patient remains conscious throughout but is calmed by breathing in a mixture of nitrous oxide and oxygen.

● In extreme cases a **general anaesthetic** may be available, but can only be administered in a hospital setting.

● One solution chosen by many people is to have a **valium** injection in the arm to relax them. So although they are awake they are so relaxed they don't feel a thing. The only problem is you have to be accompanied as it can take several hours for the effects to wear off. This type of injection isn't addictive.

SELF-HELP
Practise the drill for instant relief from a panic attack (see p.287).
Visualization
1. Imagine you are going to the dentist and visualize the trip from the moment you are leaving your house until you get to the dentist's door. Note your reactions. Use relaxation (see right) to reduce anxiety. As you familiarize yourself with what you see, venture closer, observing and coping as before.
2. Visualize being in the reception, waiting room or surgery. Imagine that your dentist says you need to have some tests. Stay with this and observe your reactions even though you may want to escape. Observe what you are thinking – perhaps you are imagining some complicated

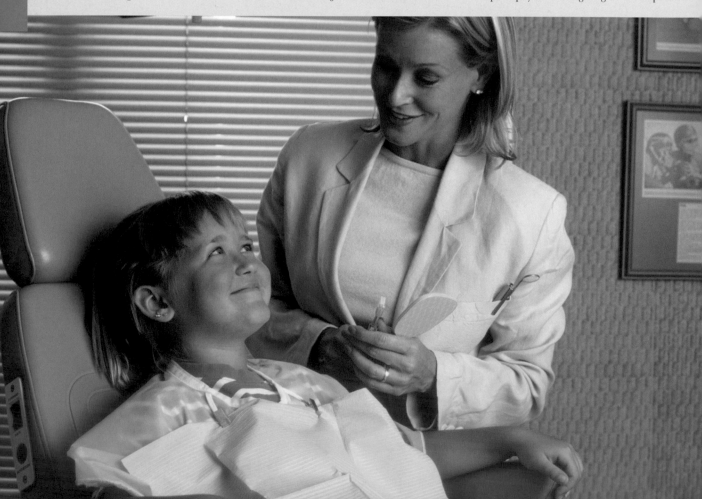

treatment. If your mind is racing along these lines, again don't stop. Stay with the thoughts until they no longer have any effect.

● The British Dental Health Foundation (BDHF) suggests one of the best ways to find **a dentist sympathetic to nervous patients** is through a friend's recommendation. Doctors can sometimes provide useful guidance on where to find sympathetic dentists. Or contact several local dental practices and explain you are nervous and ask what treatment is available for someone like you.

● To start with, just book a consultation appointment so you can discuss your fears before making any commitment to treatment. Try to take someone with you for moral support.

The BDHF can provide more information on what's available to relieve any pain and discomfort and has a variety of **free brochures**, including "Don't be Afraid", "Going to the Dentist", "Treatment Options" and "Caring for Your Teeth".

● Try and get hold of a **relaxation tape**. Play it at home and take it to the dentist with you.

● **Hypnotherapy** can work wonders for some people. You may require several sessions so it can be expensive. If you would like to explore this avenue, I suggest you get in touch with the British Society of Medical and Dental Hypnosis as it is crucial to find a qualified hypnotist and they can provide a list.

Relaxation exercises

Head: Sit in a chair with arms, shoulders and head supported. Clench fists, hold tension and relax. Repeat until hands feel relaxed. With mouth open, take a deep breath, hold it for five seconds and let the air out. Repeat six times. You will feel more calm and relaxed.

Legs: Stretch both legs out, holding them in the air. Point toes away from yourself, holding the tension. Pull toes to point towards yourself and tense leg muscles. Relax, letting legs flop onto the floor. Repeat until legs feel loose and relaxed.

Stomach: Contract stomach muscles and take a deep breath and hold the tension. Relax, letting breath out. Repeat five times

Arms: Clench fists, hold tension and relax. Stretch arms up (as if to touch the ceiling) and tense muscles, reaching as high into the air as possible. Relax, letting arms drop to sides. Repeat until your arms feel quite loose and relaxed.

Shoulders: Shrug shoulders so that they touch your ears. Then let them drop and relax. Repeat five times. Push shoulders forwards and inwards to meet each other, making a "hump" in your back (pushing arms forwards). Push shoulders backwards and inwards, arching your back. Hold the tension and then relax, falling back into the chair. Repeat five times.

Neck: Move head to left, hold tension. Turn head to right and hold tension. Press head forwards with your chin on your chest and tense back of neck. Relax, allowing head to fall back onto chair. Repeat five times.

Head and face: Raise eyebrows, tense and then frown and tense. Repeat until scalp and forehead are relaxed. Close eyes very tightly. Screw up eyes and hold tension. Relax, letting eyelids drop and close eyes. Clench teeth, feel the tension and then relax, letting the jaw drop slightly. Screw mouth into a whistling shape or "O", then tense lips as if to make an "E" sound. Relax mouth.

● Concentrate on breathing deeply and regularly, letting breath out when breathing out.

● Let yourself sink, relaxed, into the chair. Remain like this for about 10 minutes – and let yourself enjoy it.

● Pick your favourite relaxing scene and fill your mind with it.

Remember

● When you have finished relaxing, slowly open your eyes.

● Never jump up and rush around immediately.

● Use relaxation on any part of your body that feels tense during the day.

● Deep breathing is useful anywhere to help you feel calm.

● Begin by relaxing when you are on your own. Soon you will find you can do it quite easily with other people around you.

● Begin by doing each exercise in turn. Later you will find that you can just sit down and relax in a moment, doing a few exercises.

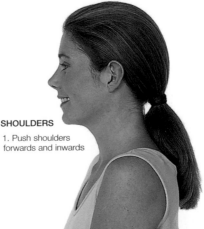

ARMS

Stretch arms up and tense muscles

SHOULDERS

1. Push shoulders forwards and inwards

2. Push shoulders backwards and inwards

continued from page 485

■ While it is a myth that your teeth suffer during pregnancy, your gums certainly do – one of the effects of the high level of circulating oestrogen and progesterone that occurs during pregnancy is softening of the gum margins. For this reason alone, you should visit your dentist two or three times during pregnancy to make sure all is well.

■ There is unequivocal evidence to show the sort of diet we eat affects the health of our gums and teeth, and that dental decay is caused in the main by sweet, sugary foods containing sucrose. Such foods include most refined foods and sweet drinks, sweets, chocolate and ice cream. If you want to have healthy teeth do not have sweet, sugary foods or drinks between meals – within 20 minutes of taking such foods, damage to your gums and teeth has already begun.

■ Dentists agree that "**safe snacks**" would include any fresh, raw fruits and vegetables, potato crisps, nuts or cheese. Cheese is a particularly useful and healthy food for the mouth, gums and teeth, as it stimulates the production of saliva and it is a very good way to end a meal. Saliva helps prevent the production of plaque acid, which is caused by bacterial fermentation of sugar in the diet (the initial process that starts off tooth decay).

■ There is clear evidence that fluoride, in all its forms, protects the teeth against decay and it is most effective if the fluoride is actually incorporated in the teeth during their development. By far the best way of taking fluoride, of course, is in drinking water. Also make sure that you always use fluoride toothpaste and consult your dentist about giving fluoride tablets or drops to your children to protect their developing teeth.

■ The arch villain of tooth decay is **plaque acid**, which corrodes the outer protective enamel of the teeth and eventually works its way through to the inner living part of the tooth, the pulp cavity (causing pulpitis).

■ Smoking upsets the natural bacterial flora of the mouth; it causes unpleasant mouth odour and stains the teeth, mouth, and even the skin surrounding the lips, an unpleasant yellowish colour. It also increases the risk of gum disease and mouth cancer.

■ Certain drugs can affect the health of the gums and teeth. Anti-epileptic drugs, such as hydantoins, can make the gum margins red, soft and swollen. Some drugs used to treat heart conditions can also cause the gums to swell. Tetracyclines, if taken by a pregnant mother, may be deposited in her baby's developing teeth and may stain the teeth a yellowish colour.

Dental caries

GRADUAL, PROGRESSIVE DECAY OF A TOOTH IS KNOWN AS DENTAL CARIES.

Dental caries usually starts as a small cavity in the enamel (the hard, protective outer covering of a tooth).

If left untreated, the decay eventually penetrates the outer layer of enamel and attacks the dentine (the softer material that makes up the bulk of a tooth). As the tooth decay progresses, the pulp (the living core of the tooth that contains the nerves and the blood vessels) may be affected. If the pulp is exposed to decay and becomes infected, it may die.

WHAT ARE THE CAUSES?

■ Tooth decay is usually caused by a build-up of **plaque** (a deposit of food particles, mucus and bacteria) on the surface of the teeth. The bacteria in plaque break down the sugar in food to produce an acid that erodes the tooth enamel. If sugary foods and drinks are taken regularly and the teeth are not cleaned thoroughly soon afterwards, a cavity is likely to form eventually.

■ The condition is especially common in children, adolescents and young adults as they are more likely to have a diet high in sugar and fail to clean their teeth regularly.

■ Babies who frequently fall asleep with a bottle of juice in the mouth may also develop severe caries, especially in the front teeth, called "bottle mouth".

WHAT MIGHT BE DONE?

■ Your dentist will examine your teeth with a probe and a mirror to look for areas of decay. An X-ray may also be taken to reveal decay

that may be developing beneath the surfaces of the teeth.

■ If you have superficial dental caries that is restricted to the surfaces of the enamel, your dentist may only apply fluoride to the area and advise you to be more careful about oral hygiene.

■ If tooth decay has penetrated further into the enamel, or if it has affected the dentine, your dentist will probably need to fill the affected tooth. An injection of local anaesthetic is often used to numb the tooth and nearby gum to prevent you from feeling pain. When the area is numb, the decayed parts of the tooth are drilled out, and the cavity is cleaned and filled to stop further decay.

■ If you have pulpitis (inflammation of the pulp) and it is found that the pulp cannot be saved you may need root canal treatment.

CAN IT BE PREVENTED?

Your teeth and gums should be brushed and flossed regularly to keep them clean and free from plaque. You can also help prevent dental caries from developing by resisting the temptation of sugary foods and drinks and eating safe snacks.

See also:
• **Root canal** p.489
• **X-rays** p.426

Toothbrushes

The dental profession is fairly well united on the sort of toothbrush you should use and the frequency with which you should use it. Here are some guidelines.

■ The toothbrush should have a short handle so that it is easy to control, so that you know exactly where the head of the brush is and so that it doesn't waggle about in your mouth.

■ The handle of the brush should be straight, without any bends in it, so that again you can direct the head accurately.

■ The head of the brush should be fairly small and the bristles ideally should be fairly short.

■ Choose nylon bristle, not pure bristle, because it resists splitting and bending better than natural material.

■ Make sure that the heads of the bristles are absolutely flat. On no account choose a toothbrush with a serrated edge.

■ The bristles should not be too hard; choose one labelled "medium".

■ Brush your teeth twice a day. Buy a new toothbrush at least every six weeks, or as soon as the bristles become misshapen.

■ Use a fluoride toothpaste.

Dental abscess

AN ACCUMULATION OF PUS IN OR AROUND THE ROOT OF A TOOTH IS KNOWN AS A DENTAL
ABSCESS. A DENTAL ABSCESS CAN BE EXTREMELY PAINFUL AND MAY CAUSE THE AFFECTED
TOOTH TO LOOSEN IN ITS SOCKET.

WHAT ARE THE CAUSES?

An abscess usually develops as a complication
of dental caries, which gradually destroys the
layer of enamel on the outside of the tooth
and the inner dentine, allowing bacteria to
invade the soft central core or pulp of the
tooth. Eventually, a dental abscess may form,
which is agonizingly painful and may cause the
gum adjacent to the tooth to swell and become
very tender (a gum boil).

An abscess may also form as a result of
certain forms of gum disease (periodontitis).
Periodontitis is usually caused by a build-up
of dental plaque (a deposit including food
particles, mucus and bacteria) in a pocket that
forms between a tooth and gum.

WHAT ARE THE SYMPTOMS?

The main symptoms of a dental abscess
develop gradually and may include:
- throbbing pain in the affected tooth
- severe pain on touching the affected tooth
and on biting or chewing
- loosening of the affected tooth
- red, tender swelling of the gum over the
root of the tooth
- release of pus into the mouth.

If the abscess is not treated, the infection
may make a channel from the tooth to the
surface of the gum, and a painful swelling,
known as a gum boil, forms. Should the gum
boil burst, foul-tasting pus is released and the
pain decreases. In some cases the channel may
persist, which leads to a chronic abscess that
discharges pus periodically. If the infection
spreads to surrounding tissues, your face may

become swollen and you may develop a fever.
If you suspect you have an abscess, you should
consult your dentist as soon as possible.

WHAT CAN I DO?

If there is a delay before you are able to see
your dentist, you can try taking painkillers
such as paracetamol, which may relieve pain.
Rinsing your mouth with warm saltwater may
also help decrease the pain and possibly
encourage a gum boil to burst. If a gum boil
does burst, wash away the pus thoroughly with
more warm saltwater.

WHAT MIGHT THE DENTIST DO?

- Your dentist will ask you about your teeth
and gums. He or she may take an X-ray of your
mouth to confirm the diagnosis.
- If the abscess has been caused by tooth
decay, your dentist will always try to save the
tooth. Under local anaesthesia, a hole is drilled
through the top of the tooth to release the pus,
which will have the effect of relieving the pain.
If there is a gum boil, a small cut may be made
in the boil to drain the pus. The cavity is then
cleaned with an antiseptic solution.
- To treat an abscess caused by gum disease,
your dentist may use a probe to scrape out the
plaque from the pocket between the affected
tooth and gum. Afterwards, the pocket is
washed out with an antiseptic solution.
- Pockets are treated with several weeks of
intensive oral hygiene, including frequent
brushing, flossing and the use of antiseptic gel
on the floss. Most can be eradicated.

TREATMENT

Root canal

Sometimes, decay invades and destroys
the pulp, containing nerves and blood
vessels, at the centre of the tooth, and
root canal treatment may be performed.
The pulp is removed and an antiseptic
solution is used to sterilize the cavity. If
infection within the tooth is severe, a
temporary filling may be inserted for a
few days before the cavity is sterilized
again. The root canals and the decayed
area of the tooth are then filled.

- Whatever the cause of the abscess, you will
probably be prescribed a course of antibiotics.
- Once the infection has cleared up, you may
need root canal treatment (see box, above).
- If it is not possible to save the tooth, an
extraction is the only remaining option.
- An extracted tooth can be replaced with a
denture, bridge or an implant.

WHAT IS THE OUTLOOK?

Most treatment is successful, but a small area
of infection may persist and further treatment
may be required.

See also:
- **Dental caries p.488** - Gingivitis p.493

Malocclusion (poor bite)

IDEALLY, THE UPPER FRONT TEETH SHOULD SLIGHTLY OVERLAP THE LOWER FRONT TEETH
AND THE MOLARS SHOULD MEET EVENLY. HOWEVER, PERFECT TEETH ARE RARE AND MOST
PEOPLE HAVE SOME TEETH THAT ARE OUT OF POSITION.

Imperfections are not usually a pressing
problem unless appearance is adversely
affected or biting and chewing are impaired.

A poor bite may occur if teeth are crowded
and overlap each other, making them crooked.
Another cause is misalignment of the jaws, so
that the upper front teeth protrude excessively
in front of the lower teeth, or the lower jaw
juts out in front of the upper jaw. The back
teeth may prevent the front teeth from
meeting, a condition known as an open bite.

WHAT ARE THE CAUSES?

Malocclusion often runs in families and usually
develops in childhood when the teeth and jaws
are growing. The condition is usually caused
by a discrepancy between the number and size
of the teeth and the growth of the jaws.
Protrusion of the front teeth may also be
caused by children who persistently suck their
thumbs beyond about age 6. If the primary
teeth are lost early (before age 9 or 10)
because of decay, the secondary molars that

are already in position may move forward to
take up some of the space meant for the new
front teeth. The new teeth then become
crowded and misaligned.

WHAT ARE THE SYMPTOMS?

The symptoms develop gradually from about
age 6 onwards. They may include:
- out-of-line, crowded or abnormally
spaced teeth

continued on page 492

FOCUS *on* cosmetic dentistry

If you want to have a perfect white smile when you are 20, you (and your parents) will need to start working on it when you are a baby. It is no good thinking that primary or milk teeth are unimportant simply because children start to lose them around the age of 6.

Strong, well-positioned milk teeth guide the secondary or permanent teeth as they erupt and grow to take up their lifelong positions in the jawbones. If the milk teeth are overcrowded, the permanent ones may grow in crookedly. If a gap has been left by the removal of a decayed milk tooth, the permanent teeth on either side of the gap will not be encouraged to grow upright.

It is therefore worthwhile taking good care of milk teeth from the moment that they appear. Never offer a child a bottle filled with fruit juice as a pacifier – its sugar content rapidly decays the teeth and encourages a "sweet tooth" in later life. It is helpful to give a baby hard foods to chew on as soon as he or she develops the liking for **chomping,** since chewing movements exercise the jaw muscles and help to make the teeth grow in straight.

The chances of serious tooth decay can be **minimized by attention to diet** (avoiding a lot of sweet and starchy foods), careful tooth-brushing with the right kind of toothbrush (see p. 488) and regular visits to the dentist. The use of fluoride either in the form of tablets or drops or as toothpaste also helps stop decay.

WHITENING THE TEETH

According to the best dental opinion, no good "cosmetics" for the teeth can be bought over the counter. **Toothpastes** that claim to whiten teeth usually do so by two methods.

The first is really an optical illusion: the toothpaste contains a red pigment that turns the gums deep pink, so that the teeth look whiter in comparison.

Toothpastes that use the second method, and claim to give a polished, gleaming smile, make the teeth shine by use of abrasives (including one known as "**jeweller's rouge**"). These substances are much too harsh to use on teeth – they work by scratching the surface enamel, which may be damaged or worn away through prolonged use of such toothpastes. Since there has been a move away from using abrasives on stainless steel kitchen sinks and ceramic baths and basins, it seems astonishing that we should continue to consider using them on our teeth.

The best and safest way to give your teeth a new look is to visit a **dental hygienist**. To keep your gums and teeth healthy you should go at least every six months – every three months is even better. The hygienist will remove from between the teeth **calculus** (hardened plaque), which irritates the gums and makes them bleed. The hygienist does this by **descaling** your teeth and giving them a good polish. This treatment makes everyone's teeth look several shades whiter, particularly smokers'.

WHAT THE COSMETIC DENTIST CAN DO

It is possible for a good, skilled cosmetic dentist to alter completely not just the look of

Repositioning teeth

In cosmetic dentistry much can be achieved by the use of simple methods and materials. It is quite possible to move the roots of teeth within the jawbone by perhaps a fraction of a **millimetre**, if they are pushed or pulled in one direction for any length of time. Even such a tiny adjustment makes a great difference to the overall effect. Very often, sufficient force can be applied to a **misaligned** tooth simply by the expert use of elastic bands. For more severe deformities, wires and braces can be fitted to manipulate the teeth over a period of months into the desired position.

your teeth or your smile, but also the set of your mouth and therefore, to some degree, your facial expression. If, for instance, your teeth have been ground away over the years either because you are a "night grinder" or simply because you have especially strong masticating muscles, your jawbones will tend to come closer together. This accentuates the folds on either side of your mouth and may have an **ageing** appearance. A cosmetic dentist can open up the distance between the jawbones by repositioning or crowning the teeth, thereby stretching out the skin in your laughter lines. This procedure can also relieve pain and tenderness in the joints of the jaw, which become over-stressed when the teeth are ground away.

Cosmetic dentistry can also change the shape, colour and arrangement of your teeth to give a more pleasing appearance.

CAPS AND CROWNS

A broken, ugly or severely **malpositioned** tooth can be given a new appearance and a new lease of life by capping or crowning (the two terms are synonymous). This is usually done by filing the tooth away to form a "peg" onto which the cap is cemented. Even a tooth that has snapped off or has had to be removed at the line of the gum margin can be capped. In such cases one or more "posts" onto which the cap can be fixed are drilled into the remnants of the tooth.

Caps and crowns are made of a variety of materials. The most modern ones are composed of extremely strong porcelains or metals covered in porcelain, which come in a number of **colours** so that the finished cap will exactly match the rest of the teeth. The cap can be made in any shape to conform to the size and contour of the original tooth – indeed its shape may even be slightly imperfect in order to maintain a natural appearance.

REPLACEMENT TEETH

If one or more teeth have to be extracted, or if they are lost, they can be replaced by one of three different types of artificial teeth: a bridge, dentures or a dental implant.

A bridge consists of one or more artificial teeth that are fixed permanently in the mouth, usually by being attached to adjacent natural teeth. This may require the adjacent teeth to be crowned.

A denture can be removed and may replace any number of teeth. Dentures have a metal or

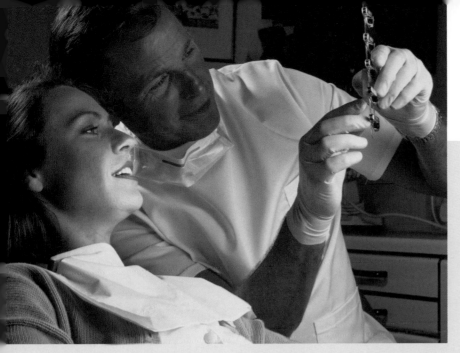

BUCK TEETH

Ideally, buck teeth should be treated before the age of 14 by a **paediatric orthodontist** who will use braces and wires to pull the teeth into line with the rest. If you reach adulthood with buck teeth, cosmetic dentistry can sometimes correct the deformity by the use of caps or crowns. The **malpositioned teeth** are filed away and the caps fitted to follow the normal line.

Cosmetic dentistry at its best is highly creative and good practitioners will rise to almost any challenge to find an inventive way of correcting tooth deformity. One of the most beautiful and effective examples I have seen was the correction of malpositioned teeth in a person with a cleft palate. Because of the cleft, there were fewer teeth than is normal; in addition, the teeth had moved round the jaw so that the front teeth were off-centre. The dentist transformed the appearance by using each of the existing teeth as the basis for a cap, but moving the position of every cap on its tooth a **millimetre** or so along in the direction that brought them all back to centre.

plastic **baseplate** and stay in place by resting on the gum ridges or are held in place by clasps that fit onto the natural teeth. They can be removed for cleaning, either with a sterilizing solution or with a brush.

An implant is a permanent and effective method of replacing a single tooth. A hole is drilled in the jaw at the site of the missing tooth, and a screw is firmly fixed into the hole. A few weeks later when the site has healed, an artificial tooth is fitted to the top of the screw.

"SHORTENING" OR "LENGTHENING" TEETH

In some people with periodontal disease the gums recede, exposing the root surfaces of the teeth. This can make the teeth very sensitive to hot and cold foods and make the crown of the tooth look very long. (Because this appearance is seen more frequently in the elderly, it has given rise to the expression "long in the tooth".) If excellent oral hygiene can be achieved it is possible to reposition the gum surgically to cover the exposed root surfaces and improve the appearance. Alternatively it may be possible to crown or reshape the teeth to hide the appearance.

Some people have the reverse problem – the gums grow too far up the teeth so that they are, or appear to be, too short, or heavy grinding or clenching of the teeth may wear the teeth away. Again it may be possible to improve the appearance by crowning the teeth.

See also:
• Malocclusion p.489

Cosmetic teeth whitening

Cosmetic teeth whitening is a non-invasive procedure that uses a bleaching agent to lighten the colour of the teeth. Your dentist begins by making a mould of your teeth, from which a plastic tray that fits over your teeth is made. Your dentist then shows you how to fill this tray with a bleaching gel. You will be instructed to wear the tray at home for a few hours each day or possibly overnight. The length of treatment depends on the gel that is used and the degree of lightening to be achieved, but it usually lasts from a week to 10 days. A similar technique may be used to lighten teeth in the dentist's surgery.

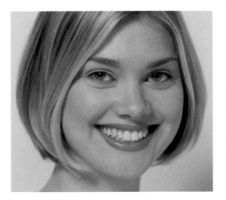

Before teeth whitening

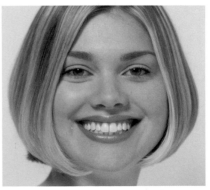

After teeth whitening

continued from page 489

- excessive protrusion of the upper teeth in front of the lower teeth
- a protruding lower jaw
- front teeth that do not meet.

Some children have some mild symptoms, but these are often temporary and tend to result from a growth spurt.

In severe cases of malocclusion, speech and chewing may be affected. An abnormal bite may be painful or cause discomfort in or around the jaw joint. A severe malocclusion may also affect the facial appearance.

WHAT MIGHT BE DONE?

- The dentist will look for malocclusion as part of a dental check-up.

- If malocclusion is found, a specialist dentist called an **orthodontist** may take casts of the teeth to study the bite in detail. The orthodontist may also take X-rays of the teeth, especially if some of the teeth have not erupted.
- Treatment is usually only necessary if malocclusion is severe and causing difficulties when eating and speaking or affecting appearance.
- If the teeth are overcrowded, some of them may be extracted.
- Rough or irregular teeth are often reshaped or capped.
- If required, the teeth may then be aligned using an orthodontic appliance such as a brace.
- Surgery is very rarely necessary.

It is best to treat malocclusion during childhood, when the teeth and jaw bones are still developing. However, if malocclusion is caused by a severe mismatch in the size of the jaws and teeth, surgery may be needed and treatment may be delayed until adulthood.

See also:
- Temporomandibular joint disorder p.494

TREATMENT

Orthodontic treatment

Orthodontics is the correction of crowded or unevenly spaced teeth. Orthodontic treatment is usually performed on older children and adolescents while the teeth are still developing, although adults can also benefit.

Casts of the teeth are taken before an orthodontic appliance, also called a brace,

is applied to move or straighten the teeth gradually. In some cases, it is necessary to extract one or more teeth to make space for others. The treatment is usually long-term and may take several months or years to complete, with regular visits to the orthodontist for check-ups.

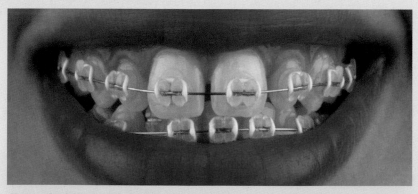

Close up of a child's mouth fitted with a fixed dental brace.

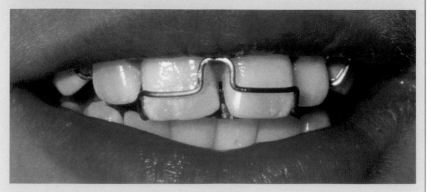

Close up of a child's mouth fitted with a removable dental brace.

TYPES OF MALOCCLUSION

There is a wide range of malocclusions, which can be divided into a small number of groups depending on the position of the first molars. Some common types of malocclusion are shown below.

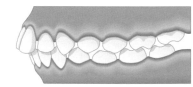

Misalignment of the molars, causing a slight overbite

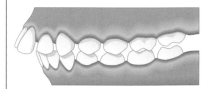

Overbite (also known as overjet), with the molars misaligned

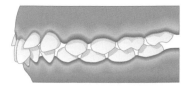

Incisors retroclined (no overlap with lower teeth); lateral incisors proclined (leaning forwards)

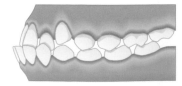

Underbite (also known as underjet), with the molars misaligned

GUM DISORDERS

Healthy gum forms a tight seal around the base of the crown of a tooth and protects the sensitive root area below from bacterial infection and corrosion. If the gums are damaged or form pockets, the teeth are more likely to decay. Most gum disorders are caused by plaque (a deposit of food particles, mucus and bacteria on the surfaces of the teeth) and can be prevented by good oral hygiene.

Most adults have some degree of gum disease which, if left untreated, may eventually lead to loss of teeth. Good oral hygiene is essential to help prevent gum disorders. During regular dental check-ups, most dentists and oral hygienists provide information on the correct way to brush and floss teeth and on general mouth care.

Gingivitis and **periodontitis**, both of which can lead to loosening and loss of teeth, are caused, in the main, by poor oral hygiene. Inadequate teeth cleaning leads to build-up of **plaque** on the teeth. If the plaque is not removed, it causes the gums to become inflamed

(gingivitis). In more serious cases, pockets form in which bacteria can erode tooth enamel and cause tooth decay and inflammation of the bony membrane around the tooth (periodontitis). The teeth may be affected and loosen or come out, either

because the periodontal tissues are inflamed and detach from the teeth or because the gums recede, exposing the roots and leading to tooth decay.

Gingivitis (gum disease)

MILD INFLAMMATION OF THE GUM MARGINS (GINGIVITIS) IS VERY COMMON AND OCCURS IN ABOUT 9 OUT OF 10 ADULTS. HEALTHY GUMS ARE PINK AND FIRM. IN GINGIVITIS, THE GUMS BECOME PURPLE-RED, SOFT AND SHINY AND BLEED EASILY, ESPECIALLY WHEN BRUSHED.

The condition is usually caused by build-up of plaque (a deposit of food particles, mucus and bacteria) where the gum meets the base of the tooth.

Gingivitis can be made worse by taking some drugs, such as phenytoin for epilepsy and antihypertensives. These drugs may cause overgrowth of the gums, making the removal of dental plaque difficult. Some contraceptive drugs can also make the symptoms worse. Pregnant women are particularly susceptible to gingivitis because of dramatic changes in their hormone levels.

If gingivitis develops suddenly in acute form, it is known as "**trench mouth**", usually occurring in teenagers and young adults. The condition sometimes develops from chronic gingivitis and is caused by an abnormal growth of the bacteria that normally exist harmlessly within the mouth. Trench mouth is more common in people who are stressed or run down and in people with AIDS.

WHAT ARE THE SYMPTOMS?
The symptoms of gingivitis develop gradually and usually include:
- purple-red, soft, shiny, swollen gums
- gums that bleed when brushed.

If gingivitis is not treated, a pocket develops between the tooth and the gum in which more dental plaque can form. Bacteria in the plaque may cause the inflammation to spread. Eventually, chronic periodontitis or receding gums may develop. In severe cases, one or

more teeth may be lost.

Symptoms of trench mouth usually develop over 1–2 days and may include:
- bright red gums that are covered with a greyish deposit
- crater-like ulcers on the gums
- gums that bleed easily
- bad breath and a metallic taste in the mouth
- pain in the gums.

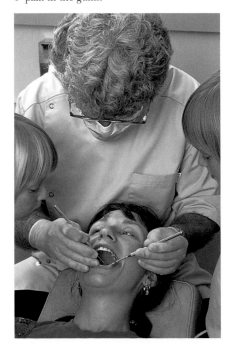

As trench mouth progresses, the lymph glands in the neck may become enlarged and you may develop a fever.

WHAT IS THE TREATMENT?
- Gingivitis is treated and prevented by effective tooth-brushing and oral hygiene to remove plaque from around the gum margin.
- If you have gingivitis, your dentist will probably scale your teeth to remove the plaque and **calculus** (hardened plaque). The procedure involves using an **ultrasonic scaler** to remove the calculus and scraping away at resistant areas with a hand tool. After scaling, the teeth are polished. Regular follow-up visits to the dentist may be necessary to monitor the condition of your gums. Your dentist may also recommend using an antiseptic mouthwash.
- If you have trench mouth, your dentist will clean carefully around all the teeth. He or she will also prescribe antibiotics and an antiseptic mouthwash. Analgesics may be prescribed to relieve pain. Once your teeth have been scaled and cleaned, your gums will gradually return to normal.

See also:
- **Caring for your teeth and gums p.485**

Receding gums

HEALTHY GUMS FORM A TIGHT SEAL AROUND THE TOOTH WHERE THE CROWN OF THE TOOTH MEETS THE ROOT. IF THE GUMS RECEDE, THE ROOT OF THE TOOTH BECOMES EXPOSED, CAUSING THE ATTACHMENT BETWEEN THE TOOTH AND THE SOCKET TO WEAKEN.

When the gum recedes, the tooth may eventually become loose and, in severe cases, may have to be extracted by the dentist.

If the roots are exposed, the teeth may be sensitive to hot, cold or sweet substances. Since the roots are softer than the enamel on the crown of the tooth, they are also more susceptible to decay.

Periodontitis affects many people over 55 and is a major cause of tooth loss. In this condition, the periodontal tissues that secure teeth in their sockets become inflamed, and the teeth loosen. Eventually, teeth may fall out. The damage from periodontitis is irreversible, but further inflammation can be prevented with treatment and by improving oral hygiene.

WHAT ARE THE CAUSES?

■ Severely receding gums are usually a symptom of chronic gingivitis or periodontitis.
■ These disorders are usually a result of **poor**

oral hygiene and a **build-up of plaque** (a deposit of food particles, mucus, and bacteria) and calculus (hardened plaque) between the base of the teeth and gums. The gums will eventually become inflamed and recede, exposing the roots of the teeth.
■ Vigorous, abrasive tooth brushing along the margins of the gums, particularly in a horizontal direction with a hard toothbrush, may also cause the gums to recede.
■ Toothpastes containing abrasives contribute.

WHAT MIGHT BE DONE?

■ Improving your oral hygiene is important in order to stop the gums from receding further.
■ Your dentist or oral hygienist will probably use a procedure known as scaling to remove plaque and calculus from your teeth. Scaling should help prevent your gums from receding any further.

■ She will also advise you on your tooth brushing and flossing techniques to avoid further damage to the exposed roots.
■ Your dentist or oral hygienist may also suggest that you use a desensitizing toothpaste or fluoride mouthwash, which will also reduce the risk of decay.
■ If your teeth are very sensitive, the dentist may treat them with a desensitizing varnish or an adhesive filling material.
■ Gum-grafting procedures may be used to help cover exposed root surfaces and prevent further recession of the gums.
■ If severely receding gums cause your teeth to loosen, they can sometimes be fixed to teeth that are more firmly anchored in the jawbone.

See also:
• **Caring for your teeth and gums p.485**
• **Gingivitis p.493**

Temporomandibular joint disorder

THE TEMPOROMANDIBULAR JOINT CONNECTS THE MANDIBLE (LOWER JAWBONE) TO THE PART OF THE SKULL KNOWN AS THE TEMPORAL BONE. THE JOINT ALLOWS THE LOWER JAW TO MOVE IN ALL DIRECTIONS SO THAT THE TEETH CAN BE USED TO BITE OFF AND CHEW FOOD EFFICIENTLY.

In temporomandibular joint disorder, the joint, the muscles and the ligaments that control the joint do not work together properly, causing pain. The condition is three times more likely to occur in women.

Temporomandibular joint disorder is most commonly caused by **spasm** of the chewing muscles, often as a result of **clenching the jaw** or **grinding the teeth**. Clenching the jaw and grinding the teeth may be increased by stress. A poor bite (malocclusion) places stress on the muscles and may also be the cause of temporomandibular joint disorder, as may an injury to the head, jaw or neck that causes displacement of the joint. In some cases, arthritis is a cause.

WHAT ARE THE SYMPTOMS?

You may notice one or more of the following symptoms:
● headaches
● tenderness in the jaw muscles
● aching pain in the face
● severe pain near the ears.

In some cases, pain is caused by chewing or by opening the mouth too widely when yawning. There may be difficulty in opening the mouth, locking of the jaw, and clicking noises from the joint as the mouth is opened or closed.

WHAT MIGHT BE DONE?

■ Your dentist may take X-rays of your mouth and jaws.
■ He may also arrange for you to see a specialist for treatment and investigations such as CT or MRI.
■ Treatment is aimed at eliminating muscle spasm and tension and relieving pain.
■ There are several self-help measures that you can adopt, including applying a warm, wet towel to the face, massaging the facial muscles, eating only soft foods and using a device that fits over the teeth at night to prevent you from clenching or grinding your teeth.
■ Taking analgesics, such as aspirin and paracetamol, may also help relieve pain.
■ Your doctor may prescribe muscle-relaxant

drugs if tension of the muscles used for chewing is severe.
■ If stress is a major factor, relaxation techniques may help.
■ If your bite needs to be adjusted, your dentist may recommend wearing a fixed or removable orthodontic appliance for a period of time.

WHAT IS THE OUTLOOK?

In approximately 3 out of 4 people with temporomandibular joint disorder, symptoms improve within three months of treatment. However, if symptoms do not improve, further treatment may be required. In a few cases surgery to the joint may be necessary.

See also:
• **Malocclusion p.489** • **MRI p.409**
• **Rheumatoid arthritis p.429**

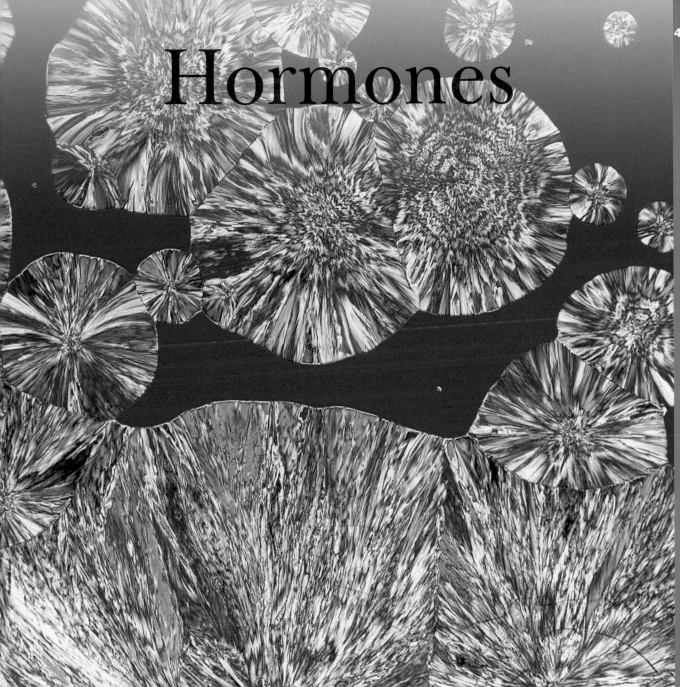

Hormones

Image shows a polarized light micrograph of crystals of the hormone progesterone

Miriam's overview

When I was a medical student hormones were a difficult concept for me to get my head around. They're defined as:

"Chemical messengers which are formed in one part of the body, usually a hormone gland, passed into the bloodstream to be carried to a distant part of the body where they exert an effect". But that definition fails to describe their intricacy.

They control most of the vital functions of the body. They certainly regulate every aspect of metabolism. And they keep all our organs in working order.

What's more, each hormone is bespoke. It's like a laser beam, focusing on one small area of our overall health. Together hormones are like an orchestra and by a myriad ingenious checks and balances they play in tune most of the time. Naturally they require a conductor and we have one, the pituitary gland in the brain, a tiny organ that has the power to switch hormones on and off.

If a rogue hormone gland gets out of control we soon know about it. An overactive thyroid gland or adrenal gland makes us ill. An underactive pancreas gives us symptoms of diabetes; and failing ovaries, the menopause. We label this kind of hormonal failure a hormone deficiency state and correct it with hormone supplements as different as insulin for diabetes and HRT for the menopause.

"together *hormones* are like *an orchestra*"

So hormones are very potent body regulators, some so powerful that they are life-giving and curative. We have harnessed hormones from the adrenal glands, the steroids, to arrest inflammation as different as arthritis and psoriasis.

The sex hormones we've synthesized into potent forms to control basic mechanisms such as ovulation to give us virtually 100 percent effective contraception.

INSIDE your metabolism

Hormones are chemicals that influence or change the activity of particular cells in the body. They are produced by a number of different **glands** and **organs** and are carried in the bloodstream to reach their target cells. The production of hormones is regulated by feedback mechanisms, which help to ensure that the correct levels of hormones and other substances are maintained in the blood. The **pituitary gland**, a pea-sized organ located at the base of the brain and regulated by the **hypothalamus**, orchestrates most of the body's hormone secretion.

Major hormone-secreting glands and organs include the **thyroid**, **parathyroid** and **adrenal** glands, the **pancreas** and the **testes** in men and **ovaries** in women. Other organs that secrete hormones include the **kidneys**, the **heart** and the **stomach**.

hormone-secreting glands and cells

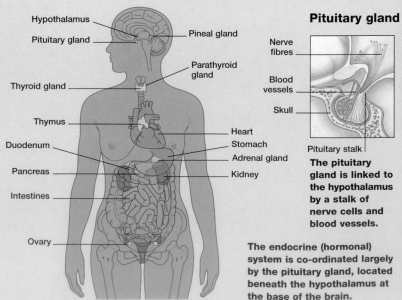

Hypothalamus
Pituitary gland
Pineal gland
Parathyroid gland
Thyroid gland
Thymus
Heart
Stomach
Duodenum
Adrenal gland
Pancreas
Kidney
Intestines
Ovary

Pituitary gland

Nerve fibres
Blood vessels
Skull
Pituitary stalk

The pituitary gland is linked to the hypothalamus by a stalk of nerve cells and blood vessels.

The endocrine (hormonal) system is co-ordinated largely by the pituitary gland, located beneath the hypothalamus at the base of the brain.

THE MENOPAUSE

Most women reach the menopause between the ages of 40 and 55 in the UK. The average age is 51. The production of sex hormones slows down; the ovaries stop producing eggs; and monthly periods become less frequent and eventually stop altogether, so after the menopause a woman can no longer get pregnant. The menopause is an oestrogen-deficiency state and the symptoms that arise are due to lack of oestrogen. Most of them are cured by taking oestrogen in the form of hormone replacement therapy (HRT). The symptoms most commonly associated with the "change" include hot flushes and night sweats; dryness and soreness of the vagina and consequently some pain on intercourse; anxiety, depression, irritability and tiredness; an inability to sleep at night; a fall in sexual interest; dry skin and thinning hair; and urinary and bladder problems due to the thinning of the bladder lining.

Women going through the menopause have a tendency to put on weight – particularly around the waist, "middle-age spread". This change in shape with loss of the waistline is a sign that carries an increased risk of heart disease, a side effect of the menopause along with stroke, osteoporosis and Alzheimer's disease. All of these long-term health hazards of the menopause are ameliorated by HRT.

I believe in women managing their menopause and taking steps to have the menopause they want. There are many tools all women can use in taking responsibility for their own menopausal health. The single most effective tool available is HRT.

SELF-HELP

As well as vitamins and herbal remedies available for menopausal women, there are a number of useful things that you can do to help yourself.

To cope with hot flushes, for example, try to keep the room temperature fairly low and wear loose rather than tight clothing (cottons are good). At night it may be useful to have blankets that you can peel off easily if you get very hot. And keep spare night clothing by the bedside in case you have a night sweat. Avoid strong coffee, alcohol and salt. A glass of cold water may help.

If you feel that you are getting hot and red, then you may also be able to help yourself by "thinking cold". Imagine that you are standing in several inches of snow, or wandering around at a ski resort or taking part in an Arctic expedition. Your skin temperature will fall in response to your imagination and the amount of flushing that takes place will be kept to a minimum.

Finally, even though you feel bright red during a flush, do remember that the flush will probably be hardly noticeable to people around you.

To cope with a dry vagina and make intercourse more comfortable, try using an oil or jelly. You can buy special products from your local pharmacy or you can use an unscented body oil or baby oil. (Avoid anything too thick or greasy or lubricants containing alcohol or medicaments.) Remember that saliva makes a useful and effective lubricant.

Annoying or persistent menopausal symptoms merit a visit to the doctor since HRT is considered by many doctors to be safe and effective for most women who have problems. HRT can ease the symptoms women find most troublesome and, despite some controversy in the past, the majority of doctors now agree that replacing missing hormones is sensible, natural and acceptable. Where necessary the treatment can be continued for several years. Indeed I personally see no reason to stop.

Finally, remember that although most women do get one or two symptoms, many women go through the menopause with no unpleasant symptoms at all.

Coping with the menopause the non-hormonal way

SOME WOMEN SAIL THROUGH THE MENOPAUSE WITHOUT ANY PROBLEMS BUT MOST EXPERIENCE SYMPTOMS RANGING FROM MILD TO VERY SEVERE.

Hormone replacement therapy can make all the difference – but what are the options if HRT is unsuitable for you or your personal preference is not to interfere with nature? The good news is there is a lot you can do to help yourself, and homeopathic and herbal treatments can go a long way to relieving symptoms.

HOMEOPATHY

This is a form of natural healing based on the principle that a substance that produces the same symptoms as an illness will, in a very dilute form, help to cure that illness.

Homeopathic remedies are derived from mineral, animal or vegetable matter. The homeopathic view of menopausal problems is that they are a manifestation of existing imbalances that can only be treated with regard to the mental and physical make-up of an individual. Women are encouraged to prepare for the menopause by looking at their overall health and developing a positive attitude before its onset.

If you would like to treat your symptoms homeopathically, it is a good idea to consult a homeopathic practitioner. If you decide to treat yourself, bear in mind the following things.
■ You should stop taking a remedy as soon as your symptoms start to improve.
■ If your symptoms are not relieved after six doses, seek medical advice.
■ Homeopathic remedies should be kept in a cool, dark place away from smells.
■ Some substances, such as coffee, peppermint, menthol and camphor, counteract the effects of homeopathic remedies and should be avoided.
■ Some homeopathic pills are coated in milk sugar and you should avoid them if you are allergic to milk.

FOCUS *on* HRT

Hormone replacement therapy (HRT) is controversial but still the main proven method of treating troublesome symptoms that arise during the menopause. It's also an important preventive medicine since it reduces the risk of certain life-threatening or painful conditions such as bowel cancer and osteoporosis.

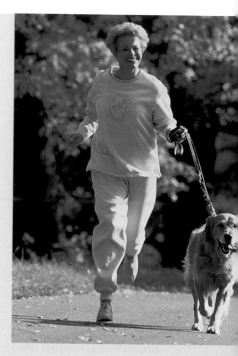

HRT is not right for everyone but knowing the advantages and disadvantages and gathering as much information as possible will help you make an informed choice about managing your menopause with your doctor.

There is hardly an organ in a woman's body whose health is not maintained by **oestrogen**. So most organs in a woman's body can benefit from oestrogen supplements when her ovaries fail at the end of her fertile life.

WHAT IS THE TREATMENT?

HRT is a combination of the female hormones oestrogen and synthetic progesterone **(progestogen)**. Oestrogen is given to maintain the health of vital organs such as the brain, bones and also the female sex organs. It also keeps the lining of the vagina and other body tissues elastic, the brain active, relieves anxiety and promotes sleep. It's helpful in preventing osteoporosis and possibly Alzheimer's disease.

Progestogen causes the uterine lining to shed, which means with some types of HRT you will still have a monthly period, but there are other no-bleed forms for you to choose from. When hormonal medication was first prescribed in the 1960s and 1970s only oestrogen was used. It was then discovered that women on this treatment had a slightly higher risk of uterine cancer than non-users. Since then, progestogen has also been prescribed since it eliminates the risk of uterine cancer and can even protect against it.

HOW DO I TAKE IT?

Types of HRT
Tablets – Most HRT is prescribed in tablet form, is highly effective in combating physical and emotional symptoms, and can be stopped immediately if it isn't right for you. It may be unsuitable if you have a history of high blood pressure, blood clotting, liver trouble, breast lumps or breast cancer, and diabetes. Some women experience breast tenderness and nausea and you may get breakthrough bleeding if you forget to take a tablet.
Creams – An applicator delivers measured doses

of oestrogen-impregnated cream directly into the vagina. It reduces genital itching, thinning, discomfort and urinary problems.
Pessaries – Pellets deliver low doses of oestrogen directly into the vagina, reducing vaginal dryness and pain when urinating. Both creams and pessaries are easy to use but doses are too low to deal with general menopausal symptoms or to act as a preventive medicine.
Transdermal (skin) patches – A low dose of hormone enters the body through the skin. Patches need to be changed every three to four days. A very few women develop red, itchy skin underneath the patch and this may get worse in a hot climate.
Skin gel – The lowest and most physiological form of HRT is delivered from a gel rubbed into the skin of the thighs and upper legs. It has the fewest side effects and you can alter the dose yourself. It's the form I favour.
Implants – A pellet containing a **six-month supply** of oestrogen is inserted under the skin of the abdomen or buttocks. Tablets of **progestogen** are usually taken as well. Implants give excellent relief from physical symptoms and protection against osteoporosis, but insertion requires minor surgery.

WAYS OF TAKING IT

Continuous therapy – The most common method. Oestrogen is absorbed daily either by taking a tablet or by wearing a skin patch twice a week. Progestogen is taken in pill form or in a combination skin patch for 12–14 days. More than 90 percent of women will have a monthly bleed, but many women find periods dry up after a few months.
Combined continuous therapy (no-bleed HRT) – Continuous daily doses of oestrogen with a very low dose of progestogen. Some women bleed at first but this usually stops after a few months. This method is popular with women on long-term treatment and women who start HRT when they're older, say, after osteoporosis develops.
Cyclical therapy – Oestrogen is taken from the first to the 21st day of the cycle and

progestogen for the last 12 or 13 days; both medications are stopped on the 21st day. Most women will have a withdrawal bleed between the 22nd and 28th day, but it usually stops over time. Alternatively, progestogen may be taken once every three months. This means that you have four bleeds a year.
SERMs – A non-oestrogen form of HRT is called **raloxifene** and is one of a group of drugs called SERMs (Selective oEstrogen Re-uptake Modulators). It protects the bones and has no risk of breast cancer. But it doesn't treat hot flushes, dry vagina or bladder symptoms as well as conventional HRT does. Nor does it protect against Alzheimer's disease.

HOW LONG DO I TAKE IT?

Treatment is usually continued for between two and five years as the body gradually adjusts to oestrogen deficiency. However, HRT must be taken for at least five years if it is to prevent bone loss. If you stop after a short time, symptoms such as hot flushes may return in a more severe form. Since there is a small increased risk of breast cancer after five years and again after 10 years, many doctors would say 10 years is the longest you should take HRT. However, the increase in risk is about the same as delaying your first child until after 30 and I, personally, am prepared to live with that risk to enjoy the benefits of HRT.

GALLBLADDER DISEASE

Between ages 50 and 75, 3 women in 100,000 not on HRT are estimated to die from complications of gallbladder disease. This figure doubles to 6 women in 100,000 among women on HRT.

WOMEN AT RISK

Women who fall into one or more of the following categories may be advised by their doctors not to take HRT, though if your menopausal symptoms are very severe you and your doctor can weigh up the pros and cons.
- High blood pressure.
- History of thrombosis.
- Diabetes.
- Chronic liver disease.
- History of breast, vaginal, cervical or endometrial cancer.

THE LATEST PERSPECTIVE ON THE RISKS OF HRT

In July 2002, a US study was published suggesting an increased risk of invasive breast cancer (by 26 percent), heart attacks (by 29 percent) and strokes (by 41 percent) on long-term HRT. Since then, however, the study has been criticized, not least by the very same scientists who worked on the study, who have said that "HRT brings more than 80 percent benefit for women who take it, versus really very tiny risks." Even so, several points need to be made to clarify the report's findings.
- When we assess the risk of breast cancer we do so against a baseline of 1.0 – every woman has a risk of breast cancer of 1.0. That means the risk of getting breast cancer for every woman is 1.0 per 1,000 women over 10 years.
- If, for some reason, that risk goes up to 1.50 per 1,000 women over 10 years that increase is reported as a 50 percent increase.

So, in simple terms, the 26 percent increase in risk of breast cancer in the US study means that the risk went from 1 woman in 1,000 to 1.26 women in 1,000 over a 10-year period, which by any accounting is not a huge jump. All this must be interpreted in the light of the study being flawed.

RESULTS

The results are not a surprise, British studies in 1997 and 1998 revealed similar figures and we didn't panic then.

We didn't panic for good reason: the increased risk is no more than the increased risk you put on yourself if you're overweight, put off your first child until you're over 30, drink too much alcohol, or have no children.

Among 10,000 women the new figures represent 8 extra cases of breast cancer, 8 extra strokes, and 7 extra heart problems over the period of a year.

BENEFITS OF HRT

Some benefits are confirmed in this study:
- A 37 percent reduction in bowel cancer.
- A 33 percent reduction in hip fracture.
- A 24 percent reduction in all fractures.
Add to this the emerging evidence that HRT can probably prevent Alzheimer's, and proof that HRT is 98 percent effective in treating menopausal symptoms such as hot flushes, night sweats and dry vagina. It keeps women's genital organs healthy, including the bladder, so protects against cystitis. Then there's the sound sleep, strong muscles, extra stamina and mental tonic effect that many women claim.

ALTERNATIVES TO HRT

If you're worried about HRT, keep in mind there are alternatives with no increase in breast cancer risk.

- Not yet available in the US, tibolone relieves symptoms and doesn't affect the breast.
- Another group of drugs, SERMs, doesn't help symptoms but appears to strengthen bones and protects you from heart disease.

THE LATEST RESEARCH

- In February 2003 a UK study of 13,000 women stated that women with diabetes should not take HRT, and found no increased risk of heart disease on HRT but no protection either.
- In March 2003 a US study reported no improvement in quality of life on HRT, though the authors admitted there were limitations to the study.

LIVING WITH THE RISK

I personally have decided not to sacrifice the benefits of HRT and to live with any perceived risk. I'm reassured that, despite the frightening headlines, the researchers state that, for each individual woman, the risks of HRT are still very low.. It's only when you lump thousands of women together that they become a concern. I, personally, will live with that, in exchange for vigour, an active brain, a certain fearlessness and a zest for life.

How HRT can help

- **Hot flushes and night sweats** – More than 90 percent of women find complete relief when they are prescribed oestrogen regardless of the form it takes; over 98 percent report that their symptoms have lessened.
- **Vaginal dryness, soreness and painful intercourse** – Can be relieved.
- **Intellectual problems** (poor concentration/ability to make decisions) – may improve within a month or so.
- **Sleep** – Research indicates that women may dream less when they are oestrogen deficient. As this type of sleep is important to your sense of well-being HRT should help make you feel rested after sleep. Take your HRT last thing at night for a really sound sleep.
- **Libido** (sexual drive) – This varies from woman to woman. Testosterone – the

male hormone – is also manufactured by the ovaries and is thought to be largely responsible for the female sex drive. Daily low doses of testosterone – or a testosterone implant – can bring about a subtle return of sexual vitality without side effects.

Other benefits

- **Osteoporosis** – This is a bone-thinning process that occurs in postmenopausal women. It can result in fractures, curvature of the spine and severe back pain. HRT is thought to be an important form of protection against osteoporosis.
- **Reduces risk of developing cancer of the colon by a third and may delay the onset of Alzheimer's disease.**

with immunosuppressant drugs is needed afterwards. However, some people are given a pancreas transplant at the same time as a kidney transplant. A method is currently being devised to transplant insulin-secreting cells isolated from a normal pancreas, but this technique is still at an experimental stage.

Injecting insulin

If you need regular injections of insulin, you will be shown how to inject yourself. You can use a syringe and needle, but many people prefer insulin pens, which are easier to use and more discreet. Insulin can be injected into any fatty area, such as the upper arms, abdomen or thighs. Insert the needle quickly into a pinch of skin and then inject the insulin slowly. You should try not to use exactly the same site each time for the injection. After about age 10, children with diabetes can be taught how to inject themselves.

Insulin pen: This device for carrying and delivering insulin holds an insulin cartridge and has a dial that lets you set the required dose. Disposable needles attach to one end.

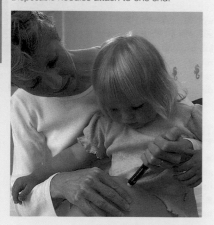

TREATMENT FOR TYPE II DIABETES

Many people with this form of diabetes can control their blood glucose levels by **exercising** regularly and following a **healthy diet** to maintain ideal weight.

■ You should follow general guidelines for a healthy diet and seek the guidance of a dietitian if necessary. Try to keep fat intake low, and obtain energy from complex carbohydrates (such as bread and rice) to minimize fluctuations in the blood glucose level. The diet should have a fixed calorie content. The proportions of protein, carbohydrate and fat must be consistent to keep a balance between food intake and medicine.

■ You must also check your blood glucose regularly. If the glucose level is higher or lower than recommended, you may need to alter your diet or adjust your insulin or drug dose with the help of your doctor. Effective monitoring is especially important if you develop another illness, such as influenza, and in other situations, such as exercising or planning to eat a larger meal than usual.

■ When diet is not sufficient to control your blood sugar, one or more drugs may be

prescribed. You will probably begin with oral drugs, such as **sulphonylureas**, which stimulate the pancreas to release insulin, or **metformin**, which helps body tissues absorb glucose. You may also be given **acarbose**, which slows the absorption of glucose from the intestine and prevents fluctuations in the blood level. If oral drugs are ineffective, you may need insulin injections.

WHAT IS THE OUTLOOK?

If cardiovascular complications develop, diabetes mellitus can cause high blood pressure and heart attacks. However, advances in monitoring blood glucose levels, combined with a healthy lifestyle, have made diabetes easier to control, allowing people to lead a more normal life. Self-help groups exist for affected people.

> **See also:**
> • **The heart and atherosclerosis p.222**
> • **Cataracts p.472** • **Cystitis p.378**
> • **High blood pressure p.226**
> • **Acute, chronic and end-stage kidney failure p.380**

TEST

Monitoring your blood glucose

You can monitor your blood glucose level using a **digital meter**. The method of use varies, depending on the type of meter, but usually involves applying a drop of blood to a test strip impregnated with a chemical that reacts with glucose. Checking your blood glucose **at least once a day** or as often as your doctor recommends allows you to monitor your treatment to confirm that it is effective and to alter it as necessary.
1. Before starting, wash your hands thoroughly and dry them. Once your hands

are clean, obtain a drop of blood by using a spring-loaded pricking device on a fingertip.
2. Cover the chemically impregnated target area of the test strip with the drop of blood. Wait for one minute (or as long as is recommended by the instructions that come with the meter).
3. Finally, wipe or wash the excess blood from the strip and insert the strip into the digital glucose meter. The metre analyzes the blood and gives an instant reading of the glucose level.

Hyperthyroidism and Graves' disease

WHEN THE THYROID GLAND PRODUCES AN EXCESS OF HORMONES, MANY OF THE BODY'S FUNCTIONS ARE STIMULATED AND METABOLISM SPEEDS UP.

An excess of thyroid hormones, known as hyperthyroidism, is one of the most common hormonal disorders. It's most common in women between ages 20 and 50 and can run in families.

About 3 out of 4 cases of the condition are due to Graves' disease, an **autoimmune**

disorder in which the immune system produces antibodies that attack the thyroid gland, resulting in overproduction of thyroid hormones. Graves' disease tends to run in families and is thought to have a genetic basis. In rare cases, hyperthyroidism

may be associated with other autoimmune disorders, in particular the skin disorder **vitiligo**, and **pernicious anaemia**, a disorder of blood formation. In some cases thyroid nodules, often called "hot" nodules, secrete hormones, leading to hyperthyroidism.

Inflammation of the thyroid gland may also temporarily produce the symptoms of hyperthyroidism.

WHAT ARE THE SYMPTOMS?

In most cases, symptoms of hyperthyroidism develop gradually over several weeks and may include:
- weight loss despite increased appetite and food consumption
- rapid heartbeat, which is sometimes also irregular, felt as palpitations
- tremor (persistent trembling) affecting the hands
- warm, moist skin as a result of excessive sweating
- intolerance to heat
- anxiety and insomnia
- frequent bowel movements
- swelling in the neck caused by an enlarged thyroid gland (goitre)
- muscle weakness
- in women, irregular menstruation.

People with hyperthyroidism caused by Graves' disease may also have bulging eyes, a condition called exophthalmos.

HOW IS IT DIAGNOSED?

If your doctor suspects you have hyperthyroidism, a blood test to check for abnormally high levels of thyroid hormones and for antibodies that can attack the thyroid gland will be arranged. Your doctor will also feel around your neck for lumps caused by general enlargement of the gland. If swelling is detected in the area of the thyroid gland, you may have radionuclide scanning to check for a hot nodule.

WHAT IS THE TREATMENT?

- Symptoms of hyperthyroidism can initially be relieved by **beta-blocker drugs**, which reduce tremor and anxiety but do not affect thyroid hormone levels.
- There are three main treatments aimed at reducing the production of thyroid hormones.
- The most common is **anti-thyroid drugs**, such as **carbimazole** and **propranolol**, which are used when hyperthyroidism is due to Graves' disease and work by suppressing production of thyroid hormones. These drugs need to be taken daily for 12–18 months, after which the thyroid gland often functions normally.
- **Radioactive iodine** may be the most effective treatment for thyroid **nodules** that secrete hormone, and is also commonly used to treat Graves' disease. Treatment involves drinking a dose of radioactive iodine in solution or swallowing a radioactive iodine capsule. The iodine is absorbed and

accumulates in the thyroid gland, destroying part of it.
- Rarely, if drug treatments are ineffective, surgical removal of part of the thyroid gland may become necessary.

WHAT IS THE OUTLOOK?

Many people recover fully following treatment. However, hyperthyroidism may recur, particularly in people who have Graves' disease. If the treatment involves surgery or radioactive iodine, the remaining part of the thyroid may not be able to produce sufficient hormones, leading to hypothyroidism (see below). It is therefore important for thyroid hormone levels to be monitored regularly after treatment so that hormone supplements can be given if needed. The autoimmune form of hyperthyroidism may "burn out", leaving behind a hypothyroid state.

See also:
- Anaemias p.236
- Arrhythmias p.231
- Autoimmune disorders p.323
- Radionuclide scanning p.508
- Vitiligo p.454

Hypothyroidism

IN HYPOTHYROIDISM, ALSO KNOWN AS MYXOEDEMA, THE THYROID GLAND DOES NOT PRODUCE ENOUGH THYROID HORMONES. THESE HORMONES ARE IMPORTANT IN REGULATING THE BODY'S METABOLISM. A DEFICIENCY CAUSES A SLOWING DOWN OF MANY OF THE BODY'S FUNCTIONS.

Hypothyroidism is more common in women, particularly over age 40, and runs in families.

WHAT ARE THE CAUSES?

- A common cause of hypothyroidism is **thyroiditis**. The most common type of thyroiditis leading to hypothyroidism is an **autoimmune disorder** known as **Hashimoto's thyroiditis**, in which the body produces antibodies that attack the thyroid gland, damaging it permanently. Other forms of thyroiditis may lead to temporary or permanent hypothyroidism. Thyroiditis occurs in women after the birth of a baby in about 10 percent of cases, but is usually a temporary condition.
- **Treatments for an overactive thyroid gland** that involve **radioactive iodine** or **surgery** can also lead to permanent hypothyroidism. These treatments destroy part of the gland, and the tissue that remains may not produce sufficient hormones.
- **Insufficient dietary iodine**, which is essential for the production of thyroid hormones, can cause hypothyroidism but is rare in developed countries.

- In rare cases, hypothyroidism is due to the pituitary gland releasing insufficient amounts of **thyroid-stimulating hormone** (TSH), which stimulates the thyroid gland to secrete its own hormones. The underproduction of TSH is often due to a pituitary tumour.

WHAT ARE THE SYMPTOMS?

The symptoms of hypothyroidism vary in severity, usually develop slowly over months or years and may initially go unnoticed. Symptoms include:
- fatigue, which may make even minimal physical activity difficult
- weight gain
- constipation
- hoarseness of the voice
- intolerance to cold
- swelling of the face and puffy eyes
- generalized hair thinning
- in women, heavy menstrual periods.

Some people with hypothyroidism develop a swelling in the neck (a goitre) due to an enlarged thyroid.

WHAT MIGHT BE DONE?

Your doctor may arrange for you to have blood tests to measure the levels of thyroid hormones and to check for antibodies that act against the thyroid gland.

WHAT IS THE TREATMENT?

Treatment is aimed at the underlying cause. Permanent hypothyroidism may be treated with **replacement synthetic thyroid hormones**, which you will need to take for life. The symptoms should begin to improve about three weeks after drug treatment starts. Hormone treatment must be monitored regularly to ensure that the correct dosage is maintained. If a pituitary tumour is the cause, further tests will be done and the tumour may be removed surgically or treated with radiotherapy.

Temporary hypothyroidism does not usually need to be treated, but short-term hormone replacement may be given in some cases, for instance if thyroiditis occurs after birth. A deficiency in dietary iodine can be treated with supplements or an improved diet.

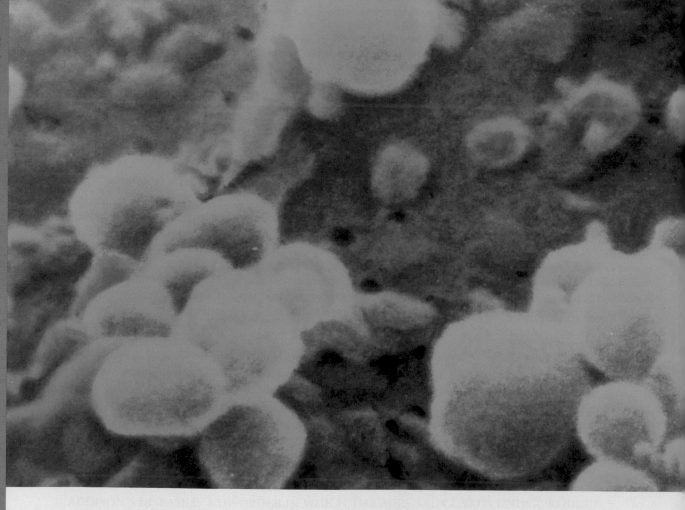

Children's conditions

Image shows a coloured scanning electron micrograph of the measles virus

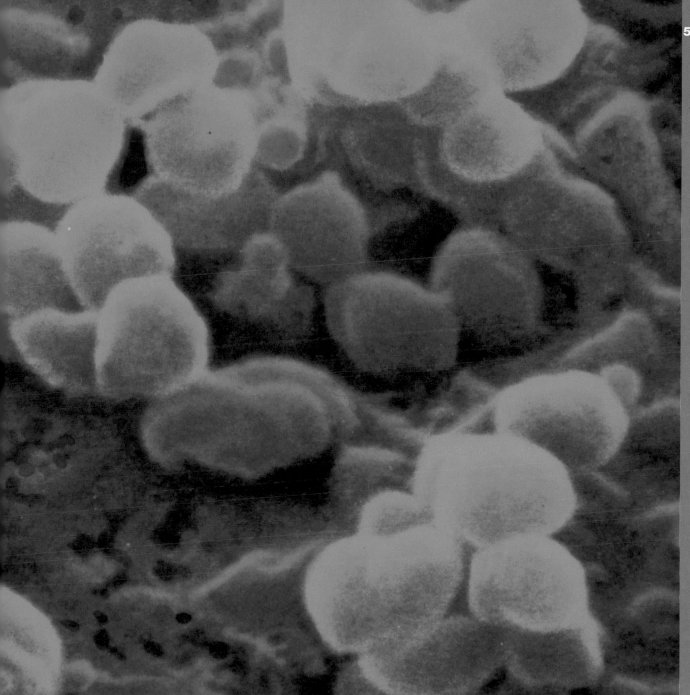

BEHAVIOUR AND DEVELOPMENT

UPPER AIRWAY CONDITIONS IN BABIES AND CHILDREN

OTHER PROBLEMS IN BABIES AND CHILDREN

Miriam's overview

I have three guiding principles when approaching illness in children.

● Children are not little adults. It follows that illness in children has to be looked at in a different way from illness in adults – children's illness isn't adult illness in miniature. So childhood asthma, childhood diabetes, childhood migraine are different from their adult equivalents and must be managed appropriately.

Then again, there are childhood diseases for which there is no exact adult equivalent. Cystic fibrosis, hydrocephalus, undescended testes are a few examples. These conditions are outside the orbit of any discussion of adult diseases.

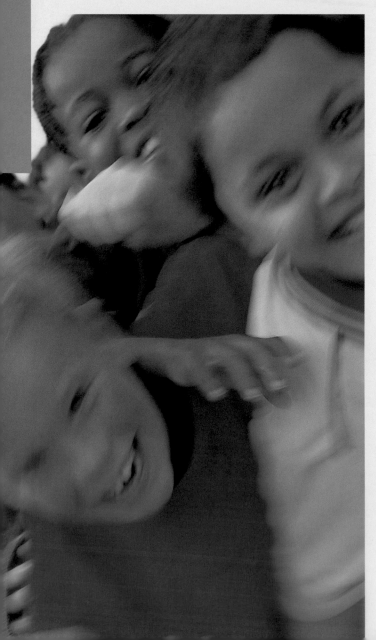

● As a junior doctor I very quickly learned there was one person whom I could not ignore when faced with a sick child. That person is you, Mum. No one in the world (not even Dad) knows your child as you do. You are sensitive to small, subtle signs of being off colour when no one else notices and even when drawn to their attention, no one else can spot. Armed with this knowledge you should understand that your child's wellbeing depends more on you than anyone else. Even though doctors and nurses may be sceptical of what you're saying you must insist if you're convinced your child is ill or sickening for something. Never be put off. Don't take no for an answer. Hang on until you get the attention and treatment you want for your child. If you don't look after your child's interests no one else will.

"if you *don't look after* your child's interests *no one else will*"

● Ill children can go downhill very quickly so prompt medical attention is mandatory – delay could always be costly so never hesitate to seek urgent medical advice if you're worried. Better safe than sorry. No doctor will mind if all they're called upon to do is reassure you that all is well.

A child's condition can deteriorate rapidly for several reasons.

● One of the most important is that children are built on a much smaller scale than adults so organs that are far enough apart to resist spread of infection in us are so close together in children that any infection of one part often has to be treated as an infection of the whole. The ear, nose, throat, sinuses and the chest are such a system: any infection of one, in a small child, threatens involvement of all.

● The immune response in children lags behind that of adults so a baby may develop a very high temperature quite suddenly, made worse by the fact that children can't regulate their temperature as efficiently as can adults.

The corollary of this is that children recover very fast too, faster than adults, because their bodies are resilient and heal quickly. A cause for celebration is that a sick, pale, limp child can be up, running around and asking for beans on toast in half an hour.

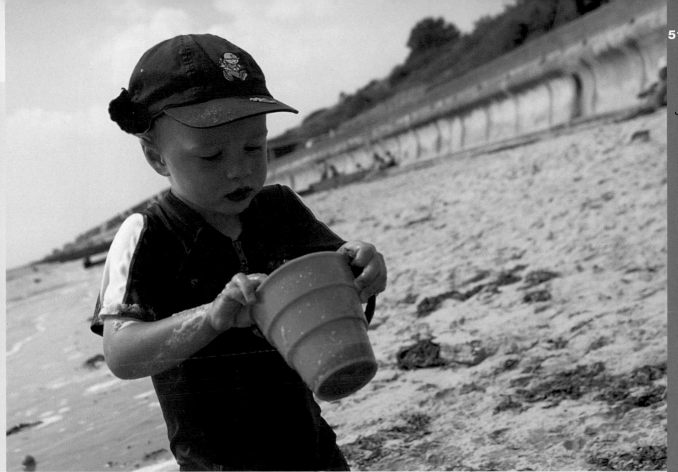

Genetic tests

The nucleus of each cell in your body normally contains 23 pairs of chromosomes – 22 pairs of autosomes and one pair of sex chromosomes (XX in women, XY in men). Each chromosome is made up of a number of genes, which are chemical codes that control the way every cell in the body functions. A faulty gene or chromosome may result in a disease or disorder. A wide range of genetic abnormalities can now be identified, and more sophisticated genetic tests are being developed all the time. Some of the best known genetic tests are the screening tests used to detect Down's syndrome and other chromosomal disorders during pregnancy. In these tests, the number of chromosomes and their structure are analyzed to determine whether the correct number of chromosomes is present and whether any of the chromosomes is abnormal.

Other genetic tests look specifically at the genes that make up each chromosome. For certain genetic conditions, such as cystic fibrosis and sickle-cell anaemia, the exact genetic abnormality and the way in which it is inherited are known.

Genetic tests are usually performed on white blood cells taken from a blood sample or on cells from tissue taken by gently scraping the inside of the cheek. In antenatal tests, the cells are taken from the amniotic fluid (by amniocentesis) or from the placenta (by chorionic villus sampling).

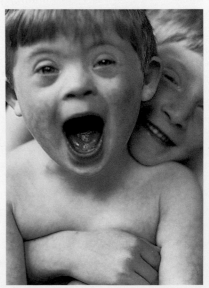

Genetic tests can identify many genetic conditions including Down's syndrome, in which 47 chromosomes are present instead of the usual 46.

CARING FOR A SICK CHILD

Most parents seem to know instinctively when their child is sickening for something. For example, your child may not be as lively as she usually is, she may refuse her food, she may be clingy.

The problem is that mums and dads can't always diagnose exactly what's wrong with their child, nor can they necessarily recognize whether the symptoms are serious.

Calling the doctor

AN ILL CHILD IS ALWAYS A DISTRESSING SIGHT AND THE SITUATION CAN BE EVEN MORE TENSE
IF YOU CANNOT DECIDE WHETHER TO CALL OUT THE DOCTOR.

There are some circumstances, for example after a serious injury, when medical help obviously should be sought immediately. There are, however, many more situations where the seriousness isn't quite as clear-cut. This is where the worry starts: "Are my child's symptoms nothing to worry about or are they potentially serious?"

You must remember that most doctors won't mind if you seek their advice. Always follow your instincts and if you're ever in doubt contact your doctor. If your child's already undergoing treatment from the doctor and you're worried about his progress call your doctor again. Only take your child to the casualty department if you become very worried about their symptoms or if they show any signs of meningitis (see p.405).

WHAT TO TELL YOUR DOCTOR
■ Your child's age.
■ Whether your child has a temperature.

Emergencies

Always get your child to the nearest hospital by ambulance or car if you notice any of the following:
■ Your child has stopped breathing.
■ Your child is breathing with difficulty and his lips are going blue.
■ Your child is unconscious.
■ Your child has a deep wound that is bleeding badly.
■ Your child has a serious burn.
■ Your child has a suspected broken bone.
■ Your child has a chemical in his eyes.
■ Your child's ear or eye has been pierced.
■ Your child has been bitten.
■ Your child has eaten a poisonous substance.

If so, what it is; how long he has had it; have there been any fluctuations and, if so, what they were. If your child has a fever, did it come on quickly?
■ Are your child's neck glands swollen?
■ Has your child vomited or had diarrhoea?
■ Does your child have a rash?
■ Has your child complained of any kind of pain? If so, where is it?
■ Has your child suffered from dizziness or blurred vision (particularly if he's recently had a bump on the head)?
■ Has your child had a convulsion? If so, how long did it last?
■ Has your child lost consciousness?
■ Did your child eat the last meal offered and has he eaten within the past three hours?

WHAT TO EXPECT FROM YOUR DOCTOR
Once the doctor has arrived he should examine your child thoroughly and give you an honest opinion of what's wrong. If your doctor doesn't know what's wrong, he should tell you what further tests are necessary to get a clear diagnosis. He should also advise you on the implications of the illness or condition. If, for example, your child has an acute attack of sinusitis or a middle ear infection, your doctor should tell you that your child may need antibiotics to eradicate it completely. On the other hand, your doctor should not give you medicine if he's sure there's nothing wrong. He would be wrong to give you something simply because you have gone to the surgery expecting to be treated. Respect him for not being pressured into giving you a prescription.

That said, he should answer all your questions – so persist until you are completely satisfied. If medicine is required, the doctor should give you as much information as possible about what he has prescribed. He should also tell you whether to give it before or after a meal, whether there may be side effects, whether there are any special precautions to take and he should warn you about possible complications and danger signs to look out for.

THINGS TO ASK YOUR DOCTOR
If your child has a recurrent condition, such as cold sores or boils, ask your doctor what you can do yourself if you notice any symptoms occurring. You can also ask your doctor for any home nursing tips.

If your child has a chronic condition, find out if there's anything you can do at home to help it. For example, with infantile eczema there's quite a lot you can do, such as adding oil to the bath water, using special soap, gently rubbing in moisturizing ointments and creams, even when the skin is clear. If your child has an infectious disease, ask about the incubation period – could friends be infected too? – the length of time your child will be infectious and how long he will have to stay away from school.

PICK UP THE PHONE NOW
These are the circumstances under which you should **always** call the doctor.

TEMPERATURE
■ Raised temperature over 39°C (102.2°F).
■ Raised temperature with drowsiness and a purplish rash.
■ Raised temperature with a convulsion, or if your child has had convulsions in the past.
■ Raised temperature with a stiff neck and headache.
■ Temperature below 35°C (95°F) with cold skin, drowsiness, quietness and listlessness.
■ Temperature that drops, rising again suddenly.
■ Temperature of more than 38°C (100.4°F) for more than 24 hours.

DIARRHOEA
■ Diarrhoea that lasts longer than six hours.
■ Diarrhoea accompanied by pain in the abdomen, a temperature or other obvious signs of illness.

NAUSEA AND VOMITING
■ Vomiting that lasts longer than six hours.
■ Prolonged, violent vomiting.
■ Nausea plus dizziness and headaches.
■ Nausea and vomiting accompanied by right-sided pain in the abdomen.

LOSS OF APPETITE
- If your baby goes off food suddenly, or is under six months and doesn't seem to be thriving.
- If your child usually has a hearty appetite, but refuses all food for a day and seems listless.

- Loss of appetite with pain and discomfort.
- Headaches, along with feeling sick and dizzy.
- If your child complains of blurred vision, especially after a head bang.
- Severe griping pains at regular intervals.
- Pain in the right side of the abdomen and feeling sick.

BREATHING
- If your child's breathing is laboured and his ribs draw in sharply with each breath.
- If your child is wheezing.

Taking your child's temperature and pulse

IN CHILDREN, NORMAL BODY TEMPERATURE RANGES FROM 36°C (96.8°F) TO 37°C (98.6°F). ANY TEMPERATURE OVER 37.7°C (100°F) IS CLASSED AS A FEVER. HYPOTHERMIA DEVELOPS IF THE TEMPERATURE FALLS BELOW 35°C (95°F).

Body temperature will vary according to how active your child has been and the time of day: it is lowest in the morning because there is little muscle activity during sleep, and highest in the late afternoon after a day's activity.

An abnormally hot forehead could be the first indication you have that your child has a temperature. To be accurate, however, you must take your child's temperature with a thermometer. Because the temperature control centre in the brain is primitive in young children, the temperature can shoot up more rapidly than in adults. When a fever is present, you should take your child's temperature again after 20 minutes, just in case it was only a transitory leap. Never regard a high temperature as the only accurate reflection of whether your child is ill or not; a child can be very ill without a high temperature or quite healthy with one.

THERMOMETERS
There are two main types of thermometer that are used for children: **digital** and **liquid crystal**. The old-fashioned mercury thermometer is rarely used for children these days.
Digital thermometers are easy to use with

children of all ages and are safer than mercury thermometers to use orally since they are unbreakable. Digital thermometers are battery-operated, so be sure to keep spare batteries on hand. Some digital thermometers, known as ear sensors or aural thermometers, are designed to read the temperature from the inside of the ear and can obtain a temperature reading in a few seconds. If you use an ear sensor, be sure to use the same ear each time you take your child's temperature, as the exact temperature between the ears varies.

Liquid crystal thermometers have a heat-sensitive panel on one side and panels with numbers on the other side. When the sensitive side is placed on the forehead, the numbers (your child's temperature) light up. Liquid crystal thermometers are not as accurate as mercury or digital thermometers but are safe and easy to use.

Mercury thermometers are the most accurate means of assessing temperature but should only be used for older children. Made of glass, they register the temperature when the mercury expands up the tube to a point on the scale. There are two different ways to

take a child's temperature with a mercury thermometer, under his armpit or under his tongue, as long as you can trust your child not to bite the thermometer. To read a mercury thermometer, hold it between your finger and thumb and turn it until you can see the point on the scale.

TAKING YOUR CHILD'S PULSE
The pulse is the wave of pressure that passes along each artery every time the heart beats. You can feel the pulse wherever an artery lies close to the skin. The most common site for taking the pulse is at the wrist (radial pulse). The pulse can also be taken in the neck (carotid pulse), although this is normally only done if you suspect the heart has stopped beating altogether, and on the inside of the upper arm (brachial pulse).

The pulse rate will vary with age. It is normally faster after exercise and slower after resting. A young baby's heart will beat about 160 times a minute; by the time he is one year old it will beat about 100–120 times per minute and by the time he is about seven or eight years old, it will have slowed down to the

Taking your child's temperature

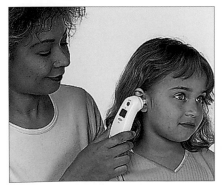
Using an ear sensor (aural thermometer)

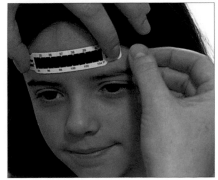
Using a liquid crystal thermometer

Tips

- Never take your child's temperature if he has just been running about.
- Never leave your child alone with a thermometer in his mouth.
- If using a mercury thermometer, make sure there is no break in the mercury – it will affect the reading.
- If your thermometer is cracked, throw it away immediately.

Taking a radial, brachial and carotid pulse

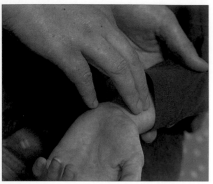

Radial pulse
The radial pulse is found on the inside of the wrist below the thumb. Use your index and middle fingers to find it and not your thrumb, which has a pulse of its own.

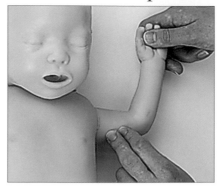

Brachial pulse
The brachial pulse is found on the inside of the upper arm in the groove between the biceps and triceps muscles (on the front and back of the arm). Use your index and middle fingers to find the pulse.

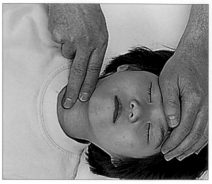

Carotid pulse
The carotid pulse is found at the top of the neck just to the right or left of the windpipe. Use your index and middle fingers to find it and not your thumb, which has its own pulse.

adult rate of 80–90 beats per minute. A normal pulse is regular and strong; any abnormality, such as a fast, weak pulse or a slow pulse, may indicate that your child is ill.

When taking your child's pulse, use the first two fingers, not your thumb, which contains a pulse of its own. Count the beats over a 15-second period and multiply this figure by four

to get the rate per minute. If your child is under one, it is generally easier to find the brachial pulse, located on the inside of the upper arm.

Giving your child medicine

WHEN YOU TAKE YOUR CHILD TO THE DOCTOR HE MAY PRESCRIBE
SOME FORM OF MEDICINE FOR HER.

Ask for as much information as possible about the medicines: ask if there are likely to be any side effects, whether there are foods that should be avoided or special precautions that should be observed while your child is taking the medication, and clarify whether to give the medicine before or after a meal.

Most medicines for young children are made

up in a sweetened syrup to make them more palatable and can be given with a spoon, tube or dropper. Droppers and tubes are often more suitable for babies who haven't learnt to swallow from a spoon. Some medicines for older children are supplied as tablets or capsules.

On most occasions your child will be co-operative but there may be the odd occasion

when she simply refuses to take her medicine. It is very important that your child takes the medicine prescribed when she is ill. In fact, I think that this is one occasion when bribery is justified. So don't hesitate to give the medicine with ice cream or another favourite food. Very occasionally a child will resist physically; there really is no alternative but for you to be forceful.

Giving medicine

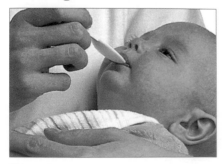

Using a spoon
Hold your baby in a semi-reclining position, gently pull his chin down with your finger and place the spoon on his lower lip. Raise the angle of the spoon and trickle the medicine into his mouth. Don't let the medicine run directly into his throat or he may choke.

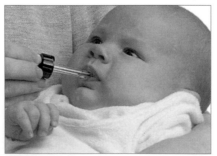

Using a dropper
Hold your baby in the crook of your arm and put the filled dropper into the corner of his mouth. Squeeze the bulb slowly and gently to release the medicine. Don't let the medicine run directly down your baby's throat or he may choke.

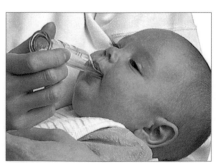

Using a medicine tube
Hold your baby in the crook of your arm and put the filled tube into the corner of his mouth. Raise the angle of the tube slowly and gently to release the medicine. Don't let the medicine run directly down your baby's throat or he may choke.

Tips for giving medicines

Giving medicines to babies

■ Enlist the help of another adult or older brother or sister.

■ If you are on your own, wrap a blanket around your baby's arms so that you can stop him struggling and hold him steady.

■ Only put a little of the medicine in his mouth at a time.

■ If your baby spits the medicine out, get the other person to hold his mouth open while you carefully trickle the medicine into the back of his mouth. Then, gently but firmly, close his mouth.

Giving medicines to older children

■ Suggest that your child holds her nose while taking the medicine, so lessening the effect of the taste.

■ Don't forcibly hold your child's nose, as she may inhale some of the medicine.

■ Mix liquid medicine with another syrup such as honey.

■ Don't add liquid medicine to a drink, as it will just sink to the bottom of the glass or stick to the sides and you won't be sure that your child has had the whole dose.

■ Show your child that you have her favourite drink ready to wash the taste of the medicine away; do this even if you do not normally allow her to have this drink.

■ Help your child to clean her teeth after taking any liquid medicine to prevent syrup sticking to her teeth.

■ Crush tablets (never capsules, however) between two spoons and mix the powder with something sweet, such as honey, jam or ice cream.

Giving drops

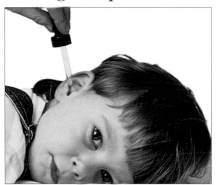

Ear drops
Ask your child to lie on his side. Using a dropper and ear drops that have been warmed to body temperature, squeeze the bulb and let the drops fall into the centre of his ear.

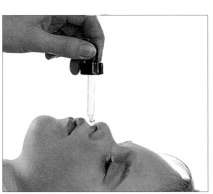

Nose drops
Ask your child to lie on his back with his head tilted backwards. Using a dropper and nose drops that have been warmed to body temperature, squeeze the bulb and let two or three drops fall into each nostril.

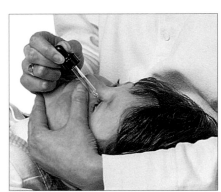

Eye drops
Ask your child to lie on her back. Gently pull down the lower lid of the affected eye and squeeze the dropper's bulb, letting one or two drops fall inside the eyelid.

On the whole, older children do not generally mind medicine too much and often want to pour it out for themselves rather than let you give it to them. I have listed a few tips (see box, above) that may help if your child is difficult. For example, tablets can be crushed and mixed with jam or ice cream. Capsules, however, should not be broken.

GIVING DROPS

Ear, nose or eye infections are generally treated with external drops. It is always easier to administer drops to a baby or young child if you lay her on a flat surface before you begin and enlist some help to keep her still and hold her head steady. An older child will probably be more cooperative and you will only need to ask her to tilt her head back or to the side, while you put the drops in.

Tips for giving drops

Giving drops

■ Warm nose drops and ear drops by standing the container in a bowl of warm, not hot, water for a few minutes, so that your child doesn't get too much of a shock when the liquid drops into his nose or ear.

■ Be careful not to let the dropper touch your child's nose, ear or eye, or you will transfer the germs back to the bottle. If the dropper does touch your child, make sure you wash it thoroughly before putting it back into the bottle.

■ Proprietary drops should not be used for longer than three days without consulting a doctor – if they are used for too long, they can cause irritation and inflammation that is worse than the condition you were treating.

Your medicine chest

You should always keep some medicines in the house in case of emergency in the middle of the night when you may not be able to get to a chemist easily. Keep them somewhere obvious so that you can find them quickly when you need them. Never mix different pills up in the same container and never keep any leftover prescription medicines. Keep all medicines well out of reach of children, in a high, locked cupboard, if necessary. You should also have a first-aid kit (see p.565). Keep all the equipment in a clean, dry, airtight box and put it somewhere it can be found in an emergency.

The items listed below would all be useful to have in emergencies and are therefore well worth keeping in the house.

Medicine cabinet
■ Digital or liquid crystal thermometer – keep two for safety.
■ Junior paracetamol tablets.

■ Liquid paracetamol – infants: from three months to six years or junior: from six to 12 years.
■ Calamine lotion.
■ Mild antiseptic wipes.
■ Cotton wool.
■ Mild antiseptic cream.
■ Gauze dressings – keep dry and paraffin-coated ones.
■ Surgical tape.
■ Crepe bandages for sprains and strains.
■ Open-weave bandages.
■ Triangular bandage.
■ Safety pins, scissors and blunt-edged tweezers.

Useful household items
■ Packet of frozen peas, or ice cubes in plastic bags for cold compresses.
■ Newspaper (folded it can make a splint).
■ Elastic belt to support a strain/sprain.
■ Rehydration fluid to replace fluid lost after vomiting or diarrhoea.

■ Bicarbonate of soda to add to a bath to relieve itching.
■ Salt to add to a bath to clean wounds and deter infection.
■ Vinegar to mix with water to soothe jellyfish stings.

Medicines to avoid
The following items, commonly given as useful, should be avoided:
■ Any proprietary product containing a local anaesthetic, such as amethocaine or lignocaine, because they can cause allergies. They are most generally found in creams for mouth ulcers or insect stings.
■ Any skin creams containing antihistamines (unless prescribed by your doctor); they can cause skin allergies.
■ Any proprietary product that contains aspirin.
■ Mouth washes, gargles, eye drops, nose drops and ear drops, unless recommended by your doctor.

Nursing a sick child

YOU DON'T NEED ANY SPECIAL SKILLS OR MEDICAL KNOWLEDGE TO LOOK AFTER YOUR SICK CHILD. IT HELPS IF YOU RELAX THE RULES AND TRY TO HIDE YOUR ANXIETY FROM HER. DON'T INSIST THAT SHE EATS WHILE SHE IS ILL, BUT DO ENCOURAGE HER TO DRINK LOTS OF FLUIDS.

As well as whatever treatment the doctor recommends, the following routines will help your child to feel more comfortable while she is ill.
■ Air your child's room and bed at least once a day.
■ Leave a bowl by your child's bed if she is vomiting or has whooping cough.
■ Leave a box of tissues by your child's bed.
■ Give small meals frequently; your child may find large portions off-putting.
■ Give paracetamol elixir for pain relief.

SHOULD YOUR CHILD BE IN BED?
At the beginning of an illness when your child is feeling quite poorly she will probably want to stay in bed and she may sleep a lot. As she starts to feel better she will still need bed rest, but she will want to be around you and she may want intervals of playing. The best way to accommodate this is to make up a bed on the sofa in a room near where you are working so that she can lie down when she wants to. Don't insist that your child goes to bed just because she is ill – children with a fever, for instance, don't recover faster if they stay in bed. When your child is tired, however, it is

time to put her to bed. But don't just leave her alone. Make sure that you visit her at regular intervals (every half an hour), and find the time to stay and play a game, read a book, or do a puzzle.

When she's on the road to recovery make sure that enough happens in her day to make the distinction between night and day. If she hasn't been watching television, let her watch it before bedtime.

GIVING DRINKS
It is essential that your child drinks a lot when she's ill – when she has a fever, diarrhoea or is vomiting – because she will be dehydrated and will need to replace lost fluids. The recommended fluid intake for a child with a fever is 100–150 millilitres per kilogram (1–2 fluid ounces per pound) of body weight per day, which is the equivalent of 1 litre (2 pints) per day for a child who weighs 9 kilograms (20 pounds).

Encourage your child to drink by leaving her favourite drink at her bedside (preferably not sugary, fizzy drinks such as cola), by putting drinks in glasses that are especially appealing, and by giving her bendy straws to drink with.

OCCUPYING YOUR CHILD
Illness is an occasion when you can completely indulge your child. When she is not resting, spend time playing games and talking to her. Relax all the rules and let her play whatever games she wants to, even if you've previously disallowed them in bed. If your child wants to do something messy like painting, just spread an old sheet or a sheet of polyurethane over the bed. If you can, move a television into her room temporarily – this will keep her entertained and make her feel special as well.

Let her do some painting; read aloud to her; get out some of her old toys and play with them together; sing songs or make up a story together; ask her to draw a picture of what she is going to do when she feels better; and, unless she has an infectious illness, let some friends visit her for a brief period during the day. As your child gets better let her play outside, but if she has a fever discourage her from running around too much.

VOMITING
Your child will probably find vomiting a distressing experience and you should try and make her as comfortable as possible. Get her

to sit up in bed and make sure there is a bowl or a bucket within easy reach, so that she doesn't have to run to the toilet. If your child's hair is in the way, tie it back. When she is being sick hold her head and comfort her. Afterwards help your child to clean her teeth, or give her a peppermint to suck to take the taste away.

When your child hasn't vomited for a few hours and she's feeling hungry, offer her bland foods, such as mashed potato, but don't encourage her to eat if she doesn't want to. More important than eating is maintaining a constant level of fluids. Give your child lots of water, or use a proprietary rehydration solution that you can buy at the chemist – be sure to follow the instructions on the packet carefully when you make it up. Avoid drinks such as milk, but give fruit juice diluted with water.

TREATING A HIGH TEMPERATURE
The first sign of a raised temperature is often a hot forehead, but to check that your child is

Immunization timetable

What is given?	How is it given?	When is it given?
POLIO	Drops	At 2, 4, 6 months and 4–6 years
HIB, DIPHTHERIA, TETANUS, PERTUSSIS, MENINGITIS C	Injection	At 2, 4, 6, 12–15 months and 4–6 years (no Hib)
MEASLES, MUMPS, RUBELLA (MMR)	Injection	At 12 months and 4–6 years

feverish take her temperature (see p. 515). Call your doctor if the fever is over 39°C (102.2°F), lasts more than 24 hours or if there are accompanying symptoms. Temperatures over 37.7°C (100°F) should be taken very seriously in children under six months.

Try to cool your child down by taking off her clothes and getting her to lie in bed. Cover her with a cotton sheet and take her temperature every hour or so. Changing the sheets on her bed regularly will help keep her comfortable. Try giving her paracetamol elixir (aspirin is dangerous for children). It's still important for her to drink lots of fluid as she will be perspiring a lot.

Your child in hospital

YOU WILL BE DOING YOUR CHILD A GREAT FAVOUR IF YOU ENCOURAGE HIM TO THINK ABOUT HOSPITALS AS FRIENDLY PLACES. TRY TO TAKE HIM WITH YOU IF YOU ARE VISITING A FAMILY FRIEND OR RELATIVE – PROVIDED THE PERSON DOES NOT MIND AND VISITING REGULATIONS ALLOW IT.

PREPARING YOUR CHILD
If your child has to go into hospital, for an operation, for example, and you are given some warning, prepare him by discussing as many aspects of it as possible. Talk about it with the rest of the family as well and get him generally used to the idea.

Answer all his questions honestly. Don't make promises that you can't keep and don't tell lies. If he is having an operation, he will probably ask you if there will be any pain or discomfort after the operation. If you say that nothing is going to hurt and it does, he will simply get a shock and will not trust you in future. Explain that there will be some discomfort but that it will not last long.

Another good way to prepare him for a hospital stay is to read him a book about someone who goes into hospital. You could also buy him a toy stethoscope and play doctors and nurses with him. Encourage him to be the doctor or nurse and suggest that he makes up a hospital bed for his favourite teddy bear or toy.

IN HOSPITAL
Few children's wards are frightening places. However, hospitals have found that it is very important for parents to be with their children as much as possible while they are in hospital and, because of this, almost all now allow parents to stay with their child, particularly if

he is very young. Many hospitals have sleeping facilities for parents with children up to the age of six.

When you are there, ask the ward sister and nurses how you can help with the daily routine. You will be encouraged to bath and change your child, and to help with his feeding. You can read books and play games with him and any other children in the ward who want to join in. If the ward has a teacher, ask if you can help with your child's schoolwork. If he is well enough and will be in hospital for a while, ask his own teacher to give you the work he would normally be doing at school.

If you cannot be with your child all day, try to arrange a rota so that someone he knows well is with him all the time.

BACK HOME FROM HOSPITAL
It's quite normal for a child to behave a little oddly when he comes out of hospital. Firstly, your child's sleeping and eating patterns may have changed. Hospital meals, and certainly bedtimes, tend to be earlier than you'd have them at home. Secondly, because your child has been away from his domestic discipline, you may find that he will make a fuss about small points like brushing his teeth. Don't be too hard on him at first, give him time to readjust to being at home before you insist that he fits in with the old routine.

What to take into hospital

If you can, you and your child should pack his case together a few days before he has to go in.
- Three pairs of pyjamas.
- Dressing gown and slippers.
- Three pairs of ankle socks.
- Hair brush and comb.
- Sponge bag with soap, flannel, toothbrush, toothpaste.
- Bedside clock.
- Portable radio or cassette player with headphones.
- Favourite books and portable games.
- Favourite picture or photograph to put by his bedside.

CONGENITAL CONDITIONS

Congenital conditions are those that are present from birth; they may also be genetic, meaning that they are caused by a defective gene.

Many congenital conditions such as congenital hip dislocation or phimosis are relatively minor, while others, such as some congenital heart defects, are more serious.

The good news is that many congenital conditions are now treatable and children who receive early treatment can expect to lead normal lives.

Cerebral palsy

CEREBRAL PALSY IS THE NAME GIVEN TO DAMAGE TO THE BRAIN THAT OCCURS EARLY IN LIFE AND RESULTS IN A LACK OF FULL CONTROL OF PHYSICAL MOVEMENT.

In most children, the damage occurs in pregnancy though in a few others, during a difficult labour, the baby may suffer from a lack of oxygen. However, it is usually not possible to determine the exact cause of cerebral palsy. It may result if a premature baby has severe breathing problems, with bleeding in the brain and lack of oxygen both contributing to the condition. Non-congenital causes include serious head injury and meningitis.

WHAT ARE THE SYMPTOMS?
Because the more sophisticated voluntary control centres of the brain do not function in the first months of life, cerebral palsy may not be apparent at birth. After a few months it may show itself if the child is slow to sit up, is generally unsteady or cannot grasp and hold things. Cerebral palsy may affect only one side (for example, the right arm and leg), both legs

with the arms hardly affected at all, or all four limbs and the trunk. Walking is delayed but usually possible. If the limbs tend to be stiff and fixed in certain postures the child is technically termed "spastic". If he is prone to frequent, purposeless writhing movements he is said to be "athetoid".

Cerebral palsy is not a progressive disease that gets steadily worse. And it's quite common for children with cerebral palsy to have normal intelligence and normal social capabilities.

WHAT IS THE TREATMENT?
The treatment for cerebral palsy consists of trying to develop the child's physical, mental and social capabilities to the full. Therefore it is important that the child is fully assessed by a specialist and a physiotherapist so that he can be given treatment at an early age. Stretching exercises will prevent fixed deformity of the

limbs; orthopaedic appliances such as calipers, and in some cases surgery, can improve mobility; and treatment, such as speech therapy, can compensate for the physical disability.

Where there is no mental handicap, the outlook is extremely good. Children adjust quite well to severe lack of motor function as long as their intellectual capacity is good and they can make themselves understood.

WHAT CAN I DO?
The reaction of the family is of great importance. Parents must guard against feeling sorry for the child. If there are other children in the family the child must be treated as far as possible in the same way as they are, although this may be hard for parents. As with all disabled children the emphasis should be on what the child can do rather than on what he cannot.

Congenital heart disease

CONGENITAL HEART DISEASE MEANS THAT ONE OR MORE DEFECTS OF THE HEART ARE PRESENT AT BIRTH.

WHAT ARE THE SYMPTOMS?
Minor congenital heart defects may not cause symptoms. If symptoms are present, they may include the following things.
■ Shortness of breath, leading to difficulty in feeding.
■ Slow weight gain and growth.

■ Bluish coloration to the tongue and lips, if oxygen levels in the blood are low.
■ Susceptibility to chest infections or infection of the lining of the heart.

WHAT IS THE TREATMENT?
Many heart defects correct themselves or need

no treatment. Only about 1 in 3 children requires surgery. Affected children are usually monitored through childhood and if necessary surgery is performed when the child is older and the operation is easier. A heart transplant is now a possibility for children with multiple heart defects. Chest infections need to be treated promptly and if the child has dental treatment or surgery antibiotics are necessary to prevent infection of the lining of the heart. Some children will need drugs such as diuretics to control the symptoms of a heart defect.

WHAT IS THE OUTLOOK?
Septal defects may close naturally or be corrected surgically. Surgical advances over the last 20 years mean that even very severe defects can often be corrected.

Types of congenital heart disease

■ Septal defects (usually a hole in the inner wall that divides the heart, known as the septum; often called a "hole in the heart").
■ Patent ductus arteriosus (failure of a small blood vessel in the heart, known

as the ductus arteriosus, to close soon after birth, preventing normal circulation).
■ Valve defects (any abnormality occurring in one or more of the four heart valves).
■ Multiple defects (rarely, several heart defects occur together).

Congenital hip dislocation

CONGENITAL HIP DISLOCATION IS A TERM THAT COVERS A WIDE RANGE OF PROBLEMS WITH
THE HIP JOINT IN NEWBORN BABIES. THESE PROBLEMS ARE SIX TIMES MORE COMMON IN GIRLS
THAN IN BOYS AND SOMETIMES RUN IN FAMILIES, SUGGESTING A GENETIC FACTOR.

In mild cases, the hip joint moves excessively when manipulated; in moderate cases, the head of the femur (thighbone) slips out of the hip socket when manipulated but can be eased back in; in severe cases, the dislocation is permanent with the head of the femur lying outside the hip socket. Simple manipulation of your baby's hips to test for congenital hip dislocation is usually done shortly after birth and by your health visitor during routine development checks.

Hip dislocation occurs more often in the left hip and rarely affects both hips. In cultures where babies are regularly carried astride their mothers' backs, hip dislocation rarely persists.

WHAT ARE THE SYMPTOMS?
Mild forms of hip dislocation may cause no symptoms. Otherwise, symptoms include:

- asymmetrical creases in the skin on the backs of the baby's legs
- inability to turn the affects leg out fully at the hip
- shorter appearance of the affected leg
- limping when older if the condition is not treated early.

SHOULD I CONSULT THE DOCTOR?
Consult your doctor as soon as possible if you suspect that there is a problem with your baby's hips. If hip dislocation is not corrected early, it may lead to permanent deformity and early onset of osteoarthritis.

WHAT IS THE TREATMENT?
If your doctor suspects congenital hip dislocation he may arrange for ultrasound scanning to confirm the diagnosis. The less severe forms of the condition often correct themselves during the first 3 weeks of life. If the problem persists, the hip joint may be positioned in a harness for 8–12 weeks to hold the head of the femur in the hip, allowing the hip socket to develop normally. In older babies the hip may have to be held in a cast for up to 6 months to correct the problem. If treatment is unsuccessful surgery may be necessary. If hip dislocation is treated promptly most babies develop normal hip joints and there is no lasting damage.

Cystic fibrosis

CYSTIC FIBROSIS IS A RARE DISEASE THAT IS PRESENT AT BIRTH AND
INHERITED FROM BOTH PARENTS.

If the mother and father are healthy, but each carries one defective gene for cystic fibrosis, each child conceived has a 25 percent chance of inheriting two defective genes and being born with the disease.

Cystic fibrosis causes several glands in the body to be defective, particularly the glands in the lining of the bronchial tubes. Instead of producing the normal thin mucus, the bronchial glands produce a thick, sticky phlegm that creates blockages in the air passages and this in turn leads to lung infections. When small parts of the lungs collapse pneumonia results. This is a common and recurrent infection in cystic fibrosis sufferers.

In cystic fibrosis, the pancreas fails to produce certain enzymes that are vital to digestion. These enzymes break down food so that it can be absorbed easily by the body. When these enzymes are missing food is poorly digested, which leads to diarrhoea and foul-smelling stools. Because the body does not absorb many of the nutrients that are essential to good health the child with cystic fibrosis tends to be small, underweight and fails to thrive. Bouts of diarrhoea may alternate with constipation that can actually block the intestine.

Parents with an affected child who are planning a further pregnancy are offered genetic counselling.

WHAT ARE THE SYMPTOMS?
- Recurrent chest infections with a cough and some breathing difficulty.
- Diarrhoea, alternating with constipation.
- Greasy and foul-smelling bowel motions.
- Failure to thrive.
- Swollen abdomen and wasted limbs.

WHAT IS THE TREATMENT?
There is no cure for cystic fibrosis, but early detection of the condition lessens the chance of permanent damage to the lungs. Simple tests on the blood or stools of a newborn baby can be carried out, but the definitive test for cystic fibrosis is a sweat test because there is an increased salt level in the sweat of sufferers. This will be done on all brothers and sisters of a child with cystic fibrosis, or if a baby has recurrent bouts of pneumonia or fails to thrive. The tests are carried out when the baby is about three months of age.

Respiratory infections are treated with antibiotics; sometimes a spray form is used for speedy inhalation. Other treatments include inhaling enzymes to help dissolve lung secretions, or a heart-lung transplant.

The gene for cystic fibrosis has been identified and gene therapy will almost certainly be a future option.

WHAT CAN I DO?
A child with cystic fibrosis has to have a special low-fat diet, with vitamin supplements and enzyme replacements, which can be taken by mouth. Physiotherapy and breathing exercises must be done daily to loosen and drain mucus from the lungs. Exposure to moist air and a cold steam vaporizer can also help the lungs.

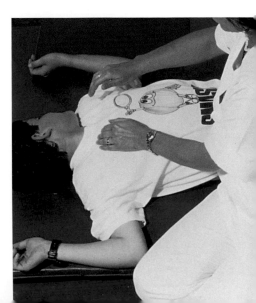

People with cystic fibrosis need daily chest physiotherapy to keep the lungs free of mucus.

Pyloric stenosis

IN CONGENITAL PYLORIC STENOSIS THE RING OF MUSCLE (PYLORUS) THAT LINKS THE STOMACH TO THE DUODENUM THICKENS AND NARROWS, PREVENTING THE STOMACH FROM EMPTYING. THE CAUSE IS NOT KNOWN BUT WHEN THE BABY IS ABOUT ONE MONTH OLD THE SYMPTOMS BEGIN.

Food builds up in the stomach, which contracts powerfully in an attempt to force the food through the thickened pylorus. Because this is impossible milk is vomited up violently after a feed. This is known as projectile vomiting and the unpleasant-smelling milk curds and mucus can be thrown for up to two yards (a metre or two). Projectile vomiting should not be confused with posseting, in which a baby naturally regurgitates milk after a feed. Pyloric stenosis is much more common in boys.

Pyloric stenosis is serious. Vomiting eventually leads to dehydration and a failure to thrive.

WHAT ARE THE SYMPTOMS?
- Projectile vomiting after a feed, beginning at around four weeks of age.
- Failure to thrive.
- Weakness and listlessness.
- Lack of bowel movements.

SHOULD I SEE THE DOCTOR?
Consult your doctor immediately if your baby vomits violently after every feed.

WHAT IS THE TREATMENT?
If pyloric stenosis is supected, your doctor will refer your baby to hospital. A paediatrician will examine your baby's abdomen during a feed to see if the enlarged pylorus can be felt. If pyloric stenosis is diagnosed, a simple surgical operation will be performed, giving a complete cure.

WHAT CAN I DO?
Stay with your baby in hospital. After the operation you will be advised to feed your baby gradually increasing amounts of milk. 48 hours after the operation, his feeding routine should be back to normal.

Down's syndrome

DOWN'S SYNDROME IS THE MOST COMMON CHROMOSOMAL ABNORMALITY. CHILDREN WITH DOWN'S SYNDROME HAVE 47 CHROMOSOMES INSTEAD OF THE NORMAL 46 IN EACH CELL. THE EXTRA CHROMOSOME, CHROMOSOME 21, USUALLY COMES FROM THE MOTHER'S EGG.

The incidence of Down's syndrome babies rises sharply with maternal age, but various forms of screening in pregnancy can identify the condition in the fetus and a termination can be performed if the parents wish. Chorionic villus sampling or nuchal scanning (scanning of the fetal neck) can be carried out between 9 and 13 weeks of pregnancy. At around 20 weeks, an amniocentesis test is usually offered to pregnant women of 35 or over. Blood tests (known as the triple test) can also be carried out at this stage.

A new screening test for Down's syndrome can identify more than 90 percent of cases after only 12 weeks of pregnancy. It's done six to eight weeks earlier than the triple test and will detect 30 percent more cases. It works by combining several of the methods to detect Down's syndrome described above. The 5 percent of patients deemed most at risk are then offered a definitive diagnosis procedure, such as chorionic villus sampling or amniocentesis.

WHAT ARE THE SYMPTOMS?
- Small, upward-slanting eyes; nose with a wide bridge; short, broad hands with a deep crease across the palm; gap between the first and second toes.
- Some degree of learning difficulty.

WHAT IS THE TREATMENT?
The degree of learning difficulty varies widely in children with Down's syndrome, and a few may be within the normal intelligence range. Modern theories reject the idea that all children with Down's syndrome should be educated in special institutions. The education of a child with Down's syndrome must be determined by the specific learning difficulty of the child, but children with Down's syndrome are usually educated in mainstream schools. As with all children the emphasis should be on what the child can do rather than what she cannot.

Almost all children with Down's syndrome will learn to walk and talk and some will learn to read and write. They will need extra help to fulfil their potential, but with this help many will go on to lead semi-independent lives.

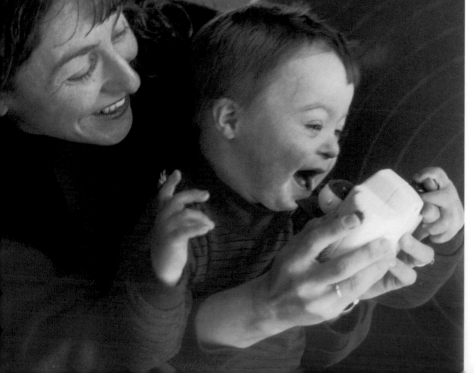

Muscular dystrophy

MUSCULAR DYSTROPHY IS A GROUP OF GENETIC CONDITIONS IN WHICH
MUSCLES BECOME WEAK AND WASTED.

The two main types of muscular dystrophy almost exclusively affect boys. The most common type of this condition is Duchenne muscular dystrophy, which causes serious disability from early childhood. A second, much rarer type of the disorder is Becker muscular dystrophy. The onset of this condition is slower and the symptoms start later in childhood. Other extremely rare forms of muscular dystrophy can affect both girls and boys.

Both Duchenne and Becker muscular dystrophies are caused by an abnormal gene carried on the X sex chromosome. Girls may carry the defective gene but do not usually have the disorder because they have two X chromosomes, and the gene on the normal X chromosome compensates for the defect in the gene on the other.

WHAT ARE THE SYMPTOMS?
The symptoms of Duchenne muscular dystrophy usually appear around the time a child would begin to walk. Late walking is common; often an affected child does not begin to walk until about 18 months and then will fall more frequently than other children. The more obvious symptoms may not appear until the child reaches age 3–5 and may include:

- waddling gait
- difficulty climbing stairs
- difficulty getting up from the floor
- characteristically, using the hands to "walk up" the thighs
- large calf muscles and wasted muscles at the tops of the legs and arms
- mild learning disabilities (especially in the Becker type).

The symptoms are progressive and a child may be unable to walk by the age of 12. The symptoms of Becker muscular dystrophy are similar but usually do not appear until about age 11 or later. The disease progresses more slowly; many of those affected are still able to walk until their late 20s or later.

WHAT IS THE TREATMENT?
If your doctor suspects muscular dystrophy he may arrange for a blood test to look for evidence of muscle damage. Electromyography, which records electrical activity in muscles, may be performed. A small piece of muscle may be removed under general anaesthesia for microscopic examination. Tests may be done to find out if the heart is affected, including recording electrical activity in the heart (ECG) and ultrasound scanning.

The treatment for muscular dystrophy is aimed at keeping a child mobile and active for as long as possible. A team of professionals such as a physical therapist, doctor and social worker can provide support for the whole family. Physical therapy is important to keep limbs supple and supportive splints may be used.

Duchenne muscular dystrophy is usually fatal before age 20; the outlook in the Becker type is better, with affected people often surviving into their 40s.

Phenylketonuria

PHENYLKETONURIA (SOMETIMES ABBREVIATED AS PKU) IS AN INHERITED
CHEMICAL DEFECT THAT CAN CAUSE BRAIN DAMAGE.

Children with phenylketonuria lack the enzyme that breaks down **phenylalanine**, a substance that occurs naturally in most food containing protein. As a result, phenylalanine is converted into harmful substances that build up in the blood and may damage the developing brain.

Although phenylketonuria is rare, all newborn babies are screened for it because of the risk of serious brain damage, which can be prevented by following a special diet that is low in phenylalanine. The baby's heel is pricked with a small needle to obtain a few drops of blood for testing; results are available in a few days.

WHAT ARE THE SYMPTOMS?
At birth some babies with phenylketonuria have a red, itchy rash similar to eczema but most affected infants appear healthy. If an affected baby is not tested as a newborn and the condition is left untreated, symptoms develop gradually over a period of 6–12 months and include:

- vomiting
- restlessness and sometimes seizures
- stale, unpleasant skin odour

- delay in development.

Left untreated, phenylketonuria may lead to serious brain damage resulting in severe learning disabilities.

WHAT IS THE TREATMENT?
If your baby is diagnosed as having phenylketonuria, he will probably be prescribed a special formula or milk substitute that is rich in protein but contains little phenylalanine. Your child will have to follow a diet low in phenylalanine for life; this is especially important for women with the condition who might become pregnant. With early diagnosis and treatment, affected children develop normally and attend regular schools.

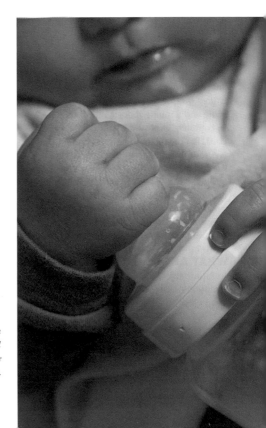

Special formula for phenylketonuria
Babies who have phenylketonuria need a special formula low in phenylalanine, a substance that is present in most proteins.

Clubfoot (talipes)

CLUBFOOT (ALSO CALLED TALIPES) IS A CONDITION IN WHICH A BABY IS
BORN WITH ONE OR BOTH FEET TWISTED OUT OF SHAPE.

Babies are often born with their feet in awkward positions, and there are two types of clubfoot: **positional clubfoot**, in which the twisted foot is flexible and can be manipulated into normal position, and **structural clubfoot**, in which the twisted foot is rigid.

In positional clubfoot, the foot is of normal size but is twisted, possibly due to compression of the baby in the womb. Most cases are mild and correct themselves. Structural clubfoot is a more serious condition in which the foot turns downwards and inwards and is usually abnormally small in size. In about half of babies with structural clubfoot, both are affected. The condition is twice as common in boys and can run in families, which suggests a genetic factor. Both types of clubfoot are usually diagnosed during the routine examination after a baby is born.

WHAT IS THE TREATMENT?

Positional clubfoot may not need treatment. If it does, physical therapy may help straighten the foot, and a cast may be used to move the foot into position. A normal position is usually achieved within three months. Structural clubfoot requires physical therapy and a cast for a long period. In 6 out of 10 cases this treatment is successful. If it is not surgery may be needed between the ages of 6 and 9 months. Surgery is usually successful and enables most children to walk normally.

Cleft lip and palate

A CLEFT LIP AND PALATE ARE SPLITS IN THE UPPER LIP AND THE ROOF OF THE MOUTH THAT ARE
PRESENT FROM BIRTH. THEY MAY OCCUR SINGLY OR TOGETHER AND OCCUR WHEN THE UPPER
LIP OR ROOF OF THE MOUTH DOES NOT FUSE COMPLETELY IN THE FETUS.

In many cases the cause is unknown, but the risk is higher if certain anticonvulsant drugs are taken during pregnancy or if the mother is a heavy drinker. Cleft lip and/or palate sometimes runs in families. Both conditions can be very upsetting for parents, but plastic surgery usually produces excellent results.

If a baby is severely affected, he may find it difficult to feed at first, and if the condition is not treated early, speech may be delayed.

Children with a cleft lip and/or palate are also susceptible to persistent build-up of fluid in the middle ear (glue ear) that impairs hearing and may delay speech.

WHAT IS THE TREATMENT?

A cleft lip is usually repaired surgically by the time a child is three months old, and a cleft palate between the ages of 6 and 15 months. While waiting for surgery, a plate may be fitted into the roof of the mouth if a baby has feeding problems. After surgery, a child may have a hearing test to check for hearing impairment caused by a build-up of fluid in the ear. A child may also need speech therapy when he begins talking. Plastic surgery usually produces excellent results and allows a child's speech to develop normally.

Squint (strabismus)

IT IS QUITE COMMON FOR THE EYES OF NEWBORN BABIES TO MOVE INDEPENDENTLY
OF EACH OTHER UNTIL THE AGE OF 6 WEEKS. AT ABOUT THIS TIME, THE BABY'S
EYES SHOULD BECOME PERMANENTLY ALIGNED.

If alignment doesn't happen, and one or both eyes wander, it is known as a squint or crossed-eyes. This condition is most commonly caused by an imbalance of the eye muscles. It may also be associated with other vision defects such as long or short sight. The brain compensates for the wandering eye by blocking out what it sees.

Your health visitor will check your child's vision at the 6-week, 3-month, 2-year and 3-year development assessments.

WHAT ARE THE SYMPTOMS?

With a squint, the eyes appear to be looking in different directions.

SHOULD I CONSULT THE DOCTOR?

Consult your doctor as soon as possible if the squint persists after your baby is three months old. A squint that persists is serious because the child could lose sight from that eye.

WHAT IS THE TREATMENT?

■ Your doctor will treat the condition by blacking out the strong eye with a pad or patch. This forces the muscles of the wandering eye to work and become stronger. The treatment usually corrects the laziness in the eye within four or five months.

■ If your child is older, an eye specialist will teach your child a series of simple eye exercises to help strengthen the eye muscles.

■ If you child's squint is associated with some vision defect and spectacles are required, you will be referred to an optician.

■ If the squint persists, surgery may be performed to correct muscular imbalance. This will not be contemplated until your child is at least two years old.

WHAT CAN I DO?

■ Have your child's eyes checked annually.
■ If you are concerned about your child's eyes, ask to be referred to an ophthalmologist for another opinion.

BEHAVIOUR AND DEVELOPMENT

In recent years both doctors and the media have paid increasing attention to behavioural disorders in children, especially attention deficit disorder (ADD) and hyperactivity (together called ADHD). More and more children are being diagnosed with behavioural disorders, correctly or not. Diagnosis of autism spectrum disorders also seems to be increasing, probably because the criteria are recognized more than they used to be. Dyslexia and other developmental disorders also concern parents, but much can be done to help.

Attention deficit hyperactivity disorder (ADHD)

FOR WANT OF A LABEL, SOME DIFFICULT BUT COMPLETELY NORMAL CHILDREN ARE SAID TO BE HYPERACTIVE. TO MY MIND THIS IS UNJUSTIFIED.

The word "hyperactive" is the broad term formerly used to describe children who have attention deficit disorder (ADD) and attention deficit hyperactivity disorder (ADHD) – behavioural conditions that include disruptive behaviour, poor attention span, sleeplessness and excitability. Contrary to parental belief, certain food colourings and flavourings have never been proven to contribute to hyperactivity and sympathetic handling by parents can improve the behaviour of most children. Only a few degrees of hyperactivity in children are abnormal or serious or need medical treatment.

WHAT ARE THE SYMPTOMS?
- Disruptive behaviour.
- Restlessness.
- Short attention span.
- Sleeplessness.
- Foolhardiness and unpredictability.

SHOULD I SEE THE DOCTOR?
Consult your doctor for advice if you find your child difficult to live with, or if his behaviour is interfering with his schooling. Your health visitor may also be able to offer advice.

WHAT IS THE MEDICAL APPROACH?
It is difficult to find two doctors who agree on the origin, features or even the fact that there is such a thing as hyperactivity. If minor behavioural problems are combined with any form of learning disability, such as dyslexia, the confusion is compounded. Your doctor may refer your child to a child psychiatrist to establish whether or not the child has ADD/ADHD. If learning difficulties are also present, these are more likely to be detected when your child starts school. Your doctor will not prescribe any drugs unless a definite diagnosis is made.

I, personally, am against the use of drugs such as Ritalin without very careful assessment by several doctors, especially as so many children respond to kinder cognitive and behavioural therapies.

WHAT CAN I DO?
- The essential approach for parents with hyperactive children is sensitive handling and it's best if you both adopt the same approach so that your child gets consistent guidance.
- Learn to live with your child by treating him as an exciting, unpredictable but nevertheless normal child. While your child is young this will be exceedingly difficult, but by the time he goes to school he should have learned to concentrate.
- You will need to be more vigilant if your child is foolhardy and more inventive at providing games so that he doesn't become bored.

Dyspraxia and DAMP

DYSPRAXIA AND DAMP, WHICH STANDS FOR DEFICIT IN ATTENTION, MOTOR CONTROL AND PERCEPTION, ARE TWO CLOSELY LINKED CONDITIONS.

Dyspraxia means simply clumsiness but the medical definition would be the partial loss of the ability to perform skilled, co-ordinated movements in the absence of any defect in motor or sensory functions.

The nervous system is the body's information gathering, storage and control system and it's organized like a computer that controls a highly complex machine. Disorders of the nervous system may result from damage to, or dysfunction of, its component parts. "Motor" is a term used to describe anything that brings about movement, such as a muscle or nerve. It is usually applied to nerves that

stimulate muscles to contract and thereby produce movement, including muscles which control speech. "Perception" is the interpretation of a sensation. People receive information about the environment through the five senses – taste, smell, hearing, vision and touch – but the way in which this information is interpreted depends on other factors too.

HELP FOR YOU AND YOUR CHILD
Drug therapy is usually used for those children with dyspraxia who fail to respond to psychotherapy. In long-term therapy drug

treatment should be gradually withdrawn every year to determine if it's still necessary.

It's important to realize that, if your child is experiencing difficulties, he should be praised for what he can excel at, rather than have attention drawn to what he can't do so well. Patient families and teachers can do a lot to make up for a child's lack of skills.

Coping strategies can go a long way to making the situation easier and, with remedial and other help, many children with dyspraxia manage very well in mainstream education.

FOCUS *on* autistic disorders

Autistic children have problems communicating with people and relating to them in a meaningful way and autism spreads over a wide spectrum of conditions. Autism affects about 1 in 500 children. It always develops before the age of 3, but can be detected as early as 18 months old.

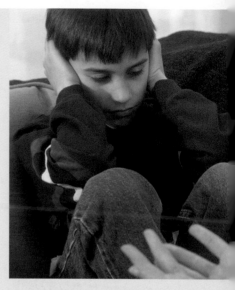

Autistic children are not physically disabled in the same way that a child with cerebral palsy may be, and they look like normal children.

THE FACTS
● The whole spectrum of autistic disorders touches the lives of more than 500,000 families throughout the UK.
● Autism cannot be cured, but research has shown that early intervention through specialist education can make a crucial difference to an autistic child's development.
● At the higher-functioning end of the spectrum is a condition called **Asperger syndrome**; people with it are often highly intelligent but are seen as being socially a bit odd.
● At the lower-functioning end of the spectrum are those who compulsively injure themselves, or who never learn to speak or become toilet trained.
● There is no evidence linking the measles, mumps and rubella (MMR) vaccine to autism.

THE AUTISTIC CHILD
The autistic child is one who is seemingly isolated in his or her own world, who makes no gestures, no eye contact and doesn't speak; who resists change, doesn't play imaginatively or show interest in other children, and is locked into inappropriate, repetitive routines. They have no in-built tools of communication. What they all **share** is a way of perceiving the world that is very different from how you or I perceive it.

The various forms of autism can be grouped into autistic spectrum disorder, a life-long disability. The exact causes are still not known but genetic factors are important, as are certain conditions affecting development of parts of the brain to do with reasoning, social interaction and communication. Typically, a trio of impairments is seen:
1. Difficulty in communicating and relating to others.
2. Lack of imaginative play.
3. Obsessive and ritualistic behaviour.

UNDERSTANDING AUTISM
Autism is four times more likely to occur in boys than girls and knows no racial, ethnic or social boundaries. Family income, lifestyle and educational levels don't affect the chances of its happening.

Autism is said to be as common as **1 in 500 children**, but if you include the whole spectrum it may be as common as **1 in 9**.

Within the spectrum of autism are those with severe learning disabilities at one extreme, and those with high ability who become **fully independent** adults at the other.

Early diagnosis is vital and typical behaviour can usually be seen between birth and three years old. But because there are many forms, children with autism may not be diagnosed and so cannot benefit from the **specialized education** that could help them later on.

The nature of autism, especially the difficulties with social interaction and relating to others, creates particular pressures for the parents, brothers and sisters. And because it's not physically visible, it's hard to promote understanding and awareness in the wider community.

THE PARENTS
Being the parent of an autistic child can be hard, leading to frustration and low morale. You may find that professional help isn't always adequate as these statistics show.
● 65 percent of parents see three or more professionals before they get a firm diagnosis, 25 percent see five professionals or more.
● Multiple diagnoses are often given to parents. Over time, the diagnosis often changes from a general and incomplete one to a more specific diagnosis on the autistic spectrum.
● 45 percent of parents state that autism is explained inadequately or not at all at the time of diagnosis; 81 percent state that there's either no assessment of severity or a vague one.
● 45 percent of parents are dissatisfied to some degree with the diagnostic process, with

Daily Life Therapy

Daily Life Therapy was developed in Japan in the 1960s as a way of teaching children with autism in mainstream schools with emphasis on very positive encouragement for all activities and very high praise for all achievement. The overall aim is for children to develop physically, emotionally and intellectually and therefore achieve social independence and dignity.
Daily Life Therapy has three key objectives:
● to **stabilize** the emotions and build up self-confidence through achievement
● to establish a routine to daily life through physical exercise, which will also build physical strength and control
● to stimulate the intellect with maths, language, communication and social skills.

The approach concentrates on a few basic lessons, so simplifying what's expected from each child. Many activities are group-orientated so that learning isn't only from teacher to child but from child to child as well, often by one child imitating another.
Daily Life Therapy isn't without its critics, who see the group approach as being based on Japanese culture, which might not sit easily in the West. Others are worried about the training element of Daily Life Therapy.

Developmental delay

THE UNDERACHIEVING CHILD OFTEN SHOWS CERTAIN
CHARACTERISTICS FROM BIRTH, WHICH CAN
BE DIFFICULT TO PIN DOWN AT FIRST.

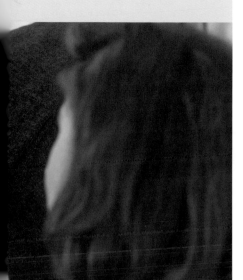

20 percent being very dissatisfied.
- 45 percent of parents report they aren't given any advice about where to go for help/support/counselling after the diagnosis.
- 50 percent of parents say the support they receive at the time of diagnosis is inadequate.

GETTING THE RIGHT HELP

Whatever the age at diagnosis – whether the person is two or 22 years old – the right type of help can make a great difference. Proper assessment can help secure services and support that could improve the quality of life in tangible and practical ways. People with autism and Asperger syndrome need **specialized pre-school help and education**, **respite care** or **support in finding employment** and benefits they have a right to, including **mobility allowances**.

THE GOOD NEWS

The earlier that diagnosis of autism is made, the better the chances are of a child receiving the specialist education and support that can really make a difference.
- Autism professionals **worldwide** agree that early intervention is crucial. Therapies such as the intensive behavioural programmes pioneered in the US have achieved extraordinary results.
- Staying power is essential. In one study of autistic children under the age of 5, nearly 50 percent of children who received 40 hours a week of therapy over two years achieved normal intellectual and educational skills. In contrast, only 2 percent who received 10 hours a week reached the same standard.

Parents often think they simply have a very good and quiet baby. This can, however, signify an unresponsive baby. If you ever find yourself saying any of the following, you should ask your doctor if all is well.

"She is always a very good and quiet baby and hardly ever cries."

"We hardly know we have him; he never gives us any trouble."

"Sometimes she just lies in her pram without moving at all, and she sleeps a lot."

"He is as good as gold, a marvellous baby and no trouble, unlike his brother."

"She hardly makes a sound; she seems to live in a world of her own."

"He only just seemed to come alive when he was about eight months old, he never moved much when he was younger than that."

HOW CAN I RECOGNIZE IT?

What distinguishes developmental delay is a slowness that affects **all** the milestones. Lateness in achieving one or two milestones is common and not abnormal. Nearly always the first sign is a lateness in noticing things and in smiling. Occasionally this is so pronounced that even blindness may be suspected. Because the child may appear to take such little notice of what is going on around him both sight and hearing may be questioned.

Sometimes your child may be late in learning to chew, which may lead to difficulty in eating solids or lumpy food. Some of the milestones may last longer than they should. For instance the **grasp reflex** should be lost around 3 to 4 weeks old but may persist beyond three months or hand regard may go on for as long as 20 weeks. Similarly taking all objects to the mouth, **mouthing**, which is quite normal for children between 6 and 12 months, may go on for longer in affected children.

The desire to throw things over the pram, **casting**, usually stops around 16 months but may go on longer if a baby is mentally slow. And while normal, bright or even exceptionally intelligent children can have attention problems, **lack of concentration** and **interest** may indicate impaired mental ability, as may aimless overactivity. **Pointless overactivity** may not show up for a time and children who were excessive sleepers when they were very young undergo a remarkable transformation and are now unable to concentrate. They may flit from one activity to the other – even flitting physically around the room transiently interested in many tiny things – and this can escalate into almost frenetic

activity that is very difficult to live with. This is particularly true of the autistic child.

WHAT CAN BE DONE?

There is no question that an underachieving child can be helped from a very early age by parental interest, attention, stimulation with songs, chatter, books, games and educational toys. A generally stimulating environment based on listening, discussion and questioning will help your child reach his optimum potential.

This is borne out by a meticulous study on infant intervention schemes carried out by Craig Ramey in North Carolina in the 1980s. Infants who entered the study were those from very poor families whose mothers had low IQs and they were enrolled in special day-care programmes eight hours a day, five days a week. (This does not mean to say that your child has to have such intensive help and education, it simply shows the effect of an education programme.) The children entered the programme from 6 to 12 weeks of age until they were five years old when they began kindergarten in an ordinary school.

The programme was stimulating and emotionally warm, very much the kind of special family characteristics that help children to develop. At the same time there was a control group from similar backgrounds that did not receive the specially enriched programmes but did receive nutritional supplements and medical treatment while being brought up at home.

WHAT THE STUDY SHOWED

The results were unequivocal. At all ages the enriched day-care improved IQ scores significantly over the control group who were reared at home before attending school without an enrichment programme. Furthermore, the difference between children who had attended a pre-school enrichment programme remained significant after a further eighteen months of regular school.

These results do not mean that impaired mental ability can be cured simply by giving children heavy doses of especially stimulating education in infancy. What they show is that the intellectual power of children who begin life with few advantages can be increased if richer stimulation is provided. To me, the importance of these findings is that parents who have children with slightly less mental power than their peers can only help if they try to provide an **enriching environment** in their own homes from infancy onwards.

Dyslexia and learning disabilities

DELAYED SPEECH DEVELOPMENT OFTEN OCCURS BEFORE LEARNING AND READING DISORDERS.
THERE IS SOME EVIDENCE THAT LEARNING DISABILITIES MAY START AS EARLY AS TWO YEARS.

Delayed reading and dyslexia

Delay in learning to read is usually part of a wider spectrum of learning disorders including difficulty in spelling, writing and learning languages, for example. This compound disorder of language, often called dyslexia, may be defined as a reading age of two years or more below the mental age.

Delayed reading may simply be a variation of normal. However, a child who is mentally slow is more often retarded in learning to read than in any other part of school lessons. Common features that go along with late reading are a short attention span, aimless overactivity, defective concentration, impulsiveness, aggressiveness and clumsiness. Your child's visual perception should also be tested.

The label dyslexia is bandied about very loosely these days, but a child should never be labelled dyslexic unless the diagnosis has been made with the help of expert, psychological advice. Nearly always there is a family history of the same complaint, or at least a learning disorder. Dyslexia is four times more common in boys and nearly

always occurs in both of twins. Sometimes there are problems of laterality, which means left- or mixed-handedness, and a tendency to read from right to left or to reverse letters.

Dyslexia is made worse by many factors including young age of the parents, poverty and unemployment, lack of suitable reading material in infancy, lack of to-and-fro conversation, domestic friction, child abuse, sexual abuse, a one-parent family or any cause of insecurity. School factors will include poor teaching, lack of motivation and school absences. Poor teaching or critical teaching may convince a child that he cannot read, and so he stops trying, then teachers are liable to label him as a poor reader and he becomes one so his inability to read turns into a self-fulfilling prophecy.

Dyslexia must have something to do with Western society because it is ten times more common in the West than it is in the East, despite the fact that China has 10,000 letters in common use out of a total of about 50,000.

Learning disabilities very often occur along with poor coordination, repetitive movements, poor memory and the inability to do formboards and drawing.

WHAT MIGHT BE DONE?

Many children grow out of their dyslexic difficulties without special help though some may have slight spelling difficulties for all of their lives. However, do seek special help. Your child's teacher at school or your local headteacher will put you in touch with a psychologist or a special teacher who is experienced in remedial teaching for dyslexic children. Your child may have to attend special classes in the evening several times a week for several years.

Your support and enthusiasm for your child's special lessons, progress and achievements is irreplaceable; you must bear in mind that whatever type of remedial teaching is being used, your child cannot help it and is not just being naughty or stupid. Please tell your child that many famous and eminent people who have gone on to achieve much have experienced exactly the same problem as he. Auguste Rodin, one of the greatest sculptors of all time, was described as "the worst pupil in the school". His father said, "I have an idiot for a son" and his uncle said, "He is ineducable". Rodin never mastered spelling throughout the whole of his life but this did not prevent him excelling at his chosen profession.

The British Dyslexic Association (see Useful addresses, p.567) will give you support, advice and information about local schools and self-help groups where your child's problem and your own difficulties will be treated sympathetically and patiently. It will also provide you with leaflets and books which will help you to understand and care for your child.

Encopresis

IF A CHILD FREQUENTLY PASSES SOLID STOOLS IN HIS PANTS OR IN INAPPROPRIATE PLACES AFTER
HE HAS BOWEL CONTROL, HE IS SUFFERING FROM ENCOPRESIS.

Encopresis that starts in a child who has bowel control should be regarded as a symptom of a problem rather than of slow development. It often starts as the result of some emotional disturbance in the child's life, such as the arrival of a new baby, separation of parents, moving house to a new location and losing contact with friends or divorce. Seen in this way, encopresis should never be punished

or derided. Occasionally, children persist in soiling their pants from infancy onwards. This soiling may be a reaction against over-fussy or over-authoritarian toilet training, something that I'm strongly against.

In a child of four or five, a common cause of encopresis is chronic constipation. Holding of the stools, not wanting to pass them, leading to constipation, may also be a feature. This again

can be the result of a parent placing too high a store on a baby or child passing a stool regularly into a potty. Encopresis is not a serious problem. Never blame your child. First, look at yourselves.

SHOULD I CONSULT THE DOCTOR?

Pure constipation is easy to treat so consult your doctor as soon as possible if you think your child has chronic constipation. If you can find no reason for the involuntary soiling, your doctor may be the best person to discover the cause of tension in the family.

WHAT IS THE TREATMENT?
■ If your child is constipated, your doctor may prescribe a mild laxative, specially formulated for babies and children, which is safe for short-term use.
■ Your doctor or health visitor will advise you on how to reduce the constipation in the future.

■ Where there is some emotional reason for the encopresis, your doctor will assess the situation after discussion with you and your child. If he feels that further counselling is needed, your doctor or health visitor may refer you and your child to a psychotherapist.

WHAT CAN I DO?
■ NEVER punish your child or show disgust if he soils his pants; this will only make matters worse.
■ Watch for signs of poor school performance.

Your child may become a target of scorn because of the odour if he soils himself at school. Be sympathetic and helpful, he really doesn't want to soil his pants, so provide him with spare underpants and take his teacher into your confidence.
■ Make sure your child has a diet that is rich in dietary fibre and liquids and takes regular exercise.

UPPER AIRWAY CONDITIONS IN BABIES AND CHILDREN

The middle ear, throat, sinuses, nose and larynx can be thought of as one single and interconnected system in children, because the tubes and passages that connect each component are very short. Given that in certain places only a few millimetres separate one area from another (for example, the throat connects to the middle ear via the Eustachian tube, which in babies is exceedingly short), it follows that bacteria or viruses treat these spaces as one. So a throat infection can spread almost immediately to the middle ear and cause otitis media (infection of the middle ear).

Similarly an infection of the throat will descend very quickly to the lungs and small airways (bronchioles) because, to an invading virus, the throat and the lungs are the same space in a child. And the younger the child the quicker the spread because distances are so tiny.

As children grow, the air passages lengthen and widen and organisms can no longer leapfrog around the upper airways. In adults the spread of infection is rarer because the ear, nose and throat are anatomically separate. Because of this unifying anatomy in children, there's logic in grouping conditions of the upper airways together, a malfunction of one component nearly always having a knock-on effect on another.

Colds in children

THE COMMON COLD IS CAUSED BY A VIRUS THAT ENTERS THE BODY THROUGH THE NASAL PASSAGES AND THROAT AND CAUSES INFLAMMATION OF THE MUCOUS MEMBRANES LINING THESE PASSAGES.

The body's defences take around 10 days to fight off the common cold virus.

A common cold is not serious, but because it lowers the body's resistance, complications such as **bronchitis** and **pneumonia** have been known to arise. A cold should be regarded more seriously in a baby because minor cold symptoms, such as a blocked nose, can cause her to have feeding problems.

WHAT ARE THE SYMPTOMS?
■ Sneezing.
■ Runny or blocked nose.
■ Raised temperature.
■ Coughing.
■ Sore throat.
■ Aching muscles.
■ Irritability.
■ Catarrh.

SHOULD I CONSULT THE DOCTOR?
Consult your doctor immediately if you think your child has developed a secondary infection. If your baby is having trouble sleeping at night or feeding, consult your doctor or health visitor.

WHAT IS THE TREATMENT?
■ Your doctor will treat any secondary infection to the cold.
■ Your doctor may prescribe nose drops to ease feeding. Use them as directed, as over-use can damage the lining of the nose.
■ Your doctor may prescribe a cough suppressant or an expectorant to ease a bad cough.

WHAT CAN I DO?
■ Ease your baby's breathing by placing a pillow under the cot mattress to raise her head.
■ Give your child plenty to drink.
■ Make nose-blowing easier by blowing one nostril at a time.
■ If possible, create a humid atmosphere in your child's bedroom so that the raw lining of the nose does not become dry.
■ Smear Vaseline on to your child's nose and upper lip if constant blowing has made them sore.
■ Capsules of camphor sprinkled on to clothing and bedding will ease your child's breathing during the night.
■ A hot bedtime drink of freshly squeezed lemon juice and water will ease your child's sore throat and clear her nasal passages.

The flu

IF YOUR CHILD IS OF SCHOOL AGE, THE CHANCES OF ESCAPING AN INFECTION WITH THE COLD OR FLU VIRUS ARE SLIM. THE FLU IS USUALLY QUITE EASY TO DISTINGUISH FROM A COLD. IN THE FIRST PLACE, IT'S MORE SERIOUS AND IT STRIKES MORE QUICKLY.

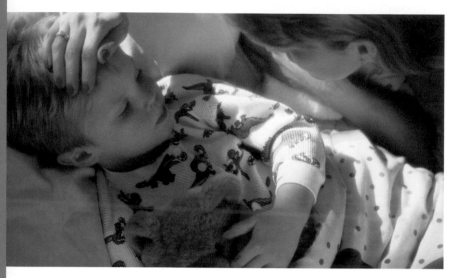

Your six-year-old may be a picture of health one minute and pale, listless and sweaty the next. Here are a few things to bear in mind.

■ The illness usually lasts around three or four days. Unless there's a secondary infection, treatment of the symptoms is all that's necessary most of the time.

■ The flu virus has the ability to mutate readily to new forms, which means it can spread rapidly around the world in epidemics most winters.

IS IT SERIOUS?

It's rare for serious complications to crop up with the flu in children. However, sometimes secondary infections such as **pneumonia**, **otitis media** (middle ear infection), **bronchitis** or **sinusitis** may result.

WHAT ARE THE SYMPTOMS?

■ Runny nose.
■ Sore throat.
■ Cough.
■ Temperature above 38°C (100.4°F).
■ Shivering.
■ Aches and pains.
■ Diarrhoea, vomiting and nausea.
■ Weakness and lethargy.

WHAT SHOULD I DO FIRST?

1. Keep children with flu at home. Don't make them stay in bed unless they want to, instead encourage them to play quietly. Strenuous sports should be avoided during viral illnesses. Use cotton sheets – they are much more comfortable for a child with a temperature. Change the sheets regularly, particularly if your child has a fever – clean sheets feel better.

Leave a box of tissues on the bedside table.
2. While your child has a temperature do your best to keep him at an even temperature, even if that means he lies on the sofa downstairs with you.
3. When your child is ill it's the time to relax all the rules, to put a TV in the bedroom and give special treats. Don't forget illness makes your child feel insecure, so read him stories, play games and give him lots of cuddles.
4. Try to avoid contact with other children outside the family to avoid spreading infection. Avoiding contact with children in the family isn't usually practical.
5. Most children with a fever don't want to eat so, while you should offer food, you should never force your child to eat if he seems unwilling. As long as children are getting plenty of liquid, they can survive perfectly well for two or three days on very little. When the illness is over, your child's appetite will return. As soon as it does, take advantage and let him eat as heartily as he wants to.
6. While you needn't worry if your child eats very little for a day or so, make sure that he gets plenty of fluids to drink. School-age children should drink around four pints (two litres) a day when they have a viral infection – this means six to eight glasses of water or other drinks. For toddlers and younger children who still prefer a bottle, you should make sure that they have a bottle of water or other clear fluids always on hand. Feel free to give them their favourite drink, just so that you can be sure they're getting enough fluid.
7. Take your child's temperature twice a day, and when you are worried about how hot he feels. A raised body temperature is a natural

defence against viral infection, as viruses can't multiply at high temperature. **For this reason, it isn't recommended any longer to bring a high temperature down with tepid sponging, unless it's very high** (over 40°C/104°F).
8. If a rash appears just after the onset of flu symptoms, your child may have measles, so tell your doctor.

SHOULD I CONSULT THE DOCTOR?

Yes, if:

● your child's temperature is consistently higher than 39°C (102.2°F), or your child is unable to manage a good fluid intake. The symptoms of moderate dehydration are a dry cough, highly concentrated (dark yellow) urine or poor output of urine and general lethargy

● you're concerned that a secondary bacterial infection is developing – a worsening cough, or a cough that produces coloured sputum (yellow or green), a pus-like discharge from the nose or an earache

● your child isn't starting to improve within 48 hours.

WHAT MIGHT THE DOCTOR DO?

■ If there's a secondary infection, your doctor may prescribe an **antibiotic**.

■ Recently some **new drugs** have been developed that show promise in reducing the duration and symptoms of flu, but their place in the treatment of straightforward cases isn't yet clear. Your doctor may consider using one of these drugs if it's a severe case of flu or if your child has other health problems.

WHAT CAN I DO TO HELP?

■ **Vaccination** can prevent influenza, but it must be repeated each autumn because of the virus's ability to mutate to new forms. An **annual influenza injection** should be considered for children with a serious chronic medical problem such as **asthma**, **diabetes** or **cystic fibrosis** and for children who are immuno-suppressed, such as transplant recipients or cancer patients. The best time for your child to have a flu jab is between **September and November** to prepare him for the winter. Ask your child's school what plans they have for a vaccination programme or speak to your GP.

■ Let the **school** know that your child has the flu, so that classmates can be diagnosed and treated if necessary.

■ Your child can return to school when the fever and other symptoms have settled down and he's feeling well again.

Croup

CROUP IS THE NAME GIVEN TO THE SOUND MADE WHEN AIR IS BREATHED IN THROUGH
A CONSTRICTED WINDPIPE, PAST INFLAMED VOCAL CORDS.

Croup usually occurs in young children up to the age of about 4, who are susceptible because their air passages (bronchi) are narrow and become blocked with mucus when inflamed – often because of a virus such as a common cold, or an infection such as bronchitis. In rare cases, croup can be caused by an inhaled foreign body. In older children the condition is less serious and is known as laryngitis. The first attack of croup can come on quickly, usually at night, and may last a couple of hours. Your child will have a croaking, barking cough and laboured breathing.

If your child has a severe attack of croup, he could develop breathing difficulties. This should be treated as an emergency.

WHAT ARE THE SYMPTOMS?
- Croaking cough.
- Laboured breathing when the lower chest caves in at every inhalation.
- Wheezing.
- Face colour becoming grey or blue.

SHOULD I CONSULT THE DOCTOR?
Consult your doctor immediately if your child's skin turns grey or blue and he has to fight for breath. Consult your doctor as soon as possible to tell him that your child has had an attack of croup.

WHAT IS THE TREATMENT?
- In a serious attack, your doctor will give your child oxygen.
- If necessary, your doctor will prescribe antibiotics to eradicate any underlying infection.
- Your doctor will give you advice on what to do should your child have another attack.
- If the attack is caused by an inhaled foreign body, your doctor will remove it.

WHAT CAN I DO?
If any further attacks occur, stay with your child and follow your doctor's instructions.

Cough

A COUGH IS EITHER A SYMPTOM OF AN ILLNESS OR THE BODY'S WAY OF REACTING
TO AN IRRITANT IN THE THROAT OR AIR PASSAGES.

A cough may bring up phlegm from the chest and clear mucus from the air passages, for example, during an attack of asthma or whooping cough (this is known as a productive cough).

A dry cough, which produces no phlegm, serves no useful purpose and its cause is not always obvious. The irritation provoking the cough may be mucus from chronically infected sinuses or nasal discharge from a common cold, both of which dribble down and tickle the back of the throat. A dry cough may also be the body's way of bringing up a foreign body stuck in the windpipe. Coughing may be caused by "passive smoking". If adults around your child smoke, the smoke may irritate your child's throat and cause a cough. Children may also adopt a cough as an attention-seeking device, when it becomes a tic or mannerism.

A cough is not usually serious, although it can be irritating. However, a cough that causes breathing difficulties such that your child turns blue around the lips and gasps for breath is serious and should be treated as an emergency.

SHOULD I CONSULT THE DOCTOR?
Consult your doctor as soon as possible if your child's cough doesn't get better after three or four days, or if your child is not getting any sleep at night, or if you cannot remove a foreign body from your child's throat. Consult your doctor immediately if your baby develops a hacking cough or if your child's coughing is

accompanied by rapid, laboured or wheezy breathing. This could be croup or asthma.

WHAT IS THE TREATMENT?
- If your child's cough is part of an infection such as otitis media, tonsillitis, or croup, your doctor will prescribe antibiotics to clear up that infection.
- If your child is suffering from a viral infection, your doctor will advise you on how to relieve the symptoms and help your child to cough up the phlegm.
- If the cough is part of an asthmatic condition, your doctor may prescribe bronchodilator drugs that help to widen the air passages.
- Your doctor may prescribe nose drops to administer sparingly to your child before he goes to bed. These drops ease congestion and prevent mucus from dribbling down the back of your child's throat.
- Your doctor may prescribe a cough medicine: either a cough suppressant (to reduce irritation and soothe the throat) or an expectorant (to encourage the coughing up of phlegm).

WHAT CAN I DO TO HELP?
- Keep your child quiet and warm to help prevent any minor infection from spreading into the lungs and causing a serious condition such as bronchitis.
- Don't let your child run around too much during the day. Breathlessness can bring on a coughing fit.
- Encourage your child to lie on her stomach

or her side at night so that mucus will not dribble into her throat.
- Keep the air in your child's room moist by leaving a window open. Don't overheat the room.
- Don't smoke at home and don't take your child into smoky atmospheres.

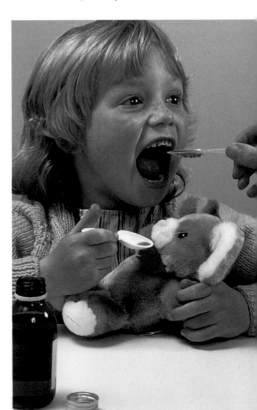

Tonsillitis

POSITIONED AT THE BACK OF THE THROAT, THE TONSILS ARE THE BODY'S FIRST LINE OF DEFENCE.
THEY TRAP AND KILL BACTERIA, PREVENTING THEM FROM ENTERING THE RESPIRATORY TRACT.

In the process the tonsils can become infected, causing tonsillitis. The adenoids at the back of the nose are usually affected as well. Babies under the age of about 1 year rarely suffer from tonsillitis. It occurs mainly among school-age children when the relatively large tonsils and adenoids are exposed to infectious microbes. As resistance to infectious microbes increases, attacks should lessen. Most children do not get tonsillitis after the age of 10. Tonsillitis is not serious unless repeatedly accompanied by infection of the middle ear.

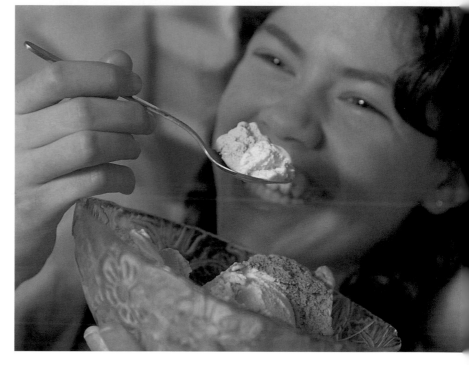

WHAT ARE THE SYMPTOMS?
■ Sore throat, possibly bad enough to cause difficulty in swallowing.
■ Red and enlarged tonsils, possibly covered in yellow spots.
■ A temperature of over 38°C (100.4°F).
■ Swollen glands in the neck.
■ Mouth-breathing, snoring and a nasal voice.
■ Unpleasant breath.

SHOULD I CONSULT THE DOCTOR?
Consult your doctor as soon as possible if you suspect tonsillitis.

WHAT IS THE TREATMENT?
■ Your doctor may take a throat swab to identify the infection. He may prescribe antibiotics for bacterial tonsillitis.
■ He will examine your child's ears to check for any infection and may prescribe antibiotics.
■ If your child has tonsillitis frequently or if enlarged adenoids cause recurrent middle-ear infections, you may be referred to a specialist.

WHAT CAN I DO?
■ Treat your child as you would for fever.
■ Keep his fluid intake up with regular drinks.

■ Never give your child a gargle for a sore throat. It can spread infection from the throat to the middle ear.
■ Offer him foods that slip down easily but don't force him to eat.

Bronchiolitis

BRONCHIOLITIS IS AN INFLAMMATION OF THE SMALLEST AIRWAYS IN THE LUNGS (BRONCHIOLES).
IT IS USUALLY CAUSED BY A VIRUS AND OCCURS IN BABIES UNDER ONE YEAR OLD.
THE CONDITION MAY START AS A COUGH OR COMMON COLD.

The virus causes the lining of the small airways to swell and to fill with mucus. This results in breathing difficulty and the baby will have to struggle for breath. Bronchiolitis is serious because the condition can cause severe breathing difficulties.

WHAT ARE THE SYMPTOMS?
■ Rapid breathing – over 50 breaths per minute.
■ Breathing difficulties.
■ Raised temperature.
■ Blueness of the lips and tongue.
■ Drowsiness.

SHOULD I CONSULT THE DOCTOR?
Consult your doctor immediately or take your baby to the nearest hospital if he has obvious breathing difficulties or if there is any sign of blueness around his lips and on his tongue. Consult your doctor immediately if you notice any deterioration in your baby's condition following a cold or cough.

WHAT IS THE TREATMENT?
If you doctor is satisfied that your baby's infection is a mild one, he will advise you on nursing procedures so that you can look after your baby at home. However, most babies with this condition are usually admitted to hospital overnight for observation.

WHAT CAN I DO TO HELP?
■ If your baby is admitted to hospital, stay with him overnight. Your presence will reassure him.
■ Try to keep your baby away from other children and adults who have coughs and colds.

Glue ear

GLUE EAR IS A CONDITION THAT RESULTS WHEN THE EUSTACHIAN TUBE AND MIDDLE EAR ARE
FILLED WITH FLUID, OFTEN AS A RESULT OF A THROAT INFECTION.

The Eustachian tube, which runs from the throat to the ear, produces large quantities of fluid as a response to chronic infections such as sinusitis, tonsillitis, or, most commonly, infection of the middle ear. If the tube in either ear is blocked by inflammation, the fluid cannot drain and becomes glue-like, impeding the efficient vibration of sound, causing loss of hearing.

Glue ear should be treated seriously because it can lead to permanent loss of hearing in the affected ear, and can cause problems with speech development and learning.

WHAT ARE THE SYMPTOMS?
■ A feeling of fullness in the ear.
■ Partial loss of hearing or deafness in one or both ears.

SHOULD I CONSULT THE DOCTOR?
Consult your doctor as soon as possible.

WHAT IS THE TREATMENT?
■ Your doctor will examine your child's ears with a special instrument called an otoscope.
■ In mild cases, your doctor will prescribe antibiotics to clear up the infection, and she may also prescribe vasoconstrictor drugs, which promote drainage by reducing swelling in the Eustachian tubes.
■ In severe and recurrent cases, your child will probably be referred to an ear, nose and throat specialist for a hearing test. He may be admitted to hospital to have the fluid drained off under a general anaesthetic and grommets

may be inserted. These are tiny plastic tubes that allow mucus to drain away. They either fall out after several months when the ears are healthy again, or can be removed by the specialist. If glue ear is a result of repeated infections or enlarged adenoids, the underlying problem will also be treated to prevent recurrences.

WHAT CAN I DO?
■ If your child has had grommets inserted, he should wait until two weeks after the operation to go swimming and should not dive. Some ear, nose and throat specialists advise against swimming altogether when grommets are in place.
■ Try to keep the ear as dry as possible.

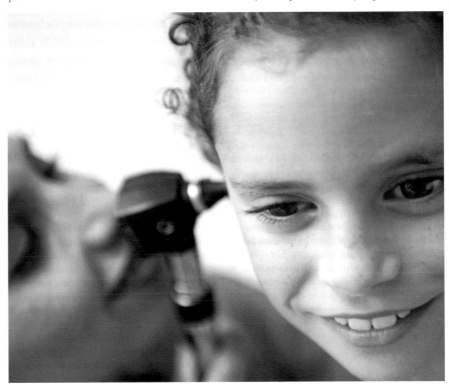

Infectious diseases in children

DISEASE	POSSIBLE SYMPTOMS
Chickenpox A common and mild viral disease.	Red, itchy spots that become fluid-filled blisters and then scabs. Headache and slight fever.
German measles (rubella) A viral infection that is usually mild in children.	Small red spots, first behind the ears, then spreading to the face and all over the body, slight fever, and enlarged lymph nodes at the back of the neck.
Mumps A fairly common viral illness that is seldom serious in children.	Tender, swollen glands below the ears and beneath the skin. Fever, headache, dry mouth and difficulty chewing and swallowing. Less common symptoms are painful testicles in boys and swollen ovaries in girls.
Measles A highly infectious and potentially serious viral illness.	Brownish-red spots appear behind the ears and then spread to the rest of the body. White spots in the mouth (Koplik's spots) are the diagnostic sign. The child is feverish, has a runny nose, a cough and a headache. He may have sore eyes and find it hard to tolerate bright lights.
Whooping cough (pertussis) A bacterial infection that clogs the airways with mucus.	A cough with a distinctive "whoop" sound as the child tries to breathe, common cold symptoms (see p. 533), and vomiting. Coughing may stop your child from sleeping.
Hepatitis A viral infection causing inflammation of the liver. There are two common types, A and B. Type A is more common in children than B.	Loss of appetite, jaundice and flu symptoms. In severe cases, your child may pass dark brown urine and pale stools.
Scarlet fever A bacterial infection whose effects are similar to those of tonsillitis, but accompanied by a rash. It is not very common, and rarely serious.	Enlarged tonsils and a sore throat, a high temperature (up to 40°C or 104°F), abdominal pains, vomiting, a rash of small spots that starts on the chest then spreads and merges, but does not affect the mouth area, and a furry tongue with red patches.
Roseola A relatively rare viral infection whose symptoms resemble those of scarlet fever.	A fever with a temperature of 39–40°C (102.2–104°F) for about three days. After this, red or pink spots appear on the trunk, limbs and neck. The rash fades after about 48 hours.
Diphtheria A serious and highly contagious bacterial infection. It is now very rare because of widespread immunization.	The tonsils are enlarged and may be covered by a grey membrane. Your child may have a mild fever, a cough, a sore throat, breathing difficulties and headaches.
Tuberculosis A highly infectious bacterial infection that most commonly affects the lungs, but can also affect the kidneys, meninges, joints, bones and pelvis if long-term.	Persistent coughing (with blood and pus in the sputum if the lungs are affected), chest pain, shortness of breath, fever (especially at night), poor appetite, weight loss and tiredness.
Poliomyelitis A viral infection of the spinal cord and nerves that can cause paralysis.	High temperature, sore throat, headache, vomiting, weakness, paralysis of muscles, usually in the lower limbs or in the chest.
Impetigo A highly contagious bacterial skin infection most often seen around the lips, eyes and ears.	Tiny blisters around the nose and mouth or ears, which ooze and harden to form crusty, yellow-brown scabs.

TREATMENT	COMPLICATIONS
Apply calamine lotion to the rash, keep your child at home, and discourage scratching. Your doctor may prescribe an anti-infective cream.	In very rare cases chickenpox may lead to encephalitis (inflammation of the brain) and, if aspirin is taken, Reye's syndrome (see p.541), a serious illness whose symptoms are vomiting and fever.
There is no specific medical treatment. You can give your child paracetamol elixir if he has a fever and you should try and keep him in isolation.	The biggest risk is to pregnant women who come into contact with a child with German measles, since it causes birth defects. There is a slight risk of encephalitis.
There is no specific medical treatment. You should keep your child away from school, give him paracetamol elixir and plenty of fluids, and liquidize his food.	Occasionally, meningitis, encephalitis and pancreatitis. Sometimes, one of the testicles is affected and decreases in size. If both testicles are affected, this can lead to infertility, but this occurs very rarely.
Keep your child in bed for the duration of the fever, keep him away from school and give him paracetamol elixir and plenty of fluids. Your doctor may prescribe eye drops for sore eyes and antibiotics for secondary infections.	Ear and chest infections, vomiting and diarrhoea may occur a couple of days after the appearance of a rash. There is also a slight risk of pneumonia and encephalitis. The lungs and ears may be permanently damaged if antibiotics aren't given.
Your doctor may prescribe antibiotics, and in severe cases your child may need to go to hospital for oxygen therapy and treatment for dehydration. Encourage your child to bring up phlegm by laying him over your lap and patting his back as he coughs, don't let him exert himself and keep him away from cigarette smoke.	The main danger is dehydration due to persistent vomiting. Sometimes a severe attack of whooping cough can damage the lungs and make your child prone to chest infections. Secondary infections, which are rare, include pneumonia and bronchitis.
Your child should be isolated and rest in bed for at least two weeks. Be meticulous about hygiene – hepatitis is highly contagious – and give him plenty of fluids. If he won't eat, add a spoonful of glucose to his drinks.	Some children suffer post-hepatitis symptoms for up to six months. These may include moodiness and lethargy.
Your doctor may prescribe antibiotics. Home treatment includes giving your child plenty of fluids and liquidizing food to make it easier to eat. Give paracetamol elixir to lower temperature.	If your child is sensitive to the streptococcus bacterium it may cause complications, including nephritis (inflammation of the kidneys) and rheumatic fever (inflammation of the joints and heart). These are rare.
Keep your child rested and sponge him to reduce his fever if it's very high. Give paracetamol elixir to lower his temperature.	If your child's temperature is very high, he may have febrile convulsions (see p.538).
Diphtheria is very serious because of the possibility of breathing difficulties and your child should be hospitalized immediately. He will be given strong antibiotics and may be given a tracheostomy to help him breathe – that is, a small tube will be inserted temporarily into the windpipe to bypass the blockage in the throat.	Without treatment diphtheria can cause other serious complications: pneumonia and heart failure.
Tuberculosis is a serious disease if left untreated but is rare nowadays due to widespread immunization. The disease can usually be treated at home. Your doctor will prescribe antibiotics.	The main complications of tuberculosis of the lungs are pleural effusion, in which fluid collects between the lung and chest wall, and pneumothorax, in which air is present between the lung and chest wall.
Quiet and bed rest are important; physiotherapy may be necessary. Polio has become rare in recent times due to immunization.	If the disease progresses it can cause paralysis, particularly in the muscles of the lower limbs and chest.
Your doctor will prescribe an antibiotic cream or oral antibiotics.	Impetigo rarely has serious side effects, but because it is highly contagious it should be treated immediately.

Teething

TEETHING IS THE TERM USED TO DESCRIBE THE SYMPTOMS THAT MAY ACCOMPANY THE ERUPTION OF A BABY'S FIRST TEETH. TEETHING USUALLY BEGINS AT ABOUT THE AGE OF 6 OR 7 MONTHS, WITH MOST OF THE FIRST TEETH BREAKING THROUGH BEFORE YOUR BABY IS 18 MONTHS OLD.

Your baby will produce more saliva than usual and will dribble; he will try to cram his fingers into his mouth and chew on his fingers or any other object that he can get hold of. He may be clingy and irritable, have difficulty sleeping, and he may cry and fret more than usual. Most of these symptoms occur just before the teeth erupt. It is important to realize that the symptoms of teething do not include bronchitis, nappy rash, vomiting, diarrhoea or loss of appetite. These are symptoms of an underlying illness, not teething. Teething itself and the symptoms associated with it are never serious. No serious symptoms, for example earache, should ever be explained away as teething.

WHAT ARE THE SYMPTOMS?
- Increased saliva and dribbling.
- Desire to bite on any hard object.
- Irritability and increased clinginess.
- Sleeplessness.
- Swollen red area where the tooth is being cut.

SHOULD I CONSULT THE DOCTOR?
You needn't consult a doctor unless your child's symptoms cannot be attributed to teething.

WHAT IS THE TREATMENT?
Your doctor will give you advice on how to cope with the symptoms of teething and may prescribe a mild analgesic to relieve the pain.

WHAT CAN I DO?
- Nurse your baby often. A teething baby needs comfort and closeness. The arrival of teeth doesn't mean a necessary speeding-up of the weaning process. Babies with teeth can still be breast-fed, with no discomfort to the mother.
- Distract your child with a chilled teething ring (never freeze it or your baby may get frostbite) or a piece of carrot – something with a firm texture. Never leave him with food in case he chokes.
- Try not to resort to giving your baby paracetamol. Over the course of the teething process, doses of such pain relievers could become too large. Only use pain relief on your doctor's advice.
- Rub the swollen gum with your finger. Try to avoid teething jellies that contain local anaesthetics as they have only a temporary effect and can sometimes cause allergy.
- If your child refuses food, encourage him to eat by giving him cold, smooth foods such as yoghurt, ice cream or jelly.

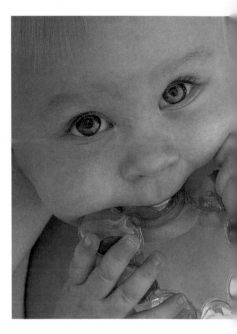

Intussusception

INTUSSUSCEPTION IS A CONDITION THAT OCCURS WHEN PART OF THE SMALL INTESTINE TELESCOPES INSIDE THE INTESTINE AHEAD OF IT, RATHER LIKE A FINGER OF A GLOVE BEING TURNED INSIDE OUT. THE FOLDED INTESTINE SWELLS AND THIS CAUSES A BLOCKAGE.

In an effort to overcome this blockage, the affected intestine goes into spasm, causing pain and vomiting. There is no known cause for intussusception but it mostly affects baby boys under 12 months of age who have previously been in excellent health. The baby may suddenly cry out as the muscular spasm begin and may vomit and be pale and feverish. In between spasms he may appear quite normal and pass normal bowel motions for the first few hours. However, as the attacks continue the bowel motions characteristically look like redcurrant jelly because they consist mostly of blood and mucus.

Though rare, intussusception is a serious condition. Never leave it untreated.

WHAT ARE THE SYMPTOMS?
- Severe abdominal pain, possibly accompanied by screaming.
- Vomiting.
- Paleness.
- Slight fever.
- Bowel motions containing blood and mucus that resemble redcurrant jelly.

SHOULD I CONSULT THE DOCTOR?
Consult your doctor immediately if your baby has a number of attacks or abdominal cramps, or if you notice any blood or mucus in your baby's bowel motions.

WHAT IS THE TREATMENT?
Your doctor will refer your baby to hospital and he will possibly have a barium enema to confirm the diagnosis of intussusception. This is a painless investigation in which fluid is pumped into the intestines through your baby's rectum; the condition of the intestines can then be seen on X-ray. The barium enema sometimes causes the condition to right itself; if it does not, your baby will have an operation when the intestine will be manoeuvred back into its normal position.

See also:
• Contrast X-rays p.353

Colic

COLIC, AS APPLIED TO A BABY UNDER FOUR MONTHS OF AGE, DESCRIBES A CRYING SPELL,
DURING WHICH THE BABY'S FACE BECOMES VERY RED AND BOTH LEGS ARE DRAWN
UP TO HIS STOMACH AS IF HE IS IN GREAT PAIN.

This crying spell usually comes in the early evening; during the rest of the day the baby is generally contented. The crying can reach screaming pitch and last from one to three hours. It doesn't usually respond to soothing techniques that work at other times. Colic is so common that it is regarded by paediatricians as normal, but for parents it can be difficult to endure. The cause of the apparent spasmodic crying is not known. It is often at its worst at three months of age but disappears by four months. Recent research has failed to confirm that colic is caused by pain, even though it looks like your baby is in pain.

The fact that your baby is contented during the rest of the day means that this crying bout is not related to a serious physical problem. Colicky babies are usually healthy and thriving.

WHAT ARE THE SYMPTOMS?
■ Your baby cannot settle in the early evening and cries no matter what you do to calm him.
■ He becomes red-faced and draws his legs up into his stomach as if in pain.
■ He may wake from a short sleep with a startled cry.

SHOULD I CONSULT THE DOCTOR?
Consult your doctor as soon as possible if you find you cannot cope with the nightly crying sessions.

WHAT IS THE TREATMENT?
Colic rarely requires treatment with drugs. Your doctor will reassure you that your baby is healthy and that he will grow out of the colic eventually.

WHAT CAN I DO TO HELP?
■ Make sure you look after yourself. You will be better able to cope if you get as much sleep as you possibly can during the day while your baby sleeps.
■ Invite good friends in to share that time of the evening with you; a relaxed atmosphere may calm both you and your baby.
■ Talk to other parents who have had colicky babies. Once you realize that colic attacks do pass you may find them easier to bear.
■ Consult your health visitor for valuable advice and support.

Appendicitis

THE APPENDIX IS A SHORT BLIND TUBE STICKING OUT FROM THE JUNCTION OF THE SMALL AND
LARGE BOWELS. APPENDICITIS OCCURS WHEN THE APPENDIX BECOMES PARTLY OR WHOLLY
BLOCKED AND A BUILD-UP OF BACTERIA CAUSES AN INFECTION.

The appendix then becomes inflamed and swollen and may need to be removed surgically. An appendectomy is a common emergency operation among children. However, appendicitis in babies under the age of 12 months is rare.

If appendicitis is diagnosed early it is not a serious condition. However, if treatment is delayed for any reason the build-up of pus in the blocked appendix can cause it to burst. This condition is known as **peritonitis** and requires immediate attention.

WHAT ARE THE SYMPTOMS?
■ Abdominal pain, starting around the navel, then moving down to the lower right abdomen.
■ Mild temperature, rarely over 38°C (100.4°F).
■ Loss of appetite.
■ Vomiting, diarrhoea or constipation.

SHOULD I CONSULT THE DOCTOR?
If you suspect that your child has appendicitis consult your doctor immediately. If the appendix has burst any delay could allow the infection to spread to the rest of the intestines.

WHAT IS THE TREATMENT?
Your doctor will examine your child's abdomen and ask you to describe the symptoms. He will probably arrange for your child to be admitted to hospital to confirm the diagnosis and for surgical removal of the appendix, if this is considered necessary.

WHAT CAN I DO TO HELP?
■ Arrange to stay with your child at the hospital overnight.
■ Encourage your child to rest and eat normally when he returns home from hospital, usually about five days after the operation. Your child should recover fully after two to three weeks.

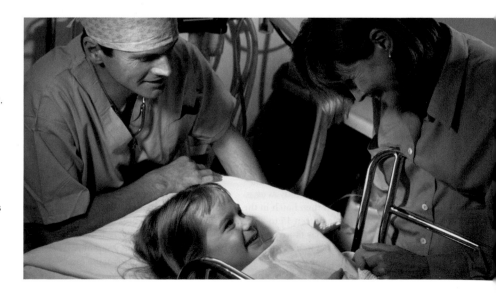

Kawasaki disease

KAWASAKI DISEASE IS A PROLONGED FEVER DURING WHICH THE HEART AND BLOOD VESSELS
MAY BE DAMAGED. IT IS MORE COMMON IN CHILDREN UNDER AGE 5, IN BOYS
AND IN PEOPLE OF ASIAN, AFRICAN OR CARIBBEAN DESCENT.

First observed in Japan in the 1960s, Kawasaki disease is now being diagnosed more often in Western countries. Heart damage occurs in about 1 in 5 of all cases of the disorder. Early diagnosis is important because Kawasaki disease can be life-threatening.

WHAT ARE THE SYMPTOMS?

Symptoms develop over about two weeks and include:

- prolonged, constant fever lasting more than five days
- sore or itchy, watery eyes
- cracked, swollen and painful lips
- sore throat
- swollen glands in the neck, under the arms and in the groin.

After about a week of fever the following symptoms may develop:

- reddening of palms of hands and soles of feet, with peeling skin on tips of fingers and toes
- blotchy pink rash over the entire body.

SHOULD I CONSULT THE DOCTOR?

Consult your doctor immediately if your child develops a fever that cannot be lowered by taking paracetamol elixir.

WHAT IS THE TREATMENT?

■ If your doctor suspects Kawasaki disease your child will be admitted immediately to hospital because treatment is most effective if started within 10 days of the onset of the disease.
■ Your child will probably have blood tests to look for evidence of Kawasaki disease.
■ Echocardiography may be done to look for damage to the heart and blood vessels.
■ Intravenous immunoglobulin may be given to fight the infection and reduce the risk of inflammation of the heart muscle (myocarditis).

■ High doses of aspirin may be given until the fever subsides, with lower doses following for a period of several weeks.

Most children with Kawasaki disease recover completely within three weeks but need regular follow-up visits to the doctor, and sometimes echocardiography, for a few months. Any inflammation of the heart muscle usually disappears after several months. Children who have had Kawasaki disease have a slightly increased risk of developing coronary artery disease later in life.

WHAT CAN I DO?

Care for your child as you would for a child who has just come home from hospital.

See also:
- **Your child in hospital p.519**

Juvenile rheumatoid arthritis

JUVENILE RHEUMATOID ARTHRITIS (JRA) IS PERSISTENT INFLAMMATION OF ONE OR MORE
JOINTS THAT OCCURS ONLY IN CHILDHOOD.

Juvenile rheumatoid arthritis is the result of an abnormal response of the immune system, leading to inflammation, swelling and pain in the lining of one or several joints. Although the cause is not understood, juvenile rheumatoid arthritis sometimes runs in families, suggesting a genetic factor may be involved. In mild cases, mobility is rarely affected. In severe cases, there may be reduced mobility and eventually joint deformities.

Juvenile rheumatoid arthritis is divided into three types according to the number of joints affected by the disease and the specific symptoms involved.

WHAT ARE THE TYPES AND THEIR SYMPTOMS?
SEVERAL JOINTS ARE AFFECTED

This type affects more girls than boys and occurs at any age. Symptoms include inflammation, stiffness and pain in five or more joints. Those joints commonly affected include the wrists, fingers, knees and ankles.

FEW JOINTS AND SOMETIMES OTHER PARTS OF THE BODY ARE AFFECTED

This type affects both sexes equally and usually occurs during early childhood. Symptoms include inflammation, stiffness and pain in four or fewer joints, and girls are at high risk of an eye condition known as **uveitis**. The joints commonly involved include those in the **knees, ankles** and **wrists**.

THE JUVENILE FORM OF ADULT RHEUMATOID ARTHRITIS

This type is also known as Still's disease and affects boys and girls equally at any age during childhood. Any number of joints may be affected, but, although they are painful, they do not become swollen. The other symptoms of the disease include **fever, swollen glands,** and a **non-itchy rash**. Some children recover totally.

SHOULD I CONSULT THE DOCTOR?

Consult your doctor as soon as possible if your child complains of pain in his joints, if his joints are swollen or if you otherwise suspect that your child may have JRA.

WHAT IS THE TREATMENT?

If the doctor suspects that your child has a type of juvenile rheumatoid arthritis, he may arrange for X-rays of the affected joints and blood tests to look for particular antibodies associated with the condition.

The goal of treatment for JRA is to reduce inflammation, minimize joint damage, and relieve pain. If your child is mildly affected, he or she may only need to take **non-steroidal anti-inflammatory drugs** (NSAIDs) to reduce inflammation and relieve pain. In more severe cases your child may be prescribed **oral steroids**, or she may be treated with locally acting steroids **injected into the affected joints**. Sometimes, inflammation can be reduced by using **antirheumatic drugs**, such as gold-based drugs or penicillamine.

Other treatments may include **physiotherapy** to maintain joint mobility and sometimes, **occupational therapy. Splints** may be used for support and to help prevent deformity. **Special devices** are also available and may help with daily activities such as dressing. If damage to the joints is severe and has caused deformity, **joint replacement** may be necessary.

WHAT IS THE OUTLOOK?

Juvenile rheumatoid arthritis usually clears up in a few years. Severely affected children may be left with deformed joints, and some may develop rheumatoid arthritis in adult life.

Moles

MOLES ARE CAUSED BY AN OVERPRODUCTION OF PIGMENTED SKIN CELLS CALLED MELANOCYTES.
THEY CAN FORM ANYWHERE ON THE SKIN, AND THERE ARE SEVERAL TYPES.

WHAT ARE THEY?

Moles are flat or raised growths on the skin, which are rough or smooth and vary in colour from light to dark brown. Freckles, by contrast, are multiple, small, brown-coloured spots on the skin that are usually harmless.

Moles may exist from birth, or appear during childhood and early adolescence; nearly all adults have about 10–20 moles by the age of 30. Most moles are non cancerous, but in rare cases a mole may undergo changes that make it cancerous.

NB Alterations in the shape, colour or size of moles are not always a sign of cancer, and changes during puberty or pregnancy are usually normal. However, any change in moles should always be evaluated by a doctor.

WHAT MIGHT BE DONE?

You should consult a doctor immediately if you have a mole that is more than 1cm (⅜in) in diameter and is growing rapidly. A mole that changes shape or colour, becomes itchy or inflamed or starts bleeding should also be investigated by a doctor.

If your doctor suspects that a mole is cancerous, he or she may recommend that you have it removed and examined for cancerous cells (a biopsy). Non-cancerous moles can also be removed either for cosmetic reasons or if they are being chafed by clothing.

> **See also:**
> • **Tissue tests p.259**

Children's teeth

DENTISTS HATE TAKING OUT TEETH, EVEN BABY ONES, BUT OCCASIONALLY
AN ORTHODONTIST WILL DECIDE TO TAKE OUT A MILK TOOTH TO PREVENT
OVERCROWDING WHILE THE PERMANENT TEETH EMERGE.

Most orthodontists feel that they have to "educate" parents as well as treating the children, because parents often demand corrective treatment for malpositioned teeth long before it should be given. There is no point considering cosmetic dentistry for a child until she is eight years old, since she will not have the requisite number of teeth on which to fix a brace or wire. Most dentists would prefer to wait until a child is about 12 years old before undertaking orthodontic treatment because if this is given too early other faults may occur. In addition, many problems improve naturally if left to the correcting effects of chewing and the position of the tongue, cheeks and lips.

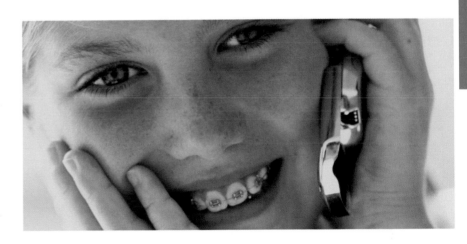

Reference 5

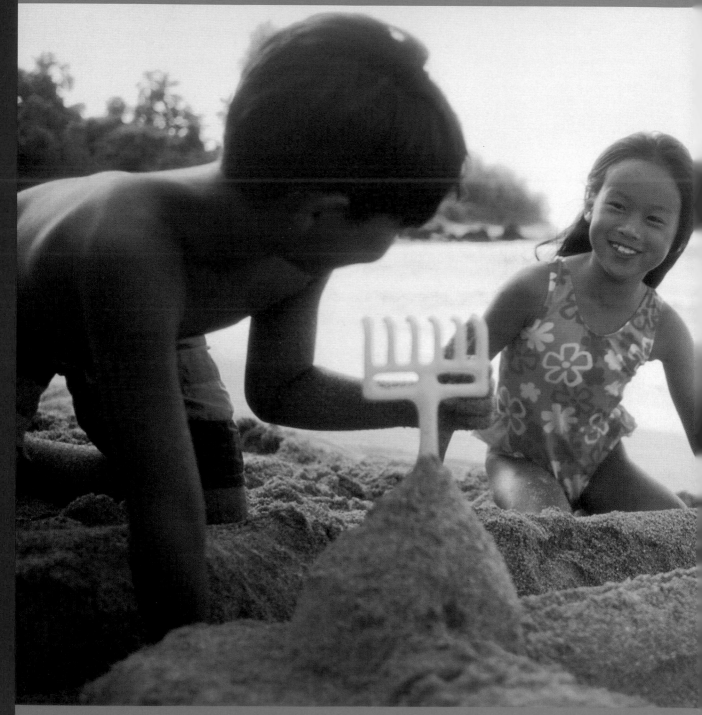

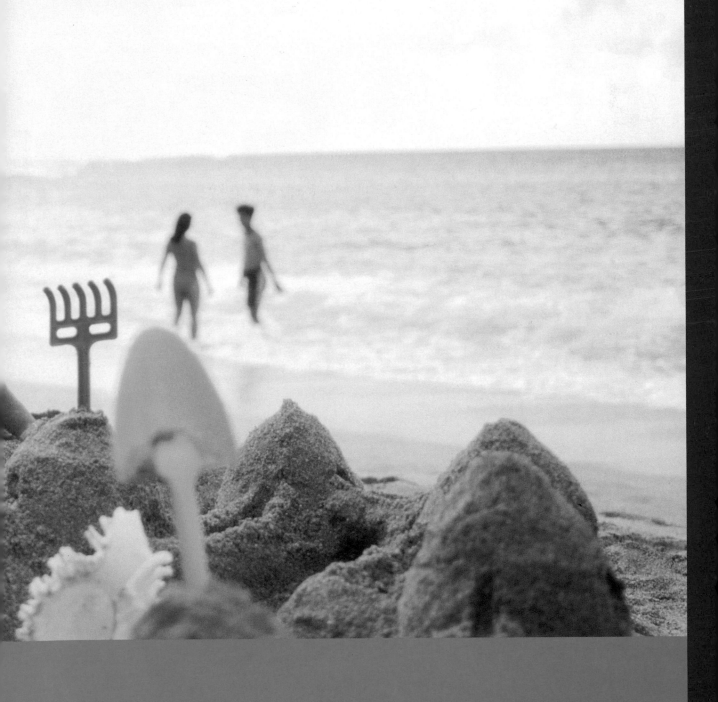

FIRST AID

In an emergency situation you need to assess what has happened and what you need to do, and you must stay as calm and be as methodical as possible while you do so. You need to consider:

• Risks to yourself.

Do not put yourself at risk. If you are injured too, you will not be able to help anyone. Be aware of your limitations; do only as much as you feel able to do.

• Risks to the injured person.

If you can't eliminate a hazard, try to move it away. Move the injured person only as a last resort.

• Risks to bystanders.

• What help you need.

• Resources you can use to help.

The recovery position

The recovery position prevents an unconscious person's tongue from falling back and blocking the throat and allows liquids to drain from the mouth, making it less likely that the person will inhale vomit. If you suspect that the person has a spinal injury, use the log roll technique if you have help (see p.562).

FOR A BABY UNDER ONE YEAR
If a baby is unconscious but is breathing and has signs of circulation (see below), cradle him in your arms with his head tilted downwards. This will prevent him from choking on his tongue or inhaling vomit.

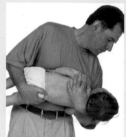

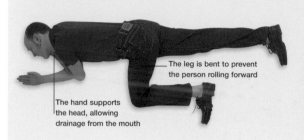

The leg is bent to prevent the person rolling forward

The hand supports the head, allowing drainage from the mouth

The ABC of resuscitation

Once you have determined that it's safe, you can quickly assess the state of the injured person and give emergency aid if necessary. Determine whether or not he is conscious by asking what has happened and gently shaking his shoulders.

You must also assess whether he:

• has an open **airway**

• is **breathing**

• has signs of **circulation**.

A good way to remember what to do is the ABC of resuscitation (see below).

A = airway
Open the airway by gently tilting the injured person's head back and lifting the chin.

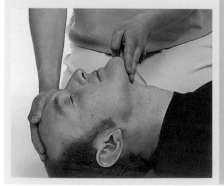

B = breathing
Check to see if he's breathing by looking at the chest to see if it's rising and falling, listening for sounds of breathing, and feeling for breath on your cheek. Do this for up to 10 seconds before you decide that breathing is absent.

If the injured person is **not breathing**, you can keep his blood supply oxygenated by giving **rescue breaths** (see p.555)

Place an injured person who is **breathing** but unconscious in the **recovery position** (see above) to ensure that his airway remains open.

NEVER delay in getting help that you need.

C = circulation
Spend up to 10 seconds looking for evidence of circulation, such as breathing, movement, coughing and a healthy colour of the skin. If **circulation is absent**, you can use **chest compressions** to keep the blood circulating around the body (see p.555). You need to do these along with rescue breaths to keep the blood oxygenated.

If the injured person is **not breathing**, you can keep his blood supply oxygenated by giving **rescue breaths** (see p.555)

Rescue breathing
Body tissues, and especially tissues in the brain, need oxygen to keep their cells alive. Although the air that you breathe out contains only about 16 percent oxygen, it's still enough to maintain life if it's

blown into the lungs of someone who has stopped breathing due to illness or injury. If there are no signs of circulation (see above), you need to perform chest compressions (see p.555) as well; together the two are known as cardiopulmonary resuscitation or CPR.

Mouth-to-mouth rescue breaths

1. With the injured person lying flat on his back, open the airway by placing one hand on the person's forehead and gently tilting the head back.

2. Remove any obvious obstruction from the mouth and lift the chin.

3. Pinch shut the nostrils of the injured person (inset). Take a full breath; place your lips around his mouth to provide a good seal.

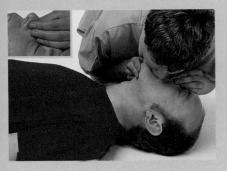

4. Blow into the person's mouth until you see his chest rise. It will take about two seconds for full inflation.

5. Remove your mouth from his and let the chest fall completely – this will take about four seconds. Repeat the procedure once more and then check for signs of circulation (see p.554).

■ **If there are no signs of recovery,** such as return of skin colour or any movement, begin CPR (see below) immediately.

■ **If there are signs of recovery,** but no breathing, give 10 breaths per minute and check for signs of circulation every 10 breaths.

■ **If spontaneous breathing returns,** put the person in the recovery position (see p.554).

RESCUE BREATHING FOR A BABY UNDER ONE YEAR

1. Seal your mouth tightly around the baby's mouth and nose and breathe out into his lungs.

2. Give two breaths, trying to provide 20 breaths every minute. Look for signs of recovery, such as breathing, coughing or return of colour to the skin.

RESCUE BREATHING FOR A CHILD AGED 1–7

1. Pinch the nostrils closed. Seal your lips around his mouth and breathe out into the lungs until the chest rises.

2. Give two breaths, trying to give 15 breaths every minute. Look for signs of recovery, such as breathing, return of skin colour or movement.

Cardiopulmonary resuscitation (CPR)

■ **If there are no signs of circulation** (see p.554), you need to keep the blood circulating around the injured person's body using artificial circulation, which you can provide by chest compressions. You must combine these with rescue breaths to keep the blood oxygenated (see above). Together these are known as cardiopulmonary resuscitation (CPR). Two people can perform CPR together.

1. Kneel beside the injured person, who should be on his back on a flat surface.

2. Find one of the lowermost ribs using the first two fingers of the hand that is closest to the person's legs. Slide your fingers along the rib to the point where the lowermost ribs meet the breastbone. Place your middle finger here (inset) and your index finger above it on the lower breastbone.

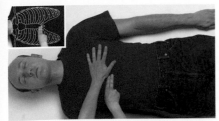

3. Put the heel of your other hand on the breastbone; slide it down until it reaches your index finger. This where you should apply pressure to compress the chest.

4. Put the heel of your first hand on top of the other hand; interlock your fingers (inset).

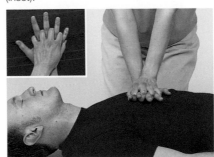

5. Leaning right over the injured person, keep your arms straight and press down vertically to depress the breastbone up to one-third of the depth of the chest (about 4–5cm/1½–2in for an average adult). Remove the pressure but leave your hands in position.

6. Compress the chest 15 times, trying to do so at a rate of 100 compressions per minute. Then give two breaths (see above) before calling for an ambulance. Continue this procedure, alternating 15 compressions with two breaths until help arrives, the casualty recovers or you become exhausted.

CPR FOR A BABY UNDER ONE YEAR

1. With the baby on his back on a flat surface, put the tips of your first two fingers on the lower breastbone. Press down at this point to a third of the depth of the baby's chest. Do this five times, aiming at a rate of 100 compressions per minute.

2. Give one full rescue breath into the baby's nose and mouth (see above).

3. Alternate five chest compressions with one breath for one minute before calling an ambulance. Continue giving CPR alternating five compressions with one breath while you are waiting for help to arrive.

CPR FOR CHILDREN AGED 1–7

1. Place your hand on the child's chest as you would for an adult (see left), but use the heel of one hand only to compress the chest to a third of its depth. Do this five times aiming for a rate of 100 compressions per minute.

2. Give one full rescue breath.

3. Alternate five chest compressions with one breath for one minute before calling an ambulance. Continue giving CPR alternating five compressions with one breath while you are waiting for help to arrive.

Choking

Choking happens when an object or piece of food gets stuck at the back of the throat, blocking it or causing the throat muscles to go into spasm. Young children and babies are prone to choking since they often put things in their mouths. Choking always requires prompt action. Be prepared to resuscitate if the person stops breathing.

Choking in a conscious adult

1. Tell the person choking to cough, but if he can't cough up the object first time don't persist.

2. Bend him forwards from the waist and give him five sharp slaps between the shoulder blades. Use the flat of your hand to do this. Check the mouth and remove any obvious obstructions.

3. If back slaps don't dislodge the object, use up to five abdominal thrusts. Stand behind the person and put your arms around his trunk. Link your hands below his ribcage and pull inwards and upwards sharply.

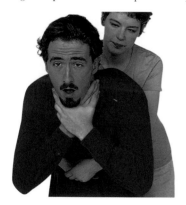

4. Alternate using back slaps and abdominal thrusts until the object is ejected. After three cycles phone for an ambulance.

■ **If the person becomes unconscious,** lay him face upwards on the floor and follow the steps for unconscious choking (below).

Choking in a conscious baby of up to one year

■ **If at any point the object clears** or the baby becomes unconscious, open the airway and check breathing (see p.554).

1. Lay the baby face down against your forearm, supporting the back and chin. Give up to five sharp slaps on his back.

2. Check the baby's mouth and remove any obvious obstruction with a finger. NEVER feel around in the throat.

3. If this fails, turn the baby face up on your arm or lap. Give up to five sharp thrusts into the chest one finger's breadth below the nipple line with your fingertips. NEVER use abdominal thrusts on a baby. Check the baby's mouth.

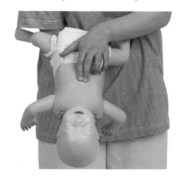

4. If the object has not cleared, repeat steps 1–4 three times and then take the baby with you to phone for an ambulance. Repeat steps 1–4 until help arrives.

■ **If the baby loses consciousness at any time,** follow the steps below.

Choking in a conscious child aged 1–7

1. Bend the child forwards so that his head is lower than his chest. Give him up to five sharp back slaps between his shoulders.

2. Check his mouth and remove any obvious obstruction with one finger.

3. If this doesn't work, stand (or kneel, if necessary) behind him. Make a fist and place it against his lower breastbone. Grasp the fist with your other hand and press it into his chest using a sharp inward thrust. Give up to five of these chest thrusts.

4. Check his mouth and remove any obvious obstruction using a single finger, as in step 2 above. If choking still persists after you have done this, go on to step 5.

5. Make a fist and put it against the child's central upper abdomen. Grasp your fist with your other hand. Press into his abdomen with a sharp upward thrust up to five times. Check his mouth using one finger and if the object has still not cleared, go on to step 6.

6. Repeat steps 1–5 three times and then phone for an ambulance. Keep repeating steps 1–5 until the ambulance arrives.

■ **If the child loses consciousness at any time,** follow instead the steps for choking in an unconscious child (below).

Choking in an unconscious adult, child or baby

FOR ADULTS AND CHILDREN AGED 8 AND OVER

1. Open the airway and check breathing (see p.554). If there is no breathing, give rescue breaths (see p.555). Make five attempts to do two effective breaths.

2. If the person's chest rises during these attempts, continue rescue breaths. If the chest does not rise, do 15 chest compressions and alternate these with two attempted rescue breaths.

3. After each set of 15 chest compressions, check the mouth to see if the obstruction has cleared using one finger to remove any obvious obstruction.

■ **Follow this procedure for one minute** and then, if it has not already been done, phone for an ambulance.

■ **If at any stage the person begins to breathe normally,** you should put him in the recovery position (see p.554). Phone for an ambulance.

FOR BABIES AND CHILDREN AGED 1-7

1. Open the airway by gently tilting the head back. Pick any obvious obstruction out of the mouth and lift the chin.

2. If there is no breathing, give two rescue breaths (see p.555). Check circulation and if there is no circulation, alternate five chest compressions (see p.555) with one rescue breath. Do this for one minute before taking the baby with you to phone for an ambulance.

Asthma attacks

In an asthma attack the muscles of the air passages go into spasm and the linings of the airways swell. This makes the airways narrow and breathing becomes difficult. Sometimes there is a "trigger", such as an allergy or a cold, for an attack; other times there is no obvious reason for an attack coming on.

People who have been diagnosed with asthma usually carry "reliever" inhalers, which are used to relieve an attack and usually have blue caps. Sometimes they also carry "preventer" inhalers, which are used regularly to help prevent attacks and usually have brown or white caps. Plastic "spacers" are sometimes fitted to inhalers to help people breathe in the medication correctly.

If you are with someone who is having an asthma attack, do the following:

1. Keep calm and be as reassuring as you can. Ask the person to use their reliever inhaler and help them to do so if necessary; you may need to fit a spacer to the inhaler. Remember that, although asthma can be frightening, a reliever inhaler usually has an effect within a few minutes.

2. Let the person get into the position they feel is most comfortable; this is often sitting down. DO NOT make the person lie down. Encourage the person to breathe slowly and deeply.

3. If the attack is a mild one and eases within 5 or 10 minutes, ask the person to take another dose from his reliever inhaler. Immediate medical help is not vital, but he should tell his doctor about the attack.

4. If this is a person's first attack or if it is a severe attack and the inhaler has no effect after 5 or 10 minutes, the person is getting worse and breathlessness makes talking difficult, phone for an ambulance. Help him use his inhaler every 5 or 10 minutes, and monitor and record his breathing and pulse regularly.

5. If the person stops breathing or loses consciousness, open his airway and check breathing and circulation (see p.554). Be ready to resuscitate if necessary. Phone for an ambulance.

DO NOT use a preventer inhaler (brown or white cap) during an asthma attack.

Croup

Croup is an attack of breathing difficulty in a baby or a child that is caused by inflammation in the larynx and windpipe. The child may make a barking noise when he coughs and wheeze when trying to breathe. It can be frightening but an attack usually passes without any lasting harm. Croup often occurs at night.

If an attack of croup does not clear or is severe, if your child's skin takes on a bluish tinge, or if croup is accompanied by feverish illness, phone the emergency services and ask for an ambulance immediately.

If you are with a child who is having an attack of croup, do the following:

1. Sit the child up and reassure him. Make sure his back is supported against something.

NEVER stick your fingers into the child's throat, and do not panic, as you will only frighten the child and worsen the attack.

2. Either create a steamy atmosphere by using a humidifier or boiling a kettle in the child's room or move the child into the bathroom and run the hot tap or the shower. Sit him down and encourage him to relax and breathe in the steam. Be sure you keep the child well away from the hot water.

3. When the child is put back to bed, create a humid atmosphere in the bedroom by using a humidifier, boiling a kettle or hanging a wet towel over a radiator. The humidity may prevent an attack from recurring.

4. Call your doctor or phone for an ambulance if the steam doesn't bring relief or if the attack is severe.

Anaphylactic shock

Anaphylactic shock (anaphylaxis) occurs when the body has a serious, general allergic reaction to something. Medical attention is urgently required and first aid is limited to helping breathing and minimizing shock until medical help arrives.

A person who develops anaphylactic shock may have widespread red blotches on the skin, obvious difficulty breathing and swelling in the face and neck. An injection of epinephrine (adrenaline) eases the symptoms, and people with severe allergies usually carry injectable epinephrine (an Epi-Pen) with them. If an affected person has an Epi-Pen, help her to use it as soon as signs of anaphylactic shock become apparent.

1. Phone the emergency services and ask for an ambulance immediately. Say that you suspect anaphylactic shock.

2. If the person is conscious, help her sit up in a position that helps breathing the most.

3. If the person is unconscious, put her in the recovery position and monitor her breathing, pulse and level of response regularly. Be prepared to resuscitate if necessary.

Seizures

A seizure (also known as a convulsion or fit) occurs when disturbance in the function of the brain causes involuntary contraction of muscles in the body. There are many causes of seizures, including head injury, certain diseases or conditions that affect the brain (such as epilepsy) or shortage of oxygen to the brain.

In babies and young children, high fever may cause seizures (see Febrile convulsions, below). Seizures usually cause consciousness to be lost or impaired, and in any seizure in which consciousness is lost, follow the treatment rules for unconsciousness (see below).

Epileptic seizures

There are two basic types of epileptic seizures: petit mal and grand mal. Petit mal seizures are also known as absence seizures, because people who experience them do not lose consciousness completely but enter into a state like daydreaming. Grand mal seizures involve unconsciousness and uncontrollable twitching or jerking of the limbs.

PETIT MAL (ABSENCE) SEIZURES

1. Help the person experiencing the seizure to sit down; remove any sharp objects or hot drinks from the nearby area.

2. Talk to her calmly but don't ask her unnecessary questions. Stay with her until the seizure has passed and she is behaving like her normal self again.

■ **If the person is unaware of her absence seizures,** suggest to her that she see her doctor.

GRAND MAL SEIZURES

1 If the person is falling, try to ease his fall if you can. Clear the space around him and ask any bystanders to stand back.

2 Loosen his clothing and put something soft under his head if possible.

3 Once the seizures have stopped, put him in the recovery position (see p.554). Check his breathing, pulse and level of response and stay with him until he is fully recovered.

■ **If a person is unconscious** for more than 10 minutes or the convulsions last for more than 5 minutes, phone for an ambulance. You should note down the time the seizure occurred and its duration.

Febrile convulsions

Babies and small children are prone to seizures when their core body temperature rises very high, as in a fever. Febrile convulsions are frightening but are not usually dangerous or indicative of epilepsy.

1. Put pillows or other soft objects around the child so that she won't harm herself. Undress her down to underwear.

2. Sponge her with tepid (not cold) water (cold water makes blood vessels constrict and drives body temperature up).

Start at her head and work down the body.

3. Ensure that her airway is open and put her in the recovery position once the seizure stops.

4. Phone for an ambulance.

> **DO NOT** lift or move a person having a convulsion unless he is in danger.
>
> **DO NOT** put anything into his mouth or attempt to restrain him in any way.

Unconsciousness

Unconsciousness occurs when the brain's normal electrical activity is interrupted, for whatever reason. A number of different conditions and accidents can cause unconsciousness, including fainting due to low blood sugar or low blood pressure, epilepsy and head injury. If a person is unconscious, follow these rules:

1. Open airway, check breathing and be ready to resuscitate (see p.555). Place him in the recovery position.

2. Examine the person for injuries, but in doing so you should not move him unnecessarily.

3. Check his response level regularly. In doing so you should consider whether he can open his eyes, can obey commands

The recovery postition

or respond to a pinch, and answer sensibly a simple question such as "what is your name?".

■ **Even if the person regains full consciousness** and remains well, he should see his doctor as soon as possible. If he does not recover or his condition deteriorates, Phone for an ambulance and continue monitoring the person's response level until help arrives.

Concussion

Concussion occurs when the brain is shaken a little in a fall or a violent blow. Although there may be a brief or partial loss of consciousness, it is followed by complete recovery. Concussion can only be safely diagnosed after the person has made a complete recovery.

You should bear in mind that all head injuries are potentially serious and should be assessed by a doctor.

1. If the person is unconscious following a head injury, put her in the recovery position (see p.554). Watch her closely; while you are doing this you should also remember to monitor and record her breathing, pulse and response level regularly. If the person remains unconscious, phone and ask for an ambulance.

2. If the person regains consciousness, you should continue to watch her carefully, looking for any change in her level of response, even if she has apparently made a full recovery.

3. Advise the person to see her doctor, even if she appears to have made a full recovery. It is particularly important for her to see a doctor if she experiences headache, sickness or tiredness afterwards.

Bleeding

Minor bleeding can be distressing but is not usually cause for alarm; it can usually be controlled or stopped by applying direct pressure to the wound and does not need medical attention. More severe bleeding needs prompt action to control blood loss and requires immediate medical attention.

Minor bleeding

First aid for minor injuries that break the skin helps to minimize the risk of infection developing and aids healing. However, you should always seek medical advice if:
● a foreign object, such as a piece of glass or gravel, is embedded in a wound
● the wound is a puncture wound or a bite
● a previous wound shows signs of becoming infected, for example if it becomes red and sore or if there is pus in it.

TO TREAT MINOR EXTERNAL BLEEDING:
1. Wash your hands well in soap and water before you treat the wound. Put on disposable gloves if available.

2. If there is dirt on the wound, rinse it under running water; alternatively, use an antiseptic wipe. Pat the wound dry with clean gauze. Cover the wound with clean gauze.

3. Elevate the part of the body that has been wounded above the level of the heart. Don't touch the wound directly and support the elevated part with one hand.

4. Clean the area around the wound with soap and water. Pat dry and remove the gauze. Apply an adhesive dressing.

Severe bleeding

Severe bleeding is very upsetting and frightening, but bear in mind that blood loss is rarely so great that the heart stops beating. It is, however, likely that the injured person will be in shock and may lose consciousness. Try to remain calm.

TO CONTROL SEVERE BLEEDING, DO THE FOLLOWING:
1. Put on disposable gloves if available. Remove clothing from the area of the wound, cutting it off if necessary.

2. Apply direct pressure on the wound with your fingers or palm. Use a clean dressing if one is to hand, but don't waste time looking for one. If an object is embedded in the wound, apply pressure firmly on either side of it.

3. Carefully raise the injured area so that it is above the level of the person's heart. Lay her down to reduce blood flow to the wound.

4. Apply a sterile dressing, but leave any original dressing in place. Make the bandage tight, but not so tight that it prevents circulation. Apply another bandage on top if blood is seeping through.

5. Phone for an ambulance and treat the injured person for shock (see p.560). Make sure that the bandages you have applied do not impede circulation.

> **NEVER apply a tourniquet; it can actually worsen bleeding and can cause tissue damage and possibly gangrene.**

A foreign object in a minor wound

1. Do not try to remove objects embedded in a wound. Small pieces of glass or gravel may be picked off the surface of a small wound, but if you try to remove objects more deeply embedded you may damage the tissue further and make bleeding worse.

2. Control bleeding by applying pressure to the wound on either side of the object using a piece of clean gauze. Elevate the injured part if possible.

3. Cover the wound with clean gauze and put pads made of gauze or cotton wadding around the object so that you are able to put a bandage over it without pressing directly on it. If you can't build the pads high enough, put the bandage around the object instead.

4. Arrange for the person to go to hospital as soon as possible.

Nosebleeds

Nosebleeds happen when blood vessels inside the nose get broken. A nosebleed can be alarming, but it is only dangerous if a great deal of blood is lost. However, if the fluid that comes out of the nose appears thin and watery following a head injury, this is a serious condition that may indicate that cerebrospinal fluid is leaking from the area surrounding the brain.

1. Ask the person to sit down and put his head forward. NEVER put the head back during a nosebleed as the blood running down the throat can cause vomiting.

2. Ask the person to breathe through his mouth and pinch his nose below the bridge. Help him if he cannot do this himself. Ask him not to speak or try to clear his nose, since these things can interfere with blood clotting. Give him a tissue or handkerchief to hold against his nose to mop up any blood.

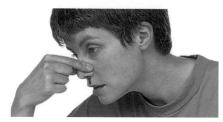

A young child can lean over a bowl and spit into it if this helps.

3. Ask the person to stop pinching his nose after 10 minutes. If the bleeding continues, repeat the procedure for another 10 minutes and check again. If after 30 minutes the person's nose is still bleeding, take the person to a hospital casualty ward with his head in the forward position.

4. When the bleeding has stopped, ask the person to stay leaning forward; gently clean the area around the nose. The person should rest for a few hours and should not blow his nose, which could cause bleeding to start again.

Shock

Shock occurs if the supply of blood to the body's vital organs is reduced. This may occur for a variety of reasons: if the heart doesn't pump blood normally (as in a heart attack); if blood vessels dilate, reducing blood pressure (as in anaphylactic shock); or if blood or other bodily fluids are lost through injury, burns, diarrhoea or vomiting.

NB The type of shock a person experiences in stressful situations where there is no physical injury is called psychogenic shock and is a separate condition needing different treatment.

SIGNS OF SHOCK
- Rapid pulse.
- Pale, sometimes bluish skin.
- Sweating and cold skin.

IF SHOCK DEVELOPS FURTHER
- Weakness and dizziness.
- Nausea and possible vomiting.
- Thirstiness.
- Rapid and shallow breathing.
- A weak pulse.

IF SHOCK CONTINUES
- Restlessness and possible aggressiveness.
- Yawning and gasping for air.
- Unconsciousness.
- Failure of the heart to beat.

TREATING SHOCK
1. Lay the person down (on a coat or a blanket if outdoors or on a cold surface), and keep her head low. Talk to her reassuringly.

2. Raise the person's legs; this will help the blood supply to the vital organs.

3. Loosen any tight clothing; the person may be wearing, such as a tie, a tight collar, cuffs or a belt.

4. Keep the person warm by covering her with coats or blankets. DO NOT put any direct source of heat near the casualty or use an electric blanket or hot water bottle. Phone for an ambulance. Record the person's breathing, pulse and response level and be prepared to resuscitate if necessary (see p.555).

A person in shock should not smoke, eat, drink or move around unnecessarily. Don't leave a person in shock on her own. If she become unconscious, be prepared to resuscitate.

Eye injury

All eye injuries should be considered potentially serious. They require prompt medical attention to minimize the risk of infection or scarring of eye tissues, which may lead to permanently impaired vision. The injured eye may appear bloodshot or may bleed or leak clear fluid.

1. Lay the injured person on his back, keeping his head still.

2. Tell the person not to move his eyes, as movement of the uninjured eye will also cause movement of the injured one.

3. Ask the person to hold a sterile dressing over the injured eye, which will help keep his from moving it and will help prevent infection.

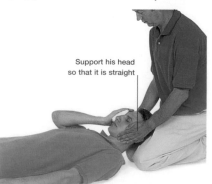

Support his head so that it is straight

4. Take the person to a hospital casualty department immediately.

> **DO NOT** touch an injured eye or attempt to remove any object embedded in it.

Foreign objects in the eye

While a speck of dust or a contact lens that is floating on the surface of the eye may be easily removed, anything that is actually stuck to the eye or embedded in it should not be touched. Take the person to a doctor or a casualty department.

1. Ask the person not to touch or rub her eye. Ask her to sit down and face a light source. Then gently pull back the upper and lower eyelids and look carefully at the eye.

2. If there is a foreign object floating on the surface of the eye, wash it out by pouring clean water over it, or by using an eyebath filled with clean water.

3. If this doesn't work, you can try to lift it out with a moist cotton swab, or a dampened corner of a tissue or clean cloth. DO NOT try to do this if the object is stuck in place.

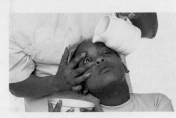

4. If the object is under the upper eyelid, ask the person to pull the upper eyelid over the lower one. This often dislodges the object.

Foreign objects in the nose

Young children are especially prone to this situation. They may put small objects up their noses, which can cause injury, infection or blockage. Do not try to remove an object from the nose yourself, as you may cause further injury or push the object further in. Instead keep the person calm and quiet, encourage him to breathe through his mouth, and take him to a hospital casualty department immediately.

Foreign objects in the ear

An object in the ear may cause temporary deafness or may injure the eardrum. Do not try to remove any object in the ear yourself, as you may worsen the injury. However, if an insect has flown or crawled into the ear, you can try rinsing it out using the following method.

1. Ask the person to sit down and stay calm.

2. Gently pour a glass of clean, tepid water into the ear, which may wash the insect out.

3. If this doesn't work, take the person to a hospital casualty department.

Broken bones and soft tissue injuries

If a person is unable to move an injured part of the body, or if the injured area is misshapen or very painful, you should suspect a bone fracture. Soft tissue injuries, such as injuries to joints, ligaments, tendons and muscles, may also cause severe pain and swelling and may sometimes be difficult to distinguish from fractures.

Bone fractures

There are two basic types of bone fracture: open fractures, in which the skin is broken and the bone is exposed, and closed fractures, in which the skin near the bone is not broken and bone doesn't protrude from the skin. An open fracture is more likely to become infected than a closed fracture, because the bone is exposed to bacteria in the air. A closed fracture will often have extensive bruising and swelling on the skin covering and near the site of the break.

TO TREAT AN OPEN FRACTURE:
If possible, get a helper to steady and support the injured area while you work.

1. Cover the wound with a clean dressing and apply pressure to control bleeding,

if necessary. However, you should NOT press down directly on a protruding bone.

2. Put some clean padding over the dressing and around it. Do not touch the wound with your fingers.

3. Keep placing padding around the wound until it is possible to put a bandage over the pads without pressing directly on the bone.

4. Fasten the dressing and padding firmly, but do not make it so tight that circulation might be impaired. Immobilize the injured part by taping or tying it gently but firmly to an adjoining part of the body (i.e. an arm against the trunk of the body, a leg against the other leg).

5. Phone the emergency services and ask for an ambulance. Check the circulation beyond the bandage regularly, and observe the injured person for shock (see p.560).

TO TREAT A CLOSED FRACTURE OR A DISLOCATED BONE:

1. Ask the injured person to stay still, and gently immobilize the injured part by taping or tying it firmly to an adjoining part of the body (i.e. an arm against the trunk of the body, a leg against the other leg).

2. Phone for an ambulance. Look for signs of shock and check the circulation beyond the injured area regularly.

Muscle strains and tears

Remember "RICE" (Rest, Ice, Compression and Elevation) when treating soft tissue injuries, such as muscle strains or sprains. If the injury isn't better in 24 hours, consult a doctor.

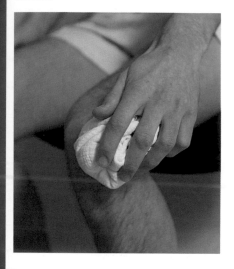

1. Apply an ice pack (ice cubes in a plastic bag, or a bag of frozen vegetables such as peas) to lessen swelling and relieve pain.

2. Wrap the injured area firmly but not too tightly using a layer of thick, soft material (such as cotton wadding) on the inside and an elastic bandage on the outside.

3. Raise the injured area to reduce blood flow to it.

4. If the injured person is still in pain, go to the casualty ward at the nearest hospital. Otherwise, he should continue resting the injured area and see a doctor if the injury seems no better after 24 hours.

> **DO NOT try to put a dislocated bone back into its socket.**

Back injury

The main danger in any back injury is damage to the spinal cord. If the spinal cord is damaged, paralysis or loss of sensation may occur below the damaged area. For this reason any back injury must be treated very carefully.

If you suspect a back injury, DO NOT move the affected person unless she is in danger or she is unconscious and her airway is not open. If you must move a person with a back injury, use the following procedure for "log roll":

1 Keep the person's head, trunk and toes in a straight line throughout the procedure.

2 While one person supports the neck, get helpers to straighten her limbs and roll her, as if she were a log, onto a stretcher on her back. Get five people to help if you can.

Slings

A sling is used to support an injured arm. You can improvise a sling with a shirt or jacket if necessary.

1. Hold the injured arm so that the hand is above the elbow, if this is possible. (If it is not possible, don't force the arm into this position.) Put one end of the sling through at the elbow and pull it around to the person's opposite shoulder. Open out the bandage so that its bottom is level with the person's little fingernail on the hand of the injured arm.

2. Bring the lower end of the sling over the person's forearm so that it meets the other end at the shoulder of the injured arm.

3. Tie a knot and tuck the ends in under it to act as padding.

4. Fold the point of the sling (by the injured elbow) forwards and tuck it into the sling. Pin it in place with a safety pin. If you don't have a safety pin, twist the point and tuck into the back of the sling.

5. Check the circulation in the person's fingers regularly. If they seem cold or numb, undo the sling and loosen any bandages.

Roller bandages

Roller bandages can be used to hold dressings in place or to provide compression for soft tissue injuries. The method of application is slightly different for each of these purposes.

To hold a dressing in place:

1. Put the end of the bandage below the injured area and, working outwards, make two straight overlapping turns to anchor it.

2. Wind the bandage from the inside to the outside of the limb in spiralling turns, working up the limb and over any dressings.

3. Use one straight overlapping turn to finish, and fasten the end of the bandage using clips, safety pins or adhesive tape.

To compress a soft tissue injury to a joint:

1. Hold the injured limb in a comfortable position. Flex the joint if possible.

2. Place the end of the bandage on the inside of the joint. Fix the bandage by winding it around the joint one and a half times.

3. Wind the bandage once around the limb just above the joint. Make a diagonal turn and wrap the bandage down just below the joint.

4. Continue wrapping in this manner, above and below, overlapping the bandage in a figure of 8 so that it extends a short way up and down the limb.

5. Use two straight turns to finish, and fasten the end of the bandage using clips, safety pins or adhesive tape.

6. Check circulation by pressing on a finger or toenail (colour should return right away) every 10 minutes. If the bandage is too tight, undo it and wait until circulation is normal before reapplying it more loosely.

Burns

Before you treat a burn, you must try to determine its depth and extent. Deep and/or extensive burns are likely to cause shock (see p.560) because they cause the body to lose essential tissue fluids. They also destroy the skin, which is the body's natural barrier to bacteria in the environment, and so infection is also a risk.

There are three types of burn: superficial, partial-thickness and full-thickness.

1. A superficial burn involves the outermost layer of skin only; the skin looks red, swollen and tender. Medical help is needed if the burn covers more than 5 percent of the body surface.

2. A partial-thickness burn affects the underlying layer of skin, the epidermis, and looks raw and blistered. Medical attention is needed.

3. A full-thickness burn affects all layers of skin and possibly nerves, fat tissue and muscle. The skin looks yellow, pale or charred. Urgent medical attention is essential.

Blisters

Blisters form on skin damaged by heat or friction. The "bubble" appearance of a blister is due to tissue fluid, called serum, entering the area just below the skin's surface. If left alone the serum is re-absorbed by the tissue, new skin forms and the outer layer of dead skin falls off.

Blisters usually need no treatment. Do NOT burst them, because this interrupts the healing process and could cause infection. If a blister breaks on its own, cover the area with a sterile dressing and leave it until the area has healed.

Minor burns

These are superficial burns that will heal naturally after first-aid treatment. (NB You should always seek medical advice if you are not sure how serious an injury is.)

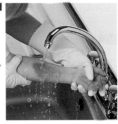

1. Run the burned area under cold water for at least 10 minutes. If there is no water available, any cold, harmless liquid such as canned drinks will work just as well.

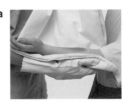

2. Cover the area with a sterile dressing or a piece of clean material that is not linty or fluffy. Bandage it loosely in place.

3. If blisters appear, DO NOT break them. This could introduce infection into the wound.

> **DO NOT apply lotions, butter or other fats to the wound. This could cause infection and further tissue damage.**

Severe burns

Your main aim in treating a severe burn is to cool the burn. You must also make sure that the person affected is able to breathe and you must get emergency help.

1. Make sure the casualty is lying down. Cool the burned area by pouring cold liquid on it for 10 minutes or until emergency help arrives.

2. Gently remove any clothing or jewellery from the injured area, unless it is sticking to the burn, cutting it off if necessary.

3. Cover the injured area with a clean, lint-free dressing (if a dressing isn't available you can improvise with a piece of a clean sheet or plastic kitchen film).

4. Phone the emergency services and ask for an ambulance. Reassure the injured person while you wait for help to arrive.

Heatstroke

In heatstroke the body's ability to control its own temperature fails and the body becomes dangerously overheated. It can occur rapidly, within a matter of minutes, and may cause unconsciousness. A person affected by heatstroke may be dizzy and have a headache, and may seem restless or confused. Her skin may be dry but hot and flushed, and she may have a rapid pulse.

1. Make sure the affected person is in a cool place. Indoors is best, but at least move her into the shade. Take off as much outer clothing as possible. Phone for an ambulance.

2. Cover the person in a cold, wet sheet and keep wetting it. Take her temperature frequently and continue this procedure until her temperature has fallen to 38°C (100.4°F).

3. When her temperature has fallen to this level, remove the wet sheet and cover her with a dry one. Reassure her until help arrives.

Sunburn

Sunburn is usually a mild burn caused by over-exposure to sunlight, although it can be severe, in which case the skin will be very red and blistered and heatstroke (see left) may be present. Sunburn can happen even on overcast days and may be due to the reflection of the sun's rays from snow or sand.

1. Cover the affected skin with a light towel or with light clothing. Take the affected person indoors or at least into the shade.

2. Cool the skin by pouring cold water over it or sponging carefully with cold water. If there is blistering, seek medical advice.

3. Give the affected person cool water to drink. Calamine lotion or after-sun cream may soothe the affected area if the burning isn't severe.

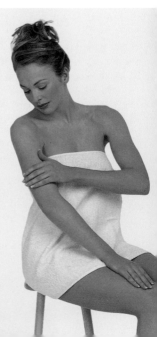

Bites and stings

Insect bites and stings may be painful but are relatively harmless compared to animal and human bites, which must always receive medical treatment. However, certain snakes and spiders, especially those encountered abroad, may be highly poisonous and if you are in doubt as to the seriousness of a bite, you should seek medical attention.

Insect bites and stings

1. To remove a sting such as a wasp or bee sting, gently scrape the affected area with a blunt-edged knife or a credit 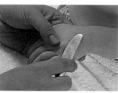 card until it comes out. Do not use tweezers to remove the sting since this can squeeze the poison sack and inject more of it into the skin.

2. Apply a cold cloth to the area. If swelling becomes worse or persists, call a doctor.

■ **If someone is stung in the mouth,** let the person suck on an ice cube or something cold and phone for an ambulance.

■ **To remove a tick,** grasp the tick as close to the person's skin as possible using fine tweezers. Using a slight rocking action, gently dislodge the tick from the skin. Keep the tick in a container and take it to a doctor for analysis, as ticks can carry diseases, such as Lyme disease (see p.354).

Snake bites

The adder is the only poisonous snake that is native to the mainland United Kingdom, and its bite rarely causes death. However, some people keep exotic snakes as pets and their bites may be more severe. If a snakebite occurs, try to put the snake in a secure container or make a note of what it looks like; this may help identify the snake so that the correct antivenom may be given. If the snake has escaped, tell the police.

1. Ask the injured person to lie down. Try to keep him as calm and still as possible to help prevent the venom from spreading.

2. Wash the wound gently and pat it dry.

3. Compress the area above the wound lightly with a bandage and immobilize the injured area as you would for a broken bone (see p.561).

> **DO NOT put a tourniquet above the wound, cut the wound open with a knife, or try to suck out the venom.**

Animal and human bites

Puncture wounds caused by an animal's teeth can carry germs deep into the flesh. Human bites can introduce infection if they break the skin and can also cause crush injuries. Any contact between teeth and skin that breaks the skin must receive prompt first aid and then medical attention.

1. If there is serious bleeding, control it by putting direct pressure on the wound and raising the injured part above the level of the heart, if possible.

2. If the bite is not bleeding seriously, wash the wounded area with soap and water and pat it dry.

3. Cover the wound with a sterile bandage.

4. Take the person to a casualty ward and tell the staff what type of animal caused the bite.

Poisoning

Most homes contain everyday substances that are potentially poisonous, such as detergents, bleach and paint solvents. Medicine cabinets also may contain over-the-counter and prescription drugs and remedies that are poisonous if taken in excessive doses. Gardens may contain poisonous plants.

Children are especially at risk of poisoning, and hazardous substances should be locked away or, at the very least, kept well out of their reach. NEVER store hazardous substances in anything but their original containers, particularly old soft drink bottles which could mislead a child.

Household poisons

If a household poison, such as bleach or detergent, has been swallowed, NEVER attempt to induce vomiting.

1. If the person is unconscious, check that his airway is open and that he is breathing. Be prepared to resuscitate if necessary (see p.555).

2. Phone for an ambulance. Say what substance has been swallowed, if you can. If the person is conscious and his lips have been burnt by a corrosive substance, give him sips of cold water or milk.

Drug poisoning

If you suspect a drug overdose, whether accidental or deliberate, DO NOT attempt to induce vomiting, which rarely helps and may make things worse.

1. If the person is unconscious, check that his airway is open and that he is breathing. Be prepared to resuscitate if necessary (see p.555).

2. Phone for an ambulance. If the person has vomited, keep a sample of the vomit to help identify the drug. Look for empty drug containers and if you find one, send it to hospital with the person.

Poisoning from plants

Children are most at risk from poisonous plants, since they may be attracted by their berries or seeds and may eat them. Teach your children from an early age never to eat anything they find outside unless an adult says that it's safe.

If you suspect that someone has swallowed a poisonous plant DO NOT induce vomiting, which rarely helps and may make matters worse.

1. If the person is unconscious, check that his airway is open and that he is breathing. Be prepared to resuscitate if necessary (see p.555).

2. Phone for an ambulance or call a doctor.

3. Try to find out which plant has been swallowed, and if possible what part of it was eaten. Keep pieces of the plant and a sample of any vomit to give to the paramedic or doctor.

Plants that cause poisoning if swallowed

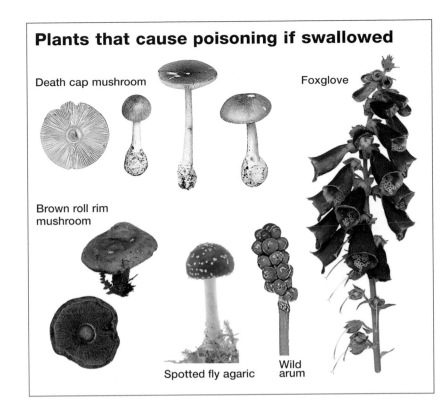

Death cap mushroom

Foxglove

Brown roll rim mushroom

Spotted fly agaric

Wild arum

Your first-aid kit

Every household should keep a well-stocked first-aid kit on hand at all times. In addition, it's a good idea to keep a first-aid kit in your car. Keep the kit in an easily accessible location with everything clearly marked.

YOUR KIT SHOULD INCLUDE:

- 20 adhesive dressings in assorted sizes
- 6 medium sterile dressings
- 2 large sterile dressings
- 2 extra-large sterile dressings
- 2 sterile pads
- 6 triangular bandages
- 2 crepe or elasticated roller bandages
- 6 safety pins
- disposable gloves
- scissors
- tweezers
- cotton wool
- non-alcoholic cleansing wipes
- notepad, pencil, writable tags
- plastic face shield.

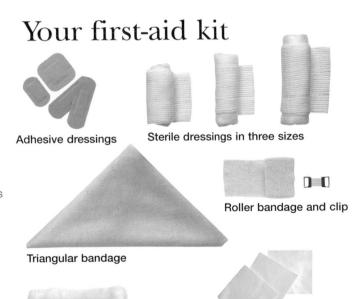

Adhesive dressings

Sterile dressings in three sizes

Sterile pads

Roller bandage and clip

Triangular bandage

Cotton wool

cleansing wipes

Safety pins, scissors and tweezers

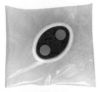

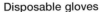

Disposable gloves

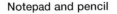

Notepad and pencil

Face shield

Travel health

Travel is part of most people's lives these days – whether for business or holiday – and it's easy to forget that, even with routine immunizations, risks to health during travel are still very real. On top of that, obtaining health care in other countries can be much more complicated than it is in the UK, and can end up being extremely expensive if you travel without the proper level of insurance.

There are however many ways you can minimize your risk of getting ill and/or facing large medical bills when you travel. Be sure to take the following precautions:

● **Find out if the country you're travelling to** has a reciprocal health care agreement with the UK – this means you can be treated in their healthcare system free of charge or at minimal cost. All European Economic Area countries (European Community countries plus Iceland, Lichtenstein and Norway) have reciprocal agreements with the UK. You will need to fill out and travel with Form E111, which you need to apply for in advance of your travel. Contact your GP or the Department of Health to find out how to apply. It's still advisable to have some insurance even when travelling to countries with reciprocal healthcare agreements; check with a travel agent for more details.

Some other non-EEA countries have reciprocal agreements with the UK, but note that most countries, including the US, Canada, Switzerland, India, Japan and all African, Central and South American and Middle Eastern countries do not. You will need travel insurance to cover your medical expenses if you need to be treated in these countries; check with a reputable travel agent for advice about how much insurance you (and your family) will need.

● **Check with your GP** about whether you and your family will need immunizations for the countries you plan to visit. You should do this at least two months before you travel as some immunizations need time to take effect. You should still check with your GP if you need to travel suddenly, since some protection may be better than none at all.

● **Be very careful in the sun.** Over-exposure to the sun can cause sunburn and heatstroke, and children are especially at risk. Don't go out in the sun at midday, stay in the shade when you can, and use a high-factor sunscreen at all times. Make sure your children wear a high-factor sunscreen and headgear that also protects the back of the neck. Drink plenty of fluids, but make sure they're safe – canned and bottled drinks are usually best.

● **Be on guard against insect and animal bites.** Even in areas where malaria is not a problem, ticks can be a carrier of disease. If you go walking in areas of high grass or woodland, make sure you wear long trousers and socks, and keep your arms covered too. Make sure that your children are also adequately dressed. Use insect repellents. If you've been prescribed anti-malarial tablets, make sure you take them regularly.

Bites from animals can cause very serious, and sometimes fatal, illness if they are not promptly treated. Be extremely cautious of all animals, even those that appear to be tame, and teach your children to be cautious too. If someone does get bitten by an animal, seek medical advice immediately.

● **If the water at your destination may not be safe to drink**, drink only bottled or canned drinks. Use disinfectant tablets if you need to use the water to wash food or clean your teeth. Don't ask for ice in your drinks, or use ice to keep food cool.

● **Make sure hot food is piping hot** and cooked all the way through. Avoid uncooked food such as raw fruits or vegetables; if you must eat them, peel them yourself. Avoid eating shellfish, especially any shellfish that is eaten raw, such as oysters. Do not drink unpasteurized milk.

● **Never swim alone**, and always make sure that children are supervised by an adult who is a good swimmer. Don't leave children alone near any water – a young child can drown in a paddling pool or even a large puddle.

● **Be extra vigilant** when driving, walking or cycling on foreign roads. Make sure you know which direction the traffic is travelling, especially when crossing roads – most countries drive on the right instead of the left. Be aware of local traffic laws.

● **If you are taking a long-haul flight**, get up and walk around at least once an hour or so to keep your blood circulating freely – this reduces the risk of developing deep vein thrombosis (see p.235).

● **If you haven't been to the dentist recently**, have a dental check-up before you travel. Dental care can be difficult to find and very expensive in some countries.

Useful addresses

AIDS

Sexual Health and National AIDS Helpline
Tel: 0800 567 123

Terrence Higgins Trust
52-54 Grays Inn Road
London WC1X 8JU
AIDS treatment phoneline: 0845 9470047
Counselling: 020 7835 1495
Email: info@tht.org.uk
Website: www.tht.org.uk

Alopecia

Hairline International
The Alopecia Patients' Society
Lyons Court, 1668 High Street, Knowle
West Midlands B93 0LY
Tel: 01564 775281
Website: www.hairlineinternational.co.uk

Skin Care Campaign
Hill House, Highgate Hill, London N19 5NA
Website: www.skincarecampaign.org

Alzheimer's disease

Alzheimer's Society
Gordon House, 10 Greencoat Place
London SW1P 1PH
Helpline: 0845 300 0336
Email: info@alzheimers.org.uk
Website: www.alzheimers.org.uk

Arthritis

Arthritis Research Campaign
Copeman House, St Mary's Court,
St Mary's Gate, Chesterfield
Derbyshire S41 7TD
Tel: 01246 558033
Email: info@arc.org.uk
Website: www.arc.org.uk

Asthma

National Asthma Campaign
Providence House, Providence Place
London N1 0NT
Helpline: 0845 7010203

British Lung Foundation
78 Hatton Gardens, London EC1N 8LD
Tel: 020 7831 5831
Email: blf@britishlungfoundation.com
Website: www.lunguk.org

Attention deficit disorder (ADD)/Attention deficit hyperactivity disorder (ADHD)

ADDNet UK
Website: www.btinternet.com/~black.ice/addnet

Autism

The National Autistic Society
393 City Road, London EC1V 1NG
Tel: 020 7833 2299
Email: nas@nas.org.uk
Website: www.nas.org.uk

Birthmarks

Changing Faces
1 & 2 Junction Mews, London W2 1PN
Tel: 020 7706 4232
Email: info@changingfaces.co.uk
Website: www.changingfaces.co.uk

Disfigurement Guidance Centre
P.O. Box 7, Cupar, Fife KY15 4PF
Fax : 01337 870310
Website: www.dgc.org.uk

Blindness

Royal National Institute for the Blind
224 Great Portland Street, London W1N 6AA
Tel: 020 7388 1266
Website: www.rnib.org.uk

Cerebral palsy

SCOPE
P.O. Box 833, Milton Keynes MK12 5NY
Tel: 0808 800 3333
Email: cphelpline@scope.org.uk
Website: www.scope.org.uk

Cancer

Cancer BACUP
3 Bath Place, Rivington Street
London EC2A 3JR
Tel: 020 7696 9003
Website: www.cancerbacup.org.uk

CancerHelp UK
Institute for Cancer Studies
The University of Birmingham, Edgbaston
Birmingham B15 2TA
Email: cancerhelp@crc.org.uk
Website: www.cancerhelp.org.uk

Macmillan Cancer Relief
Information line: 0845 601 6161
Email: information_line@macmillan.org.uk
Website: www.macmillan.org.uk

Cosmetic surgery

British Association of Aesthetic Plastic Surgeons (BAAPS)
The Royal College of Surgeons
35-43 Lincoln's Inn Fields, London WC2A 3PN
Tel: 020 7405 2234
Email: info@baaps.org.uk
Website: www.baaps.co.uk

Cot death

Foundation for the Study of Infant Deaths
Artillery House, 11-19 Artillery Row
London SW1P 1RT
24-hour helpline: 020 7233 2090
Email: fsid@sids.org.uk
Website: www.sids.org.uk/fsid

Stillbirth and Neonatal Death Society (SANDS)
28 Portland Place, London W1N 4DE
Helpline: 020 7436 5881
Email: Support@uk-sands.org
Website: www.uk-sands.org

Counselling

British Association for Counselling (BAC)
1 Regent Place, Rugby, Warwickshire CV21 2PJ
Tel: 01788 550899
Email: bac@bac.co.uk
Website: www.counselling.co.uk

Relate
Herbert Gray College, Little Church Street
Rugby, Warwickshire CV21 3AP
Tel: 01788 573241
Email: enquiries@national.relate.org.uk
Website: www.relate.org.uk

Cystic fibrosis

Cystic Fibrosis Trust
11 London Road, Bromley, Kent BR1 1BY
Tel: 020 8464 7211
Email: enquiries@cftrust.org.uk
Website: www.cftrust.org.uk

Deafness

Royal National Institute for Deaf People

19-23 Featherstone Street, London EC1Y 8SL
Tel: 0808 808 0123
Textphone: 0808 808 9000
Email: informationline@rnid.org.uk
Website: www.rnid.org.uk

Depressive illness

Association for Post-Natal Illness

145 Dawes Road, London SW6 7EB
Helpline: 020 7386 0868
Email: info@apni.org
Website: www.apni.org

Depression Alliance

35 Westminster Bridge Road, London SE1 7JB
Tel: 0207 633 0557
Website: www.depressionalliance.org

The Samaritans

Kingston Road, Ewell, Surrey KT17 2AF
Helpline: 08457 909090
Email: jo@samaritans.org
Website: www.samaritans.co.uk

Diabetes

Diabetes UK (formerly British Diabetic Association)

10 Queen Anne Street, London W1G 9LH
Tel: 020 7323 1531
Email: info@diabetes.org.uk
Website: www.diabetes.org.uk

Down's syndrome

Down's Syndrome Association

155 Mitcham Road,
London SW17 9PG
Tel: 0208 682 4001
Website: www.downs-syndrome.org.uk

Drugs

National Drugs Helpline

Tel: 0800 77 66 00

Dyslexia

British Dyslexia Association

98 London Road, Reading
Berkshire RG1 5AU
Tel: 0118 966 2677
Email: info@dyslexiahelp-bda.demon.co.uk
Website: www.bda-dyslexia.org.uk

Dyspraxia

The Dyspraxia Foundation

8 West Alley, Hitchin
Hertfordshire. SG5 1 EG
Helpline: 01462 454 986
Website: www.emmbrook.demon.co.uk/dysprax

Eating disorders

Eating Disorders Association

103 Prince of Wales Road
Norwich NR1 1DW
Helpline: 01603 621414
Email: info@edauk.com
Website: www.edauk.com

Eczema

National Eczema Society

Hill House, Highgate Hill
London N19 5NA
Helpline: 0870 241 3604
Website: www.eczema.org

Ekbom (restless legs) syndrome

Ekbom Support Group

18 Rodbridge Drive, Thorpe Bay
Essex SS1 3DF
Tel: 01702 582002
Email: gill@ekbom-88.demon.co.uk
Website: www.patient.org.uk/illness/e/ekbom_syndrome.htm

Epilepsy

British Epilepsy Association

New Anstey House
Gate Way Drive, Yeadon
Leeds LS19 7XY
Tel. 0808 800 5050
Email: helpline@bea.org.uk
Website: www.epilepsy.org.uk

Family planning

Family Planning Association

2–12 Pentonville Road
London N1 9FP
Tel: 020 7837 5432
Website: www.fpa.org.uk

British Pregnancy Advisory Service (BPAS)

Tel: 08457 3040 30
Website: www.bpas.org

Food allergies

The Anaphylaxis Campaign

P.O. Box 275, Farnborough
Hampshire GU14 7QY
Tel: 01252 542 029
Email: anaphylaxis.campaign@virgin.net
Website: www.anaphylaxis.org.uk

Heart disease

The British Heart Foundation

14 Fitzhardinge Street, London W1H 6DH
Tel: 020 7935 0185
Email: internet@bhf.org.uk
Website: www.bhf.org.uk/index.html

Herpes infection

Herpes Viruses Association (SPHERE)
41 North Road, London N7 9DP
Tel: 020 7609 9061
Website: www.herpes.org.uk

Impotence

Impotence Association

PO Box 10296, London SW17 9WH
Tel: 020 8767 7791
Email: theia@btinternet.com
Website: www.impotence.org.uk

Infertility

CHILD – The National Infertility Support Network

Charter House, 43 St Leonard's Road
Bexhill on Sea, East Sussex TN40 1JA
Tel: 01424 732361
Email: office@child.org.uk
Website: www.child.org.uk

Issue

114 Lichfield Street, Walsall WS1 1SZ
Tel: 01922 722888
Email: info@issue.co.uk
Website: www.issue.co.uk

Irritable bowel syndrome (IBS)

Irritable Bowel Syndrome Network

Northern General Hospital, Herries Road
Sheffield, South Yorkshire S5 7AU
Tel: 0114 261 1531

Digestive Disorders Foundation

3 St Andrews Place, London NW1 4LB
http://www.digestivedisorders.org.uk/leaflets/ibs.html
Website: www.digestivedisorders.org.uk

Lupus

Lupus UK
St James House, 1 Eastern Road
Romford
Essex RM1 3NH
Tel: 01708 731251
Website: www.geocities.com/HotSprings/2911

Miscarriage

Miscarriage Association
c/o Clayton Hospital
Northgate, Wakefield
West Yorkshire WF1 3JS
Helpline: 01924 200799
Email: miscarriageassociation@care4free.net
Website: www.miscarriageassociation.org.uk

Multiple sclerosis

Multiple Sclerosis Society
MS National Centre
372 Edgware Road
London NW2 6ND
Tel: 020 84380700
Helpline: 0808 800 8000
Website: www.mssociety.org.uk

Muscular dystrophy

Muscular Dystrophy Campaign
Helpline: 020 7819 1821
Website: www.muscular-dystrophy.org

Osteoporosis

National Osteoporosis Society (NOS)
Camerton, Bath BA2 0PJ
Helpline: 01761 472721
Email: info@nos.org.uk
Website: www.nos.org.uk

Polycystic ovary syndrome

Verity (Polycystic Ovaries Self-Help Group)
52-54 Featherstone Street
London EC1Y 8RT
Email: enquiries@verity-pcos.org.uk
Website: www.verity-pcos.org.uk

Prostate problems

Prostate Help Association
Langworth, Lincoln LN3 5DF
Email: philip@pha.u-net.com
Website: www.prostatecancer.org.uk

Psoriasis

The Psoriasis Association
Milton House, 7 Milton Street
Northampton NN2 7JG
Tel: (0604) 711129

Rape

Lifeline
The Old Bakehouse, Main Road
Hullnad Ward
Ashbourn, Derbyshire DE6 3EA
Tel: 01262 674505

Sexual problems

Institute of Psychosexual Medicine
12 Chandos Street
Cavendish Square
London W1G 9DR
Tel: 020 7580 0631
Website: www.ipm.org.uk

Sexuality

Gay Switchboard
Tel: 020 7837 7324
Web: www.switchboard.org.uk

Spina bifida and hydrocephalus

Association for Spina Bifida and Hydrocephalus
42 Park Road
Peterborough PE1 2UQ
Tel: 01733 555988
Email: postmaster@asbah.org
Website: www.asbah.org

Stroke

The Stroke Association
Stroke Information Service
Stroke House, 123–127 Whitecross Street
London EC1Y 8JJ
Tel: 020 7566 0300 or 0845 3033100
Email: info@stroke.org.uk
Website: www.stroke.org.uk

Testicular cancer

Everyman – Action Against Male Cancer
Tel: 0800 731-9468
Email: everyman@icr.ac.uk
Website: www.icr.ac.uk/everyman

Tinnitus

Action for Tinnitus Research
1 The Square Business Centre,
Manfield Avenue, Walsgrave, Coventry CV2 2QJ
Tel: 0181 316 6116
Email: tinnitus@tinnitus-research.org
Website: www.tinnitus-research.org

Travel health

The Department of Health
Richmond House, 79 Whitehall
London SW1A 2NS
Tel: 0207 210 4850
Email: dhmail@doh.gsi.gov.uk
Website: www.doh.gov.uk/traveladvice

Women's health issues

Women's Health
52 Featherstone Street
London EC1Y 8RT
Tel: 0845 125 5254
Email: health@womenshealthlondon.org.uk
Website: www.womenshealthlondon.org.uk

Australian useful addresses

AIDS

Australian Federation of AIDS Organisations (AFAO)
PO Box 876
Darlinghurst NSW 1300
Tel: 02 9281 1999
Website: www.afao.org.au

National Association of People Living With HIV/AIDS
Tel: 02 9281 2511
www.napwa.org.au

Alopecia

Alopecia Areata Support Association of Victoria Inc.
PO Box 89
Camberwell VIC 3124
Tel: 03 9513 8580

Alzheimer's disease

Alzheimer's Association National Dementia Behaviour Advisory Service
Tel: 1800 639 331
Email: www.alzheimers.org.au

Arthritis

Arthritis Foundation of Australia
Tel: 1800 011 041
Website: www.arthritisfoundation.com.au

Asthma

Asthma Foundation
Tel: 1800 645 130
Website: www.asthma.org.au

Attention deficit disorder (ADD)

VIC   Vic Active Inc.
Tel: 03 9650 2570

ACT   ADD Support Group
Tel: 02 6290 1984

NSW   Hyperactivity and Attention Deficit Association
Tel: 02 9411 2186

QLD   ADD Information and Support Services
Tel: 07 3817 2429

SA   ADD Information Service
Tel: 08 8221 5166

Autism

Autism Council of Australia
VIC   Tel: 03 9885 0533

Cerebral palsy

Cerebral Palsy Support Network
Tel: 03 9348 2677
Website: www.cpsn.info

Cancer

The Cancer Council Australia
Level 4, 70 William Street, East Sydney
NSW 2011
Tel: 02 9380 9022
Website: www.cancer.org.au

Cancer Helpline & Information Service
Tel: 13 11 20
Website: www.accv.org.au

Continence

Continence Foundation of Australia
National Continence Helpline
Tel: 1800 330 066
Website: www.contfound.org.au/

Cot death

SIDS (Sudden Infant Death Syndrome)
Tel: 1300 308 307

Counselling

National Association for Loss and Grief
VIC   Tel: 03 9351 0358
NSW   Tel: 02 9976 2803
ACT   Tel: 02 6259 3940
WA   Tel: 08 9385 4748
Website: www.grieflink.asn.au

Lifeline
Tel: 02 6282 6511

Relationships Australia
Tel: 1300 364 277

Coeliac disease

Coeliac Society of Australia
Tel: 02 9411 4100

Cystic fibrosis

Cystic Fibrosis Australia Inc.
51 Wicks Road, NSW 2113
TeL: 02 9878 5250
Website: www.cysticfibrosisaustralia.org.au

Dementia

Dementia Helpline
Tel: 1800 639 331
Website: www.alzheimers.org.au

Depressive illness

Lifeline
Tel: 13 11 14, 03 9662 9030, 02 6282 6511

SANE Australia
Tel: 1800 688 382
Website: www.sane.org

Diabetes

Diabetes Australia
Tel: 1800 640 862
Website: www.diabetesaustralia.com.au or www.dav.org.au

Down's syndrome

Down Syndrome Association
ACT   Tel: 02 6290 0656
NSW   Tel: 02 9683 4333
NT   Tel: 08 8985 6222
QLD   Tel: 07 3356 6655
SA   Tel: 08 8365 3510
TAS   Tel: 03 6244 0490
VIC   Tel: 03 9486 2377
WA   Tel: 08 9358 3544
Website: www.dsav.asn.au

Emphysema and lung support

Quality of Life Through Patient Support
Tel: 1800 654 301
Website: www.lungnet.org.au

Epilepsy

National Epilepsy Association of Australia
PO Box 879
Epping NSW 1710
Tel: 02 9856 7075, 1300 36 6162
Website: www.epilepsy.org.au

Hearing problems

The Western Australian Deaf Society Inc
16 Brentham Street
Leederville WA 6007
Tel: 08 9441 2677
Website: www.wadeaf.org.au

Haemophilia

Haemophilia Foundation Australia Inc (HFA)
213 Waverley Road
East Malvern VIC 3145
Tel: 03 9572 5533
Website: www.haemophilia.org.au

Head injury organizations

Head Injury Council of Australia Inc
Tel: 1800 626 370, 02 6290 2253
Website: www.headinjurycouncil.org.au

Heart disease

Heart Foundation of Australia
Cnr. Denison Street and Geils Court Deakin
ACT 2600
Tel: 1300 36 27 87
Website: www.heartfoundation.com.au

Hepatitis C infection

Hepatitis C Helpline
Tel: 1800 032 665

Herpes infection

Australian Herpes Management Forum
P O Box N159
Grosvenor Place NSW 2000
Tel: 02 9291 3358
Website: www.herpes.on.net

Kidney disease

Kidney Foundation, Australia
GPO Box 9993 (in your capital city)
Tel: 08 8334 7555, 1800 682 531
Website: www.kidney.org.au

Miscarriage

Stillbirth and Neonatal Death Support (SANDS)
Suite 208/901 Whitehorse Road, Box Hill
Tel: 03 9899 0218

Multiple sclerosis

Multiple Sclerosis Australia
Tel: 02 9955 0700
Website: www.msaustralia.org.au

Muscular dystrophy

Muscular Dystrophy Australia
Tel: 1800 656 632
Website: www.mda.org.au/

Osteoporosis

Osteoporosis Australia
Level 1, 52 Paramatta Road
Forest Lodge, NSW 2037
Tel: 02 9518 8140, 1800 011 041
Website: www.osteoporosis.org.au

Palliative care

Palliative Care Australia
Tel: 02 6232 4433
Website: www.pallcare.org.au/

Parkinson's disease

Parkinson's Australia
Tel: 1800 644 189
Website: www.parkinsons.org.au

Prostate problems

Cancer Council of Australia
Level 4, 70 William Street, East Sydney
NSW 2011
Tel: 02 9380 9022
Website: www.cancer.org.au

Spina bifida and hydrocephalus

Spina Bifida information line
Tel: 1800 819 775

Spinal cord injury

Australian Quadriplegic Association (AQA)
Tel: 03 9489 0777
Website: www.aqa.org.au

Paraplegic and Quadriplegic Association of Victoria
Tel: 1800 805 384
Website: www.paraquad.asn.au

Stroke

Stroke Recovery
National Stroke Foundation
Tel: 1800 787 653
Website: www.strokefoundation.com.au

Testicular cancer

Anti-Cancer Council of Victoria
Tel: 13 11 20
Website: www.accv.org.au

Cancer Council of Australia
Level 4, 70 William Street
East Sydney, NSW 2011
Tel: 02 9380 9022
Website: www.cancer.org.au

Thalassaemia

Thalassaemia Society
VIC   Tel: 03 9888 2211

Tinnitus

Australian Tinnitus Assoc (NSW) Ltd
9 Ice Street
Darlinghurst NSW
Tel: 02 8382 3331
Website: www.tinnitus.asn.au

Tinnitus Association of Victoria
Better Hearing Advisory Centre
5 High Street, Prahran, Vic 3181
Tel: 03 9510 1577

Index

Acknowledgements

DK would like to thank the following people for their contribution to the book:

CONSULTANTS

Directory: Professor M.W. Adler, Dr Robert Allan, Dr Robin Blair, Professor Charles Brook, Dr Christopher Davidson, Mr J.M. Dixon, Professor Andrew Doble, Dr Tony Frew, Mr Michael Gillmer, Professor Terry Hamblin, Dr Paresh Jobanputra, Professor P. Kendall-Taylor, Dr David Kerr, Professor P.T. Khaw, Professor Leslie Klenerman, Professor David Mabey, Dr Hadi Manji, Dr Martin Partridge, Professor Robert Peveler, Dr J.A. Savin, Professor Martin H. Thornhill

Dietary information: Lyndel Costain **First aid:** Dr Vivien Armstrong

Thanks also to: Laboratory Spa and Health Club in London, Corinne Asghar, Angela Baynham, Sue Bosanko, Peter Byrne, Ellie King, Alyson Lacewing, Mary Lyndsay, Ruth Midgley, Michelle Pickering, Esther Ripley, and Sally Smallwood for additional photography

The publisher would like to thank the following for their kind permission to reproduce their photographs: (Abbreviations key: t=top, b=bottom, r=right, l=left, c=centre)

Britesmile 491 (bc, br); Corbis Stock Market 486; Corbis Stock Market/Ariel Skelley 425 (c); Corbis Stock Market/Darama 104 (br), 127 (br); Corbis Stock Market/David Raymer 184 (bc), 198 (bl); Corbis Stock Market/David Woods 327; Corbis Stock Market/DiMaggio/Kalish 185 (bl), 199 (tr); Corbis Stock Market/Ed Bock 163 (cr), 179 (bl); Corbis Stock Market/George Disario 77 (bl); Corbis Stock Market/George Shelley 191 (b); Corbis Stock Market/John Henley 175 (bl); Corbis Stock Market/Jon Feingersh 530-531; Corbis Stock Market/Jose Luis Pelaez Inc. 45 (tl), 92 (tr), 197 (b), 342 (c) ; Corbis Stock Market/Jules Perrier 63(bl); Corbis Stock Market/Michael Keller 136 (tl), 138 (tr); Corbis Stock Market/Norbert Schäfer 82 (b, c), 99 (bl), 100 (tl); Corbis Stock Market/Tom & DeeAnn McCarthy 105 (br), 124 (tr); Corbis Stock Market/Tom Stewart 93 (bl); Corbis/Martin Hughes 162 (tl), 168 (tl); Eyewire 157 (cla, ca), 226 (bl), 285, 345 (b), 537 ; ImageState 114 (tr), 162 (cr), 176 (tr); ImageState/AGE Fotostock 7 (cb), 85 (tl); ImageState/Stock Image 171 (br), 500 (tl); Masterfile UK 164 (tr), 166 (tl); Masterfile UK/Brian Kuhlmann 42 (tl), 47 (tcr); Masterfile UK/Dan Lim 39 (bc), 57 (cl); Matt Meadows 401 (br); Meningitis Research Foundation 405 (tr, cl); Photodisc 157 (tl), 294, 310, 329 (t), 417; Photonica/Neo Vision 411; Powerstock Photolibrary 144 (tr), 163 (t, c), 169 (cr), 301 (tr); Rex Features 156 (cb, b, c); Science & Society

Picture Library/Science Museum 473 (b); Scott Camazine 412 (b, cl); SPL 353 (bc, br), 392 (b); 541 (tl); SPL/Alfred Pasieka 474, 495; SPL/Antonia Reeve 406; SPL/Biophoto Associates 397; SPL/BSIP 319 (tl); SPL/BSIP VEM 372; SPL/BSIP, Laurent 344 (b); SPL/BSIP, LA/Filin.Herrera 442 (t); SPL/BSIP, Sercomi 219; SPL/Chris Priest 146 (br), 245 (cr), 549 (br); SPL/CNRI 382; SPL/Conor Caffrey 334 (b); SPL/David Parker 243 (br), 263; SPL/Department of Clinical Radiology, Salisbury District Hospital 412 (bl); SPL/Dr Linda Stannard UCT 330; SPL/Dr. P. Marazzi 337 (b); SPL/Faye Norman 376 (bl); SPL/Gaillard, Jerrican 466 (t); SPL/Geoff Tompkinson 331 (b), 401 (tr); SPL/Gusto 387 (tr), 482 (cr); SPL/Hattie Young 493 (b, c); SPL/J. C. Revy 423 (cl, c, cr); SPL/James King-Holmes 391 (c); SPL/John Greim 431; SPL/John Radcliffe Hospital 318 (t, c), 405 (tl); SPL/Lauren Shear 513 (br); SPL/Mark Clarke 315 (b, c), 317 (r); SPL/Martin Dohrn 462; SPL/Matthew Munro 383; SPL/Mauro Fermariello 521 (br); SPL/Mehau Kulyk 218 (b, c), 231 (cr), 240; SPL/NIBSC 510-511; SPL/Oscar Burriel 308; SPL/Peter Menzel 395 (tr); SPL/Philippe Plailly/Eurolios 225 (br); SPL/Prof. P. Motta/Dept of Anatomy/University "La Sapienza", Rome 419, 424; SPL/Quest 8 (cl), 309, 347, 443; SPL/Robin Laurance 522 (bl); SPL/Samuel Ashfield 277; SPL/Saturn Stills 23 (bl), 506 (cl); SPL/Sheila Terry 535 (br) ; SPL/Simon Fraser 224 (b); SPL/Tim Beddow 284; SPL/Tissuepix 483; SPL/Will & Deni McIntyre 409; SPL/Y. Beaulieu, Publiphoto Diffusion 381(c); Stone/Getty Images 3, 6: (tr, c), 7 (tc), 8 (bl), 14-15, 17 (tr), 20, 21 (tr), 22 (tr), 25 (tl), 26 (bl), 27 (bl), 29 (tr), 32 (b), 34-35, 38 (tr, cr), 44 (br), 46 (bcl), 48 (tr), 51 (br), 53 (tr), 70 (bl), 80, 83 (cl,

b, c), 90 (tr), 91 (br), 98 (tr), 101 (tr, bl), 102, 105 (cl), 115 (tr), 117 (t), 120 (bl), 126 (tl), 129 (t), 133 (t), 136 (tc, br), 137 (b, c), 141 (bl), 143 (bl), 153 (bl), 154 (bl), 155 (br), 157 (tc, tr), 158 (tr), 160, 167 (br), 184 (br), 187 (b), 195 (bl), 198 (tr), 200 (tl, br), 201 (b), 204-205, 216-217, 220 (b), 228, 254, 286 (b), 290 (tl), 418, 427 (b), 444, 475, 478, 479 (c), 491 (tl), 501, 524 (b), 527 (br), 547 (br), 552-553; TCL/Getty Images 6 (cl, br), 16, 19 (tr), 28, 36, 38 (tl), 39 (cl, br), 41 (b), 47 (bcl), 50 (c), 52 (br), 53 (c), 55 (cr, bl), 57 (br), 58, 72 (bl), 75 (t), 111 (tr), 119 (tr), 131, 136 (tr, c), 139 (br), 149 (b), 178 (tl), 179 (t, c), 182, 184 (tl, bl, cl), 190 (tl), 192 (bl), 196 (br), 203, 229 (tr), 266, 289, 292 (b), 297 (tr), 315 (tr), 325 (tr), 356 (cl), 373 (b), 433 (bl), 455 (br), 534 (tl); Telegraph Colour Library 74; The Image Bank/Getty Images 33 (tr), 38 (cl), 39 (tc), 49 (c), 54 (tl), 66 (br), 86 (tl, br), 97 (br), 104 (cr), 116 (tl), 118 (tl), 121 (b), 125 (t), 134, 158 (tl), 159, 162 (tc, cl, bl), 163 (tl), 167 (br), 172 (tr), 173 (bl), 176 (bl), 180 (tl), 188 (tl), 194 (tr), 202 (tr), 291, 302 (br), 420, 440 (t), 484, 551; The Photographers' Library 502 (tr); The Wellcome Institute Library, London 324, 526 (br)

Back jacket

Corbis Stock Market/Jon Feingersh (cl); ImageState/Blackdog Productions (tr); SPL/Hank Morgan (clb)

All other images © Dorling Kindersley.

For further information see:
www.dkimages.com

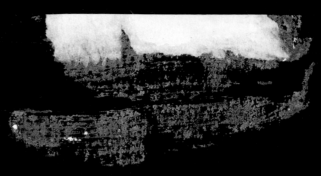

ADVERTISING TODAY

ADVERTISI

NG TODAY

WARREN BERGER

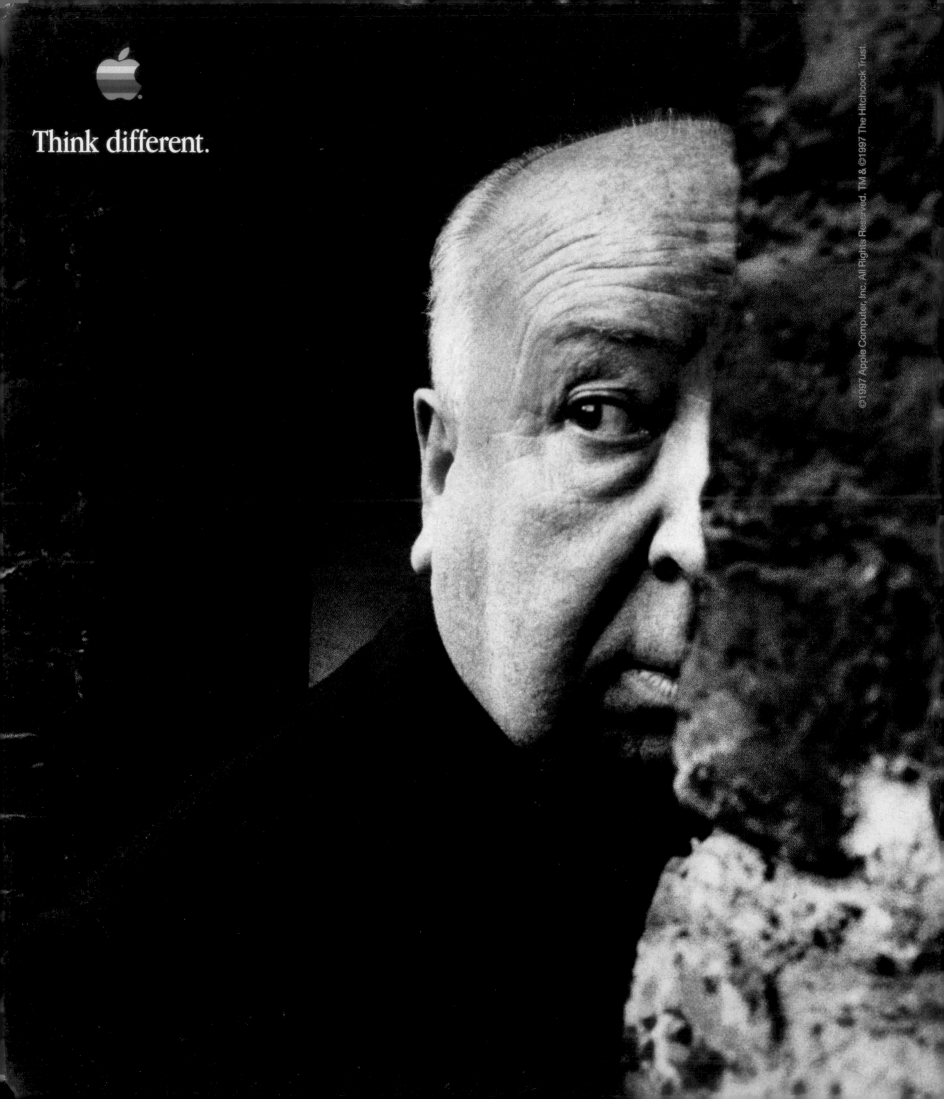

Think different.

CONTENTS

1. INTROD
WHY ADV
MATTERS.

DUCTION:
ERTISING
HONESTLY.

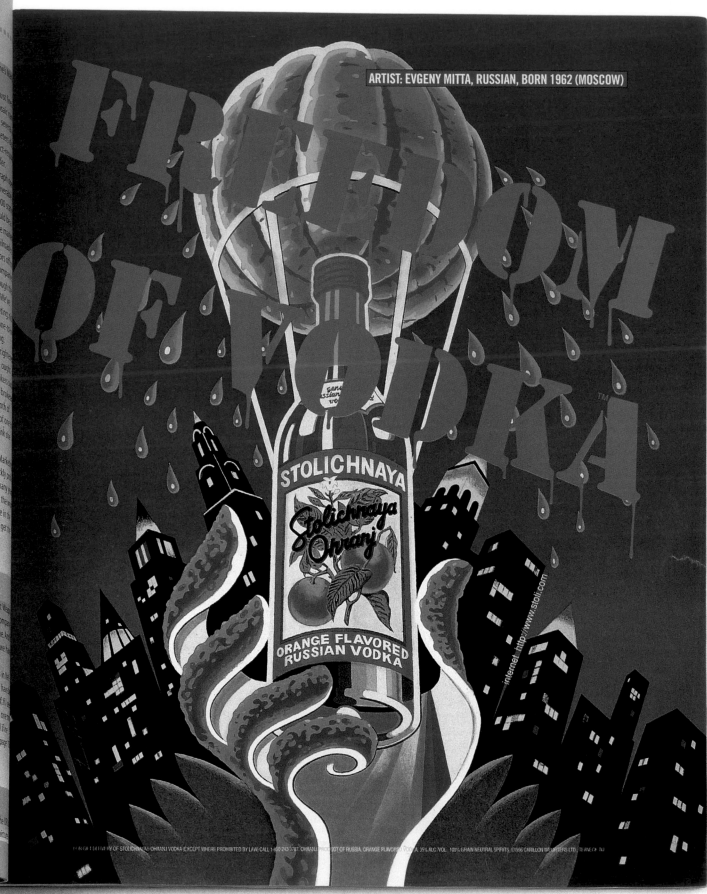

ARTIST: EVGENY MITTA, RUSSIAN, BORN 1962 (MOSCOW)

STOLICHNAYA

Stolichnaya
Ohranj

ORANGE FLAVORED
RUSSIAN VODKA

internet http://www.stoli.com

strategies ("One-on-One with One-to-One's
Rogers," *Wired* 4.03, page 152).

These principles have been working just
more than 100 years under the more prosaic
direct marketing, though only in the last
have software and other high-tech marketers
ered the cost-effective benefits that direct-
media and lead-generation strategies offer.

In 1886 Richard Sears, a railroad telegraph
tor, found himself with a supply of undelivered
pocket watches. He also had a list of 20,000
masters, each of whom, he reasoned, would be
logical prospect for an accurate watch. He mar-
the watches "one-to-one" to his fellow railroad

As direct marketing has blown the doors off
marketing, a parade of individuals and companies
have attempted to divert the stream through their
own little marketing mill by renaming it. We've
had relationship marketing, target marketing,
marketing, customer bonding, and, yes, one-to-
marketing, long before Rogers came along.

And before Weinberger becomes too frightened
by Rogers's so-called learning brokers, he ought
to check out the activities of major list brokers such
as Worldata Inc. with its WebConnect link broker
service and Direct Media's CatalogLink, both of
which are designed to facilitate the kind of one-to-
one communications Rogers seems to think he
discovered.

As for the issue of privacy, the Direct Marketing
Association has been addressing that prickly problem, with increasingly better results, for many years.
"Junk mail," I often say, "is an offer sent to the wrong
person." The DMA and most everyone else in the
industry is working hard to make sure we get to the
right person, the first time.
George Duncan
duncdirect@aol.com

Barksdale's Barking
To quote Jim Barksdale ("Netscape's Secret Weapon,"
Wired 4.03, page 154): "I don't know of a company
that's created a brand quicker than we have. And by
the way, over a period of a year and a half we have
never run an ad."

Now, I can truly admire the pride he has in Netscape's accomplishments, but he must not have been
surfing the Web during that year and a half. If I see
that "Download Netscape Now" banner on one more
site's ad space I think I'll go looney. Oh, and if he
means print ads, please ask him to turn to page 151
of *Wired Scenarios* 1.01.
Jet Thompson
art@sensenet.com

Our Hubble Apologies
Tired: *Wired* magazine. For not publishing the full
the Hubble Space Telescope Eagle Nebula picture

Perhaps the first question to be asked of a book about advertising is: *Why?*

Why create an enduring document for something as ephemeral and disposable as advertising? Why take the time to analyze a form of communication that often consists of not much more than a cheery jingle and a simplistic slogan? And above all, why charge good money for a book stocked with imagery that is, each day, foisted upon all of us free of charge and against our will?

Here are two answers. One, because advertising matters. Two, because some advertising matters more than the rest.

The second statement is easier to defend, so let's start there: Almost everyone, including advertising's most dedicated practitioners, freely acknowledges that the vast majority of it is banal, unimaginative, mind-numbing. We've all winced at those hyperactive car commercials heralding a "sale-a-bration!" at the local dealership . . . and

the detergent ads in which stains on shirts magically disappear for the hundredth time (though no one cared or believed it the first time). We've flipped through endless fashion-magazine ads so posed and lifeless they seem to bore even the models appearing in them. And we've all seen quite enough of Snuggles, the Fabric Softener Bear. We encounter these all-too-familiar images hundreds of times daily—mere static that we ignore or tune out.

But then along comes something that reminds us how powerful advertising can be: A swing-dancing Gap clothing commercial that manages to be visually arresting and exhilarating, even upon the tenth viewing; a sobering anti-drunk-driving ad that brings home, just for a moment, the specific horror of a traffic accident; an elegant Nike print campaign that somehow expresses our own unspoken feelings about personal achievement (and maybe inspires us to actually take that jog we've

been meaning to take). This rare strain of advertising—it probably amounts to no more than 5 percent of all ads, if that much—is the kind that breaks through the clutter by virtue of its style, cleverness, and originality. That 5 percent is the focus of this book. The other 95 percent shall be left on the cultural scrap heap, where it belongs.

As to the first point, that advertising matters, a more detailed case can and should be made. Because even with the acknowledgment that some ads are better than others, there is still a prevailing sense that advertising, as a whole, adds little of value or substance to the culture—and that it is therefore not worthy of the kind of thoughtful appreciation or analysis one might devote to, say, architecture. But this view seems out of step with the reality of today, wherein advertising is even more pervasive than the architecture that surrounds us (and sometimes, the commercials are also better

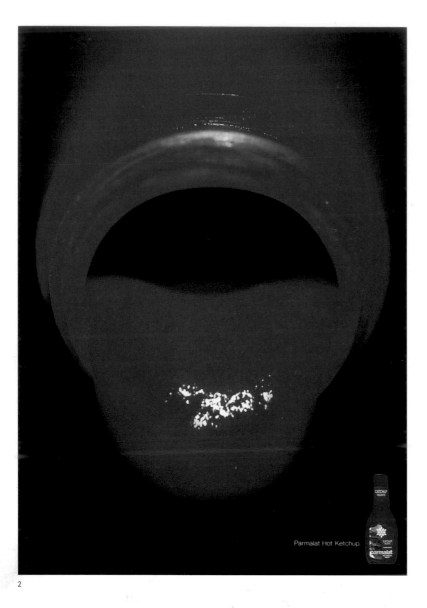

Parmalat Hot Ketchup.

2

designed than the buildings). Advertising almost certainly has a greater influence on our lives. The typical television viewer watches more than 40,000 commercials a year, and—contrary to popular belief—usually pays attention. A recent survey by the Starch Roper research firm found that people today actually like watching commercials more than ever before, no doubt because ads have evolved to become far more watchable in recent years. But entertainment value aside, today's ads also inform and guide many of the important decisions we make— not just the cars we drive but whether we take entrepreneurial risks or choose to lead a healthy lifestyle or plan ahead for retirement or donate to charity. The ways in which ads are affecting and shaping our attitudes, lifestyles, and culture are too numerous to tally.

But let's count off a few anyway. What follows is a list of nine reasons advertising truly matters, and why, therefore, the very best of it is worthy of further examination.

1. ADVERTISING IS ONE OF THE PISTONS THAT DRIVE THE GLOBAL ECONOMY. More than $400 billion a year is spent on advertising worldwide; beyond that, the economic impact of advertising touches just about every consumer-product industry, from cars to candy bars. There is much more to be said about this, but since this book is about the aesthetic and cultural aspects of advertising, we'll leave further financial analysis to the economists and the bean counters.

2. "IT MAY BE THE MOST POWERFUL ART FORM ON EARTH." So says Mark Fenske, a highly regarded American copywriter known for his groundbreaking advertising for Nike and other brands. While Fenske is clearly a biased source, he makes a point that is contentious but worth

considering. "Art is something that reinterprets for people the life they're leading; it allows you to experience what you know about life," Fenske says. "And because advertising deals with the minutiae of everyday life, any art that comes out of it is going to be particularly relevant and powerful." While some fine arts have become increasingly esoteric and removed from people's everyday experience, Fenske argues, advertising can—in rare instances— make a revealing statement "about something that happened to you that very day." Perhaps that morning, you were distraught to discover there was no milk in the refrigerator. Subsequently, you saw a "Got Milk?" commercial vignette that captured and crystallized the feelings of that experience; you found yourself empathizing with the poor fellow who can't enunciate the words "Aaron Burr" because there's no milk to wash the cookies from his

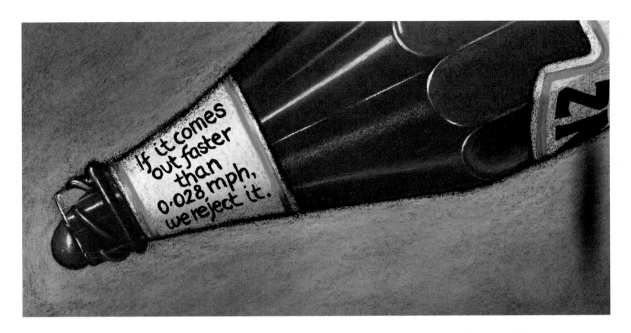

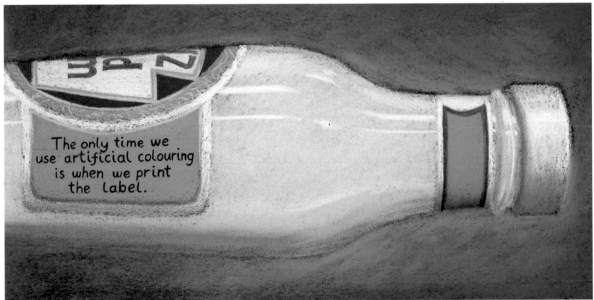

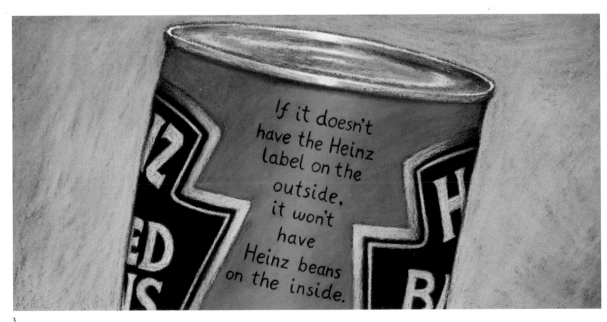

3

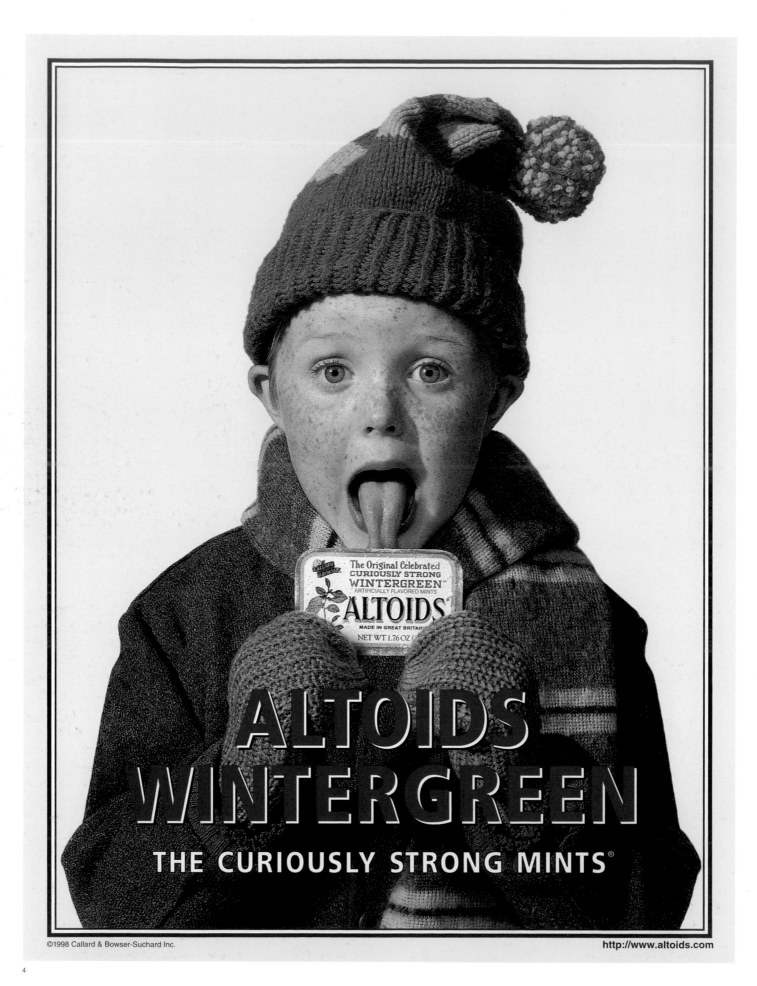

ALTOIDS
WINTERGREEN

THE CURIOUSLY STRONG MINTS®

http://www.altoids.com

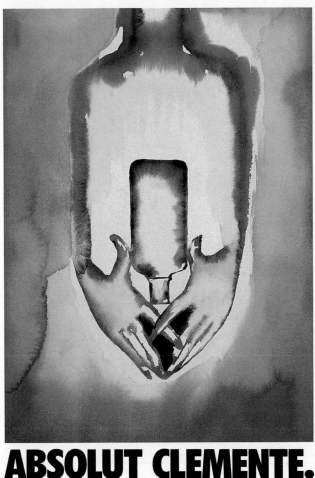

ABSOLUT CLEMENTE.

ABSOLUT® VODKA. PRODUCT OF SWEDEN. 40 AND 50% ALC/VOL (80 AND 100 PROOF). 100% GRAIN NEUTRAL SPIRITS. ABSOLUT COUNTRY OF SWEDEN VODKA & LOGO. ABSOLUT, ABSOLUT BOTTLE DESIGN, ABSOLUT
CALLIGRAPHY AND ABSOLUTVODKA.COM ARE TRADEMARKS OWNED BY V&S VIN & SPRIT AB. ©1999 V&S VIN & SPRIT AB. IMPORTED BY THE HOUSE OF SEAGRAM, NEW YORK, NY. ARTWORK BY FRANCESCO CLEMENTE.
ENJOY OUR QUALITY RESPONSIBLY.

5

mouth. At that moment, Fenske and others
maintain, the ad becomes a form of popular art.

It is still controversial to call advertising
art—though less and less so, now that major
museums around the world house permanent
collections of ads, and Absolut vodka posters
are framed and hung on walls like paintings.
But there remains a large contingent that
insists advertising cannot be art for the simple
reason that it is conceived for commercial
purposes, and controlled and financed by
corporations. Of course, many artists through
the years have been commercially motivated,
and Renaissance painters were financed and
controlled by patrons like the Medicis—who
were apt to demand that certain details be
inserted into the artwork, much the way a
business client often insists that the logo be
made more prominent in an ad. And all of that
was happening long before the lines between
art and commerce really started to blur.

Today, artful filmmakers like Woody Allen
and Spike Lee shoot ads in their spare time,
top photographers are sponsored by camera
companies, and serious novelists sometimes
negotiate the Hollywood film rights to their
work before the ink is dry on the page. In the
current environment, is there any point in trying to ferret out the commercial intentions or
ambitions that may lurk in the heart of someone embarking on the creative process?

Within the ad industry itself, the question of
whether advertising is, or ever can be, an art
form is a highly divisive issue. Many advertising
professionals think it's dangerous for ad creators
to begin to think of themselves as artists—
because it may lead them to forget that their
primary purpose, always, is to sell the product.
"Advertising can be a popular art form—but that
should happen by coincidence, not design," says
the American ad executive Andy Berlin. Greg
DiNoto, who runs the New York ad agency

DiNoto Lee, says, "Persuasion—advertising—can
be art, but ultimately that's for the consumer and
the world at large to decide. Advertisers get into
trouble when they attempt to make art that per-
suades, instead of persuasion that might be art."

Indeed, the challenge for advertising creators
is always to maintain a delicate balance—producing something pleasing to the audience that
also serves the business purpose of the client.
It is one of the trickiest tightropes in all the
creative world. Sometimes ads lean too much in
the direction of art or entertainment, and stray
too far from the original selling purpose and the
product. When that happens, the viewer is likely
to love the commercial—but will have no idea,
afterward, whose commercial it was. At that point
an ad can still be artful but must nevertheless be
judged a failure. "When the art becomes an end
in itself, the advertising becomes pointless," says
the Singapore-based ad creator Neil French. "It's
still art, but it ain't advertising."

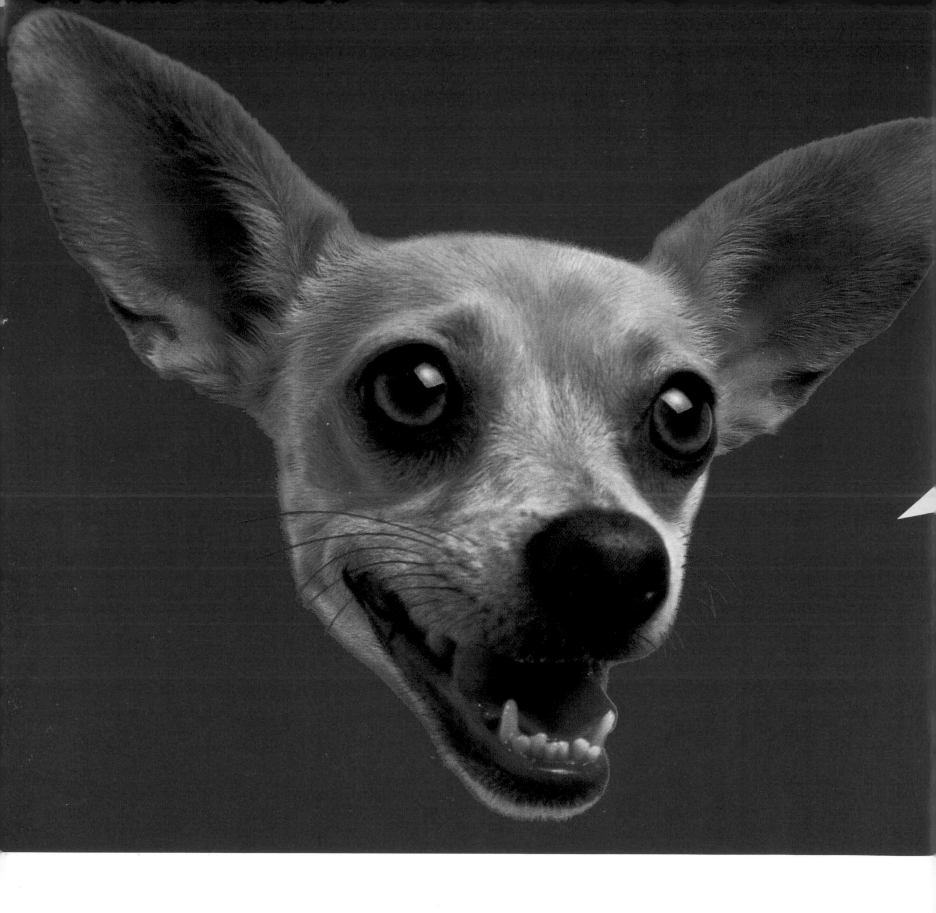

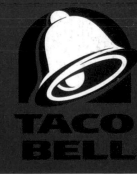

6. **TACO BELL**
TBWA/CHIAT/DAY,
LOS ANGELES, 1997
The Chihuahua became a pop-
culture phenomenon in this
campaign for a Mexican-food
chain (though not everyone
approved of the dog's Spanish
accent).

WHY ADVERTISING MATTERS. HONESTLY.

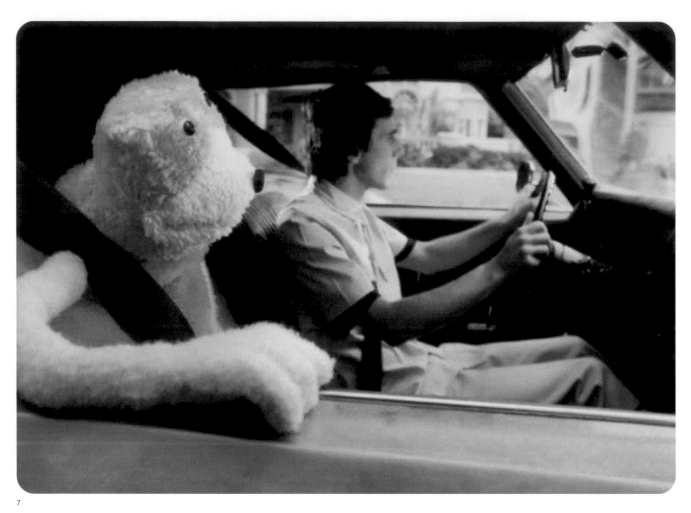

7

**7. LEVI STRAUSS EUROPE –
STA-PREST**
BARTLE BOGLE HEGARTY,
LONDON, 1999
The British equivalent of the
Taco Bell Chihuahua, "Flat Eric"
was a mysterious orange
puppet that had Europe talking
in 1999 (though the puppet and
his partner never spoke a word).

8. LITTLE CAESARS PIZZA
CLIFF FREEMAN & PARTNERS,
NEW YORK, 1995
The campaign presented absurd
scenarios such as the "Training
Camp" commercial, in which
pizza deliverymen were sent to
boot camp.

There are many people, both inside and outside the ad industry, who view advertising as much more of a science, grounded in sophisticated research, focus-group studies, and formulaic selling approaches. And, certainly, all of those elements do figure prominently in the creation of ads. But the real mystery of advertising is that it so often defies science and measurement. With all the vast amounts of money and effort devoted to research, analysis, and testing (in the U.S. last year, companies spent more than $100 million researching and testing their own ads), often the most powerful advertising springs from pure intuition—from one person or perhaps two, sitting quietly in a room somewhere and dreaming up off-the-wall ideas. "Just do it," the Nike tag line that is one of the most powerful single lines of ad copy produced in advertising in the past twenty years, was penned by a soft-spoken writer in Oregon named Dan Wieden—with no help

from studies or research committees. Wieden sat down at his desk one day, and, in a matter of minutes, just did it.

Most of the advertising in this book was created that way—by one or two people relying on gut feelings while endeavoring to say something original and insightful about a product (and sometimes a very mundane product, at that). Copywriters and art directors usually fail at this task, and produce the expected—the messages that are obvious and don't stand out from the clutter (ad people call this nondescript advertising "wallpaper"). But the best ad creators seem to know instinctively what will resonate. "They have a talent they're born with, and they happen to wander into advertising, where that particular talent begins to grow and flower," says the celebrated British advertising writer Tim Delaney. "It isn't easy to measure this intuitive talent, or even to explain how it works. At the root of it is the ability to somehow fathom and

piece together all sorts of disparate information about people and products, and then come up with an idea that captures the imagination of the public or the individual. It's more magic than anything else."

However, even Delaney is not sure it should be called art. "Persuasion can certainly be thought of as an art form—particularly when it brings together a combination of creative elements that are not entirely logical," he says. "But I think an art form should be an altogether pure thing that tries to illuminate what's really important, like the meaning of life. Advertising does sometimes shine a torch on certain truths, but they're usually more mundane truths—for example, the way you feel deep down about your car." But that's good enough for the American art director George Lois, who believes Pablo Picasso's observation that "art is the lie that tells the truth" can be applied to great advertising. "Almost all

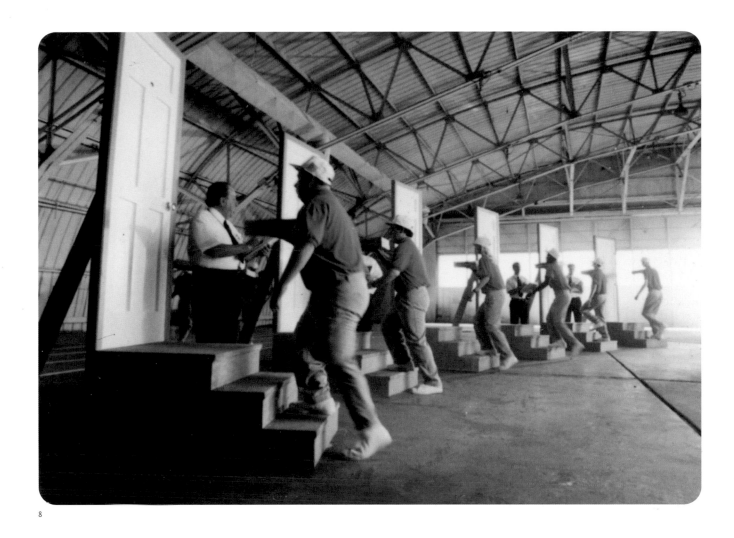

8

3. IT IS SHAPING THE POPULAR CULTURE.

products are comparable in quality," Lois has noted, "but when advertising is great advertising—when it's inventive, irreverent, audacious, and loaded with chutzpah—it literally becomes a benefit for the product, and Picasso's 'lie' becomes the truth. Food tastes better, clothes feel better, cars drive better."

Given its utilitarian nature, perhaps the best way to think of advertising is as a kind of folk art, rather than a fine art. "There used to be a lot of pride taken in the creation of very utilitarian things," observes Dan Wieden of Wieden + Kennedy. "In fact, we dig them up all over the world now; we look at vases and bowls and forks and spoons from different eras and cultures. At the time, they were basically commodities—but the person making them cared enough about them to put something special into them, and that made them art. I think the same thing, perhaps, could be true for this slimy business."

In the late 1990s, the aforementioned Gap "Khakis Swing" commercial seized on a burgeoning trend, swing dancing, and turned it into a raging phenomenon in America. Around the same time, a series of commercials created by the Los Angeles agency TBWA/Chiat/Day for Taco Bell restaurants managed to turn a Chihuahua into a media star that was soon appearing on talk shows, T-shirts, and magazine covers, while also stirring political protest (Hispanic groups thought the talking dog's Spanish accent was offensive). Meanwhile, the catchphrases that had seemed to be on everyone's lips around that time—"Just do it," "Think different," "I've Fallen and I Can't Get Up"—were far more likely to have come from ads than from books or even movies.

This is not just an American phenomenon. In Germany, a series of British-made Levi's ads featuring a mysterious, lifelike puppet called

Flat Eric became so wildly popular that Levi's stopped running the ads (because the brand, seeking "hipness," wanted to be talked about by some people but not everybody). In England, commercials for a soft drink called Tango featured an orange-painted man who slapped everyone's ears; so naturally, people on the streets of London started slapping one another's ears, like the orange Tango man. In Australia and New Zealand, a recent Toyota commercial had one word of dialogue repeated over and over—the profane term *bugger*. Subsequently, "the swear word became something of a national obsession," says local journalist Paul Panckhurst, and it started showing up in newspaper headlines on a regular basis. Meanwhile, in Brazil these days, advertising jingles are sung in pubs. "Advertising has become so entrenched in the Brazilian culture that it is one of the preferred topics of conversation in bars, along with soccer and politics,"

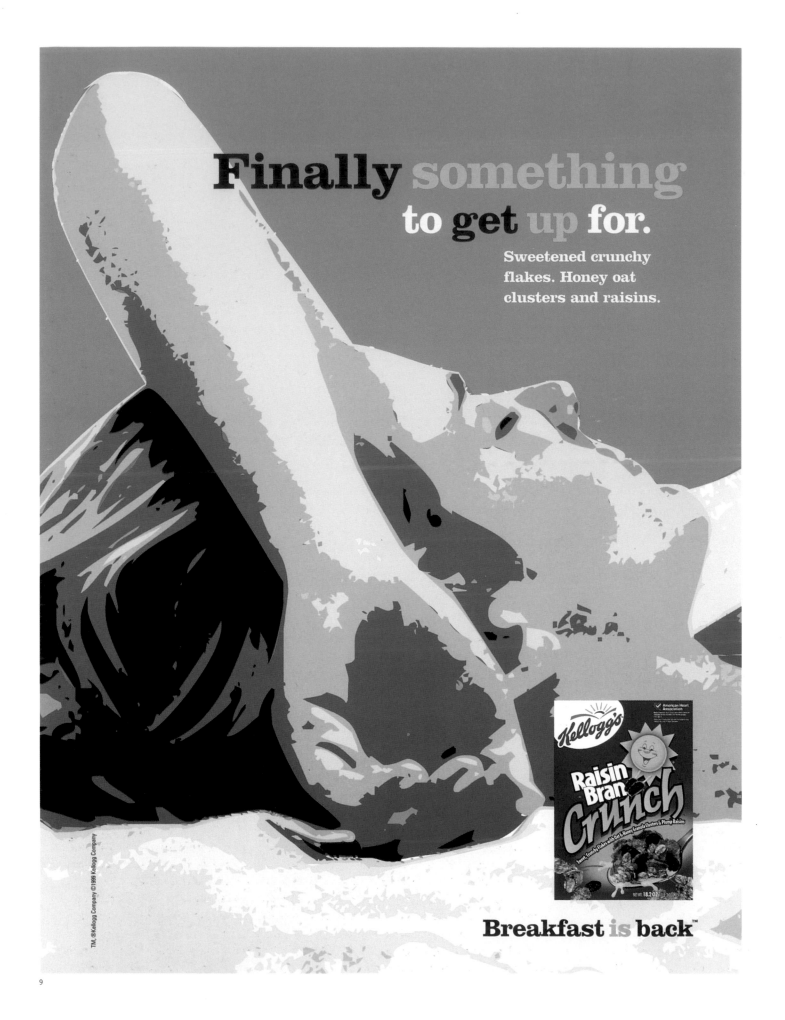

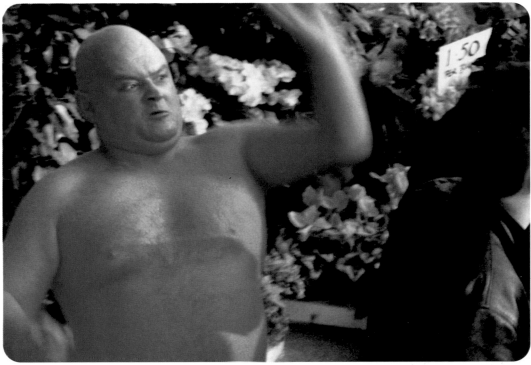

10

9. **KELLOGG'S**
J. WALTER THOMPSON,
NEW YORK, 1999
Providing the tired masses with
a reason to get up in the morning.

10. **TANGO**
HOWELL HENRY CHALDECOTT
LURY, LONDON, 1992
The weird orange character in
these soft-drink ads slapped
people's heads. Soon, imitators
were doing likewise on the
streets of London.

says Sergio Caruso of the Brazilian agency
Carillo Pastore Euro RSCG. Caruso adds that
"the names of some of Brazil's advertising
people have become part of the layman's
repertoire," and "more Brazilians now want to
become advertising people than doctors,
engineers, or journalists."

All of this is not necessarily an encouraging
sign for civilization. Brazil undoubtedly needs
good doctors a lot more than it needs clever
ad-makers. And this would probably be a better
world if all of us were more apt to quote
Shakespeare than Chiat/Day. On the other
hand, ads are providing at least *some* piece of
common culture in a media world that is
becoming increasingly fragmented. Popular
commercials may be among the last pieces of
shared communication, which is perhaps why
people talk about them so much. The latest car
ads are the bridge that crosses over from the
Lifetime women's cable channel to the ESPN

sports channel to the business magazines,
connecting all of those disparate audiences.

More and more, advertisers aren't just a
central part of the cultural mix, they're a
determinant. Once upon a time, television
shows and magazines tried to appeal to the
public first—then sold that popularity to
advertisers. In recent years, that priority has
changed somewhat. Today, the TV programs we
see and the publications we read are more likely
to be conceived and engineered with specific
advertising demographics in mind. And so,
when television seems to be overtaken by
programming geared to teenagers, or when
every new magazine seems to be targeting
young "lads" with raging hormones, blame it
on advertising. These days, a show or a
magazine is deemed a hit not so much because
the public says so as because advertisers say
so—and are willing to pay a higher rate to
sponsor it, which begets more shows and

magazines that are similar. In effect, advertising
today isn't just influencing the culture—it is
programming it.

4. IT IS ENDLESSLY ENTERTAINING. (SOMETIMES.)
Beginning with the Creative Revolution that
swept through advertising in the 1960s, many of
the creators of ads have made a conscious effort
to imbue their work with cleverness, humor,
emotion, and style. Commercials also began to
take on a more cinematic flavor, telling stories
that could be powerful. As more than one media
critic has observed, the ads were sometimes
better than the shows they interrupted. Why
wouldn't they be? Each small story had a point
and a message. And with each ad, the creators
could start with a clean slate—they didn't have
to beat the same old sitcom story line to death
again every week.

The rise of entertainment-driven advertising
in recent years may have provided countless

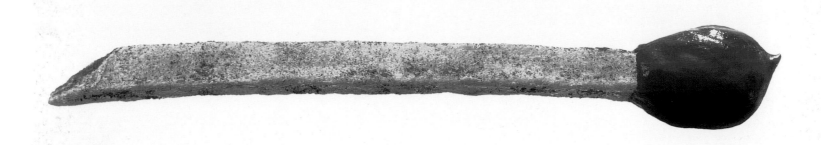

Fiery Fries. **BURGER KING**

11

amusing moments for the audience, but it has been a source of constant controversy within the industry itself, owing to the schizophrenic nature of advertising. Should the ad's primary purpose be to entertain or to tout the product? Is it possible to do one without compromising the other? These questions have divided the ad business into two rival camps, the hard-sellers against the "creatives." The former tends to believe that ads should always focus on providing compelling reasons to buy, and should hammer that sales pitch home through volume and repetition. But the creatives believe this is pointless because today's media-savvy audience tunes out such overt sales pitches; the only way to engage such an audience, they contend, is by offering them a laugh or a moving moment—in hopes that the audience will come away feeling good about the brand that brought them that good feeling. Lately, the creative camp has been winning the advertising war—or, as one industry

pundit commented recently, "The creatives have taken over the asylum."

Is this a good thing? For the business itself and the brands that subsidize it, it's anybody's guess whether entertaining soft sell works better than old-fashioned hard sell; there are studies that can prove either side of the argument. (In fact, there are studies in advertising that can prove anything; as one might imagine, advertisers are masterly at constructing an argument to promote any viewpoint.) Interestingly, when it comes to measuring most commercials' direct impact on actual sales results—which can be influenced by an almost infinite number of factors aside from ads—advertisers don't seem to know much more than they did a century ago, when the businessman John Wanamaker famously commented, "I know half of my advertising is wasted—I just don't know which half."

However, a case can be made that we, the audience, are better off when creative advertising

prevails. Today's more entertainment-driven soft-sell ads—even the ones that end up being a bit oblique or bizarre—are probably the least offensive form of advertising. They recognize that they are intruding in our homes and offer something in return: a joke, a story, a pretty picture. And in so doing, they tend to avoid some of the more negative aspects of advertising, such as battering us with silly slogans or denigrating the competition (political ads, which generally are not produced by ad agencies, demonstrate how bad advertising can be when it is devoid of all creativity—all that's left is the lies, the slander, and the pandering).

But as shoppers and consumers, wouldn't we be better off if ads dispensed with the distracting stories and eye-catching designs, and simply provided us with the straight facts about products—the features, benefits, and reasons to buy? Probably not. Conventional ads that rattle on about features and benefits and

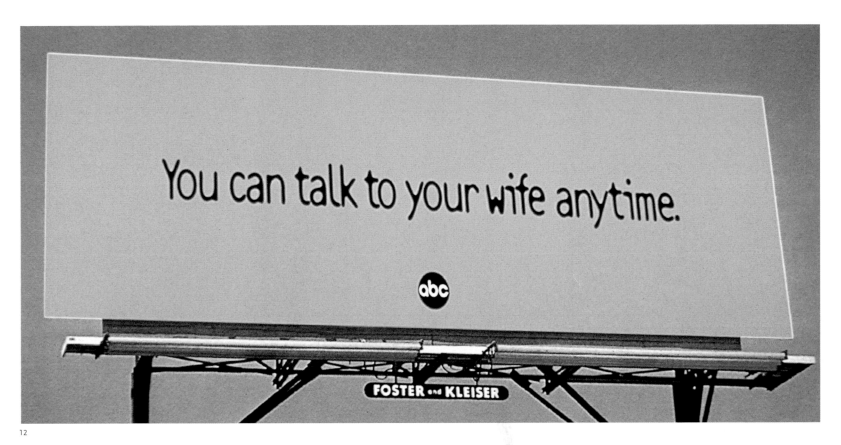

12

11. BURGER KING
SAATCHI & SAATCHI,
SINGAPORE, 1997
This ad turns a mere french fry
into something incendiary.

12. ABC TELEVISION
TBWA/CHIAT/DAY,
LOS ANGELES, 1997
The campaign argued that it was
acceptable to watch TV, even if it
meant neglecting other domestic
or more cerebral duties.

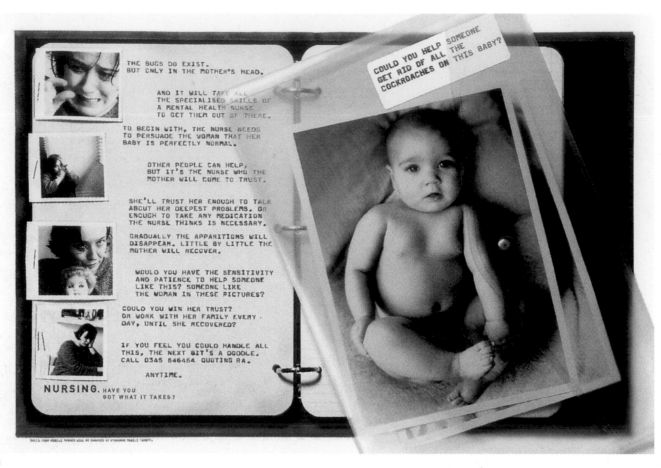

13

13. **BRITISH DEPARTMENT OF HEALTH**
SAATCHI & SAATCHI, LONDON, 1997
Tackling the tough issue of mental illness, the campaign challenged people to empathize and to devote their lives to helping.

14. **PARTNERSHIP FOR A DRUG-FREE AMERICA**
DDB NEEDHAM, CHICAGO, 1988
The gun-up-the-nose imagery in this ad shocked some, but cocaine usage dropped sharply following the appearance of this campaign.

15. **NIKE**
WIEDEN + KENNEDY, PORTLAND, 1992
This campaign, written by women for women, touched on deep feelings and became a source of inspiration.

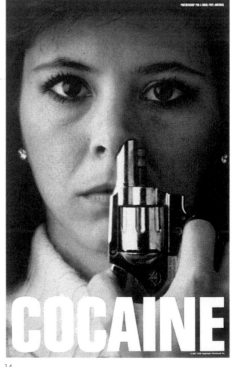

14

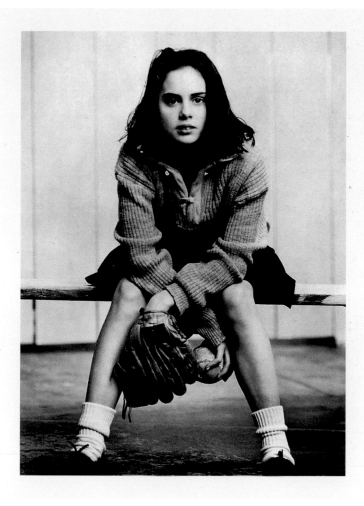

Did you ever wish you were a boy?

Did you? Did you for one moment or one breath or one heartbeat beating over all the years of your life, wish, even a little, that you could spend it as a boy? Honest. Really. Even if you got over it.

Did you ever wish that you could be a boy just so you could do *boy things* and not hear them called *boy things*, did you want to climb trees and skin knees and be third base and not hear the boys say, Sure, play, but that means you have to *be* third base.

Oh *ha ha ha*.

But did you ever wish you were a boy

just because there were *boys*, and there were *girls* and they were *them*, and we were, well,

we weren't them, and we knew there must be a difference because everybody kept telling us there was. But what was it?

You never knew. Like you *knew* that you were a girl *(you run like a girl you throw like a girl you girl you)* and that was great, that was swell, but you (continued)

15

"rack-and-pinion steering" often must resort to exaggeration and hyperbole. Worse than that, they're boring. Advertisers can't help it: In today's parity marketplace, most products are comparable in quality. But you can't say that in an ad without riling the client (who, like a proud parent, frequently harbors the illusion that his baby really is better than everyone else's). For a shopper seeking hard, reliable facts on a product, advertising will never be a good resource; better to read articles in *Consumer Reports* or other unbiased sources. Look to the ads for humor and style—those are about the only worthwhile things they can provide.

Some cultural watchdogs have a problem with ads that try to entertain or be stylish and artful; they see this kind of advertising as the wolf in sheep's clothing, distracting us with humor or beauty, while actually manipulating us to buy, buy, buy. But that suggests a

somewhat condescending view of the savvy media citizens of the twenty-first century. It's a viewpoint that would have us believe that only the tweedy academics and cynical journalists have figured out what's really going on—while the rest of us poor sheep are still being herded around by devious advertisers. The reality is that today even the average couch potato has an advanced degree when it comes to decoding media images and messages, with an understanding of satire, irreverence, hyperbole. We all have built-in "rubbish detectors" that are as sensitive as that of any media-studies professor (if not more so; after all, academics don't watch much TV except when they're stooping to analyze it). As Fenske notes, today's viewers watch daily reruns of sophisticated TV programs like "Seinfeld" and "Monty Python's Flying Circus," and they get the inside references, the jokes within the jokes. And so they probably also can grasp that, for

example, an advertiser that mocks its own ad is doing so to try to gain our trust. Yes, we get it—we know there's a sell in there somewhere. But we'll play along. We want that little surprise, the tiny chuckle, the sappy greeting-card-induced tear—that moment of fun that a truly entertaining ad provides.

5. IT CAN ENLIGHTEN AND INSPIRE.

Someone once said that "Nike killed the three-martini lunch." That may be an overstatement of the transformative power of Nike ads. But maybe not. There can be no doubt that the athletic-shoe company's stirring campaigns, urging people to become more active, live healthier, go the extra mile, put in maximum effort, and overcome personal obstacles, have had a tangible impact on the lives of people around the world. In particular, Nike's ads directed toward women, with headlines like "You are not a goddess," "Ever wish you were

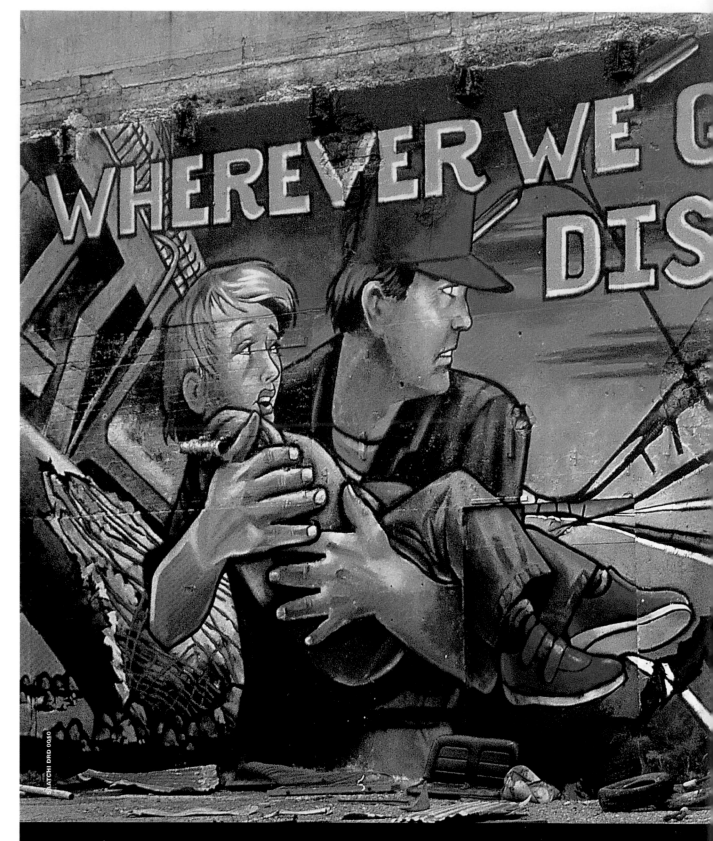

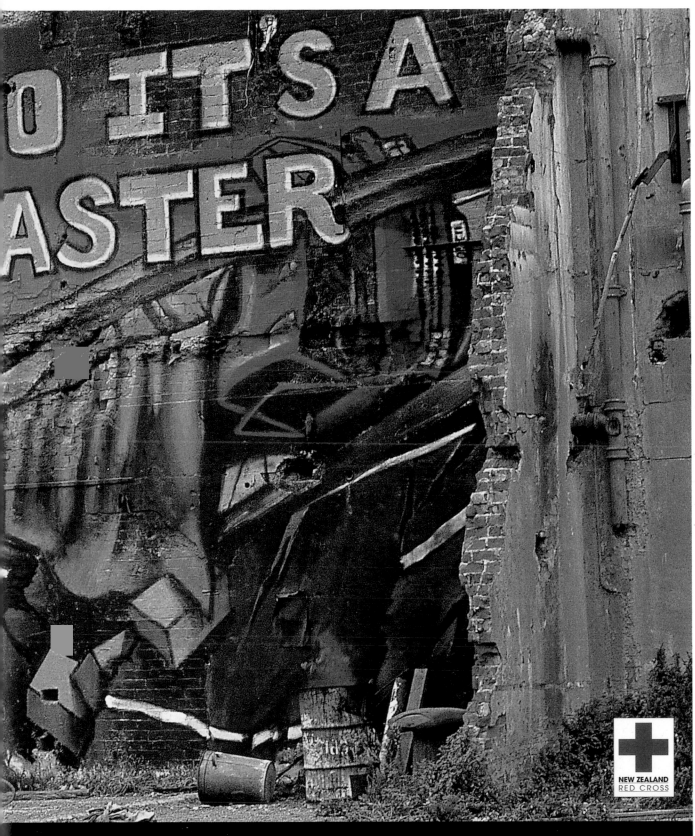

O IT'S A
ASTER

A FAMILIAR AND REASSURING SIGHT IN THE AFTERMATH OF A DISASTER. WE PREPARE OURSELVES FOR AN INSTANT RESPONSE. AND THROUGH OUR FIRST AID AND RESCUE COURSES. WE ALSO PREPARE YOU. ALTHOUGH WE MAY ASK FOR YOUR HELP NOW AND THEN. ONE DAY YOU MIGHT NEED OURS.

NEW ZEALAND RED CROSS

16. **NEW ZEALAND RED CROSS**
SAATCHI & SAATCHI
NEW ZEALAND, WELLING-
TON, 1995
An artful, dramatic visual
campaign that reminded New
Zealanders why the Red Cross
still matters.

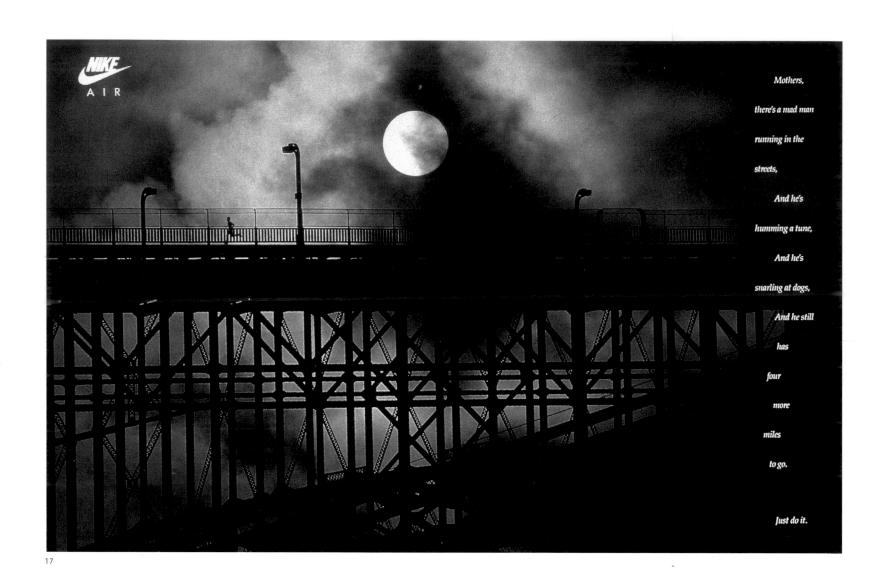

17

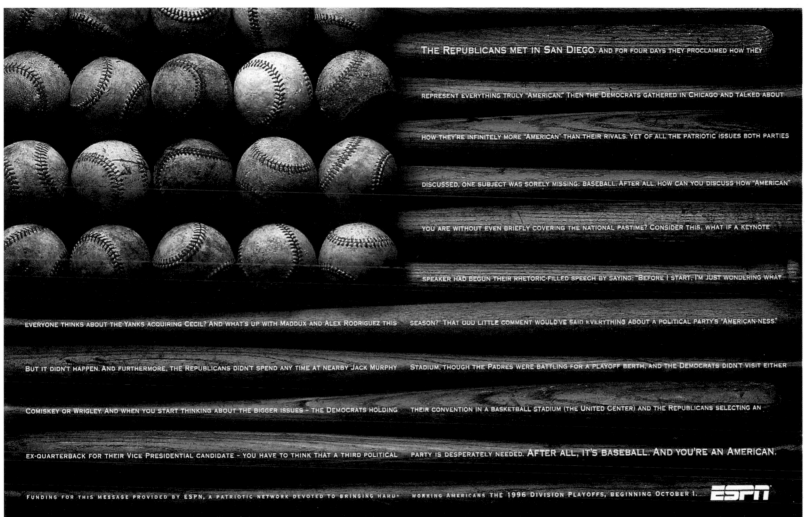

18

17. **NIKE**
WIEDEN + KENNEDY,
PORTLAND, 1990
An early ad in the "Just do it"
campaign captured the
loneliness and exhilaration of
the long-distance runner.

18. **ESPN SPORTS NETWORK**
WIEDEN + KENNEDY,
PORTLAND, 1996
The cable channel and its ad
agency recognized that sports
fans are a nation unto
themselves.

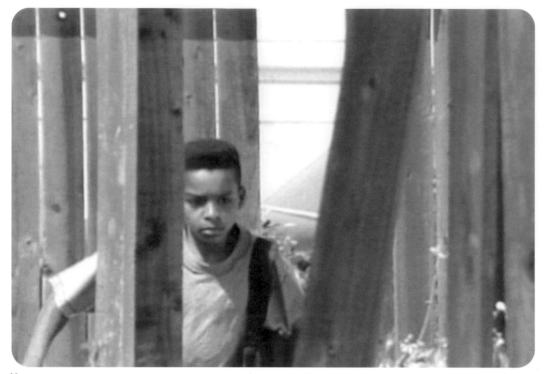

19

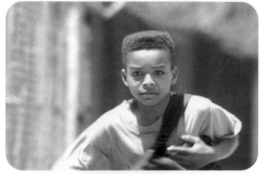

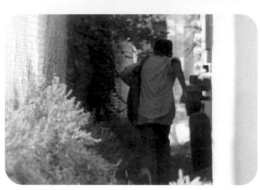

19. **PARTNERSHIP FOR A DRUG-FREE AMERICA**
GOODBY SILVERSTEIN & PARTNERS, SAN FRANCISCO, 1992
Proving it isn't easy to "just say no," the boy in this commercial was shown traveling a circuitous route, the "Long Way Home," to avoid streetcorner drug dealers.

20. **VISA**
BATEY ADS, SINGAPORE, 1996
The campaign mirrored a changing culture in Asia, with the arrival of credit cards and self-indulgence.

a boy?" and "If you let me play sports . . .," caused the company to be flooded with letters from women and girls across America, who confessed that the ads had been taped to their walls for daily inspiration.

It's not just Nike that has had this kind of effect. Over the past thirty years, public-service advertising has reminded a generation of kids that drugs cook your brain, doing so with simple indelible frying-pan imagery that packed a thousand times the power and authenticity of, say, former First Lady Nancy Reagan imploring people to "just say no." Ads have helped persuade people to buckle up, to clean up (who can forget the Native American driven to tears by litter?), to pay more attention to the kids, to consider the plight of the homeless, to drive more responsibly, to practice contraception in India, to abolish apartheid in South Africa, to support medical research, to quit smoking. (On the flip side, advertising

also has had a long history of persuading us to start smoking; and even though cigarette ads have been greatly diminished and restricted, in this particular area the industry still has much penance to do.) For those who suspect that advertising can't really influence intractable social problems, there is evidence to suggest otherwise. One particularly moving commercial from the American ad agency Goodby Silverstein & Partners, titled "The Long Way Home," showed the plight of an inner-city child forced to take a circuitous route to and from school in order to avoid having to pass by local drug dealers. The commercial had only a limited run, but follow-up studies in the markets where it aired revealed surprising shifts in the attitudes and behavior of young people exposed to the ad; it actually seemed to break through the wall. Not all "good cause" advertising is this effective, and some of it is created for self-serving reasons (see Chapter 9). But

the best of it has almost certainly changed minds and lives.

6. IT IS A MIRROR THAT REFLECTS OUR VALUES, HOPES, DREAMS, AND FEARS.
The author Marshall McLuhan called advertisements "the richest and most faithful daily reflections that any society ever made of its entire range of activities," which means we can learn a lot about our society by studying it. Advertising is often accused of telling us what to think, of manipulating attitudes and behavior—which it sometimes does. (A quick aside: Ads directed at young children and political ads have long been considered the most coldly manipulative and least artful kinds of advertising; that's why both categories have been largely omitted from this book.) But more often, advertising tries to reflect and reinforce attitudes and behavioral trends that have already begun to take hold. Ads didn't create the self-indulgent, status-obsessed spirit of the

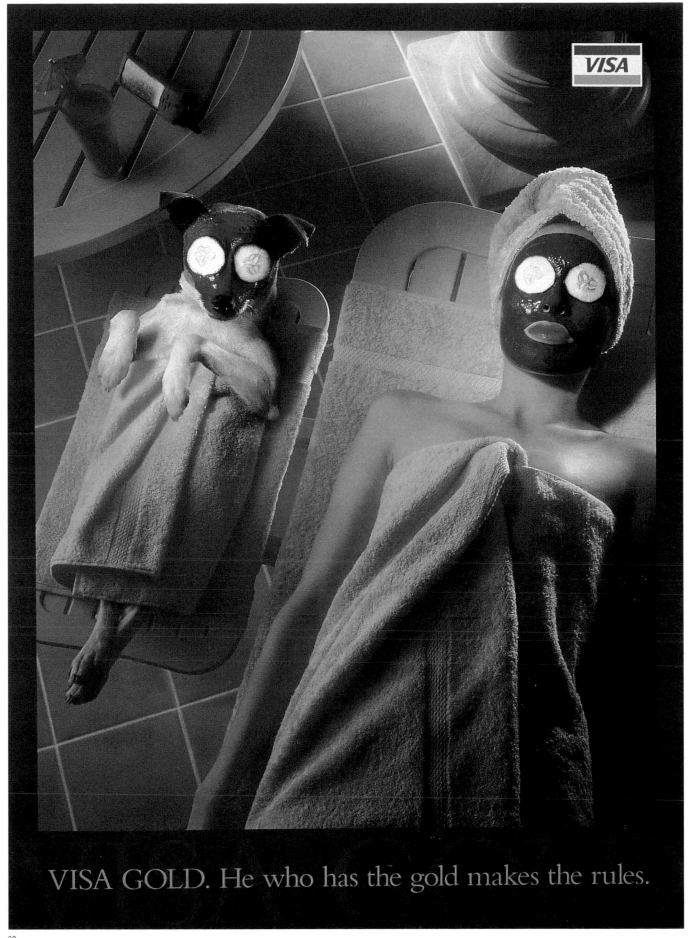

VISA GOLD. He who has the gold makes the rules.

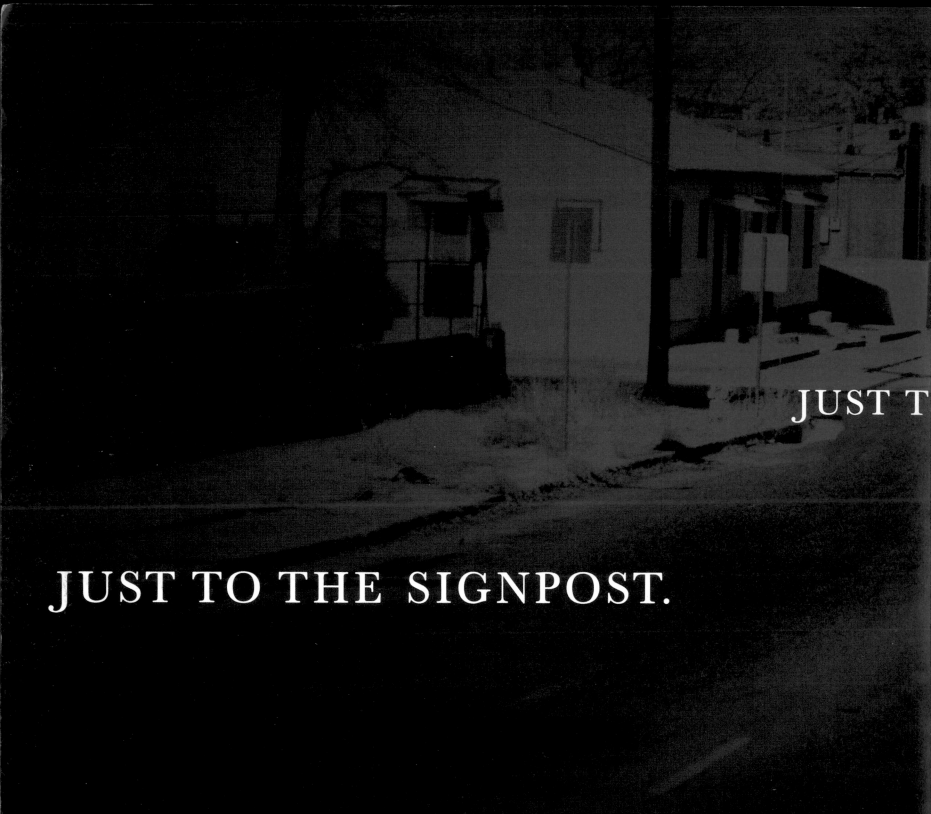

JUST TO THE SIGNPOST...

JUST TO THE TRUCK.

JUST TO THE KERB.

JUST TO THE CROSSROADS.

THE CAR.

adidas®
RUNNING

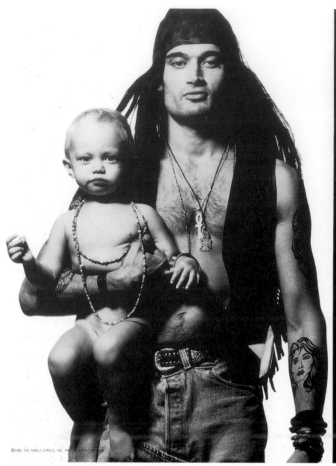

We were just driving along in the family bandwagon and

suddenly everyone else jumped on.

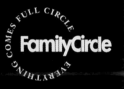

EVERYTHING COMES FULL CIRCLE

FamilyCircle

©1992 THE FAMILY CIRCLE, INC. PHOTO: ALBERT WATSON

22

Would you like to sit next to you at dinner?

The Economist

23

21. (PREVIOUS SPREAD)
ADIDAS
LEAGAS DELANEY, LONDON,
1995
Like Nike, Adidas used its ads to
urge people to go the extra mile
(and to associate this achievement with Adidas shoes).

22. **FAMILY CIRCLE MAGAZINE**
KIRSHENBAUM BOND &
PARTNERS, NEW YORK, 1992
Ads occasionally lead, but more
often mirror, social trends and
changing demographics—
though advertisers, like this
one, often claim to be ahead of
the pack.

23. **THE ECONOMIST**
ABBOTT MEAD VICKERS,
LONDON, 1998
This campaign asked pointed
questions, emphasizing the
point that reading *The
Economist* could make you a
more interesting person.

24. **BERNIE'S TATTOOING**
THE MARTIN AGENCY,
RICHMOND, VIRGINIA, 1990
A little ad, for a local tattoo
parlor, that ultimately became
a part of advertising lore and a
regional movement.

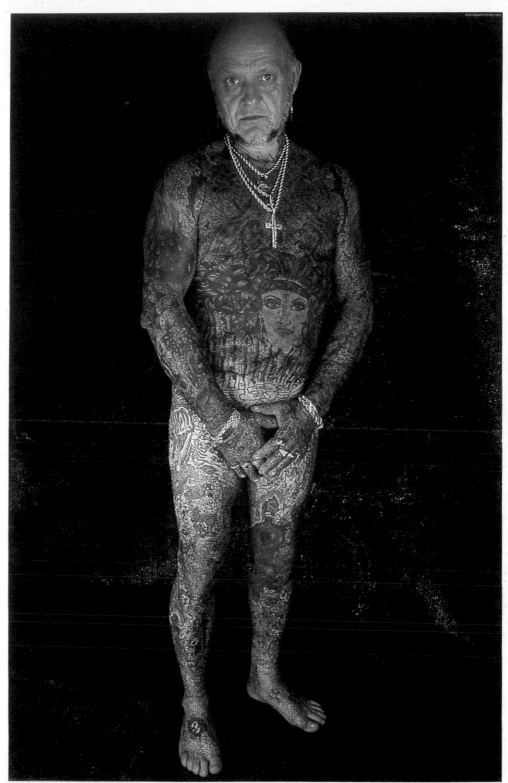

SURPRISE YOUR WIFE.

BERNIE'S TATTOOING
2924 West Avenue Bristol PA. 788-6196

24

WHY ADVERTISING MATTERS. HONESTLY.

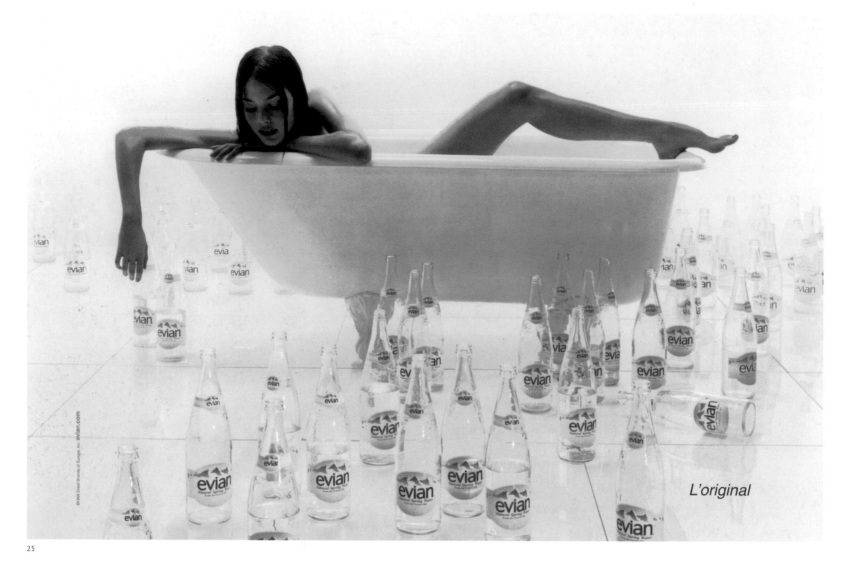

L'original

25

America in the 1980s—but the ads of that period, taken as a whole, do form a rich and revealing portrait of that species known as the "Yuppie." Similarly, ads didn't create the renewed emphasis, a few years later, on family values—but advertising indisputably picked up that ball and ran with it.

Advertising's mirror is sometimes of the fun-house variety, distorting reality to have us believe that the life going on around us is something different from what it actually is. The clichéd Norman Rockwell approach to ads—projecting wholesome happy families, or hardworking, good-natured farmers amid lush fields, played to the sound track of "The Heartbeat of America"—still is in use in the U.S., particularly by more conventional and conservative marketers.

But if you look closely at today's ads, there is less and less of the old-fashioned imagery that tended to idealize and sanitize. Many ads

now are more realistic snapshots of the culture, not all of them pretty or comforting. A gritty series of Miller High Life ads rhapsodizing about all things macho undoubtedly reflects longings by conflicted modern men to rediscover their "inner guy." Meanwhile, the increasingly aggressive behavior depicted in ads lately— deranged stalkers, people physically attacking one another, the sorts of images that would have been unthinkable in advertising a few years back—clearly represents one more warning bell about the violence that has overtaken the culture. And as irony becomes inescapable in today's ads, one must wonder whether some pundits are right in suggesting that current society seems to be losing its capacity for smirk-free, earnest discussion. Conversely, amid all the cynicism, the reemergence of the old American ad character Mr. Whipple seems to speak to our desire to return to a more innocent past. And finally, there are

all those get-rich-quick Internet stock-trading ads that have flooded the airwaves the past couple of years (what would the famous Smith Barney pitchman John Houseman, whose ads used to sing the praises of making money "the old-fashioned way," have made of all this?). One thing is certain: Years from now, when historians want to know what it was like to live at the dawn of the new millennium, ads like these will all be precious artifacts.

7. IT KNOWS OUR SECRETS.

Decades ago, when American books like *The Hidden Persuaders* and *Subliminal Seduction* were popular, the air was rife with conspiracy theories about advertising: that it was engaging in mind-control tactics or planting concealed messages. For the most part, these were paranoid fantasies, but advertisers do have a few tricks up their sleeves. In recent years, they've become highly adept at getting inside our

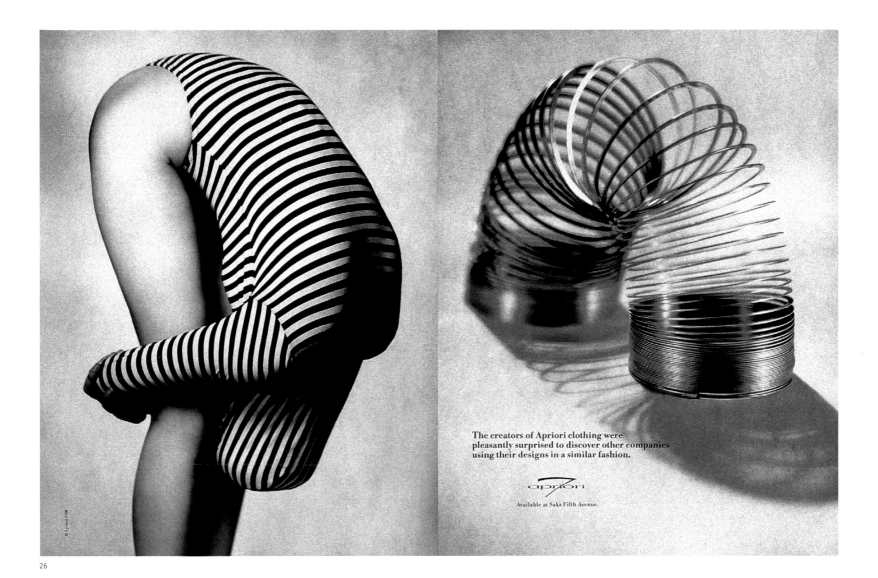

The creators of Apriori clothing were pleasantly surprised to discover other companies using their designs in a similar fashion.

apriori

Available at Saks Fifth Avenue.

26

25. EVIAN
EURO RSCG, NEW YORK
AND PARIS, 1999
This campaign encouraged consumption of Evian bottled water, "*L'original,*" in unexpected ways.

26. APRIORI ESCADA
WEISS WHITTEN STAGLIANO,
NEW YORK, 1992
Showing the playful side of fashion, this ad campaign drew parallels between stylish clothes and simple objects.

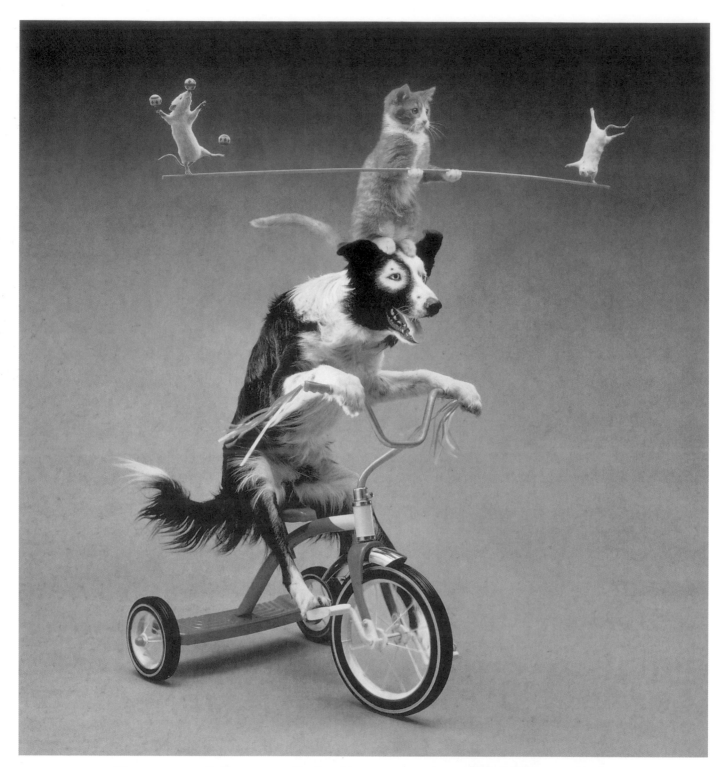

Get paid to think up stuff like this.

Some ad agency actually paid a writer and an art director to think up this crazy visual idea for an ad. But coming up with wildly creative solutions to real marketing problems is what advertising is all about. And, after 8 semesters at Art Center, you'll have a good portfolio and a good shot at landing a job in a field that's financially as well as creatively rewarding. Call us at 818-584-5035. Or write to Admissions, Art **ArtCenter** Center College of Design, 1700 Lida St., Pasadena, CA, 91103.

27

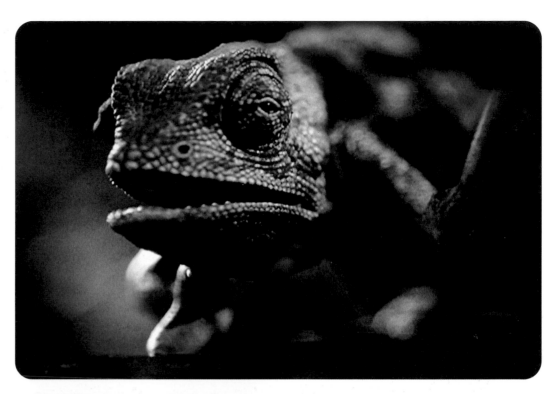

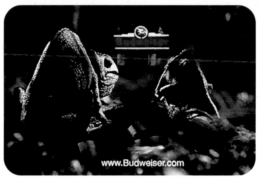

28

27. ART CENTER COLLEGE OF DESIGN, PASADENA, CALIFORNIA
FALLON McELLIGOTT, MINNEAPOLIS, MINNESOTA, 1992
This design school promoted the lure of advertising in a nutshell: people are encouraged to think of crazy ideas, which sometimes defy logic and succeed wildly.

28. BUDWEISER
GOODBY SILVERSTEIN & PARTNERS, SAN FRANCISCO, 1997
Frogs and lizards became characters in this memorable ongoing series of TV commercials; the brand name was briefly flashed on screen, lest we forgot who was telling the tale.

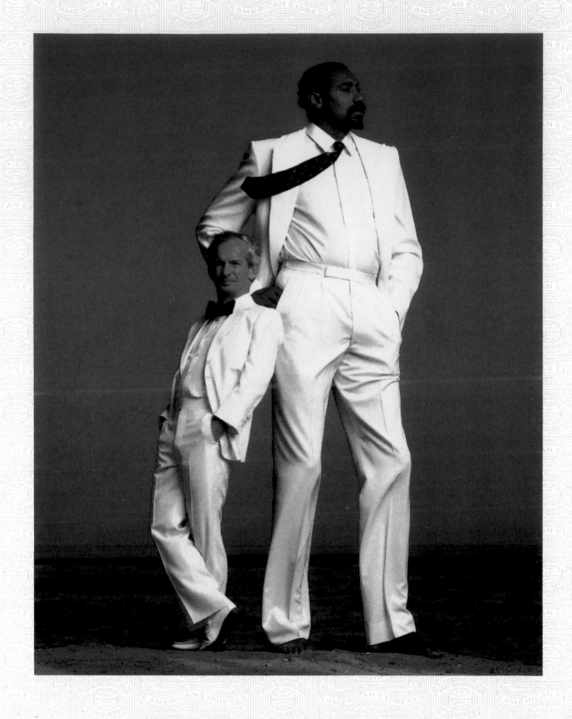

Wilt Chamberlain.   Cardmember since 1976.
Willie Shoemaker.   Cardmember since 1966.

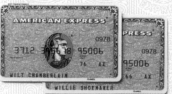

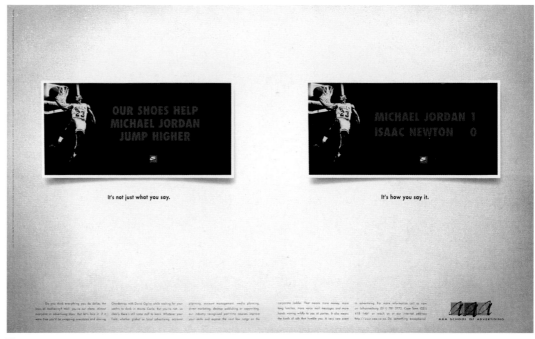

It's not just what you say.

It's how you say it.

30

heads. This may conjure up images of hypnosis and high-tech mind-reading gadgetry—and, in very rare instances, advertisers may use these tools (including skin sensors that measure a subject's response to an ad) as part of research. But most of the time, advertisers study us the old-fashioned way—just by watching. In the past fifteen years ad agencies have refined the science of cultural anthropology, largely via a process developed in the UK known as "planning." What planners do, simply, is observe people as they eat, shop, converse, and putter about the house (it's not uncommon for a planner to live with willing research subjects for extended periods of time). Planners then hand these observations over to the people who create ads—which is why you may find yourself, upon watching an ad, wondering, "How did they know I felt that way about bananas?"

On the other hand, sometimes ad creators are able to connect with our deepest feelings simply because they have an instinctive, God-given understanding of human nature. The Salk Institute in La Jolla, California, in honoring the legendary American adman Bill Bernbach, once said of him, "He could explain us to ourselves." That's reason enough to take a closer look at Bernbach's ads: not to understand him but to understand yourself. Besides, if advertising is going to study you and figure out all your secrets, shouldn't you do the same thing to it in return?

8. IT GAINFULLY EMPLOYS SOME OF OUR MOST TALENTED ACTORS, DESIGNERS, WRITERS, FILMMAKERS, WORLD LEADERS, AND PERFORMING ANIMALS.

Maybe it all started when the American ad executive Jerry Della Femina announced, "Advertising is the most fun you can have with your clothes on." In recent years, the ad business has been a magnet for young talent. More and more advertising schools have popped up all over the world, attracting the best art directors and writers. Talented filmmakers—who years ago wouldn't have touched ads for fear of sullying their reputations—now jump at the chance to make "thirty-second movies." No one—not Jerry Seinfeld, not Madonna, not the Dalai Lama, not the hottest new hip-hop star of the moment—is too cool or too important to appear in an ad these days. And never, ever before have there been so many ripe career opportunities for talking dogs and loquacious lizards.

9. IT IS INESCAPABLE AND CANNOT BE KILLED.

Recently, Pizza Hut stamped its logo on a rocket to the moon. This is understandable—on this planet, it seems there is no place left in which to squeeze an ad. There are ads in bathroom stalls, ads stamped on fruit, ads in the bottom of your cocktail glass, ads under your feet as you amble down the street (a favorite: the Kirshenbaum & Bond lingerie ad

WHY ADVERTISING MATTERS. HONESTLY.

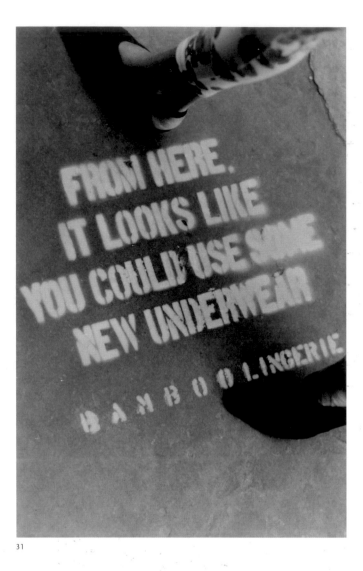

31

stenciled on New York sidewalks that read, "From here, it looks like you could use some new underwear"). Ogilvy & Mather now practices what it calls "360-degree branding"— the idea that you, the consumer, shall encounter the brand everywhere you turn in the course of your day. That is the new mission of advertising. The proliferation of ads used to be a Western phenomenon, but now ads are ubiquitous in China; they are planted in all kinds of unexpected places throughout South Africa (big practitioners of "guerrilla advertising"); and they're running wild throughout Tahiti.

For a while, in the mid-1990s, a rumor began to spread that advertising was an endangered species. The Internet was surely going to kill it (*Wired* magazine, to make this point, featured a cover with the New York ad creators Richard Kirshenbaum and George Lois blindfolded before a firing squad). But by the late 1990s, it became clear that the Silicon Valley whiz-kids

were as hooked on advertising as everybody else; they quickly poured huge sums of their newfound money into the coffers of conventional ad agencies, to make old-fashioned TV commercials about their Web sites. The ad executives laughed all the way to the bank, just as they had when doomsayers predicted that the VCR or the remote control or the expansion of cable would spell the end of advertising. One can state this loud and clear: Advertising will change, will mutate, will reinvent itself. But for the foreseeable future, it isn't going away. (Except for the occasional little jaunt to the moon and back.)

The prospect of being more and more enveloped by 360-degree advertising, with no escape hatch in sight, is hardly cause for a "sale-a-bration." But it only reaffirms the point that quality and good taste in advertising really *do* matter, and they matter more and more as ads continue to proliferate. Cognizant of this,

the American ad executive Jeff Goodby believes that advertisers have an environmental obligation. "If people are going to have to encounter this every day," he says, "then I think we have a responsibility to produce something that has a certain amount of style or wit. I don't want to add to the cultural pollution that's out there." As evidenced by Goodby's work throughout this book, he has done more than his share to improve the advertising landscape, as have Bernbach, Wieden, Delaney, Lee Clow, John Hegarty, Oliviero Toscani, Bob Barrie, Nizan Guanaes, and others. This book celebrates their work and supports the hope that many others, who continue to weave the cocoon that surrounds us, will follow their good examples.

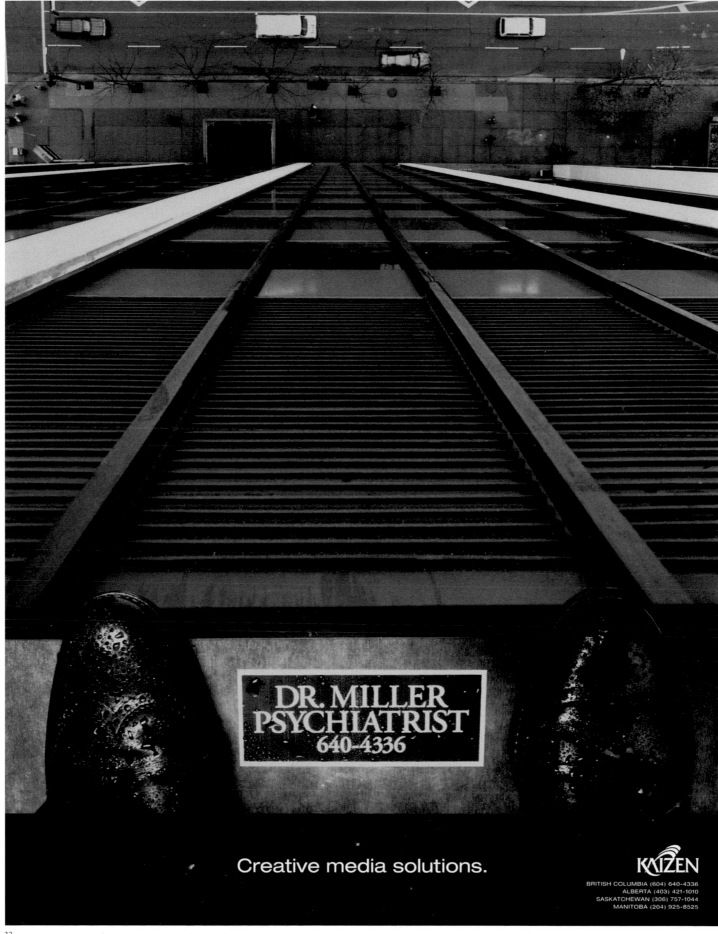

2. WHE
GOT S

N ADS
MART.

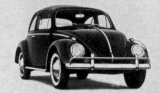

Think small.

Our little car isn't so much of a novelty any more.

A couple of dozen college kids don't try to squeeze inside it.

The guy at the gas station doesn't ask where the gas goes.

Nobody even stares at our shape.

In fact, some people who drive our little flivver don't even think 32 miles to the gallon is going any great guns.

Or using five pints of oil instead of five quarts.

Or never needing anti-freeze.

Or racking up 40,000 miles on a set of tires.

That's because once you get used to some of our economies, you don't even think about them any more.

Except when you squeeze into a small parking spot. Or renew your small insurance. Or pay a small repair bill. Or trade in your old VW for a new one.

Think it over.

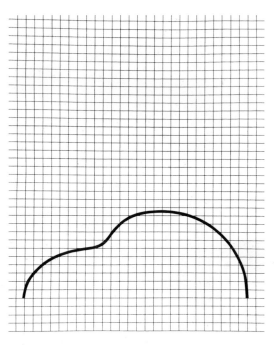

Is the economy trying to tell you something?

2

1. **VOLKSWAGEN**
DOYLE DANE BERNBACH,
NEW YORK, 1960
"Think small." This ad from
1960 launched advertising's
Creative Revolution.

2. **VOLKSWAGEN**
DOYLE DANE BERNBACH,
NEW YORK, EARLY 1970s
First, DDB had the nerve to
shrink the car in the ads; in this
one, they didn't show it at all.

magine that the year is 1960, and you are reading the February 22 issue of *Life* magazine. Toward the front of the publication, amid colorful advertising images of Chevrolets and soft drinks, you come upon a stark, black-and-white full-page advertisement for the Volkswagen Beetle automobile. Something about this ad catches your eye and stops you from turning the page. Maybe it's because the picture of the car is so tiny; cars in ads are not supposed to be mini-mized this way. You read the headline: "Think small." Again, something seems amiss: This is a time in America when "bigger is better" is the credo, when Cadillacs rule the road and a prosperous population is living large. Why think small? You seek an explanation in the copy at the bottom of the page, which tells you, in effect, that this car is not for everyone. Other ads in this magazine are urging you to keep up with the Joneses, but this one is issuing a challenge: Go against the flow. Forget about appearances. Use

your head. It's a message that seems almost insurrectionist in these Eisenhower times (John F. Kennedy had not yet been nominated for president of the U.S. as you were reading this), but it's couched in language that is understated, self-deprecating, with a wry sense of humor. One ad winkingly refers to the German car being "as American as Apple Strudel." You savor the last line, squint at the small picture of the Beetle one more time. Only then do you finally turn the page, unaware that you've just absorbed the advertising equivalent of "the shot heard round the world."

The Volkswagen campaign of the 1960s, created by the New York ad agency Doyle Dane Bernbach, was the launching point of a revo-lution in advertising. If you were one of the magazine or newspaper readers who happened upon that infamous "Think small." ad, and the equally stirring ads in the series that followed, it may not have persuaded you to run out and buy a Beetle—even the most compelling advertising

rarely sends people scampering to the store (though Volkswagen's sales did increase substantially that year). However, the ad may well have caused you to adjust your thinking about a funny-looking foreign car, and maybe about cars in general, and social conformity, and heaven knows what else. And maybe it changed the way you would approach some ads from now on: No longer could you assume that an ad was obvious and one-dimensional, a mere sales pitch. Now, suddenly, there were ads with an unspoken message and a complex personality; ads that were capable of engaging you in a dialogue, and that challenged you to keep up with their level of wit and intelligence.

Advertising wasn't supposed to be this complicated. Before Doyle Dane Bernbach and others ignited what would be called the Creative Revolution, ads were primarily populated by cute characters and icons—the Jolly Green Giant; Snap, Crackle & Pop; Speedy, the Alka-Seltzer

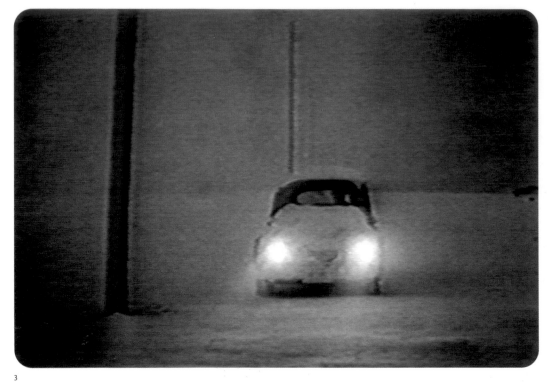

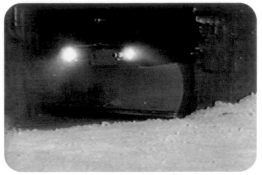

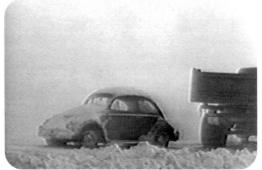

3

3. **VOLKSWAGEN**
DOYLE DANE BERNBACH,
NEW YORK, 1963
"Snow Plow," one of the first
cinematic, storytelling
commercials, revealed how the
man who drives the snow plow
manages to get to the snow
plow: in a VW Beetle, of course.

4. **EL AL AIRLINES**
DOYLE DANE BERNBACH,
NEW YORK, 1957
Tearing up the page: DDB's art
directors broke the established
rules of layout and design.

mascot; and dancing cigarettes—accompanied by cheery jingles and slogans ("You'll wonder where / the yellow went / when you brush your teeth / with Pepsodent"). And to drive these messages home, the advertiser's hammer was simple repetition; the advertising of old wasn't trying to engage you so much as beat you into submission with a smile and a song that just kept coming back.

To be sure, there were some advertising mavericks who tried to buck this simplistic approach and imbue their work with more style and subtlety. David Ogilvy, for example, founder of New York–based Ogilvy & Mather, introduced the world to more intriguing, enigmatic advertising characters, like the eye-patched Hathaway man in the 1950s. Still, the prevailing force in the ad industry pre-1960 was Rosser Reeves, head of Madison Avenue's Ted Bates Agency, who believed that advertisers should follow simple formulas that were foolproof in manipulating consumers. The idea was to identify a compelling

reason people should buy a product—Reeves called this the "Unique Selling Proposition"—and then harp on that point, over and over. Reeves's mission, and that of advertising as a whole, was simply to "get a message into the heads of as many people as possible at the lowest possible cost." Was there any style or substance to the message? That hardly seemed to matter at the time; to the disciples of the Reeves approach, advertising was, beneath the warm and fuzzy images and slogans, a cold and efficient science of the business world.

Bill Bernbach, on the other hand, had a different take. A writer from the Bronx who worked at several Madison Avenue agencies before opening his own in 1949, Bernbach believed that advertising was "fundamentally persuasion," and that persuasion was more art than science. While many advertisers swore by the power of redundancy, Bernbach felt that consumers would be more apt to respond to

novelty. The impact of an ad, he reasoned, "is a direct result of how fresh and original it is, because you react strongly to something you've never seen or heard before." To come up with those fresh ideas, Bernbach felt that ad creators had to approach their task in the manner of artists—trusting their intuition, rather than relying on formulas and research.

Bernbach had another insight that would fundamentally change advertising in years ahead. In his early days, at the William Weintraub agency, he worked alongside the great graphic designer Paul Rand. In developing ideas with Rand, Bernbach became convinced that writers and art directors should brainstorm while working on an ad campaign (previously, most ads were created in more of an assembly-line fashion: "A copywriter would write a headline and then slip it under the art director's door, expecting a layout in return," recalls DDB veteran Bob Levenson). Bernbach felt that "if two good people

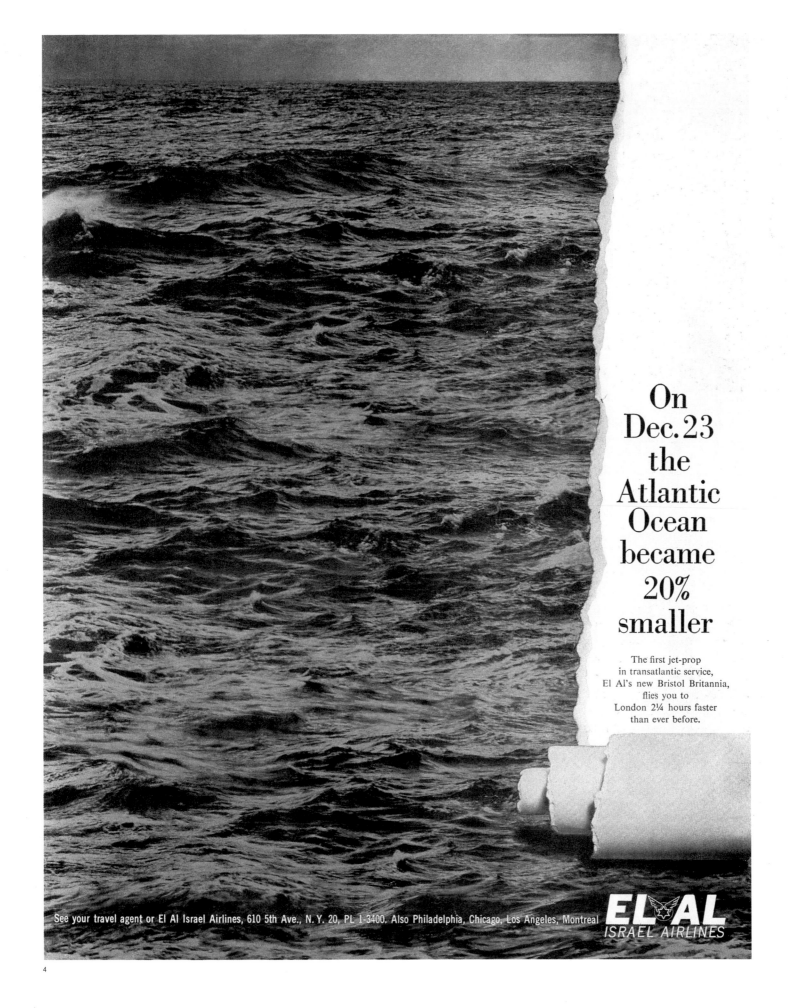

On Dec. 23 the Atlantic Ocean became 20% smaller

The first jet-prop in transatlantic service, El Al's new Bristol Britannia, flies you to London 2¼ hours faster than ever before.

See your travel agent or El Al Israel Airlines, 610 5th Ave., N. Y. 20, PL 1-3400. Also Philadelphia, Chicago, Los Angeles, Montreal

EL AL
ISRAEL AIRLINES

4

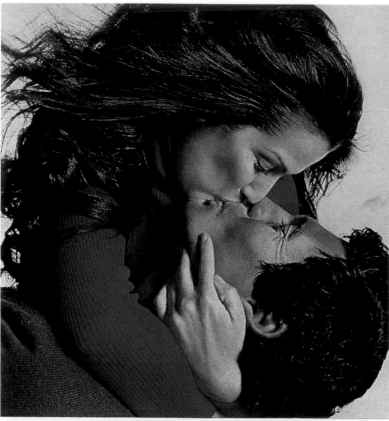

It lets me be me:

In hair color, as in make-up, clothes, love, work…a woman wants to be herself. Not somebody else's idea of what she is, or should be. That's what women like about Nice'n Easy." Whether you want to color or conceal, to change a little or a lot, Nice'n Easy assures you of beautiful coverage, healthy-looking hair and honest color that becomes part of you.

No wonder, now more than ever, it sells the most. Nice'n Easy. From Clairol.

Nice'n Easy

5

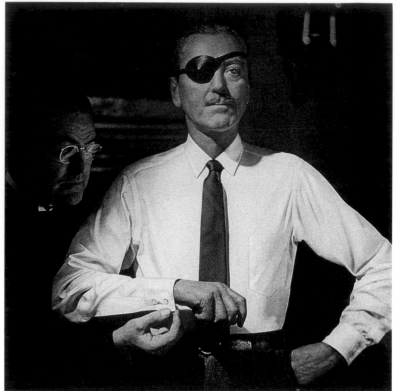

Hathaway's batiste broadcloth shirt is 100 per cent lightweight cotton. It weighs a third less than ordinary broadcloth.

Hathaway announces the first summer-weight broadcloth

THIS NEW HATHAWAY shirt is the world's first *batiste broadcloth*. It is the best news in lightweight shirts since Hathaway brought out batiste Oxford fifteen summers ago.

Until now, nobody has been able to reduce the weight of broadcloth without sacrificing some of its luster and softness. The secret of how this has at last been done remains overseas with our weavers. And they have a right to it. They spent ten years of trial and error perfecting this revolutionary broadcloth.

More news. Hathaway has put a *two-button cuff* on the batiste broadcloth shirt. If you are now wearing an ordinary single-button cuff, notice how the corners tend to cross at an angle. A *pair* of buttons keeps the corners squared —so that your cuff forms a perfect circle around your wrist. Very neat-looking—particularly under a jacket.

About $9. White, blue, Scotch Dawn, Cactus or Sahara. Solid or stripes.

For names of stores, and a free copy of Hathaway's informative little *Dictionary of Shirts and Shirtings*, write C. F. Hathaway, Waterville, Maine. Call OXford 7-5566 in New York.

6

5. CLAIROL NICE 'N EASY
DOYLE DANE BERNBACH,
NEW YORK, 1971
Written by DDB's Phyllis Robinson, this campaign was a breakthrough in terms of preaching individualism to women.

6. HATHAWAY
OGILVY & MATHER,
NEW YORK, 1960
David Ogilvy put an eye patch on "the man in the Hathaway shirt," suggesting to readers that there was an untold story behind the ad.

7. LEVY'S RYE BREAD
DOYLE DANE BERNBACH,
NEW YORK, 1967
DDB's campaign featuring ethnic faces "helped people feel comfortable with America's diversity," noted the journalist Michael Kinsley.

8. OHRBACH'S
DOYLE DANE BERNBACH,
NEW YORK, 1959
Early DDB print ads, like this one for a New York clothing retailer, showed the clean and spare design that would later distinguish the Volkswagen campaign.

You don't have to be Jewish

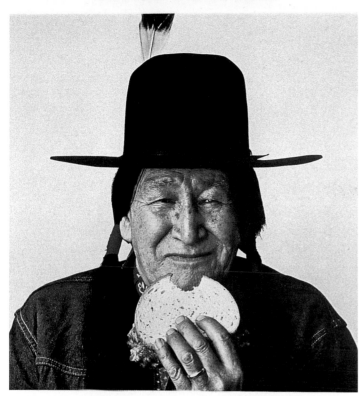

to love Levy's
real Jewish Rye

7

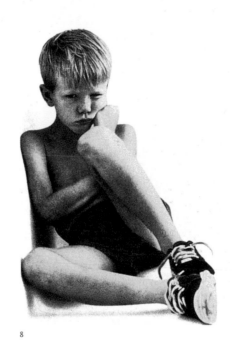

8

get together, an art director and a copywriter, sometimes you don't know who's writing the copy and who's doing the art because you get excited about the thought—which is the important thing."

This simple notion of doubling up writers and art directors—which is status quo today—had a groundbreaking, profound effect on the creative process of advertising: It served to knock down the wall between copy and art, and between the literal and the visceral aspects of advertising. In this new unified approach, creative teams sought out not just the clever line or the pretty picture but a seamless union of the two in the form of the big idea or "concept" that would resonate.

Bernbach's New York agency, formed with business partners Ned Doyle and Maxwell Dane, was stocked with creative people who had artistic sensibilities. The copywriter Phyllis Robinson idolized author Dorothy Parker; the art director Bob Gage had studied under renowned designer

Alexey Brodovitch of *Harper's Bazaar;* Helmut Krone, meanwhile, was a designer's designer, with a unique vision of how an advertising page might look. Still, Doyle Dane Bernbach was not a place to indulge artistic whims; Bernbach believed that selling the product was the first order of business. And the doctrine at the agency was that there was no room for cleverness or ornamentation that was not directly tied to selling the product (Bernbach once remarked that if you're going to show a man upside down in an ad, it should be for a reason—such as to show that the pockets in his pants keep his money from falling out). Research certainly played a role at the agency; Bernbach's teams immersed themselves in the cultures of the companies they worked for, and also studied the products closely. But as they sought to forge an emotional connection between those products and the people who might use them, DDB's creative teams were encouraged to trust their own intuition and instincts. "Listen to

the ideas percolating up from your unconscious," Bernbach advised his creative troops.

They did, and the results were astounding. Prior to the VW campaign, the agency had made a name for itself with playfully designed ads for Ohrbach's department store, and with its campaign for Levy's bread, which would eventually proclaim that "you don't have to be Jewish to love Levy's" (featuring the faces of Native Americans, Asians, and African-Americans, this advertising was years ahead of its time, and "helped people feel comfortable with America's ethnic diversity in a way that any number of human relations commissions could not," wrote the journalist Michael Kinsley). The agency's ads for El Al Airlines broke all the rules of airline advertising—they didn't show planes, stewardesses, or flight schedules. One ad, making the point that El Al's flights were 20 percent less expensive, showed a picture of the ocean, with part of the image ripped away. The headline read, "On Dec. 23, the Atlantic Ocean

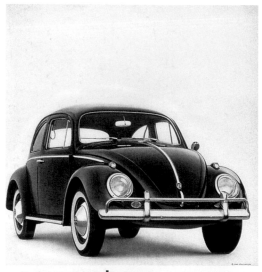

Lemon.

This Volkswagen missed the boat.

The chrome strip on the glove compartment is blemished and must be replaced. Chances are you wouldn't have noticed it; Inspector Kurt Kroner did.

There are 3,389 men at our Wolfsburg factory with only one job: to inspect Volkswagens at each stage of production. (3000 Volkswagens are produced daily; there are more inspectors than cars.)

Every shock absorber is tested (spot checking won't do), every windshield is scanned. VWs have been rejected for surface scratches barely visible to the eye.

Final inspection is really something! VW inspectors run each car off the line onto the Funktionsprüfstand (car test stand), tote up 189 check points, gun ahead to the automatic brake stand, and say "no" to one VW out of fifty.

This preoccupation with detail means the VW lasts longer and requires less maintenance, by and large, than other cars. (It also means a used VW depreciates less than any other car.)

We pluck the lemons; you get the plums.

9

9. **VOLKSWAGEN**
DOYLE DANE BERNBACH,
NEW YORK, 1960
The famous "Lemon" ad: Copy that seems at first glance like criticism actually praises the German carmaker for its high standards.

10. **VOLKSWAGEN**
DOYLE DANE BERNBACH,
NEW YORK, 1964
A typical example of the wry, self-deprecating humor that distinguished the early VW series from other ads.

became 20% smaller." (Bob Levenson recalls that when he first saw that ad as a young man riding the Manhattan subway, it struck him that "it was the perfect blend of words and pictures, and I hadn't seen anything like it." Shortly thereafter, he applied for a job at DDB). These early campaigns "lit the fire of the Creative Revolution," says Robinson. "Clients and creative people started coming to the agency, saying, 'Whatever you're doing, I want to get in on this.'"

But the Volkswagen campaign was the real breakthrough for DDB—and for advertising as a whole. Initially, there were reservations among Bernbach's employees (a significant number of whom were Jewish) about even working on the German account, recalls Robinson. "Some people at the agency didn't want to have anything to do with it," she says. But Bernbach maintained that Hitler and the old Germany were history, and it was time to move on. George Lois, then a young art director at the agency and part of the

anti-Volkswagen faction, recalls that Bernbach at one point showed him a newspaper article about Israel buying military parts from Germany— the point being, if Israel could now do business with the Germans, so could DDB. Lois, along with writer Julian Koenig and art director Helmut Krone, was part of the agency team that traveled to Germany to visit the Volkswagen factories, prior to beginning work on the ads. "You have to remember this wasn't that long after World War II, and I felt almost embarrassed to be walking around in that place," Lois says. But at the same time, the visitors couldn't help noticing the obvious dedication and passion of the car's German engineers—who seemed to take pride in the smallest details of their work. The result of their labor was a car that was unorthodox in its look and design, highly efficient and practical, small but indomitable.

Sometime during the factory visit it began to occur to Koenig that the car's perceived

drawbacks—the things that made it different from the more bloated American cars—were in fact its strengths. All that was required was the boldness to state that without apology, which Koenig did with his "Think small." headline. His partner Krone, a noted perfectionist, initially had trouble figuring out how to visually maximize the impact of this idea. He eventually produced a layout in which the tiny car seemed almost adrift in a sea of white space—a total departure from the cluttered ads of the day. The two-word headline was punctuated with a period (Krone's idea), and even that little period was, itself, a statement— a kind of anti-shout. "Bernbach took the exclamation point out of advertising," Krone would later remark, "and I put in the period." The "Think small." ad seemed to violate every advertising dictum of the day, and in doing so had a profoundly liberating effect within the advertising creative community. The ad would subsequently be held up as a banner for the new advertising, a

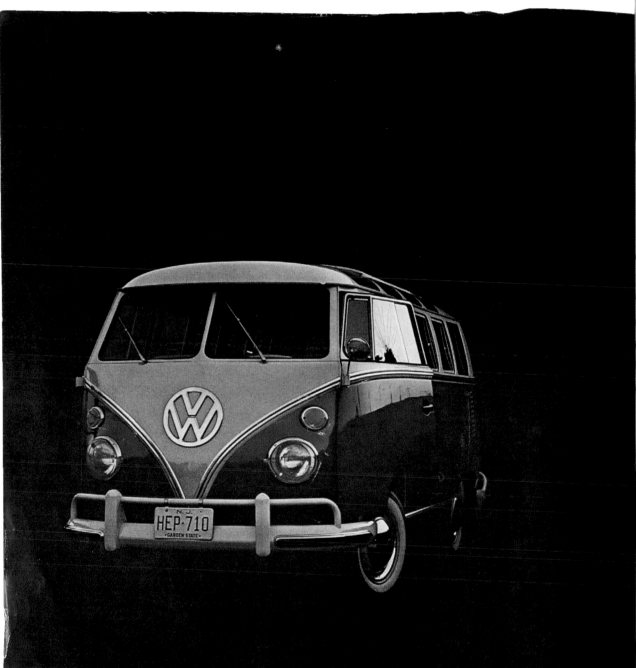

Somebody actually stole one.

We were tickled pink to hear that somebody wanted a Volkswagen Station Wagon badly enough to go out and steal one.

It wasn't so long ago that we practically couldn't give them away.

So when Martin Carlson reported his loss to the police, we took it as a triumph.

In its own way, the VW Station Wagon is one of the world's best getaway cars.

You can escape north or south of the border. (The VW engine can't freeze up or boil over because it's cooled by air.)

You can go farther in a VW than in any police car (24 mpg is our average).

You have 21 windows to spot anyone who's tailing you.

And it carries more loot (170 cu. ft.) than the biggest regular wagon you can steal.

Sadly, the whole theory blew apart when Mr. Carlson found his VW abandoned in the very spot he had left it.

Maybe everyone isn't ready for it, after all.

Not even crooks.

Nine Ways to
Improve an Ad

Rule: Show the product.
Don't turn it into a postage stamp or a test of failing eyesight. Show it. Boldly. Dramatically. Excitingly. Like this:

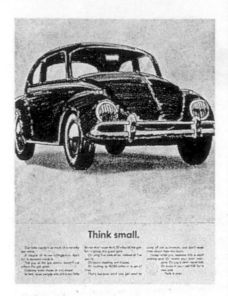

Think small.

There. See the difference already? Now, I'll admit the headline no longer makes complete sense—but that brings us to another obvious improvement.

Rule: Don't use negative headlines.
"Think Small" may be very clever, very witty...but what an idea to leave in the minds of everyday readers.

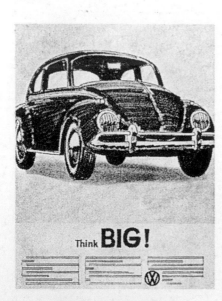

Think **BIG!**

"Think BIG!" Now I ask you—isn't that better? Isn't it more positive, more direct? And note, too, the interesting use of type to punch home the excitement of the idea.

Well that brings us to still another improvement—and one of the most important rules in advertising.

Rule: Whenever possible, mention your product name in the headline.
Which the people who thought up this ad could have done so very, very easily.

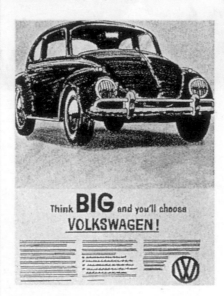

Think **BIG** and you'll choose **VOLKSWAGEN!**

See how the ad is beginning to jell? How it's really starting to come alive.

Let's see another way we can breathe some life into it—with a warming touch of humanity.

Rule: Whenever possible, show people enjoying your product.

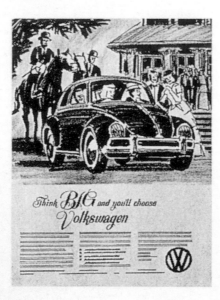

Think *BIG* and you'll choose *Volkswagen*

That's more like it. A gracious mansion. A carefree band of dancers. And best of all, a proud pair of thoroughbreds.

Now for an improvement to correct a fault in the product itself. You'll note that the VW, unfortunately, is totally lacking in news. From year to year, while other cars bring out a host of exciting changes—it stays its own dowdy self.

Rule: Always feature news in your advertisement. And if you have no news, invent it. Like this:

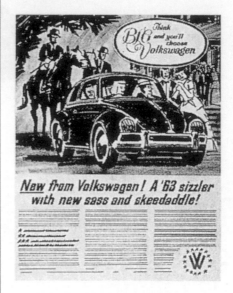

New from Volkswagen! A '63 sizzler with new sass and skeedaddle!

How's that for news?

Rule: (One of the most obvious of the bunch) **Always give prominent display to your product logo.**

And I don't mean an arty jumble of initials no one can read; I mean a proud unashamed logo like this:

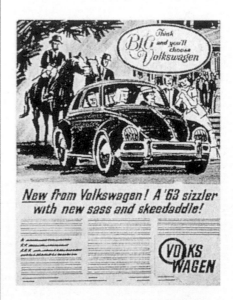

New from Volkswagen! A '63 sizzler with new sass and skeedaddle!

There. Now they know who's paying for the ad!

Rule: Avoid all unpleasant connotation about your product.

Which brings us to a somewhat delicate area: the country of origin of the Volkswagen car. Now I don't have to dwell on the subject of World War II and its attendant unpleasantness for you to grasp my meaning. Let's simply say that it might be wise to "domesticate" the car, so to speak.

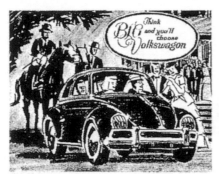
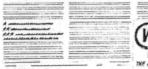

VOLKSWAGEN—THE ALL-AMERICAN CAR!

And in a flash, apple strudel turns into good old apple pie!

Rule: Always tell the reader where he can buy your product.

Where can you buy a Volkswagen?

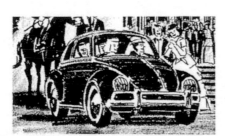

"At your friendly authorized Volkswagen dealer." Note the warmth of words like "friendly." And the use of "Authorized" to make sure that prospects don't stumble into places that are unauthorized.

One rule to go. The most important rule of all.

Rule: Always localize your ads.

And mind the way you spell the dealer's names.

There you have it. No clever, precious, self-conscious waste of space like the ad we started with; but an honest hard-hitting, two-fisted ad like this that really sells.

I said "sells." ∎

The dandelion is one of nature's prettiest villains. It's not only good to eat, there was a time when people took it as medicine.

But here in Marysville, Ohio, where we have our main grass research farms, it's just another weed.

In fact, it's a bully. It pushes the good grass out of the way and takes the food in the soil for itself. This is one weed that doesn't die every year. It's a tough perennial with roots that go down as far as 2 feet.

And that pretty yellow blossom turns into a white puffball full of seeds that the wind carries all over your lawn.

You can't stop dandelions from coming in, the way you can with crabgrass.

You have to get this pest to get rid of it. But it's easy to lick.

Leave one bit of its root and the dandelion will be back.

We'll get these dandelions out of your lawn and that's a promise.

And don't make it hard on yourself by trying to dig it out. Leave one bit of that root and back she'll come.

But just spend 30 minutes with your spreader and our *Turf Builder® Plus-2*. Your dandelion population (and a lot of other weeds) will be on the way out in a matter of days. That's our promise.

And the *Turf Builder®* in this is our own slow-release fertilizer. It will also feed your lawn for up to 2 months.

In fact, if you also spend 30 minutes with our straight Turf Builder®— say once in July and once again in September—

your grass will be so thick there won't even be room for weeds to come in. Good thick turf helps crowd weeds out.

Your Scotts retailer can tell you all about weeds. (We've probably even had him out here to see how we do it.) But you can call us toll-free if you like: (800) 543-1415. From Ohio: (800) 762-4010, from the Dakotas and Nebraska West call: (800) 543-0091.

You might also like to get our quarterly, Lawn Care®. It's free and it's filled with good things to know about grass.

Just write us here in Marysville, Ohio. You don't need a street address. We've been here since just after the Civil War.

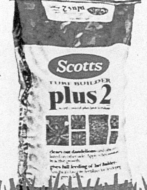

14

Avis is only No.2 in rent a cars. So why go with us?

We try damned hard.
(When you're not the biggest, you have to.)

We just can't afford dirty ash-trays. Or half-empty gas tanks. Or worn wipers. Or unwashed cars. Or low tires. Or anything less than seat-adjusters that adjust. Heaters that heat. Defrost-ers that defrost.

Obviously, the thing we try hardest for is just to be nice. To start you out right with a new car, like a lively, super torque Ford, and a pleasant smile. To know, say, where you get a good pastrami sandwich in Duluth.

Why?

Because we can't afford to take you for granted.

Go with us next time.

The line at our counter is shorter.

TIME, FEBRUARY 1, 1963

15

Who do you think of first when you think of rent a cars? Certainly not Avis.

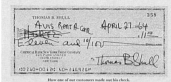

It must be nice to be a household word. Like Jell-O, Coke or Kodak.

But we're not. Avis is only No. 2 in rent a cars, and it's always the big fellow you think of first.

So we have to try harder. Hoping the people who stumble on us will come back for more.

(We probably have the world's most fussed-over Fords. Spick and span and nicely in tune.)

And when someone calls us by the wrong name, we turn the other cheek.

After all, it doesn't matter what you call us.

Just so you call.

16

14. SCOTTS LAWN PRODUCTS
DOYLE DANE BERNBACH,
NEW YORK, MID-1960s
The designer Helmut Krone constantly experimented with "the new page." Here he surrounded the text with a grass border.

15 AND 16. **AVIS**
DOYLE DANE BERNBACH,
NEW YORK, 1963
In a bit of marketing jujitsu, DDB turned a problem (the fact that Avis lagged behind Hertz in the rental car market) into an asset by arguing that "No. 2 tries harder."

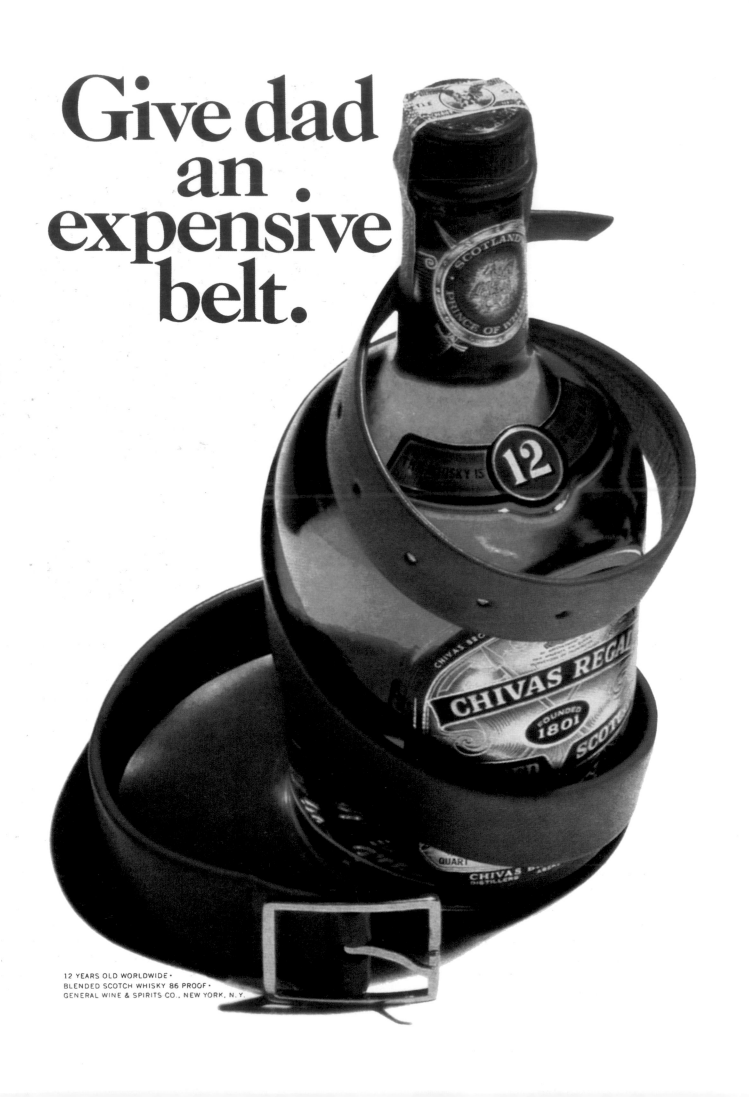

Give dad an expensive belt.

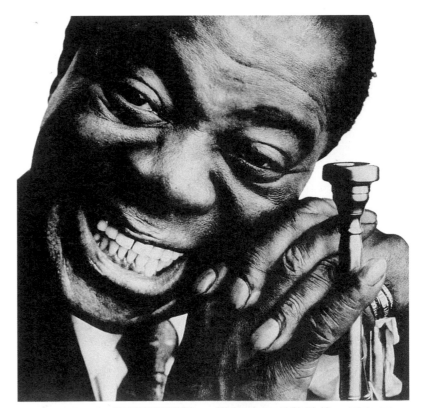

FIRST SHOWING OF A NEW POLAROID LAND FILM. This is an enlargement of an actual 60-second picture of Louis Armstrong. It was taken with a new film, just introduced, which is twice as sharp as the previous film. With this latest development, the Polaroid Land Camera not only gives you pictures in 60 seconds, but pictures of exceptional clarity and brilliance. Polaroid Land Cameras start at $72.75. The new film can be identified by a star on the box.

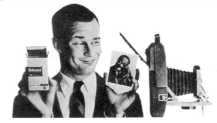

18

about being a runner-up, and the task was made more difficult when Bernbach prescreened the "We're No. 2 idea" with a panel of consumers and found that it did not score well. "But he stuck with the idea anyway," Levenson recalls. When it ran, it was a hit with the public and became one of the most famous ad campaigns in history.

The campaigns for Volkswagen, Avis, and other clients were popular and effective for years—because the agency's creative teams found ways to freshen them, to add new twists and surprises. DDB's art directors constantly experimented with new designs. Bob Gage was the first to try to "explode the page," says Robinson, referring to his bold use of white space, photography, and type treatments; "You would have to look to Toulouse-Lautrec's posters to find another artist with as wide an influence on the printed advertising message," she says. Gage's disciple, Krone, was forever trying to create "the new page," in which he would violate any rules he seemed to have estab-

lished in previous ads—replacing large pictures with small ones; moving the headline from top of page to the bottom. Krone used design elements to suggest a feeling about a brand (something that is quite common in ads now but was not at the time). He created a grass border around ads for Scotts lawn products; for Porsche he made some of his ads resemble pages from a technical engineering report. Krone understood that an ad's design didn't just dress up the concept—it could be the concept. The agency's writers, meanwhile, continually used language or scenarios that hadn't been seen in advertising before. One memorable VW commercial was set in a funeral procession and involved the reading of a will (in it, the deceased has decided to leave his wealth to the only relative who is fiscally responsible—the one who drives a VW, of course). At the time, says Roy Grace, "a funeral was the worst thing you could have in a commercial—and that's why it was so right." Similarly, for Chivas Regal, simply using a

line like "Give Dad a little belt for Christmas" was a risqué use of vernacular in advertising. Not everyone approved of what the agency was doing at the time, recalls Grace. "A lot of mainstream advertisers didn't understand it, couldn't do it themselves, and became very vocal about saying that we were wasting clients' money by using humor that supposedly wasn't appropriate for ads," he says. "Even David Ogilvy was still saying at the time that ads shouldn't be using humor."

But the the mid-1960s, DDB was not the only agency producing this new style of more candid and provocative advertising. In effect, Bernbach helped trigger a new wave of "advertisers with attitude," who took a more hard-hitting approach in their ads. Lois and Koenig had left DDB to form Papert Koenig Lois, which took the wry wit of DDB and infused it with more of a street-smart edge; the same could be said of one of PKL's own young hires, Carl Ally, who soon left and formed Carl Ally Inc., which emerged as a third leader in

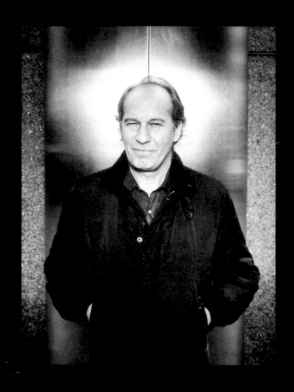

INTERVIEW: GEORGE LOIS

George Lois burst onto the advertising scene in the early 1960s, at the dawn of advertising's Creative Revolution, as a feisty art director at Doyle Dane Bernbach. He went on to start his own competing agency, Papert Koenig Lois, nearly as influential as DDB in those days. Lois is associated with some of advertising's most famous campaigns—from "I want my Maypo" to "I want my MTV"—but his contributions didn't end there. As the designer of some of *Esquire* magazine's unforgettable covers—artist Andy Warhol drowning in a soup can, boxer Muhammad Ali posed as Saint Sebastian, and others—Lois showed that his ability to convey powerful messages was not limited to pitching products.

YOU'VE CALLED DDB "THE FIRST CREATIVE AGENCY." WHAT MADE THAT SO?

To preface, there was a lot of great advertising before Bernbach, mostly in the form of great copy lines—"They laughed when I sat down at the piano" or "I'd walk a mile for a Camel." But almost never was there a marriage of real visual design that worked with the copy. Bernbach had an epiphany. It came out of his early work with the great designer Paul Rand. He saw Rand create advertising that had modern, humanistic imagery. He couldn't hire Rand, but he brought in Bob Gage and other great art directors, then put them in the same room with great writers—which had never been done—and they worked toward a common cause. And somehow, one plus one equaled three, and it changed everything. It created a new kind of advertising, with a new attitude, a new power, a new simplicity.

WHAT WAS THE ATMOSPHERE LIKE AT DDB?

When I first got there I knew I was in Nirvana. I loved knowing there was great talent around me. You could stick your head in almost any door and you knew the guy was doing great work. But the best thing about it was Bernbach—he truly understood what a great idea was, and he could sell that idea to a client. I have to say, there was a kind of arrogance that developed at DBB because they knew how good they were, and there was a lot of competitiveness. But there wasn't one day that I didn't love it there.

ANY MEMORIES OF THE VOLKSWAGEN CAMPAIGN "THINK SMALL."?

I remember that when we came back from visiting Germany, [DDB copywriter] Julian Koenig was going crazy. He had this headline, "Think small.," but he told me Helmut [Krone] didn't want to do a layout for it. Meanwhile Bernbach had some other idea; he was trying to get Helmut to do a close-up of a wheel with a reflection of a family in it—which would have been just terrible. And that went on for a week, and then finally Helmut did a "Think small." layout. And the advertising came out and everyone went crazy.

HOW DID YOU GO FROM DESIGNING ADS TO *ESQUIRE* COVERS, AND HOW WAS THAT DIFFERENT?

I was running my agency PKL, and the publicity we got back then was unbelievable. I got a call one day from [*Esquire* editor] Harold Hayes, asking me to help with covers. I did one cover on a weekend, it was a hit, and I did another. And I did that for the next ten years, on weekends, while running my ad agency. It was a different process, because when I do advertising, I always think in words, like "I want my MTV." What I want is a mnemonic slogan, a great copy line, that is impossible to ignore—and then I marry that with a great visual. With the *Esquire* covers the thinking was all visual—you just have a theme, like avant-garde in pop art, and the visual idea of Warhol in the soup can comes out of that.

SOME PEOPLE MIGHT BE WILLING TO CONSIDER THOSE MAGAZINE COVERS ART, BUT PERHAPS NOT YOUR ADS. WHY IS THAT?

Oh, yes, that's true. In fact, I was at a memorial service for the designer Saul Bass and I met Steven Spielberg and Martin Scorsese, who were big fans of the old *Esquire* covers. They asked what I've been doing since then, and I told them I'm an advertising man. And I could see they thought, "Advertising?" Like I sold out or something.

When I wrote a book years ago and called it *The Art of Advertising,* a lot of art directors were really disturbed that I would use that word. And I said, "F—- you, I'm an artist; I don't care what you think you are." The major thing in advertising is that it's got be cause and effect; the idea must work on people. But I do it my way, and I try to make it bright, inventive, surprising

thinking, and do it in a way that architecturally looks the way I want it to look. To me, that's an art. Maybe it's not art with a capital *A*, but it's some kind of art.

WHAT HAS SURVIVED FROM THE CREATIVE REVOLUTION, AND WHAT HAS BEEN LOST?

It's all been lost. With the influx of communications schools, everybody in America has been through marketing courses that teach advertising as a science, not an art—that you can construct an ad in a scientific way and test it to make sure it works. And if you try to tell these people advertising is an art, they look at you askance. So we've lost the great clients who instinctively reacted to things as human beings.

Also, now it's considered uncool to do advertising to younger people that actually sells. Because they know so much about marketing, and know you're trying to sell them, so advertisers now think, "We better not ask them for the sale." What you get is hip, ambiguous advertising. Witness all this dot-com crap—95 percent of it, you don't understand what the company even does. If you actually try to sell something, a dot-com client will say to you, "No, young people don't want to be sold to." Are you kidding me? A great idea is a great idea. And people do want to be sold to. Great advertising in and of itself becomes a benefit of the product. You have to use ideas and imagery to bring a vitality to a brand, an attitude that makes people fall in love with the product because they love the advertising. And you must do that unabashedly.

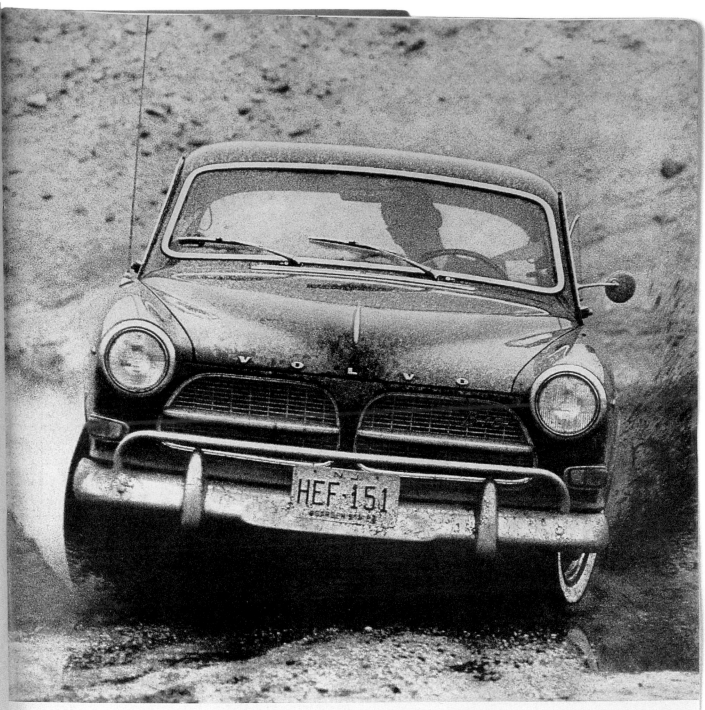

Drive it like you hate it.

When Volvo came to the U. S. from Sweden in 1956, Chevy was the "hot one," Ford was the "safe one" and Volkswagen was just catching on as the "funny one."

We'd like to say that Volvo immediately caught on as the "tough one." It didn't.

At first only the "car nuts" bought it. They figured that if a Volvo could hold up under Swedish driving (no highway speed limits), survive Swedish roads (80% unpaved), withstand Swedish winters (30° below), that a Volvo would hold up under anything.

They figured right. Volvos were driven right off showroom floors onto race tracks where they proceeded to win more races than any other compact ever made.

Volvos are still winning races. But that isn't why they're bought today. Volvos are now being used and misused as family cars. They're safe. And on the highway they run away from other popular-priced compacts in every speed range, yet get over 25 miles to the gallon like the little economy cars.

Volvo is now called the "tough one." And it's the biggest-selling imported compact in America today.

You can drive a Volvo like you hate it for as little as $2330.* Cheaper than psychiatry.

*Mfr's suggested retail price East Coast POE. Gulf and West Coast POE slightly higher. Overseas delivery available. See the Yellow Pages for the Volvo dealer nearest you.

R5

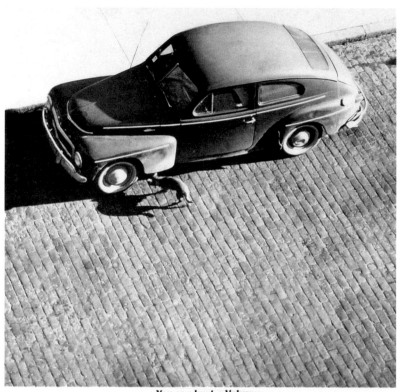

You can hurt a Volvo,
but you can't hurt it much.

This Volvo was bought new in Ann Arbor, Michigan, in 1956. Its owner paid $2345 for it, complete. He has raced it, pulled a camping trailer halfway across the country with it, his kids climb all over it, and it's seldom under cover. It has 80,261 miles on it. The head has never been off, the brakes have never been relined, the original tires lasted 55,000 miles, the clutch hasn't been touched, the valves have never been adjusted (much less ground), and it will still top 95 mph. Total cost of repairs exclusive of normal maintenance: One hood latch, $4.50. One suspension rod, $40.00. Not all Volvos will do this. But Volvos have a pretty good average. One enthusiastic owner in Wyoming wrote us that he has driven his Volvo over 300,000 miles without major repair. We think he's exaggerating. It's probably closer to 200,000 miles.

Volvo 122s compact. Like the Volvo above, it runs away from other popular-priced compacts in every speed range, gets over 25 miles to the gallon like the little economy imports, is virtually indestructible.

20

19. AND 20. **VOLVO**
CARL ALLY INC., NEW YORK,
MID-1960s
Ally became Bernbach's rival,
and his Volvo campaign
challenged VW. According to
Ally's ads, the little German car
might be smart and cute, but the
Swedish car was a lot tougher.

PLAYBOY.

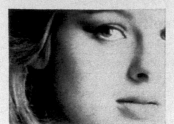

Rome P. 54

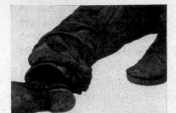

Red Line P. 38

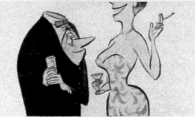

Party P. 46

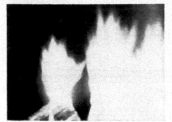

Outer Space P. 80

CONTENTS FOR THE MEN'S ENTERTAINMENT MAGAZINE

HUGH M. HEFNER *editor and publisher*

A. C. SPECTORSKY *associate publisher and editorial director*

ARTHUR PAUL *art director*

JACK J. KESSIE *managing editor*   VINCENT T. TAJIRI *picture editor*

FRANK DE BLOIS, JEREMY DOLE, MURRAY FISHER, TOM LOWNES, SHELDON WAX *associate editors;* ROBERT L. GREEN *fashion director;* DAVID TAYLOR *associate fashion editor;* THOMAS MARIO *food & drink editor;* PATRICK CHASE *travel editor;* J. PAUL GETTY *consulting editor, business and finance;* CHARLES BEAUMONT, RICHARD GEHMAN, WALTER GOODMAN, PAUL KRASSNER, KEN W. PURDY *contributing editors;* ARLENE BOURAS *copy editor;* RAY WILLIAMS *editorial assistant;* BEV CHAMBERLAIN *associate picture editor;* DON BRONSTEIN, MARIO CASILLI, POMPEO POSAR, JERRY YULSMAN *staff photographers;* REID AUSTIN *associate art director;* PHILIP KAPLAN, JOSEPH H. PACZEK *assistant art directors;* WALTER KRADENYCH, ELLEN PACZEK *art assistants;* JOHN MASTRO *production manager;* FERN HEARTEL *assistant production manager* • HOWARD W. LEDERER *advertising director;* JULES KASE *eastern advertising manager;* JOSEPH FALL *midwestern advertising manager;* VICTOR LOWNES III *promotion director;* NELSON FUTCH *promotion manager;* DAN CZUBAK *promotion art director;* HELMUT LORSCH *publicity manager;* BENNY DUNN *public relations manager;* ANSON MOUNT *college bureau;* THEO FREDERICK *personnel director;* JANET PILGRIM *reader service;* WALTER J. HOWARTH *subscription fulfillment manager;* ELDON SELLERS *special projects;* ROBERT S. PREUSS *business manager and circulation director.*

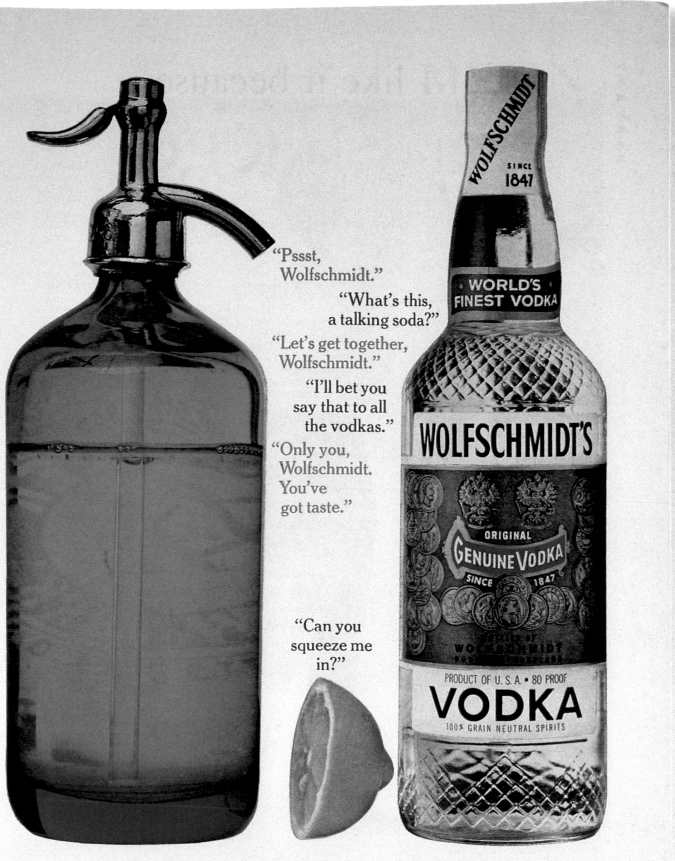

"Pssst, Wolfschmidt."

"What's this, a talking soda?"

"Let's get together, Wolfschmidt."

"I'll bet you say that to all the vodkas."

"Only you, Wolfschmidt. You've got taste."

"Can you squeeze me in?"

Pssst: Want to try something delicious this summer?

Try the Wolfschmidt Pssst! (Wolfschmidt vodka, soda, ice and lemon squeezed in.) Soda has never tasted this good before. Wolfschmidt makes it possible. It has the touch of taste that marks genuine old world vodka. More?
GENERAL WINE AND SPIRITS COMPANY, NEW YORK 22, N.Y., MADE FROM GRAIN, 80 OR 100 PROOF. PRODUCT OF U.S.A.

21. **WOLFSCHMIDT VODKA**
PAPERT KOENIG LOIS,
NEW YORK, 1962
In the early 1960s, the sassy art director George Lois believed ads should have an attitude; this series featured sexy banter between vodka and mixers— perfect for placement in a "men's entertainment magazine."

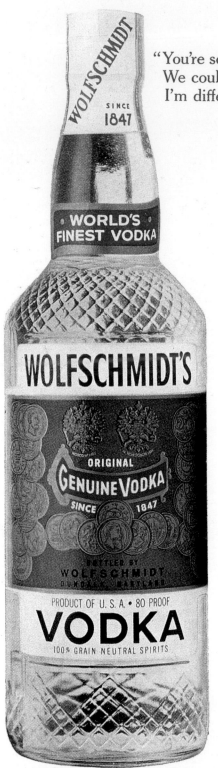

"You're some tomato.
We could make beautiful Bloody Marys together.
I'm different from those other fellows."

"I like you, Wolfschmidt.
You've got taste."

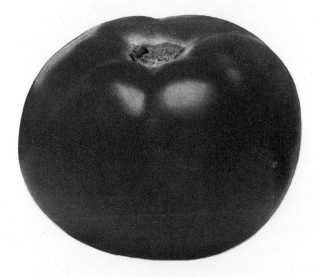

Wolfschmidt Vodka has the touch of taste that marks genuine old world vodka. Wolfschmidt in a Bloody Mary is a tomato in triumph.Wolfschmidt brings out the best in every drink. General Wine and Spirits Company, N.Y. 22. Made from Grain, 80 or 100 Proof. Prod. of U.S.A.

22

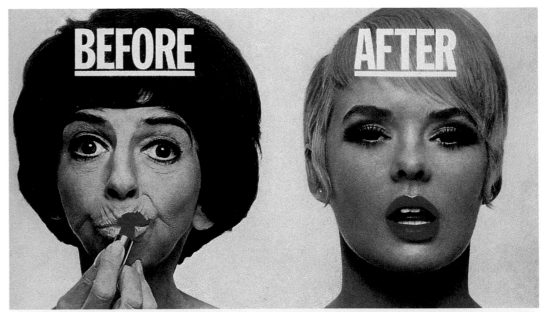

A Coty Cremestick turned Alice Pearce...into Joey Heatherton.

And you thought lipsticks weren't important, eh?
Another Cremestick trick: they're moisturizing,
but they're never greasy.
And zip! They're on in a stroke.
Ask Alice Pearce.

Some luscious Cremestick colors:

23

22. WOLFSCHMIDT VODKA
PAPERT KOENIG LOIS,
NEW YORK, 1962
Another in the classic series of
George Lois ads in which the
vodka and a potential companion
engage in cocktail-party
seduction.

23. COTY CREMESTICK
PAPERT KOENIG LOIS,
NEW YORK, LATE 1960s
Mocking the conventional
"before and after" approach to
cosmetics advertising, PKL
transformed an ordinary woman
into actress Joey Heatherton,
one of the original Golddiggers
on the "Dean Martin Show."

the Creative Revolution. Marty Cooke, now a creative director with M&C Saatchi and a veteran of DDB, says the agencies PKL and Ally "were the Rolling Stones to DDB's Beatles . . . they were more aggressive, more cynical." That was perhaps a reflection of the personalities involved in these two spin-off agencies: Lois was known almost as much for his New York tough-guy manner as for his designer's eye; he referred to his advertising as "poison gas" and remarked that his mission was to "spray it and watch people fall." Once, when faced with a resistant client, Lois threw open the window in a skyscraper office and threatened to jump out if the client didn't approve his campaign. Carl Ally was just as volatile: A former fighter pilot, he lived by the slogan, posted in his office, "Comfort the afflicted, afflict the comfortable."

That toughness was evident in the ads created by both agencies, including PKL's saucy, sexy ads for Wolfschmidt vodka, in which the randy bottle propositioned tomatoes and oranges. (Lois would

also become famous for creating the line "I want my Maypo," which, a couple of decades later, he recycled for a new client, as "I want my MTV.") Ally, meanwhile, shot back at Bernbach on behalf of Hertz ("No. 2 says he tries harder. Than who?"). And like DDB, Ally sang the virtues of a small foreign car, the Volvo—but Ally made the little car seem not so much smart and cute as just plain tough. "Drive it like you hate it" was one Ally headline.

One of the key writers in Ally's stable was a former juvenile delinquent from Chicago named Ed McCabe, who'd worked his way up from a mailroom job and who wore bandages on his arms to conceal his tattoos. After writing a number of stellar campaigns for Ally, McCabe struck out on his own, starting Scali McCabe Sloves—where he continued to create groundbreaking ad campaigns for Perdue chicken (he introduced one of the least photogenic ad spokesmen ever seen in Frank Perdue, and turned him into a major celebrity),

Hebrew National ("We answer to a higher authority"), and Maxell tape. McCabe epitomized the Young Turk of advertising's creative world: He brought a Hemingwayesque quality to ad copywriting, punching out staccato copy that often seemed like an outright challenge ("My chickens eat better than you do," one Perdue ad barked). Appropriately, McCabe lived fast and hard, venturing out to bars to work on ad campaigns—and sometimes not returning for weeks. A typical tale had him walking down the street talking to a Ford executive when he noticed a beautiful woman in a car stopped at a traffic light; he draped himself on the hood of the car as the shocked client watched. "My attitude," he later explained to a journalist, "was that I could wait for Ford."

The macho culture that dominated the New York–based Creative Revolution would set the tone in advertising for years to come. Even thirty-odd years later, as the new millennium arrived, creative advertising remained primarily a man's world;

NO OTHER AUDIO TAPE DE

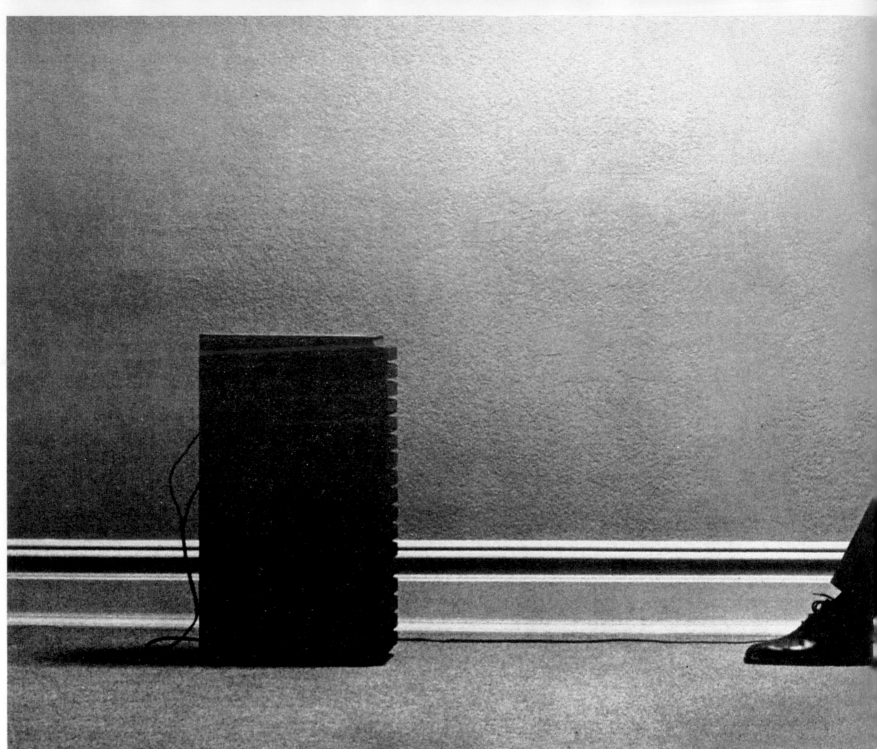

IVERS HIGHER FIDELITY.

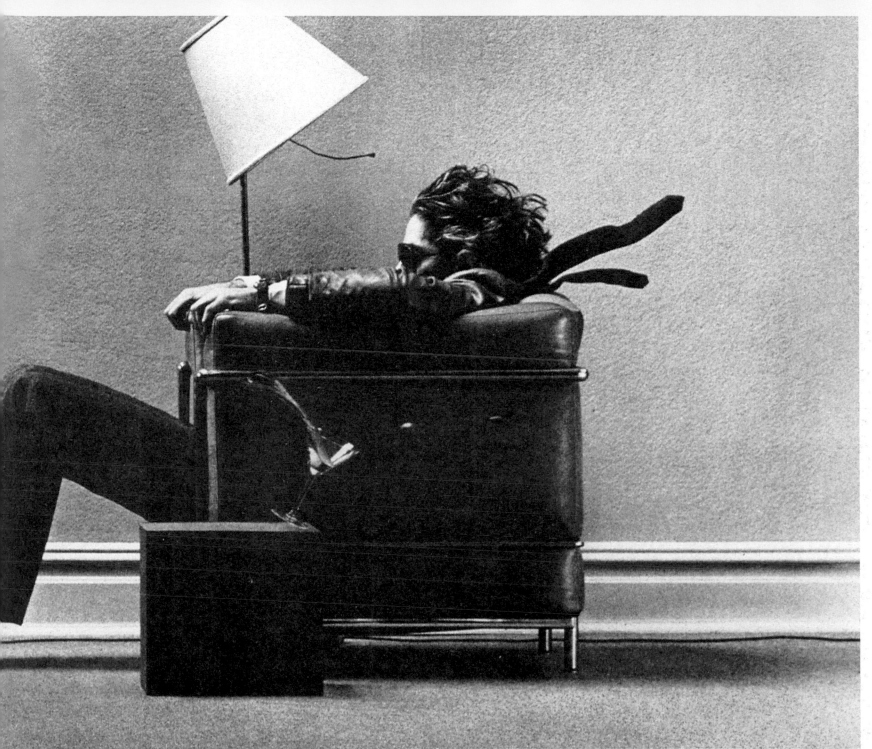

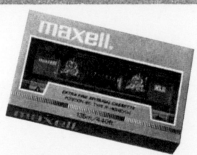

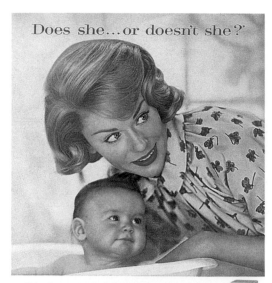

Does she...or doesn't she?

Hair color so natural only her hairdresser knows for sure!

MISS CLAIROL® HAIR COLOR BATH!

29

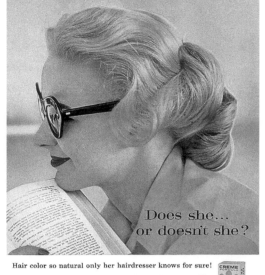

Does she... or doesn't she?

Hair color so natural only her hairdresser knows for sure!

MISS CLAIROL® HAIR COLOR BATH!

30

28. (PREVIOUS SPREAD)
MAXELL
SCALI McCABE SLOVES,
NEW YORK, 1979
Despite the headline and copy,
this image said all there was to
know about Maxell cassette
tape's powerful sound. The
poster was found on college
dormitory walls around the U.S.
in the 1980s.

29 AND 30. **MISS CLAIROL
HAIR COLOR**
FOOTE CONE & BELDING,
NEW YORK, 1961
Copywriter Shirley Polykoff
posed an intriguing question in
a groundbreaking campaign that
launched in the late 1950s.
Some ads in the series balanced
the sexually suggestive headline
with wholesome imagery.

31. **HORN & HARDART**
SCALI McCABE SLOVES,
NEW YORK, 1970s
This ad for an Automat-style
restaurant chain featured
another tough, uncompromising
headline from Ed McCabe,
whose ads tried to cut through
the often misleading boasts of
advertising.

today, the vast majority of the industry's best-known creative directors, both in the U.S. and around the world, are men. Part of the reason for that may be attributable to the tone and style of advertising that was forged in the 1960s—rooted in aggressive, cocky, blunt, in-your-face humor. "If you looked at the work we produced," Lois says, "it was usually obvious from the attitude that a man had written it." The copywriters who broke through in the 1960s "were the guys who grew up on street corners in New York, cracking jokes and making everyone laugh," says Grace. As these hardscrabble entrepreneurs opened their agencies and began to chase new accounts, there was a spirit of fraternalism, of going off to war together, that undoubtedly led to discrimination (unconscious or otherwise) against women. Then, too, ad managers on the client side were usually men—and the agency executives believed that many of these male clients would tend to feel more comfortable entrusting the stewardship of their

brands to other men. On the other hand, Lois says, many women opted not to enlist in this particularly grueling war. "It was brutal; you had to work fourteen-hour days to make it in advertising then," he says. "A lot of women didn't want to give up their lives to it."

But a few women did, and they left their mark. Robinson, the pioneering copywriter at DDB who worked on Levy's, Ohrbach's, Polaroid, and other classic campaigns, was one of them. Another was Shirley Polykoff, a copywriter at Foote, Cone & Belding who sent Clairol hair-coloring sales through the roof with the line "Does she or doesn't she?," which suggested that women could reinvent themselves without apology, and without anyone else even knowing for sure. But the single most successful woman from that period—and perhaps to this day in advertising—was Mary Wells, who initially became a star at DDB and then went on to launch her own agency, Wells Rich Greene. Wells proved that her advertising

could be as mischievous as that of any of the men; with a Benson & Hedges campaign that focused on the disadvantages of B&H's longer cigarettes, she poked fun at her own product. For Alka-Seltzer, Wells introduced the memorable line "I can't believe I ate the whole thing." And she brought a sense of playful stylishness to companies like Braniff Airlines—which, under her guidance, painted its planes in bright colors and announced "the end of the plain plane."

Though their styles and approaches differed, the leaders of the American creative scene of the 1960s had certain common attributes. All were inveterate rule-breakers—in fact, that was perhaps the defining characteristic of all of them, and it separated them from creative predecessors like Ogilvy and Leo Burnett. Burnett had exerted a profound influence on advertising and on American culture with his agency's creation of advertising icons like the Marlboro Man, the Jolly Green Giant, and Tony the Tiger, but the reliance

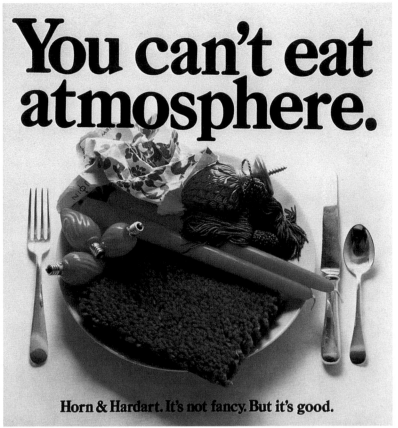

You can't eat atmosphere.

Horn & Hardart. It's not fancy. But it's good.

31

on such icons became, in itself, a formula that was followed faithfully by Burnett. Similarly, Ogilvy created brilliant soft-sell ads for clients like Rolls-Royce—one of his most memorable headlines was "At 60 miles an hour the loudest noise in this new Rolls-Royce comes from the electric clock"—but he, too, insisted that sensible ads must adhere to certain basic principles and guidelines; in fact, Ogilvy set down those rules in his best-selling handbooks on advertising. But the likes of Bernbach, Lois, Ally, McCabe, and Wells, along with a West Coast insurrectionist named Howard Gossage, had no use for such formulas. To some extent, they were products of their time: The author Thomas Frank has noted that the writers and artists driving the Creative Revolution were truly part of the 1960s spirit of the counterculture; they may have worked within the "establishment" of Madison Avenue, but they were also trying their best to overthrow that old bureaucracy and its conservative ways.

Moreover, the new advertisers—unlike many of their predecessors—had come into advertising not just to build a successful business but to make a statement. Whether or not they fancied themselves artists (some did, most didn't), they all wanted to have an impact on the culture, and all wanted to be respected for their creative abilities in the same way that, say, filmmakers were. According to McCabe, "We wanted to be able to tell our family and friends that we were in advertising and, when we told them [which ads] we were doing, watch the disdain on their faces melt into something almost like admiration."

Eventually, they succeeded. As the public gained a new appreciation of advertising, "the cocktail circuit buzz found television commercials, for the first time, more compelling than the programs," observed one publication, and advertising's creative stars "were favored guests of talk show hosts . . . and their entrances at the rococo photographers' parties of the 1960s set off

a stir the way hot young fashion designers do in trendy nightclubs today."

What grew out of this period was a cult of creativity in advertising, which became the magnet that would continue to draw young writers and artists to the business in years ahead—not just in America but around the world. The DDB revolution was, indeed, televised, and everyone was watching. One of the first places it migrated to was London, which, in the early 1960s, caught the Bernbach fever. Tim Delaney, now one of the UK's best-known creative directors, was a teenager when he first saw DDB's ads, at a gallery show in London; he became a fan for life. "The DDB approach to advertising particularly resonated in the UK for several reasons," says Delaney. "We were weaned on the BBC, which taught us to respect visual imagery, and we also had a very strong writing ethos in our national newspapers. And so we were nurtured with a certain appreciation for pictures and words, and when we saw

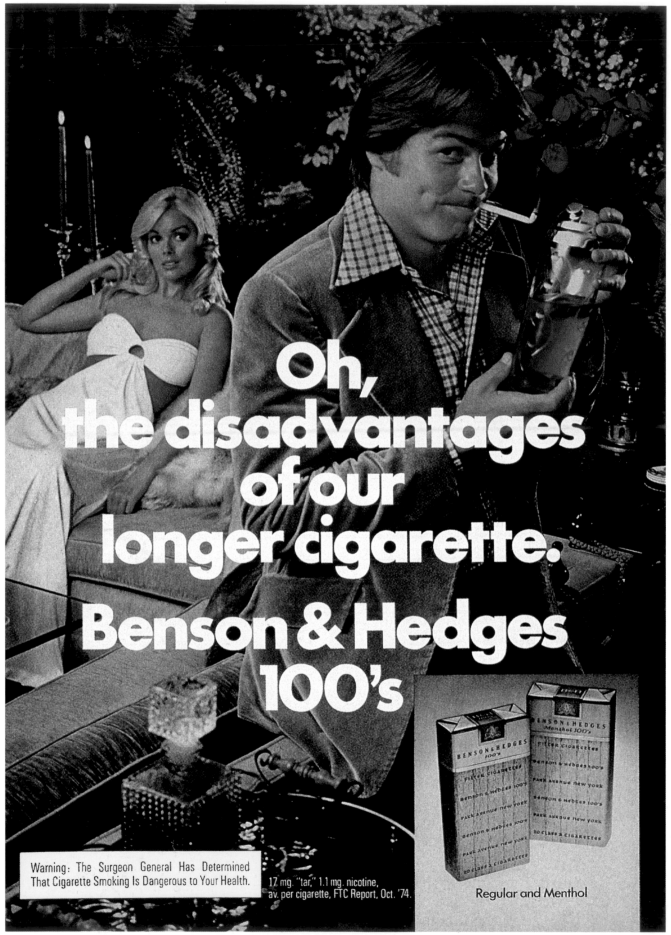

Oh, the disadvantages of our longer cigarette. Benson & Hedges 100's

Warning: The Surgeon General Has Determined That Cigarette Smoking Is Dangerous to Your Health.

17 mg. "tar," 1.1 mg. nicotine, av. per cigarette, FTC Report, Oct. '74.

Regular and Menthol

32

32. AND 33.
BENSON & HEDGES
WELLS, RICH, GREENE,
NEW YORK, 1968–75
The agency headed by Mary
Wells took a page out of
DDB's book by playing up
"the disadvantages" of
B&H's longer cigarettes.

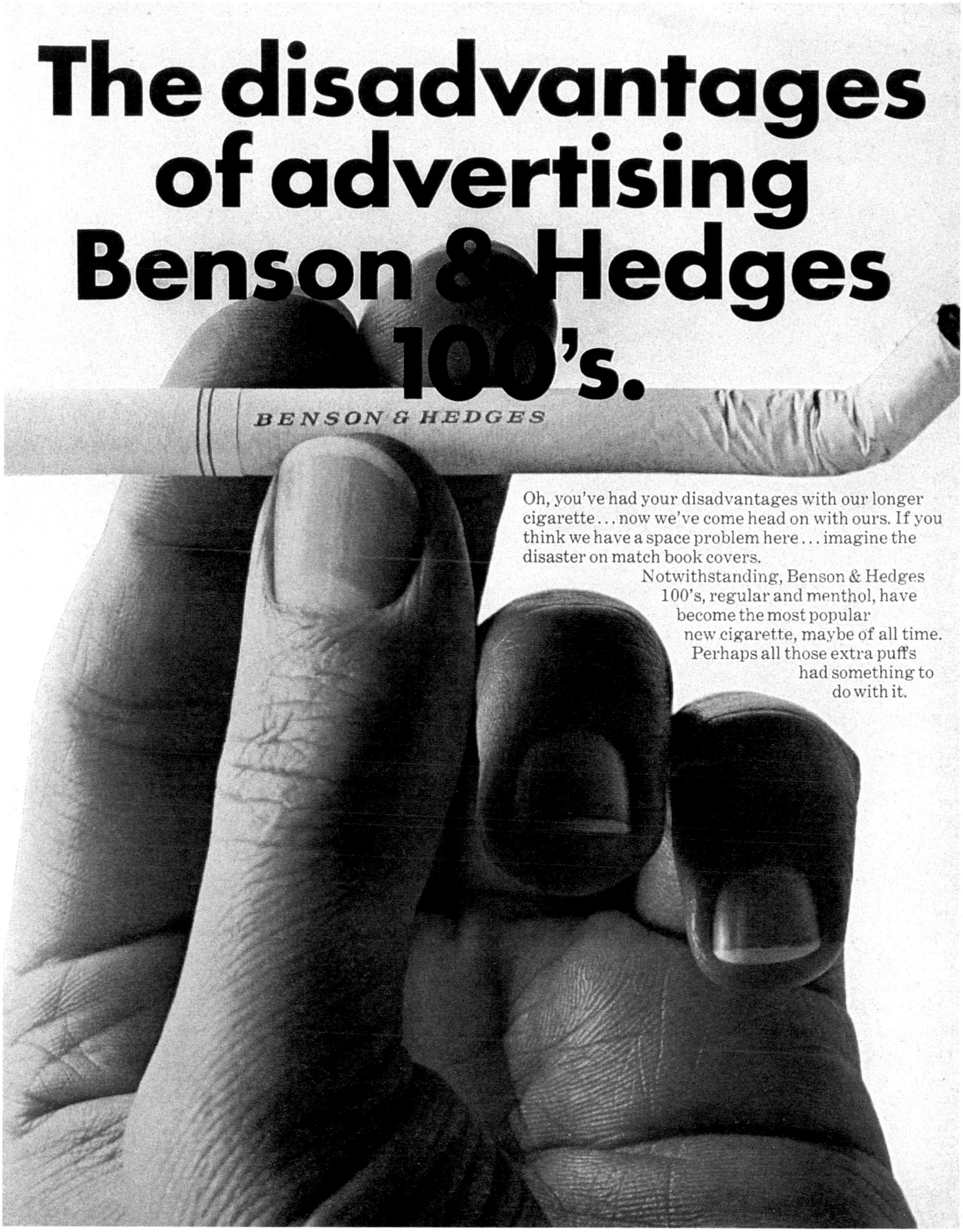

The disadvantages of advertising Benson & Hedges 100's.

Oh, you've had your disadvantages with our longer cigarette...now we've come head on with ours. If you think we have a space problem here...imagine the disaster on match book covers.

Notwithstanding, Benson & Hedges 100's, regular and menthol, have become the most popular new cigarette, maybe of all time. Perhaps all those extra puffs had something to do with it.

BENSON & HEDGES

33

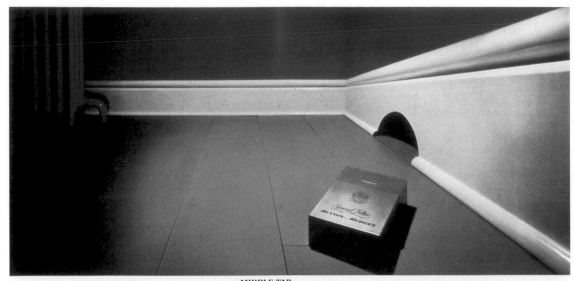

MIDDLE TAR As defined by H.M. Government
H.M. Government Health Departments' WARNING: CIGARETTES CAN SERIOUSLY DAMAGE YOUR HEALTH

34

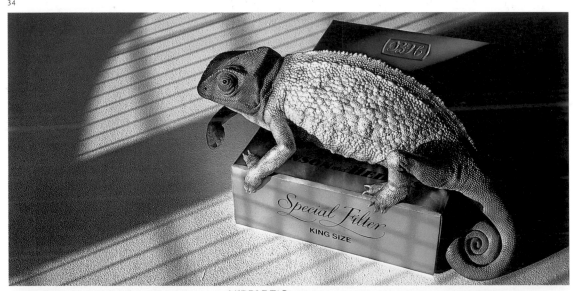

MIDDLE TAR As defined by H.M. Government
DANGER: H.M. Government Health Departments' WARNING: THINK ABOUT THE HEALTH RISKS BEFORE SMOKING

35

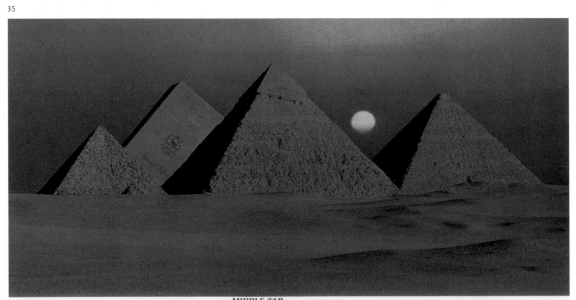

MIDDLE TAR As defined by H.M. Government
H.M. Government Health Departments' WARNING: CIGARETTES CAN SERIOUSLY DAMAGE YOUR HEALTH

36

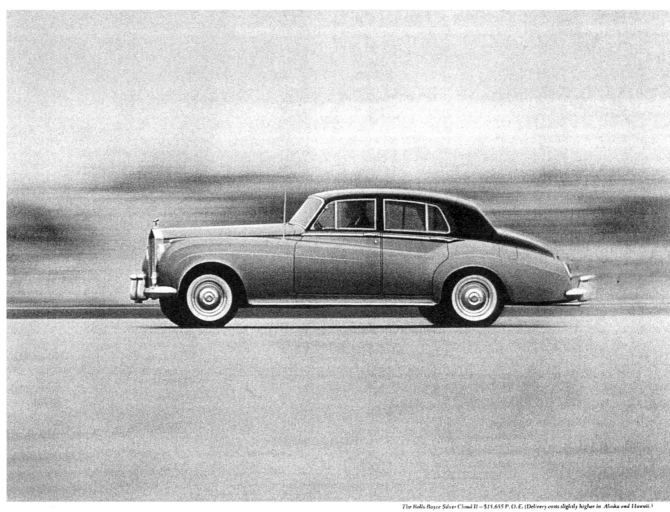

The Rolls-Royce Silver Cloud II — $15,655 P.O.E. (Delivery costs slightly higher in Alaska and Hawaii.)

"At 60 miles an hour the loudest noise in this new Rolls-Royce comes from the electric clock"

What __makes__ Rolls-Royce the best car in the world? "There is really no magic about it—it is merely patient attention to detail," says an eminent Rolls-Royce engineer.

1. "At 60 miles an hour the loudest noise comes from the electric clock," reports the Technical Editor of THE MOTOR. The silence inside the car is uncanny. Three exhaust mufflers tune out sound frequencies—acoustically.

2. Every Rolls-Royce engine is run for four hours at full throttle before installation, and each car is extensively test-driven over varying road surfaces. Every Rolls-Royce has its "History Book"—an eleven-page signed record of all operations and inspections performed on the car. This goes into the Company's permanent files.

3. The Rolls-Royce Silver Cloud II is designed as an *owner-driven* car. It has power steering, power brakes and automatic gear-shift. It is very easy to drive and to park. Women handle the car with ease.

4. The finished car spends a week in the final test-shop, being fine-tuned. Here it is subjected to ninety-eight separate ordeals. For example, the engineers use a stethoscope to listen for axle-whine. Silent operation of *every* part is the standard for acceptance.

5. The new eight-cylinder aluminium engine is even more powerful than the previous six-cylinder unit, yet it weighs *ten pounds less.* It accelerates from zero to 60 miles an hour in 11.4 seconds. (ROAD AND TRACK test report.)

6. The coachwork is given as many as *nine coats of* finishing paint—*hand rubbed.*

7. Every Rolls-Royce takes the "Monsoon Test." Windows are rolled up and the car is pelted with water and air at gale force. *Not a drop may come through.*

8. By moving a switch on the steering column, you can adjust the shock-absorbers to suit road conditions. (The lack of fatigue in driving this car is remarkable.)

9. Another switch defrosts the rear window, by heating a network of 1360 almost invisible wires in the glass.

10. The seats are upholstered with eight hides of English leather—enough to make 128 pairs of soft shoes.

11. A picnic table, fashioned of inlaid French walnut, slides out from under the dash. Two more swing out behind the front seats.

12. The engine cooling fan is *lopsided.* Its five blades are unequally spaced and pitched to take thick and thin slices of air. Thus it does its work in a *whisper.* The company goes to fantastic lengths to ensure peace and quiet for the occupants of the car.

13. There are *three* independent brake linkages. The Rolls-Royce is a very *safe* car—and also a very responsive and *lively* car. It cruises serenely at eighty-five. Top speed is in excess of 100 m.p.h.

14. The gas tank cannot be opened without the driver's consent: you unlock it electrically from a button on the dash.

15. Automatic transmission, power brakes and power steering are *standard.* So are the radio, heating and ventilating equipment, walnut panelling, seats adjustable for tilt and rake, and white sidewall tires. The Rolls-Royce people do not designate essential equipment as "optional extras."

16. The Bentley is made by Rolls-Royce. Except for the radiator shells, they are identical motor cars, manufactured by the same engineers in the same works.

The Bentley costs $300 less, because its radiator is simpler to make. People who feel diffident about driving a Rolls-Royce can buy a Bentley.

ROLLS-ROYCE AND BENTLEY

PRICE. The car shown above costs $15,655 P.O.E. Delivery costs slightly higher in Alaska and Hawaii.

If you would like to try driving a Rolls-Royce or Bentley, write or telephone any dealer listed below. For further information or complete list of U. S. dealers, write Mr. Richard L. Yorke, Vice President, Rolls-Royce Inc., Room 405, 45 Rockefeller Plaza, New York, N. Y.

NEW YORK, N. Y. J. S. INSKIP, INC.—DISTRIBUTOR	Detroit (Ferndale), Mich.	Falvey Motor Sales Company	Miami, Fla.	Waco International Salon
Atlanta, Ga. — Import Motors Ltd., Inc.	Greenville, S. C. — Judson T. Minyard, Inc.	Milwaukee (Thiensville), Wisc. — Milrace Motors Ltd.	St. Louis, Mo. — Gruet Motor Car Company
Baltimore, Md. — General Pontiac Corporation	Hartford, Conn. — Russ Seeli, Inc.	Nashville, Tenn. — E. Gray Smith	St. Paul, Minn. — Schneider Motors Co.
Boston, Mass. — Foreign Motors, Inc.	Indianapolis, Ind. — Messrs. Schaler-Waters	Pittsburgh, Penna. — Motorfair — Rolls-Royce — Pittsburgh	Schenectady, N. Y. — Van Curler Motor Co., Inc.
Bryn Mawr, Penna. — Warrington Motors Imports, Inc.	Kutztown, Penna. — Nick Ciliberti Pontiac	Providence, R. I. — J. S. Inskip, Inc.	Washington, D. C. — Flood Pontiac Company
Chicago (Wilmette), Ill. — Imperial Motors, Inc.	Louisville, Ky. — Koster-Swope Imports	Richmond, Va. — Mooers Motor Car Co.	West Palm Beach, Fla. — Taylor Imported Motors
Cincinnati, O. — Charles Raymond, Inc.	Memphis, Tenn. — Pryor Oldsmobile Company	Shaker Heights, O. — Salter Automotive Imports, Inc.	Wilkes-Barre, Penna. — Lewis Wolfe, Inc.

37

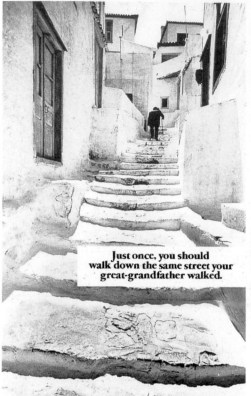

All of us come from someplace else.

Just once, you should walk down the same street your great-grandfather walked.

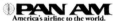

Picture this if you will.

A man who's spent all his life in the United States gets on a plane, crosses a great ocean, lands.

He walks the same streets his family walked centuries ago.

He sees his name, which is rare in America, filling three pages in a phone book.

He speaks haltingly the language he wishes he had learned better as a child.

As America's airline to the world, Pan Am does a lot of things.

We help business travelers make meetings on the other side of the world. Our planes take goods to and from six continents. We take vacationers just about anywhere they want to go.

But nothing we do seems to have as much meaning as when we help somebody discover the second heritage that every American has.

PAN AM.
America's airline to the world.

See your travel agent.

38

the work of DDB, something clicked. Particularly among a whole generation of working-class lads who gravitated toward advertising in the 1960s. They found that they could create street-smart, savvy ads just like Bill Bernbach." The British agency that emerged as the leader of the local movement, Collett Dickenson Pearce, had been greatly inspired by DDB, and hired a number of DDB's "missionaries" in England. CDP's ads for Hovis, Birds Eye, Heineken, Benson & Hedges, and Fiat Strada had all the freshness and originality of DDB's work, with perhaps even more distinctive style. And the agency didn't need to import much talent, because it was busy developing plenty of its own—including Charles Saatchi, who would go on to form the agency that bore his name, as well as the young commercial-makers Ridley Scott and Alan Parker, who eventually made their mark in the film world. In subsequent years, Delaney's own agency, Leagas Delaney, would, along with shops like Bartle Bogle Hegarty

and Abbott Mead Vickers, carry the creative flame forward in the 1980s as England became a new creative mecca. Gradually, the Creative Revolution began to spread to other parts of the world, including Australia, where agencies like Campaign Palace, with British expatriate Lionel Hunt at the creative helm, produced ads that bore the unmistakable stamp of DDB—the same look, the same wit, the same cheeky attitude. Eventually, the DDB influence even made its way to Asia, transported by expatriates from America, the UK, or Australia. One could walk into a creative agency in Singapore, says local ad man and author Jim Aitchison, and find people studying Bernbach.

Interestingly, while the fever was spreading around the world, it was beginning to subside in America. As the business recession of the 1970s squeezed advertising, and caused clients to tighten budgets and demand immediate results from the ads they did run, Mary Wells sounded what some would consider to be the death knell

for the Creative Revolution: "Hard times demand hard selling," she declared. What followed in the late 1970s and early 1980s was a period in which much of American advertising (with exceptions, of course) seemed to regress to formula and conservatism. And the mid-1980s brought a wave of mergermania to the ad industry that didn't help matters; by the late 1980s, there were few dynamic and independent creative agencies operating on Madison Avenue. Many agencies, including DDB itself, were swallowed by international conglomerates, and creativity was usually not the top priority in these business arrangements which tended to favor a more research- driven, risk-averse approach to advertising.

Still, Bernbach's conceptual, idea-driven approach to advertising couldn't be killed. It simply migrated to smaller regional American markets, where there was still room for experimentation. The rise of regional advertising in

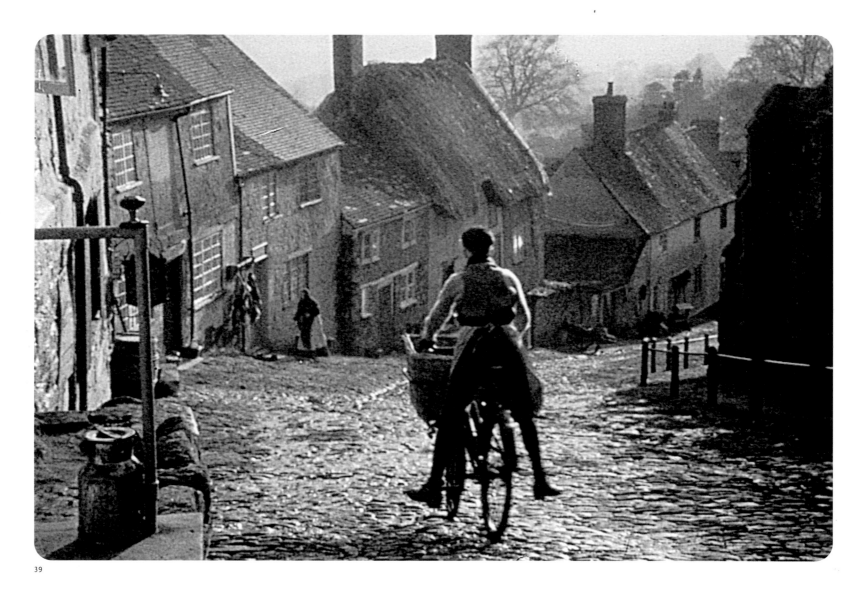

39

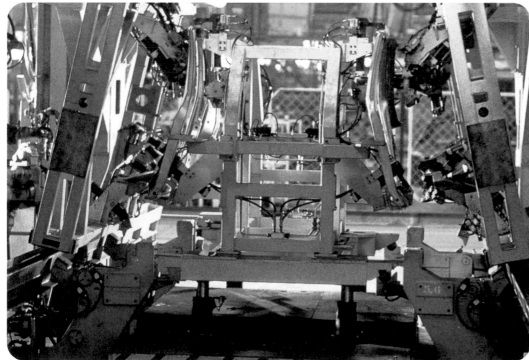

40

WHEN ADS GOT SMART.

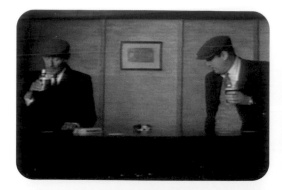

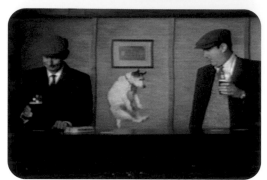

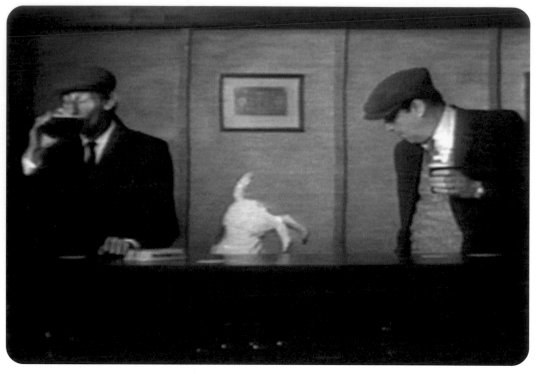

41

41. **JOHN SMITHS
YORKSHIRE BITTER**
BOASE MASSIMI POLLETT,
LONDON, 1982
In this TV commercial, "Two
Tricks," a fiesty dog amuses two
chaps enjoying pints of beer in a
British pub.

42. **ANSETT AIRLINES**
CAMPAIGN PALACE,
MELBOURNE, 1981
Lionel Hunt brought an irreverent
style to ads Down Under; this
one, in particular, caused a stir
when it first appeared.

43. **TALON ZIPPERS**
DELEHANTY KURNIT &
GELLER, NEW YORK,
EARLY 1970s
This long-running series found
endless ways to play off the
open-fly joke and the potential
vulnerabilities caused by an
inferior zipper.

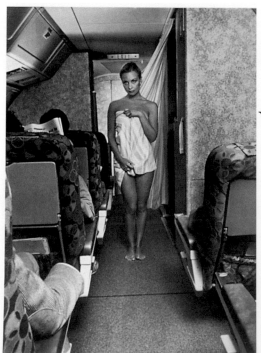

42

If the hostess was out of uniform would you know which airline you were flying with?

Until recently probably not.
But from next June you won't be
in any doubt at all.

Ansett will be offering you a real
choice of the planes you fly in, the
times you depart, and the services you
get both in the air and on the ground.

In June we start taking delivery
of our new fleet of 12 Boeing 737's
and new generation 727's and start
pensioning off our DC9's.

This means we'll soon be offering
you Boeing comfort and reliability on
all our jet routes.

Just as important, more planes
will mean far greater frequency. And
no more identical schedules.

You'll be far more likely to find
a departure time that suits you, rather
than one that just suits the airline.

And you'll check-in faster, get on
and off quicker, and get your baggage
sooner.

We'll also be offering major service
benefits that we can't reveal now for
reasons that will be obvious to readers
who are also in a highly competitive
situation. But don't wait until next June
to try the new Ansett. Our competitive
philosophy is showing up right now
in lots of little ways that already make
flying with us just that much better.

But you ain't
seen nothing yet. **ANSETT**

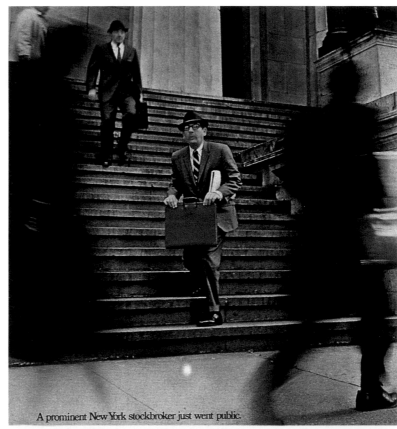

A prominent New York stockbroker just went public.

It's bad enough when the market takes a sudden plunge.

But when your trouser zipper goes down, you lose another kind of security. So for your own good, look for

the Talon Zephyr® nylon zipper next time you buy yourself a suit or a pair of slacks.

The Zephyr zipper is designed not to snag, or jam. And a little device

called Memory Lock® will make sure your zipper stays up.

So all you'll have to worry about going down are your stocks.

43

America was made possible by a number of factors, including the spread of computers, fax machines, and other technology that enabled clients to work with agencies located anywhere. But what really drove the trend was the reluctance of talented writers and art directors from around the country to go to New York—where they knew they would have to toil in large, stifling corporate environments. Seeking a more creative alternative, many began to open their own small local shops, often starting with modest hometown accounts, then building a national reputation via award-winning creative work. In Minneapolis, Minnesota; Richmond, Virginia; Portland, Oregon; and San Francisco, agencies like Fallon McElligott, the Martin Agency, Wieden + Kennedy, and Goodby Silverstein all, to some extent, carried Bernbach's tradition forward to the present. "Bernbach was my Che Guevara," says the copywriter Ernie Schenck, whose Providence, Rhode Island, agency Pagano

Schenck & Kay was one of the small regional agencies leading the late-1980s wave of new creativity. "What we learned from Bernbach," says Schenck, "is that you could create great work by isolating a single, compelling point, and you could give it an emotional resonance by putting visuals and words together in unexpected ways. Conceptual advertising totally reshaped the way we think about advertising, both as creators and consumers." Schenck's sentiments are echoed in places like Amsterdam, where the creative director Johan Kramer of the agency KesselsKramer says, "Bernbach's work understood that consumers are intelligent and recognize manipulation. All his books are here on our tables—we see them as advertising bibles."

Bernbach himself didn't live to see the second coming of the revolution; he passed away in 1982, just as Fallon McElligott was making a name for itself, and as Wieden + Kennedy was opening its doors. At the time of his death, few outside the

ad world grasped the importance of what this advertising man had accomplished, and the dominant effect he'd had on a medium that would come to dominate the culture. *Harper's* magazine was one of the few to observe this at the time, noting in 1983 that Bernbach "probably had a greater impact on American culture than any of the distinguished writers and artists who have appeared in the pages of *Harper's* during the past 133 years." What *Harper's* failed to note was that the impact extended far beyond "American culture"; Bernbach, as would eventually become clear, changed not just America but the world. He helped to forge a style and an attitude that are now part of the ad/cultural vernacular in Bangkok, in Johannesburg, in Warsaw, as well as in Ernie Schenck's Providence. As the following pages demonstrate, it is a way of thinking and communicating that crosses borders and yet needs little or no translation. The advertising concept— Bernbach's baby—is now a universal language.

3. A NEW
LANGUAGE

VISUAL
EMERGES.

When building a mousetrap," the San Francisco adman Howard Gossage once advised, "always leave room for the mouse."

Gossage's point was that when people interact with advertising, as with other forms of communication, they don't necessarily want everything spelled out for them; give them points A and B, but allow them to make the mental leap to C themselves. This is not an easy concept for a salesman to accept; it runs counter to the driving instinct to complete the sale, leaving nothing to chance. (As decreed by the *Über*salesman character in American playwright David Mamet's drama *Glengarry Glen Ross,* the first law of selling is "A-B-C: Always Be Closing.")

Bill Bernbach and other leaders of the 1960s Creative Revolution understood and accepted the "mouse" theory—indeed, they often used a "less is more" approach to selling, keeping ads simple, challenging readers to figure out the point of a headline like "Lemon." However, in many of the

ads from this period, beneath the double-entendre headline and the intriguing photograph, way down at the base of the ad, you invariably found the anchor of logic. Why should car buyers "Think small."? Doyle Dane Bernbach clearly and persuasively articulated the answer to that by citing reasons—sometimes three or four of them— in the copy at the bottom.

Bernbach had sought to tear down the wall between art and copy in advertising and had, to a large extent, succeeded in doing that (in the post-DDB world, as writers and art directors brainstormed to try to find the "big idea" that would captivate hearts and minds, that idea could come from either party, or from both simultaneously). Nevertheless, the advertising produced by Bernbach, Ally, McCabe, and others of that period was still ruled by language and logic. With few exceptions (DDB's Helmut Krone, for example, had understood early on that design could drive the idea), a print ad's art elements—the layout, the photography, the typography—usually served to amplify or clarify the headline, while the body copy closed the sale.

All of this worked fine in the world of yesteryear, when one could reasonably assume that people might read an advertisement from beginning to end, provided it was clever enough. By the 1980s, that was beginning to seem like a quaint notion. The decade that ushered in MTV and computer games seemed to trigger a realization that perhaps the visual aspects of advertising mattered as much as—if not more than—the verbal. If, as the success of the newspaper *USA Today* suggested, people weren't willing to devote much time to reading news stories, why on earth would they spend time reading ads?

Moreover, there was a growing belief in advertising that logic might not be the best tool for persuading people anymore. Some considered this heresy, but it was catching on nonetheless. The classic way of approaching

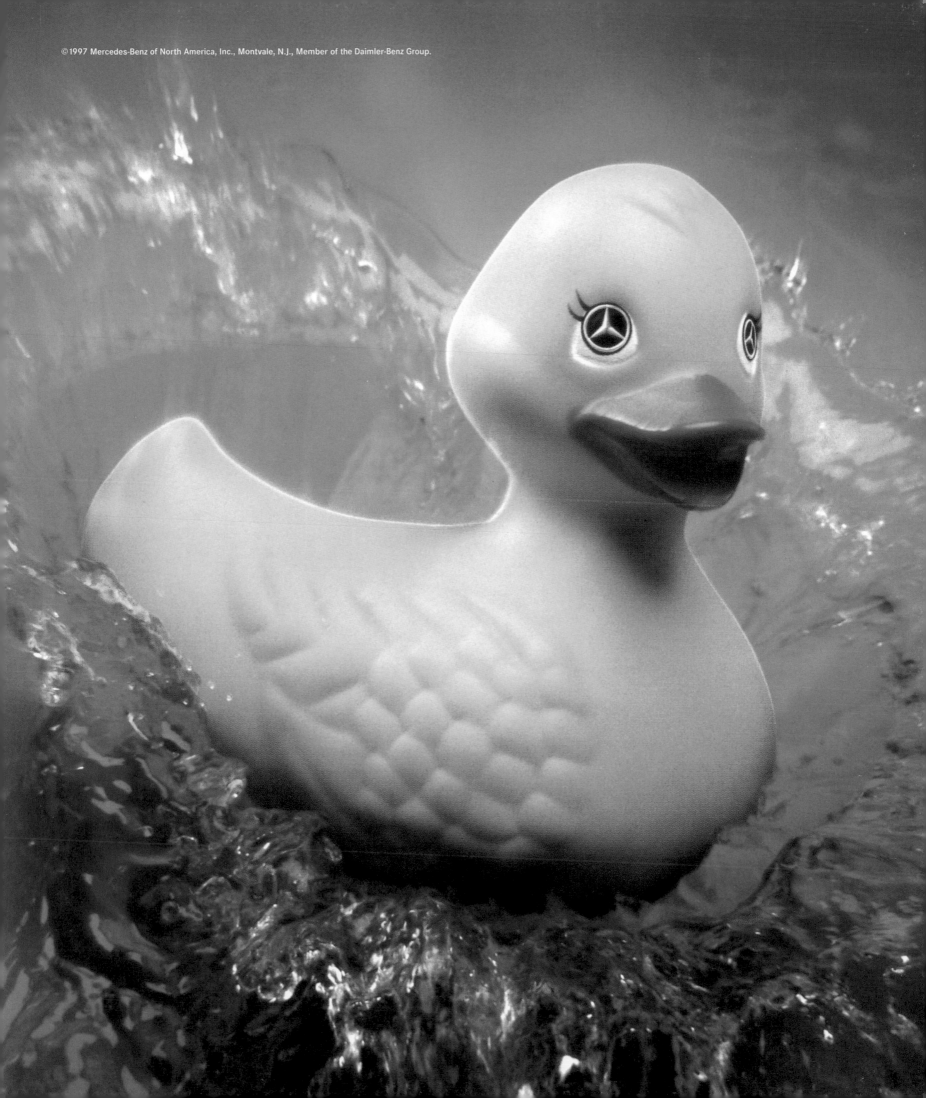

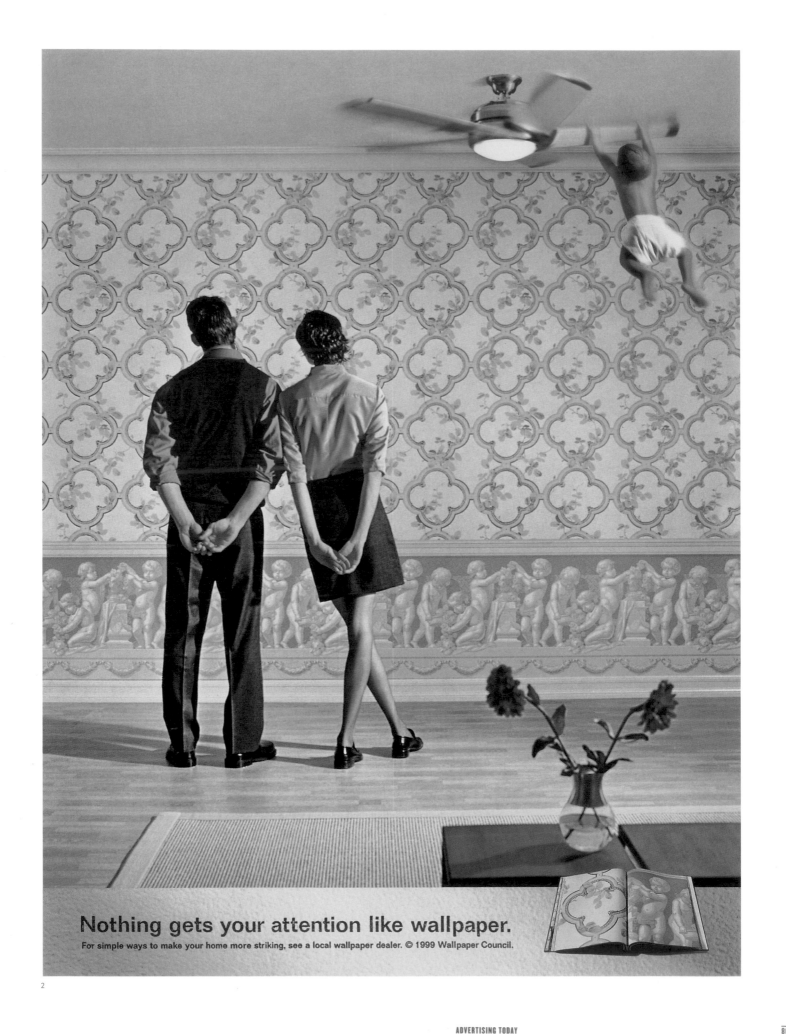

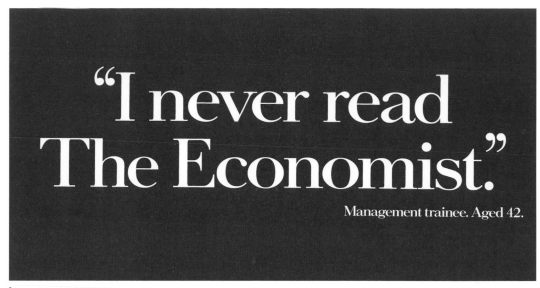

3

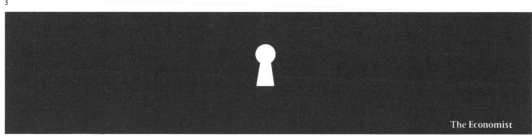

4

advertising—which had survived even Bernbach's revolution—was to find a product's point of difference, Rosser Reeves's so-called Unique Selling Proposition, and use that as the basis for making a case. Even Bernbach, who resisted Reeves's formulaic approach, still tended to build much of his advertising around the USP—by arguing, for example, that the Volkswagen was more efficient and better engineered than other cars (though Bernbach adorned the logic with wit and style, to make it more palatable).

But gradually, product parity in the marketplace—whether in the category of cars or ballpoint pens—made it increasingly difficult for an advertiser to issue a credible claim of superiority. As TBWA/Chiat/Day executive Bob Kuperman noted, "With more product parity, the differences and unique benefits became increasingly slight, and more easily copied by competitors that didn't have any of their own." So it became

necessary for advertisers to distinguish themselves by other means—one of which, Kuperman noted, was by developing a unique and powerful visual style in their ads.

Gradually, advertisers would begin to downplay persuasive copy and experiment more with innovative layout, minimalist design, unusual typography. In some cases, they would engage the audience in lively visual games and riddles that often required no words at all, and that played to emotion more than logic. In recent years, this has evolved as a modern form of communication—a visual shorthand—that can now be found posted on walls or in the pages of magazines around the world. It is expertly produced by agencies like DM9 DDB Publicidade in São Paulo, Brazil, or TBWA Hunt Lascaris, in South Africa, or Leo Burnett in Chicago. The Singapore-based advertising writer Jim Aitchison calls it "the international language of graphics." Relying on signs and

symbols, free association, and visceral reactions, it is an ideal form of communication for advertisers that are trying to cross all boundaries, and for consumers that no longer have time or patience for logical explanations.

The new visual style of print ads didn't arrive overnight. To a great extent, the 1960s sensibility in advertising lasted not only throughout the 1970s but well into the 1980s, with ads that continued to look similar to what DDB was producing earlier—the same head/photo/copy layout and the same wry sense of humor. The DDB model was so solid and so effective that advertisers were loath to meddle with it, other than to perhaps tinker with the typeface (for example, sans serif headlines gave way to Franklin Gothic in the early 1980s). Moreover, the DDB revolution had instilled in many creative people the belief that on any ad campaign, the concept reigned supreme—and that too much stylistic tinkering could undercut a great

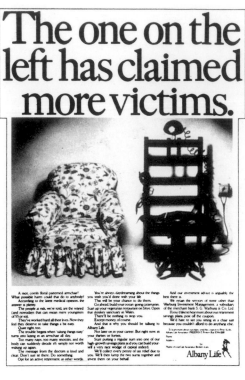

The one on the left has claimed more victims.

A nice, comfy floral-patterned armchair? What possible harm could that do to anybody? According to the latest medical opinion, the answer is plenty.

The people at rest, we're told, are the retired (and nowadays that can mean mere youngsters of 55 or so).

They've worked hard all their lives. Now they feel they deserve to take things a bit easy. Quite right too.

The trouble begins when 'taking things easy' turns into lazing in an armchair all day.

Too many naps, too many snoozes, and the body can suddenly decide it's simply not worth waking up again.

The message from the doctors is loud and clear. Don't just sit there. Do something.

Opt for an active retirement, in other words.

You're always daydreaming about the things you wish you'd done with your life.

This will be your chance to do them.

Go ahead, build your ocean going catamaran. Start up your vegetarian restaurant on Skye. Open that donkey sanctuary in Wales.

There'll be nothing to stop you.

Except money, of course.

And that is why you should be talking to Albany Life.

Not later on in your career. But right now, at your thirties or forties.

Start putting a regular sum into one of our high growth savings plans and you can build yourself a very nice wedge of capital indeed.

We'll collect every penny of tax relief due to you. We'll then lump the two sums together and invest them on your behalf.

And our investment advice is arguably the best there is.

We retain the services of none other than Warburg Investment Management, a subsidiary of the merchant bank S. G. Warburg & Co. Ltd.

If you'd like to hear more about our retirement savings plans, post off the coupon.

We'd hate to see you sitting in a chair just because you couldn't afford to do anything else.

Albany Life

5

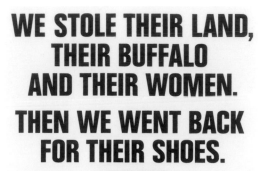

WE STOLE THEIR LAND, THEIR BUFFALO AND THEIR WOMEN. THEN WE WENT BACK FOR THEIR SHOES.

Timberland

6

idea or, worse still, might be used to mask the fact there was no idea in the ad at all. For these reasons, the now "classic" 1960s look became almost sacrosanct—and continued to yield some of the best advertising of the 1980s, even if the style was starting to seem a bit familiar. BMW's ads, created by the New York agency Ammirati & Puris, could have easily been done years earlier by DDB (except for the "It's good to be rich" 1980s mentality that pervades the campaign). Similarly, campaigns produced across the ocean by hot new 1980s British agencies like Leagas Delaney and Lowe Howard Spink, for clients like Timberland and Albany Life, bore a classic look—not that it made them any less striking. If anyone was beginning to suspect that headlines had lost their power by the 1980s, Tim Delaney could have silenced them with one of his audacious lines for Timberland; in an ad for moccasins, above a picture of a Native American, he wrote: "We stole their land, their buffalo and their women. Then we went back for their shoes."

But even among creative purists, some quiet tinkering was happening, particularly off the beaten path in America. In cities like Minneapolis, Minnesota, and Richmond, Virginia, up-and-coming regional creative agencies like Fallon McElligott and the Martin Agency were beginning to cross the bridge from more verbal, logic-driven advertising to something more visual and emotional. The revitalization of simple print ads by these "boondock" agencies came out of necessity; if Madison Avenue of the 1980s was a place where big-budget, slickly produced, star-studded Pepsi commercials were the order of the day, Richmond and Minneapolis represented a whole different universe, where modest clients—businesses with names like Bernie's Tattooing and the 7th Street Barbershop—couldn't even dream of TV commercials but could afford to do print ads (indeed, print is the most democratic form of advertising; even a local dog trainer can afford a print ad, particularly if he/she hires an attention-hungry agency that may create the ad for free, and might even help put up the posters).

Luckily for the barber shops and tattoo parlors in Minneapolis, Richmond, and Providence, the burgeoning ad agencies in those towns had become a haven for some of advertising's most talented craftsmen. The regional print world became advertising's equivalent of the independent-filmmaking segment of the movie business—a place where budgets and resources were limited but where original ideas were in great supply. To some ad creators, this represented the purest and most challenging form of advertising; its creators couldn't rely on celebrity endorsers or special-effect film techniques, as many commercials do. Nor could they bludgeon people with the redundancy made possible by big media budgets. They had to engage an audience that was rapidly turning

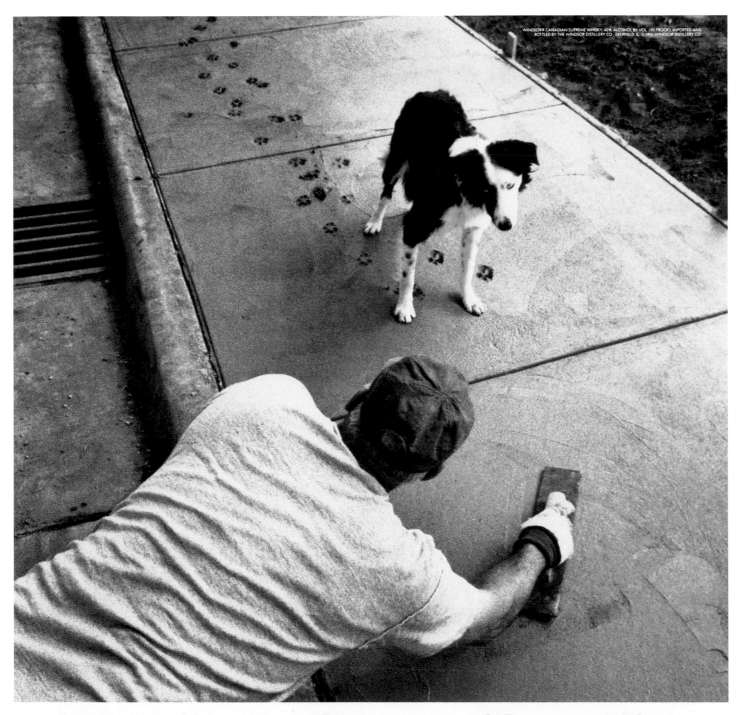

Fortunately, every day comes with an evening.

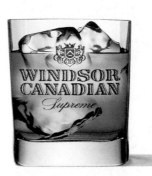

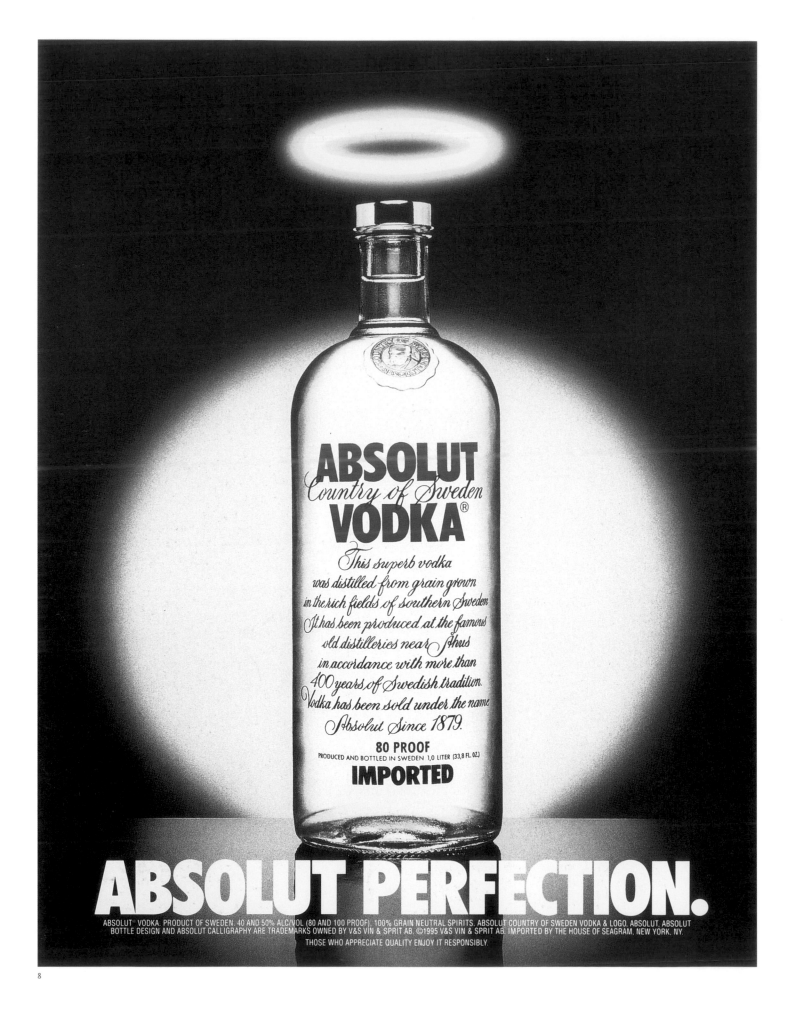

ABSOLUT PERFECTION.

8

Whose birthday is it, anyway?

The Episcopal Church believes the important news at Christmas is not who comes down the chimney, but who came down from heaven. We invite you to come and join us as we celebrate the birth of Jesus Christ.
The Episcopal Church

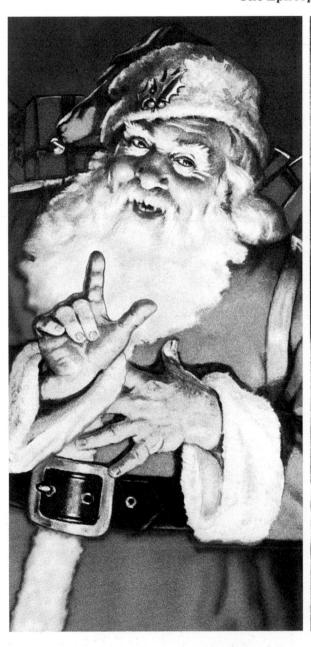 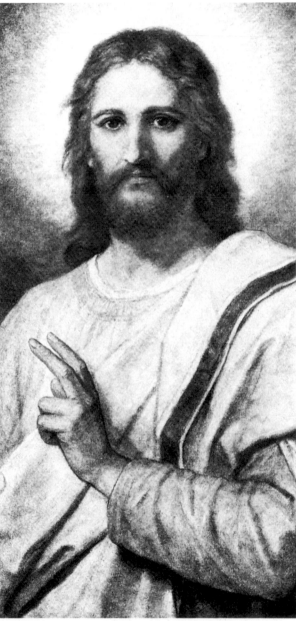

9

A NEW VISUAL LANGUAGE EMERGES.

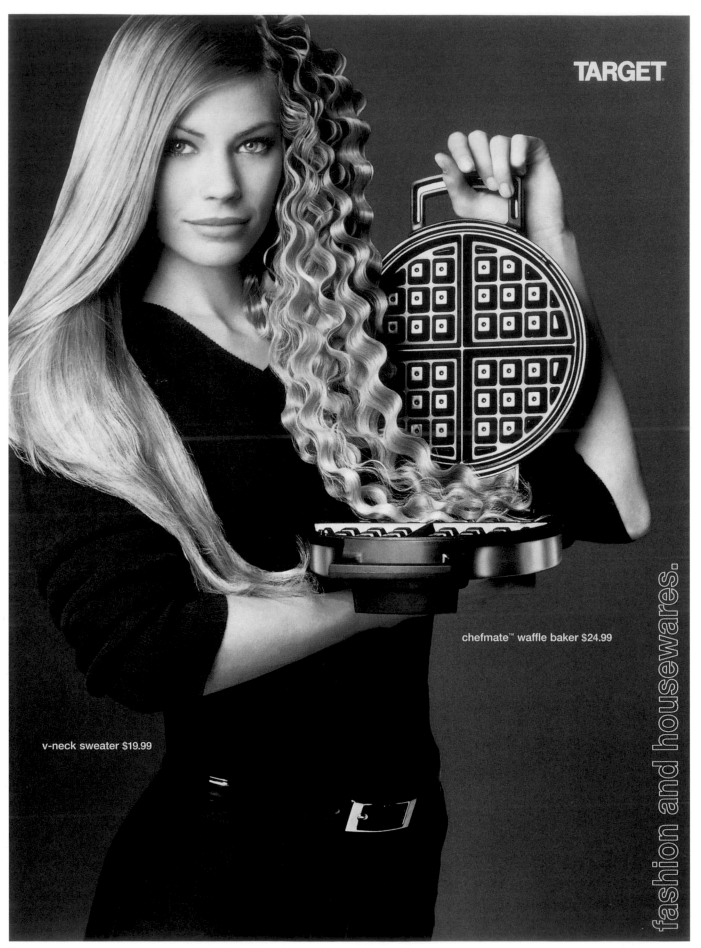

TARGET

chefmate™ waffle baker $24.99

v-neck sweater $19.99

fashion and housewares.

10

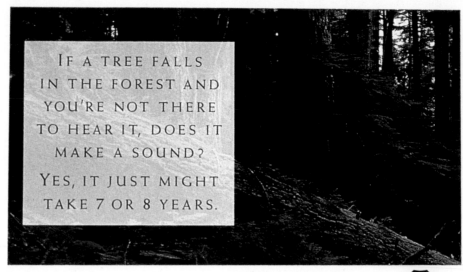

IF A TREE FALLS
IN THE FOREST AND
YOU'RE NOT THERE
TO HEAR IT, DOES IT
MAKE A SOUND?
YES, IT JUST MIGHT
TAKE 7 OR 8 YEARS.

To make a good guitar, you've got to devote a lot of time and attention to it. But then, we haven't been doing much of anything else for the last few years. Write us at 1940 Gillespie Way, El Cajon, CA 92020 to find a dealer

11

10. TARGET
KIRSHENBAUM BOND &
PARTNERS, NEW YORK, 1996
In the late 1990s, Target stores
began to use a playful visual
approach to make the point
that it sells both fashion
and housewares.

11. TAYLOR GUITARS
VITRO ROBERTSON,
SAN DIEGO, CALIFORNIA,
1992
Instead of showing the product,
a fine guitar, the ad shows the
woods where the instrument's
natural material originated.

pages or walking down the street with print ads and posters that relied on the most basic elements—writing, photography, graphic design, and that most important element of all, intrigue.

The print craftsmen demonstrated that striking imagery could be the great equalizer, bringing attention to small, obscure clients. In Richmond, the Martin Agency promoted a local tattoo parlor with a poster of a man who was naked and covered with tattoos, his hands clasped over his private parts; the headline read, "Surprise your wife." It was a piece of advertising that was seen and discussed around the country. Similarly, the Minneapolis agency Fallon McElligott, while known for its clever copy, kept those words to a minimum—many ads had not much more than one line and a stirring image. For a local barbershop, the agency used an extreme close-up of Moe of the Three Stooges, with the headline "A bad haircut is no laughing matter." For the Episcopal Church, it juxtaposed

pictures of Santa Claus and Jesus Christ, and asked, "Whose birthday is it, anyway?" An ad for Purina made a point about chemical additives in dog food by simply showing a dog poised over his dish, wearing a gas mask. The agency understood, early on, that a picture could tell an entire story, as in a Windsor Canadian liquor ad showing a laborer face-to-face with a dog that had just trekked footprints across his freshly paved sidewalk; "Fortunately, every day comes with an evening" was the ad's only copy. Fallon McElligott's art directors, like the talented veteran Bob Barrie, took the view that as the media landscape grew more complex and noisy, ads should get quieter. "It only stands to reason that the simplest messages will cut through and be remembered," says Barrie. And it is the image, Barrie noted, that has the power to stop people in their tracks.

Perhaps the biggest breakthrough campaign of the 1980s, in terms of demonstrating visual

power, was the Absolut vodka campaign from the TBWA agency, based in New York. It debuted in 1980, with a picture of an Absolut bottle and a halo, headlined, "Absolut Perfection." The co-creator Geoff Hayes came up with the idea at home one evening while watching an episode of the television show *The Honeymooners*, demonstrating that the best advertising ideas aren't necessarily inspired by elaborate research, nor from gazing upon masterpieces at the museum. In one sense, the Absolut campaign was a throwback: It prominently featured the product in its bottle—not unlike the way soft-drink ads from the past once consisted of simple pictures of the bottle, or someone drinking from it. But there was an important difference: Those old-fashioned poster-style ads showing the product were doing only that, without conveying an idea. Then, after the pretty posters, came the next generation of ads that did convey ideas, but primarily through words. Now Absolut

A NEW VISUAL LANGUAGE EMERGES.

Perception.

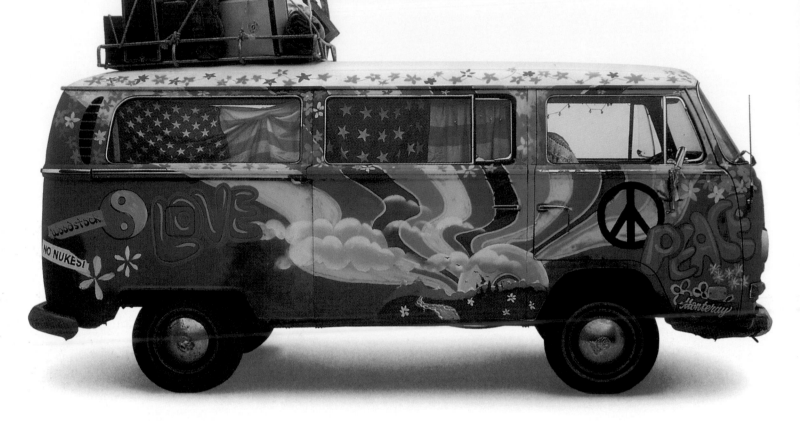

Reality.

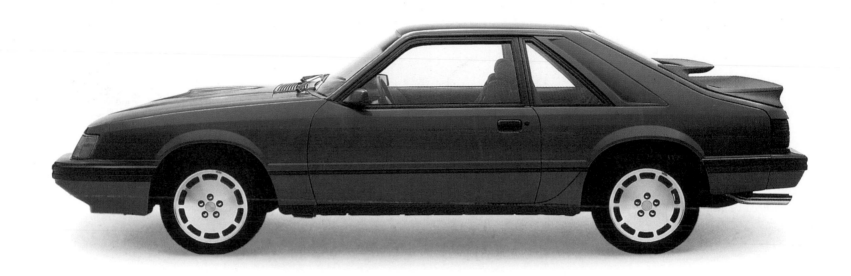

If you still think a Rolling Stone reader's idea of standard equipment is flowers on the door panels and incense in the ashtrays, consider this: Rolling Stone households own 5,199,000 automobiles. If you've got cars to sell, welcome to the fast lane. Source: Simmons 1984

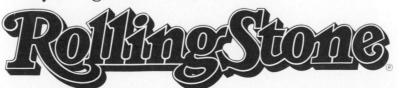

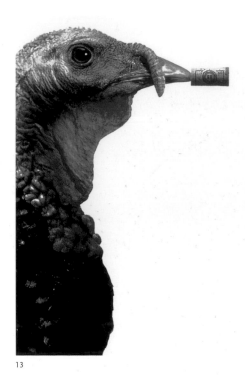

nothing like a delicious turkey for opening a bottle of rose wine **RENÉ BARBIER**

13

represented the next stage in the evolution—
using the picture to convey the idea. It was also
one of the first ad campaigns to create a visual
riddle that invited the reader to play along.
Particularly as the series evolved, often the image
of the vodka bottle was not immediately
discernible; one had to study the ad to find it, or
to make the connection between image and
headline. Absolut ads invited the audience to
become part of the communication process, and
readers eagerly joined in.

Another seminal campaign in developing
advertising's visual language came a few years
later, in the mid-1980s, from Fallon McElligott.
The agency had taken on the account of *Rolling
Stone* magazine, a publication dearly loved by its
readers but underappreciated by advertisers—
who seemed to think of those readers as pot-
smoking hippies who were not apt to buy cars
or expensive clothing. But in fact, *Rolling Stone*
knew that its readers, particularly by the

mid-1980s, did not fit that easy stereotype; many
were successful, affluent, and acquisitive. A
conventional ad might have tried to explain this
at great length, with demographic data and
statistical charts. But the creative team on the
campaign, Nancy Rice and Bill Miller, came up
with an idea that put the whole argument into
visual shorthand—a simple juxtaposition of the
"Perception" of a *Rolling Stone* reader as
compared to the "Reality." Miller jotted down
the first juxtapositions on a napkin in a coffee
shop; subsequently, Rice dressed them up into
finished ads, but the truth is they never became
much more elaborate than what Miller had put
on the napkin—just white space, with the two
pictures side by side. The power of the campaign
lay in the images that were chosen and the way
they related to each other (cigarette-rolling paper
was juxtaposed with Post-it notes; Earth shoes
were paired with Nike running shoes), and also
in the way that his campaign, like Absolut, invited

readers to connect the dots—an interactive
approach that would become a staple of print
ads in years to come. (In fact, the "Perception/
Reality" campaign is undoubtedly one of the
most widely imitated ad campaigns ever; more
than fifteen years after it was created, and years
after *Rolling Stone* stopped running it, other
advertisers continued to juxtapose contrasting
images to make the point their product is not
what you think it is.)

The success of the Absolut and *Rolling Stone*
campaigns made it abundantly clear that highly
visual print ads, rooted in a strong idea, could
have a resounding impact even in a world of
television and other media clutter. By the 1990s,
"with the expansion of electronic media, the
public was growing less and less willing to submit
to content, and advertisers were beginning to
rely more on the power of imagery," observed
the renowned art director John Doyle of the San
Francisco agency Publicis/Hal Riney & Partners.

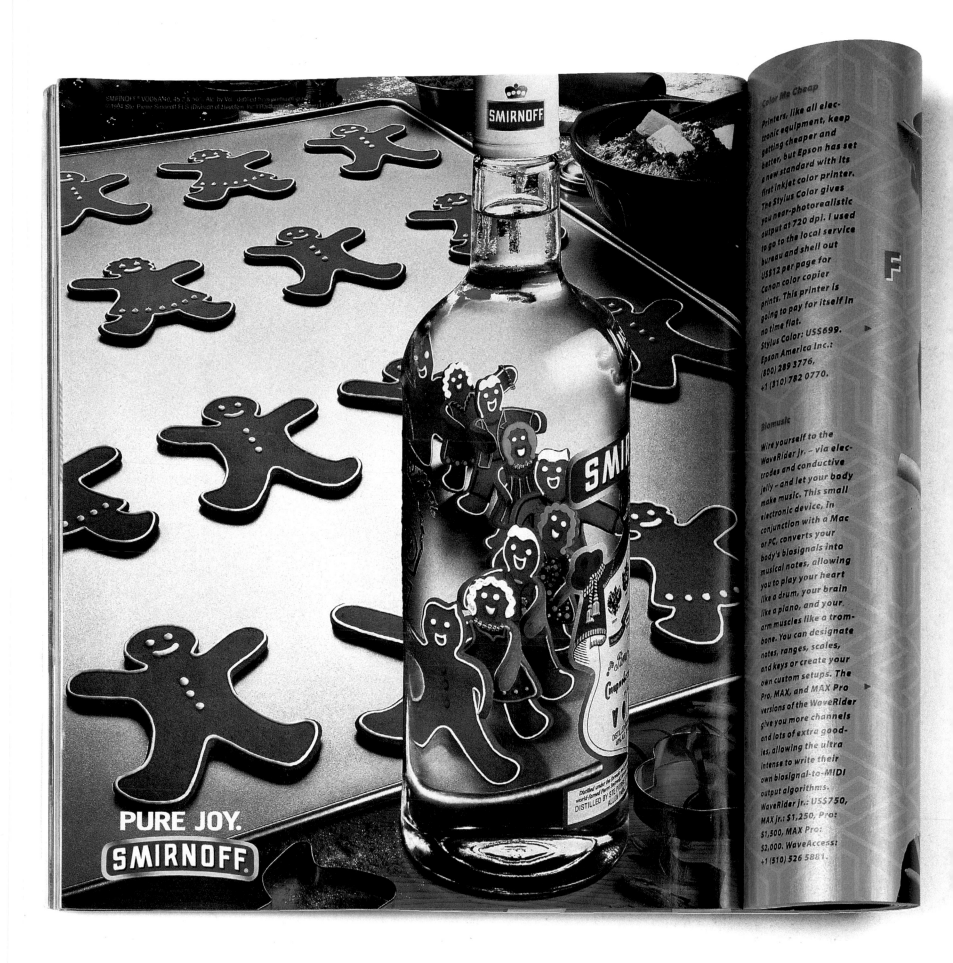

      A NEW VISUAL LANGUAGE EMERGES.

Color Me Cheap

Printers, like all electronic equipment, keep getting cheaper and better, but Epson has set a new standard with its first inkjet color printer. The Stylus Color gives you near-photorealistic output at 720 dpi. I used to go to the local service bureau and shell out US$12 per page for Canon color copier prints. This printer is going to pay for itself in no time flat. Stylus Color: US$699. Epson America Inc.: (800) 289 3776, +1 (510) 782 0770.

Biomusic

Wire yourself to the WaveRider jr. – via electrodes and conductive jelly – and let your body make music. This small electronic device, in conjunction with a Mac or PC, converts your body's biosignals into musical notes, allowing you to play your heart like a drum, your brain like a piano, and your arm muscles like a trombone. You can designate notes, ranges, scales, and keys or create your own custom setups. The Pro, MAX, and MAX Pro versions of the WaveRider give you more channels and lots of extra goodies, allowing the ultra intense to write their own biosignal-to-MIDI output algorithms. WaveRider jr.: US$750, MAX jr.: $1,250, Pro: $1,500, MAX Pro: $2,000, WaveAccess: +1 (510) 526 5881.

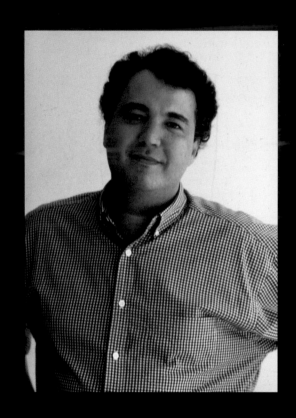

INTERVIEW: NIZAN GUANAES

Nizan Guanaes, a native of the Bahia region of Brazil, opened his own ad agency in 1989, and his ads quickly became the talk of São Paulo. But that was just the beginning; Guanaes soon led his agency, DM9 DDB Publicidade, to the top of the advertising world. When DM9 was named ad agency of the year at the International Advertising Festival in Cannes in 1998—and then again in 1999—it marked the first time ever that an agency outside the United States or Europe had earned this distinction. In 2000, Guanaes left advertising as dramatically as he'd entered it, starting a new career on the Internet. But he left a legacy. DM9's style—simple, visually striking, intellectually challenging—has become the hall-

Brazil, this country is like several countries in itself—you have some parts that are highly developed and urban, others that are rural. So you want the advertising to cross those boundaries, too. But you can't do visual advertising for every client. If you are advertising something that is very new, and complex, with a lot of features to explain, then it would be irresponsible to do this kind of visual work. On the other hand, if you have a product that people already know, and maybe you have just one point to make . . . then it's powerful.

SOME OF THESE VISUAL PUZZLES CAN BE SUBTLE— FOR EXAMPLE, YOUR AD FEATURING THE BENT NAIL

WHAT IS THE PUBLIC ATTITUDE TOWARD ADVERTISING IN BRAZIL THESE DAYS?
People love it. You find them talking about it, and even singing jingles, in bars. Brazilian advertising is funny, fresh, and light. It's related to the spirit of our people—this is a very musical, sexy, easygoing country. So you cannot have dull, serious advertising.

But at the same time, I believe this is not art—people don't meditate on advertising. Do you know anyone who runs home in the evening to watch the ads? I believe advertising is mostly irrelevant to people—and that's why I take it seriously. Because once you understand how irrelevant our work is to people, then you realize

A GUERRA DO VIETNÃ TEVE INÍCIO EM 1945 E TÉRMINO EM 1973. DURANTE ESSE PERÍODO, VÁRIOS CONFLITOS MILITARES OCORRERAM NA REGIÃO, COM ALG CARÁTER COLONIAL. MAS, DEVIDO À CRESCENTE GUERRA FRIA E À SITUAÇÃO POLÍTICA MUNDIAL, O CONFLITO EVOLUIU PARA UMA GUERRA CIVIL. DE UMA VIETNÃ TEVE DUAS FASES: O PERÍODO FRANCÊS, DE 1945 A 1954, E O PERÍODO NORTE-AMERICANO, DE 1959 A 1973. O PERÍODO FRANCÊS TEVE INÍCIO EM NÃO OCUPARAM O NORTE. POIS, PELA CONVENÇÃO DE 6 DE MARÇO DE 1946, ASSINADA POR HO CHI MINH E PELO REPRESENTANTE DA FRANÇA EM HANÓI REUNIFICAÇÃO, MAS EXIGIU A PRESENÇA DE 15 MIL HOMENS EM HANÓI. PORÉM, O ALMIRANTE FRANCÊS GEORGES THIERRY D'ARGENLIEU, NOMEADO ... DEZEMBRO DE 1946, AOS PRIMEIROS CONFLITOS ARMADOS CONTRA AS FORÇAS FRANCESAS. A LUTA CONTINUOU NOS ANOS SEGUINTES, COM ALGUNS P COMUNISTA DO SUL, OS VIETCONGUES, ALIADA ÀS TROPAS DO NORTE, RETORNA AO VIETNÃ DO SUL COM A MISSÃO DE ACABAR COM O GOVERNO PRÓ-C SE ESTENDEU ATÉ A COMPLETA INTERVENÇÃO MILITAR A PARTIR DE 65. A ADESÃO DOS EUA À GUERRA FRIA ENVOLVENDO A DISPUTA DO CAPITAL 16 DE MARÇO DE 1968, O TENENTE WILLIAM CALLEY JR. COMANDAVA UM PELOTÃO DE SOLDADOS DO EXÉRCITO DOS ESTADOS UNIDOS QUE INVADIU O PEQUE SE EM 21 DE MARÇO DE 1971 CALLEY FOI CONSIDERADO CULPADO E, EM 29 DE MARÇO, A CORTE MARCIAL O SENTENCIOU À PRISÃO PERPÉTUA. EM 31 DE NACIONAL, DOS ESTADOS UNIDOS COMO MOTIVO DE VERGONHA. A AJUDOU A ALTERAR A OPINIÃO PÚBLICA DO COMBATE À PRESENÇA AMERICANA DE PESSOALMENTE TER MATADO PELO MENOS 109 PESSOAS, FOI SIMPLES PARA OS SEUS SOLDADOS, MATEM VIET CONGUES NÃO H OUTUBRO DE 1970 NO JULGAMENTO, O OPERADOR DE RÁDIO DO PELOTÃO, CHARLES SLEDGE, DISSE QUE O TENENTE JOGAVA MULHERES E CRIANÇAS NO NESSE TIPO DE ACUSAÇÃO. ELE ESTAVA CUMPRINDO ORDENS DE SEUS SUPERIORES. ELES ERAM TODOS INIMIGOS. TODOS TINHAM DE SER DESTRUÍDOS DAR CHICLETE ÀS CRIANÇAS. ELAS SÃO PERIGOSAS. SÃO EXCELENTES PLANTADORES DE MINAS. EM 31 DE MARÇO DE 1971. A FIM DA MAIS LONGA CORTE O PAÍS FICOU DIVIDIDO EM RELAÇÃO À SENTENÇA. MUITOS CONSERVADORES CONSIDERARAM A DECISÃO INJUSTA E DIZIAM QUE CALLEY ERA UM HERÓI DE G DE 1971 A PENA FOI REDUZIDA PARA 20 ANOS DE PRISÃO. ELE CUMPRIU MENOS DE UM TERÇO DA SENTENÇA E FOI LIBERADO. ELE...

[...]

SE APROXIMAR DO NÍVEL DE DESENVOLVIMENTO DOS PAÍSES RICOS. TERMINADA A ENTREVISTA, GRAVADOR DESLIGADO, O GENERAL ESTENDEU O BR ELE SE REFERIA A SEUS INCENDIÁRIOS ARTIGOS PUBLICADOS NO VIET LAP. UM VILAREJO CHAMADO AN XA ENTROU PARA A HISTÓRIA AO SE TORNAR, A 28 DE DURANTE A GUERRA DO VIETNÃ, CASTIGADA PELOS INSISTENTES BOMBARDEIOS NORTE-AMERICANOS. MAS NA DÉCADA DE 10, ERAM OS FRANCESES OS D ENVOLVEU EM DUAS REVOLTAS, UMA EM 1885 E A OUTRA EM 1888. PARA ACABAR NA PRISÃO EM 1919, ACUSADO DE SUBVERSIVO. MORREU EM SUA CELA, ADOECEU NA CADEIA E FOI SOLTA EM SEGUIDA. MORREU DUAS SEMANAS DEPOIS DE VOLTAR PARA CASA. AS DUAS MORTES DEIXARAM MARCAS NA MEMÓRIA DE G INSTITUIÇÃO PASSARAM AINDA MAIS DOIS ESTUDANTES IMPORTANTES PARA A HISTÓRIA CONTEMPORÂNEA DO VIETNÃ: HO CHI MINH, O LÍDER REVOLUCIONA CONTINUOU AS ATIVIDADES CLANDESTINAS. O OBSTINADO ALUNO CONSEGUIU QUE A ESCOLA O ACEITASSE NOVAMENTE ATÉ SER PRESO POR LIDERAR MANIF SE TORNAR UM ADVOGADO PELA UNIVERSIDADE DE HANÓI, A ÚNICA DO PAÍS. O MILITANTE NACIONALISTA SE JUNTAVA A UMA ELITE, JÁ QUE ENTRE 1920 E 19 DO NAMORO COM NGUYEN THI MINH GIANG. OUTRA MILITANTE DO MOVIMENTO ANTIFRANCÊS. QUANDO DO CASAMENTO, EM JUNHO DE 1938, OS DOIS FIGURA DEPOIS DE FAZER UM CURSO PARA REVOLUCIONÁRIOS NA URSS, FOI PRESA, CONDENADA À MORTE E FUZILADA. EM 1940, A MULHER DE GIAP PARTIU EM VIAGE O MARIDO GIAP ORGANIZAVA O EMBRIÃO DO EXÉRCITO VIETNAMITA. ELE, AO RECEBER A NOTÍCIA, NÃO ESBOÇOU NENHUMA REAÇÃO. MAS DEPOIS RECONHE CASAMENTO, O GENERAL TEVE QUATRO FILHOS. A SEGUNDA GUERRA MUNDIAL ENFRAQUECEU O PODER COLONIAL DA FRANÇA E DEPOIS ABRIU CAMINHO PAR EM 1940, DOIS DE SEUS PRINCIPAIS AJUDANTES, PHAM VAN DONG E GIAP, FORAM PARA A CHINA APRENDER TÁTICAS DE GUERRA COM OS COMANDADOS DE NACIONALISTA. SEU PRIMEIRO COMANDANTE: VO NGUYEN GIAP. A AÇÃO DE BATISMO FOI DESLANCHADA NO NATAL DE 1944. OS 34 COMANDADOS DE GIAP E ENTÃO JÁ 5.000 E MUNIDOS DE ARMAMENTO OBSOLETO, CENTRARAM FOGO CONTRA O INVASOR JAPONÊS. OS EUA, INTERESSADOS EM ACELERAR A DERRO VIETNAMITAS ENTRAVAM EM HANÓI, VITORIOSAS E LIVRES DE JAPONESES OU FRANCESES. MAS ERA APENAS A PRIMEIRA FASE DE UMA LUTA QUE SE TORNARIA O FUGIRAM DESSE REGIME SEVERO E BRUTAL. NO CAMBOJA, AGORA CAMPUCHÉA, OS COMUNISTAS MATARAM CERCA DE 30% DA POPULAÇÃO. A REVOLUÇÃO MATOU OS SUCESSORES DE HO CHI MINH, LE DUC THO, LIDERAM KIETI, DEPOIS DE ARRESTARAM OS HABITUAIS HORRORES STALINISTAS. OUTROS, PARA UMA POPULAÇÃO CAMPONESA DESTRUÍRAM A ECONOMIA DE CONSUMO NO VIETNÃ DO SUL, CONSIDERANDO A RELÍQUIA PODRE DO CAPITAL É RICO EM RECURSOS MINERAIS. NÃO PODERIA EXPLORÁ-LOS SEM CAPITAL E TECNOLOGIA DO MUNDO CAPITALISTA. AS FÁBRICAS QUE MONTARAM LEVAR UNIDOS A PONTO DE CRISE FATAL. A GUERRA PROVOU ALGUMAS COISAS: O NACIONALISMO É A MAIOR FORÇA IDEOLÓGICA NO MUNDO NO FIM DO SÉCULO VINTE A ÚNICA LIÇÃO DA HISTÓRIA É QUE NADA SE APRENDE DA HISTÓRIA. NEM MESMO A FANTASIA DOMINANTE NOS EUA, DE QUE A TECNOLOGIA TUDO PODE, F

Folha de S. Paulo Newspaper. Illustrating life with words for 77 years.

A NEW VISUAL LANGUAGE EMERGES.

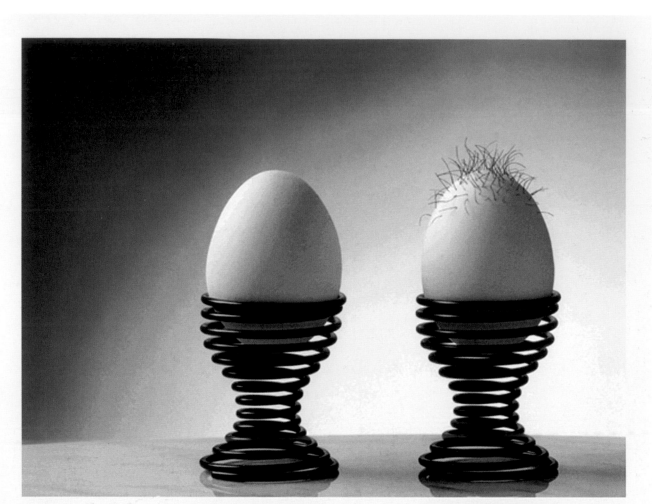

(Be careful with the Kaminomoto)

21

21. KAMINOMOTO HAIR GROWTH,
THE BALL PARTNERSHIP, SINGAPORE, MID-1980s
A before-and-after demonstration of a hair-growth product with a playful twist. The series also featured an ad that showed hair sprouting on a cue ball.

22. TRIUMPH LINGERIE
WIRZ WERBEBERATUNG AG, ZURICH, 1996
The ad becomes a game: by turning the page upside down, the reader sees a visual metaphor of the product's benefit.

23. STREN FISHING LINE
CARMICHAEL LYNCH, MINNEAPOLIS, MINNESOTA, 1995
Instead of proclaiming the fishing line as strong, the campaign showed off its strength—with a bit of playful exaggeration.

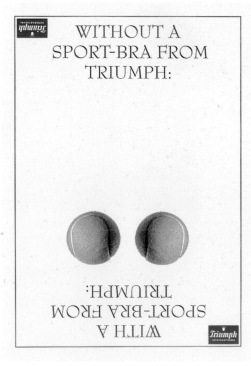

22

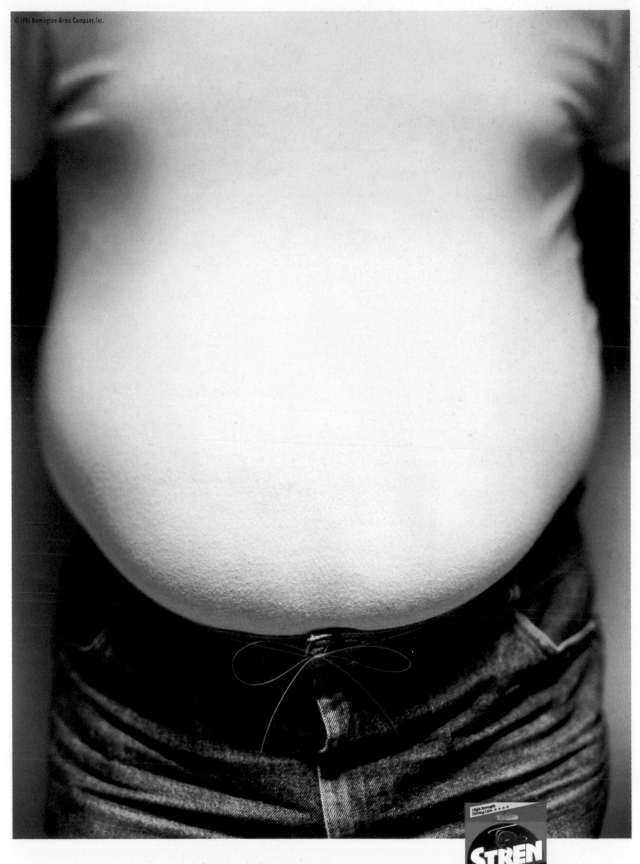

The most dependable fishing line in the world.

23

A NEW VISUAL LANGUAGE EMERGES.

24. **SÃO PAULO MUSEUM OF ART**
DM9 DDB PUBLICIDADE,
SÃO PAULO, 1998
To promote an exhibit by Botero
(who paints playfully plump
subjects), DM9 showed a bent
nail on a wall; the reader had to
deduce the rest.

25. **PREPARATION H**
BSB, HONG KONG, 1993
This less-subtle image for a
hemorrhoid ointment makes an
uncomfortable but unmistakable
point. You can almost feel
this ad—and it doesn't
feel good.

Botero
at the São Paulo
Museum of Art.
From March 17 to May 17.

24

than to their own local culture. (To some extent, Wilhelm acknowledges, universal ads are also designed to win international advertising awards as much as to influence consumers.)

Whatever the motives behind this style, it is becoming clear that ad agencies in Asia, Australia, South Africa, and particularly South America have proved highly adept at constructing visual riddles, which might also be called "picture plays"—a new version of an old advertising tool, the word play. For example, to make the point that H&R Block accountants are thorough, the company's Australian agency wove its copy into the shape of a comb. Japan's Dentsu Young & Rubicam featured an image of a safety pin, with no words, in its advertising for Volvo. A South African ad for the deaf showed a picture of a telephone handset receiver—upon closer inspection, one notices that the earpiece has no holes in it. Singapore's Ball Partnership agency used a baguette, cut

into pieces, to draw a comparison to airline flights that are interrupted by too many stops. Even a mundane product like Preparation H lends itself to this lively and playful approach: Bates Hong Kong created a suggestive series of visual analogies that captured the feeling of hemorrhoids by showing an image of a bicycle whose seat is a saw blade. On a similar note, a laxative advertiser in Uruguay used a corkscrew to make the key point about its product.

While visual-analogy ads can sometimes be obvious and unimaginative (certain symbolic objects, such as razor blades and magnets, have already been overused), the best practitioners of this style of advertising, such as the Brazilian agency DM9 DDB, which was brought to international prominence by its former creative director Nizan Guanaes, have tended to challenge the audience with the subtlety and sophistication of the picture-plays. Consider, for example, one of the agency's ads for the São Paulo Museum of

Art's Botero exhibit: The ad shows a bent nail on a wall, surrounded by broken plaster. It's left to the reader to figure out that the nail couldn't support the heft of Botero's paintings, which feature chubby figures as their subjects. Similarly interactive is a Swiss lingerie ad showing a stark image of two tennis balls, and inviting the reader to play a game that requires turning the ad upside down. And another lingerie ad, this one from the Johannesburg agency TBWA Hunt Lascaris, promoted the enlarging effects of a Wonderbra by showing a pair of sunburned feet—with only the tips of the toes reddened.

While American ads don't go in for picture-plays quite as much, the most popular campaigns in recent years have been minimalist—stripped down to a single striking image and few, if any, words. The "Think different" campaign for Apple, the relaunch of the Volkswagen Beetle, and the "Curiously Strong" series for Altoids breath mints represent three of the most

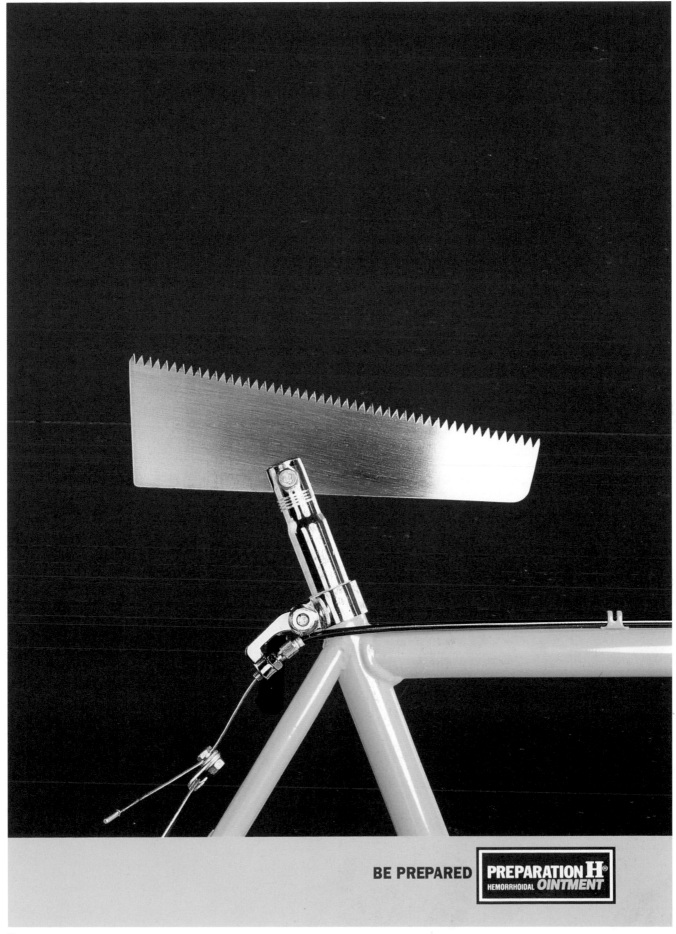

BE PREPARED **PREPARATION H** HEMORRHOIDAL *OINTMENT*

A NEW VISUAL LANGUAGE EMERGES.

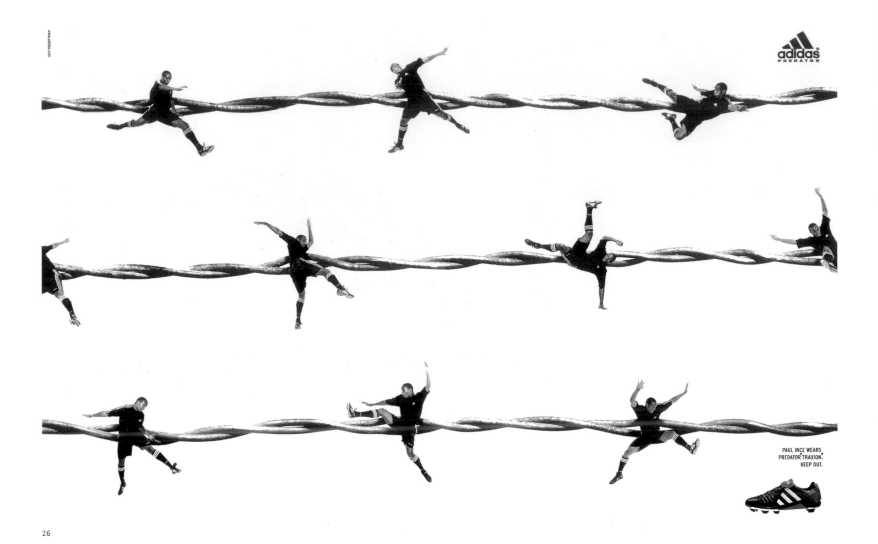

26

26. **ADIDAS**
LEAGAS DELANEY, LONDON,
1998
By the late 1990s, Delaney had
taken a more visual route,
turning images of agile soccer
players into barbed wire.

27. **SIMS SNOWBOARDS**
HAMMERQUIST & HALVERSON,
SEATTLE, WASHINGTON, 1997
The ad evokes a famous image
from the 1989 Tiananmen Square
uprising in China—but this
time, it's a lone snowboarder
defying oncoming snow plows.

28. **NIKE**
KESSELSKRAMER,
AMSTERDAM, 1996
Another example of advertising's
new visual language, this Dutch
ad is a reminder that fancy
sports equipment is not
necessary for all athletes
(but shoes are a must).

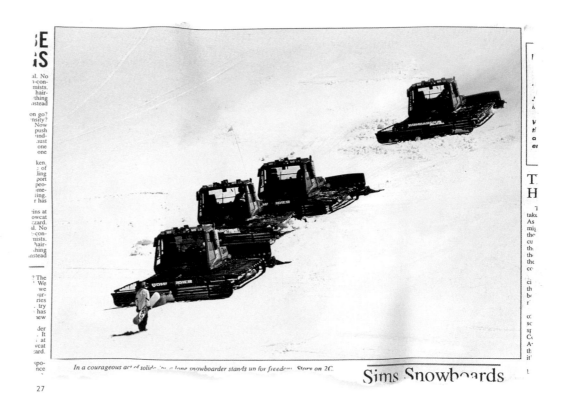

In a courageous act of solidarity, a lone snowboarder stands up for freedom. Story on 2C.

Sims Snowboards

27

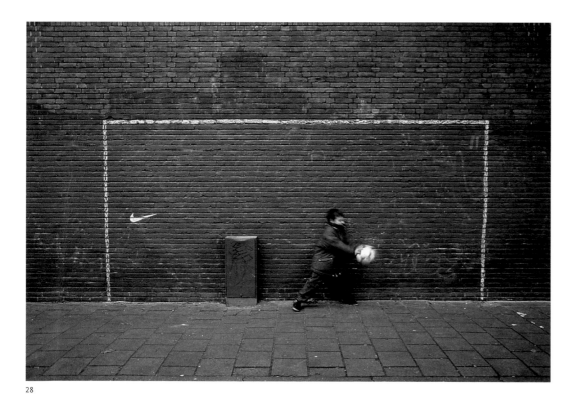

28

A NEW VISUAL LANGUAGE EMERGES.

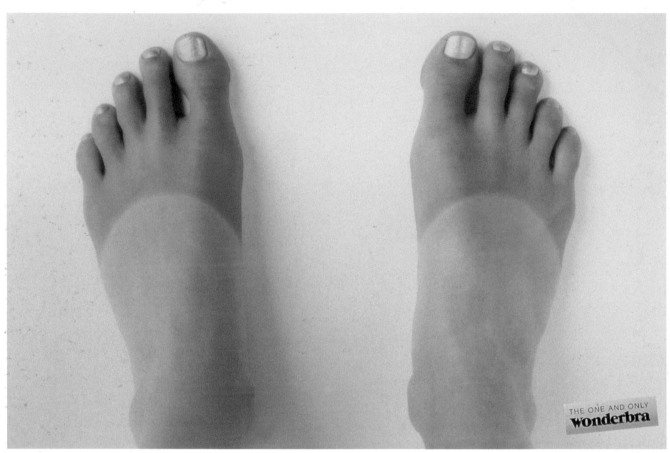

29

29. WONDERBRA
TBWA HUNT LASCARIS,
JOHANNESBURG, 1998
The "sunburned feet" ad
promoting the powers of
Wonderbra is another playful
visual puzzle; South Africa
has taken a shine to such ads
because they cross cultural
barriers easily.

30. MCDONALDS
PALMER JARVIS DDB,
VANCOUVER, 1997
This Canadian campaign used
the visual power of the company's
"Golden Arches" symbol in new
and surprising ways.

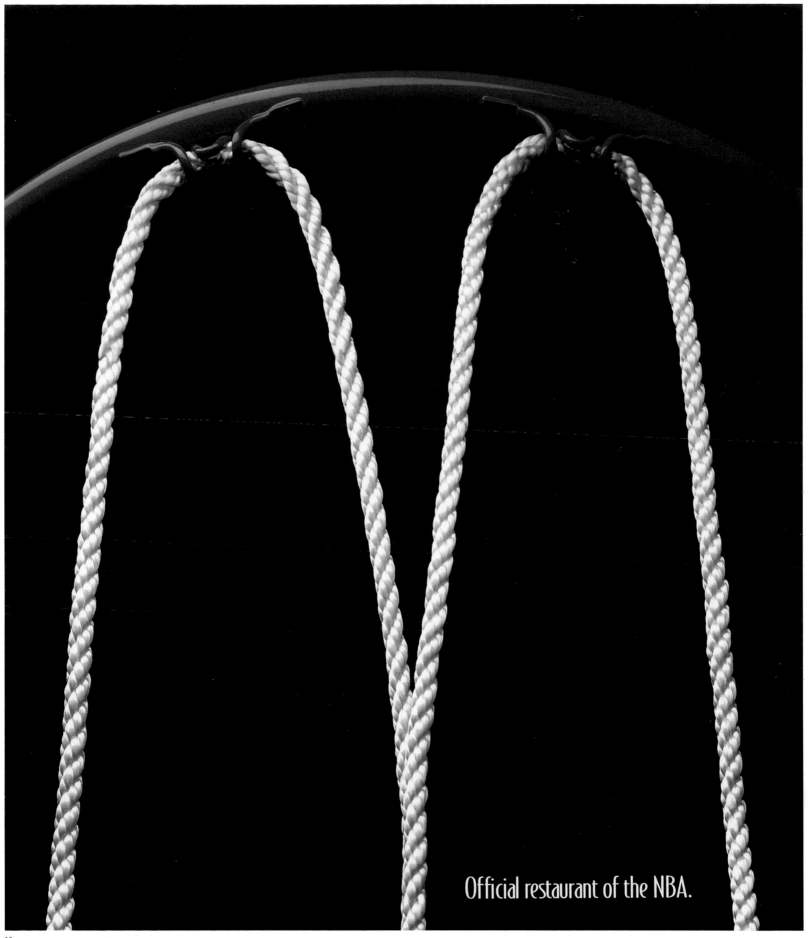

Official restaurant of the NBA.

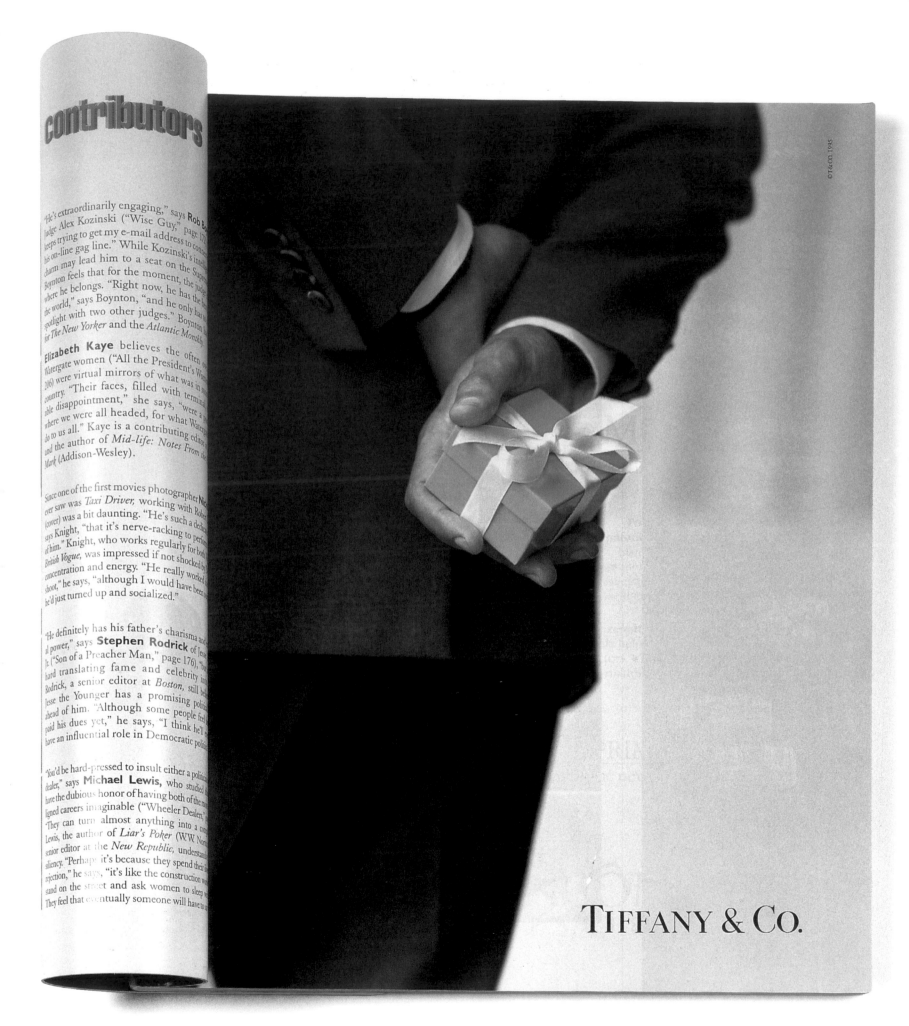
"He's extraordinarily engaging," says **Rob B...** Judge Alex Kozinski ("Wise Guy," page 17... keeps trying to get my e-mail address to con... his on-line gag line." While Kozinski's intell... charm may lead him to a seat on the Supre... Boynton feels that for the moment, the judg... where he belongs. "Right now, he has the be... the world," says Boynton, "and he only has... spotlight with two other judges." Boynton... for *The New Yorker* and the *Atlantic Monthly.*

Elizabeth Kaye believes the often o... Watergate women ("All the President's Wom... 206) were virtual mirrors of what was in... country. "Their faces, filled with termin... able disappointment," she says, "were a... where we were all headed, for what Water... do to us all." Kaye is a contributing editor... and the author of *Mid-life: Notes From th...* *Mark* (Addison-Wesley).

Since one of the first movies photographer Ni... ever saw was *Taxi Driver,* working with Rob... (cover) was a bit daunting. "He's such a ded... says Knight, "that it's nerve-racking to perfor... of him." Knight, who works regularly for both *British Vogue,* was impressed if not shocked by... concentration and energy. "He really worked... shoot," he says, "although I would have been... he'd just turned up and socialized."

"He definitely has his father's charisma and... al power," says **Stephen Rodrick** of Jes... Jr. ("Son of a Preacher Man," page 176), "... hard translating fame and celebrity int... Rodrick, a senior editor at *Boston,* still bel... Jesse the Younger has a promising politi... ahead of him. "Although some people feel... paid his dues yet," he says, "I think he'll... have an influential role in Democratic politic...

"You'd be hard-pressed to insult either a politi... dealer," says **Michael Lewis,** who studied... have the dubious honor of having both of the m... ligned careers imaginable ("Wheeler Dealer,"... "They can turn almost anything into a cr... Lewis, the author of *Liar's Poker* (W.W. No... senior editor at the *New Republic,* understan... saliency. "Perhaps it's because they spend their... rejection," he says, "it's like the construction w... stand on the street and ask women to sleep w... They feel that eventually someone will have to...

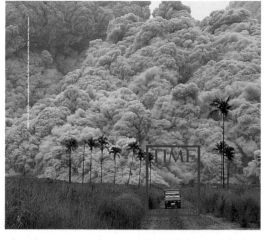

If you think watching a volcano
in a movie is frightening, imagine
watching one in a rearview mirror.

The world's most interesting magazine.

33

32

successful American print campaigns of the 1990s, and all speak the new succinct language of visual advertising. Meanwhile, the smaller campaigns from the regional agencies have continued to rely on imagery: The best ones have included a wordless series from Minneapolis's Carmichael Lynch for Stren fishing line, in which we see the product tested in memorable ways; an ad from the Seattle, Washington, agency Hammerquist Saffel & Halverson for Sims snowboards, which captures the rebel spirit of the product by evoking the 1989 Tiananmen Square uprising in China with an image of a snowboarder defiantly standing in the path of snowplows; and a long-running Fallon McElligott series for *Time* magazine, which uses a simple red box, strategically placed in certain photos, to make a point about the magazine's ability to cut to the essence of news events.

If any countries have been resistant to the visual movement, they are probably Germany and the UK, where copy-driven advertising is still popular. "Germans are analytical and like information from their advertising," explains Guido Heffels—though some of the country's cutting-edge creative agencies are bucking that trend. The UK, meanwhile, has always had a fondness for clever and witty copywriting— but even so, there's a growing recognition by top creative directors like John Hegarty, of Bartle Bogle Hegarty, that such a strategy may have to change now, with the growing emphasis on global communication. Hegarty says the language-driven advertising "obviously becomes a problem if you're going to talk to lots of people in different countries. Consequently, we now have to think of advertising as being more driven by the image. This doesn't mean you can't use words—only that you have to think about the words you're using in a different way. You have to think about reducing your ideas down, so that even people who don't understand the particular language can capture an essence of what the idea is about." Hegarty has practiced what he preaches in his own advertising for Boddingtons Cream Ale—in which the creamy quality of the beer is conveyed by, for example, visualizing ice cream cones made of beer (this campaign is featured in Chapter 11). Another recent acclaimed British ad featured nothing more than a picture of a parked Mercedes-Benz with skid marks in the street alongside the car, suggesting the car's effect on passersby.

While such ads can be baffling, the audience for today's advertising seems to relish the challenge of figuring out what's the product, what's being said, and where's the punchline. "Younger people tend to read this visual shorthand faster, because they're used to looking at a barrage of images," says Myrna Davis of the Art Directors Club of New York. "We've shown some of these ads to older art directors, and they shake their heads. But younger people look at it,

34

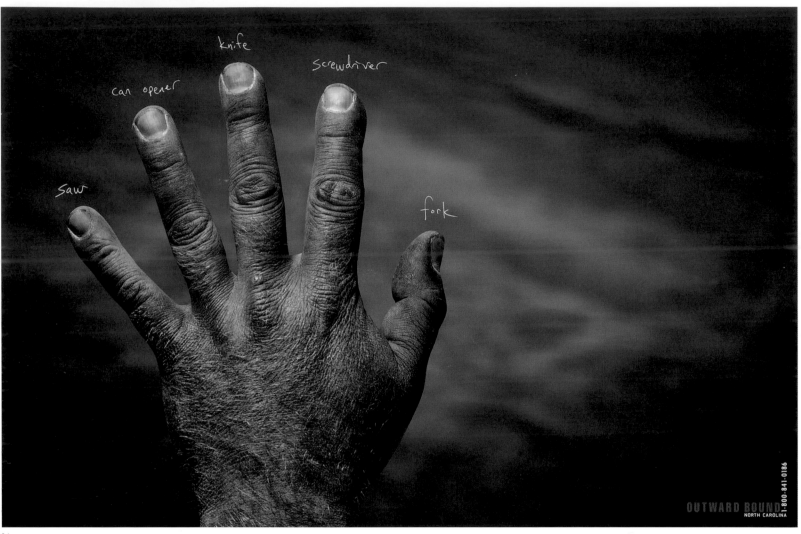

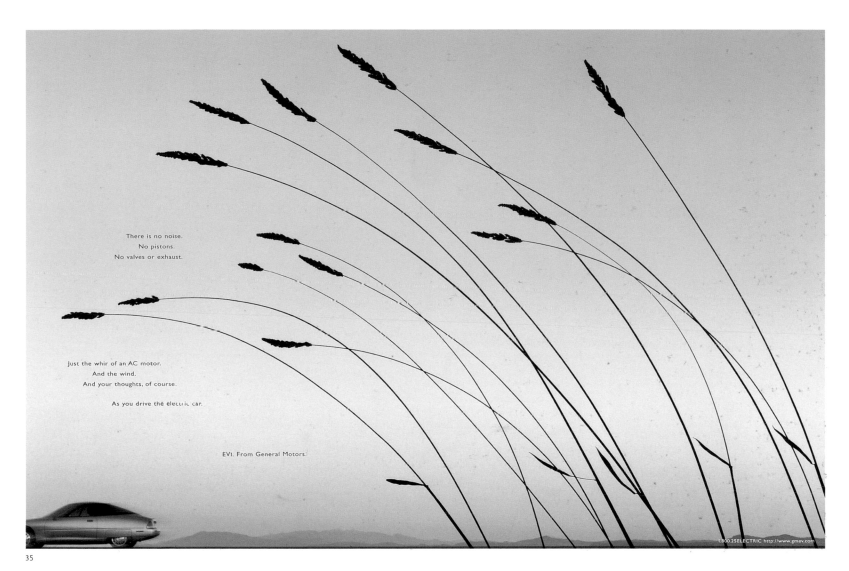

There is no noise.
No pistons.
No valves or exhaust.

Just the whir of an AC motor.
And the wind.
And your thoughts, of course.

As you drive the electric car.

EV1. From General Motors.

1.800.25ELECTRIC http://www.gmev.com

35

34. OUTWARD BOUND
LOEFFLER KETCHUM
MOUNTJOY, CHARLOTTE,
NORTH CAROLINA, 1997
To promote this wilderness
survival program, ads used
simple imagery to show how a
few days in the woods can change
the way you look at things.

35. GENERAL MOTORS EV-1
HAL RINEY & PARTNERS,
SAN FRANCISCO, 1996
A series of ads for the EV-1
electric car conveyed the
picture of serenity, making the
clean, quiet car seem at one
with nature.

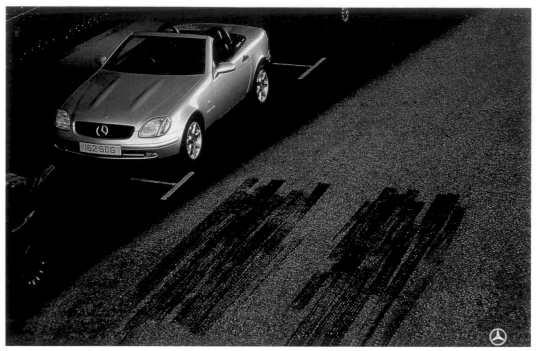

36

and say right away, 'Oh, yes, I get it.'" To this segment of the audience, Davis says, "a lot of the information that used to seem essential in ads now just seems too literal and unnecessary."

Is there no place left, then, for the word-smith in advertising? In fact there is and no doubt will be in the future. As ad historians note, every time someone pronounces ad copy dead, it makes a comeback; advertising loves to contradict itself. However, the ad writers of today are not so much persuaders and closers as they are storytellers; their writing strives to evoke emotion in the same way that powerful imagery does. Resorts to logic are minimized, in favor of reciting from-the-heart poetry for Nike, or spin-ning yarns about the people who work in the factories for Dr. Martens shoes. And even these ads are becoming rarities in the new landscape.

There are those within the business who worry about the diminishing role of copy in advertising and blame it on short attention

spans and MTV. But the trend can also be viewed as a step forward for advertising—a movement away from overexplaining, from the salesman's tendency to talk endlessly about product features and benefits that are not all that special or different from those of the competition. It has been a struggle for adver-tising's creators to distill and edit down their communications; the client almost always wants to say more, not less. As BBH's Hegarty points out, "Most advertising tries to say too much and ends up doing less. Writing less and saying more requires confidence and courage." If that's so, the new visual language is not only bolder but braver.

At the same time, it provides a fascinating shorthand for what is happening in the culture at any given moment. You could read a long-winded essay about the violence in today's video games—but all you need to see is the American agency Crispin Porter + Bogusky's "bloody

windshield" ad to get the point. You could listen to endless pontification on the baby boomers' desperate attempts to cling to their youth—or just look at that Mercedes "rubber duck" ad. Moreover, these ad signposts don't just tell us about our own particular culture; as Amster Yard's Weiss observes, this new strain of advertising acknowledges that people around the world share certain ideas, values, and interests—something that "old" advertising never believed. "Advertising used to try to identify differences in cultures, and then create ads for each group based on those differences," Weiss says. "Now advertising tends to look for the likenesses in cultures—and then communicates those ideas visually." Perhaps the best thing about the new visual language of advertising, however, is that it invites us to solve the puzzle and take part in the process of advertising—leaving room, as Gossage said, for the mouse.

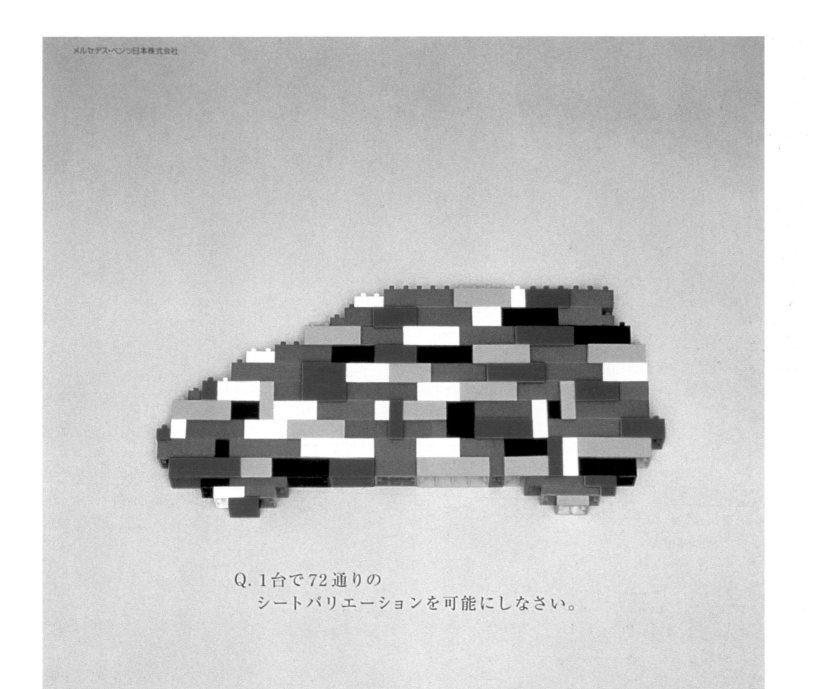

メルセデス・ベンツ日本株式会社

Q. 1台で72通りの
シートバリエーションを可能にしなさい。

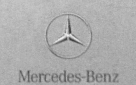

Mercedes-Benz

A NEW VISUAL LANGUAGE EMERGES.

4. THE CI
NEW W
COMMI

NEMATIC
AVE OF
RCIALS.

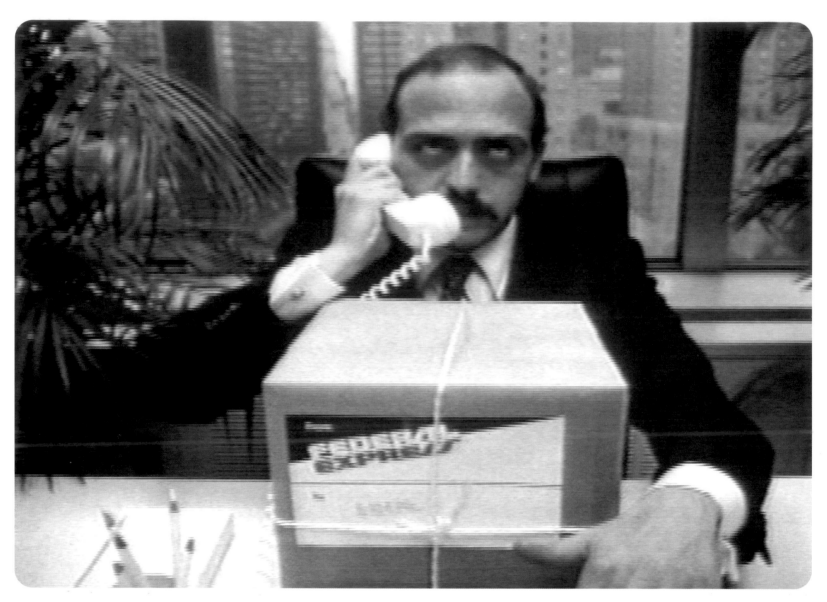

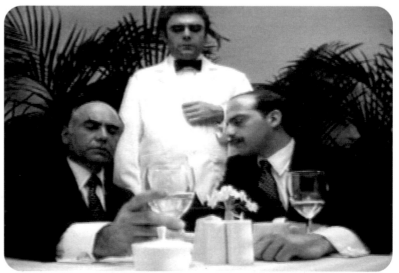

1. FEDERAL EXPRESS
ALLY & GARGANO,
NEW YORK, 1981
Director Joe Sedelmaier brought
quirky characters to life in thirty
seconds, including this courier
company's "fast-talking man" in
the early 1980s.

2. ALKA-SELTZER
DOYLE DANE BERNBACH,
NEW YORK, 1970
Howard Zieff, who directed
some of the earliest cinematic
commercials during the 1960s,
scored a huge hit with the
"Spicy Meatball" ad of the 1970s.

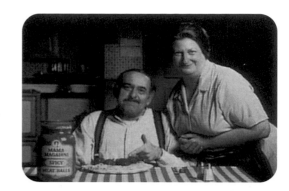

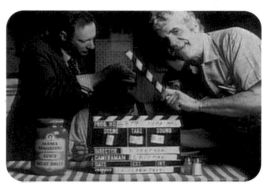

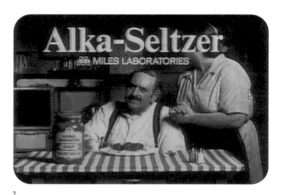

2

The power of a great print ad often lies in its simplicity: one central idea, elegantly or cleverly expressed. It is advertising in its purest form, and it can be highly effective. But it is not a story.

It was in the medium of television that advertisers were able to take the message and add movement, layers, characters, and stories that came to life in a minute or less. Gradually, the best commercials seemed to transcend television, becoming more cinematic in style and scope. Unlike so many episodic TV shows, a commercial could tell a complete tale, with a point to it. At the same time, a commercial's characters, seen only in brief glimpses, might have a certain mystery about them (what exactly *was* the relationship between those two slackers who put that smelly old chair in the back of their Volkswagen?), which could help to make them more memorable than those legions of cookie-cutter sitcom characters who come and

go each television season. As for style, a high-quality commercial's elaborate sets, innovative camerawork, and at times stupefying special effects tend to have much more in common with film than with television.

It wasn't always so. Commercials in their early days could be charming but were the most rudimentary type of TV fare: In many cases, advertisers were simply presenting on-camera testimonials and demonstrations (the demos, in rare instances, could be dramatic, as in Timex's "Takes a licking and keeps on ticking" campaign, which shot live footage of stunts such as cliff diving), or dancing cartoon characters. Commercials were often shot live, with little or nothing added in the way of production values. With no real story or film style, the early commercials were essentially just print ads brought to TV, often shot by industrial-film directors and TV-show cameramen.

But that began to change during the Creative

Revolution of the 1960s. As agency copywriters and art directors began coming up with richer, more complex concepts that evolved beyond conventional sales pitches, testimonials, and demonstrations, they saw the need to bring the ideas alive, visually, in commercials. That would require talented commercial directors, and the first wave of them included a number of still photographers, led by Howard Zieff. They were visual stylists who "began to bring the beautiful, lush look of print ads to commercials," noted the longtime *Advertising Age* journalist Anthony Vagnoni, a student of the commercial-production world. Vagnoni notes that these photo artists also had a great eye for casting characters; rather than using models or celebrities, they brought to the screen talented actors and quirky faces, such as the owlish Jack Gilford, who became the star of Cracker Jack commercials. Moreover, what quickly became apparent was that this new generation of commercial directors had a latent

THE CINEMATIC NEW WAVE OF COMMERCIALS.

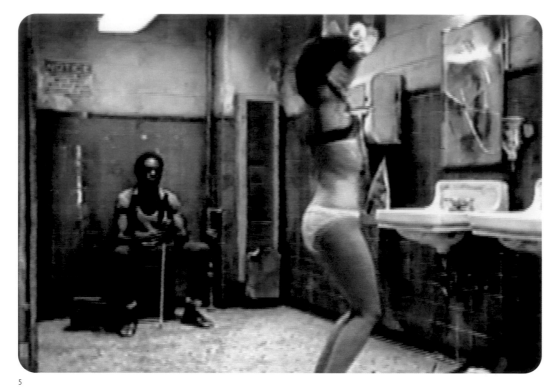

5

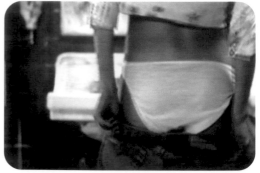

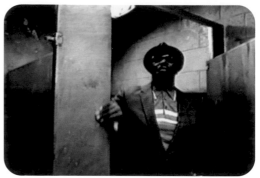

5. **LEVI STRAUSS EUROPE**
BARTLE BOGLE HEGARTY,
LONDON, 1996
By the 1990's European directors
like Tarsem Singh were telling
stories without dialogue. In
"Washroom," a woman on the
run must make a quick-change
and assumes the man in the
room is blind (he is not).

6. **SMIRNOFF VODKA**
LOWE HOWARD SPINK,
LONDON, 1993
Tarsem Singh created a wordless ad in which people and
objects are magically transformed when viewed through the
looking glass of a vodka bottle.

date—a singing, dancing Michael Jackson extravaganza that borrowed its style from a Giraldi music video done previously for Jackson.

While the Hollywood-style blockbuster commercial was taking center stage in America, an art-film style of commercial-making was emerging in Great Britain, led by a group of cinematic auteurs like Ridley Scott (best known at the time for directing the 1982 film *Blade Runner*), his brother Tony Scott, Alan Parker, Adrian Lyne, and Hugh Hudson. A number of these directors cut their teeth producing commercials in the basement of the renowned British ad agency Collett Dickenson Pearce, where they developed a different sensibility from that seen in American commercials; British ads could be darker, moodier, more experimental. They were being made by directors who had one foot in the film world. While Americans like Sedelmaier, Horn, and Levine were dedicated

full-time to commercials, the British directors easily traversed the boundaries between movies and ads. In the UK, it seemed, there was no stigma attached to shooting ads, as there was still in the U.S. at that time—perhaps because by the 1980s, commercials in England were generally considered wittier and more stylish than most American advertising, and had earned the respect of the public and the film community. The same would eventually happen in America, with Hollywood embracing ad directors—but not until later, in the 1990s. And the Brits, interestingly enough, would play a significant role in making commercials respectable in Hollywood.

Ridley Scott, in particular, became a pivotal figure in this phenomenon. Scott had first made his mark in British commercials with his stylish work for Benson & Hedges cigarettes. Gradually, his commercials began having an impact in other countries, too: One of his most famous

was a 1979 commercial titled "Share the Fantasy," for Chanel Nº 5 perfume. The spot was awash in atmospheric mystery: As a woman sat poolside, a man appeared at the far end and began to swim toward her, while a voice-over purred, "I am made of blue sky and golden light, and I will feel this way forever." The ambiguity of the commercial (was the man real?) seemed to work in its favor, if you didn't find it too pretentious. American commercial producers took notice, and before long Scott and other British directors were being brought over to inject art-film style into American ads.

One of Scott's most important new clients in America was an upstart computer company named Apple. The company's co-founder Steve Jobs and its stellar Los Angeles ad agency, Chiat/Day, sensed that a seminal moment had arrived in America. The computer revolution was beginning to take hold, and Apple was ready to

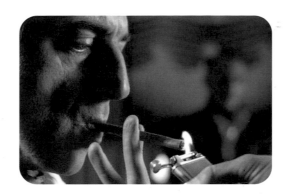

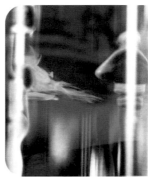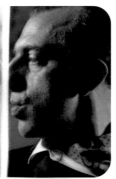

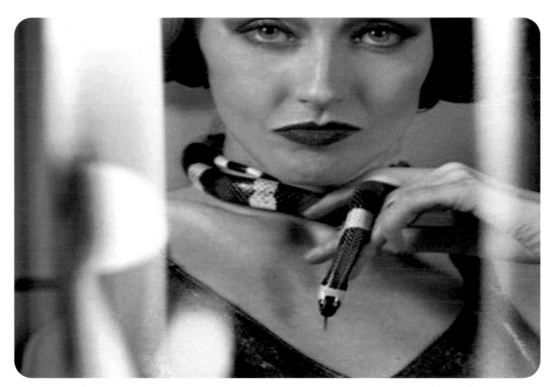

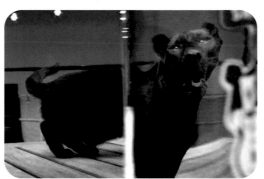

6

THE CINEMATIC NEW WAVE OF COMMERCIALS.

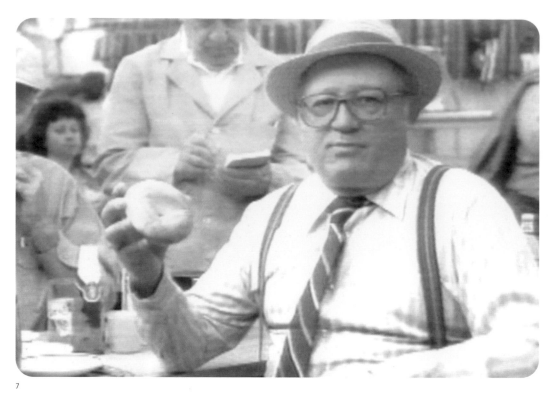

7

7. **BARTLES & JAYMES**
HAL RINEY & PARTNERS,
SAN FRANCISCO, 1985
Director Joe Pytka introduced
two deadpan characters named
Frank and Ed to promote these
wine cooler drinks in the U.S. in
the mid-1980s.

8. **HBO NETWORK**
BBDO, NEW YORK, 1996
In this Emmy Award-winning Joe
Pytka commercial, famous lines
from movies (as in "I'm mad as
hell and I'm not going to take
it anymore!" from *Network*)
sprang from the mouths of
animals like this chimpanzee.

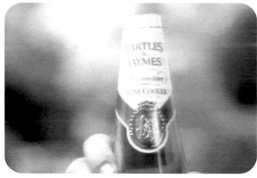

stake its own claim with an important new product, the Macintosh. At the same time, the advertising world was stirring from the creative dormancy of the late 1970s, with Chiat/Day proclaiming itself the pirate leader of the new creative movement in the 1980s. And the final ingredient in this combustible mix was Scott, an audacious filmmaker who saw no reason that an American commercial couldn't aspire to cinematic art. From all of this would emerge a commercial that ran just one time nationally—but would change advertising forever.

Viewers of pro-football's Super Bowl in January 1984, by now used to dramatic albeit coherent and generally upbeat commercials, had to be taken aback by what appeared onscreen midway through the game. The commercial opened on a futuristic, dreary scene, reminiscent of Scott's *Blade Runner,* but it quickly became apparent that it was referencing George Orwell's novel *1984:* It showed an

auditorium full of expressionless people with shaved heads mesmerized by a giant TV screen image of a Big Brother character ranting about "pure ideology" and "unification of thought." Gradually, a heroine appeared, toting a sledgehammer and running from masked authority figures; she eventually burst into the auditorium and hurled the hammer at the screen, smashing the image of Big Brother. The spot closed with the line "On January 24th, Apple Computer will introduce Macintosh and you'll see why 1984 won't be like *1984.*"

The commercial was as much of an advertising breakthrough as Volkswagen's "Think small." had been twenty years earlier, though in different ways. If Bernbach's campaign had been a triumph of logic, wit, and subtlety, "1984" relied on emotion, abstractness, and over-the-top theatricality. VW advertising always left the audience with a smile, but here was a commercial that was mysterious (was Big

Brother intended to represent IBM? If so, what nerve!), dark and gritty in tone. And yet it worked, driving $4.5 million in sales within six hours. Meanwhile, the commercial was like an adrenaline rush for advertising's creative community: In effect, the creators of the spot, Chiat/Day's Lee Clow, Steve Hayden, Brent Thomas, and Jay Chiat, were the hammer-throwers shaking up the advertising establishment. And, like the hunted character in the spot, they found themselves in peril: The client, nervous about the spot beforehand, never gave approval, but the agency and Scott completed it anyway. There were calls to fire Chiat/Day, and even a last-minute attempt by Apple to pull the plug on the spot just prior to the game. It ran only because Apple was unable to sell off the Super Bowl airtime it had purchased. The artfulness of the ad, and the sense of intrigue and legend surrounding it, all helped to fuel the cult of creativity that blossomed in advertising in the

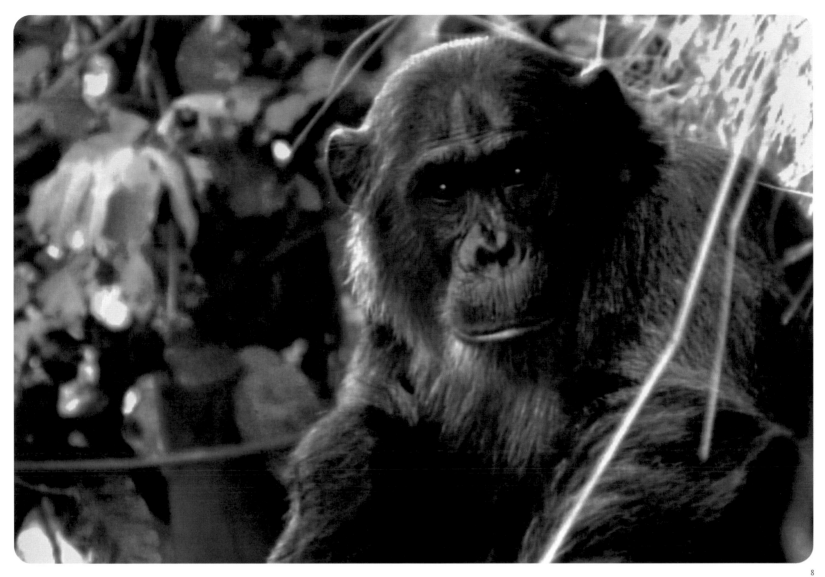

late 1980s, as young artists flocked to the offices of Chiat and other creative agencies.

The commercial had a couple of other important aftereffects: It established the Super Bowl as the premiere showcase of advertising in the United States. And it made it clear that a commercial, like a popular film, could become a national cultural event. But to create such an event, it was generally agreed, you needed not just a big idea but a big-time director like Scott. Ridley, much in demand after "1984," could do only so much ad work, however, particularly since he was pursuing a film career. By the late 1980s, a new generation of cinematic stylists and storytellers began to fill the vacuum and create the mini-movies that would often debut on a certain Sunday in January, between the punts and passes.

Leading the pack was Joe Pytka, who gradually supplanted Scott as the director that every advertiser wanted to hire. If Scott was advertising's auteur, Pytka, a native of Pittsburgh,

Pennsylvania, became the ad world's Spielberg, blending stylistic film vision with a common touch. There was nothing, it seemed, he couldn't do. He shot lush, warm-and-fuzzy vineyard landscapes for Gallo wine, but for the same client he produced a hilarious bit of banter between a couple of deadpan characters named Bartles and Jaymes. (On all of these spots, Pytka worked for the West Coast adman Hal Riney—one of the ad-agency pioneers in the advancement of richly cinematic commercials.) Pytka could evoke an ethereal world of streams and frolicking French schoolchildren for Perrier, or he could present cold, hard-edged slice-of-life scenes for the John Hancock insurance company. He was a master storyteller, as evidenced by the 1985 Pepsi spot "Archaeology"; in it, an archaeologist of the future embarks on a dig and uncovers a relic—which, it gradually becomes clear, is a Coke bottle. But Pytka could also do song-and-dance bits, built around musical stars like Ray Charles

(the famous "Uh-huh" commercials for Pepsi) or celebrity athletes like Bo Jackson, whom he immortalized in the frenetic commercial "Bo Knows." Lacking a star, Pytka could succeed with chimpanzees; a memorable HBO ad featured apes mouthing famous lines from movies, such as "I'm mad as hell and I'm not going to take it anymore," from the 1976 film *Network*. And if you couldn't afford a trained animal, Pytka could make an interesting ad out of an egg frying in a pan: he did just that in the memorable public-service commercial that declared, "This is your brain on drugs. Any questions?". All of this made him an advertiser's dream, though he was also, quite often, an agency or client's worst nightmare: Continuing in the Sedelmaier tradition, Pytka demanded complete control over his commercials, and—as an intimidating man who was a muscular six-foot-six with a shock of wild hair—he was known to frighten clients or agency creatives who tried to interfere too much.

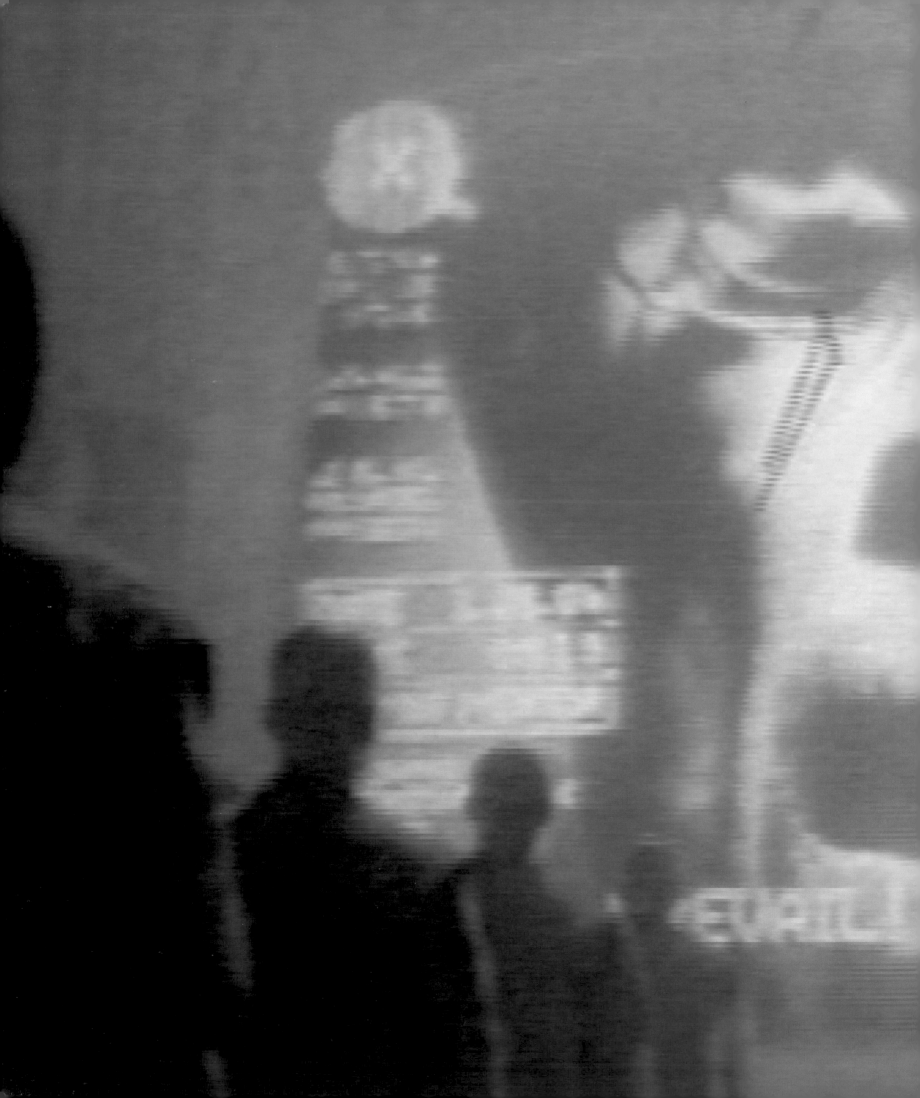

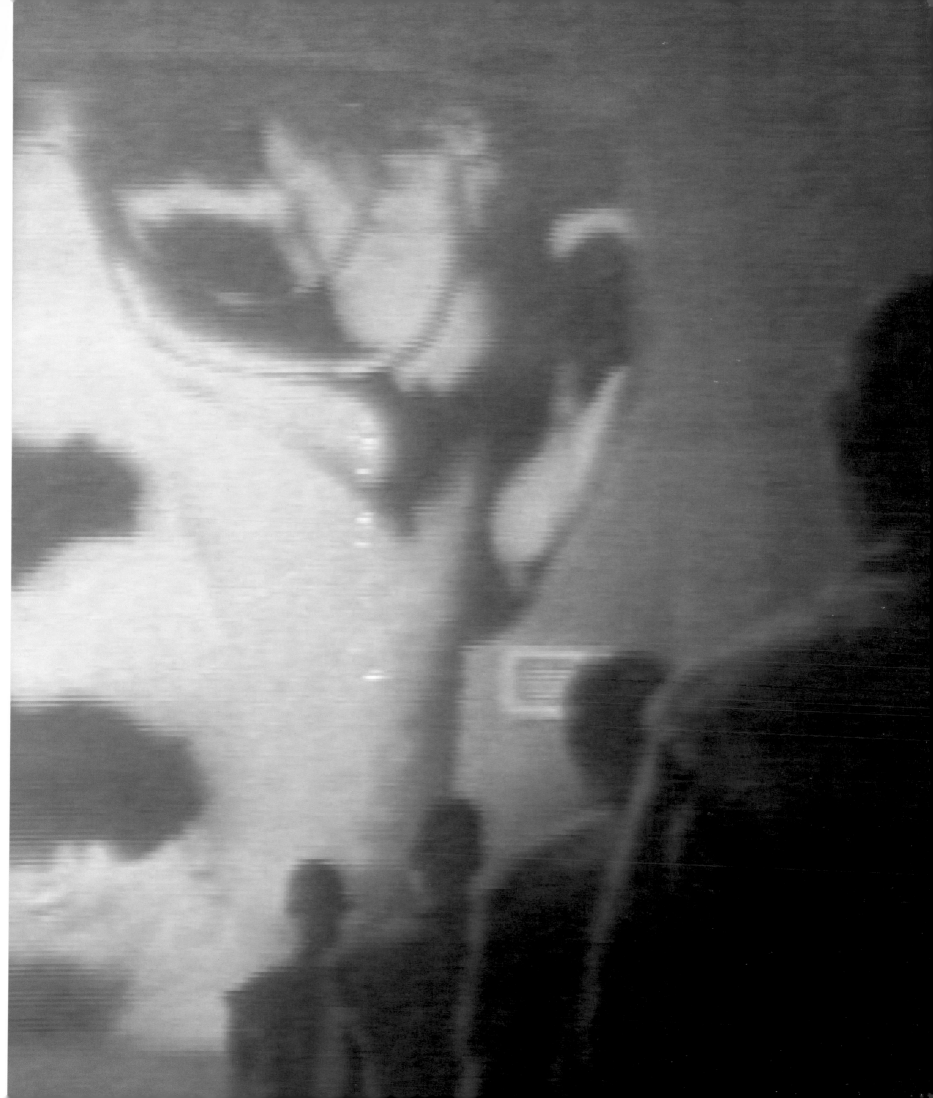

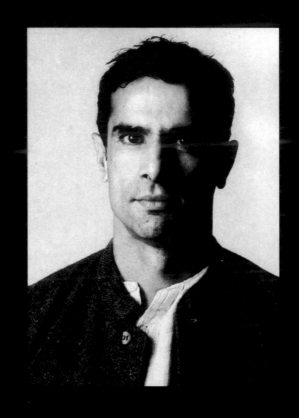

INTERVIEW: TARSEM SINGH

Born and raised in India, Tarsem Singh became one of the most sought-after commercial directors in Europe during the 1990s. His highly cinematic, storytelling commercials for Levi's, Nike, Coca-Cola, and other brands include some of the most stylistic and memorable ads ever put on film. Intended for a visually sophisticated modern international audience, Tarsem's commercials rarely feature any type of sales pitch—or any dialogue at all. And they can be mysterious and unsettling. One chilling Smirnoff ad used a vodka bottle as a window to the inner nature of characters walking through the scene (a normal-looking passerby was revealed to be a serpent when viewed through the bottle). For Nike in Amsterdam, Tarsem staged an epic soccer game between the forces of good and evil—and created perhaps the most frighteningly realistic Mephistopheles ever to show his face in an ad. In 2000, the director released his first feature film, *The Cell*.

DOES COMMERCIAL DIRECTING TODAY REPRESENT THE STATE OF THE ART IN TERMS OF FILM TECHNIQUE?

Yes, it's usually ahead of where feature films are. Movie effects that people say are cutting-edge as in *The Matrix,* are actually happening in advertising at least five or six years beforehand. It used to be that a lot of the directing technique coming into advertising started out in music videos—but right now the budgets for music videos seem to have gone lower and lower, so a lot of the technical stuff has gone out of them.

YOU RECENTLY MADE YOUR FIRST MOVIE. DO YOU THINK COMMERCIAL DIRECTORS MAKE GOOD FILM DIRECTORS?

Not necessarily. The classic problem of people coming from advertising and trying to do films is that the sum is less than the parts. A commercial director may shoot a lot of great scenes, but the whole movie doesn't seem to be greater than the scenes. There are exceptions. If you look at [director Ridley Scott's film] *Alien*, the small scenes are great but the whole film is also a great film that climaxes.

YOUR COMMERCIALS HAVE OFTEN BEEN WORDLESS AND AT TIMES RATHER SURREAL. IS THAT YOUR PREFERRED STYLE?

They have been more visual than anything else. That was the kind of work I wanted to do, and it's the reason I went to Europe as opposed to doing ads in America. In America, the emphasis is first on comedy and second on dialogue. I wasn't interested in doing commercials that were all about dialogue. And the only place that allowed you to work visually is Europe—because there, when you create an ad it has to be able to run two hundred miles away, where people don't speak the same language. So the idea has to be done visually. When I started working on Levi's in Europe, I found that this was the kind of advertising they were looking for. And it kind of became like the days of silent cinema. What I also like more about European advertising is that you're usually doing the sixty-second format, not thirty seconds. I think sixty seconds is the amount of time needed to at least get some sort of feeling into something.

HOW MUCH DO YOU THINK THAT COMING FROM INDIA HAS INFLUENCED YOUR STYLE?

I would say quite a bit. I came to America when I was twenty-five. Before that all my upbringing was Indian. I ended up with the techniques of the West. But the color and eye coordination of the Indian cinema—which are very vibrant—have somehow come creeping into my work. It's not something I was aware of until I sat back and watched my reel and thought, "You know what? This doesn't look very American." And somehow that's come from my background being what it is. I never sat down and said, "I'm Indian, so this will have to be done a certain way."

WOULD YOU SAY THERE'S A MYSTICAL SIDE TO YOUR WORK THAT COMES OUT OF THAT BACKGROUND? SOME OF YOUR COMMERCIALS SEEM OTHERWORLDLY.

I've been an atheist since fifth grade. So I wouldn't say there's a mystical side to what I do. But the visual aspects of religious themes interest me, not religion itself. If it's something you grow up around, as I did, then it

probably influences you even if you aren't aware of it. In the West, I have a slightly different perspective than the next guy because my upbringing is so different from the people here.

TO WHAT EXTENT ARE TOP DIRECTORS SUCH AS YOURSELF IN CONTROL OF THE ADVERTISING PROCESS? ARE YOU GIVEN A LOT OF FREEDOM BY THE AGENCIES AND THE CLIENTS?

I have been, which is great for me. If the commercial is visual, I want the agency to present the idea to me in one line. If you can give me the idea that simply, then it's my job to plot it out and create the storyboards. I've never done a commercial where someone gave me a step-by-step storyboard and then I just shot it. I tell them, "No, you need to put your idea down in one line, and I'll make the visuals work for it." For instance, on the Smirnoff ad, the agency gave me a brief that said, "Smirnoff is an alternative world inside a bottle." That's the kind of brief I'm looking for. I can bring everything to it.

ARE CLIENTS EVER CONCERNED THAT YOUR WORK IS TOO ABSTRACT?

Almost never. Because I don't think a client would come to me for hard sell. My commercial reel is such that you wouldn't think of me if you had to do a commercial about getting a cold and it's just full of people coughing. And I made a conscious effort in the beginning of my career, starting with the show reel I made in school, to let people know the kind of work I do. If you're looking for hard sell, a million guys can do that. I wanted to position myself as something else.

DO YOU THINK OF ADS AS BEING AN ART FORM?

I think *art* is a four-letter word. I never use it for anything; it means too many different things to me. There are some photographs that I think are artistic and some commercials I think are artistic, but I don't know what that word really means. It's used so loosely that anytime someone calls something art, I just think it's the kiss of death.

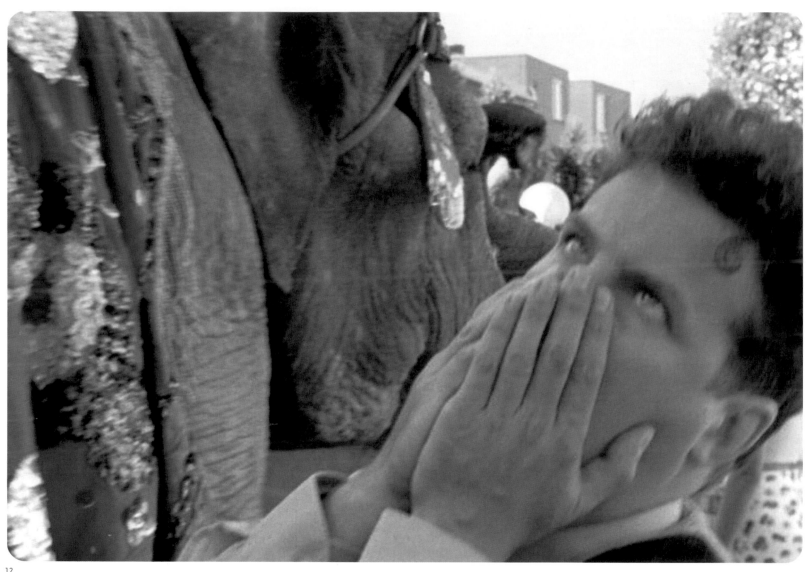

12

12. ROLOS
AMMIRATI PURIS LINTAS,
AMSTERDAM, 1995
Director Rogier van der Ploeg
spun a tale of a lifetime in thirty
seconds: A bratty child is mean
to an elephant, and many years
later, the elephant gets even.

13. COCA-COLA
FALLON McELLIGOTT,
MINNEAPOLIS, MINNESOTA,
1994
Another "silent film" from
director Tarsem Singh, this time
featuring a swimming elephant
who journeys to a float, deposits
some peanuts, takes a Coke,
and leaves.

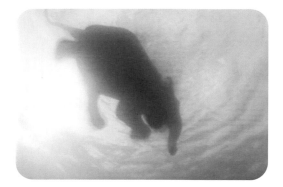

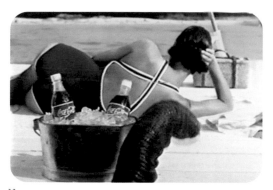

13

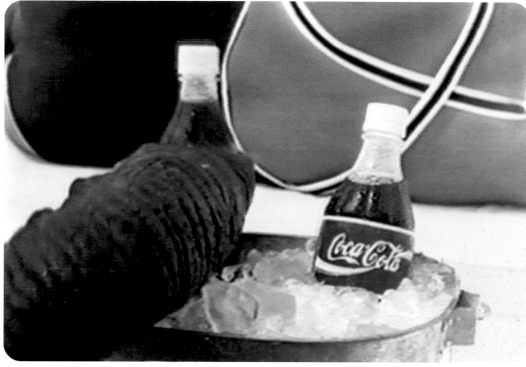

as by the surrealism of Salvador Dalí and David Lynch. And so one could expect just about anything in a Tarsem commercial; for an MTV Asia promotion, he once filmed a live animal sacrifice, shot with an overhead camera as a slaughtered lamb bled to death and traditional Indian music played in the background (the spot never ran). His subsequent work was more tranquil, though no less mesmerizing: For Coca-Cola, he constructed an entire commercial around muted scenes of an elephant swimming, with much of the ad shot from beneath the water. As advertising was becoming more of a global form of communication in the 1990s, Tarsem was the ideal international ad director; his wordless, dreamlike commercials needed no translation—which is not to say they didn't leave some viewers baffled.

In Europe, where Tarsem was doing much of his best work, a number of other directorial talents flourished. The French, always at the forefront in cinema trends, produced some important "new wave" commercials, most notably from the director Jean Paul Goude, whose Perrier commercial featuring a feral woman and a lion facing off over a bottle of water became the talk of the Cannes advertising festival. In Germany, home-bred filmmakers like Wim Wenders tried their hand at commercial-making, with the kind of interesting results one would expect. And Dutch directors like Rogier van der Ploeg proved adept at visual storytelling with commercials like the Rolos candy classic "Elephant"—in which a bratty young boy taunts an elephant and then pays the price many years later when the elephant in a passing parade, spots the grown-up man in the crowd and remembers.

Back in the UK, some of the directors who earlier had helped launch the wave of cinematic commercials continued to flourish, including Hugh Hudson—who produced the most winning smile ever seen in an advertisement. Hudson

choreographed four thousand people, wearing red, white, and blue caps, to form a giant living face shot from overhead by an airborne camera; the movements of the crowd then change the image, by adding first a smile and then a wink; further movement transforms the face into a living map of the world, to make the point that British Airways "brings people together" from around the world. Not all British commercials were as feel-good as that one; the work of Tony Kaye—who emerged as one of the hottest British directors of the late 1980s and early 1990s—could be downright disturbing and at times bewildering. One of Kaye's best-known commercials, for Dunlop tires, featured a nightmarish fantasy in which a car driving alone on the road is terrorized by a Buddha-like demon and his evil army, as they set all manner of deadly traps and obstacles in the car's path. In *Advertising Age*, Vagnoni called the commercial "arguably the most surreal, abstract bit of

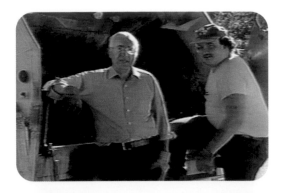

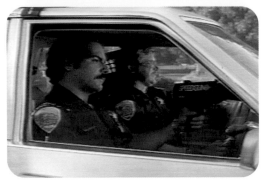

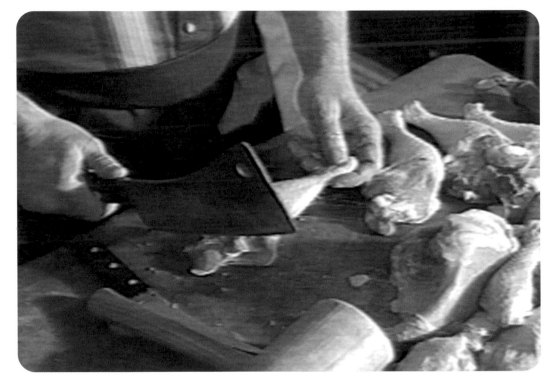

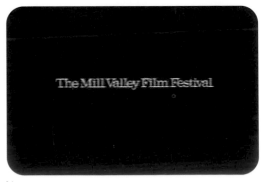

14

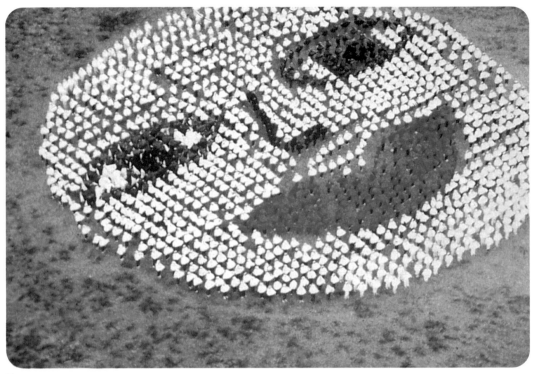

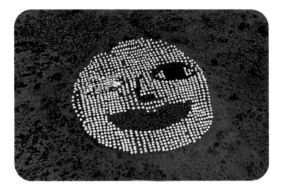

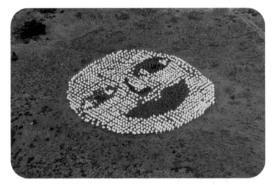

15

**14. MILL VALLEY
FILM FESTIVAL**
GOODBY BERLIN &
SILVERSTEIN,
SAN FRANCISCO, 1983
This early 1980s commercial
was among the first to blend
satire with cinema verité-style
camerawork. A decade later,
the "mockumentary" approach
was much in vogue.

15. BRITISH AIRWAYS
SAATCHI & SAATCHI,
LONDON, 1990
"Happy Face," directed by Hugh
Hudson, was an amazing bit of
choreography in which thousands
of people form a human face,
then make the eye wink.

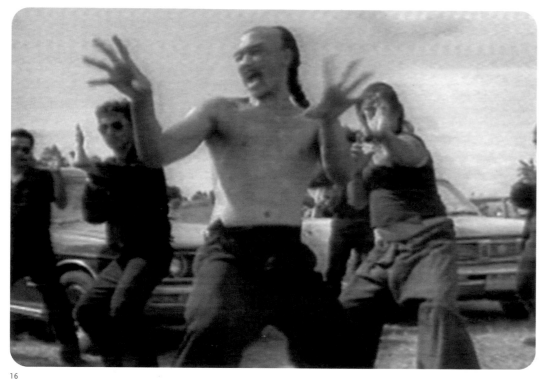

16

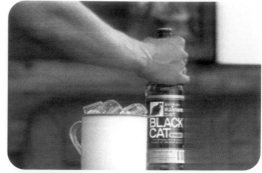

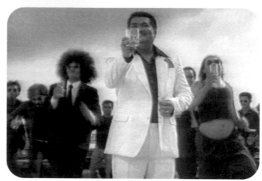

16. **BLACK CAT WHISKEY**
OGILVY & MATHER, BANGKOK, 1996
This commercial brought the kung-fu theatrics of Asian film to ads, in a wild story about gangsters and street rumbles.

17. **HEINEKEN**
BATES HONG KONG, 2000
The American film director Oliver Stone shot this Asian commercial in which a key bit of dialogue is obscured by the sound of a blender. Stone is one of many film directors who have "crossed over" into advertising.

impressionism ever produced by a major agency for a major brand." The stunning visual power of the ad did not happen by accident; Kaye shot the commercial in black-and-white, then computer-colored it, frame by frame, to achieve the most vibrant effect. To some this was evidence of Kaye's genius, while to others it demonstrated that commercials were perhaps becoming overstylized and self-indulgent (it didn't help that Kaye was yet another enfant terrible of the ad-directing fraternity, known for spending huge sums in production, refusing to compromise on the content of his ads, and engaging in eccentric behavior; once, when he was chosen to give the prestigious Design & Art Directors president's lecture in London, Kaye stunned the audience by appearing onstage dressed as a Hasidic Jew and singing "My Way").

By the mid-1990s, it was clear that Kaye, Tarsem, and others had ushered in what Vagnoni called "the age of the visual stylist—

in which the commercial is no longer so much about great storytelling or memorable characters, but instead is all about sumptuous images that stay in your mind."

Hollywood soon realized that the power of those images could extend beyond commercials and into feature films. By the late 1990s, Kaye, Tarsem, David Fincher, and the fast-rising ad director Kinka Usher were being signed up for movies. The lines between Hollywood and Madison Avenue were coming down; not only were commercial directors making films, but highly regarded filmmakers like Joel and Ethan Coen, Oliver Stone, and Errol Morris were bringing their talents to ads. Some worried about the effect the commercial directors might be having on feature films; the director Michael Bay, who made the transition from directing Coke and Levi's ads to shooting big-budget Hollywood blockbuster movies like *Armageddon,* was cited by some as living proof that ad

directors would suck the substance right out of films. "The problem is that in commercials, you're trained to tell a story visually in thirty seconds," commented film director Barry Sonnenfeld. "So these guys are very good at creating a visual style and using special effects and quick-cut editing. But there's not much room in commercials for emotion or character development or plot. They often don't know how to deal with any of that."

At the same time, esteemed filmmakers were often criticized for what seemed like half-hearted efforts in advertising. Pytka, who once compiled his own reel of obscure commercials shot by Martin Scorsese, Jean-Luc Godard, and Federico Fellini, noted that the ads were "were uniformly dreadful." Why? According to Pytka, film directors often underestimate how difficult it is to make a good commercial. "They don't take it seriously," he says. "They treat the ad like a jokey scene in a movie." (There have been

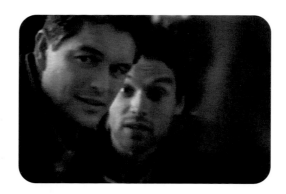

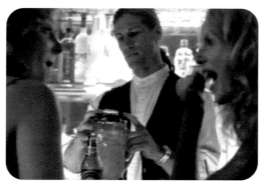

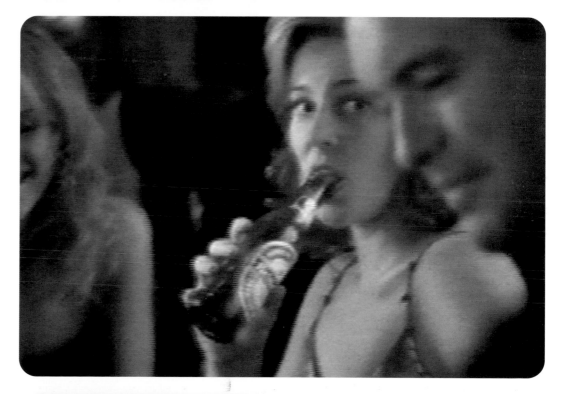

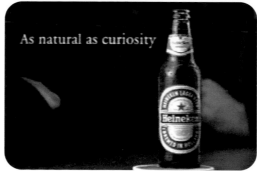

17

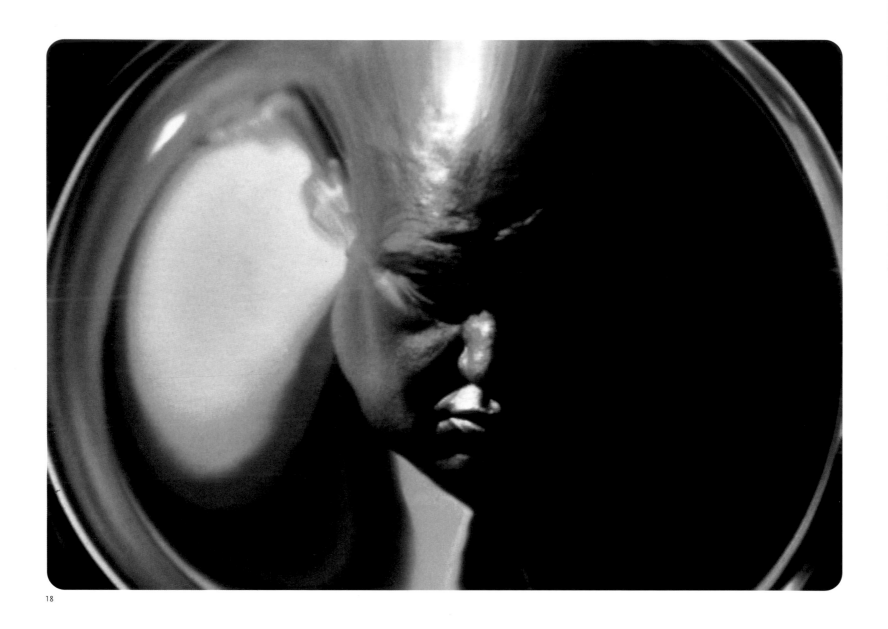

18

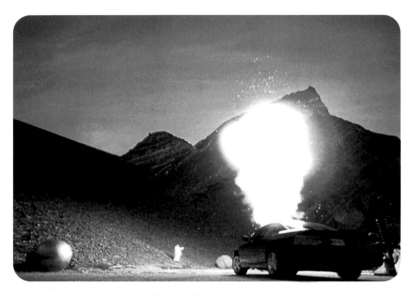
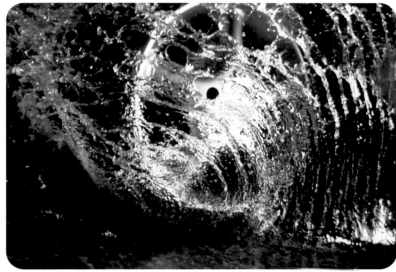
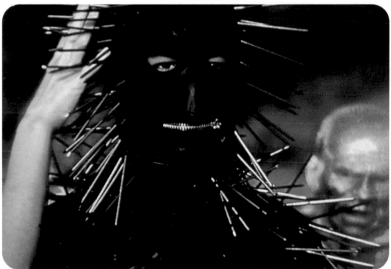
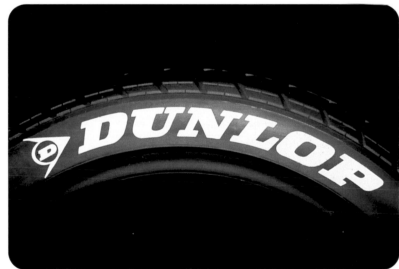

18. **DUNLOP**
ABBOTT MEAD VICKERS,
LONDON, 1993
This tire ad, from the controversial British director Tony Kaye,
featured a surreal, nightmarish
fantasy: A car on a lonely road is
terrorized by demons.

THE CINEMATIC NEW WAVE OF COMMERCIALS.

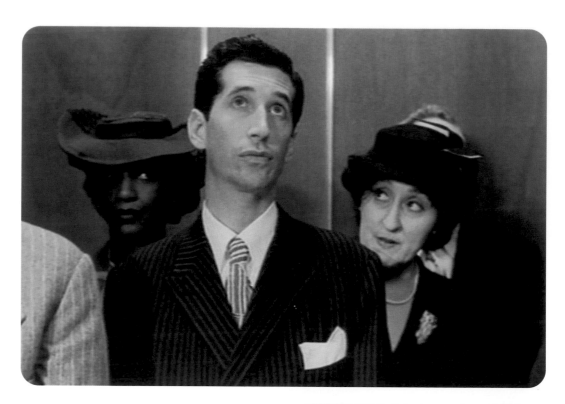

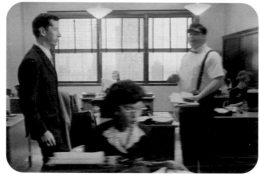

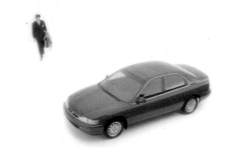

Simplify.
HONDA

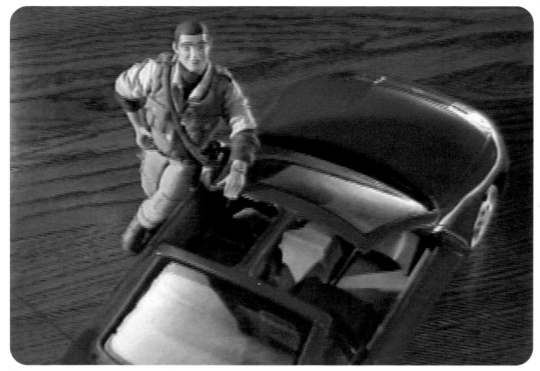

20

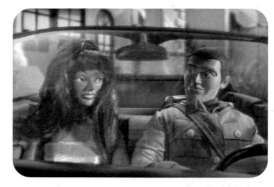

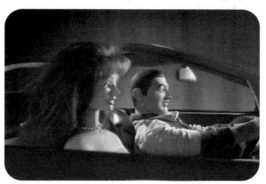

19. **HONDA**
RUBIN POSTAER &
ASSOCIATES, LOS ANGELES,
1996
Directed by Joel and Ethan Coen,
and reminiscent of their film *The
Hudsucker Proxy*, this ad features
a harried businessman who
flees to a pristine white place.

20. **NISSAN**
TBWA/CHIAT/DAY,
LOS ANGELES, 1996
"Toys" answered the question:
What would happen if G.I. Joe
hooked up with Barbie? Kinka
Usher directed it more like a
music video than an ad.

exceptions: Errol Morris's recent black-and-white commercials for Miller High Life, celebrating duct tape and all things macho, have been highly praised, as has a Honda commercial by the Coen brothers that re-created the visual style of their film *The Hudsucker Proxy*.)

Regardless of whether the new highly visual ad directors came from the world of film or cut their teeth on sales pitches, some in the ad creative community felt that these directors' emphasis on style was not necessarily good for advertising. The American creative director Greg DiNoto credits advertising's star directors with producing memorable ads but noted that their flashy approach "has hurt advertising, too, by making otherwise vacuous concepts all sparkly and beautiful and seductive and easy for agencies to sell to advertisers. All show and no go." The joke around the ad industry, by the mid-1990s, was that when an advertiser lacked an idea, the fallback plan was "Get me Pytka."

That criticism notwithstanding, the commercials that most resonated with the public in the late 1990s were style-driven, not concept-driven. The Gap's minimalist white-background commercials with swing dancers and country line dancers and sullen models singing "Mellow Yellow" to the camera were devoid of what most ad people would call a concept—they were pure style, and their effectiveness derived from the way director Matthew Rolston framed his shots, as well as from the sophisticated film techniques he used, such as stop-action film sequences in the "Swing" commercial. That technique subsequently ended up in the 1999 movie *The Matrix*, demonstrating that now the movies were borrowing tricks and techniques from the cinematic ads, instead of the other way around.

Another of the most arresting and talked-about commercials of the late 1990s was Kinka Usher's "Toys" for Nissan—in which dolls resembling G.I. Joe and Barbie race around the

living-room floor in a tiny car. Again, the spot was loved not so much because it was a strong idea as because Usher had produced a marvelous little movie, one that could be watched again and again. That commercial—and countless others like it—proved that in the new cinematic world of advertising, style *was* substance.

Meanwhile, if "Toys" exemplified the perfect advertising mini-movie, it also exhibited other traits of the new and improved commercial of the 1990s, beyond just cinematic flair. The ad borrowed from pop culture (the sound track was a song from the American rock-music group Van Halen) and from other forms of expression; it looked more like a music video than an ad. It had a hip, ironic sense of humor. And it buried the sales pitch so deeply that it was impossible to find it. All of which raised the question: Was this any way to sell cars? In the mid-to-late-1990s, advertising had not only "gone Hollywood"—it had gone thoroughly postmodern, as well.

5. NIKE
POSTMO
REVOL

AND THE
DERN AD
UTION.

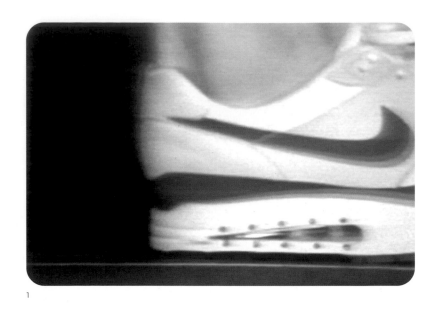

1.**NIKE**
WIEDEN + KENNEDY,
PORTLAND, 1987
The "Revolution" commercial
took the Beatles song of the
same title as its soundtrack, and
featured rapid-fire, grainy scenes.

In the 1960s and 1970s, the creative insurrectionists in New York had begun to subvert some of the conventions of advertising, replacing empty slogans and jingles with more candid and provocative statements, and injecting a strong sense of attitude and style into ads. It proved both popular and effective, and subsequently the heirs to Doyle Dane Bernbach—including British and Australian agencies that had studied Bernbach and adopted his conceptual approach, as well as the American regional agencies like Minnesota's Fallon McElligott—managed to spread the ad revolution, and in many ways advance it with their own refinements.

But they didn't radically change the new advertising model that DDB had helped invent, and by the mid-1980s, there was a restlessness in advertising, a sense that the sound concepts and clever headlines of modern ads had lost some of their ability to surprise. By this time, the consumer audience was evolving, becoming more media-literate with the arrival of MTV and other cable channels, booting up personal computers for the first time, growing hungry for sensory material that challenged it in new ways. Because of these factors—and perhaps also because advertising tends to reinvent itself every so often with bold new packaging—the business was ripe for another revolution. And Dan Wieden had the perfect anthem for it.

Wieden, a quiet Northwesterner who ran a small agency in Portland, Oregon, with his partner David Kennedy, did not seem like much of a rebel. In fact, he hadn't set out to change advertising; he drifted into the field reluctantly and apathetically, after he'd tried writing Beat poetry. "I never liked advertising," Wieden acknowledged years later. He had no taste for the glad-handing ways of the business, nor for the inanity of much of the work the industry produced. And so when he eventually began forming his own small agency, it was not surprising that Wieden would surround himself with others who shared his "anti-advertising" sensibility. His partner Kennedy, a talented art director, was a castoff from several larger agencies. One of Wieden's first hires was Jim Riswold, a perennial college student who read Nietzsche, worshiped the gender-bending rock star David Bowie, and was known to lie on the floor in his office, meditating. Wieden's agency was a small group of advertising misfits located somewhere northwest of nowhere, registering not even a blip on Madison Avenue's radar. Until, that is, the debut of Wieden + Kennedy's first major national TV commercial for its new client Nike, appropriately titled "Revolution."

The commercial featured rapid-fire, grainy scenes that seemed to have been edited almost randomly. For consumers used to seeing slickly produced commercials with linear story lines, there was the shock of the raw; you had to

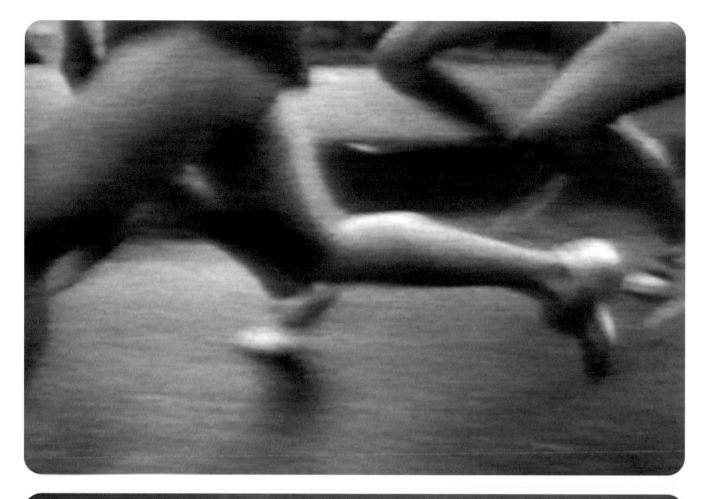

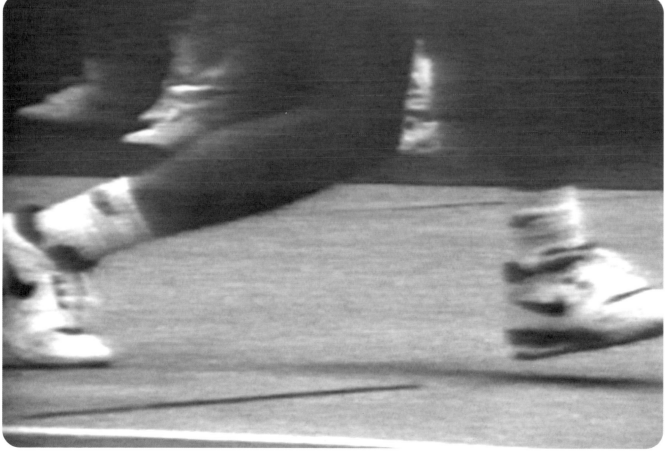

NIKE AND THE POSTMODERN AD REVOLUTION.

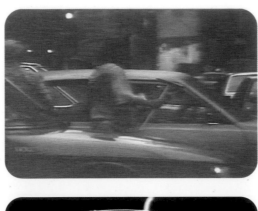

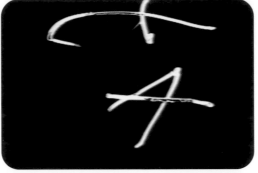

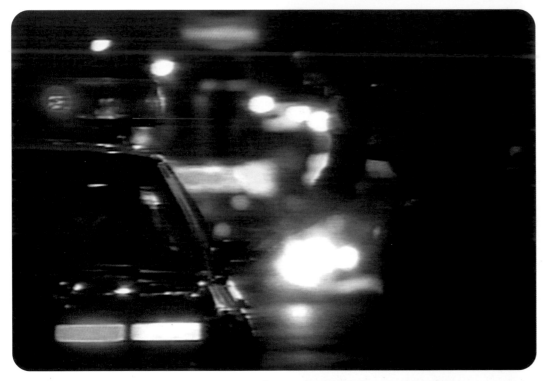

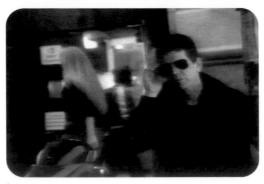

2

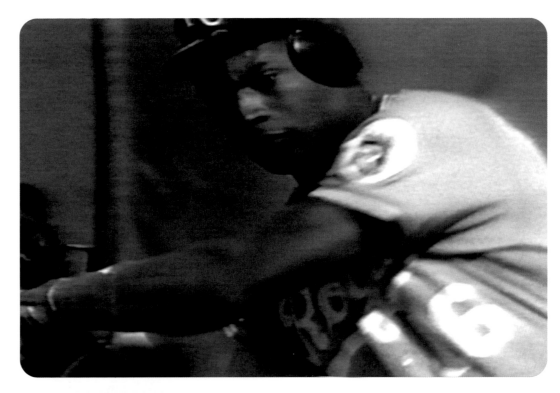

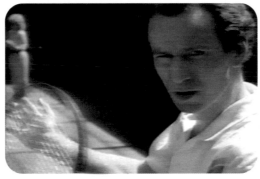

3

squint to see what was going on. There was no voice-over, and in fact the commercial contained no words at all, a radical departure (*Where was the sales pitch?*). Perhaps the most striking thing about it was the sound track: Wieden + Kennedy played the famous Beatles song "Revolution," which immediately stirred controversy. From a legal standpoint, there was haggling and an eventual lawsuit over rights to the song (which had been purchased from Michael Jackson, who had previously obtained rights to some of the Beatles' music). But the real debate triggered by the spot was not so much legal as cultural: What right did advertising have to co-opt a Beatles song, and particularly this song, which was an anti-establishment, countercultural anthem?

It was only the beginning of a debate that would continue for years, with Wieden + Kennedy in the thick of it. With the "Revolution" ad, the agency signaled to the world that adver-

tising in the late 1980s and subsequently in the 1990s was about to stake new ground—right at the center of American and world culture. In the ads that followed from W+K and other hip agencies, there was a tendency to borrow freely from sources that previously had been off-limits to advertising—not just rock-and-roll but literature, film, art, history. These new complex commercials were dubbed "postmodern advertising" by some journalists and academics because they seemed to share many of the identifying characteristics of postmodern art and architecture—they mixed old and new styles, borrowed from other forms of communication, blended high and low culture, deconstructed themselves, were filled with inside references, and often adopted an ironic and self-aware tone.

"Revolution" was the noisiest shot, but in fact, Wieden had been experimenting with a new kind of advertising a couple of years earlier

for a smaller client, Honda Scooters. Partly by accident and partly from gut instinct, the agency created a commercial in 1984 that seemed to break the mold at the time—though the ad is now largely unknown or forgotten outside advertising circles. Like "Revolution," the Honda Scooter ad used grainy film footage and a hip sound track (in this case, Lou Reed's provocative "Walk on the Wild Side") with no sales pitch. The star, Reed—an underground American rock musician with a bad reputation and a complete lack of affect—was about as unlikely a commercial endorser as one might find. The ad came about more or less by happenstance: Riswold was a fan of the musician and wanted to use him, for fun. As for the rough, cinema-verité film look, it was patched together in the editing room—partly because of problems with the original film that was shot. Wieden recalls that when his producer Larry Bridges finished editing the spot and

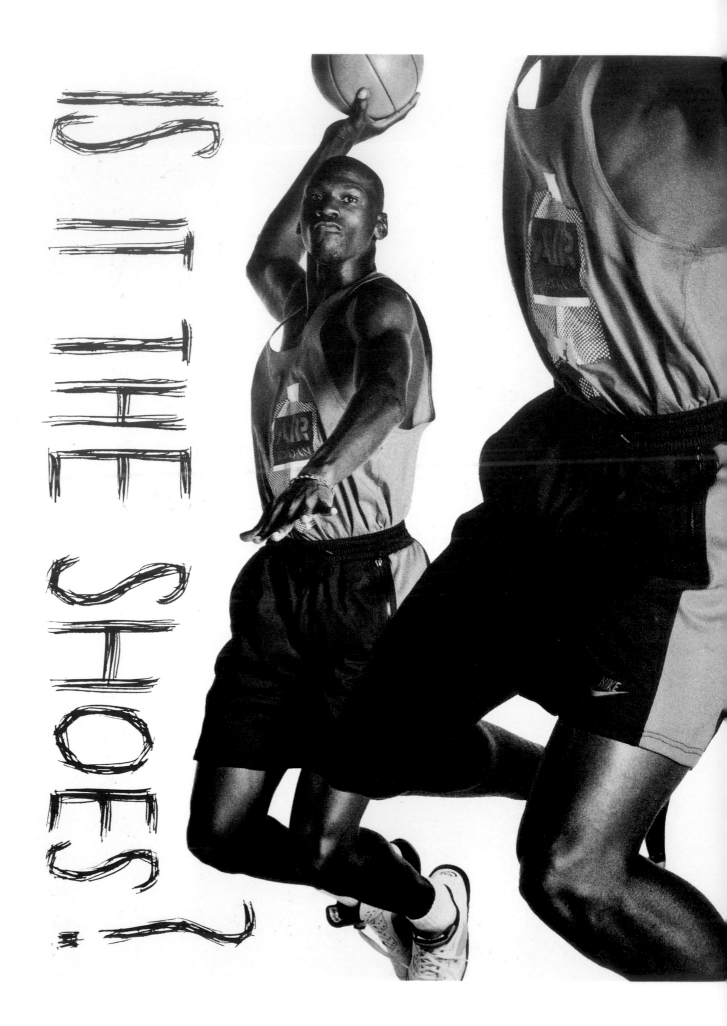

IS IT THE SHOES?

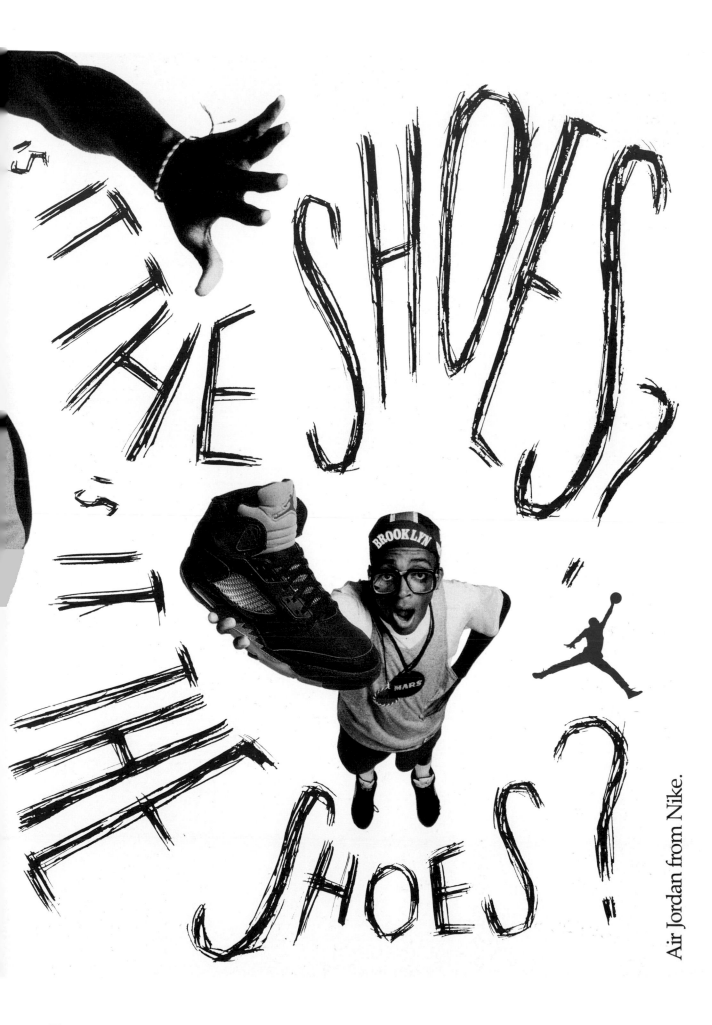

IS IT THE SHOES? IS IT THE SHOES?

Air Jordan from Nike.

NIKE AND THE POSTMODERN AD REVOLUTION.

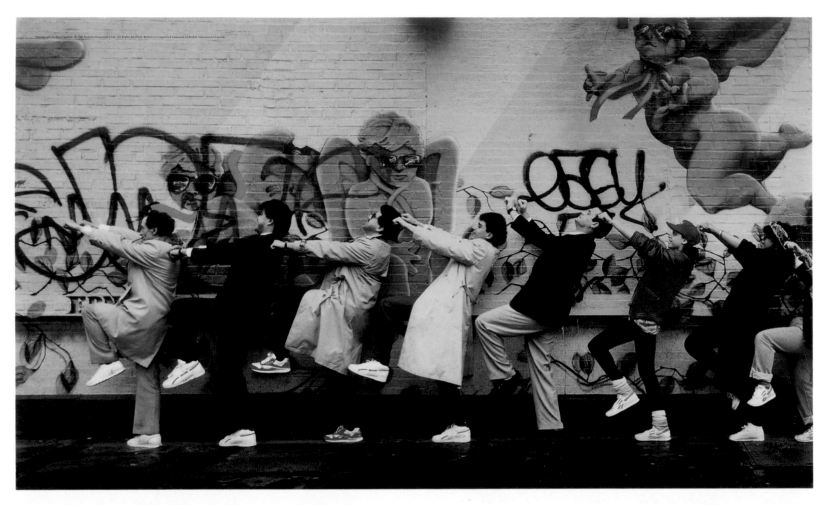

REEBOKS LET U.B.U.

Reebok 🏴󠁧󠁢󠁥󠁮󠁧󠁿

5

showed him the rough cut, "We just looked at each other and said, 'Jiminy Christmas, what the hell is that?' We knew we'd stumbled on a different way of communicating in sixty seconds." The author Randall Rothenberg has described the Lou Reed spot as a seminal work that may have been the first postmodern ad (though Chiat/Day's slightly earlier "1984" commercial also had its share of "po-mo" qualities, including an oblique message, an artistic film style, and a story line that borrowed from author George Orwell). In any case, the commercial didn't have much impact on the marketplace—W+K subsequently lost the account—but its style and originality very much impressed Nike and led to the far more well-known "Revolution" ad.

After "Revolution," Wieden and Nike's collaboration took off as they produced, over the next few years, a series of dazzling ads all connected by a single line of copy that Wieden

had written in about fifteen minutes in his office one day. The line, "Just do it," was one of the most ambiguous advertising slogans ever penned. What did it mean? Just do what? (There were all kinds of far-fetched theories; the American journalist John Leo suspected that Nike's message might contain some dark agenda, commanding urban kids to go wild and wreak havoc—an interpretation that astounded and mildly offended Wieden when he was told of it.) Ad conspiracy theorists aside, most people grasped the essence of what Wieden was saying: Be active, get off your couch, stop talking about doing something and get started on it. Wieden had written a simple and stirring call to action, though it was left to the individual to decide what specific action to take.

Like the Doyle Dane Bernbach advertising of old, Nike commercials were usually rooted in a strong, surprising idea, and they were invariably clever. But that was where the similarities

ended. With DDB, the big idea was almost always linked directly to product or company attributes—smaller is better, number two tries harder, and so on. With Nike ads, the big idea was often only tangentially connected to the product—and the idea was just the starting point in the creation of an elaborate, complex, and hyperstylized piece of work that, by completion, didn't look much like a commercial at all. In the ad "Bo Knows" (dreamed up by Riswold and a few others in a bar), the idea was rooted in the fact that one of Nike's endorser athletes, Bo Jackson, had made headlines by playing two professional sports simultaneously. Riswold then mused, "What if Jackson tried to play every sport? And then what if he tried to go beyond sports, taking on, say, guitar-playing? Would he succeed at everything?" The frenzied commercial, directed by Joe Pytka, showed Jackson's sometimes comical attempts at tennis, hockey, basketball—with cameo critiques by other

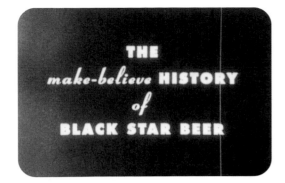

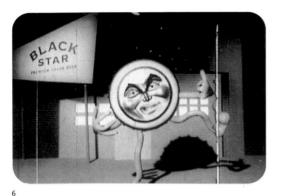

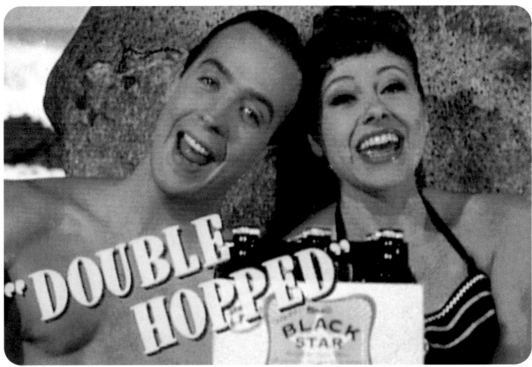

6

5. **REEBOK**

CHIAT/DAY, NEW YORK, 1988
The postmodern style began to
show up in other ads, including
those of Nike's competitor,
Reebok. But the U.B.U. campaign
was considered too strange at
the time.

6. **BLACK STAR BEER**

WIEDEN + KENNEDY,
PORTLAND, 1992
Wieden + Kennedy also took a
postmodern approach with some
of its other brands; campy Black
Star beer ads were designed to
look old-fashioned and fake.

athletes, some of whom are clearly skeptical of the whole endeavor. The commercial ends with Jackson playing a guitar riff miserably, prompting the rock-and-roll musician Bo Diddley to declare, "Bo, you don't know diddley." The commercial then closes with the Nike logo and the words "Just do it" flashed onscreen. Like most Nike ads, the commercial didn't seem to be promoting anything, other than the growing legend of a particular athlete; Nike shoes are not mentioned in the commercial at all. The spot bore other hallmarks of Nike advertising: inside references to sports, rock music, and pop culture; a willingness to poke fun at the endorser Jackson; a jagged and uneven film style that was almost dizzying. But "Bo Knows" was nearly impossible for television viewers to ignore. The American filmmaker Spike Lee observed at the time that, along with the much-hyped release of the movie *Batman*, the commercial had taken American culture by storm in 1989.

Lee himself would soon be swept into the Nike ad whirlwind, as he began appearing in commercials pairing himself and the basketball star Michael Jordan, with Lee playing a character, Mars Blackmon, he'd created in his first film, *She's Gotta Have It*, in 1986. In the commercials, Lee's character became a kind of anti-spokesman, badgering the star Jordan, making ludicrous statements (Mars insisted that it "must be the shoes" that enabled Jordan to defy gravity, inviting the audience to laugh at this silly proposition), and even calling attention to the advertising process itself: In one ad, Mars yells out the window, "Shut up, we're shooting a Nike commercial." For an ad to acknowledge its status as an ad wasn't entirely novel; in earlier times, everyone from Groucho Marx to the radio pitch-characters Bert and Harry Piel sometimes joked about doing ads as they were doing them. And the self-mocking pitchman was used perhaps most famously in the mid-

1980s with the character Joe Isuzu, whose outrageous claims and promises in ads were acknowledged, in subtitles, to be lies. But Nike ads brought self-referential advertising to a new level, telling the audience, in effect, "We know this is an ad, and you know this is an ad—so let's have fun with it." As Wieden said, such ads were "like pulling back the curtain and showing the little man behind Oz."

On one level, that made the ads more "honest" than most. But critics took a different view. The agency was accused of cannily co-opting the culture and cynically using icons of hipness to sell shoes. In his book *Where the Suckers Moon*, Randall Rothenberg suggests, in effect, that some of the creative people at W+K may have sold out their own countercultural values when they placed rebel heroes like Reed in ads. Other critics noted that the use of irony and "honest" self-deprecating humor in the ads simply served as cover, enabling the

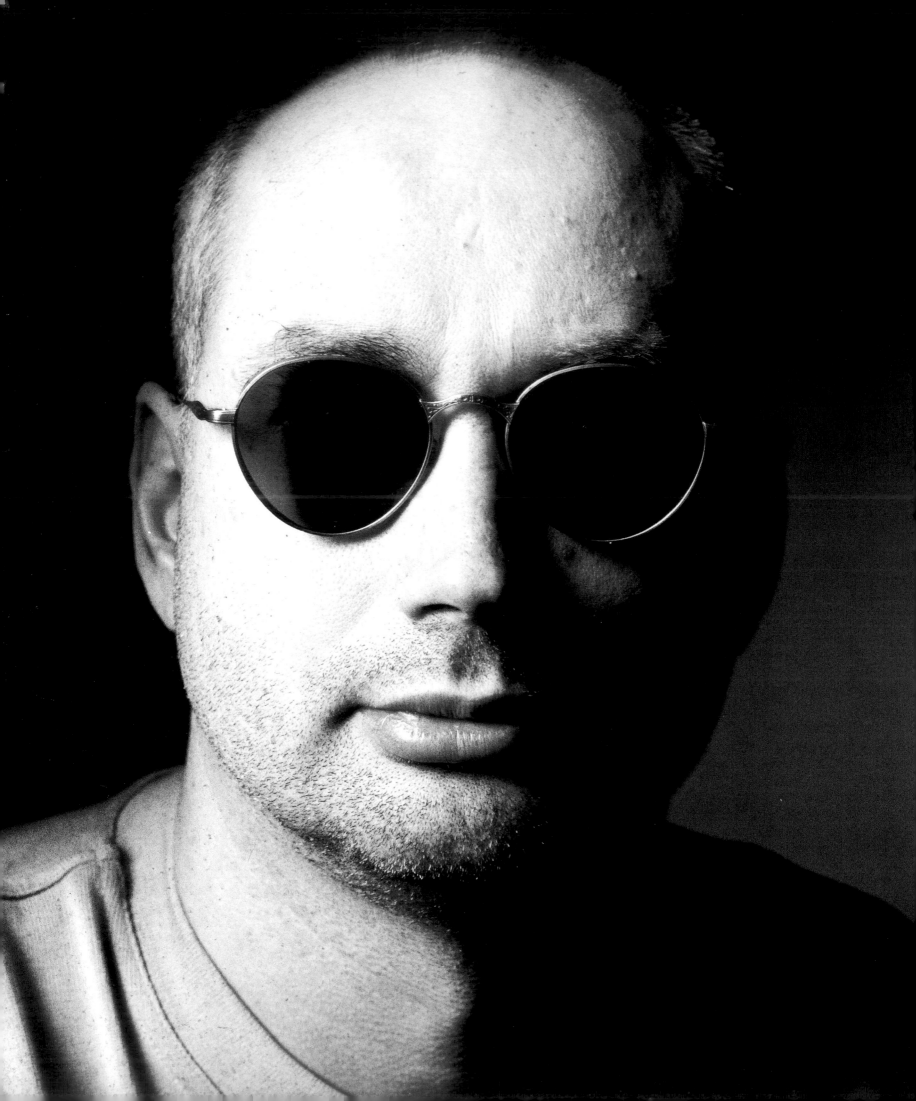

INTERVIEW: JIM RISWOLD

Few copywriters in the late 1980s and 1990s have had as much influence on advertising as Jim Riswold of Wieden + Kennedy. As the preeminent writer and creative director on the Nike account, Riswold has been credited with helping to introduce a postmodern style to ads. He has also written several of the most famous commercials of the past twenty years—including "Bo Knows," featuring Bo Jackson, and "I Am Not a Role Model," featuring Charles Barkley. And the author David Halberstam credits Riswold with helping to turn Michael Jordan into a global icon.

WHAT WAS WIEDEN + KENNEDY LIKE IN THE LATE 1980S?
It was a time when we weren't afraid to make glorious mistakes. And boy oh boy, did we make a bunch.

THE AD YOU DID FOR HONDA SCOOTERS FEATURING LOU REED HAS BEEN CITED AS A BREAKTHROUGH IN BRINGING AN "UNDERGROUND" SENSIBILITY TO ADS. WHY DID YOU CHOOSE REED?
Everybody knows celebrities have been used in advertising since time immemorial. However, what I think made the Lou Reed spot different at the time was that it used a persona non grata celebrity.

The very things that made Reed off-limits to any sane advertising professional are what appealed to me: his outspokenness, his troubles, his 24-hour sunglasses, his choice of subject matter, his grating personality, his aloofness, his coolness, his ego, his sexual ambiguity, his darkness; in short, his Lou-ness. He has the guts to stand for something, and the audacity to be Lou Reed on his terms. Maybe people who admired Mr. Reed, warts and all, saw the commercial as speaking to them. Maybe they appreciated being welcomed to the wonderful world of consumerism.

I don't know; partly I did the ad because I just wanted to meet Lou Reed.

WHY WERE THE "SPIKE AND MIKE" COMMERCIALS [PAIRING BASKETBALL STAR MICHAEL JORDAN AND FILMMAKER SPIKE LEE] SO SUCCESSFUL?
I think they gave America a glimpse of what Michael Jordan as a person was like. They were a counterpart to the Jordan we saw on sports

reports every night—Jordan the total predator, the assassin who went out and laid waste to enemy teams. Opposing teams got the killer, but the fans watching these ads got the charmer, the smile, a man of humor and intelligence.

YOU SEEM OPEN TO USING ALL KINDS OF PERSONAL INFLUENCES IN YOUR ADS—THE KIND OF MUSIC YOU LISTEN TO, WHAT YOU'RE READING AT THE TIME, OR FILMS YOU'VE SEEN. WHY DO YOU CHOOSE TO INCORPORATE ALL OF THIS INTO YOUR ADS?
I have never had an original thought in my career. Everything I have ever done has been borrowed, reformulated, regurgitated, turned upside down or inside out, played back at a different speed, and sometimes just plain stolen from either popular culture, music, history, art, literature, the back of cereal boxes, Hegelianism, an athlete's life, a bedtime story my grandmother once read me—whatever. Anything and everything is fair game when it comes to stimulus. (My lawyers have asked me to point out that this is not plagiarism; it is appropriation.)

But, hopefully, what my complete lack of originality did was open up an unlimited number of resources from which to make completely original ads. And, more important, maybe it led to more meaningful and enjoyable ways for people to hear an advertiser's message.

AS YOU KNOW, ONE CRITICISM OF MODERN ADVERTISING IS THAT IT CO-OPTS THE CULTURE—FOR EXAMPLE, BY BRINGING LOU REED OR JOHN LENNON INTO ADS, YOU'RE TAKING SOMETHING THAT WAS PURE AND AUTHENTIC, AND PUTTING THE TAINT OF COMMERCIALISM ON IT. WHAT'S YOUR FEELING ABOUT THAT?
Die-hard fans of the long-dead John Lennon hated the "Instant Karma" Nike commercial. Some brain-damaged fans of Lou Reed were up in arms that I shared their Lou with the non-brain-damaged world.

Even my mother was upset with my translation of "I am Spartacus" into "I am Tiger Woods."

To all these criticisms—yes, even to my mother's—I reply by asking these people to get off their high horses. We're not talking about sacred texts here; we're talking about a song, a book, a TV show, or a movie. These are part of popular culture, and so is advertising. It

should be allowed to draw upon all the inspirations that the rest of popular culture does. To all the Lou Reed fans I may have upset by "bastardizing" him (never mind that he could have turned down the offer to be in the ad) I reply, "I got to meet him and you didn't." And to my mother (whom I love deeply): It could've been worse; it could've been "I am Cap'n Crunch."

YOUR ADVERTISING HAS BEEN CALLED POSTMODERN. WHAT DO YOU THINK ABOUT THAT?
What does postmodernism mean?

Seriously, when I read some weighty commentary about my work, it makes me wish I were half as smart as some author thinks I am.It confounds the hell out of my intellectual sisters, who, upon reading these things, exclaim, "He's really stupid! We know; we had to grow up next to him!" While my sisters were up to their necks in Euclidean geometry, I spent my adolescence with the likes of Monty Python, Andy Warhol, "SCTV," and "Saturday Night Live." (This was before I tried to make myself smart by studying nineteenth-century German philosophy.) I learned from these people not to take anything too seriously.

There is no better place to apply this philosophy than advertising. When did advertising deem itself so damn important? Was there a sentence I missed on the tablets Moses brought down from Mount Sinai referring to the sanctity of advertising?

Thanks to the Warhols and Pythons of the world, I was fortunate enough to stumble into a career in advertising with a healthy dose of cynicism. I was doubly fortunate to work for Dan Wieden and David Kennedy, who were equally cynical about the advertising profession. That cynicism and "it's only advertising" attitude allowed us to create some truly wonderful advertising.

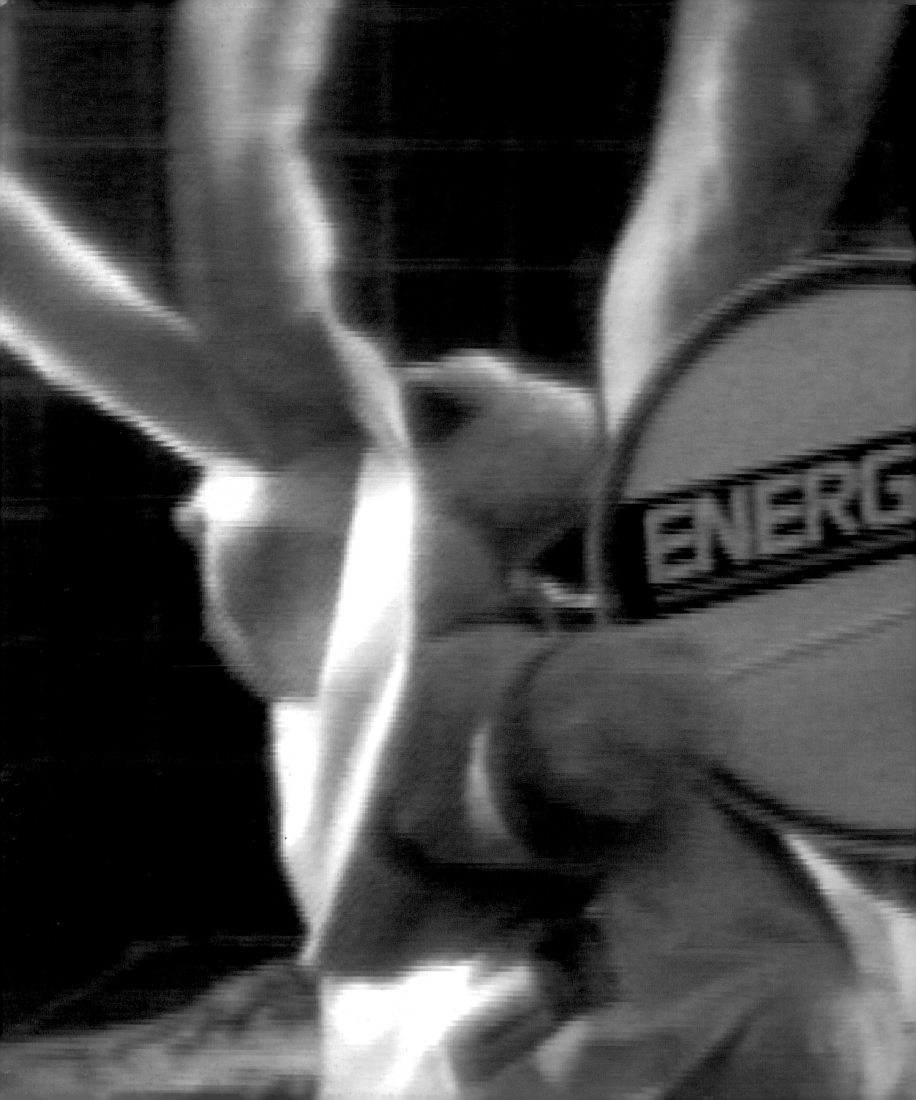

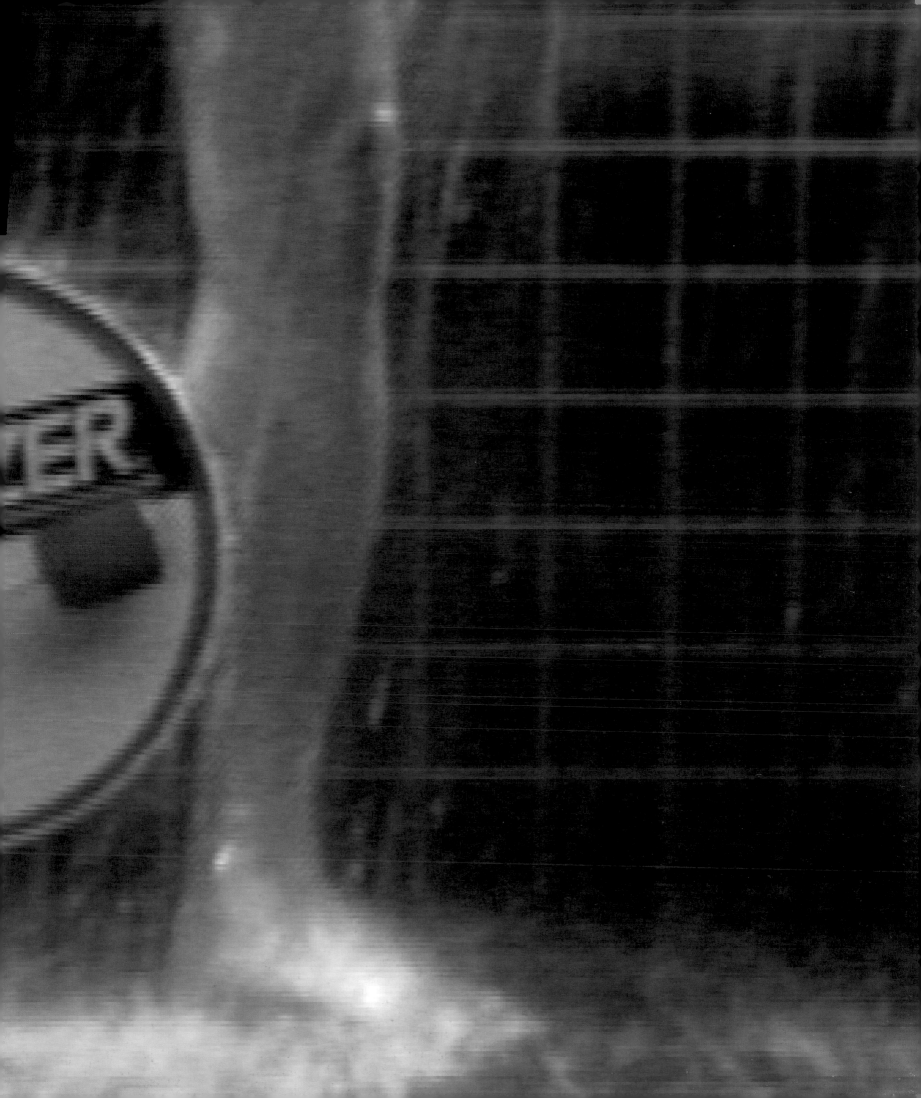

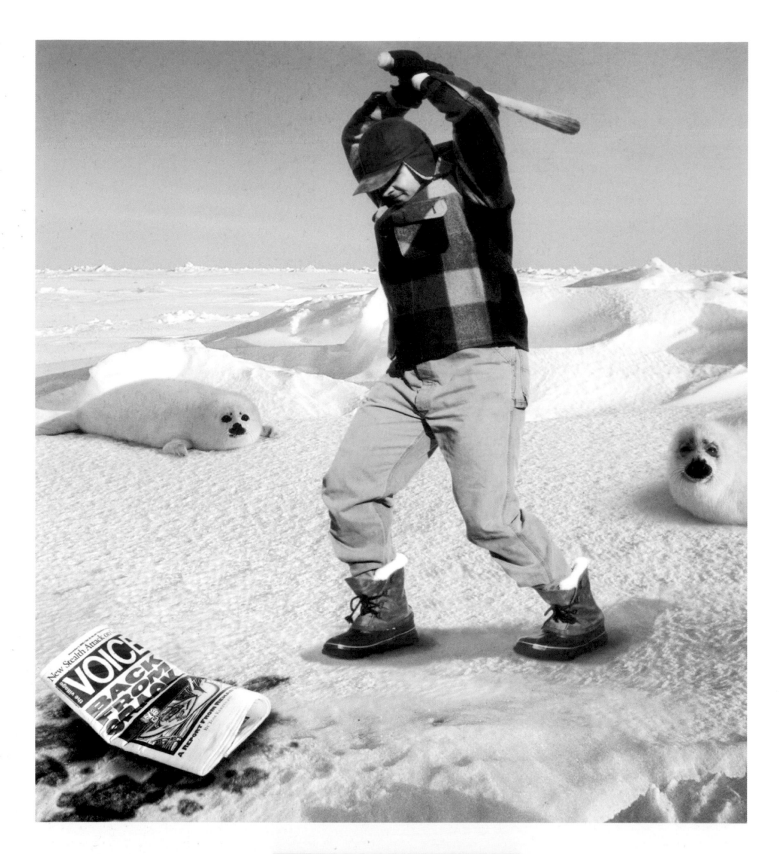

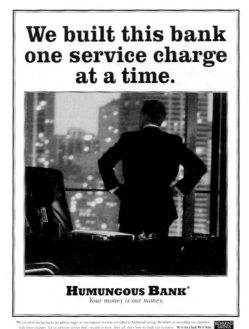

We built this bank one service charge at a time.

HUMUNGOUS BANK*
Your money is our money.

9

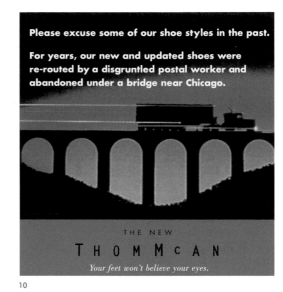

Please excuse some of our shoe styles in the past.

For years, our new and updated shoes were re-routed by a disgruntled postal worker and abandoned under a bridge near Chicago.

THE NEW
THOM McAN
Your feet won't believe your eyes.

10

7. (PREVIOUS SPREAD)
ENERGIZER
CHIAT/DAY, LOS ANGELES,
1989
In this campaign, the Energizer
Bunny appeared unexpectedly in
the middle of fake commercials
for ersatz products.

8. THE VILLAGE VOICE
MAD DOGS & ENGLISHMEN,
NEW YORK, 1996
The Mad Dogs agency
sometimes attacked the
products it was promoting;
here, New York's *Village Voice*
newspaper takes a beating.

9. RICHMOND SAVINGS BANK
PALMER JARVIS DDB,
VANCOUVER, 1987
This ad campaign promoted a
fictional bank, Humungous,
along with facetious headlines
like this one; the point was to
make the real client, Richmond
Savings, look good in comparison.

10. THOM MCAN SHOES
MAD DOGS & ENGLISHMEN,
NEW YORK, 1994
Once again, Mad Dogs makes
fun of its own client: the ads
apologize (and offer lame excuses)
for Thom McAn's previously
unstylish shoes in order
to introduce a revamped
product line.

advertising to slip past the guard of even the most savvy, cynical consumers. Yes, Nike advertising *seemed* to be offering moments of pure entertainment sans the annoying sales pitch, but in fact the pitch, the link to the product, was always lurking somewhere under the surface. As media-studies professor Mark Crispin Miller pointed out, the modus operandi of ironic advertisers like Wieden + Kennedy was to wink at the audience and flatter its intelligence with clever inside jokes—all for the single purpose of closing the sale. Seen in this light, postmodern advertising could be considered even more manipulative, and perhaps more dishonest, than the old-fashioned, straightforward advertising that didn't bother to cleverly disguise itself.

It's difficult to know, without actually crawling inside the heads of Wieden and his staff, whether the creation of Nike ads was as

cynically calculated as some critics suspect. But for their part, W+K staffers insist the agency had no hidden agenda. "My sense is that we were just having fun," Wieden says. "I think our best work has never been trying to appropriate pop culture and turn it into advertising. It was simply a reflection of people who have contemporary brains and taste, just exploring things that they liked, things that turned them on." That seems entirely credible, and in fact likely: Rather than being a result of cold calculation, the Nike postmodern style of advertising was more likely the product of near-complete creative freedom. Nike had given Wieden license to reinvent advertising—and, for the most part, didn't even subject the agency's ideas to standard focus groups or other testing. Wieden, in turn, created a free-wheeling work environment in which he encouraged his staff to be open to outside

influences beyond the narrow world of advertising (he sometimes held seminars at the agencies, bringing in artists or musicians). He hired offbeat people like Riswold, who were far more interested in film, philosophy, and rock music than in advertising. And Riswold, in turn, seemed to see the agency as a creative playground in which he could use his sandbox—Nike ads—to salute cult heroes, play under-appreciated songs, and introduce hip new artists. (Riswold came up with the Spike Lee idea after seeing a trailer for *She's Gotta Have It;* "That would be cool," he thought.)

In the end, what mattered was the results. The Nike commercials were both effective—the company vaulted past arch-rival Reebok and never looked back—and thoroughly enjoyed by the public. Moreover, they set the standard for advertising in the 1990s; as the *Adweek* columnist Barbara Lippert noted, just about every

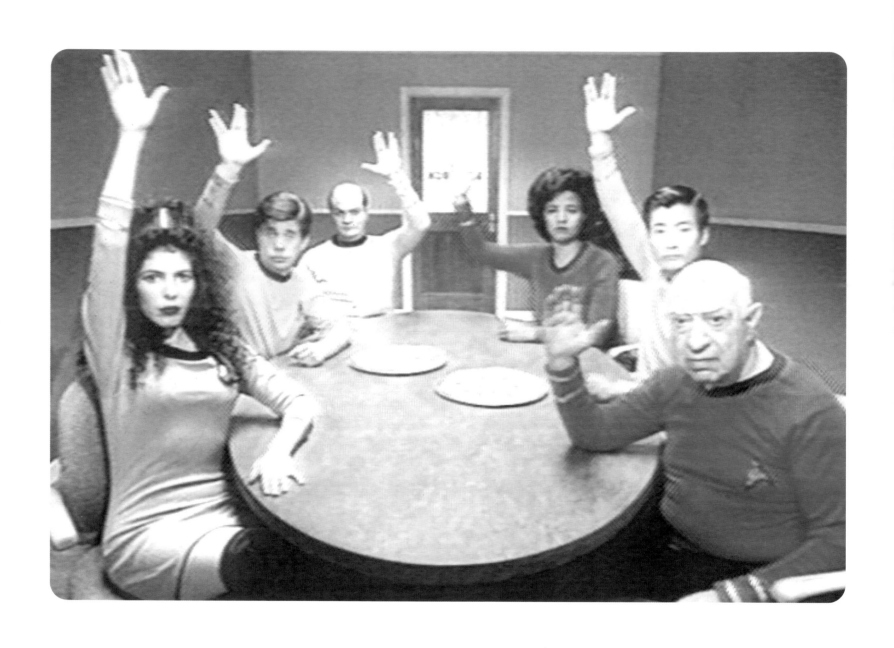

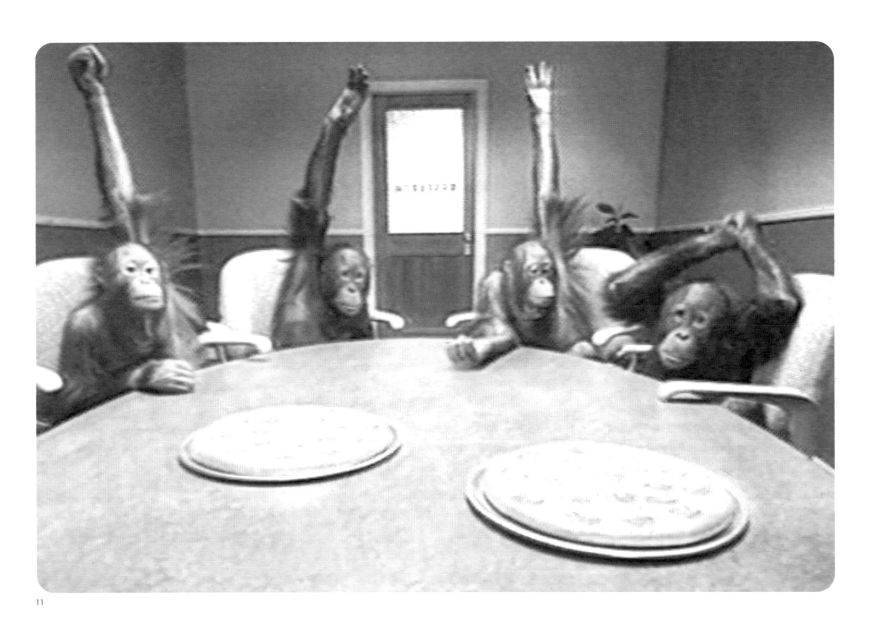

11

11. **LITTLE CAESARS PIZZA**
CLIFF FREEMAN & PARTNERS,
NEW YORK, 1994
Postmodern ads often make fun
of advertising itself; this spot
ridiculed focus groups, showing
that they tend to be comprised
of likeminded participants.

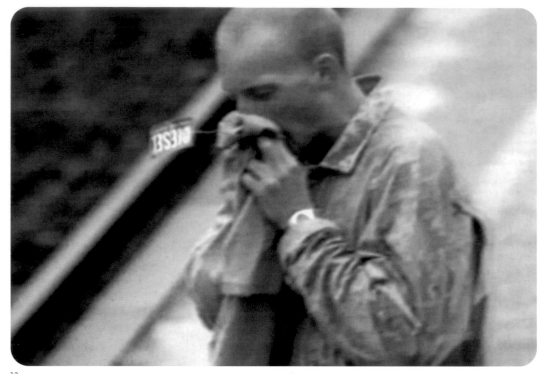

12

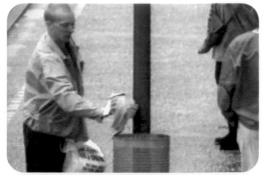

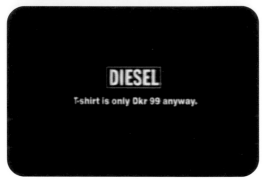

DIESEL
T-shirt is only Dkr 99 anyway.

advertiser developed a case of "Nike envy." To be fair, however, Wieden + Kennedy was not the only agency breaking new creative ground at the time. Goodby Berlin & Silverstein, a small San Francisco shop, had been among the first to experiment with cinema-verité-style documentary commercials; the agency's ad promoting a local film festival was shot with a handheld camera and had an air of authenticity that was rare in ads at the time. Goodby would later create a campaign for the Chevy's restaurant chain that would feature rough-and-tumble low-budget commercials shot and aired on TV all in the same day—the idea being that the ads should be "made fresh each day," just like the restaurant's food. The partners Jeff Goodby and Rich Silverstein—one a veteran of *Harvard Lampoon* magazine, the other from *Rolling Stone*—seemed to share Wieden's "outsider" mentality and his general distaste for most advertising. Though Goodby was not a "post-

modern agency" per se (many of its subsequent commercials, including the famous "Got Milk?" vignettes, featured more classic approaches, albeit brilliantly written and executed), it was nevertheless central in the development of the new advertising in the 1990s.

A little farther down the California coastline, Chiat/Day in Los Angeles was at the forefront of postmodern advertising, perhaps even a step ahead of Wieden. Having been the first to produce the commercial-as-art-film ("1984" for Apple) and the first to shoot a commercial-as-music-video (the rousing "I Love L.A." spot, in which singer Randy Newman cruises the city in his car, promoting Nike sponsorship of the 1984 Summer Olympics), Chiat/Day also produced a campaign for Reebok that tried to take on Nike with a style even more experimental and abstract. Under the banner of "Reeboks let UBU," the ads featured oddball characters, lines from Ralph Waldo Emerson, and the surreal

cinematic style of Italian films: "We mixed it all together to see what we'd get," says the creative director on the campaign, Marty Cooke. The result was advertising that was undeniably intriguing but also baffling. It might have been quite at home in the "Oddvertising" environment of the late 1990s (see Chapter 6), but it arrived in the marketplace a few years earlier and landed with a thud. However, another of Chiat/Day's innovative campaigns from the same period, for Energizer batteries, was a hit. The campaign introduced the Energizer Bunny, a relentless toy rabbit that managed to trample conventional advertising; commercials would start off seeming like a typically banal ad for a make-believe product—only to have the scene interrupted by the battery-powered bunny, unexpectedly and inappropriately marching into the scene.

Following the lead of these three West Coast agencies, much of advertising had by the early

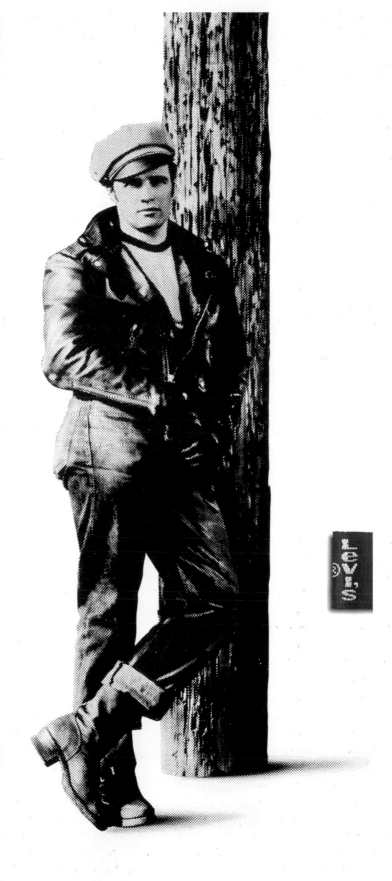

OUR MODELS CAN BEAT UP THEIR MODELS.

13

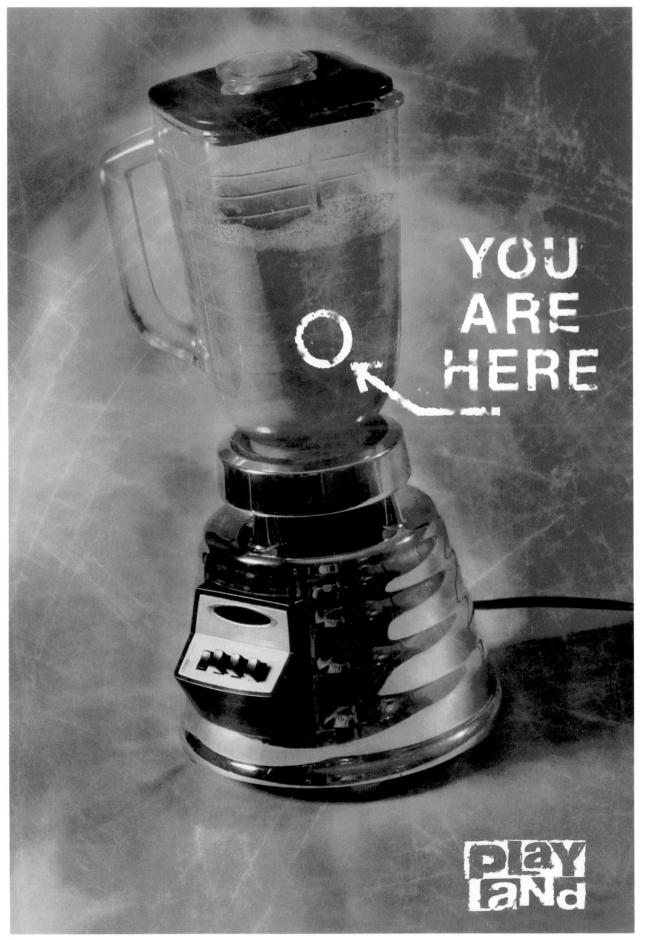

14

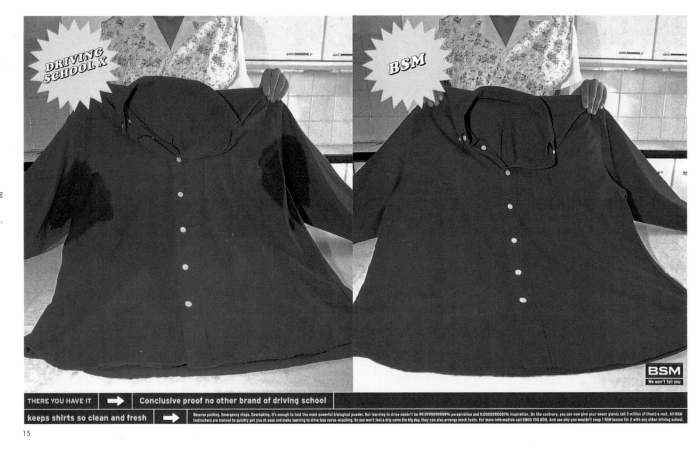

15

to mid-1990s embraced at least some elements of postmodernism: Ads were suddenly awash in irony and seized every available opportunity to break with the conventions of advertising. A new "anti-advertising" approach became the standard way to pitch products. Often, such advertising would demonstrate its candor by gently laughing at the product or brand being advertised. In its late 1990s ads for Thom McAn shoes, a brand that had been popular in the 1970s but had long since fallen out of fashion, the New York agency Mad Dogs & Englishmen created a campaign that offered lame apologies: "Please excuse some of our shoe styles in the past," one ad read. "Through a fluke computer error, the office supply store repeatedly sent us the wrong desk calendars and we still thought it was 1976." Mad Dogs' ads for *The Village Voice* also made the client the butt of its jokes; under the facetious headline "America's favorite newspaper," one ad showed a club-wielding

man attacking a rolled-up copy of the *Voice*. (Mad Dogs' creative director Nick Cohen had a history of making light of clients and products: Early in his career, when Cohen was asked to create a promotional poster for a performance of *A Midsummer Night's Dream,* his ad summed up the Shakespeare classic with the tabloid-style headline "Fairy Queen in Donkey Sex Scandal Drama.") Perhaps no client was more ruthlessly parodied in its own ads than the unfortunate Humongous Bank, whose ad agency DDB Palmer Jarvis of Vancouver portrayed the bank as a selfish entity whose own slogans were damning: "We're not just interested in money. We're interested in people with money," read one of the bank's ads. Of course, the agency could afford to be critical of Humongous Bank since the institution didn't actually exist; it was created by the agency as a humorous straw horse, on behalf of a smaller bank that was DDB Palmer Jarvis's real client.

When not joking about their own products, ads were publicly deconstructing the process of advertising. The soft drink Sprite and its agency Lowe & Partners began producing commercials that mischievously exposed the fakery of ads, from bought-and-sold endorsers to outrageous claims; the ads concluded with the line "Image is nothing. Obey your thirst." The behind-the-scenes practices of advertising, both real and imagined, were also played for laughs in a series of ads for Seagram's gin; the ads mischievously resurrected the decades-old suspicion that ads contained subliminal messages, as Seagram's challenged readers to find the secret symbols planted in these new ads. Meanwhile, a series of Little Caesars pizza ads ridiculed focus groups and the tendencies of researchers to assemble like-minded people for their studies; the commercials featured focus groups composed entirely of chimpanzees or *Star Trek* fanatics or other homogeneous oddballs.

NIKE AND THE POSTMODERN AD REVOLUTION.

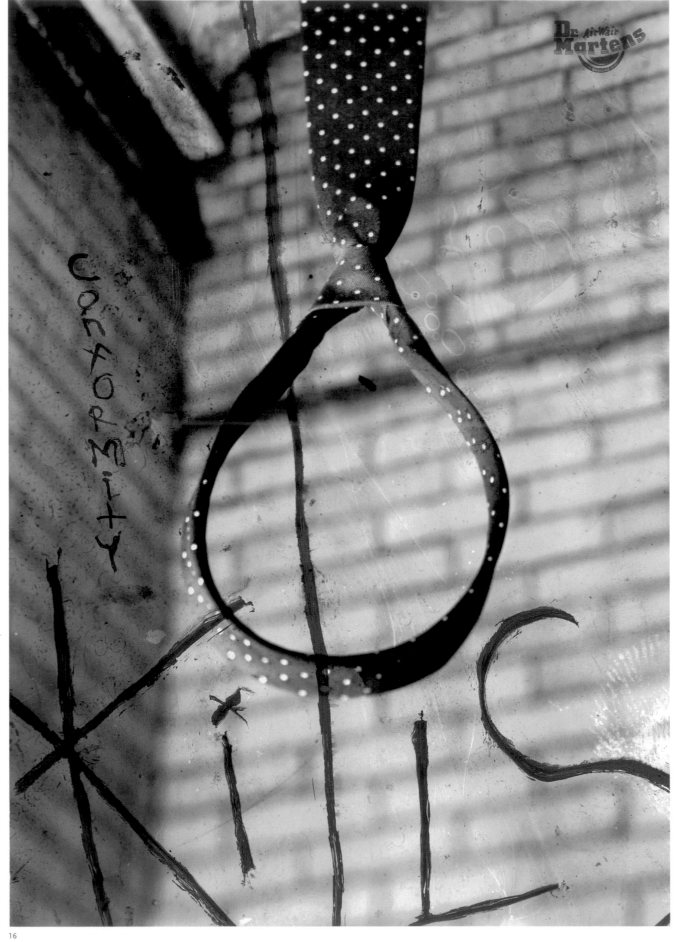

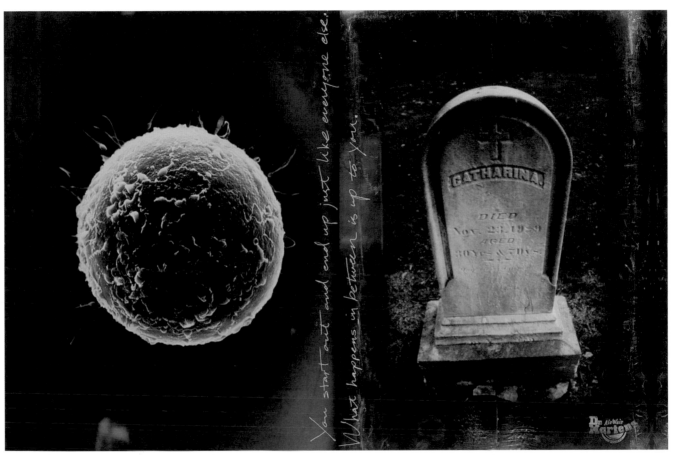

17

16 AND 17. **DR. MARTENS**
CORE, ST. LOUIS, MISSOURI,
1995
The brothers Todd and Eric
Tilford became the new "angry
young men" of mid-1990s
advertising, with harsh
headlines like "Conformity Kills"
and a rough style of design.

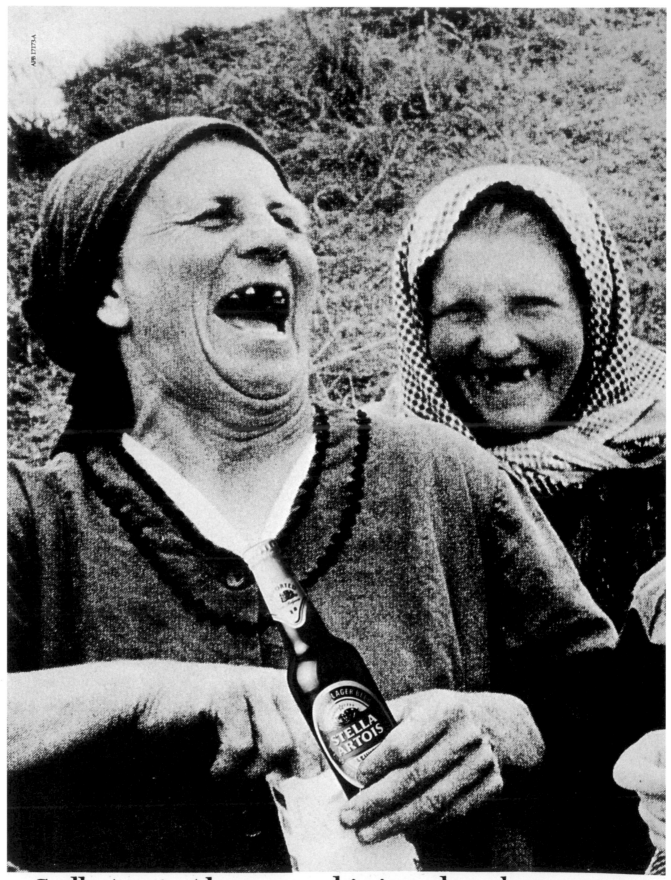

Stella Artois. About as sophisticated as a beer can get.

18. **STELLA ARTOIS**
CAMPAIGN PALACE,
MELBOURNE, 1992
An Australian campaign
opted for less glamorous
spokesmodels in the form of
gap-toothed peasants.

19 AND 20. **MEZZO MIX**
AMMIRATI PURIS LINTAS,
SWITZERLAND, 1996
An example of "don't believe
the hype" advertising in these
ads for a European soft drink:
the audience is supposed to
admire the advertiser for being
cool enough to admit that ad
promises are fake.

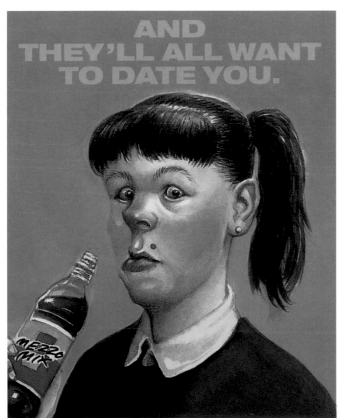

All the other girls have found boyfriends. They're having fun, going out, and even your best girlfriend would rather be with him than you. You've asked all the boys in your class, but they won't even give you a second look. All that's going to change. Drink Mezzo Mix and you'll have a boyfriend in no time. **Mezzo Mix. Coke and orange and everything will be cool.**

19

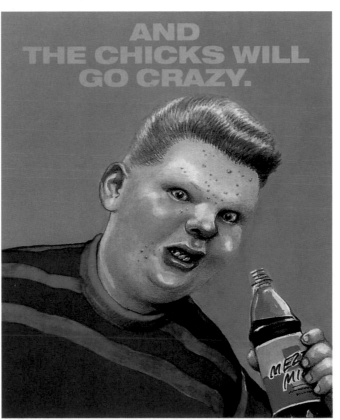

You broke into your kid sister's piggy bank to buy skin lotion, but they still call you pimple face. All you want to do is get to know a nice girl. But none of them take any notice. And if you try rappin' with them they just whisper and giggle. Don't panic. Drink Mezzo-Mix and the girls will be lining up to go with you. **Mezzo-Mix. Coke and orange and everthing will be cool.**

20

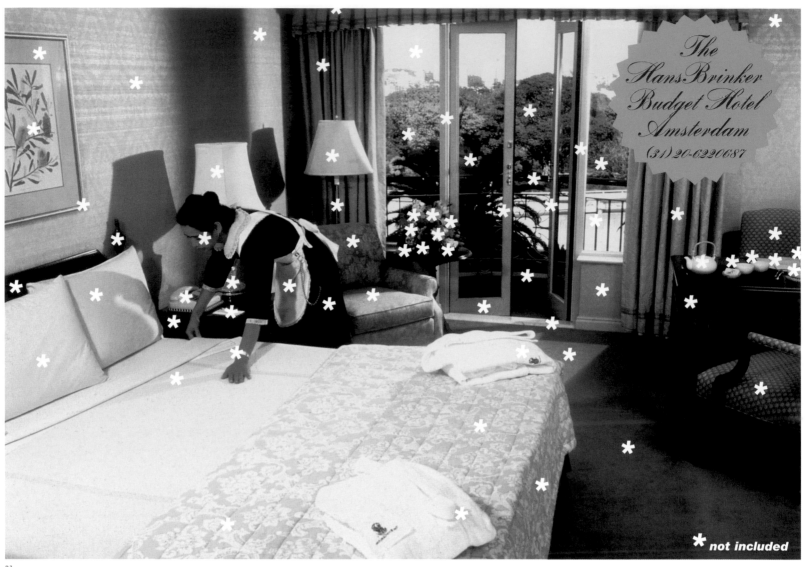

The Hans Brinker Budget Hotel Amsterdam (31) 20-6220687

* not included

21

21. HANS BRINKER BUDGET HOTEL
KESSELSKRAMER, AMSTERDAM, 1997
Postmodern ads can be surprisingly candid: this Dutch ad, for a low-budget hotel, delights in pointing out all of the hotel's deficiencies.

22. SCHLAFLY BEER
CORE, ST. LOUIS, MISSOURI, 1995
Ads by Todd and Eric Tilford often had a weathered look, intended to make them seem grittier and more authentic.

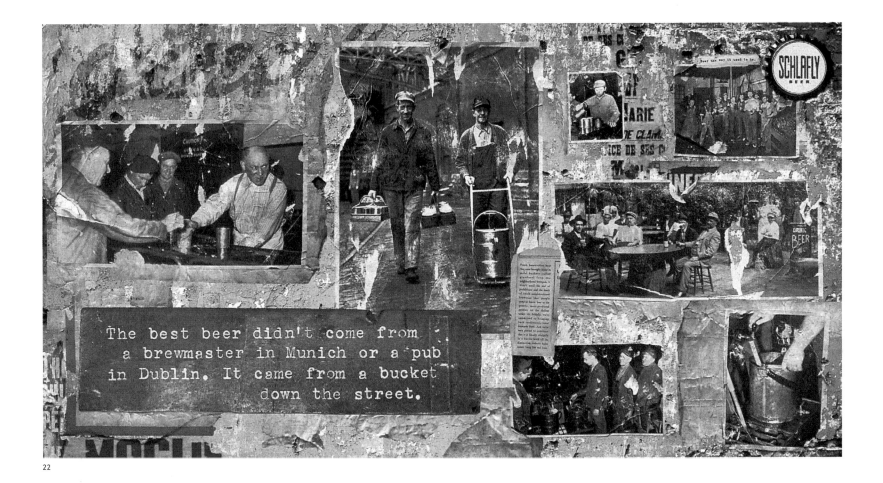

The best beer didn't come from a brewmaster in Munich or a pub in Dublin. It came from a bucket down the street.

Even the models posing in ads weren't safe from the postmodern agency's barbs: One Levi's campaign showed movie stars in tough poses and declared, "Our models can beat up your models." By the 2000 Super Bowl, one advertiser had turned its ad into a joke about the high cost of advertising during the game; the commercial, for the E-Trade on-line brokerage, was intentionally low-brow (it starred a dancing monkey wearing an E-Trade shirt) and closed with the admission "We just wasted two million bucks."

All of this self-referential irony could seem, at times, like mere navel-gazing by advertisers. One also had to wonder whether all the self-flagellation by advertisers, while a logical way to deflect public cynicism about ads, might also suggest a lingering self-loathing on the part of ad creators—many of whom noisily profess to "hate advertising" even as they make their living in it.

The dismantling of the accepted conventions of advertising was occurring not only in the U.S. but around the world. The influence of Nike, a global force by early 1990s, was felt everywhere, though particularly in Europe, where Wieden + Kennedy set up outposts starting with Amsterdam. Moreover, in some sectors of the world, a postmodern way of thinking about advertising had already developed independently. In Scandinavia, Australia, the UK, and elsewhere, advertisers had established a tradition of not taking themselves, or their products, too seriously. The British, in particular, had long embraced the philosophy that an ad's primary challenge was to entertain and amuse the public—and if that required self-deprecating humor or a bit of playful ad-bashing, so be it. One British ad for Amstel beer, by Howell Henry Chaldecott, facetiously pleaded with consumers not to buy the product. The British agency St. Luke's poked fun at

advertising research in a series of ads for Ikea, and Lowe Howard Spink used a classic scenario, the side-by-side laundry demonstration, to make a humorous point about the British School of Motoring ("driving school X," we are shown, causes severe underarm-perspiration stains in shirts).

Australia seemed to particularly embrace this new "nudge and a wink" approach to advertising. An Australian ad for Stella Artois beer used a doctored photograph to place the beer in the hands of toothless peasant women; the headline read, "About as sophisticated as a beer can get." An Australian hospital's ads adopted the blaring bargain-promising headlines of a classic retail ad in their appeal for public donations to help pay for lifesaving medical equipment (demonstrating that ironic humor might be used even in ads dealing with somber subjects). Postmodernism also played well in Switzerland, Sweden, and the

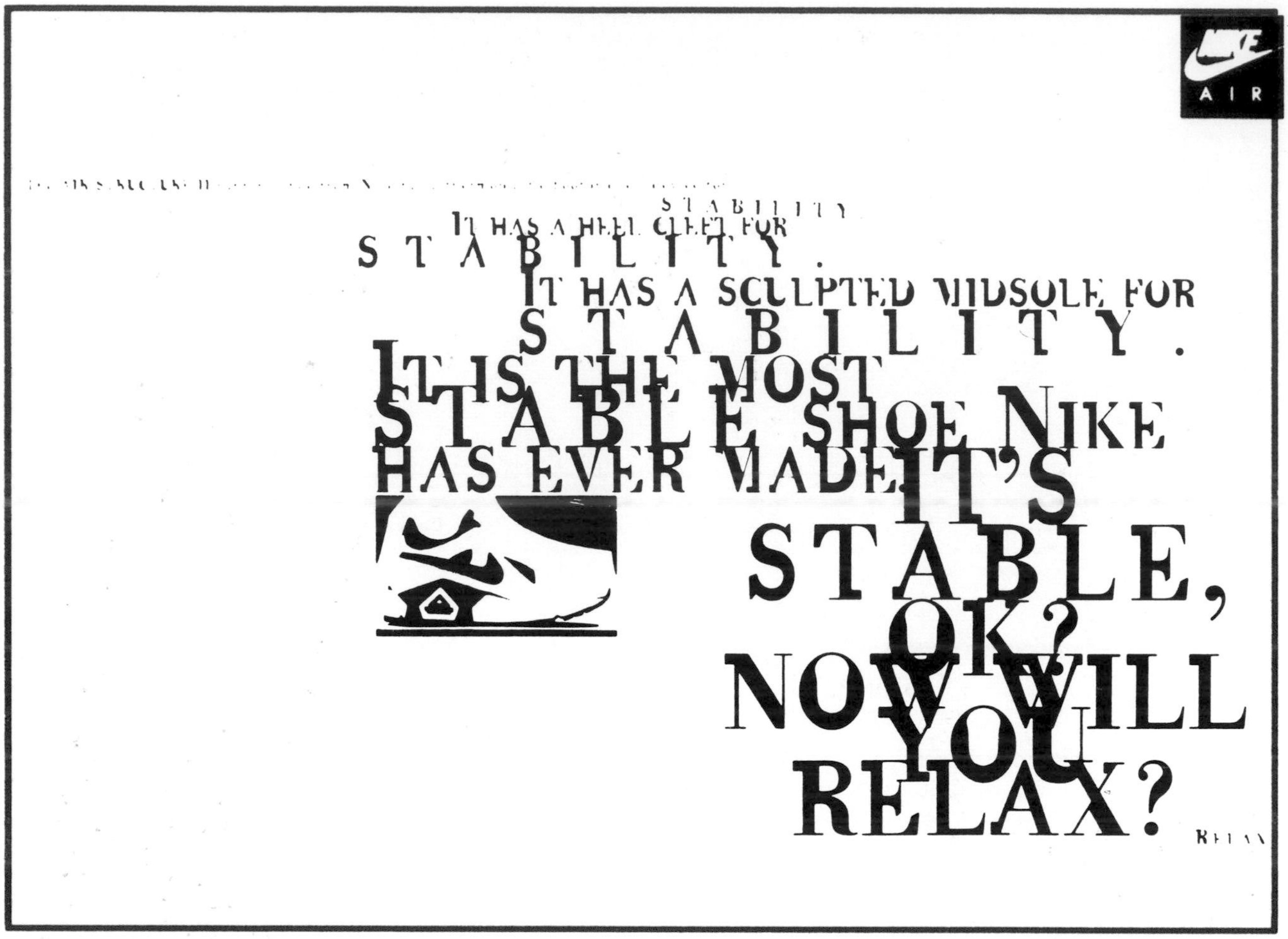

STABILITY

IT HAS A HEEL CLEFT FOR
STABILITY.
IT HAS A SCULPTED MIDSOLE FOR
STABILITY.
IT IS THE MOST
STABLE SHOE NIKE
HAS EVER MADE IT'S
STABLE,
OK?
NOW WILL
YOU
RELAX?

23

23. NIKE
WIEDEN + KENNEDY,
AMSTERDAM, 1994
Typography went wild in the
mid-1990s, as the influence of
graphic-design rebel David
Carson began to show up in
ads. Here, Carson seems to be
making the type scream.

24. NIKE
WIEDEN +KENNEDY,
AMSTERDAM, 1992
W+K art director Jelly Helm—
who would eventually leave
advertising and become a harsh
critic of it—felt the ads would
seem more real if they were
handwritten.

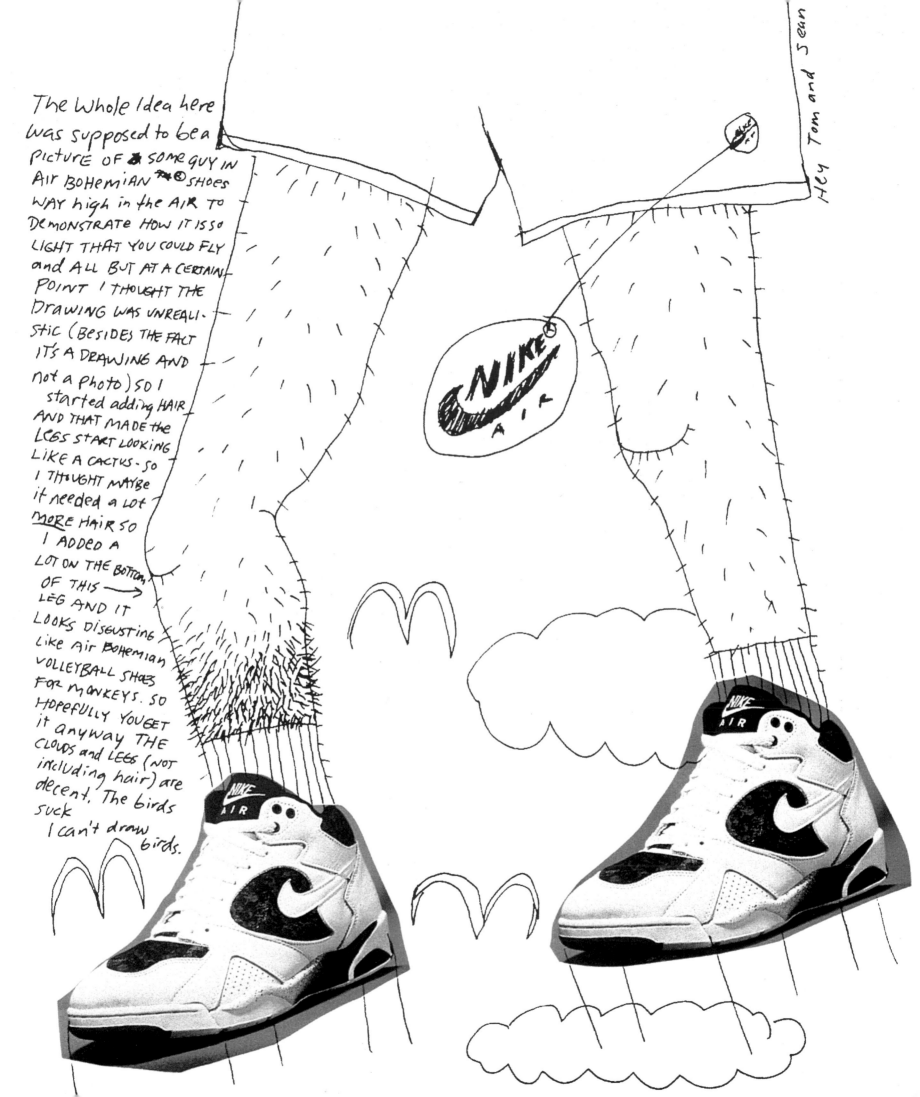

The whole idea here was supposed to be a picture of some guy in Air Bohemian ™® shoes way high in the air to demonstrate how it is so light that you could fly and all but at a certain point I thought the drawing was unrealistic (besides the fact it's a drawing and not a photo) so I started adding hair and that made the legs start looking like a cactus. So I thought maybe it needed a lot more hair so I added a lot on the bottom of this → leg and it looks disgusting like Air Bohemian volleyball shoes for monkeys. So hopefully you get it anyway the clouds and legs (not including hair) are decent. The birds suck I can't draw birds.

NIKE AIR

Hey Tom and Sean

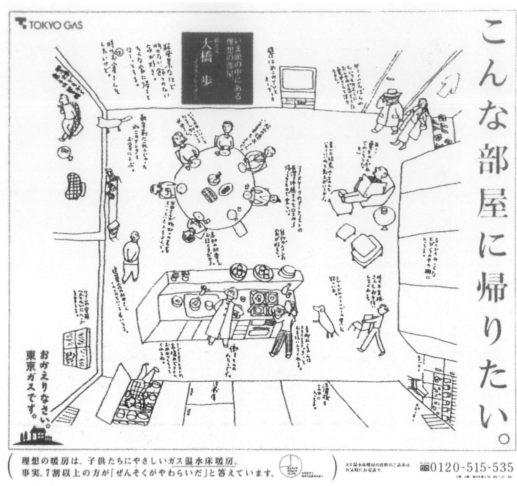

25

Netherlands, all of which had long featured irreverence in their ads. A Swiss ad for Mezzo Mix soft drink dripped with sarcasm, as it showed illustrations of unattractive kids and promised that the product would make them popular with their peers. Meanwhile, the Dutch agency KesselsKramer constructed an entire ad campaign based on the inadequacies of its client, the Hans Brinker Budget Hotel in Amsterdam. One picture shows a luxurious hotel room, full of wonderful amenities—but asterisks are stamped all over the photo, marking the large bed, the minibar, the balcony, and so forth; as we learn from the ad's fine print, the asterisk means that none of these amenities are included with a room at the Hans Brinker. Irony and anti-advertising were not embraced everywhere, however; such approaches tended to fall flat in Asia, notes the Singapore ad writer Jim Aitchison, because "people here are not as cynical about ads. If

you tried to run an ad that mocked itself, the public's reaction would be 'Why are you showing me an ad like that? It's a waste of money! Either run the ad or don't, but don't talk about the ad being an ad!'"

Littering an ad with asterisks, as the Hans Brinker ads had done, would have been unthinkable in the past—if only for purely aesthetic reasons. After all, weren't ads supposed to be visually pleasing? Not in the postmodern ad world, which seemed to adopt the philosophy that beauty isn't truth—it's just phony advertising gloss. A new school of ad designers believed that a feeling of authenticity could be achieved by presenting more jarring, rough imagery. The New York–based graphic designer David Carson—who specialized in using typography to wreak havoc in ads and magazine layouts—became a large influence in advertising in the early 1990s, and particularly had an impact on ads being produced in Amsterdam.

Carson himself designed a series of Dutch Nike ads that seemed to use type to scream at the reader. Before long, advertisers around the world were aping the Carson style, using unusual typefaces in outrageous ways. Technology was a factor in driving this trend, according to the design writers Steven Heller and Julie Lasky. "Postmodern design styles were boosted by the development and proliferation of desktop computers in the late 1980s," Heller and Lasky wrote in the book *Borrowed Design*. They noted that the newly available technology enabled postmodern designers to play easily and inexpensively with typefaces and mixed fonts, while also layering and manipulating photographs.

Again, part of the objective of all this image manipulation was to make ads that didn't look like ads—so, in effect, digital trickery was used to rough up advertising. Agencies like CORE in St. Louis and Pyro in Dallas,

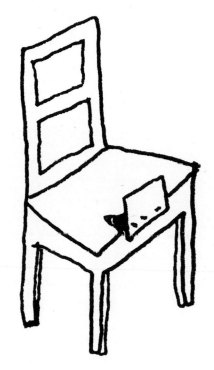

sharon Stone'schair.

Made to order furniture. Recycled timber furniture made to your own specifications. Collingwood: 9419 4866. **Ancient Modes** South Yarra: 9827 0899. Fitzroy: 9419 3418.

26

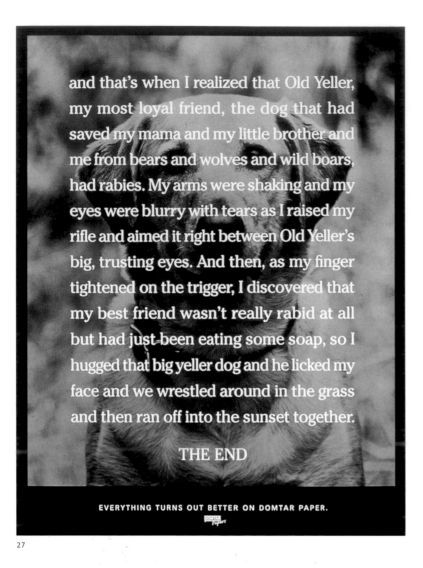

and that's when I realized that Old Yeller, my most loyal friend, the dog that had saved my mama and my little brother and me from bears and wolves and wild boars, had rabies. My arms were shaking and my eyes were blurry with tears as I raised my rifle and aimed it right between Old Yeller's big, trusting eyes. And then, as my finger tightened on the trigger, I discovered that my best friend wasn't really rabid at all but had just been eating some soap, so I hugged that big yeller dog and he licked my face and we wrestled around in the grass and then ran off into the sunset together.

THE END

EVERYTHING TURNS OUT BETTER ON DOMTAR PAPER.

27

run by the brothers Eric and Todd Tilford, seemed to revel in the obscurity of their visuals, using fractured type, and dark, blurry photographs— which somehow ended up yielding elegant, artful ads. Some in advertising dismissed this as style for style's sake, but Eric Tilford argued that the raw style of his ads was more than an affected look—it was an attempt to make the ads feel as real and weathered as the outdoorsy brands that CORE represented.

If CORE was trying to capture a weather-beaten look in its ads, others were going for more of a homemade feeling. In one series of ads created by Wieden + Kennedy's Amsterdam office, the art director Jelly Helm achieved a startling effect by using handwritten scrawl in place of type. Similarly, a series of Tanqueray gin ads from the New York agency Deutsch, featuring a character named Mr. Jenkins, featured a purposely clumsy cut-and-paste collage look; while the Sausalito agency Butler Shine & Stern created ads for Miller's Outpost that looked like a handmade school newspaper. All around the world, one could find similar examples of deconstructed ads, designed to look amateurish—including hand-drawn ads from Dentsu for Tokyo Gas. In some cases, it looked as if advertising was reverting to childhood—all stick figures and scrawled writing. Of course, this advertising was not nearly as naive as it seemed; as Myrna Davis of the Art Directors Club of New York points out, all of the deconstructed and defaced ads of the 1990s were designed to project "an attitude of hipness and street authenticity. With these ads, the attitude is the message."

While some within the advertising creative community felt that the new computer-generated looks in ads were gimmicky, the real debate at the heart of postmodernism revolved around the tendency to appropriate or co-opt.

While it was generally seen as acceptable for a postmodern artist to refer to, or borrow from, other sources (Andy Warhol, of course, was known for borrowing from the commercial world in his art), it was quite a different story when advertisers did it; understandably, questions of exploitation and commercialization were raised, particularly when the ads borrowed from sources considered sacrosanct. It wasn't enough that the Mona Lisa became a pitchwoman in a number of ads—some advertisers even took liberties with Leonardo da Vinci's rendering (Fallon McElligott fattened Mona up a bit, for a Prince spaghetti-sauce ad). Shakespeare was quoted and at times rewritten. Even *Old Yeller,* the sentimental, much-loved American children's tale, was given a new twist—a hilariously upbeat happy ending—from the Minneapolis ad agency Hunt Adkins, making the lighthearted point that "everything turns out better" when printed

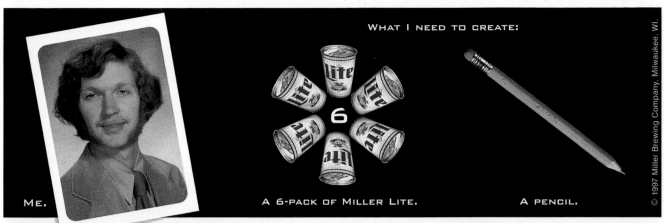

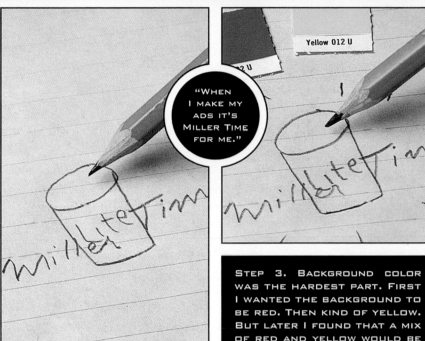

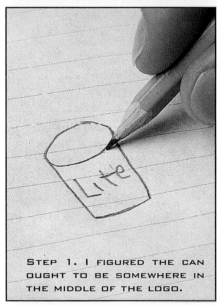

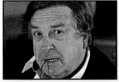

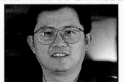

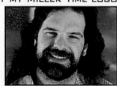

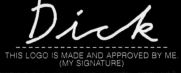

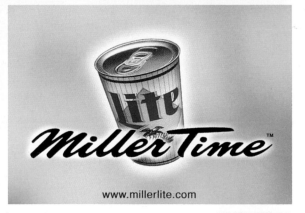

28

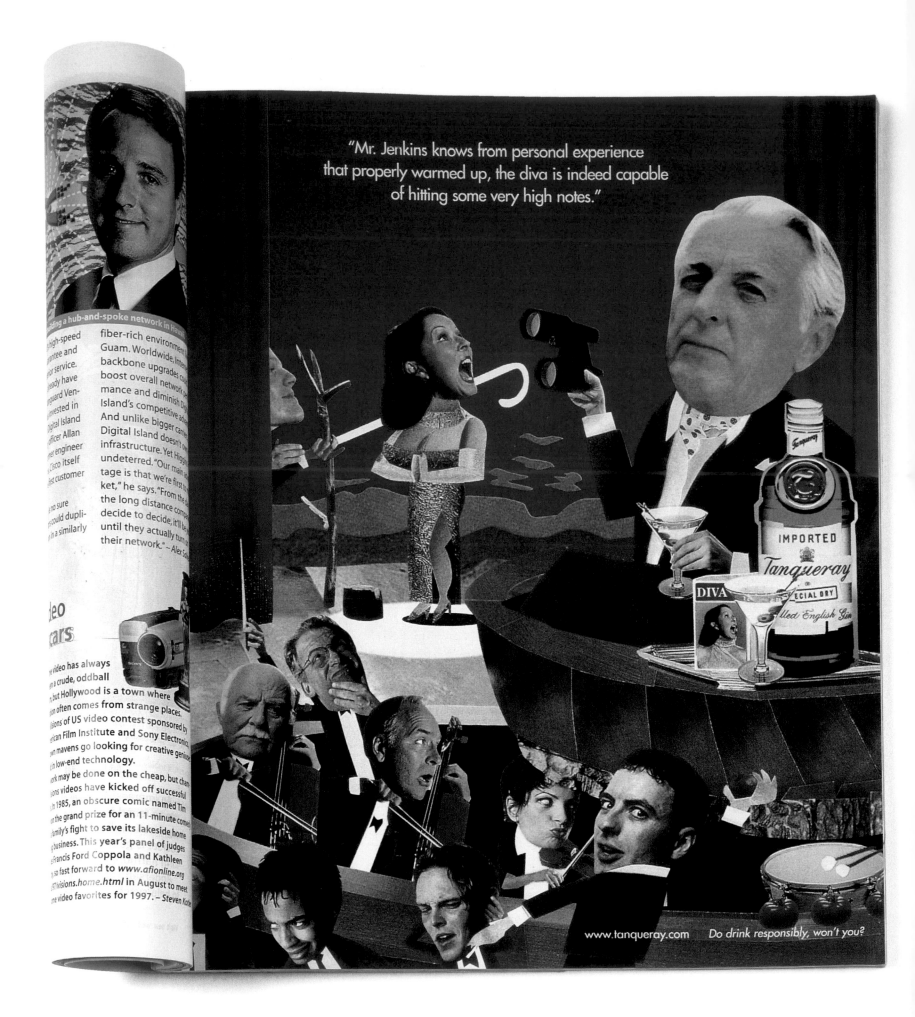

29. TANQUERAY GIN
DEUTSCH INC., NEW YORK,
1997
Tanqueray came up with its own
offbeat character, the suave Mr.
Jenkins, and placed him in the
midst of photo-collage scenes.

30. MARTINI
AMSTER YARD, NEW YORK,
1995
Ads referenced hip films, both
new and old. In the mid-1990s,
Fellini's *La Dolce Vita* was still
considered cool enough to be
appropriated by a trendy brand
of Italian liquor.

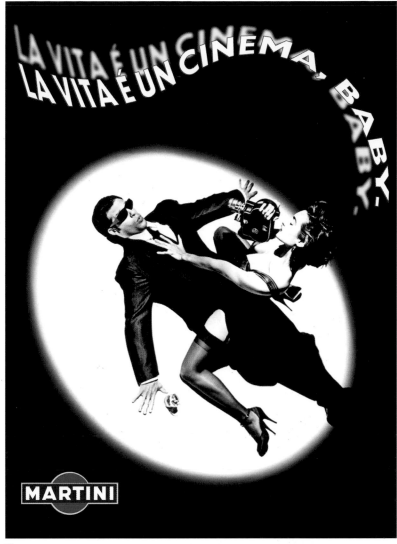

30

on a certain brand of paper. In terms of
co-opting rock music, it might have seemed
Nike's "Revolution" had gone about as far as
one could go—but then in the mid-1990s
Mercedes-Benz came out with a commercial
whose soundtrack was Janis Joplin singing,
"Oh Lord, won't you buy me a Mercedes-Benz"
(lyrics that had originally been written by the
late Joplin as an ironic statement against
status symbols). Elsewhere around the world,
Elvis Presley was given a 1990s-style goatee
by a Finland agency promoting a nightclub,
and Fellini's film *La Dolce Vita* became the
basis of a European campaign for Martini
liquor. Was nothing sacred? Apple Computer
answered that question in the late 1990s,
when its "Think different" campaign began
featuring Gandhi and the Dalai Lama in ads.

Cultural guardians did not take kindly to
all this. Michiko Kakutani, a *New York Times*
book reviewer and culture critic, wrote,

"Advertising implacably forges ahead like one
of those indestructible sci-fi monsters, noncha-
lantly co-opting the very techniques used
against it. Just as it has co-opted rock-and-
roll alienation . . . and Dadaist jokes, so it
has now co-opted irony, parody and satire."
The end result, Kakutani concluded, is "a blurring of the lines between art and commerce."
To the charges that it has co-opted the culture,
advertising's creative community has a reasonable response: The culture belongs to everyone,
including ad creators. "Advertising is a reflection
of our shared experience as human beings,"
says Bob Kuperman of TBWA/Chiat/Day. "I
see no problem with using anything that
makes up that shared experience."

The debate on this issue has continued in
the new millennium and probably will not be
resolved soon. But as the 1990s progressed,
the cultural watchdogs weren't the only ones
expressing concerns about the new advertising.

Marketing traditionalists, including the
guardians of some of the world's foremost
brands, were beginning to raise another issue:
Just how far could the postmodern approach
to advertising go before it strayed too far
from the fundamentals of selling products?
Was it possible that the growing emphasis
on "anti-sell" statements and self-conscious
style was losing touch with basic logic and
strategy? They were reasonable questions from
the people paying the bills for the world's
advertising. And they would be amplified in
the late 1990s, as many ads strayed even
further from logic and rationality—and
moved into the wide-open, anything-goes
realm of "Oddvertising."

6. THE
'ODDVEI

RISE OF
TISING."

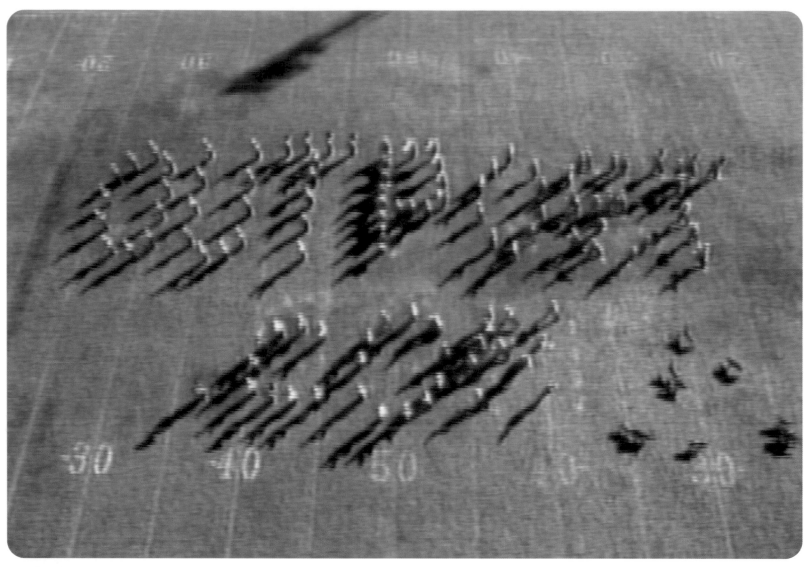

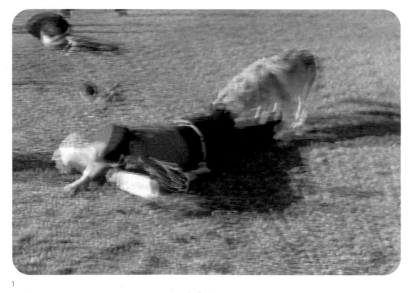

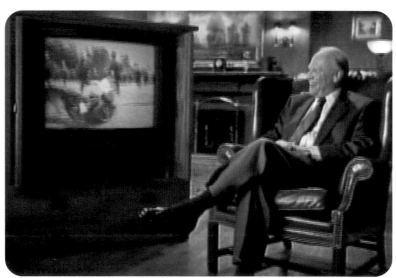

In a 1998 commercial for the Web site Outpost.com, the opening scene looks like a bit of classic advertising Americana: The camera follows a high school marching band, in full regalia, as members play their instruments and form the letters Outpost on a football field. So far so good, but as the ad's narrator explains, Outpost wanted to add something to make the commercial "more memorable." And so, the narrator deadpans, "we decided to release a pack of ravenous wolves." In the next scene, the wolves are shown attacking the band members, who drop their instruments and run for their lives. Laughing, the narrator concludes, "That's good stuff."

Welcome to the strange new world of "Oddvertising," where anything can happen in an ad—and quite often does. Beginning sometime in the mid-1990s and accelerating as the new millennium arrived, advertisers and their creative agencies increasingly began using advertisements to present extreme scenarios, offbeat characters, and at times baffling messages. Is this any way to advertise a product? Lately the answer to that question, both in America and around the world, seems to be a resounding yes.

"People have a real yearning for the unexpected in advertising now," observes the New York ad executive Cliff Freeman, the creator of the Outpost "Wolves" commercial. If it's a strange twist that viewers crave, Freeman—who has emerged as one of the leaders of the new Oddvertising—rarely disappoints. When his Outpost ads weren't unleashing wolves on marching bands, they were firing tiny rodents from a cannon. Freeman's infamous "Gerbils" commercial—not all that widely seen, yet probably one of the most influential American ads of the late 1990s—featured the same deadpan announcer, once again presiding with no shame over a shocking stunt intended to help viewers remember the Outpost name. This time, the "Outpost" letters were printed on a wall, with a hole in the O. The cannon was used to attempt to fire gerbils through the hole—although the first few shots were off-target, causing the critters to bounce off the wall (which didn't seem to bother the sadistic narrator in the least). One of the strangest aspects of the Outpost ads was that they didn't even bother to explain who the sponsor was or what products it offered; such dry, straightforward information seemingly had no place in advertising that was pure, unadulterated absurdity.

Freeman took a similar approach in some of his advertising for other clients. To promote hockey telecasts on the Fox TV network, ads posed the question, "What if other sports were like hockey?" We were then shown the outrageous answer as, in one ad, a golfer quietly and studiously lined up his putt—when suddenly a competing golfer charged onto the green and

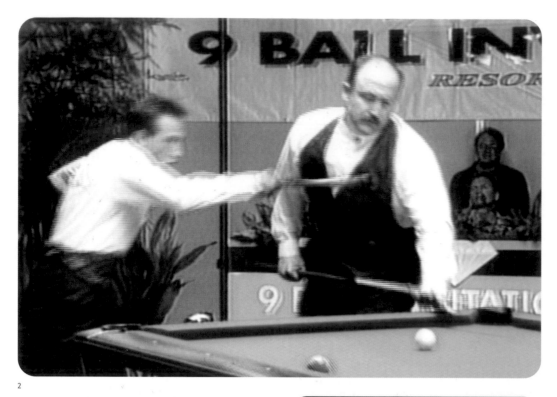

2

2. **FOX SPORTS**
CLIFF FREEMAN & PARTNERS,
NEW YORK, 1997
Wondering what it would be like
if other sports were more like
hockey, Freeman showed pool
players and golfers attacking one
another with sticks and clubs.

3. **OUTPOST.COM**
CLIFF FREEMAN & PARTNERS,
NEW YORK, 1998
Cliff Freeman strikes again;
this time, a gerbil is shot from
a cannon. The ads attracted
headlines and complaints, but
not enough paying customers.

BILLIARDS WOULD BE BETTER
IF IT WERE HOCKEY.

began attacking with his club, hockey-style. Still another Freeman ad, for the Fox Sports Web site, started out looking like a heart-wrenching public-service commercial, with a close-up view of a man's toes fumbling with a baby's diaper. Did this mean the man's hands were disabled? Not at all—the camera gradually revealed that the whole time, his fingers were busy tapping away on his computer keyboard as he visited the Fox Sports Web site.

The mischievous Freeman has not been the only one veering off the straight and narrow path of logical advertising. Bizarre ads have been surfacing all across the American advertising landscape, promoting brands large and small. In Adidas and Nike commercials, deranged sports fans were shown stalking athletes. The happy families once prevalent in commercials began to give way to the likes of the "Jukka brothers," stars of Fallon McElligott ads for MTV (like backwoods characters from the film

Deliverance, the Jukkas live in a remote cabin, watch only MTV, and occasionally whack one another on the backsides with paddles). In Budweiser's advertising, computer-generated lizards joked about committing murder. In presenting surreal or outrageous scenarios, many of the new ads typically adopted a deadpan tone of voice—with a number of ads using the format of an absurd documentary (or "mockumentary"), a style made popular by the commercials of the ESPN cable television network. Mockumentary ads could transport viewers into an imaginary world or subculture where characters behave obsessively and where the featured product or service—a sneaker, a TV channel—sometimes served as the object of obsession.

Oddvertising has marked a dramatic shift from the linear, easy-to-follow ads of old, and frequently leaves viewers shocked or mystified—though the best of these ads are usually amusing and intriguing, as well. The fever has not been

limited to American advertising. It has surfaced in the ads of the United Kingdom—which dabbled in Monty Python–style absurdity years ago but have now moved further into what the British ad executive John Hegarty calls "the new era of irrationality." One of Hegarty's own recent campaigns for Levi's exemplified the trend: Revolving around a mysterious man who is always shown accompanied by a living yellow puppet named "Flat Eric," the series of ads defied explanation. The stolid man and the frenetic puppet exchanged meaningful glances but never spoke as they traveled around, getting haircuts together, while being pursued by police for reasons never made clear. The mystery seemed to reel in viewers, as "Flat Eric" became a popular phenomenon, first in the UK and then in Germany. Another British campaign, for Tango orange drink, featured an orange-painted bald man who roamed around slapping people's ears for no good reason. And a popular ongoing

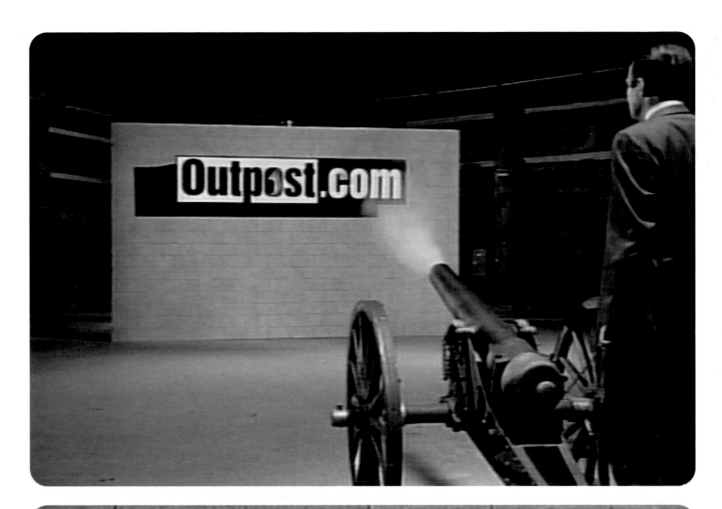

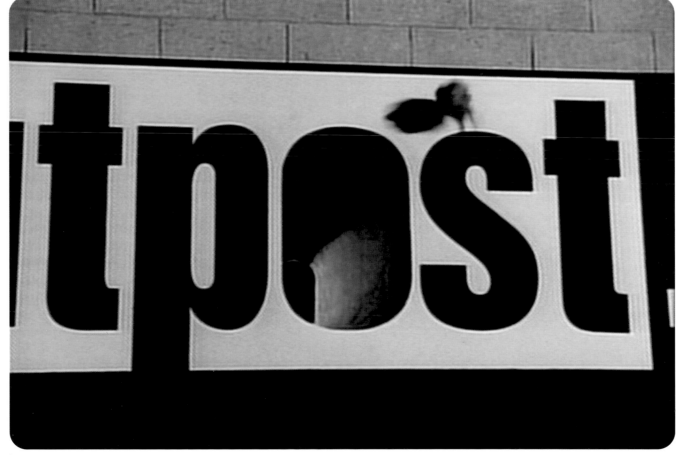

3

THE RISE OF "ODDVERTISING."

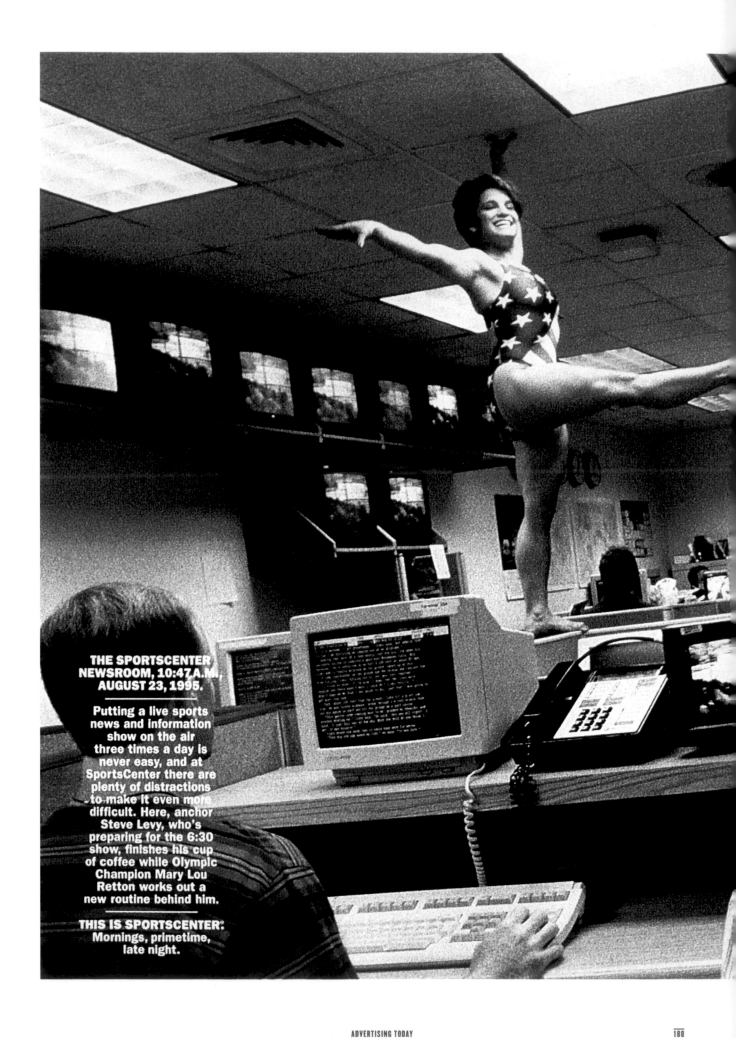

THE SPORTSCENTER NEWSROOM, 10:47 A.M., AUGUST 23, 1995.

Putting a live sports news and information show on the air three times a day is never easy, and at SportsCenter there are plenty of distractions to make it even more difficult. Here, anchor Steve Levy, who's preparing for the 6:30 show, finishes his cup of coffee while Olympic Champion Mary Lou Retton works out a new routine behind him.

THIS IS SPORTSCENTER: Mornings, primetime, late night.

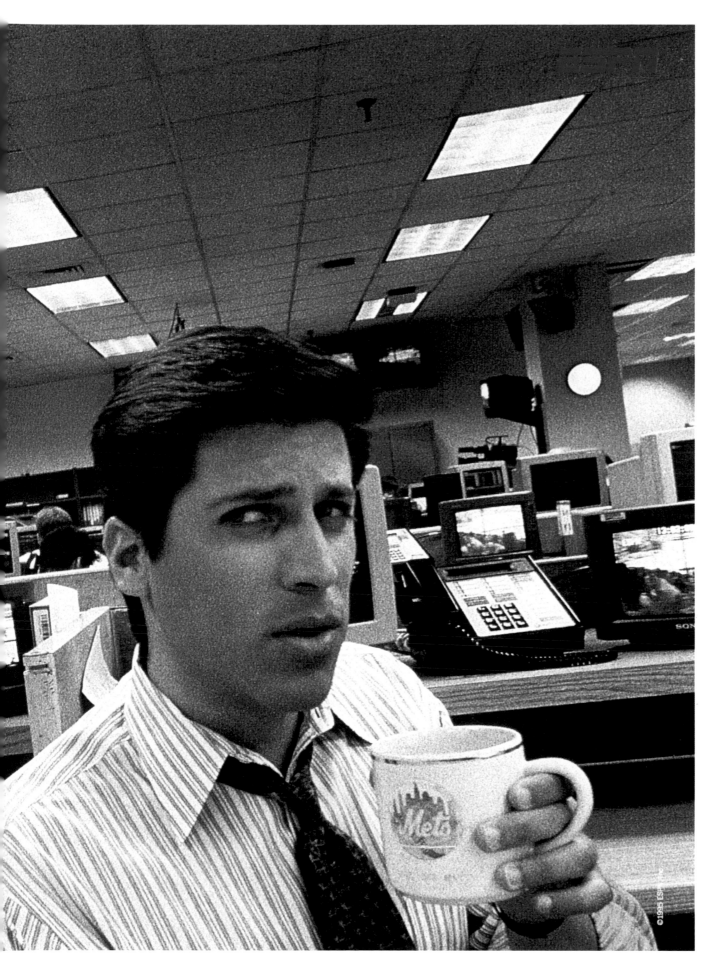

©1995 ESPN Inc.

4. **ESPN NETWORK**
WIEDEN + KENNEDY,
PORTLAND, 1995
The One Club of New York
called this the ad campaign of
the decade. Using a "mockumentary" style, it took the
audience behind the scenes
at the sports network.

THE RISE OF "ODDVERTISING."

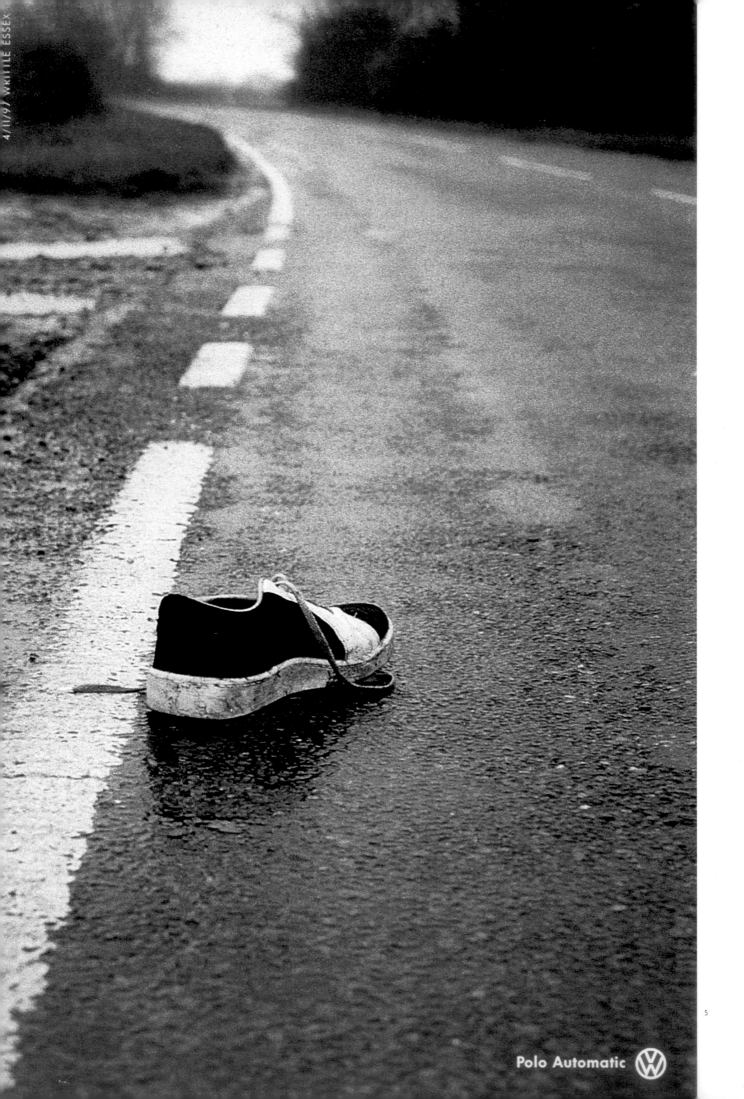

Polo Automatic W

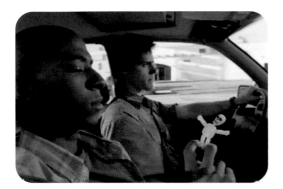

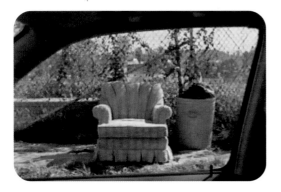

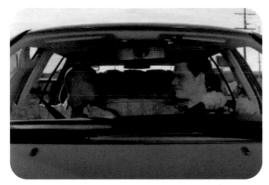

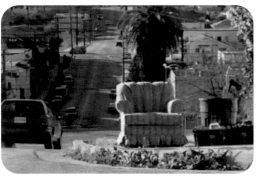

6

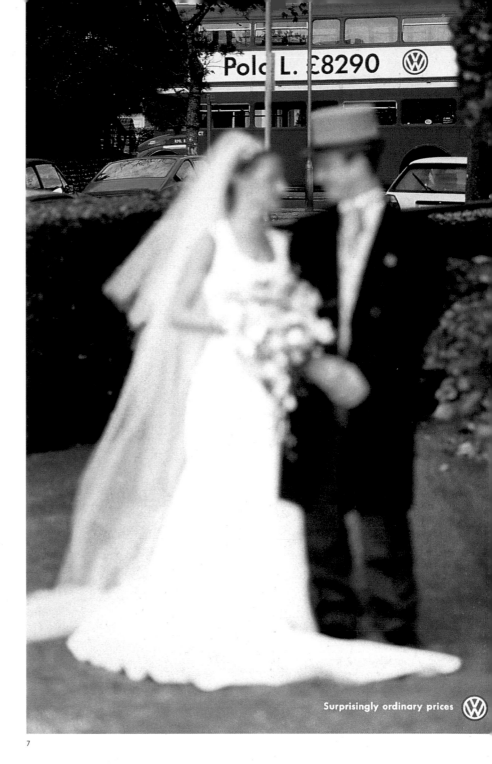

7

5. VOLKSWAGEN
BMP DDB, LONDON, 1997
This campaign baffled the UK by
showing a series of photos of a
left shoe abandoned in the road
(by drivers who had been freed
from having to step on a clutch).

6. VOLKSWAGEN
ARNOLD COMMUNICATIONS,
BOSTON, 1997
The intrigue of Oddvertising: in
this TV commercial, we don't
know who these two men are or
why they picked up this old
smelly chair on the street.

7. VOLKSWAGEN
BMP DDB, LONDON, 1998
The wedding photo was ruined
because the photographer was
focusing on VW's low prices in
the background; the same series
featured distracted pedestrians
colliding with streetpoles.

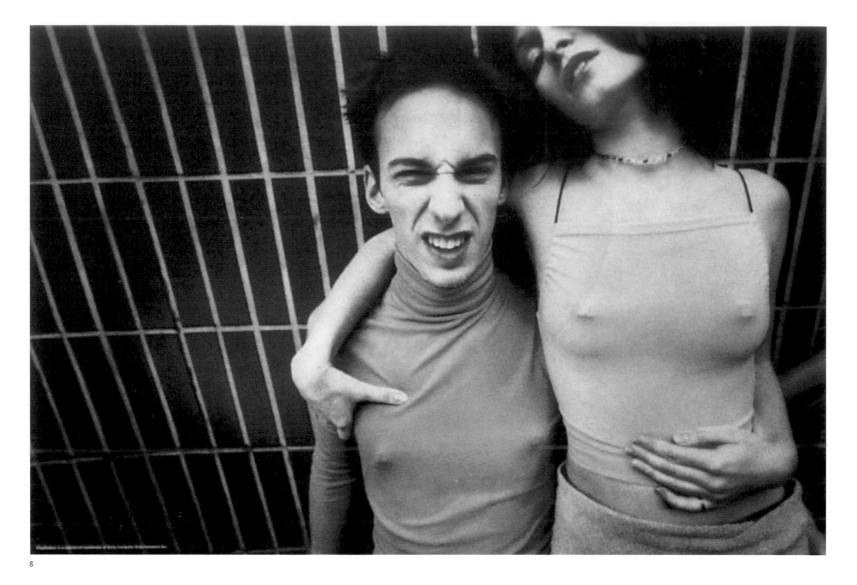

8

8. SONY VIDEO GAMES
TBWA GGT SIMONS PALMER,
LONDON, 1999
This ad, a big winner at the
International Ad Festival in
Cannes, showed hard-core video
game fanatics displaying the
look of video game control
knobs in an eye-catching way.

9. URGE SOFT DRINK
LEO BURNETT, OSLO, 1997
If you don't understand the
headline, you're not alone; the
campaign used the obscure
vernacular of skateboarding
culture.

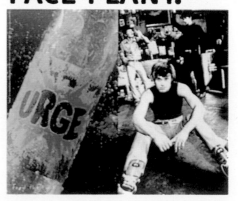

9

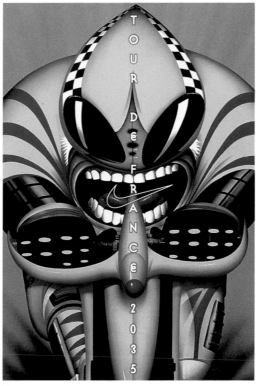

10

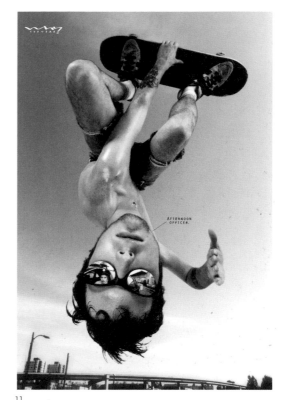

11

10. **NIKE / TOUR DE FRANCE**
KESSELSKRAMER,
AMSTERDAM, 1997
By the mid-1990s, the art used
in ads became more abstract,
impressionistic, and even a little
scary, as in this Dutch Nike poster.

11. **WHY EYEWEAR**
PALMER JARVIS DDB,
VANCOUVER, 1997
Turning the world upside down:
An old ad trick finds new life in
the era of Oddvertising.

British campaign for Volkswagen Polo depicts silent and strange little vignettes in which the characters are so surprised to learn of the car's low prices that they suddenly lose consciousness, dropping their faces into their food and walking into lampposts.

While odd advertising has been popping up around the world, some countries, such as Australia, seem particularly predisposed to it. Ads from Down Under have been over the top for years, though the new extremity of the trend can be seen in a commercial for the Australian "Ladies Masters" golf tournament—in which dominatrix female golfers tee up the ball on a man's nose and swing away (the ad ends with a shot showing a disembodied nose on the ground). One of the most popular Australian commercials of the late 1990s was a madcap bit of slapstick for Toyota entitled "Bugger!," wherein a series of mishaps involving a Toyota vehicle cause the commercial's characters to

repeatedly yell, "Bugger!"—the only dialogue in the ad.

Even markets that are generally considered more conservative have been experimenting with wild, offbeat approaches. For example, France has traditionally favored elegant, stylish advertising— which makes it all the more striking to encounter a French Orangina ad featuring a homicidal, chainsaw-wielding man dressed as a piece of fruit. And while Asia has the reputation of being a "straight-arrow" ad market, certain countries, such as Thailand, are embracing outrageousness. It's not uncommon to see wild Thai commercials starring transvestites painted silver. And Japan, whose advertising has long featured quirkiness, seems to be pushing new boundaries. An extremely popular ad campaign for Sega was not just peculiar but almost sadistic: Acknowledging that the company's past products were inferior to those of its competitors, the commercials featured a real-life

senior executive who was repeatedly humiliated on-screen as punishment for Sega's past mistakes. (In one ad, the man, Yukawa Hidekazu, overheard kids saying that "Sega video games suck." After drowning his sorrows at a bar, the drunken Yukawa got beaten up and lay sprawled on the ground while an off-camera voice said, "Come on, Mr. Yukawa, get up!") The campaign turned Yukawa into a pop celebrity in Japan.

As the Oddvertising fever spreads globally, the question arises, "Why are so many ads going a bit mad?" To some extent, eccentric behavior and quirky characters have been seen in commercials since the 1970s era of Charmin bathroom tissue's Mr. Whipple and his compulsive squeezing. The difference is really a matter of degree: Today's odd commercial characters have more of an edge to them and can seem genuinely deranged; Mr. Whipple's innocent fetish pales in comparison to the behavior of a 1990s ad character played by Dennis Hopper in Nike

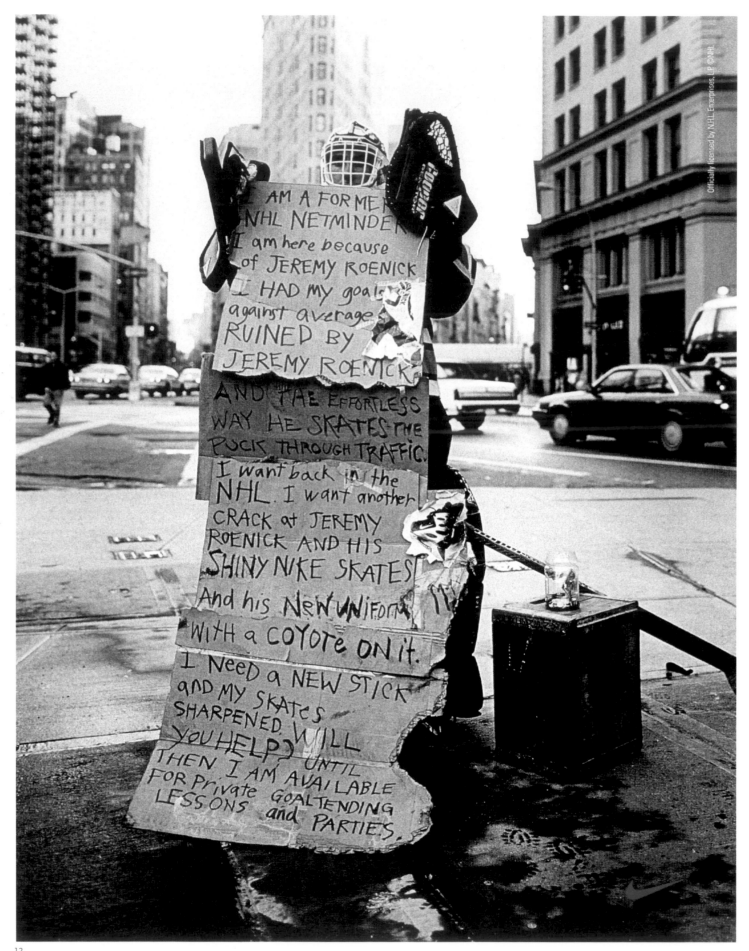

12

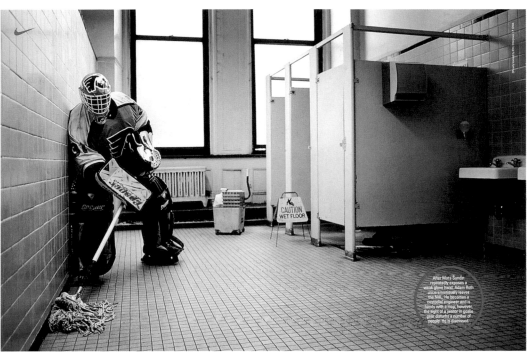

13

12 AND 13. **NIKE**
WIEDEN + KENNEDY,
PORTLAND, 1997
Telling strange tales: In this
series, a goalie loses his job and
becomes homeless—all because
Nike skates made it easier for
his nemesis to score goals
against him.

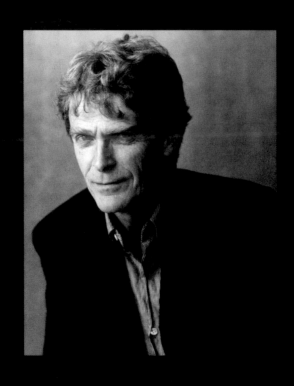

INTERVIEW: JOHN HEGARTY

As creative director at the preeminent London ad agency Bartle Bogle Hegarty, John Hegarty has had a hand in creating many of the UK's most popular and innovative ad campaigns of the 1980s and 1990s. But no Hegarty creation has had a bigger impact than Flat Eric, a puppet that appeared in a series of commercials named the best advertising of 1999 by England's *Campaign* magazine. The success of the Flat Eric ads, which rapidly spread through Europe, seemed to defy rational explanation—as did the ads themselves. They featured very little dialogue, no coherent storyline, and a series of bizarre scenarios that followed the puppet and his human companion as they cruised in a car and bopped to "dirty house" music, were pursued by police, got a haircut, and somehow ended up in a mortuary. Hegarty himself isn't entirely certain why Eric became a cultural phenomenon—though he thinks it may have something to do with advertising's new "era of irrationality."

WHEN AND WHY DID IRRATIONAL ADS LIKE "FLAT ERIC" START TO BECOME MORE POPULAR?

You have to look at the history of this. First, advertising went through a period of being dominated by the "Unique Selling Proposition," which was based on the fact that technology was playing a greater part in the manufacture of products. If you go back to the 1950s, science seemed to have the answer to everything, and advertising used that as a means of promoting brand difference—new Colgate with extra fluoride, and so forth. But after a while, it was obvious that everybody had the technology, and no one company could stay ahead of the crowd. And then we moved toward the Emotional Selling Proposition, where the emotional value—how someone felt about that brand—became the point of difference.

But more recently, I think we've entered a new period, relying on what might be called the Irrational Selling Proposition. In the 1990s, advertisers found ourselves in a situation where a lot of it just wasn't working—there was too much, and people had become acutely able to filter it out. So increasingly, you had to do things to capture people's imaginations. Often that meant talking to a young media-literate

audience in a unique way. That could involve absurdity—because absurdity might provide a stimulation that people want.

In a sense, we're now saying a brand is about fun, and it has an element of irreverence about it—and that's what you try to capture with the advertising. With "Flat Eric," what we were doing is laughing at Levi's own culture; for a long time, Levi's ads had heroes who were muscled, handsome pinups—and now we wanted to break that mold and say, "Here is a hero who's a fluffy puppet. And if Flat Eric can be a hero then you can, even if you've got a pimply face, with thick glasses." People may look at that and ask, "Where's the logic?" The logic is as simple as that—he's fun. He's not taking things seriously, and Levi's is not taking its advertising overly seriously. We know that there's a game in progress, and we want you to enjoy the game.

IS PART OF THE APPEAL THE MYSTERY OF THE ADS, THE FACT THAT WE DON'T REALLY KNOW WHAT'S GOING ON WITH THESE TWO CHARACTERS?

Yes, that's a big part of it. You don't want to spell things out too much; you want to let the audience fill out the story for themselves, though we gave them little clues and ideas to work with. When the policeman pulls them over in one ad, you see their driver's licenses—very briefly, you have to look quickly to get it—and that's how you learn that he's called Flat Eric. And on the license, if you look really closely, you can barely make out his date of birth. But it was enough that on the Internet, we started getting birthday cards for him. You give people lots of clues and allow them to get to it. The trouble with most advertising is that it completes everything for you. Which means there's nothing left for you to do, and consequently, your mind is off doing something else while the commercial is on.

ISN'T THERE A DANGER OF GOING OFF-TRACK WITH ODD ADS LIKE THIS?

Of course. The danger is that one can look at the Irrational Selling Proposition and say, "Well, this is a license to do anything." But it's not. There always should be a line of logic there—and you have to be careful how you

track that line of logic, because if you don't have that there, then you will produce stuff that has no bearing on the brand. In the case of "Flat Eric," the logic is that Levi's is spoofing its own culture.

IN THE U.S., THERE HAS BEEN A BACKLASH AGAINST SOME OFFBEAT, ENTERTAINMENT-DRIVEN ADS; SOME MARKETERS HAVE REJECTED THEM AND CALLED FOR MORE OF A HARD-SELL APPROACH.

Well, they're right in a sense. There are some people creating ads now who are trying a little too hard to be wacky or edgy. It's like everything—imitators come along and don't quite understand the process that was going on originally. And they end up with the trappings of it but not the real meaning of it. We shouldn't be trying to be wacky. However, we should be trying to be entertaining. If you do that, you involve someone in the process and draw them into your sphere of influence. And then you want to link that back to the brand in some way.

I also must say, I've always disliked these terms *hard sell* versus *soft sell*. People use the term hard sell as an argument that's turned against creativity—that creativity doesn't sell. But in fact, great creative advertising has always sold better than conventional *hard-sell* advertising. The problem with the hard-sell ad is that it doesn't intrigue me, it doesn't seduce me, it doesn't create an ambience that I want to enter into. It just shouts at me. It might make the company sales director feel comfortable, but the consumer increasingly is rejecting it. Because in the end, if it worked—if advertising were that simple—we'd all be doing it that way.

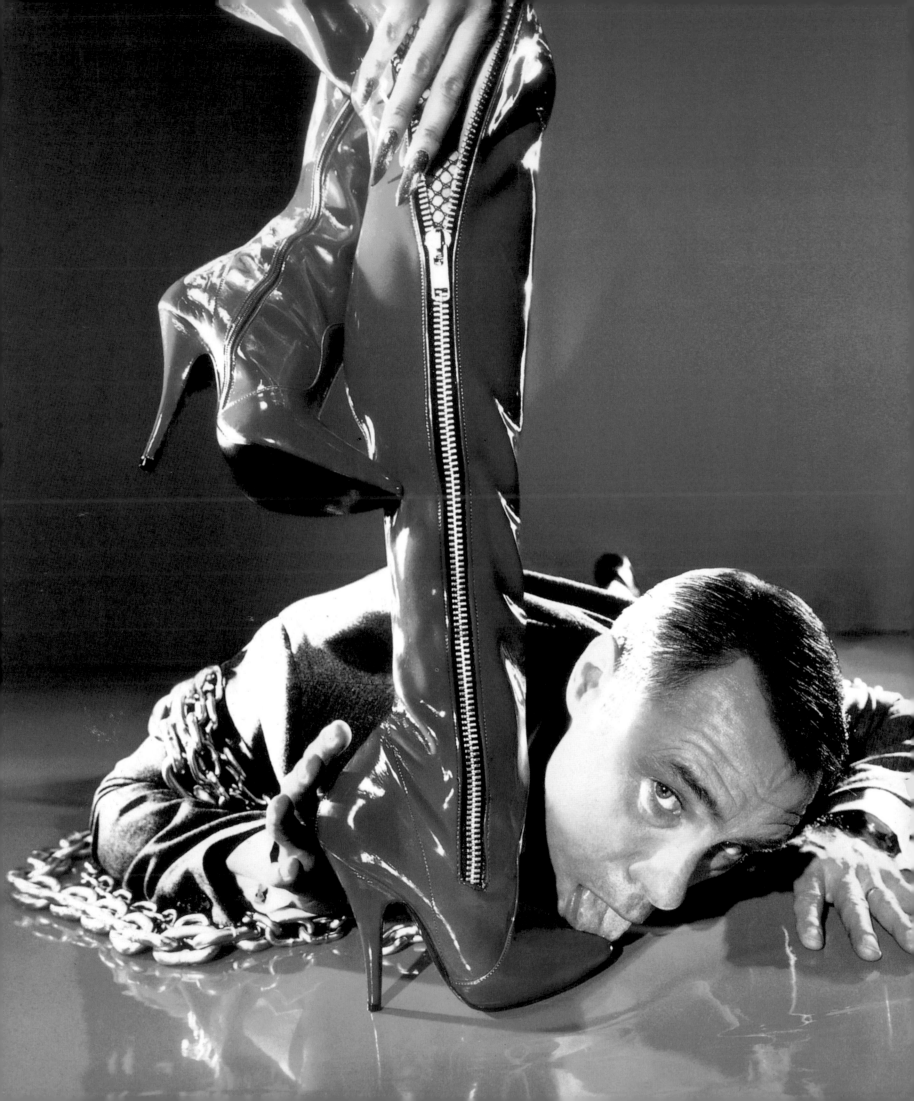

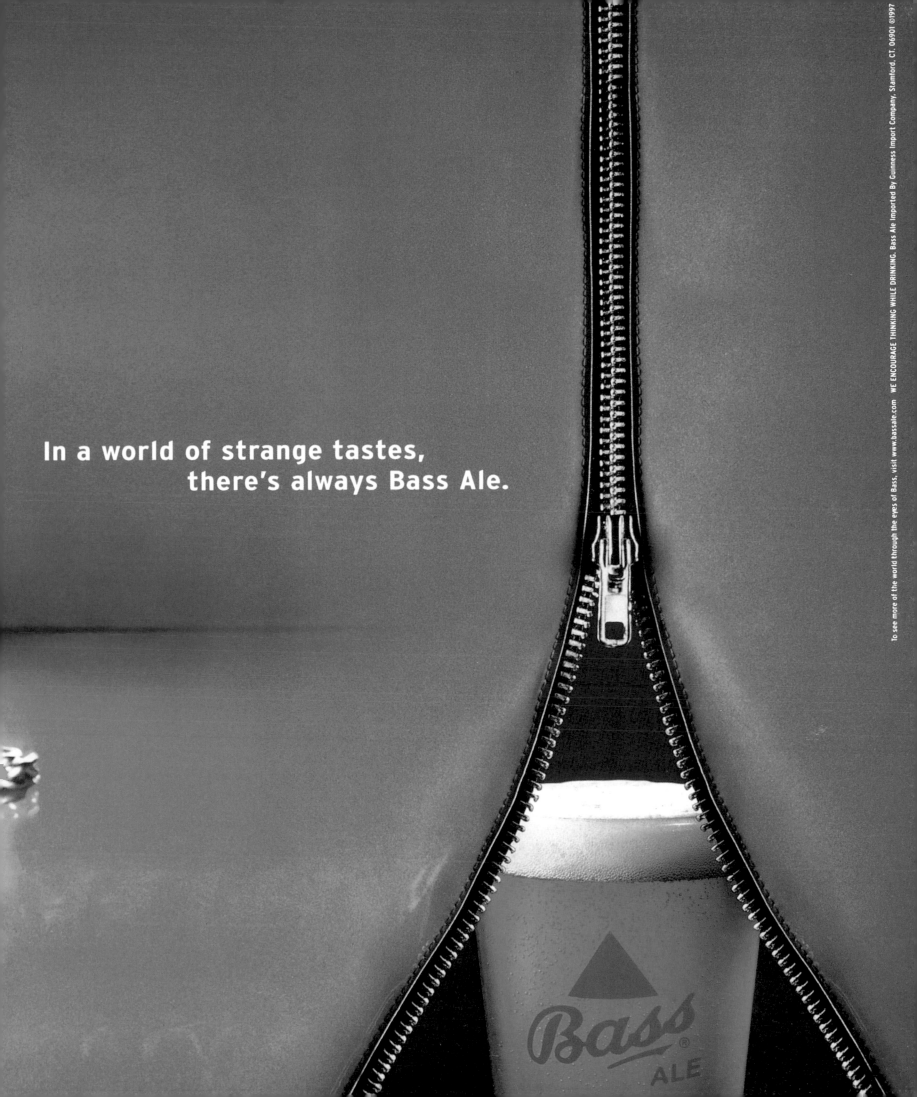

In a world of strange tastes,
there's always Bass Ale.

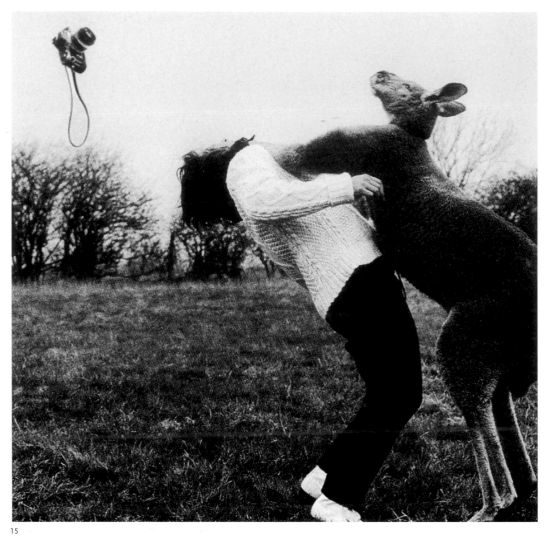

15

commercials, in which Hopper is shown stalking athletes and sniffing their shoes in the locker room when no one is looking. The other difference now is the prevalence of bizarre ads: A decade ago, they were rare and served as curiosities. The American fashion designer Calvin Klein, for example, was among the first to dabble in strangeness, producing "Obsession" ads in which emotionally tormented characters spoke in obtuse, highly artificial dialogue— which often ended up being the object of well-deserved ridicule or parody. (Klein's particular brand of Oddvertising was different from today's in that it seemed to take itself so seriously; the ads borrowed more from Ingmar Bergman than from Monty Python, and that pretentiousness drove viewers to distraction.) But in today's environment, Klein's ads begin to seem almost coherent and not all that unusual. There are now so many "offbeat" ads that the word no longer is appropriate; such ads now *are* the beat.

To some extent, the mainstreaming of oddness could be seen as just another step in the evolution that began with Doyle Dane Bernbach's reinvention of advertising. At the heart of much of DDB's work was the element of surprise— designed to give ads a twist, a look, an attitude that caught the public off-guard. That continued to be a primary objective of creative advertising in the 1980s and early 1990s, as the American ad executive Jeff Goodby notes. "It's become more and more important for advertising to be intriguing in some way, and to give people the sense that they don't know where the story is going," says Goodby. As that became increasingly difficult to do, advertisers had to resort to ever more unusual stories, situations, and characters in order to surprise the audience.

Bartle Bogle Hegarty's John Hegarty believes that in the 1990s, many advertisers began to fully realize that the public could no longer be reached with rational messages, neatly packaged

and presented. "People were just filtering it out," says Hegarty. "Increasingly, you had to do unusual things to capture people's imaginations. Lots of the old rules have gone by the boards." What campaigns like "Flat Eric" are now presenting, Hegarty says, is not so much a coherent message as "an attempt to talk to a young, media-literate audience in a unique way." The ads may seem illogical, but, Hegarty adds, "I could argue that they are logical in their own way—they're part of the irrational selling proposition that has emerged in the 1990s."

Cliff Freeman believes that a big factor driving this trend has been a profound change in the attitudes of sponsors, including larger clients like Budweiser, Miller Brewing Co., and the Mars candy company, all of whom have gravitated toward more unconventional ads. "Even the big clients are loosening up," Freeman notes. Engulfed by more competition, greater product parity, and fragmented media, "they're

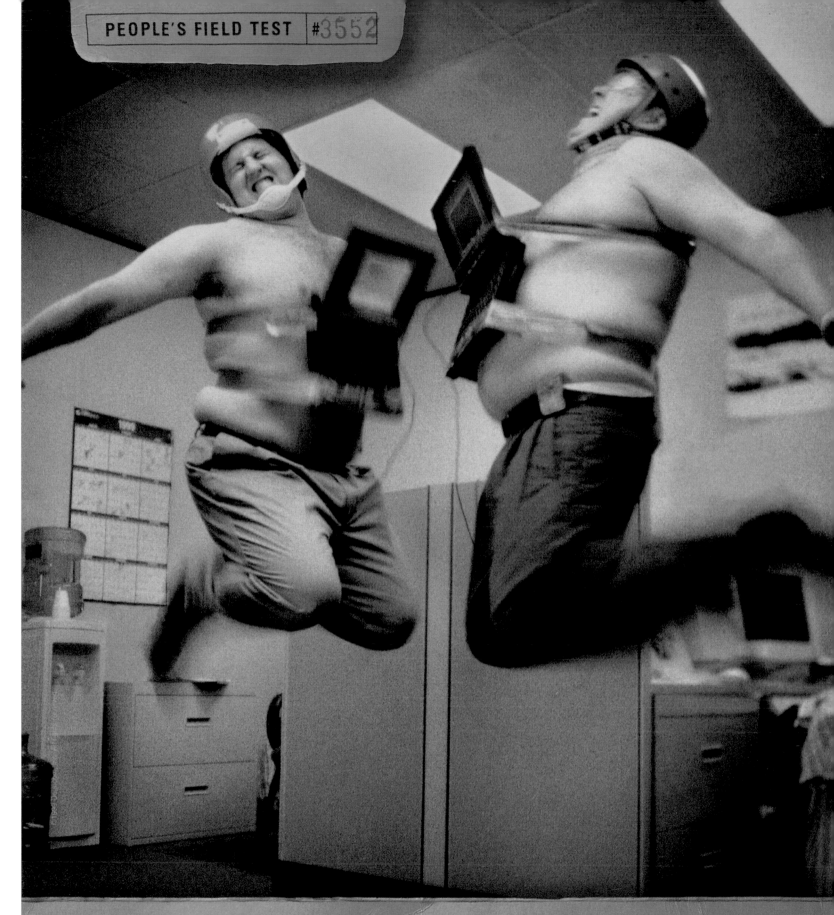

>> *LAPTOPS* >> *DURABILITY*

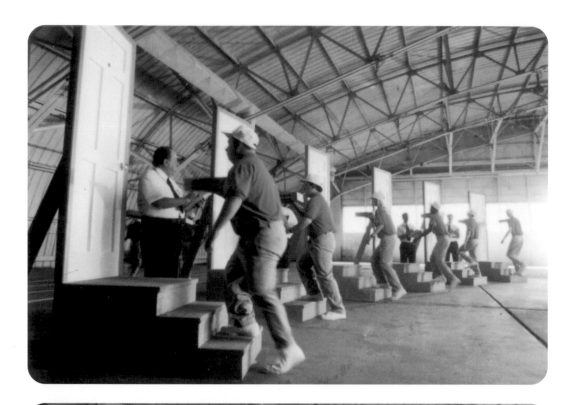

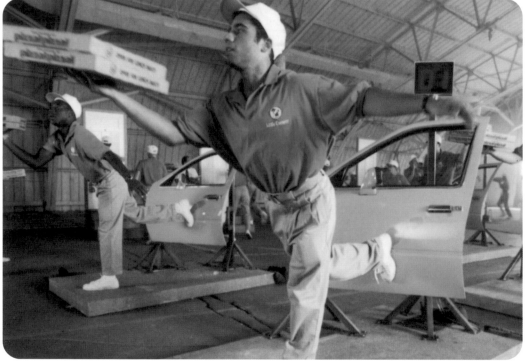

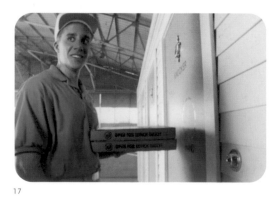

17

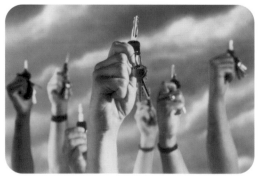

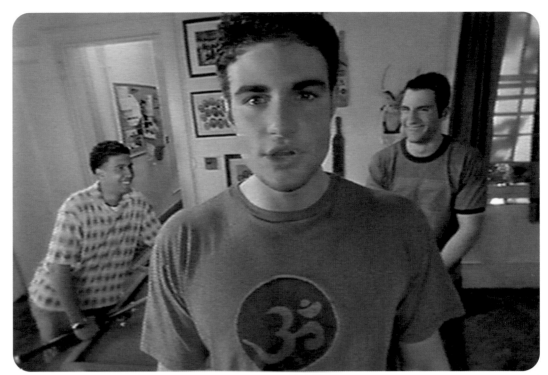

18

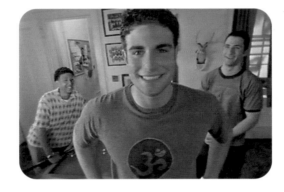

realizing that nobody can play it safe anymore,"
he says.

In fact, advertising in recent years has come
to be led by a different kind of sponsor. In the
past, large and conservative packaged-goods
companies, like Procter & Gamble, controlled
much of the airtime and set the general tone for
advertising. But today, some of the biggest
advertisers—and certainly the most influential—
are younger, more daring entrepreneurial companies like Apple Computer, Nintendo, and Nike,
who are much more inclined to produce quirky
advertising designed to project a hip image.

If there is a single category of advertiser that
most favors the shoot-from-the-hip style of
Oddvertising, it is the Internet-based companies—the so-called dot-coms—whose outrageous
imagery and messages began to flood the airwaves and the print media in the late 1990s.
The aforementioned Outpost led the charge, but
other dot-com clients were just as willing to

present bizarre scenarios. The Web site
Ecampus.com ran ads showing college students
belching, and depicted one student so strapped
for cash he cooked up his goldfish for food.
Another site, for Beyond.com, created ads
featuring a stay-at-home businessman who
paraded in front of his neighbors in the nude.
The emphasis on egregious behavior in the
dot-com ad market was partly driven by
desperation. In a crowded, rapidly growing
marketplace filled with no-name newcomers,
these companies needed to take drastic measures
to draw attention to themselves. As many of the
dot-com clients approached their agencies, they
made it very clear what was needed: Get us
noticed, by any means necessary. Outpost, for
example, specifically challenged Cliff Freeman to
"do whatever it takes to drive people to the Web
site." It was a wide-open challenge that Freeman,
and many other top creative people in advertising,
eagerly embraced. However, the result, as

The New York Times noted in mid-1999, was
often not a pretty sight: "Dot-com advertising
seems to be the place where practically no bodily
function is too private and no rude behavior is
too coarse to be featured in a spot."

The rush of these dot-com ads was the most
obvious manifestation of the booming Western
economies of the late 1990s, but those strong
global economic conditions also seemed to foster
offbeat advertising in a variety of other markets
and product categories. The American ad executive Andy Berlin believes that the boom times
emboldened advertisers, giving them confidence
to take more risks. The noted Massachusetts
Institute of Technology economist Paul Krugman
also observed a link between economics and wild
ads. "When TV commercials get funny, that's
a sign of excessive optimism," Krugman noted.
Advertisers loosen up because, Krugman says,
"when the market is very bubbly, they think they
can get away with that. The point is to get the

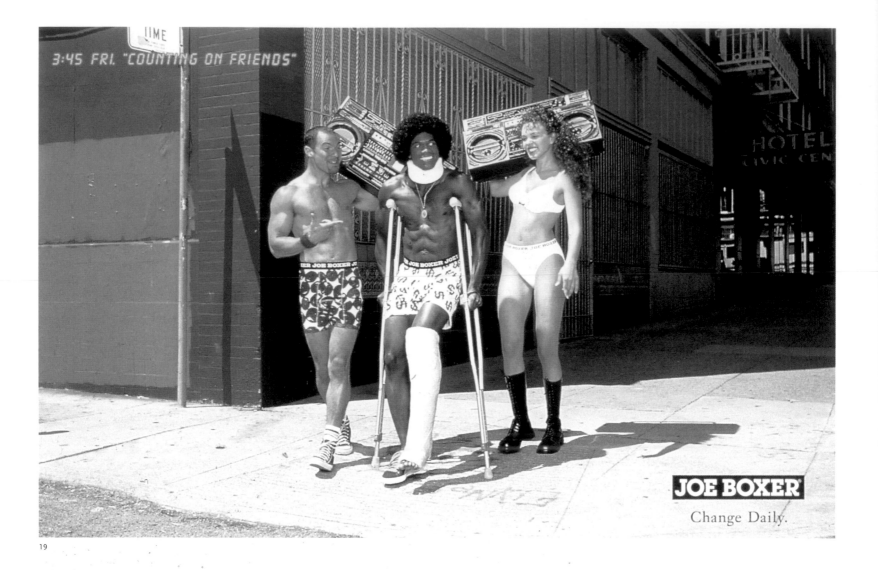

3:45 FRI. "COUNTING ON FRIENDS"

JOE BOXER®
Change Daily.

19

attention of people who have plenty of money to spend." On the other hand, "when things turn bad, they just repeat the product [name] fifteen times," Krugman says, echoing Mary Wells's famous "Hard times demand hard selling" statement. Certainly, the larger ad budgets of the 1990s allowed for the kind of ad experimentation that usually isn't attempted during leaner economic times.

While sociological and economic factors fueled the rise of Oddvertising, its spread can also be attributed to an even more powerful force in advertising: imitation. Advertising creators are never shy about jumping on bandwagons; one of the plagues of the industry is that creative people study award-show annuals to see what played well the previous year—then shamelessly begin creating similar ads themselves. In this case, several bizarre mid-1990s campaigns caught the fancy of the public and the advertising creative community, and subsequently kicked the trend into high gear.

Freeman was a pivotal player, and his impact was felt long before the Outpost campaign. In the early 1990s, his agency's highly successful campaigns for Little Caesars pizza could take the simplest, most mundane idea and turn it into wild theater of the absurd. For example, when Little Caesars decided to offer pizza delivery, Freeman created a commercial called "Training Camp," a behind-the-scenes mini-film that purported to show how the company was rigorously training its pizza deliverymen (the trainees are drilled, over and over, on how to outrun dogs and how to kick the car door shut while carrying pizzas in both hands).

Another highly influential campaign came from Wieden + Kennedy. For the cable-TV sports channel ESPN, W+K set out to create ads showing that ESPN sportscasters lived, breathed, and were completely immersed in the world of sports. Inspired by the mock-documentary film *This Is Spinal Tap,* the agency created a series

of commercials that supposedly took the viewer behind the scenes at ESPN headquarters to reveal a sports fantasy world: The channel's sportscasters casually mingled at the office with superstar athletes, as gymnasts danced atop ESPN desks, a basketball star played the piano for tips in the company lounge, and a pole vaulter used his pole to carry around neckties for the sportscasters.

With the popularity of the ESPN campaign (lauded by *TV Guide* as one of the top television ad campaigns of all time), a wave of similar mockumentary-style ads began to surface. A campaign for the Seattle Supersonics basketball team, from the agency WongDoody, showed the team's star players trying to get closer to their fans by visiting ordinary people's homes—then agreeing to help with household chores like washing the dishes. Mockumentaries weren't limited to sports ads; the format was also used to freshen up ads featuring old-fashioned characters

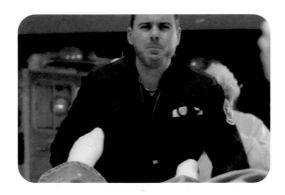

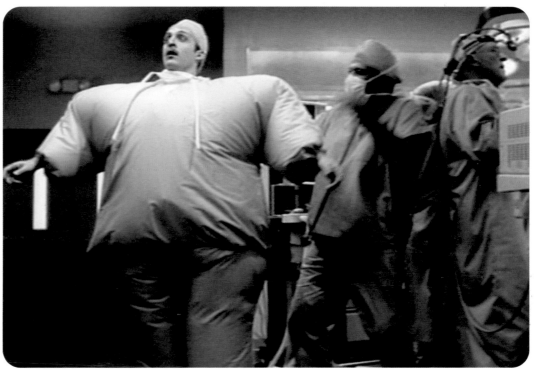

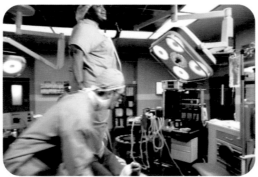

20

19. **JOE BOXER**
ODIORNE WILDE NARRAWAY +
PARTNERS, SAN FRANCISCO,
1998
For this free-spirited underwear
company, OWN+P's creative
director said he wanted to
show "slices of life"—but a bit
twisted. He explained, "We
developed a campaign we called
'Norman Rockwell on acid.'"

20. **LEVI'S JEANS**
FOOTE CONE & BELDING,
SAN FRANCISCO, 1995
The commercial "Doctors" was
set on an operating room table;
as a patient lay in critical
condition, doctors danced to
the rhythm of the EKG machine.

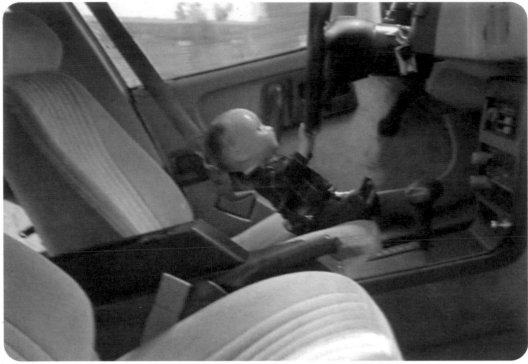

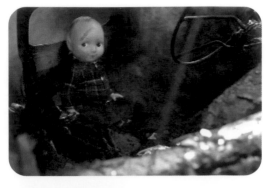

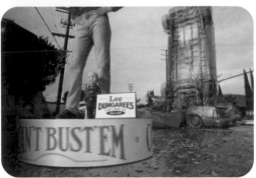

21

21. LEE JEANS
FALLON McELLIGOTT,
MINNEAPOLIS, MINNESOTA,
1998
A new kind of ad hero: Buddy
Lee, a tiny doll with a big head,
saves the day in ridiculous ways.

22. MENTOS
PAHNKE & PARTNERS,
AMSTERDAM, 1992
Tapping into the power of
"badvertising," Mentos ads
were cheesy and awkward—
and the MTV crowd loved to
laugh at them.

**23. LEVI STRAUSS EUROPE –
STA-PREST**
BARTLE BOGLE HEGARTY,
LONDON, 1999
Flat Eric, the orange puppet, was
a mystery that intrigued Europe
(in the U.S., a poor imitation
called "Bad Andy" failed to
generate the same appeal).

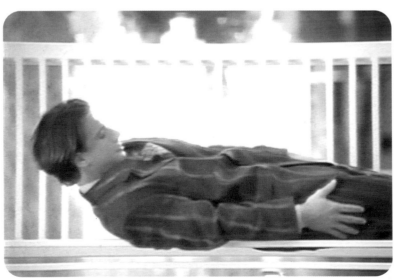

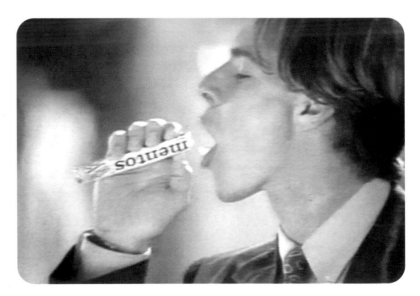

22

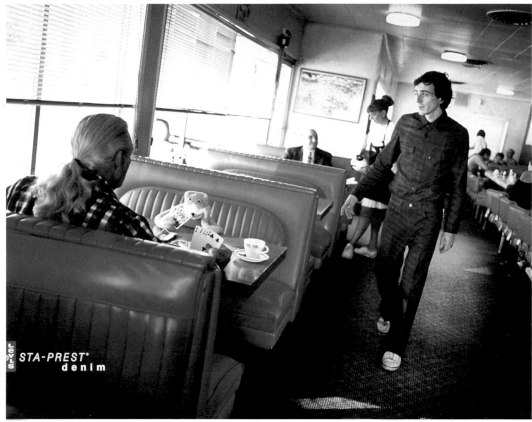

23

like Tony the Tiger. One series featured interviews in which people speculated on the existence of the animated tiger (as one man is interviewed, the viewer catches a fleeting glimpse of Tony rushing past a window in the background). A similar series of ads followed a team of people trying to track down the elusive Energizer Bunny.

Part of the appeal of the mockumentary, aside from the absurd humor, was that the ads tended to have an intentionally raw, cinema-verité film style—distinguishing them from the more polished big-budget ads that viewers were accustomed to seeing. With Oddvertising, bad can be good: Often, the more awkward and amateurish an ad seems, the better it may play to a younger audience that responds to camp and kitsch. The best example of this—and another seminal ad in the emergence of the genre—was an accidental hit campaign that came to America from Europe in the mid-1990s. The candy

Mentos arrived from Holland as a relatively unknown brand, with ads produced in-house by a Dutch production team. The ads featured ludicrous scenarios that always ended with one smiling character giving the camera an overly enthusiastic thumbs-up signal. In an age of cynicism, such pure hokiness seemed to have emerged from a time warp. Making matters worse—or in this case, better—the campaign had been exported to America complete with awkward English translation; for example, the candy was referred to as "the fresh-maker." The ads were so amateurish that it was difficult not to laugh at them, and they soon became a cult hit, joyfully ridiculed by young fans on the Internet.

Naturally, more sophisticated advertisers soon tried to imitate the "schlock as chic" appeal of Mentos, creating intentionally bad ads. Commercials for the clothing retailer Old Navy, starring a motley collection of grade-B American celebrities like the actress Morgan Fairchild,

combined silly scenarios, stiff dialogue, and hokey songs. But they lacked the innocent charm of the Mentos campaign, demonstrating that it's actually hard to make something so bad it's good. Some advertisers also tried to inject camp appeal into their ads by giving them a nostalgic, unsophisticated, and old-fashioned tone—harking back to the days when advertising was chock-full of phony optimism. One of the more successful retro-campaigns was for Altoids breath mints, invoking images and featuring graphic design that seemed to be from a bygone era. Meanwhile, Lee Jeans even resurrected an old mascot, the Buddy Lee doll, and made the doll the star of a series of mockumentary commercials.

If Mentos had successfully exported "bad is good" appeal, Diesel, another European brand, used advertising surrealism as its international calling card. Perhaps never had a single ad campaign managed to bewilder so many people all around the world: With highly stylized

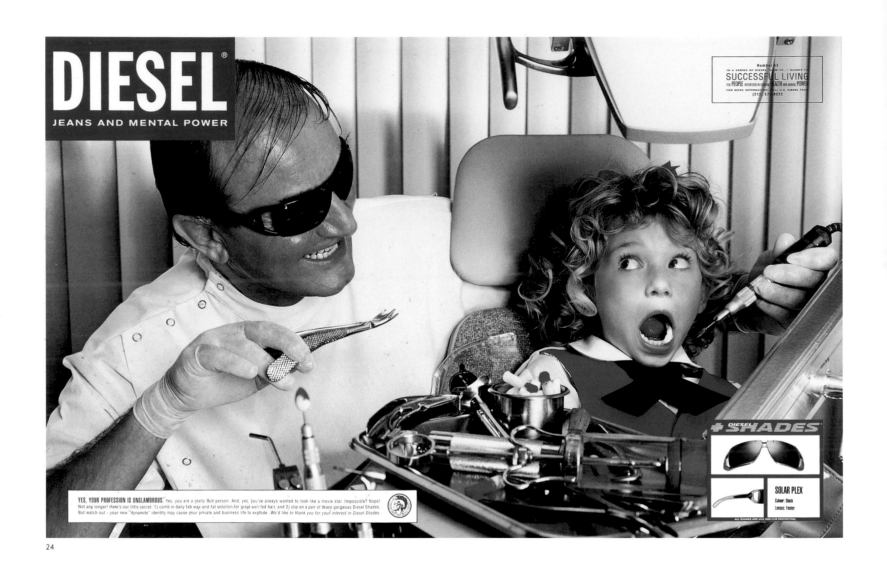

24

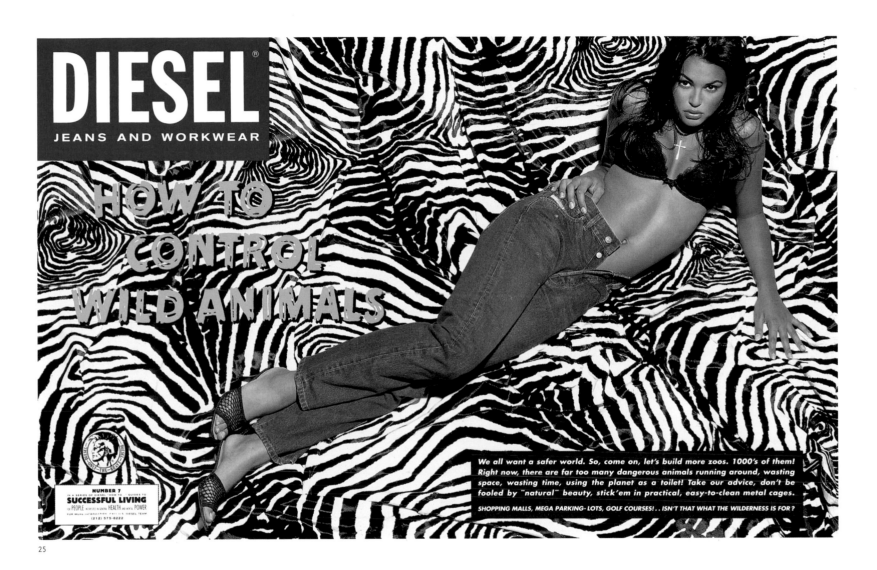

DIESEL
JEANS AND WORKWEAR

HOW TO
CONTROL
WILD ANIMALS

NUMBER 7
IN A SERIES OF DIESEL "HOW TO" GUIDES TO
SUCCESSFUL LIVING
FOR PEOPLE INTERESTED IN GENERAL HEALTH AND MENTAL POWER
FOR MORE INFORMATION CALL U.S. DIESEL TEAM
(212) 575-0222

We all want a safer world. So, come on, let's build more zoos. 1000's of them!
Right now, there are far too many dangerous animals running around, wasting
space, wasting time, using the planet as a toilet! Take our advice, don't be
fooled by "natural" beauty, stick'em in practical, easy-to-clean metal cages.

SHOPPING MALLS, MEGA PARKING- LOTS, GOLF COURSES!.. ISN'T THAT WHAT THE WILDERNESS IS FOR?

25

24 AND 25. **DIESEL**
PARADISET DDB,
STOCKHOLM, 1992–95
Absurd scenes, stylized
photography, and ironic copy
were the hallmarks of this
campaign. The ads were
mocking something, but it
wasn't clear what.

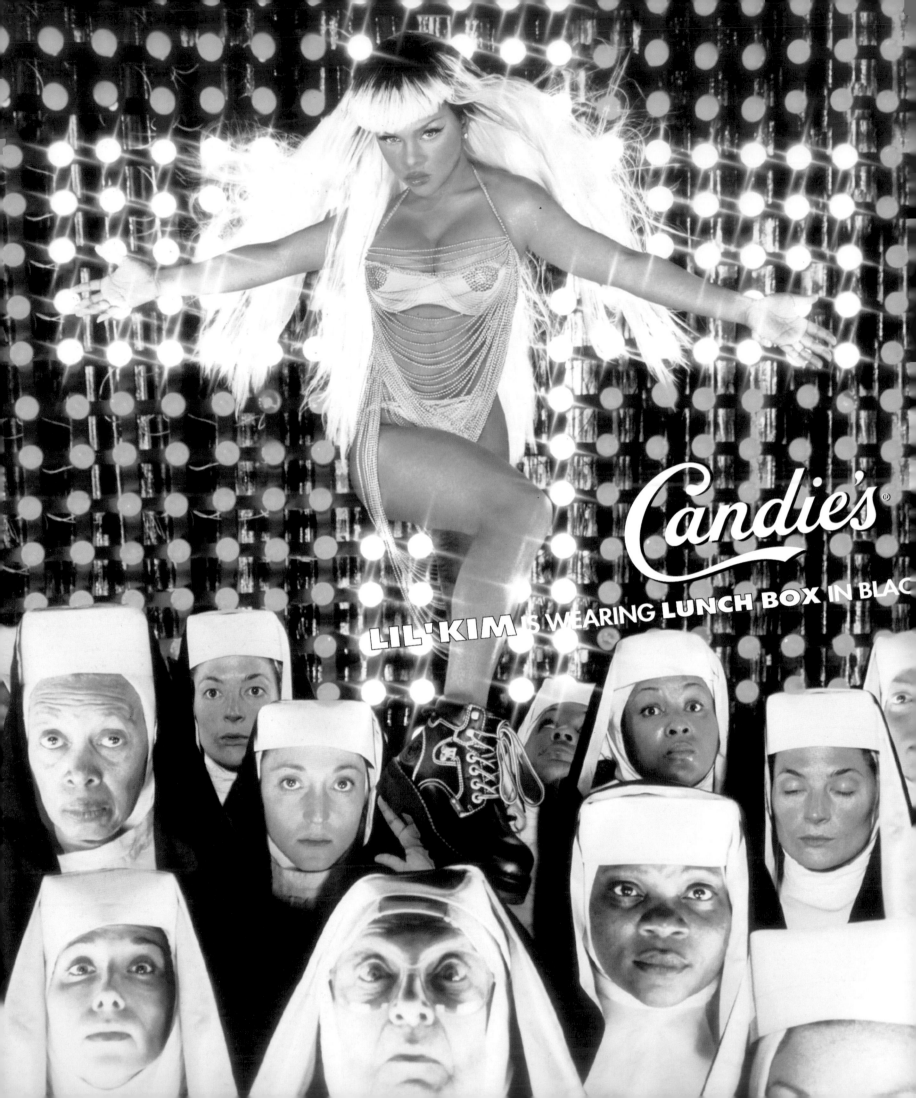

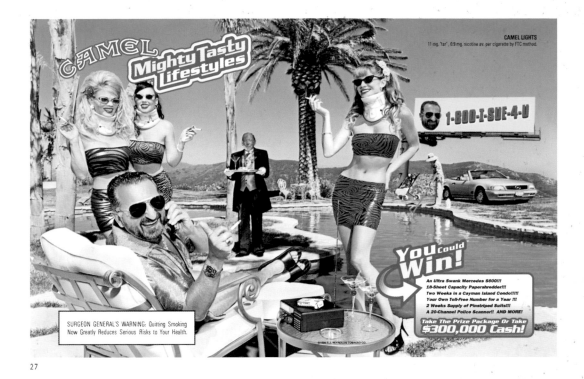

27

26. CANDIE'S
IN-HOUSE AGENCY,
NEW YORK, 1998
The photographer David
LaChapelle, who worked on
Diesel campaigns, specialized in
artificial, over-the-top imagery.
Here, he poses a sexy American
hip-hop star among nuns.

27. CAMEL CIGARETTES
GYRO, PHILADELPHIA,
1998–99
Camel used the Oddvertising
approach to make smoking
seem hip. In this ad, nothing is
to be taken seriously, including
the warning label.

images of politicians in diapers, evil dentists, and sun-worshipping senior citizens, the ads promised to dispense life lessons (how to get rich, how to get a suntan, how to control wild animals), but the copy dripped with irony. Diesel ads seemed to be mocking something—American commercialism? Vapid fashion models? The self-righteous, socially conscious ads of its competitor Benetton?—but the target wasn't particularly clear. For all their postmodern absurdity, the ads could also be maddeningly pretentious and heavy-handed in their attempts at satire, which probably only added to their abrasiveness and ultimately their effectiveness. Loved or hated, the ads for this Italian fashion company would not be ignored. The agency behind the campaign, Sweden's DDB Paradiset and its creative director Joakim Jonason, seemed to specialize in this type of overstylized, incomprehensible advertising, creating similar work for other clients in Europe.

A number of brands around the world tried to copy the Diesel style, and did so, in part, by hiring the photographer who had shot some of the ads in the campaign, David LaChapelle. LaChapelle had a knack for shooting real-life images that looked cartoonish and surreal, and he brought that style to ads for the Italian motor-scooter company Aprilia, as well as to his work for Bass Ale and Candie's clothing. One of LaChapelle's more noteworthy campaigns was for Camel cigarettes—for whom he created wild, orgiastic scenes that exaggerated the classic cigarette-ad depictions of frolicking cheerful smokers; even the Camel headline, which screamed "Mighty tasty!," was intentionally fake and campy.

But nowhere was the Diesel influence more significant than in the advertising produced by Miller Brewing Co. in the late 1990s. Miller—which had long been one of the most important advertisers in America, dating back to its famous "Tastes Great, Less Filling" celebrity campaign

that ran during the 1970s—opted to take a big gamble when it put its advertising in the hands of the creative agency Fallon McElligott. Fallon, in turn, gave the assignment to a Swedish creative team that had worked on Diesel before being hired and brought to America by Fallon. The campaign that Linus Karlson and Paul Malmstrom created for Miller Lite bore touches of Diesel's absurdity and self-referential humor. Early ads were introduced by a fictitious adman named "Dick," who was sarcastically described as "a creative superstar." The vignettes that were presented—supposedly the work of Dick—were as weird as anything previously seen in American advertising. One ad featured a cheesy magic act that concluded with the magician's female assistant suddenly sprouting mice under her arms; another was a short silent film that followed a man with no pants; a third was a singing tribute to a menacing costumed character called Evil Beaver. What did any of this

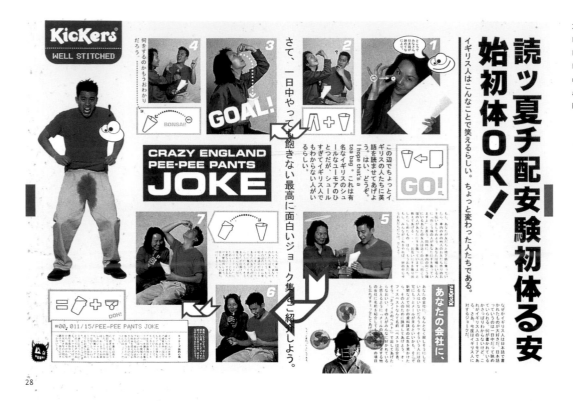

strangeness have to do with beer? It was a good question, and soon it was being asked by more than a few people.

The campaign became a lightning rod for controversial debate within the American ad industry in the late 1990s. It was one thing for a trendy European fashion brand like Diesel to embrace surreal, absurdist advertising; for a mainstream brand like Miller to do so was considered marketing heresy by some, including many of the company's beer distributors—who began to demand that Miller return to more conventional advertising.

The Miller uproar triggered a larger discussion within the ad industry about offbeat advertising. By the late 1990s, ads had so much freedom to explore and experiment that the period was one of unfettered creativity—at least, this was the optimist's view. Advertising seemed to have become a form of sponsored entertainment that could be highly expressive or individualistic. In

effect, companies were hiring offbeat storytellers to create brief skits or tales, often in an absurd style; the clients simply attached their logo onto the end of the sketch, but otherwise didn't inject much selling into the theatrics. This new advertising was certainly daring in that it was apparently unafraid to present unconventional themes and characters. And since it was unencumbered by sales pitches and logic, the story could go anywhere. Ad creator Freeman observed in 1998 that "the opportunities to try something different or unusual are probably greater now than they've ever been." And he defended the outrageousness of the new ads as a reflection of real human behavior, which was, for the first time, being depicted more honestly in advertising. "Offbeat ads might be tapping into feelings and desires to just let go," he said, "and to laugh at things we weren't supposed to laugh at in the past."

But others saw problems with the trend. The violence, antisocial behavior, profanity, and

cynicism in some of the ads seemed to have "moved beyond irreverence—it's kind of nihilistic," observed Marty Cooke, a creative director with the M&C Saatchi agency. The creative director Woody Kay of the Boston agency Pagano Schenck & Kay noted, "The increasing volume of mean-spirited humor and cynicism is a bit depressing. Humor and irony seem to have bullied sincerity and emotion into submission." And the veteran New York ad executive Jerry Della Femina described the new wild advertising's relationship to consumers as follows: "We don't sell them anymore; we stun them."

One of the biggest critics of the trend was *Advertising Age* publisher Rance Crain, who continually argued that ads were losing all touch with reason and strategy. "The technique most in vogue today is sheer unabashed outrageousness," Crain wrote, adding that "the creative people have taken over the asylum and we're all being held captive."

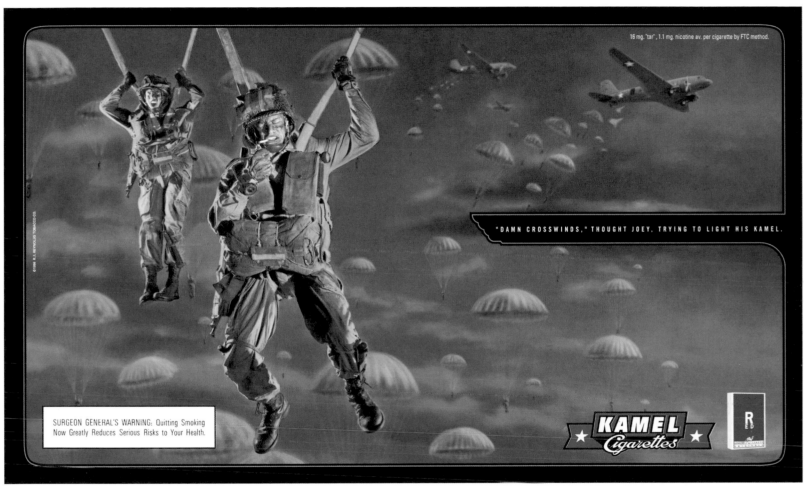

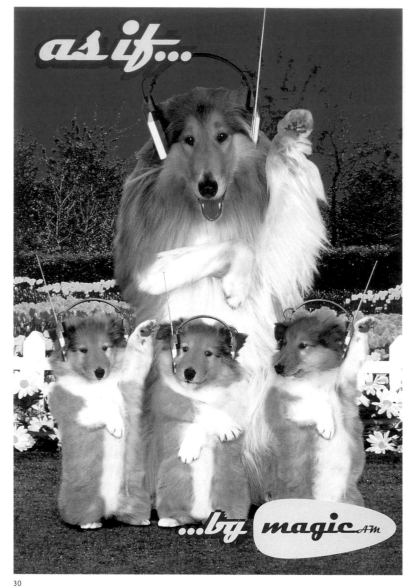

30

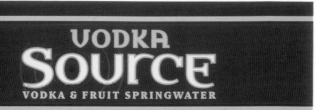

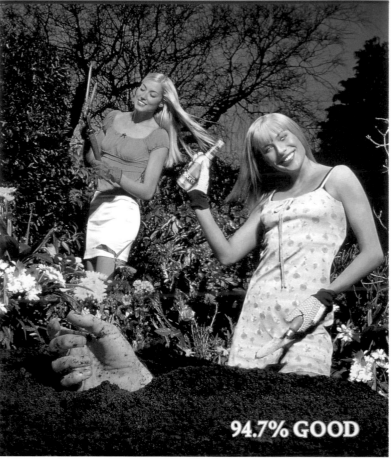

31

30. **MAGIC RADIO**
MOTHER, LONDON,
LATE 1990s
This campaign used special
effects and hyper-saturated
colors to achieve absurd results;
here, dogs appear to move to
the music on the radio.

32. **OHIO THEATRE**
MAD DOGS & ENGLISHMEN,
NEW YORK, 1991
Small clients and unusual
offerings lent themselves to off-
beat humor in ads. In this ad for
a musical, we learn what made
Frankenstein sing.

31. **VODKA SOURCE**
MOTHER, LONDON,
LATE 1990s
Murder and mayhem were
played for laughs in this campaign, which featured a couple
of perky, beautiful Swedish
women who also happened to
be cold-blooded killers.

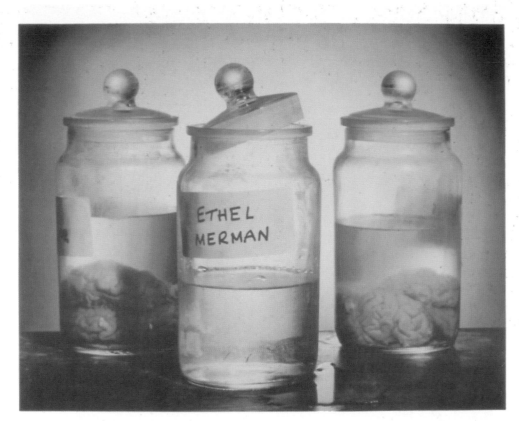

Frankenstein. The Musical. Feb 22-Mar 10. Ohio Theatre.

32

Crain and other critics particularly focused on the Miller Lite campaign, noting that the brewery's sales were not performing well during the "Dick" campaign. Similarly, Freeman's Outpost ads were cited as an example of an outrageous campaign that initially drew attention but didn't help the Web site generate much sales; the "flying gerbil" was quickly grounded. Also coming under attack was the Nissan "Toys" commercial, a highly entertaining spot in which dolls resembling G.I. Joe and Barbie come to life and ride across a living-room floor in a toy car; the ad contained no sales pitch at all, which, even in an era of soft sell, was still highly unusual for automobile advertising. Echoing Clara Peller's famous cry about the missing beef in the Wendy's burger, Crain and other marketing traditionalists screamed, "Where's the strategy?" To which creative-siders like the American copywriter Mark Fenske countered: If the strategy were easily visible to

pundits like Crain, then it would also be far too transparent to consumers. "When the strategy clearly shows through in an ad," Fenske observed, "that's about as effective as fishing with a hook that has no worm on it."

In the end, for Miller Brewing at least, dollars were the deciding factor. Because of its flagging beer sales, Miller pulled the plug on the "Dick" campaign, and by mid-1999, had returned to an updated variation on its classic "Tastes Great, Less Filling" strategy. (These new "conventional" ads didn't produce stellar sales results, either—which led some observers to wonder whether perhaps Miller's problems went beyond the advertising.)

The backlash seemed to be extending to other marketers. While offbeat ads continued to proliferate at the close of the century, a simultaneous trend saw some advertisers returning to more classic approaches. Volkswagen, in its relaunch of the Beetle, created a campaign that

borrowed some of the style and sensibility of the great DDB campaign of the 1960s. Old familiar characters—including Kentucky Fried Chicken's Colonel Sanders and Charmin's Mr. Whipple—were brought back from the dead. Camel cigarettes abandoned its wacky "Mighty Tasty" campaign, and opted for a more old-fashioned theme. And even some of the wild-and-crazy dot-coms (including Outpost, which parted company with Freeman) began to tone down their ads somewhat.

But the overall advertising landscape remained a wild and untamed frontier as the new millennium arrived. For a new generation of advertisers, it seemed to be a world of "anything goes"—though, of course, it wasn't really. As the battle-scarred veterans of advertising controversies attest in the next chapter, the fact is that even in the "brave" new world of Oddvertising, there are certain boundaries that ads can never safely cross.

THE RISE OF "ODDVERTISING."

7. PUS

THE L

HING
MITS.

1. **PERSONAL CONDOMS**
KIRSHENBAUM & BOND,
NEW YORK, 1987
By the late 1980s, advertisers
were taking more risks; K&B
was a small agency that gained
notoriety by creating cheeky ads
like this one.

2. **DEMOCRATIC NATIONAL
COMMITTEE**
DOYLE DANE BERNBACH,
NEW YORK, 1964
This ad for U.S. President
Lyndon B. Johnson used scare
tactics—an image of an atomic
explosion—to discourage voters
from choosing the opposition.
But it was a rarity, and
controversial, at the time.

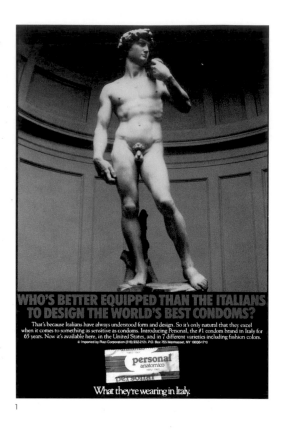

1

If one were to think of advertising as a living creature that has evolved and adapted through generations, it would seem that the species started out relying on aggression—repeatedly clubbing its hard-sell message home in those early days—then gradually developed more of a reasoning mind that could even, occasionally, express thoughts abstractly. But as this evolution took place, there was one part of "Adman" that was slow to develop: the backbone.

Fear has always been uppermost in the minds of advertisers. The guardians of the world's great brands long worried that their advertising might somehow alienate consumers or send the wrong message about a product or, worst of all, stir up controversy that could yield bad publicity for the brand. Because of this, many advertisers imposed strict limitations on what the ad creators could do, and repeatedly tested and retested ads to make sure no one could possibly be offended. In most cases, the ad creators hardly needed to

be reined in: Acutely aware that any misstep could cost them the account, they tended to be just as cautious as the brand managers.

But this approach began to change somewhat in the 1960s, as some of the Creative Revolution agencies started producing more provocative advertising—partly to draw attention to their clients and partly to make a name for themselves. Bill Bernbach was, again, at the forefront in challenging advertising conservatism; he seemed to understand early on that while controversy might not necessarily be good, it wasn't always a bad thing, either. In 1964, Bernbach produced a commercial with imagery that was unthinkable in advertising: To promote the presidential campaign of Lyndon Baines Johnson against the more militaristic candidate Barry Goldwater, Doyle Dane Bernbach showed a little girl picking petals off a daisy—then ended the spot by showing the mushroom cloud of an atomic explosion. The commercial shocked America and drew a

fair amount of criticism, perhaps justified: Was it fair or even conscionable to suggest that Goldwater wanted to blow up the world? But it hit the message home, and Americans chose the LBJ brand in November.

But even though the 1960s produced some examples of advertising derring-do, it was limited and short-lived. Subsequently, throughout the 1970s and early 1980s, "advertisers began subjecting everything we did to tests," says DDB's Roy Grace, and much of the testing was designed to weed out any possible controversial elements in ads. It wasn't until the mid-to-late 1980s, and particularly the 1990s, that attitudes toward controversy in ads truly began to change. Increasingly, some advertisers began to actually court trouble. Among certain ad agencies, it suddenly became a badge of honor to have produced ads that made clients nervous and set tongues wagging. The Los Angeles agency Chiat/Day, run by the maverick ad executive Jay Chiat and

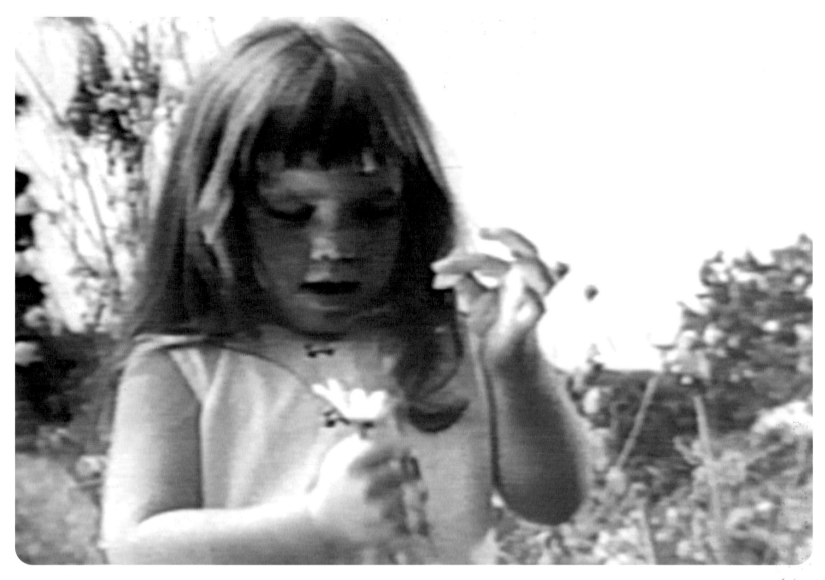

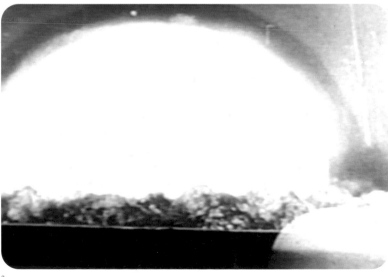

VOTE FOR PRESIDENT JOHNSON
ON NOVEMBER 3.

2

AN AUTHENTIC ITALIAN RESTAURANT WHERE NO ONE'S BEEN SHOT.

YET

Positano
250 Park Avenue South
N.Y.C.
212-777-6211

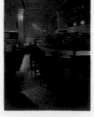

Advertising Agency: Kirshenbaum & Bond

3

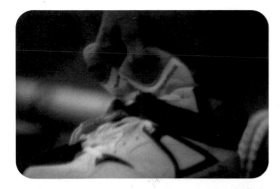
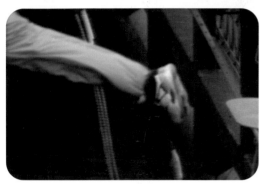

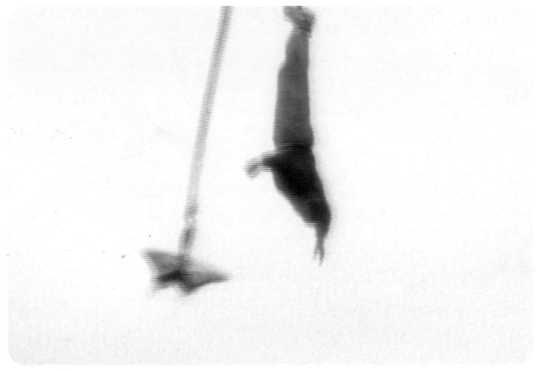

4

3. POSITANO RESTAURANT
KIRSHENBAUM & BOND,
NEW YORK, 1987
K&B wasn't afraid to use ethnic
humor in its ads; this one for a
New York restaurant makes fun
of the Mafia's reputation for
gunning down mobsters in
Italian eateries.

4. REEBOK
CHIAT/DAY, NEW YORK, 1989
Death comes to advertising:
This TV commercial showed two
bungee jumpers; only the one
wearing Reeboks survived. It was
pulled off the air after viewers
complained.

his artful creative lieutenant Lee Clow, forged
its identity as a creator of "dangerous" ads; the
agency even hoisted a pirate flag in its offices as
a warning signal to the world. The creative staff
at Chiat insisted that they never actually sought
out trouble—rather, they claimed, it was usually
a by-product of speaking more candidly and
boldly in ads. "We're not consciously trying to
stir controversy," Clow said. "But somehow,
we touch nerves."

When showing its risky ideas to clients who
were understandably nervous, Chiat/Day would
push and push (sometimes threatening to
resign the account) until eventually the client
agreed to run a daring ad—the "1984" commercial for Apple Computer being one of the more
noteworthy examples of this. Occasionally, the
controversial spots backfired on the agency and
its clients: The successful "1984" was followed
up the next year with another Apple commercial
called "Lemmings," which showed a group of

blindfolded businessmen following a Pied Piper
(IBM, perhaps?) and eventually marching off a
cliff. The ad had an impact, certainly, but this
time the effect was more depressing than exhilarating: America wasn't quite ready for depictions
of mass suicide on Super Bowl Sunday. (Even
after this experience, Chiat/Day had no fear
of showing people falling to their deaths in
commercials: A few years later, the agency
produced a Reebok ad in which two bungee
jumpers fling themselves off a cliff; the one
wearing Reeboks bounces back up on his tether,
while on the other side, all that remains is a
pair of empty sneakers on a rope. It ran for a
short time, drew heavy criticism, and then was
pulled off the air.)

But even if their controversial ads sometimes
fell flat, creative agencies and their attention-
starved clients reveled in the attention they
attracted. A controversy could turn an unknown
ad creator and his obscure clients into media

stars overnight, as Richard Kirshenbaum proved
in the late 1980s. A cofounder of Kirshenbaum
& Bond, a tiny New York agency whose early
clients included a local shoe store and an Italian
manufacturer of condoms, Kirshenbaum had to
operate on a limited budget—his small clients
couldn't afford to buy much ad space or television
time. But he found a way to thrust them in the
spotlight nonetheless. One of his condom ads
featured a full-frontal view of Michelangelo's
David, with the headline "Who's better equipped
than the Italians to design the world's best
condoms?" For his shoe client, Kenneth Cole,
Kirshenbaum created ads that ridiculed public
figures of the day, including the vice president
of the United States, Dan Quayle (one ad
showed Quayle, notorious for his poor spelling,
under the headline "Don't Forget to Vot").

Such ads prompted a blizzard of media
coverage, both for the clients and for the agency.
Kirshenbaum would subsequently describe this

PUSHING THE LIMITS.

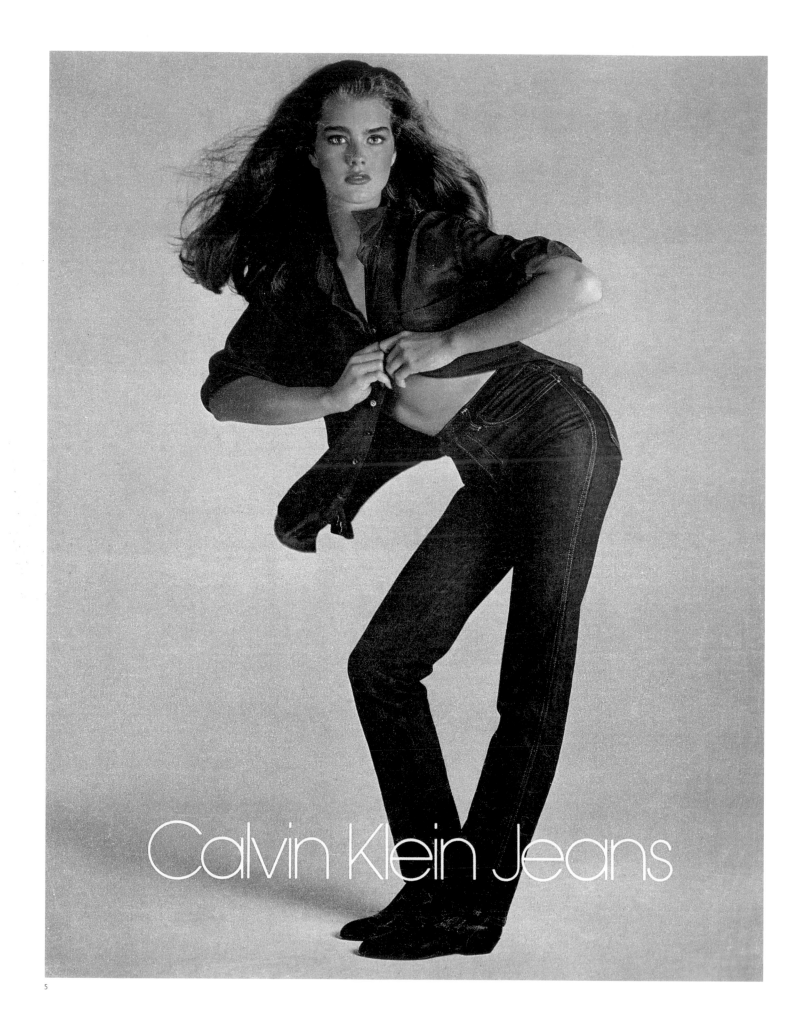

Calvin Klein Jeans

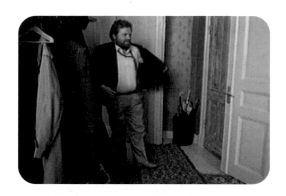

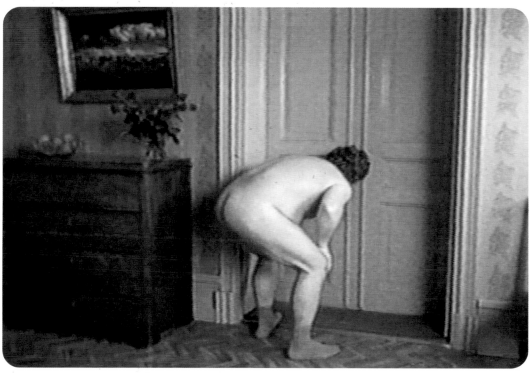

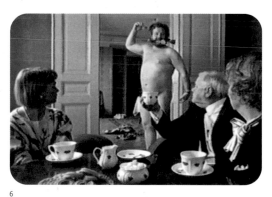

6

5. **CALVIN KLEIN JEANS**
IN-HOUSE AGENCY, NEW
YORK, 1980
Calvin Klein was constantly
pushing the boundaries; his
famous Brooke Shields ads
sexualized the teenager.

6. **BRAATHENS SAFE AIRLINE**
LEO BURNETT, OSLO, 1993
In the commercial "Naked
Lunch," a man arriving home
early from a business trip
decides to surprise his wife—
but he's unaware that her
parents are also in the house.

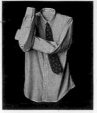

THE SUGGESTED RETAIL PRICE OF THIS SHIRT IS $125. WE HAVE A SUGGESTION FOR WHOEVER SUGGESTED IT.

We also have a suggestion for you. Come into Daffy's where you'll find men's, women's and children's fashion & designer clothing 40-75% off, every day. New York City; Manhasset, NY; Philadelphia; Elizabeth, East Hanover, Paramus and Wayne, NJ; and Potomac Mills Mall, VA.

DAFFY'S
CLOTHES THAT WILL MAKE YOU. NOT BREAK YOU.

7

7. DAFFY'S STORES
DEVITO VERDI, NEW YORK, 1996
If you can't say it, show it: A coarse gesture becomes the ad's punchline.

8. ONVZ HEALTHCARE
KESSELSKRAMER, AMSTERDAM, 1999
European advertising was more open to showing nudity, as in this Dutch commercial for a healthcare company.

---

phenomenon as "the multiplier effect"—meaning that as ads attracted heavy news coverage, their exposure level was multiplied without additional expense; an advertiser might spend a million dollars running K&B's ads and end up with $10 million worth of publicity. (This theory, of course, does not distinguish between good and bad attention, abiding by the Oscar Wilde philosophy that the only thing worse than being talked about is not being talked about.)

Agencies like Chiat/Day and Kirshenbaum & Bond weren't the only ones living on the edge in the 1980s; some sponsors were out there, too. It seemed that no one understood the multiplier effect better than fashion designer Calvin Klein, who drew early attention by putting an adolescent Brooke Shields in jeans ads and having her deliver the sexually suggestive line "Nothing comes between me and my Calvins." That was just the beginning for Klein, who, throughout the 1980s and 1990s, continued to push the

boundaries of sexual explicitness in advertising. *Advertising Age* critic Bob Garfield called Klein "the pioneer of 'shockvertising,'" noting that the designer's modus operandi was to "inflame the many in order to impress the view. Klein didn't create ads, he created Molotov cocktails—he'd toss them out there to see what would happen."

Of course, it remained risky to do this (as Klein would discover firsthand with the infamous "kiddie porn" controversy of the mid-1990s, discussed later). But by the 1990s, a growing number of advertisers could justify taking these risks because of their desperate need to generate attention in a landscape that made it hard to stand out. With the media increasingly cluttered by expanded cable channels, the Internet, and an explosion of advertising in all forms, an interesting reversal took place in the minds of at least some marketers, who now began to feel, in the words of Mary Stow of London's Howell Henry Chaldecott Lury & Partners, that "the biggest

risk is to be safe—because if you're safe you're invisible and you waste your money." One of Stow's agency partners, Steve Henry, advised fellow ad creators, "Get your work banned." To Henry, having ads occasionally struck down by the British media or government was taken as a healthy sign that the Howell Henry agency was doing its job right. It was a way of thinking that began to take hold at creative ad agencies around the world. "We try to be on the edge all the time, and sometimes a bit over the edge when a brand needs shock therapy," said Johan Kramer, of the Amsterdam-based agency KesselsKramer, whose commercials for a healthcare service featured men and women walking through the ad naked. (Actually, those ads didn't shock Kramer's fellow Dutch citizens all that much; "it's hard to be controversial here, because we're very liberal in Holland," he says.)

In fact, much of Europe, and parts of Asia, have tended to be far ahead of America in terms

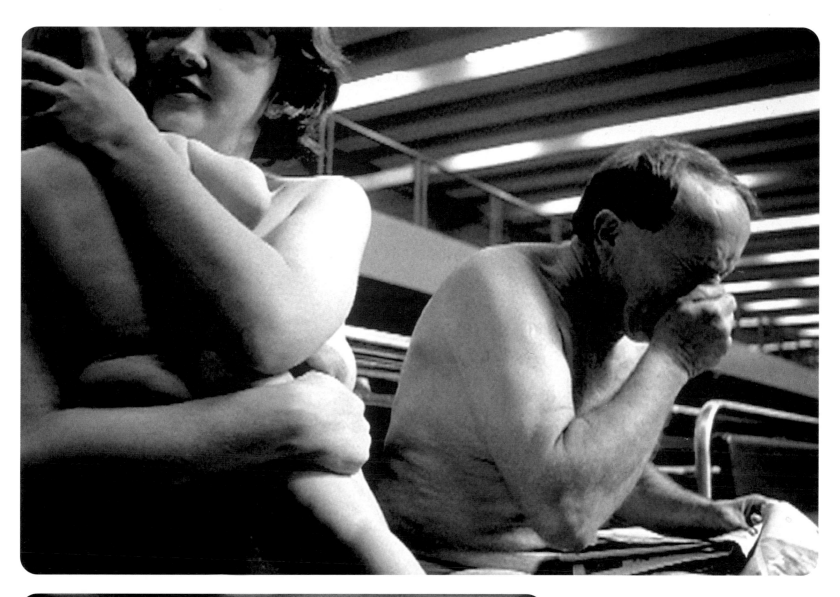

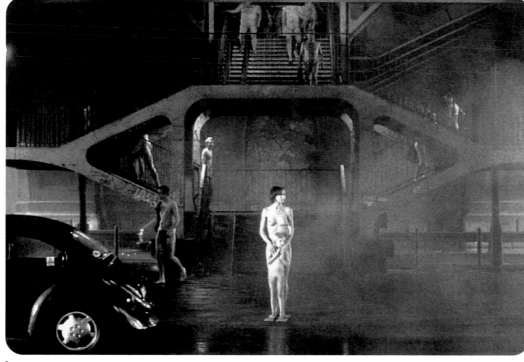

8

PUSHING THE LIMITS.

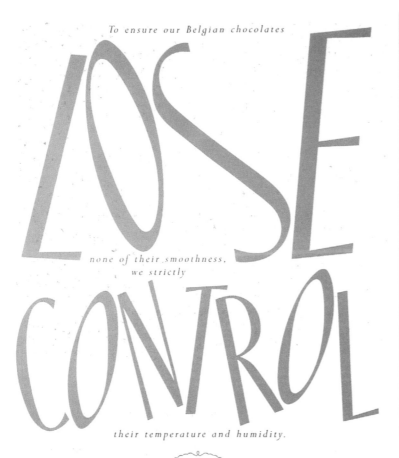

To ensure our Belgian chocolates

LOSE

none of their smoothness,
we strictly

CONTROL

their temperature and humidity.

Häagen-Dazs

REAL CREAM ICE CREAM

Dedicated to Pleasure

9

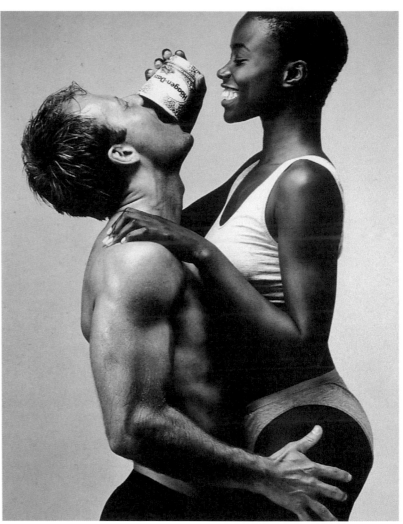

9. HAAGEN-DAZS
BARTLE BOGLE HEGARTY,
LONDON, 1991
This early 1990s campaign
shocked England by taking on
two taboos at once: not just sex,
but interracial sex.

10. LEVI STRAUSS EUROPE
BARTLE BOGLE HEGARTY,
LONDON, 1990
BBH played nudity for laughs in
this ad; it contrasted a pair of
Levi's (which become more
comfortable over time) with
something that doesn't benefit
from aging: the human body.

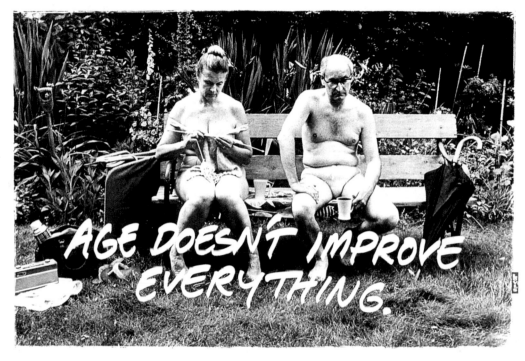

10

of pushing the boundaries of sexuality in advertising. As far back as thirty years ago, French ads were not only featuring topless women but threatening to go further: In a famous series of outdoor billboards that appeared in the 1960s, the first billboard featured a woman wearing only a bikini bottom, and promised that in the next ad the woman would be shown completely naked; sure enough, she was, although this time the picture was shot from behind. As a French advertising executive from the agency Leo Burnett recently said, when it comes to French advertising, "you can use a breast in anything, provided you can think of a vaguely plausible reason for doing so." Scandinavian advertising has tended to be even more permissive when it comes to nudity and sex, often using these as the basis for commercial storylines. One memorable Norwegian airline commercial, "Naked Lunch," featured a man who arrives home early from a business trip; peering through the keyhole, he

sees his wife sitting quietly, sipping tea. He promptly strips off his clothes and bursts into the room naked with a rose clenched in his teeth—only to discover that sitting across the room from his wife are his in-laws. Even the supposedly staid British—who still have an occasional tendency to "snicker like schoolboys" when referring to sex in ads, according to creative director Gerard Stamp of Leo Burnett in London—have lately been producing a number of ads that deal with sex and nudity in an understated, elegant manner, as in a stylishly sensuous campaign from the London agency Bartle Bogle Hegarty featuring intertwined bare bodies (promoting, of all things, Häagen-Dazs ice cream). Likewise, a number of other advertising markets that might be expected to be more conservative—including Japan and Hong Kong—are apt to feature nudity in ads quite casually, often treating it more as an aesthetic element than as a shock mechanism. Of course, showing geni-

talia is still taboo in ads, though advertisers dance around that in clever ways—as in a Spanish ad that used carefully arranged type to form a penis.

By the mid-to-late 1990s, American advertising, too, had grown more casual about showing sex and skin in ads. Print allowed more freedom than television. Partial nudity in print ads became so acceptable that top-name athletes, like the track star Michael Johnson, began appearing in the buff for Nike, and Nike also showed bare breasts in a 1999 campaign for its sports bras—eliciting a barrage of mail, according to the campaign's creator, Jeff Goodby. ("It surprised me that even today, people could still be freaked out by the idea of breasts in ads," acknowledged Goodby.) Even large, mainstream American brands seemed more willing to move beyond sexual innuendo—a longtime tool of advertisers—toward more explicitness. If nudity wasn't an option on broadcast TV,

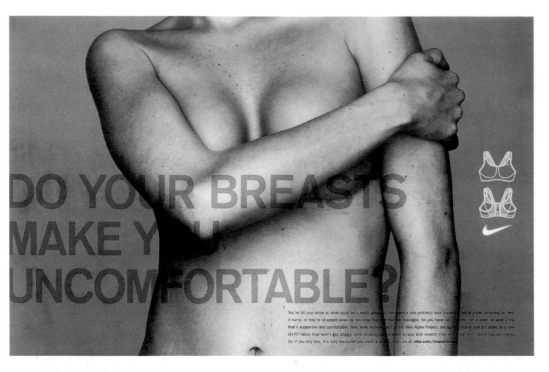

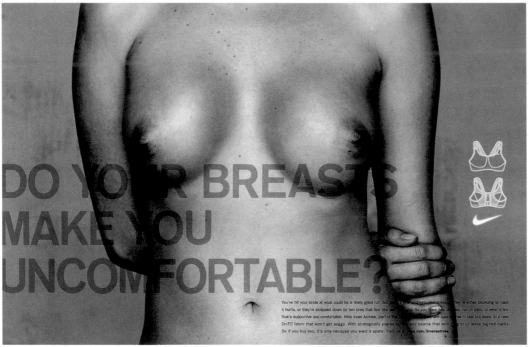

11

11. NIKE
GOODBY SILVERSTEIN &
PARTNERS, SAN FRANCISCO,
1999
The advertiser took two
approaches in this ad for a sports
bra: one covered up, one not. The
latter drew complaints, which
surprised ad creator Jeff Goodby.

12. ALTOIDS
LEO BURNETT, CHICAGO, 1998
Sadomasochism goes main-
stream: even a perky campaign
like the one in the late 1990s for
Altoids mints was not afraid to
portray a dominatrix.

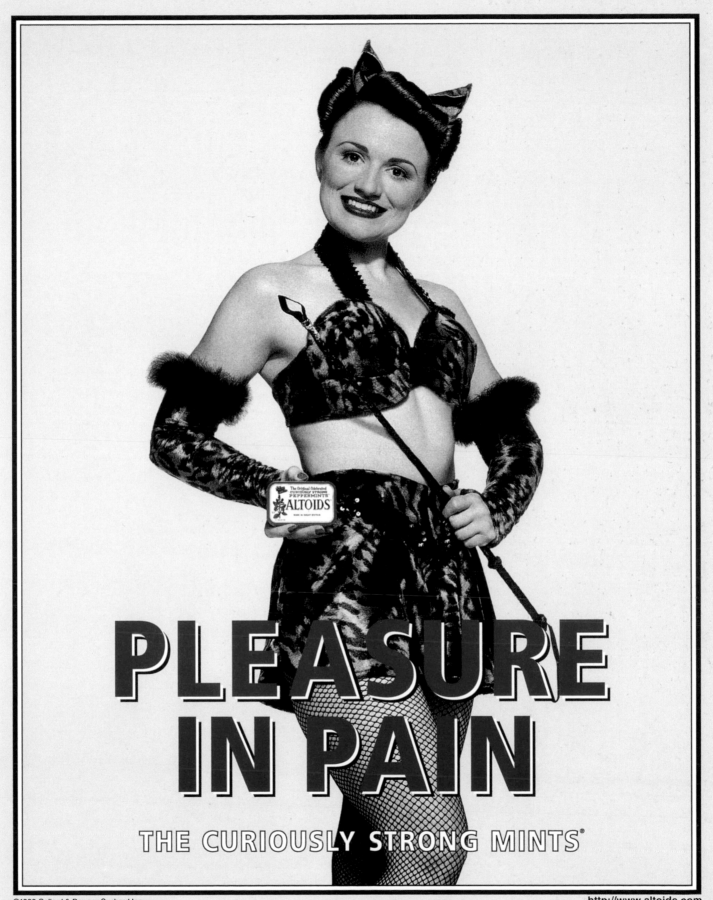

http://www.altoids.com

12

PUSHING THE LIMITS.

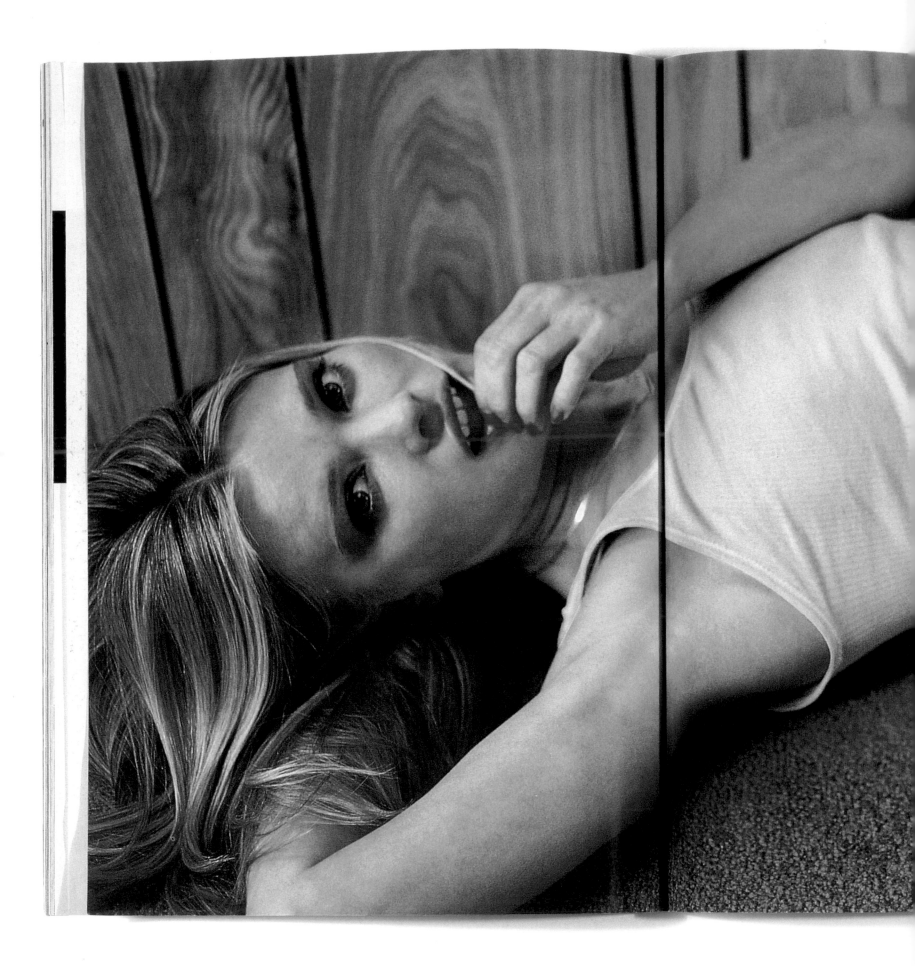

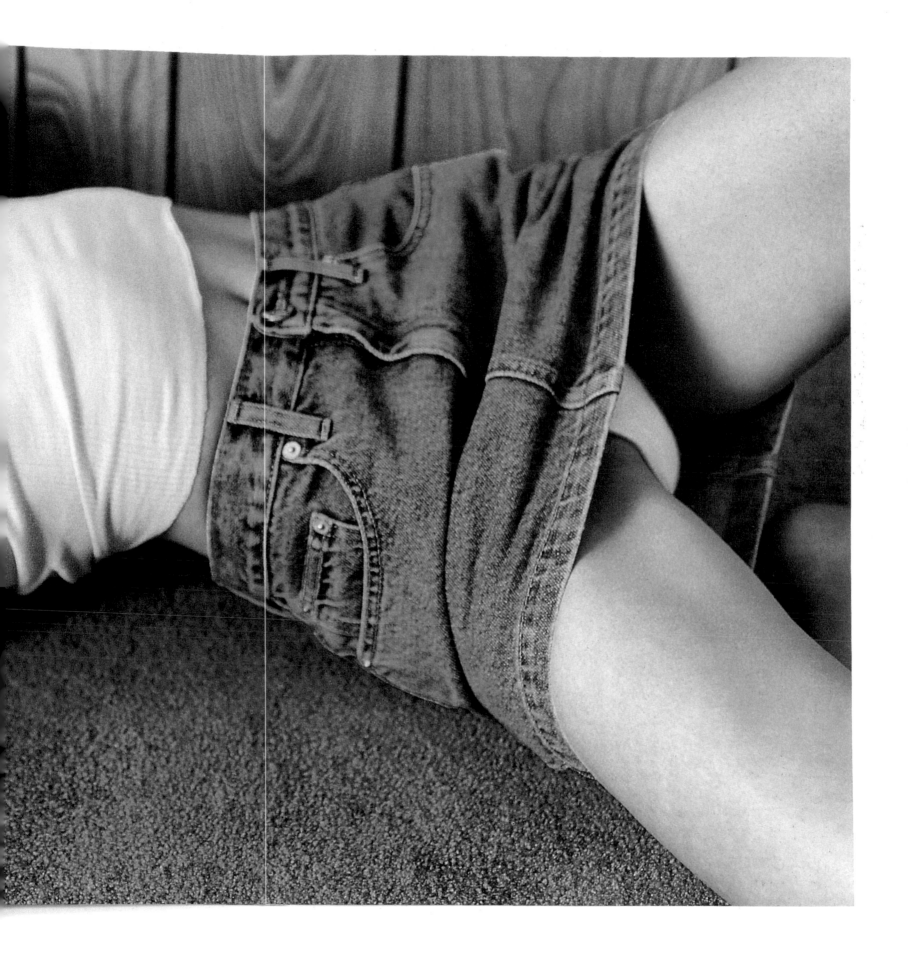

PUSHING THE LIMITS.

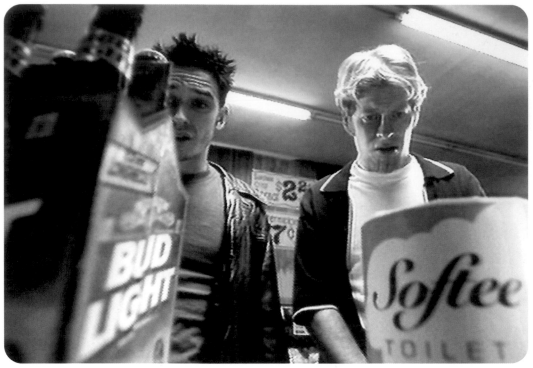

14

there were other ways to be sexually adventurous in this medium. To make the point that its hotels had gone through a dramatic overhaul, Holiday Inn produced a commercial whose main character was a transsexual—and it ran the ad during the Super Bowl, though it was subsequently pulled after viewer complaints. Clairol, meanwhile, began running commercials in which a woman groans and sighs as if having an orgasm, though she's actually just washing her hair with Herbal Essences shampoo. (The heavy-handedness of this campaign was, regrettably, a far cry from the slyly suggestive Clairol line "Does she or doesn't she?") Even playful ads for candy were willing to get a little kinky—as in an ad for Altoids mints featuring a cartoonish portrait of a dominatrix, with the headline "Pleasure in Pain," a reference to the mint's reputation for having a strong flavor.

As mainstream advertisers became more sexually daring, the fashion advertisers naturally

had to push even further: fashion ads were more likely to feature images of raw sexuality and even touches of sadomasochism, particularly in the advertising of clothing labels like Guess. Calvin Klein, meanwhile, began to tread in ever more dangerous areas. In 1995, Klein encountered his fiercest controversy when he created a series of ads featuring models who appeared to be teenagers, posing for what seemed to be a seedy pornographic-film shoot. Klein later insisted that the imagery was misinterpreted, but he came under heavy fire before pulling the ads. In the aftermath, the longtime provocateur began to tone down much of his advertising and remarked, "The country has moved to the right, and creatively I don't think this is a moment where people should take too many chances." But it wasn't so much the times, or even the place—in fact, Klein had simply stumbled upon one of the last remaining taboos, which is firmly in place even in more

permissive cultures. Two years ago, a series of French Evian ads created a stir when they showed naked images of children; these portraits were far more innocent and tasteful than Klein's porno-suggestive ads, yet they still caused a public outcry. These episodes served as a reminder, if one was needed, to all advertisers that while sex sells, and children sell, the two should never be mixed in ads.

If it was getting harder in the 1990s to shock the public merely by flashing bare skin in ads, advertisers were finding other ways to the stir the pot. Increasingly, ads began to use more frank—sometimes even profane—language, both in America and in Europe. Here again, standards tended to be a bit looser in Europe, particularly in terms of what was permitted on television. A recent Saatchi & Saatchi commercial for a small London jewelry shop ended with the line "If you don't like it, then f—- off." Another British spot, by Gold Greenlees Trott for Holsten Pils beer,

RESEARCH SAYS SEX SELLS BEER.

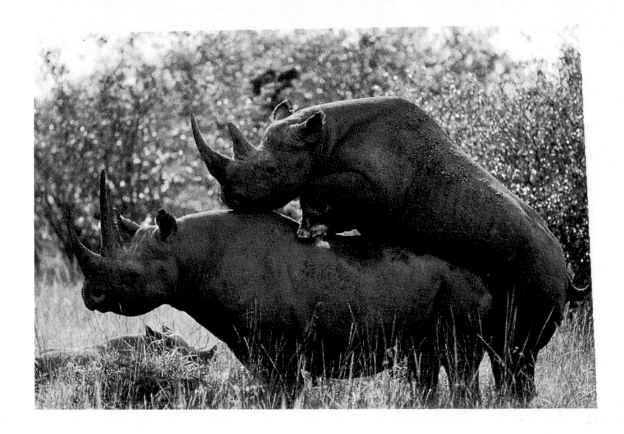

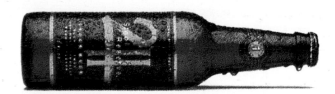

STEEL RESERVE. THE NOT-TOO-SERIOUS HIGH GRAVITY LAGER.

15

PUSHING THE LIMITS.

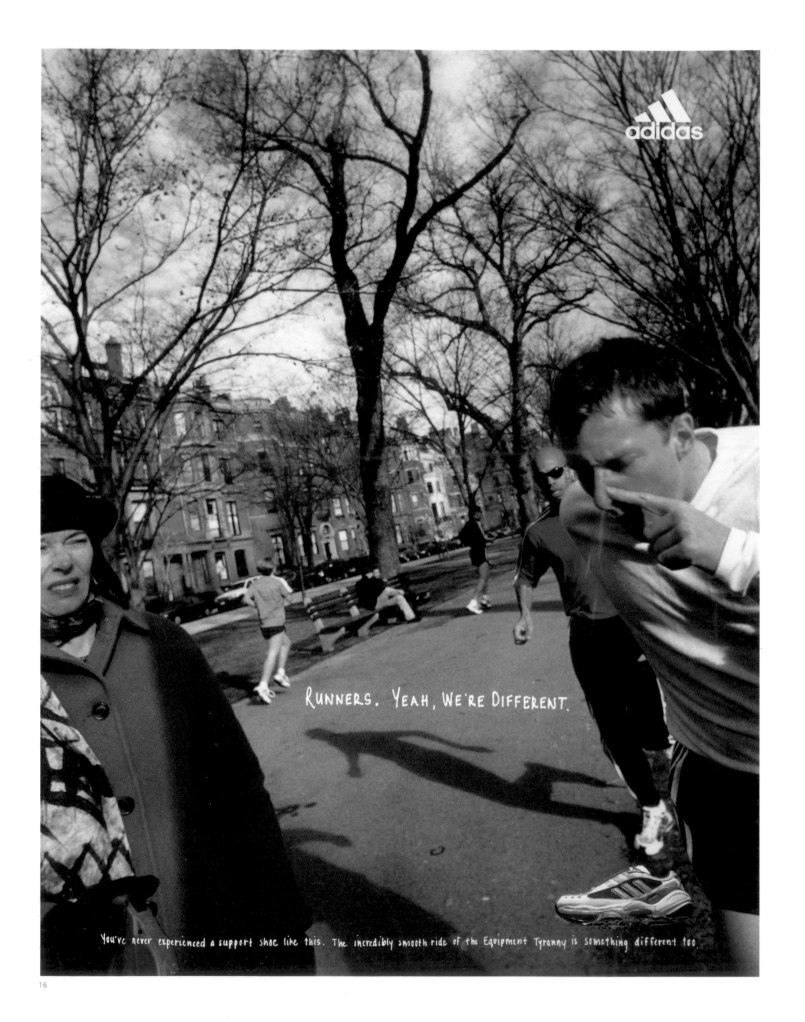

RUNNERS. YEAH, WE'RE DIFFERENT.

You've never experienced a support shoe like this. The incredibly smooth ride of the Equipment Tyranny is something different too.

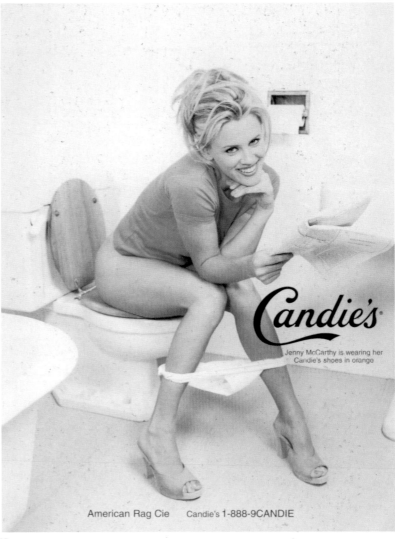

Jenny McCarthy is wearing her
Candie's shoes in orange

Candie's®

American Rag Cie   Candie's 1-888-9CANDIE

17

featured a comedian who hurled beer bottles as he cursed about additives in beer. Some advertisers have opted for substitutes for profanity, as in a popular American ad for Daffy's clothing that featured an obscene arm gesture being formed by a folded shirt sleeve.

One of the more pervasive trends, particularly in American ads, has been toward scatological humor. A growing number of late-1990s ads began to feature imagery and dialogue revolving around bodily functions. Some were mildly amusing, as in a Polaroid ad displaying photographic evidence of a neighbor's dog soiling the lawn, while others could be more shocking—for example, an Adidas ad featuring a close-up shot of a runner blowing his nose, a Candie's shoe ad showing the actress Jenny McCarthy sitting on a toilet, or a British commercial from Saatchi & Saatchi that showed a man defecating in public (the point of the spot was to persuade people in the London borough of Islington to clean up

after their pets). An ad for the Adam Sandler movie *Big Daddy* featured an image of Sandler and his young co-star urinating against a wall; as *The New York Times* noted at the time, the ad drew surprisingly few complaints from anyone, which led a number of ad executives to conclude that the culture had grown so coarse, it was now actually becoming difficult for ads to offend.

The increase in potty humor in ads has also been accompanied by a growth in the number of ads depicting violence and other antisocial behavior. To promote hockey games in the U.S., the Fox Network showed golfers and bowlers physically attacking one another; the commercials were making the tongue-in-cheek point that these sedate sports would be more lively if they featured the kind of rough action found in hockey. Other recent ads have depicted violence against animals, as in the previously noted Outpost.com ad that showed gerbils being shot through the air (Chapter 6); the ads ended by

advising angry viewers where they could "send complaints." An ad for the long-distance phone service Qwest featured a priest beating a bandaged patient in a hospital bed. For the most part, depictions of violence in ads are not particularly realistic—they tend to be more absurd and cartoonish, in the spirit of the rough horseplay typical of slapstick comedy. But they can be jarring nonetheless and have raised concerns within the ad industry. "There's increasingly a nasty undertone detectable in some of the commercials," observed the renowned British ad executive Adrian Holmes.

Even as they acknowledged the pressing need of advertisers to somehow catch the wandering eye of consumers, some observers considered the proliferation of "shockvertising" an overreaction. However, others pointed out that the new ads were no more risqué than what was being commonly found in other forms of mass communication at the time. In America,

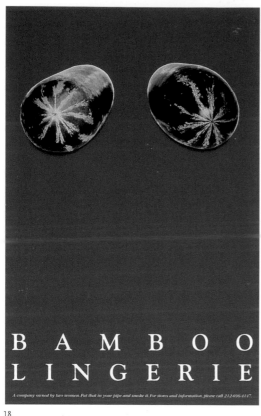

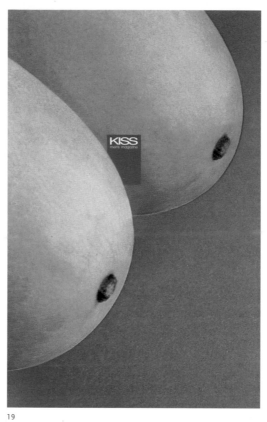

18 19

18. **BAMBOO LINGERIE**
KIRSHENBAUM & BOND,
NEW YORK, 1992
K&B had fun with stereotypes,
featuring melons in this lingerie
ad, but not everyone appreciated
the joke.

20. **DUREX CONDOMS**
McCANN-ERICKSON,
LONDON, LATE 1990s
Here, a sexy fruit gets equal
opportunity to pitch a product.
You still can't show some things
in ads, but advertisers have
ways around that.

19. **KISS MAGAZINE**
LEO BURNETT, HONG KONG,
1997
Different fruit, similar idea: this
Hong Kong advertiser used the
fruit with less irony, but
produced a striking image.

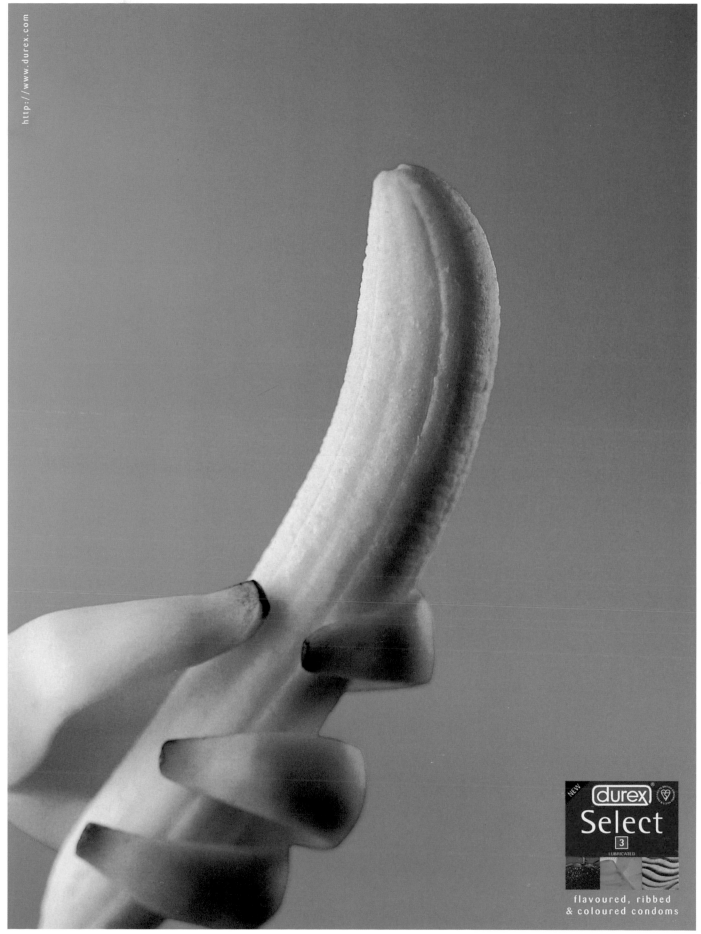

NEW
durex ®
Select
3
LUBRICATED
flavoured, ribbed
& coloured condoms

20

PUSHING THE LIMITS.

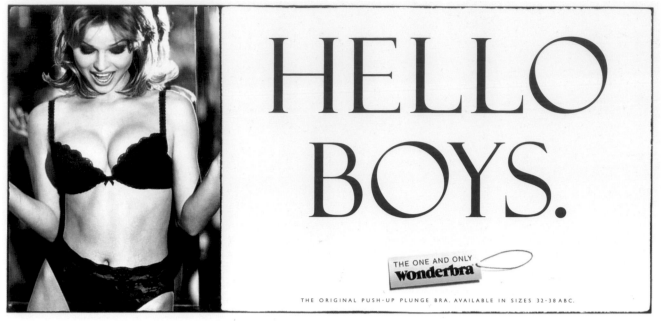

HELLO
BOYS.

THE ONE AND ONLY
wonderbra

THE ORIGINAL PUSH-UP PLUNGE BRA. AVAILABLE IN SIZES 32-38 ABC.

21

21. WONDERBRA
TBWA SIMONS PALMER,
LONDON, 1994
In the mid-1990, Wonderbra
became a leading purveyor of
cheesecake imagery worldwide.
This ad created a sensation in
the UK, partly because of that
intriguing headline.

22. EXCITE.COM
ODIORNE WILDE NARRAWAY +
PARTNERS, SAN FRANCISCO,
1997
Sex is one thing, but politics
still scares many advertisers.
This ad, however, was unafraid
to tweak U.S. President Bill
Clinton. Some thought it was
disrespectful.

the popularity in the late 1990s of crude and raunchy films like *There's Something About Mary* and TV shows like "South Park," as well as bad-boy magazines like *Maxim,* had a very big impact on advertisers. "I think when you look at the success of a movie like *There's Something About Mary,* that was a big moment in defining how far you can stretch popular culture in a commercially successful piece of entertainment," said Neal Tiles, a top advertising executive with the Fox television network. Rich Silverstein, co-founder of Goodby Silverstein & Partners, observed that at his own agency, the standards seemed to change overnight. "I'm getting scripts every day," Silverstein noted, "where I say, 'We can't do that stuff! It's advertising; you can't swear, can't have a butt joke, can't say 'penis!'" And you just wonder, "Where's this coming from?" And then you watch TV, and every joke is a sex joke. Or you look at the magazine rack

and you see that every magazine is trying to be like *Maxim*—really out there, in terms of sex. If younger people who are writing ads now are finding everything they see—from movies to music to magazines—filled with ramped-up sexual tension, then it's naturally going to find its way into advertising scripts, too. They're just trying to reflect the times. But I'm saying to them, 'It's still advertising, we can't do that!'"

Perhaps the real question is not why young ad creators are pushing these boundaries but rather why clients—who have so much to lose—are out on that edge, too. Why would so many sponsors make the sudden leap from extreme caution to reckless abandon? According to the American journalist John Leo, today's corporations "understand that in-your-face messages that shred social norms can move the merchandise by playing to the current sour, antisocial mood. Thus, the rapid spread of ads

urging us to break all the rules or just make up our own."

But there's more to the trend than just a shift in the cultural mood and standards. A significant contributor is undoubtedly the rise of "targeted marketing" in the current business world—which has all but eclipsed the traditional mass-marketing approaches for many brands. As a growing number of advertisers have narrowed their sights to focus on specific niches of consumers, a side effect has been that many of these advertisers are now less inclined to worry about whether people outside the niche might be offended by certain ads. In effect, what matters now is only the target group. And if the target group happens to be young males—the most sought-after segment among many advertisers—then the content of the ads will be geared to the sensibilities of that group, even if that means offending others in the audience. Such is the

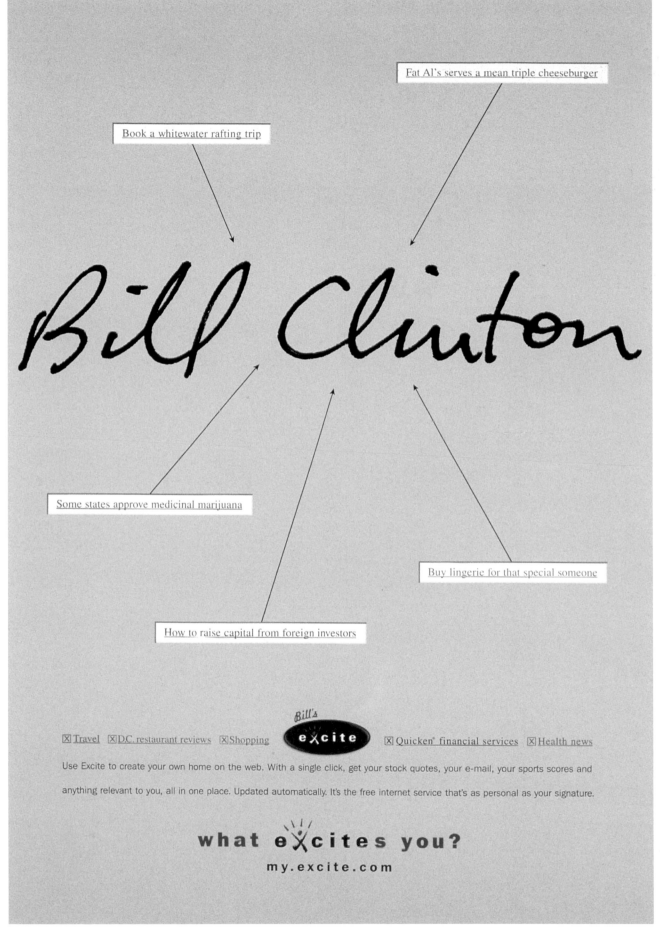

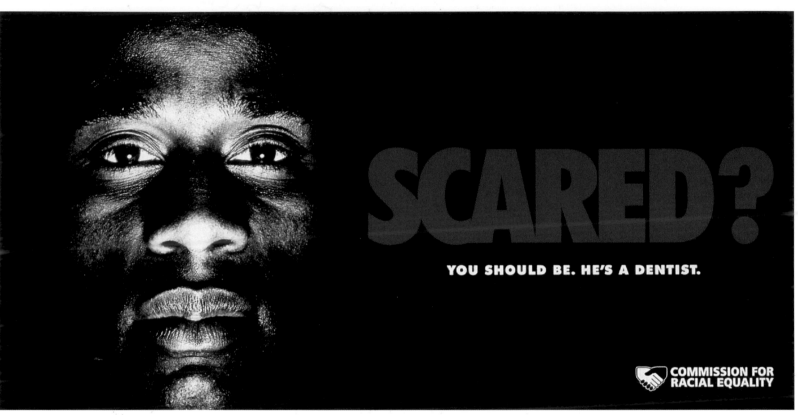

SCARED?

YOU SHOULD BE. HE'S A DENTIST.

COMMISSION FOR
RACIAL EQUALITY

23

23. COMMISSION FOR RACIAL EQUALITY
EURO RSCG WNEK GOSPER, LONDON, 1999
Race is a minefield for advertisers. This well-meaning campaign came under heavy fire for offending the people it was trying to help.

24. ATLANTA'S BLACK PROFESSIONALS
AUSTIN KELLEY ADVERTISING, ATLANTA, 1997
This ad, on the other hand, took a provocative but less abrasive stand against the "ebonics" language controversy, perhaps because the sponsor was a black professional group.

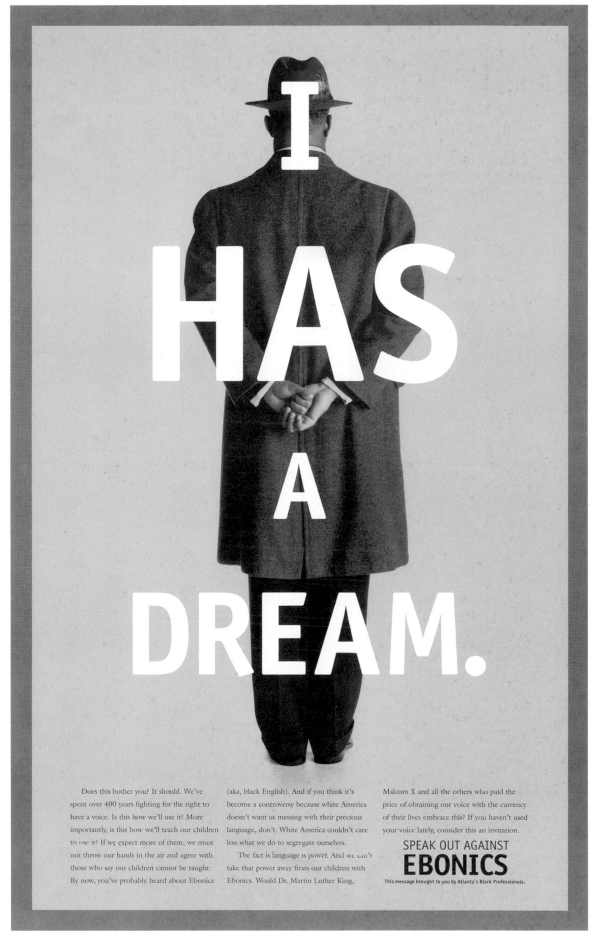

Does this bother you? It should. We've spent over 400 years fighting for the right to have a voice. Is this how we'll use it? More importantly, is this how we'll teach our children to use it? If we expect more of them, we must not throw our hands in the air and agree with those who say our children cannot be taught. By now, you've probably heard about Ebonics (aka, black English). And if you think it's become a controversy because white America doesn't want us messing with their precious language, don't. White America couldn't care less what we do to segregate ourselves.

The fact is language is power. And we can't take that power away from our children with Ebonics. Would Dr. Martin Luther King, Malcom X and all the others who paid the price of obtaining our voice with the currency of their lives embrace this? If you haven't used your voice lately, consider this an invitation.

SPEAK OUT AGAINST
EBONICS
This message brought to you by Atlanta's Black Professionals.

24

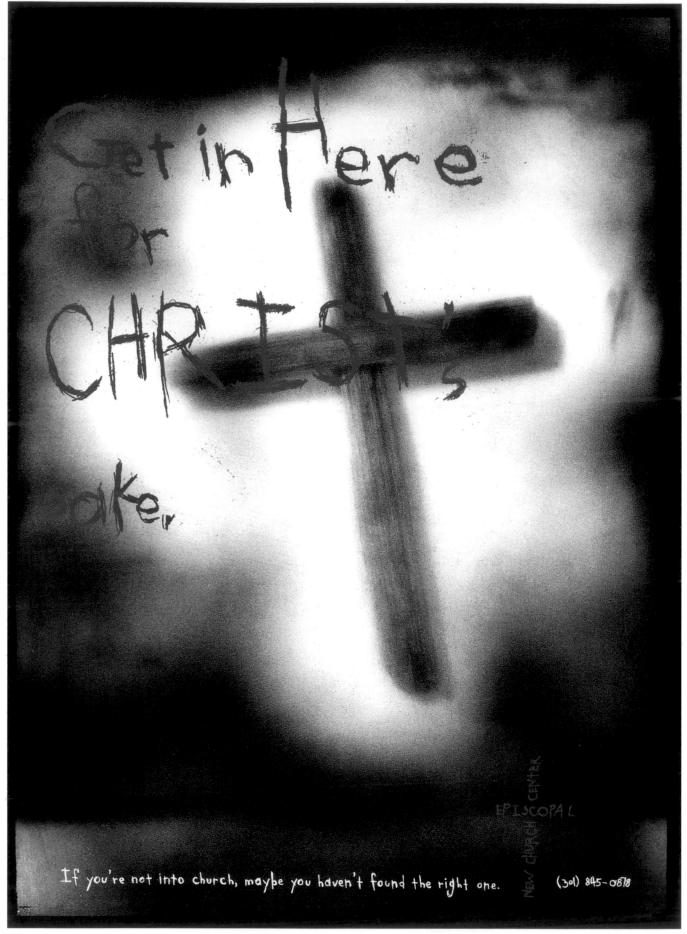

25

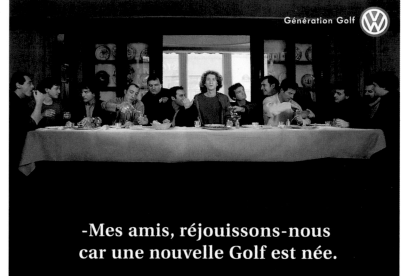

-Mes amis, réjouissons-nous
car une nouvelle Golf est née.

27

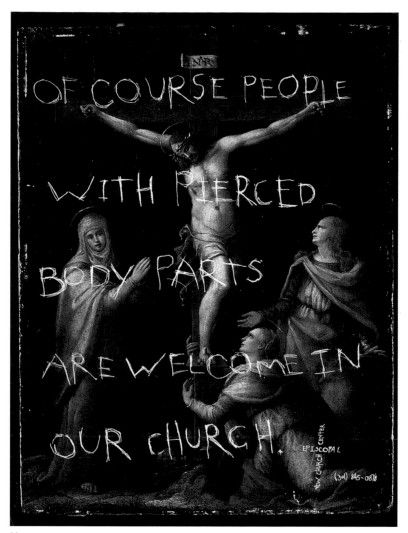

26

**25 AND 26. EPISCOPAL
CHURCH**
THE RICHARDS GROUP,
DALLAS, 1998
Religion, too, is usually consid-
ered off-limits to advertisers.
But churches have lately begun
to use hip, postmodern ads to
try to attract a younger crowd.

27. VOLKSWAGEN GOLF
DDB, PARIS, 1998
The scene resembles *The Last
Supper*, but this gathering is
rejoicing because "a new Golf is
born." French Catholic bishops
sued VW and its agency over
this ad.

case at Fox Sports, which aims its ads squarely at young males. "Our main concern when we consider our ads is whether they're right for [our] target audience," says Fox's Tiles. "Because if we try to be appropriate for everybody, then we become relevant to nobody." Tiles acknowledges that Fox gets complaints about some of its wilder, more violent ads, but "usually from people outside the demographic—mothers, older men." The company sees that situation as almost unavoidable because, Tiles says, Fox and many other of today's marketers are faced with a paradox: "We're in a mass medium in terms of how we're consumed, but we're dead set on selling to a specific demographic."

In truth, some advertisers today feel that if an ad polarizes the audience—offending some while impressing others with its bravado—that can actually work to the benefit of the brand. "Being polarizing can be a good thing," says Marty Cooke of the M&C Saatchi agency,

"because it solidifies your core base of customers. If other people don't like what you're doing, that just makes your core supporters like you even more." Calvin Klein, of course, understood this two decades ago, but today even a larger, more conservative advertiser like JCPenney is buying into the same divide-and-conquer niche strategy.

Interestingly, while advertisers now seem to be less afraid of offending the mainstream masses, they're more worried than ever about offending particular ethnic-minority groups. For the most part, the industry has largely cleansed itself of the racial stereotypes that once plagued advertising. But every so often, ads with racist imagery still surface. A noteworthy recent example appeared during the 1999 Super Bowl and promoted a footwear chain by showing a barefoot black Kenyan runner being hunted down by whites, then drugged and forced to wear sneakers. The

spot was so appalling that the client eventually tried to sue the small upstate New York agency that produced it.

The racial minefield in advertising is so treacherous that sometimes ads with good intentions can encounter problems. The London agency Euro RSCG Wnek Gosper recently tried to create a series of public-service ads encouraging people to speak out against racist imagery seen in public. In making its point, the agency tried to be perhaps a bit too clever; Wnek Gosper created a series of outrageous, deliberately racist posters, such as one billboard headlined, "Dominate the race," showing a white man stepping on the hand of a black man while climbing over him on a ladder. After posting the offensive ad around London for a short time, the agency followed up with a subsequent billboard that reprinted the original image along with this message: "What was worse? This advert or

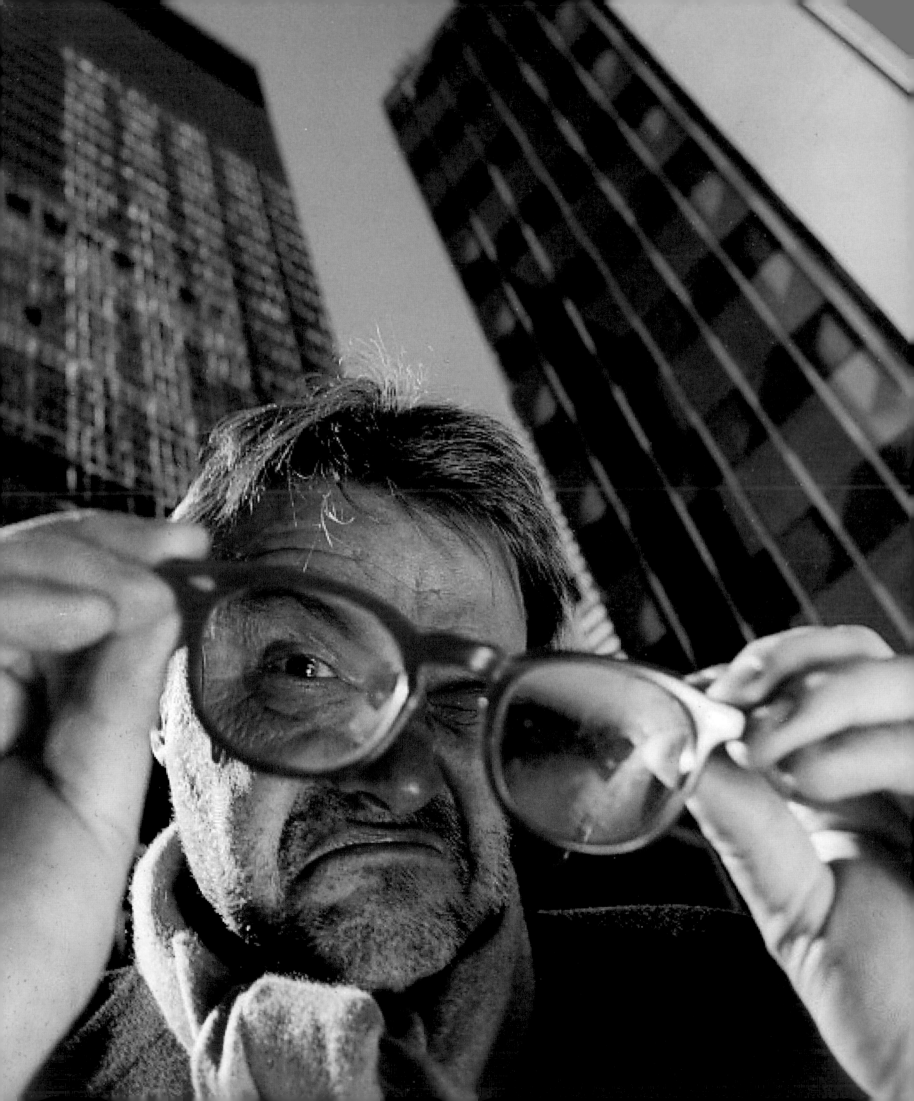

INTERVIEW: OLIVIERO TOSCANI

As the longtime creative director of advertising for the Italian clothing retailer Benetton, Oliviero Toscani was one of the first—and to this day, one of the only—advertisers to mix social commentary and marketing. Beginning in the mid-1980s, his print and outdoor ad campaigns (featuring his own photographs) presented images of interracial relationships, a bloody baby fresh from the womb, a dying AIDS patient, a priest kissing a nun, a close-up of the bloodstained clothes of a dead Croatian soldier—no subject was off-limits to Toscani. His final ad campaign for Benetton appeared in 2000 and profiled American prison inmates on death row. Toscani is currently the creative director of *Talk* magazine, and he runs Fabrica, a center for communication arts based in Italy.

WHY DO YOU CHOOSE TO ADDRESS SOCIAL ISSUES IN ADS?
I think advertising is a social message in itself. Of course—telling people what they are to consume and how they should look and what they should drive. Isn't that a social message?

BUT YOUR CRITICS SAY ISSUES LIKE AIDS, RACISM, AND WAR ARE TOO IMPORTANT, TOO SERIOUS TO BE DISCUSSED—OR THEY MIGHT SAY, EXPLOITED—IN ADS.
That's old talk. Advertising is the richest and most powerful medium today, the one where the most money is invested. If it's okay to do very powerful, socially concerned songs and sell a lot of records, and it's okay to do movies the same way, then I don't know why only advertising has to stay stupid. Advertising is the language of production and consumption—two very important activities in the history of humanity. Production means work and consumption means culture. So I don't understand why the language of advertising has to be used in the same old way. I think it's just because advertisers are not smart.

DO YOU THINK ADS ARE BECOMING LESS FEARFUL OF CONTROVERSY?
Oh yes; people now don't always do what the client asks them to do. And I think that, for example, what's happened with Benetton has proved that you can be courageous and stand for your idea, and by doing that the company got

twenty times bigger. I think people appreciate when you stand for something.

BUT IF PEOPLE DISAGREE WITH YOUR POLITICS, WON'T THEY HOLD THAT AGAINST THE BRAND?
Everybody thinks that's the case, but it is not true. There are a lot of people who, even if they don't agree with what you're saying, will appreciate that you have the courage to say it. They say, "Look, this is a company that speaks up." For any brand, the most valuable thing is to be known by people. Benetton is one of the five best-known brands worldwide. And it was all done without using television. I never use television.

WHY NOT?
I hate television. I think it's very expensive and it's not necessary. [With print ads], you pollute less. A billboard is much more interesting to me. Billboards are simple, as simple as possible. They should appeal to everybody, and everybody can see them and understand them.

YOUR ADS ALSO DON'T USE WORDS MUCH; THE PICTURE DOES THE TALKING.
We live in a world of images, we don't live in a world of words. And an image by itself can be a worldwide message—you can use the same picture everywhere, and you don't have to deal with the problem of translation.

HOW DID YOU DECIDE WHICH ISSUES TO ADDRESS IN YOUR ADS?
Totally instinct, things I felt strongly about. I don't do marketing research. I look at what the marketing research says, and if you want to have success, you do the opposite.

HAVE YOU BEEN SURPRISED BY THE DIFFERING REACTIONS IN VARIOUS COUNTRIES?
Well, every country is different; every one has its own problem. You know there are some countries that don't react at all to a picture—and that same image gets another country really mad. For example, Scandinavian countries never seem to get shocked about anything. Then if you take the ad with the newborn baby—it was a big problem all over Europe, especially in England. But in America it wasn't any problem at all. And then the soldier ad, that ran everywhere except

Germany. The HIV-positive ad upset people in France. By now, we usually know how countries will react based on their political past. For example, "Death Row" was a big problem in America, of course, whereas not in Europe at all.

SHOULDN'T YOU BE TELLING CONSUMERS AT LEAST SOMETHING ABOUT BENETTON PRODUCTS IN THE ADS?
Oh, we've done that. That's not difficult. That's something even advertising people can do. But you have to take chances. If you want to interest the world in your message, you have to talk about more than the product—you have to talk about life and death. You have to go for something that might be controversial, that might be rejected, criticized, but so what? That is why you have freedom of speech.

DO YOU SEE ADVERTISING AS AN ART FORM?
It could be an incredible art form. When you look back into history and look at Renaissance painting, that was like advertising painted in the church. The painters were called in to express a religious idea, which was like a product—so the painting was there to promote a power, a king, a religion. But those Michelangelos and Leonardos were able to transcend all of that to become art. And we should do the same. I wish advertising's art directors and creative directors, instead of trying to become more and more like salesmen, would move more in the direction of artists. Instead they listen to the marketing men, and for that they give up their art. And that's why advertising is mostly boring and ugly.

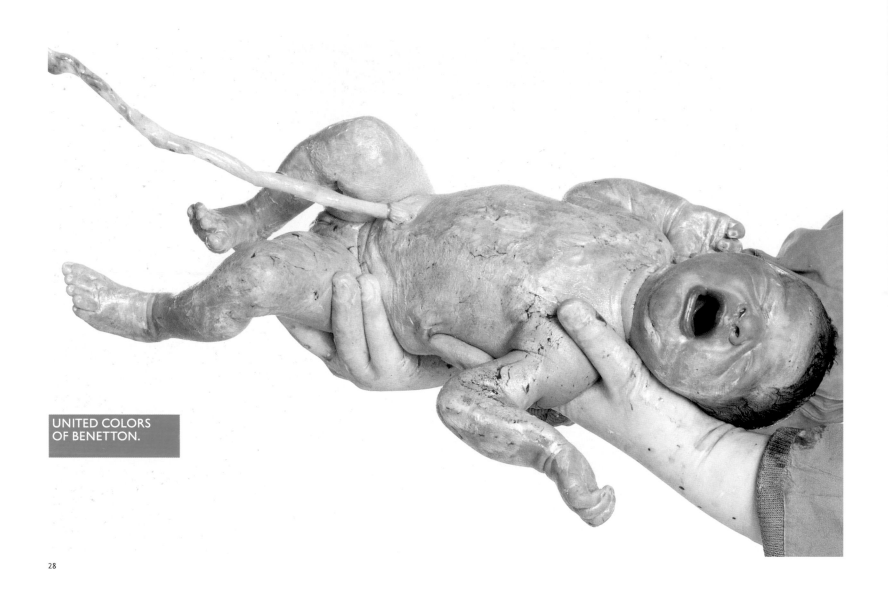

UNITED COLORS
OF BENETTON.

28

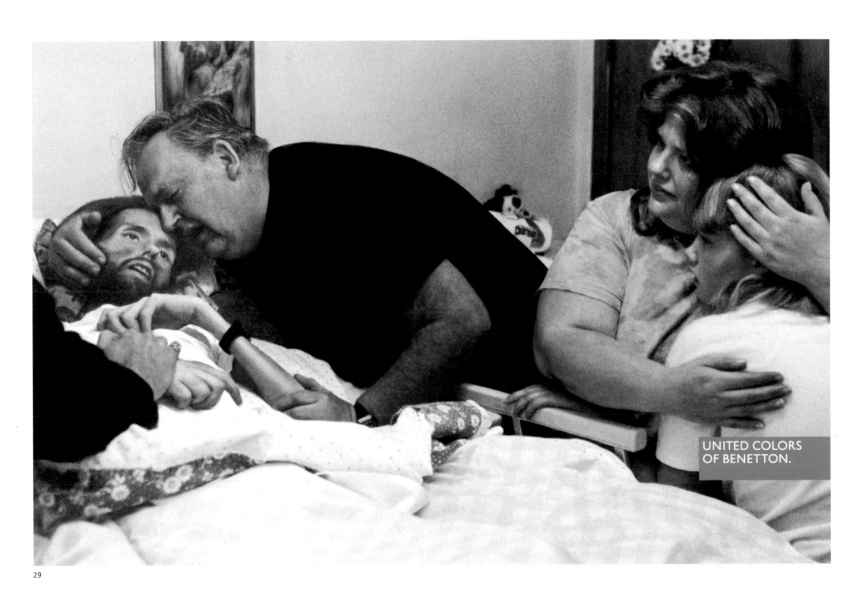

UNITED COLORS OF BENETTON.

29

28. BENETTON
OLIVIERO TOSCANI, MILAN,
1991
One of Oliviero Toscani's
early shockers featured a baby
fresh from the womb and still
bloody—England, in particular,
objected.

29. BENETTON
OLIVIERO TOSCANI, MILAN,
1992
Here, Toscani focused on
the death of an AIDS victim
surrounded by his family. Critics
felt the advertiser was exploiting
human suffering.

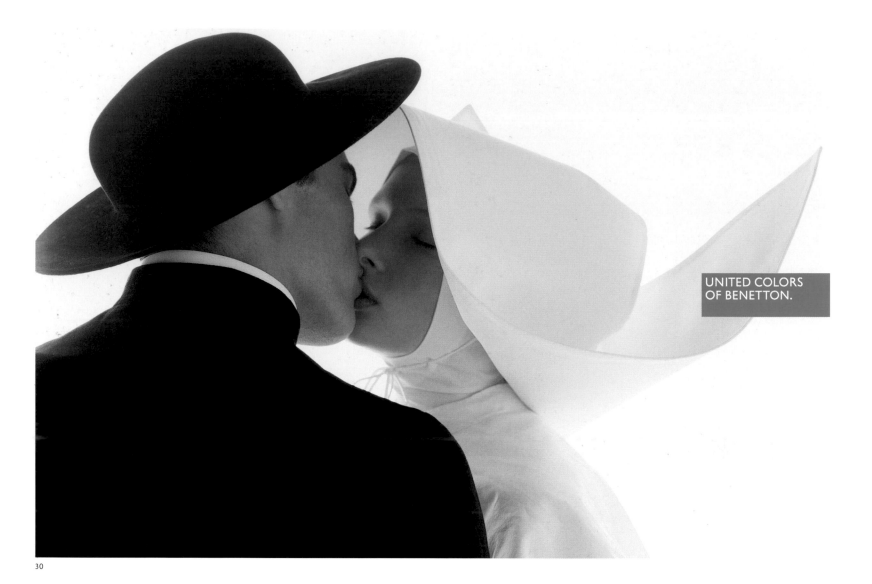

UNITED COLORS
OF BENETTON.

30

your failure to complain?" But the campaign backfired, as the advertiser was accused of endorsing racist imagery and was compelled to apologize.

Advertisers typically try to avoid misunderstandings like that by handling the subject of race very carefully in ads—perhaps too carefully, according to some critics, who believe the ad industry is currently straitjacketed by its own insecurities and fears. "Political correctness inhibits good advertising," says Rogier van Bakel, the editor of the magazine *Creativity*. He notes that because advertisers are paralyzed by fear of offending members of minority groups, the ads aimed at these groups end up being particularly bland and patronizing. Such ads "shy away from humor and candor," van Bakel says, in favor of "the feel-good, self-esteem-building variety of minority advertising."

Van Bakel and other critics believe that political correctness in advertising has also

taken some of the creative spark out of ads directed to women, many of which have shied away from irreverent humor in favor of relentlessly upbeat and "empowering" messages. But even in the enlightened and empowering 1990s, it still wasn't hard to find ads that ogled women's bodies—and sometimes got into trouble for it. A case in point was the "Swedish Bikini Team" ad campaign for Stroh's beer, which created an uproar in the U.S. in the early 1990s. The ads presented over-the-top scenarios in which a group of men, typically fishing or camping in the middle of nowhere, were unexpectedly visited by beer-toting, dancing, bikini-clad women in blonde wigs. While the campaign's creators took pains to point out that the ads were intended to be tongue-in-cheek, critics weren't buying that line; as one skeptic noted, it seemed clear that Stroh's was trying to "have it both ways," presenting titillating and sexist images of women, while also suggesting, in

very postmodern fashion, that it was all just an inside joke. The controversy seemed to have a significant after-effect on beer advertising; this onetime bastion of sexist imagery began to rely less on exploiting women's bodies in ads and more on bathroom humor (was this progress?). But as the beer advertisers reduced their own "cheesecake" quotient, the new-era lingerie brands like Wonderbra and Victoria's Secret produced ads that, at times, seemed almost indistinguishable from pinup magazine centerfolds. (Wonderbra, to its credit, at least acknowledged its own naughtiness with playful and outrageous headlines accompanying all those body shots: "Hello Boys!" screamed one billboard that briefly became the talk of London in the mid-1990s.)

If advertisers had come to tread lightly around issues of race and gender, they were even more careful when it came to religion. Those few advertisers that took on churches as

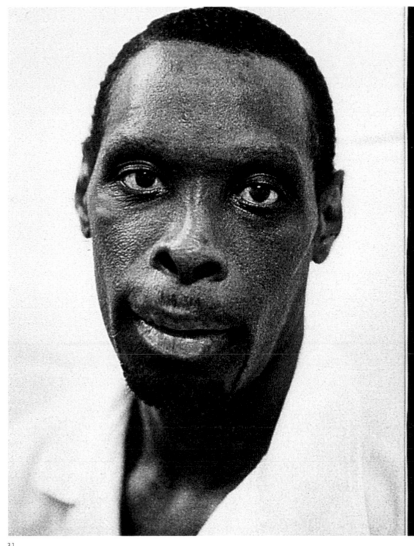

30. **BENETTON**
OLIVIERO TOSCANI, MILAN, 1991
While many advertisers avoid the minefields of race and religion, Toscani has not. He insisted there was "nothing sinful" about his ad showing a priest and nun kissing.

31. **BENETTON**
OLIVIERO TOSCANI, NEW YORK, 2000
Toscani's last campaign for Benetton featured sympathetic portraits of inmates on death row. The campaign angered some who had been victimized by crime.

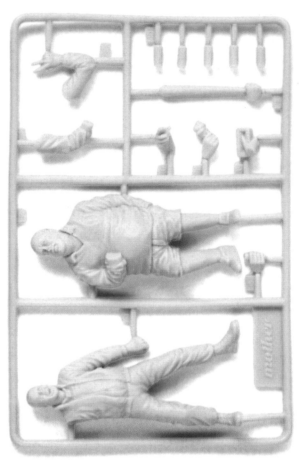

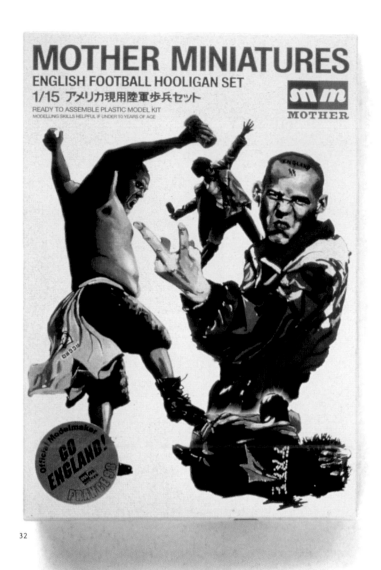

MOTHER MINIATURES
ENGLISH FOOTBALL HOOLIGAN SET
1/15 アメリカ現用陸軍歩兵セット

READY TO ASSEMBLE PLASTIC MODEL KIT
MODELLING SKILLS HELPFUL IF UNDER 10 YEARS OF AGE

MOTHER

32

clients usually opted for solemn and reverent approaches. Recently, however, some religious advertising has become a bit more humorous. One ad, produced in Texas for the Episcopal New Church, featured an image of Jesus Christ on the cross, with the headline "Of course people with pierced body parts are welcome in our church." And a series of billboards in Florida showed a light touch with the headline "Let's meet at my house Sunday before the game." It was signed, "God." Another ad in the same campaign threatened, "Don't make me come down there." The campaign was designed to encourage young people to attend church, though its creator, Charlie Robb, acknowledged that not everyone appreciated the tone of the ads. European advertising, while often more daring in dealing with sex, is as skittish as American agencies when it comes to religion: In France, a recent Volkswagen ad created an uproar by mimicking *The Last Supper;* the ad

featured people in modern dress posed in exactly the same positions as the figures in Leonardo da Vinci's famous fresco, with the headline, "My Friends, let us rejoice because a new Golf is born." French Catholic bishops sued Volkswagen and its agency.

Like religion, politics is seen as a potentially divisive domain that most advertising agencies and brand marketers avoid. Particularly in America, it's rare to find an advertiser taking a stand on any issue that isn't a reasonably safe one (for example, companies have no problem speaking out against drunk driving—a no-brainer—but hot-button topics like gun control, capital punishment, and abortion are typically avoided). One exception to this rule has been the Italy-based clothing company Benetton, whose advertising in the late 1980s and early 1990s tackled a number of controversial political and social issues, including AIDS, racism, and the ravages of war. Through the stark and

sometimes shocking imagery in his ads, Oliviero Toscani, the creative director of Benetton's advertising, clearly emerged as one of the most outspoken advertisers ever. One of Toscani's more provocative images showed a black woman breast-feeding a white baby; another showed a priest and nun kissing; still another featured the bloodstained clothes of a dead Croatian soldier; and perhaps the most controversial of all Benetton's ads showed a dying AIDS victim.

To some critics, Toscani's advertising seemed exploitive and manipulative; in effect, they argued that he was using the suffering of the world to sell clothes. Toscani's own position was that his ads were simply an attempt to raise social consciousness on certain issues, and to stir debate through the powerful and pervasive medium of advertising. But perhaps the biggest debate he stirred was on the question of whether for-profit advertising can ever

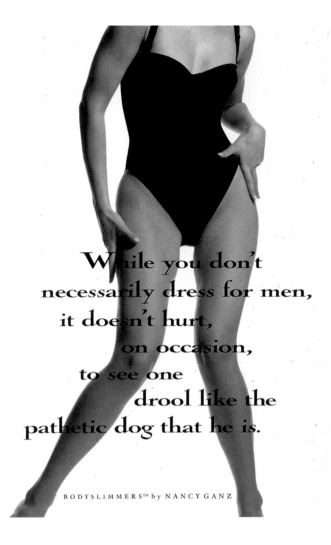

While you don't necessarily dress for men, it doesn't hurt, on occasion, to see one drool like the pathetic dog that he is.

BODYSLIMMERS™ by NANCY GANZ

33

be an appropriate forum for examining serious issues; do advertisers like Toscani have enough objectivity and moral authority to take on the role of journalist or social commentator? The question was never really resolved, though Toscani's aggressive ad campaigns eventually receded from the spotlight. Benetton and Toscani briefly seized the spotlight again in 2000 with an ad campaign opposing capital punishment. In the end, Toscani was beaten back not so much by his critics as by the cold, hard marketplace: Benetton's sales first sky-rocketed, then plummeted, during the course of its controversial campaigns. The vagaries of the fashion business notwithstanding, it's reasonable to conclude that Benetton's shock-politics approach was eye-catching in the short run but gradually turned off consumers who were already getting their fill of painful images on the evening news and didn't need to see more in ads. Still, the legacy of Benetton's

work lives on somewhat in the more recent ads by the clothing company Diesel and also among young European ad-agency creative directors like Johan Kramer of KesselsKramer, who occasionally tries to use his advertising to issue statements about discrimination and other social issues.

Challenging authority or the social structure can be particularly hazardous in some countries, but advertisers still occasionally try it. Kitty Lun, former creative director of the Hong Kong agency Euro RSCG Partnership, notes that while the general public in Asia is usually fairly accepting of sexually frank ads, such ads will often come under fire from governments or activist groups. Lun observes that a recent telecommunications campaign was banned when the commercial tried to make its point—that its mobile phone can access many different networks—by making a comparison to having multiple sex partners. The ad was clever, but "it

really offended a lot of people," says Lun. The Singapore-based ad copywriter Jim Aitchison points out that a recent local ad in which a son was disrespectful to his father became quite controversial. Meanwhile, in Eastern Europe, advertising is still relatively young and finding its voice. A Polish beer ad, for example, ridiculed corrupt Russian military figures; it had only a short run, but the ad developed a cult following in Poland.

It's rarer to find American ads that challenge authority or social convention in that manner. Interestingly, though, American ads some-times trigger social debate unexpectedly, by tapping into deep feelings people may have on a given subject. For example, the ABC television network recently ignited a controversy with a series of seemingly innocuous ads about the guilty pleasure of watching TV. The ads' creators at TBWA/Chiat/Day simply wanted to suggest that perhaps watching TV wasn't such

Before TV,
two World Wars.
After TV, zero.

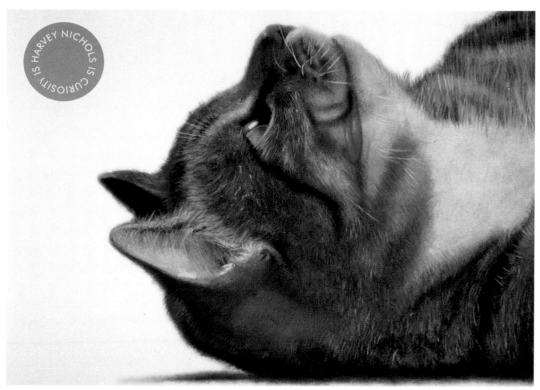

35

34. ABC TELEVISION
TBWA/CHIAT/DAY,
LOS ANGELES, 1997
Another unexpected controversy:
Critics swarmed all over this
humorous campaign because
they felt it was making light of
the mind-numbing effects of TV.

35. HARVEY NICHOLS
MOTHER, LONDON, 1998
This department store ad, on the
other hand, featured an image
of a dead cat (albeit computer-
generated), and surprisingly few
people took issue with it.

an awful thing to do, and they did so with headlines that defended TV-watching by way of ironic statements: "Don't worry, you've got billions of brain cells," one ad said reassuringly, while another noted, "You can talk to your wife anytime." In the ensuing weeks, the American media swarmed all over the ABC campaign, which was accused of being overly cynical and of promoting illiteracy. The campaign seemed to touch on strong opinions people had about two separate issues—the effects of watching TV and the use of cynical irony in ads. All of which stunned ad-agency president Bob Kuperman, who says, "We never thought the ads would cause so much intellectual masturbation."

Similarly, Nike and its agency, Wieden + Kennedy, were taken aback by the criticism of an Olympics ad that declared, "You don't win silver, you lose gold." The ad was accused of promoting a win-at-all-costs attitude that ran counter to the Olympic spirit of competition.

But agency founder Dan Wieden claimed the ad was just misunderstood: "The confusion may have been that it was thought to be Nike's voice saying these words, rather than the voice of the athlete," said Wieden. "The whole idea of the campaign was that the Olympics is war minus the killing—for an athlete, just before that gun goes off, it's a very uncompromising moment."

The ABC and Nike campaigns may be testaments to the truly unpredictable nature of ad controversy. Ad-agency executives tend to agree that it's perhaps more difficult than ever to gauge exactly what will upset today's more desensitized consumer. "It always surprises me," said Mark Waites of the British agency Mother. Waites pointed out that he once put a close-up picture of a dead cat in an ad, and braced for complaints—but they were minimal. He also ran a truly incendiary self-promotion for his agency, in which he created a mock ad offering an artificial-fireplace log designed to

look like an American flag—the idea being that America-haters could use this product for the dual pleasure of burning the U.S. flag every time they sat in front of the fireplace. "I thought that would be controversial, but people seemed to get the joke," Waites said. However, when he created another mock ad, offering collections of toy warriors designed to look not like soldiers but like English soccer hooligans, Waites was inundated with complaints by faithful football fans. The bottom line, Waites has learned, is that advertisers can never predict when controversy will rear its head. "The things you think will upset people end up being fine," he said, "and the things you don't worry about are the ones that end up causing the most trouble of all."

8. THE
OF ADVE

FACES

RTISING.

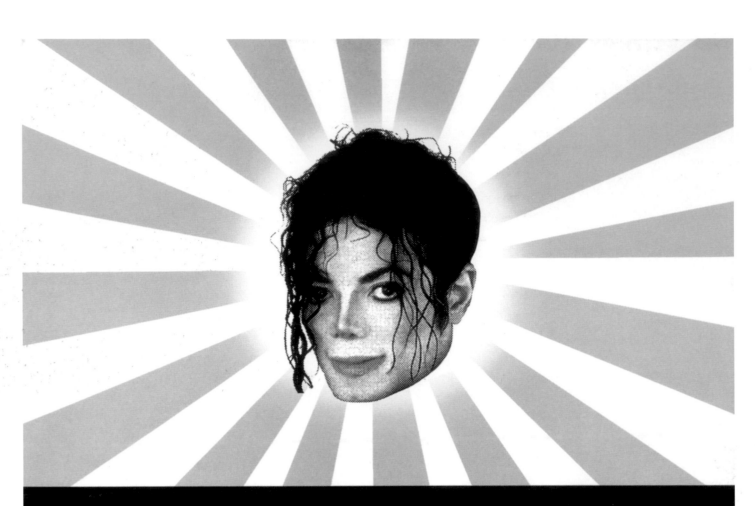

SOME PEOPLE ARE JUST TOO WHITE.

SUN WORSHIPPERS

PRIVATE TANNING BEDS • 215 SOUTH ST. 629-0040 • 1326 SPRUCE ST. 545-6703 • OPEN EVERY DAY

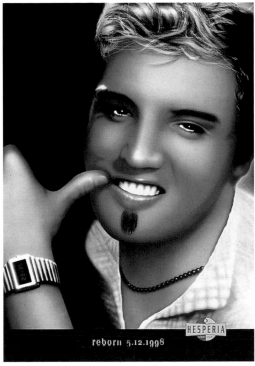

2

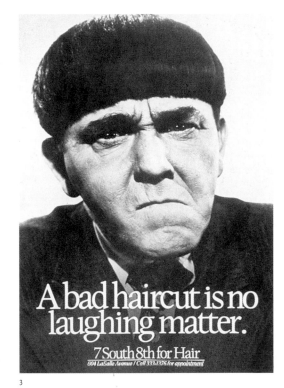

3

A

s the messages of advertising changed in recent years, so did the messengers who brought them to us.

Historically, the face that advertising turned to the world was apt to be famous, wholesome, warm, and inviting—in America, it was Bob Hope for Texaco gasoline in the 1960s, or, a decade later, Bill Cosby for Jell-O. Elsewhere around the world, popular mainstream stars, from the comic actor Paul Hogan in Australia to the soccer star Pele in South America, all played a similarly straight-forward, if somewhat disingenuous, role: Smile for the camera, hold up the product, say something laudatory. When not relying on star endorsers, many advertisers, particularly in the U.S., opted for another classic approach: hiring lesser-known actors to portray benign, lovable, fictional characters—such as Mr. Whipple, known for squeezing Charmin bathroom tissue, or the Maytag Repairman, "the loneliest man in town"— who became part of an ongoing story that

revolved around the product. It was a wink-and-nod form of communication with the audience, which knew, of course, that the Maytag Repairman wasn't real, and also suspected that Cosby probably didn't really love Jell-O all that much. Still, there was a feel-good aura surrounding such images, and those familiar faces helped infuse brands with a personality.

Indeed, the classic advertising characters and spokespersons, who continued to dominate ads well into the 1970s and early 1980s, managed to "put a human face on nearly every product," noted Robert Thompson, director of Syracuse University's Center for the Study of Popular Television. "Almost in a Walt Disney–like fashion, Madison Avenue anthropomorphized products— so that toilet paper became Mr. Whipple," Thompson said. "It was a very effective way of getting the audience to identify with people, not just products."

Fast-forward to the present, and one finds

that faces are still at the center of most advertising—though now they are as apt to be snarling as smiling. Hope and Cosby have given way to people like Dennis Rodman, the mischievous, tattooed, cross-dressing basketball star who has appeared in ads for that most wholesome of all products, milk. And while fictional characters still populate ads, they, too, have changed; no longer pleasant and benign, ad characters became "edgier," to use a favorite buzzword of ad creators. Their ranks now include the likes of Stuart, the featured character in a series of commercials for the Ameritrade on-line trading service—a rude, punkish, wild-haired office boy who bullies the boss and wreaks havoc at work. Stuart actually seems quite civilized compared with the 800 Call Collect Guy, played by the actor David Arquette in a series of ads for AT&T, who is often seen stalking and screaming at other characters in the ads. On one level, this new, slightly twisted face of advertising is yet

THE FACES OF ADVERTISING.

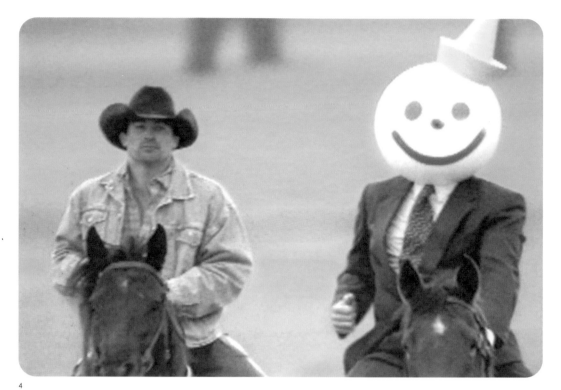

4

4. **JACK IN THE BOX**
KOWLOON W. S.C. AGENCY,
LOS ANGELES, 1998
In this late 1990s campaign for
a Southern California-based
hamburger chain, the company
spokesman had a ping pong
ball for a head and a penchant
for violence.

5. **AMERICAN EXPRESS**
OGILVY & MATHER,
NEW YORK, MID-1990s
American comedian Jerry
Seinfeld met his hero in this
commercial. Like a number
of contemporary endorsers,
Seinfeld maintains an ironic
distance from the product.

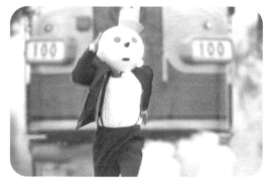

another desperate try by sponsors to somehow be heard above the din of growing ad clutter. But at the same time, it's also an attempt to associate with more contemporary, rebellious, break-the-rules attitudes and behavior.

The modern pitchman need not be stark raving mad but must, at minimum, be somewhat cynical. The comedian Jerry Seinfeld, for example, has maintained a pleasant demeanor in his ongoing ad campaign for American Express. Nevertheless, Seinfeld embodies the new-generation ad spokesperson—far removed from Hope and Cosby in attitude. Like many of the trendier spokespersons who have emerged in recent years (the sardonic American comedian Dennis Miller is another example), Seinfeld keeps his skeptical persona even in ads, and always maintains an ironic distance from the product. Today's modern endorsers rarely smile for the camera and almost never do old-fashioned testimonials praising the product. Often they simply

do their personal "shtick" in commercials, allowing the brand to tag along for the ride. If this suggests a certain reluctance on their part to commit to the product, that's perfectly acceptable—that skepticism, hesitance, and candor, along with Rodman-like personal flaws, all come together to form advertising's version of the anti-hero, the perfect postmodern pitching machine.

The evolution of the face of advertising began in the 1960s, when up-and-coming American creative agencies—some of which were staffed by ethnic New Yorkers—tried to bring more diversity and authenticity to the casting of their ads. "We wanted to show in our ads that not everyone was blond and beautiful," said Roy Grace, formerly of Doyle Dane Bernbach, now of Grace & Rothschild. That agency's ad campaign for Levy's rye bread broke new ground by featuring the faces of ordinary people, including Asian-Americans and African-Americans. By the 1970s and early 1980s, a number of advertisers

began using so-called real people in ads—though this was something of a misnomer, because the models and performers were usually actors who just happened to look like imperfect ordinary people. In any case, the ad landscape soon featured people who were balding or overweight, or others with exaggerated features that made them look sad or silly (as noted in Chapter 4, the commercial director Joe Sedelmaier specialized in ads starring unglamorous characters—including his most famous, Clara Peller, from the Wendy's "Where's the Beef?" ads).

But the ground truly shifted in the mid-1980s, as several convergent trends began to take hold. By this time, a growing number of advertisers had begun to accept the notion that old-fashioned commercials featuring benign mascot characters or overly earnest star endorsers were no longer credible or compelling to an audience that was more savvy and cynical. "The growing feeling was that consumers could

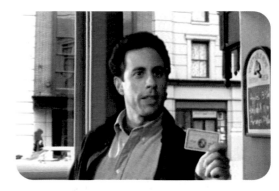

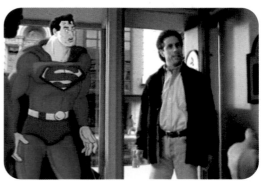

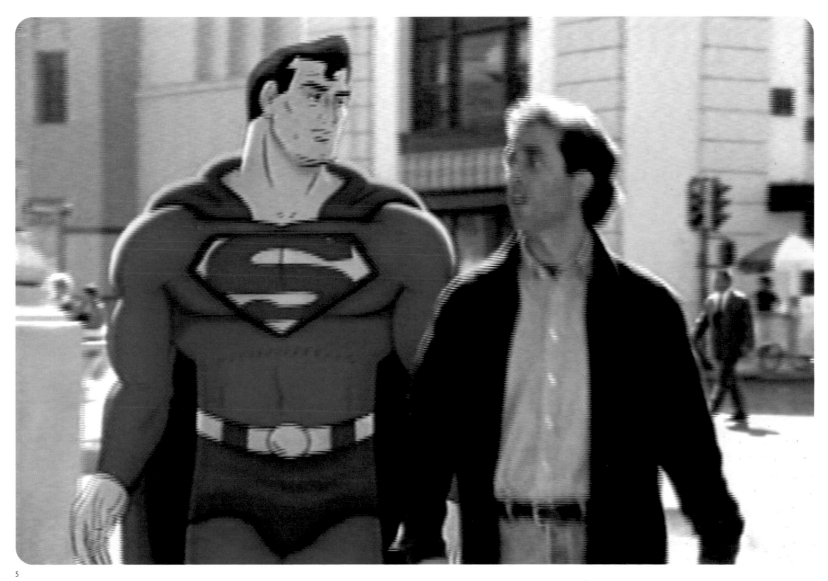

5

THE FACES OF ADVERTISING.

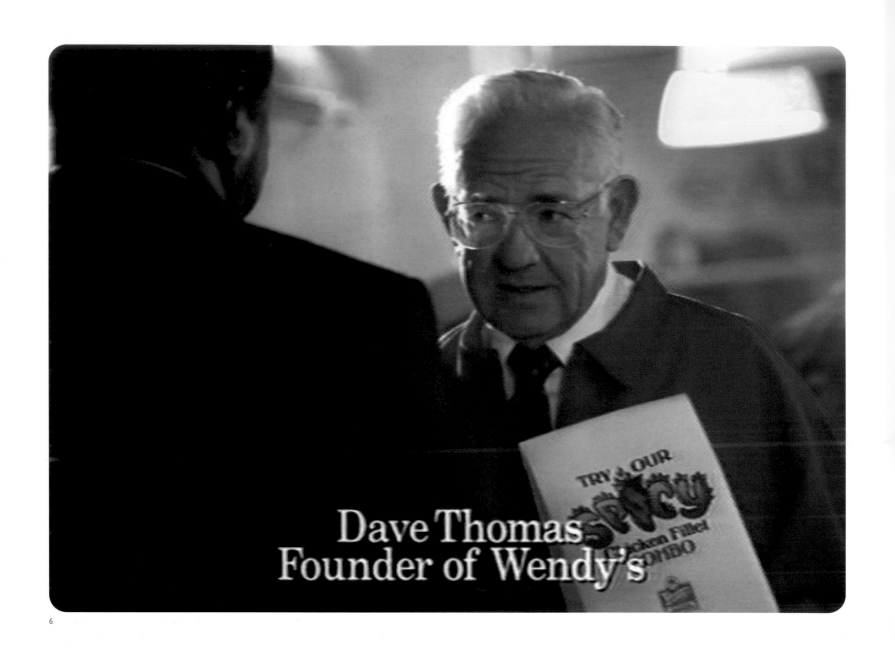

6

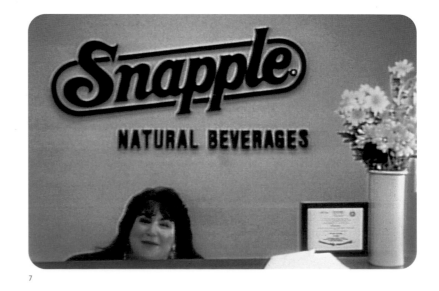

7

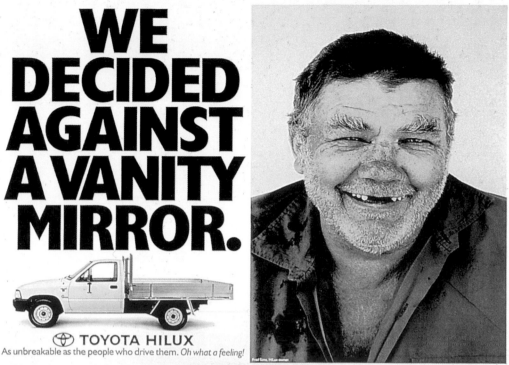

WE DECIDED AGAINST A VANITY MIRROR.

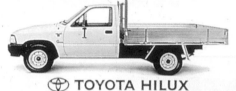

TOYOTA HILUX

As unbreakable as the people who drive them. *Oh what a feeling!*

8

6. WENDY'S RESTAURANTS
BATES WORLDWIDE,
NEW YORK, 1994
The regular guy as spokesman:
Wendy's executive Dave Thomas
wasn't smooth in these TV
commercials, but his "Everyman"
quality was effective.

7. SNAPPLE BEVERAGES
KIRSHENBAUM BOND &
PARTNERS, NEW YORK, 1994
While Pepsi ads featured glam-
orous model Cindy Crawford,
Snapple opted for Wendy the
receptionist: the anti-Cindy.

8. TOYOTA HILUX TRUCKS
SAATCHI & SAATCHI, SYDNEY,
1996
Australia came to love this face,
and the ad earned much acclaim
for Saatchi.

see right through celebrities," said Bill Oberlander, a creative director with the New York ad agency Kirshenbaum Bond & Partners. "To stand apart from all the glamour and all those big stars, ads needed to find anti-stars— people who had more character and integrity."

This accelerated the trend of finding people who didn't look like actors—and who, in some cases, weren't actors—to appear in ads. Kirshenbaum Bond produced one of the more memorable examples with its ad campaign for Snapple fruit drinks, featuring Wendy Kaufman— a heavyset woman with a strong New York accent who had been a telephone receptionist at the beverage company for years. According to Oberlander, the use of Kaufman was an attempt to run directly counter to Pepsi, which was at the time featuring the glamorous model Cindy Crawford in its commercials. "Wendy represented an attempt to zag while everyone else was zigging," Oberlander said. But

Kaufman, who developed a popular following while the ad campaign ran during the early 1990s, also was a good match for the product itself: "She was natural and real," said Oberlander, "and that's what Snapple wanted to stand for."

Increasingly, other advertisers also sought to suggest authenticity and integrity by showing "real people," who sometimes delivered their lines in an unpolished, seemingly unscripted way. One of the most successful regular-guy pitchmen to emerge during the 1990s was Dave Thomas, the top executive of the Wendy's ham- burger chain. Thomas certainly was not the first unglamorous, hardworking company boss to appear in his own ads: Frank Perdue of Perdue Chicken had paved that ground years earlier, and Perdue—whose bald, droopy-eyed, beakish head made him look as if he might actually have some chicken genes in him—proved that one didn't need a pretty face to capture the hearts of consumers. But Thomas took the anti-star

movement even further; whereas Perdue had come across as somewhat glib and clever in his ads, Thomas seemed as if he had no business being on TV. Overweight, blandly dressed, slightly marble-mouthed—the *Advertising Age* columnist Bob Garfield once called Thomas "a steer in a half-sleeve shirt"—Thomas became legendary in the ad industry for his ineptitude as a performer (one commercial script requiring him to say "*Muchas gracias*" necessitated four hours of retakes before Thomas got the line right). And yet in spite of all that, or more likely because of it, he was a huge hit with the television audience. Jim McKennan, who wrote the original commercials starring Thomas, noted that he had "an Everyman quality" that "appeals to people on all kinds of levels."

Real people could sell hamburgers and soft drinks, but, predictably, there was far less interest in featuring unattractive faces in ads for clothing and cosmetics. After all, these were the marketers

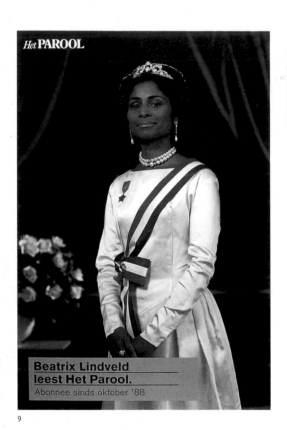

Beatrix Lindveld
leest Het Parool.
Abonnee sinds oktober '88

9

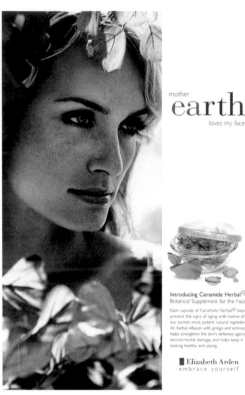

mother
earth
loves my face

Introducing Ceramide Herbal®
Botanical Supplement for the Face

Each capsule of Ceramide Herbal® helps
prevent the signs of aging with twelve of
our purest, most potent natural ingredients.
An herbal infusion with ginkgo and echinacea
helps strengthen the skin's defenses against
environmental damage, and helps keep it
looking healthy and young.

■ Elizabeth Arden
embrace yourself

10

that had, for many years, propagated advertising's so-called beauty myth by showing only
flawless faces (and bodies) in ads. But even the
beauty-myth-makers had to acknowledge that
new consumers wanted at least a bit more
authenticity in ads. Influential research studies
in the late-1990s by the firm Lubin Lawrence
revealed that women had simply had enough
of ads projecting standards of beauty that were
seen as unreal and unattainable. And while this
did not spur the makeup companies to sign up
women like Wendy Kaufman, the industry did
take a few tiny steps away from perfection. In
1999, the cosmetics company Lancôme actually
made news when one of its fragrance ads
featured a woman with freckles on her face.
At the same time, ads for Elizabeth Arden
cosmetics started portraying women who,
while physically attractive, looked less like
fashion models and more like fully functioning
human beings; the copy downplayed beauty with

lines like "My best feature is my big beautiful
sexy brain."

The trend toward bringing more natural,
authentic faces to ads became popular in many
ad markets around the world. KesselsKramer
produced one of its most popular and successful
ad campaigns for a Dutch newspaper when it
dressed up frumpy-looking, stocky, and even
buck-toothed housewives to look like royalty (the
women were chosen because they had the same
first name as Queen Beatrix of Holland). And in
Australia, one of the most wildly popular ads in
recent years featured a Toyota truck owner with
a flat nose, unshaven face, and gap-toothed grin,
appearing under the headline "We decided
against a vanity mirror." Aside from being funny
and visually arresting, the ad also made a point—
that the trucks are designed for rough customers.

Of course, even as "real people" in ads were
gaining popularity, celebrities never went out of
vogue. Advertising had been hooked on stars for

too long to give up that dependable quick fix;
many still followed the old advertising maxim
"If you have nothing to say about a product, hire
someone famous to say it." The British ad executive Frank Lowe, founder of the Lowe group of
agencies, has noted that stars "are a shortcut
to getting attention." And, in fact, they're more
than that. According to the *Journal of Consumer
Research*, as consumers process information
from an ad, they often "use information about
the celebrity to make inferences about the
product. This transfer of information from
celebrity to product is, in part, what makes the
endorsement effective."

Star-worshiping in ads is not strictly
American or even Western: In recent years,
Chinese companies have begun to associate their
products with celebrities and mythic figures
(this in spite of the fact that Chinese culture has
historically been less hero-driven than Western
culture). Hong Kong film stars have proved

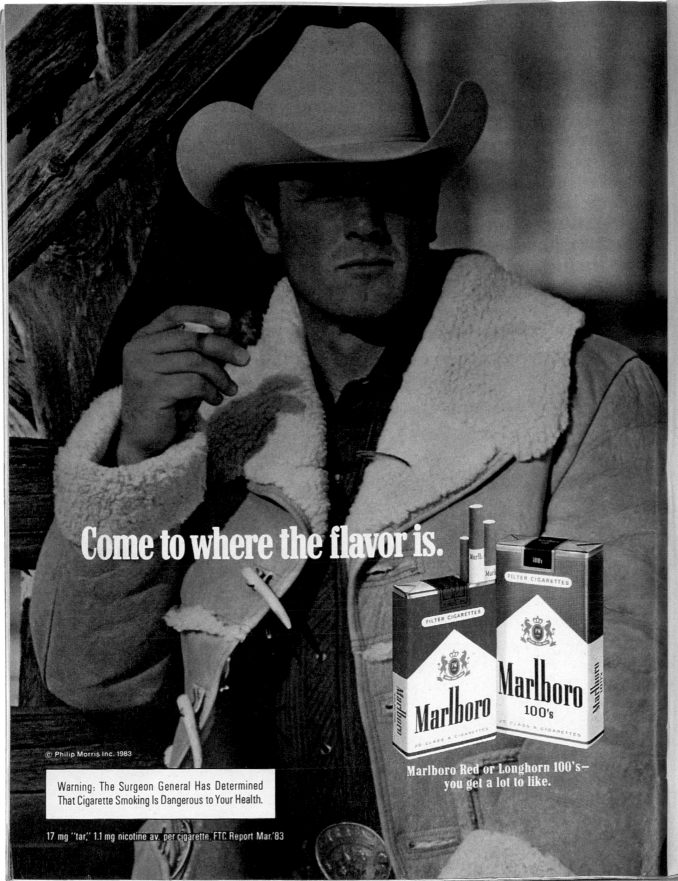

Come to where the flavor is.

© Philip Morris Inc. 1983

Warning: The Surgeon General Has Determined That Cigarette Smoking Is Dangerous to Your Health.

17 mg "tar," 1.1 mg nicotine av. per cigarette, FTC Report Mar.'83

Marlboro Red or Longhorn 100's— you get a lot to like.

ANGOLA

Deadly Rite of the

A new offensive produces the sa

Caked in grime, ragged in their new-grown beards, the South Africans had finally begun to withdraw. The last of some 2,000 soldiers were making off with booty ranging from Soviet-made guns to Russian-language maps. Some of their trucks were still decorated with Christmas tinsel. But the condition of the 30-mile-long column was hardly festive. At the village of Mupa, they had to put up a rickety bridge across a swollen river; farther south, they drove past a treasure trove of Soviet-made equipment, including recently developed AGS-17 automatic grenade launchers. After five weeks of "Operation Askari," the South Africans reported knocking out 25 Soviet-made tanks, giving chase to two Cuban battalions, and killing 400 enemy troops. Their own casualties were 21 dead, more than in any other campaign since 1975. Said Lieut. Ian Gleeson: "It was an extended operation and a hard slog."

So ended the annual deadly rite of the rainy season. Every year, before the heavy summer storms, the South Africans launch punishing raids into southern Angola to pre-empt attacks by the black nationalist guerrillas of the South West Africa People's Organization (SWAPO). And every year, once the rains provide them with foliage cover and vital water supplies, the rebels cross the border into northern Namibia, hoping to bring an end to South Africa's 17-year control of that nation. This year, for the first time, South African troops came into direct confrontation with those of Marxist Angola, supported by some of the country's estimated 26,000 Cuban soldiers and advisers. After five years of tortuous U.N. negotiation, the Angolan-Namibian situation is still at a violent stalemate: Angola refuses to dismiss its Cuban troops until South Africa withdraws; South Africa refuses to withdraw until the Cubans are dismissed. Meanwhile, South Africa will doubtless continue assisting the insurgent National Union for the Total Independence of Angola (UNITA) in its attacks against the Angolan government.

The latest offensive showed just how stagnant and how strenuous the evenly matched tug of war has become. Last August UNITA forces, reportedly supported by South African air strikes, captured the strategic town of Cangamba in southern Angola. During the following two months, SWAPO guerrillas swarmed through north-

Going thr
Fighting w

TIME, JANUARY 23, 1984

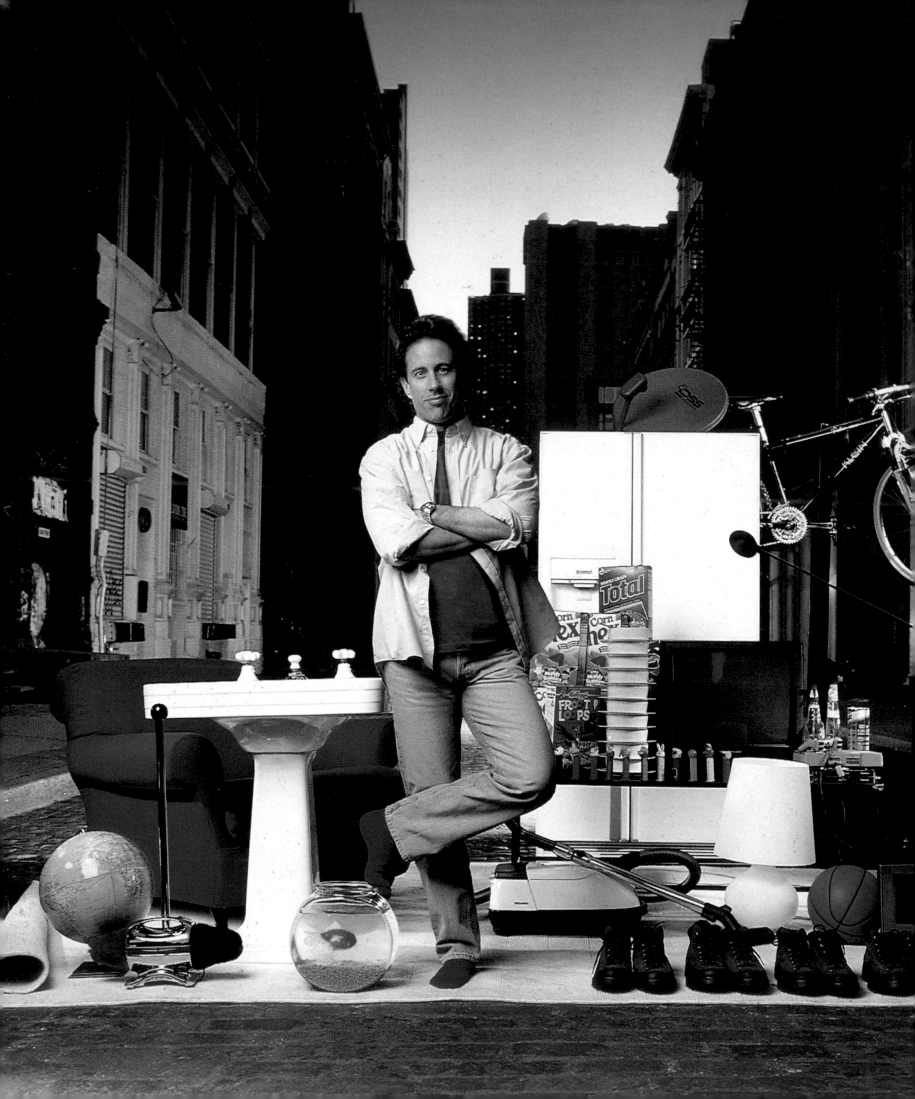

INTERVIEW: JERRY SEINFELD

His long-running TV series, *Seinfeld,* was one of the most popular and influential shows in the history of television. But the American comedian Jerry Seinfeld has also made his mark on the world of advertising in his ongoing role as the spokesman for American Express credit cards. Seinfeld doesn't just appear in the ads, he helps create them, working closely with Ogilvy & Mather creative director David Apicella. In fact, Seinfeld's interest in advertising runs so deep that he has considered starting his own ad agency.

WHY DID YOU CHOOSE TO DO ADS FOR AMERICAN EXPRESS?
I had always kind of liked the company; they had a certain dignity about them. At the time I decided to do this, [comedian] Jay Leno was doing Doritos ads, and I remember that anytime he went onstage, people would yell out, "Hey, Doritos, hey, nachos"—and I figured that was the last thing I needed. I didn't see that kind of down-side to American Express.

And creatively, they were pretty wide open. They didn't really have any set form they wanted to fit me into, and they were willing to let me get involved. And I got more and more involved as we went along. They'll usually give us a general idea of what they're trying to do with the ads— and then we'll take it from there. It's not a hard-sell campaign, obviously. They're giving us sixty seconds to create an entertaining commercial that includes the American Express card. They allow us to use the advertising time to explore the art form of the commercial.

YOU'VE TALKED ABOUT OPENING YOUR OWN AGENCY. WHAT ATTRACTS YOU TO ADVERTISING?
I've always been interested in it. In fact, I know if I weren't a comedian, I would be in advertising. I like the restrictions of it. It's kind of like stand-up comedy, which is also a very restrictive form to work in—it may seem free, but you actually have to have the utmost discipline to create something funny in a very small space. In stand-up, you have to bring up an idea, get to the funny part of it, and resolve it—in about forty seconds. Good comedy writing has a very spare, elemental feel to it. And advertising has the same kind of restriction, in that you're working with a very finite amount of

time and space. I just enjoy that smallness. It's kind of a haiku.

IN TERMS OF CELEBRITIES' WILLINGNESS TO APPEAR IN ADS, IT NOW SEEMS THAT EVEN THE MOST CUTTING-EDGE PERFORMERS ARE EAGER TO DO THEM; THE NEGATIVE BAGGAGE THAT USED TO COME WITH PITCHING PRODUCTS SEEMS TO BE ALMOST NONEXISTENT TODAY. IS THAT TRUE?
It depends on the ad. When I see celebrities in ads where I know they walked on the set, were handed a script, and just read what was written, I consider that very treacherous territory. For a celebrity, I think there is still a huge potential penalty for appearing in the wrong ad. I'm not going to mention names, but there are people doing things they should not be doing. And it's mostly because the celebrity looks at the offer simply as, "Here's how many days it will take, and here's how much they're paying." And they judge it on that basis, which to me is lunacy. The only thing that should count is, How will I appear in this exposure? Will I be entertaining and come off the way I want to come off to the public in everything I do? Just taking the money is almost always a mistake.

WE'RE SEEING LOTS OF ADS WITH OFF-THE-WALL HUMOR THESE DAYS—GERBILS SHOT FROM CANNONS AND OTHER "ODDVERTISING." ARE YOU IMPRESSED BY THE EDGINESS OF HUMOR IN ADS RIGHT NOW?
I'm very impressed by it. I think some people feel it's all kind of happened at the same time. Like that Internet company that had the great ad where they released the wild pack of wolves on the marching band. . . . I remember them being the first Internet company to have really funny, unusual ads, and everyone seemed to talk about it, and then there was just an avalanche of it. Of course, then it began to get to the point where people couldn't distinguish one ad from another—the oddity became sameness. The ad that impresses me most is for Budget rental cars, where they send people to Mount Everest, and then they show corpses at the end. I mean, come on—this is something that really happened! That is nervy to do that in an ad. I don't know how you get a client to sign off on that.

YOU USED TO JOKE ABOUT LAUNDRY-DETERGENT ADS THAT CLAIMED THEY COULD GET MESSY BLOODSTAINS OUT OF CLOTHES [THE PUNCH LINE: IF YOU HAVE MESSY BLOODSTAINS ON YOUR CLOTHES, LAUNDRY MAY NOT BE YOUR BIGGEST WORRY]. HAVE YOU OBSERVED ANY OTHER CURIOSITIES IN RECENT ADS?
Well, advertising has always been some of the easiest fodder for the stand-up comic. I'm doing a bit now about ads for prescription medicines where they don't tell you anything about the drug. Someone comes on and says, "My doctor says Lipitor." And that's it. And I'm saying, "Well, what's wrong with this guy; is he going to be all right? What's Lipitor? I'll take it—just tell me what it is!"

HOW MUCH IMPACT WOULD YOU SAY ADVERTISING HAS ON POP CULTURE, COMPARED WITH, SAY, MOVIES OR TV SHOWS?
It's an incredibly powerful forum. You can come up with a great idea for an ad, and two months later, everyone will be talking about it. The only other medium you could do that in is series television. Movies can't pick up on the culture that quickly, because the [production] pipeline's too long. I think that because advertising works so much faster than everything else and goes through so many ideas, it really forces everybody else to keep up. As a medium of the moment, of the current zeitgeist, advertising is absolutely at the forefront. And that's what attracts me to it— I love to be at that moment.

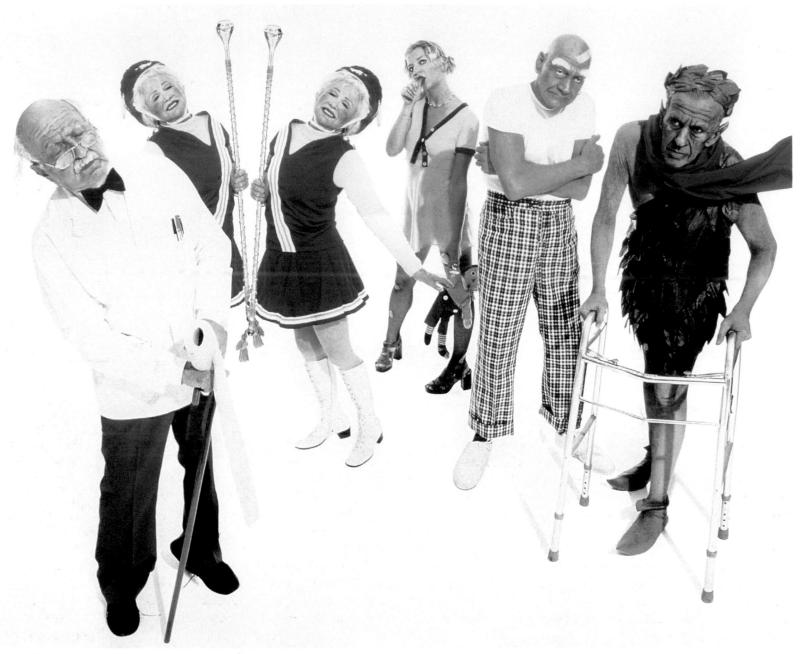

12

12. ART DIRECTORS CLUB OF NEW YORK
BILL OBERLANDER, NEW YORK, 1996
Advertising has been resurrecting its classic characters, sometimes for camp appeal. Kirshenbaum Bond art director Bill Oberlander parodied the trend by showing tired old versions of Mr. Whipple, the Doublemint Twins, the Coppertone girl, Mr. Clean, and the Jolly Green Giant.

13. VEJA MAGAZINE
ALMAP BBDO, SÃO PAULO, 1994
Nothing and no one is sacrosanct; in recent years, the Pope, the Dalai Lama, and Jesus Christ have all been featured in ads.

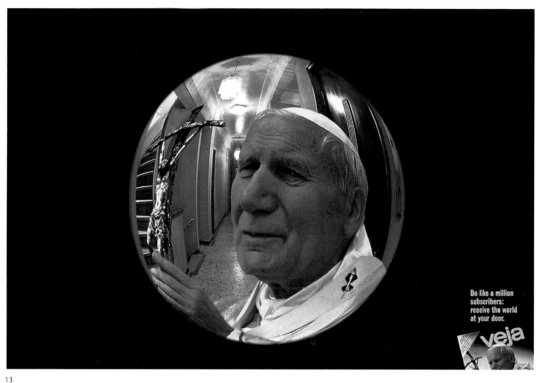

13

particularly popular, but some ads have also featured Western icons like Michael Jordan and Mickey Mouse.

But even as celebrities have maintained their longstanding appeal to advertisers, there has been a change in the kind of stars in demand. One of the more intriguing recent trends has been the rise of what might be called the "semi-star," who is only slightly famous. Increasingly, ads have featured endorsers who are known to only a small segment of the population. A recent ad campaign for American Express included the Hollywood film-studio executive David Geffen—an important figure but not necessarily a recognizable one—as well as the architect Frank Gehry (whose face is far less familiar than some of his buildings) and a leading advertising executive, Lee Clow of TBWA/Chiat/Day. The ads didn't bother to identify the subjects, leaving the audience guessing. "We wanted interest and intrigue," said an American Express spokesperson,

Emily Porter. "Being recognizable is important, but being almost recognizable plays into the mystique we wanted to create." Oberlander of Kirshenbaum Bond, whose agency's ads for Rockport shoes featured such "undiscovered heroes" as a hot young Web site designer from the company Razorfish, said, "Sometimes advertisers are looking for undiscovered talent, so you can ride their wave when they explode." Another advantage to using semi-stars is that it can lend ads an "underground" sensibility—suggesting that the advertiser is in tune with that which is too cool to be widely known.

A different way to move counter to the mainstream is for advertisers to select stars with a controversial reputation—the "bad boy" (or bad girl) approach that has made Rodman and others increasingly popular. Not long ago, this would have been unthinkable in advertising; one of the ironclad rules of the business was that advertisers should avoid trouble and, therefore, troublemak-

ers. Endorsers had to be squeaky clean and were dropped at the first hint of a scandal. But by the late 1990s, that rule was turned on its head by some advertisers. Suddenly, a scandal could actually lead to an endorsement contract. The American basketball player Latrell Sprewell found himself in demand as a spokesperson after a highly publicized incident in which he choked his coach. Monica Lewinsky, one of the most scandal-tainted figures in recent history, was quickly signed to an advertising contract by a leading American weight-loss center. And Nicholas Leeson, the rogue stock trader who was infamous for causing the financial collapse of the British bank Barings, was recently featured in the advertising for a Swedish on-line stock-trading company (in the ads, Leeson warns of the dangers of gambling on the stock market—and, of course, he would know).

Why would a company want to associate itself with scandal? To start with, the mere

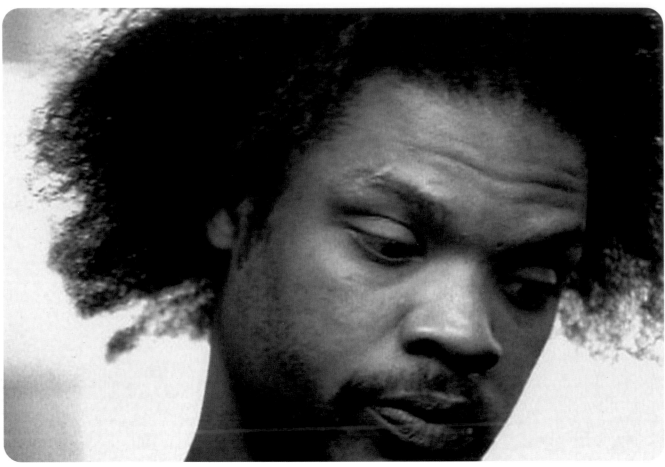

14

announcement that a celebrity involved in one will appear in ads brings instant news coverage and public attention (another example of Kirshenbaum's multiplier effect). Moreover, "if you're an advertiser and you want to say you're cutting-edge and not stodgy, then you do the opposite of what old-fashioned advertisers do," said Syracuse University's Thompson. "Putting Monica Lewinsky in your ads is a bold statement. It says, 'We're not part of the establishment.'"

The strategy seems to be particularly popular among fashion advertisers trying to show their rebel side to a youthful consumer audience. A few years back, the Philadelphia ad agency, Gyro, featured the mass murderers Charles Manson and Jeffrey Dahmer in its ads for a clothing merchant, Zipper Head (the copy: "Everyone has the occasional urge to go wild and do something completely outrageous"). The ads drew an avalanche of complaints, but they also turned a spotlight on both the brand and the agency. Is

it possible to push the boundaries beyond Manson? Believe it or not, Adolf Hitler has starred in a number of ads, including one of the most famous Brazilian commercials in recent years. The spot, for a São Paulo newspaper, opened with an extreme close-up of dots forming an unrecognizable image as the voice-over recited, "He made the economy grow . . . he invested in the arts. . . ." As the camera continued to pull back, it became clear that the dots formed the image of Hitler's face. The point of the ad: Knowing only a few facts about a person or story can be misleading if you're not shown the whole picture.

But even the more daring advertisers of today have their limits. O. J. Simpson, who had been such a huge star years ago in his work for Hertz car rental and other clients, has been persona non grata in the ad world since his infamous California murder trial. And the basketball star Magic Johnson, who announced

in 1991 that he had contracted the AIDS virus, seemed to lose some of his luster for advertisers thereafter. One of Johnson's sponsors, Converse sneakers, publicly voiced its support—but also backed off from producing new ads with Johnson after the news broke.

Perhaps no one took a greater fall from the heights of advertising stardom than the American pop singer Michael Jackson. During the 1980s, Jackson had been the featured attraction of one of the biggest ad campaigns ever, for Pepsi-Cola, and reportedly earned $15 million in the process. But after allegations of child molestation surfaced, Jackson's pitches for Pepsi dried up, and the sponsor didn't renew his contract. At the time, even the notoriously daring advertising man George Lois said of Jackson, "I'm supposed to be outrageous, and I'd be too chicken to touch him." (Actually, there were a couple of advertisers willing to feature Jackson in their ads—but now they cast him as the object of

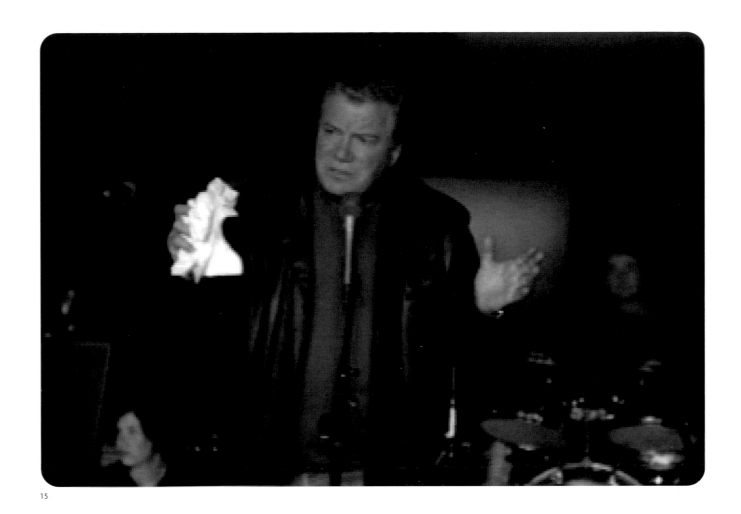

15

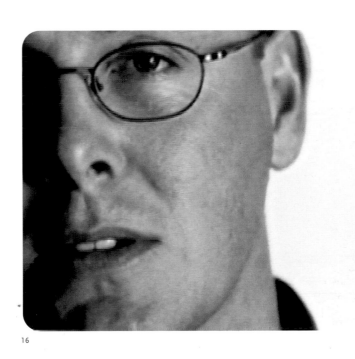

16

14. AND 1 ATHLETIC WEAR
CRISPIN PORTER + BOGUSKY,
MIAMI, LATE 1990s
After NBA basketball star Latrell
Sprewell was suspended for
choking his coach, he starred in
these commercials. "Some
thought we were glamorizing
thuggish behavior," says ad creator Alex Bogusky, "but we felt
Sprewell deserved another
chance."

16. MATTEUS.COM
TBWA, STOCKHOLM, 2000
Nicholas Leeson, the rogue
stock trader blamed for the
1995 collapse of Barings bank,
emerged from the scandal as
the new ad spokesman for an
on-line stock trading company.

15. PRICELINE.COM
HILL, HOLLIDAY, CONNORS,
COSMOPULOS, NEW YORK,
2000
Actor William Shatner, the
original Captain Kirk in the
1960s TV series *Star Trek*,
helped resurrect his career by
making fun of himself in these
ads, but Priceline's stock price
eventually plummeted.

everyone
has the occasiona
urge to go wild and d
something completel
outrageous
when you fight this urge
it builds up within yo
until one day you snap

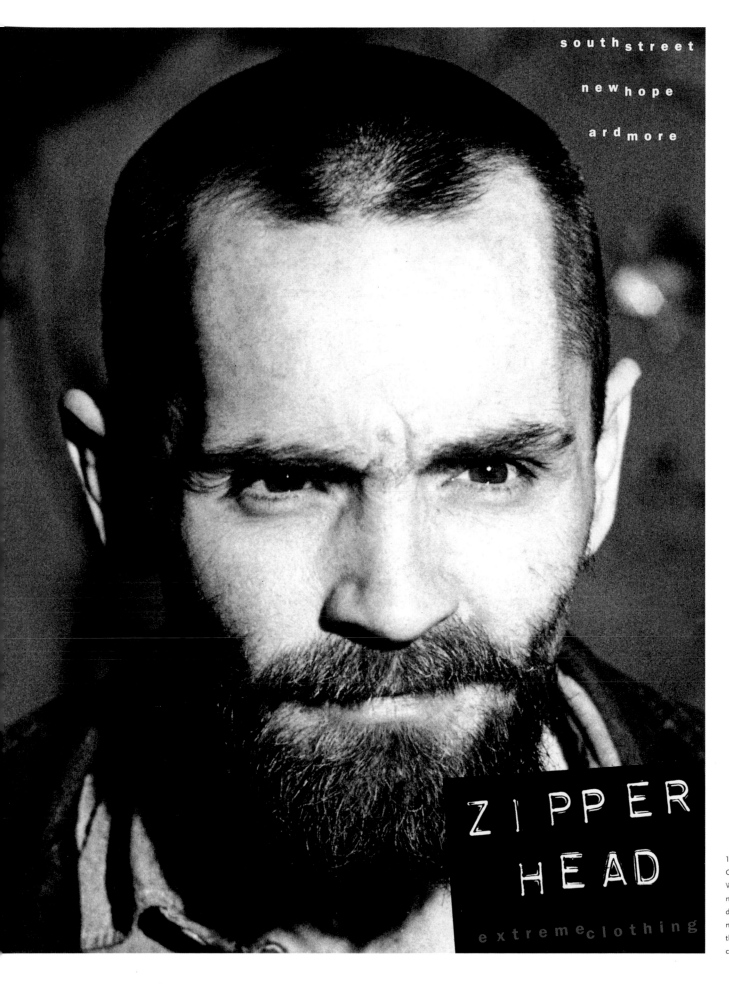

south street

new hope

ardmore

ZIPPER HEAD

extreme clothing

17. ZIPPER HEAD CLOTHING
GYRO, PHILADELPHIA, 1991
When this upstart clothier and its
mischievous agency wanted to
draw attention, they put famed
murderer Charles Manson in
their ad. It worked, but also
caused problems.

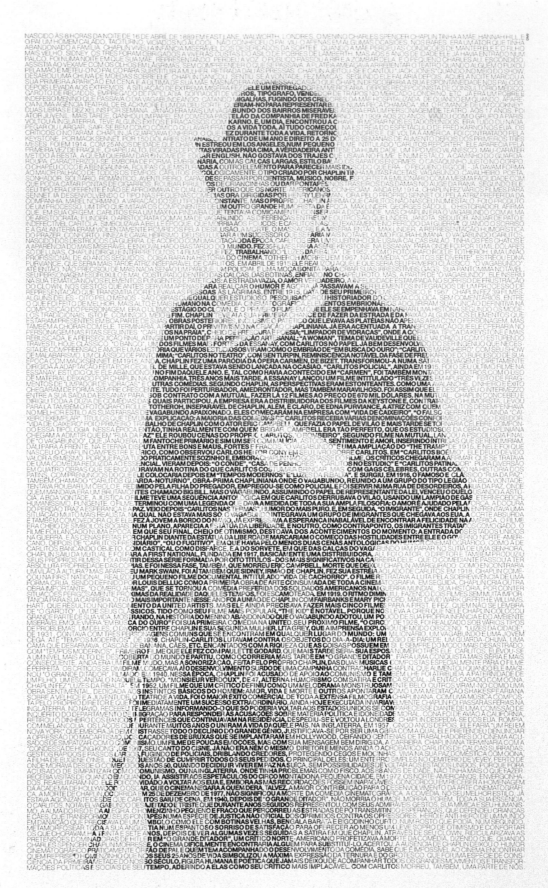

Folha de S. Paulo. Há 77 anos retratando o mundo com palavras.

18. **FOLHA DE SÃO PAULO NEWSPAPER**

DM9 DDB PUBLICIDADE, SÃO PAULO, 1998
This series used type treatments to recreate portraits of famous people, including Charlie Chaplin; one ad featured the image of Adolf Hitler.

19. **FIFTH AVENUE STAMP GALLERY**

HAMPEL STEFANIDES, NEW YORK, 1998
Rock star Jerry Garcia's colorful past as a user of hallucinogenic drugs didn't discourage this advertiser; rather, it became part of the joke.

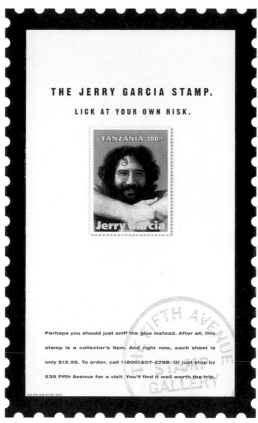

19

ridicule. One ad from the Gyro agency, the mischief-makers behind the Manson ad, promoted a tanning salon with a picture of Jackson's bleached, surgically altered face and the headline "Some people are just too white.")

While advertisers were generally more willing to take a chance on endorsers who were controversial enough to have a rebel image and an underground following, there was an evolution taking place on the other side of the bargaining table, as well—underground stars, cultural rebels, and icons of hip were becoming far more receptive to the overtures of advertisers than in the past. Suddenly, it seemed, no one was too cool or too independent-minded to consider doing a little shilling on the side.

In fact, the whole notion that appearing in ads was a form of "selling out" became almost quaint in the 1990s. Even the most anti-establishment performers—rebel rock stars or menacing hip-hoppers—were ready and eager

to pitch products. As the raucous musician Kid Rock told a newspaper reporter, "I'm about to start hitting everyone up for money. I want to be like NASCAR, where people are going to pay me to wear stuff. If they call that sellin' out, they don't understand. If I want to make a difference, I need the money. I've never seen too many hippies make a difference—no one listened to them because they didn't have any money." This represented both a new "commercial chic" attitude and a new level of greed, as the advertising executive Marty Cooke of M&C Saatchi observed. "Years ago, the idea of someone like Bob Dylan doing a commercial would have been unthinkable," Cooke said. "Now the whole purpose is to sell out. You adopt an anti-establishment stance—until you get the big commercial offer."

How did the act of appearing in an ad become so acceptable, even among cultural rebels? "In the continuum of what is hip, commercials went through a complete change in the 1990s,"

noted Syracuse's Thompson. "It used to be if a star did ads, it meant their career was over. But now for a young, cool actor or musician to do a commercial, it can be a great career move." Appearing in ads "doesn't have the stigma it once had," Liz Rosenberg, Madonna's spokeswoman, recently observed. As commercials became more stylistic, artful, and entertainment-driven in the late 1980s and early 1990s, with some beginning to seem more like miniature films than product plugs, they gradually became a more acceptable forum for many performers. If a star chose the right ad vehicle—one with a hip Nike style, perhaps directed by a Hollywood-style storyteller like Joe Pytka, with a humorous script, lively music, and a cool, ironic sensibility—the result was nothing to be ashamed of.

In fact, as Rosenberg noted, "It's a way of [gaining] exposure without having to tell your life story to a reporter all over again." Plus, she

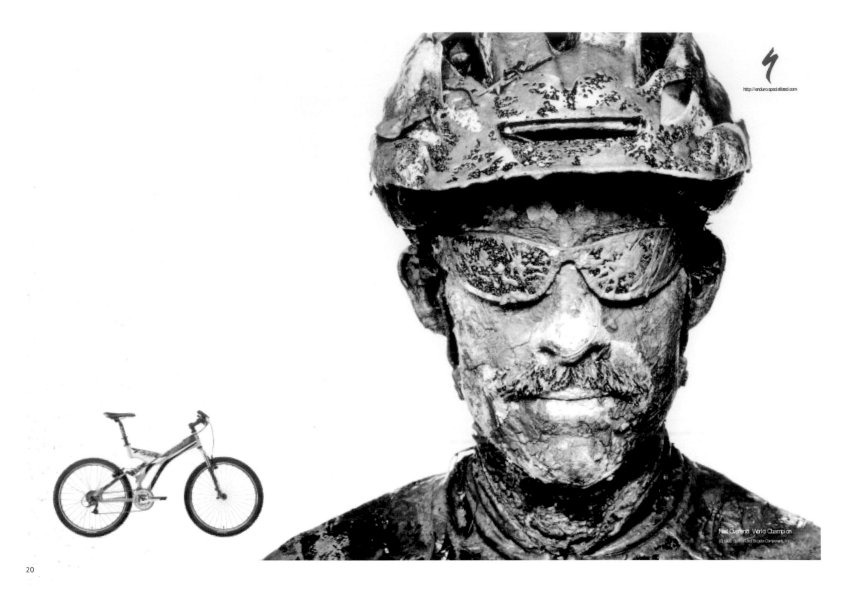

Neil Overend, World Champion
© 1998 Specialized Bicycle Components, Inc.

20

added, it was unlike an interview with the press; "you can have control over an ad shoot—and that's what artists want." Certainly, today's ad stars are far more in control of the commercial process than ever before. Most refuse to recite a sales pitch—many stars in ads don't even talk about the product at all. Stars in recent years have been wary of hyping products not only because it's "uncool" but also because it is potentially dangerous for them: The singer Pat Boone once came under fire from the U.S. Federal Trade Commission just for reading aloud lines from a script that contained unsubstantiated claims about an acne medicine. Consequently, many contemporary star-driven ads are much more about the performer than the product; the ads represent a vehicle within which to sing a hit song, do a comedy routine, or act out characters. For some stars, an ad may offer a chance to soften or lighten their public image (in his ads for the Internet company Priceline,

former *Star Trek* television star William Shatner was able to rejuvenate his popularity by making fun of his own image as a hammy actor and woeful would-be singer). For others, ads can serve to enhance and build upon the star's own growing legend.

In terms of the latter, no one has done a more masterly job than the basketball star Michael Jordan. When Jordan entered professional basketball, he announced that he wanted to be the best-marketed player in the game— and by the mid-1990s, he was the most popular advertising figure in America and one of the most popular in the world, earning ten times as much money for his ads as for his ballplaying. The phenomenal marketing success of Jordan owes much to his unparalleled playing skills and charismatic personality, but he was also helped immensely by the ongoing ad campaign created by Nike and its ad agency, Wieden + Kennedy. The ads presented Jordan as a kind of mythic

hero of the sports world, but they also showed his human side; some of them explained, in Jordan's own voice, what motivated him, how he managed to overcome self-doubt, why he loved to challenge and push himself. ("I've failed over and over and over again in my life," Jordan acknowledged in one ad, "and that is why I succeed.") Each new campaign seemed to add another chapter to his unfolding life story, which continued in ads even after he retired in 1998. In effect, Nike advertising was, and still is, Jordan's official biographer.

Jordan wasn't the only athlete that Nike tried to mythologize through ads. The football star turned baseball player Bo Jackson was presented as a multisport miracle in the memorable "Bo Knows" commercials. And the sometimes-surly basketball star Charles Barkley became a heroic clown prince in Nike ads, mugging his way through a mock-opera spot called "Barkley of Seville." When not clowning, Barkley also

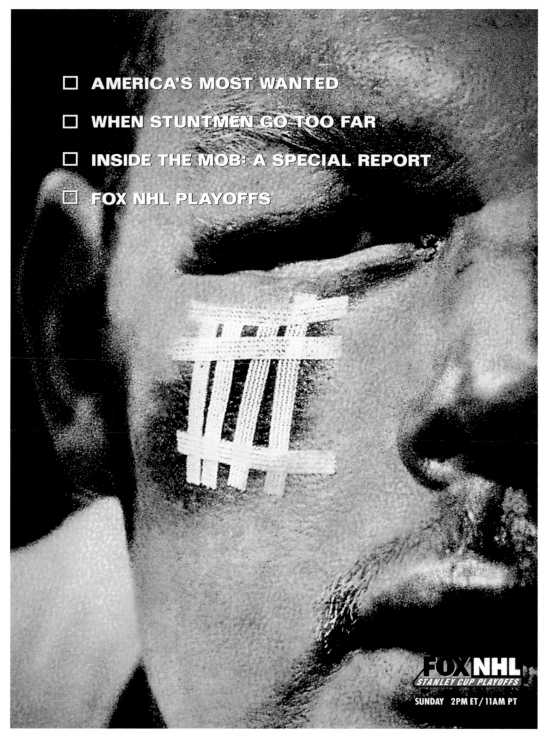

□ AMERICA'S MOST WANTED

□ WHEN STUNTMEN GO TOO FAR

□ INSIDE THE MOB: A SPECIAL REPORT

□ FOX NHL PLAYOFFS

FOX NHL
STANLEY CUP PLAYOFFS
SUNDAY 2PM ET / 11AM PT

21

20. **SPECIALIZED BICYCLES**
GOODBY SILVERSTEIN &
PARTNERS, SAN FRANCISCO,
EARLY 1990s
Who says the face of advertising
must be clean and fresh? A little
dirt doesn't hurt, especially when
the audience is outdoorsmen.

21. **NATIONAL HOCKEY
LEAGUE (NHL) ON FOX**
CLIFF FREEMAN & PARTNERS,
NEW YORK, 1999
Here, the face is battered and
bruised, though the headline
remains playful. Freeman under-
stood that violence was hockey's
Unique Selling Proposition.

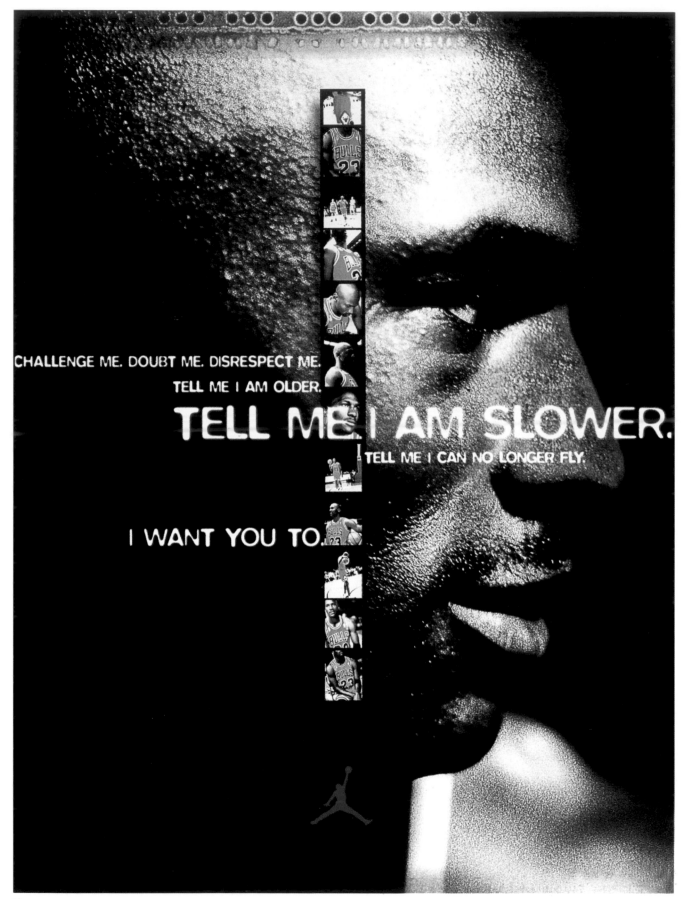

CHALLENGE ME. DOUBT ME. DISRESPECT ME.

TELL ME I AM OLDER.

TELL ME I AM SLOWER.

TELL ME I CAN NO LONGER FLY.

I WANT YOU TO.

22

22 AND 23. **NIKE**
WIEDEN + KENNEDY,
PORTLAND, 1993
Nike became Michael Jordan's
official biographer, turning him
into a mythological figure while
also showing his human
frailties. When Jordan retired in
1998, he left a gaping hole in
basketball and in advertising.

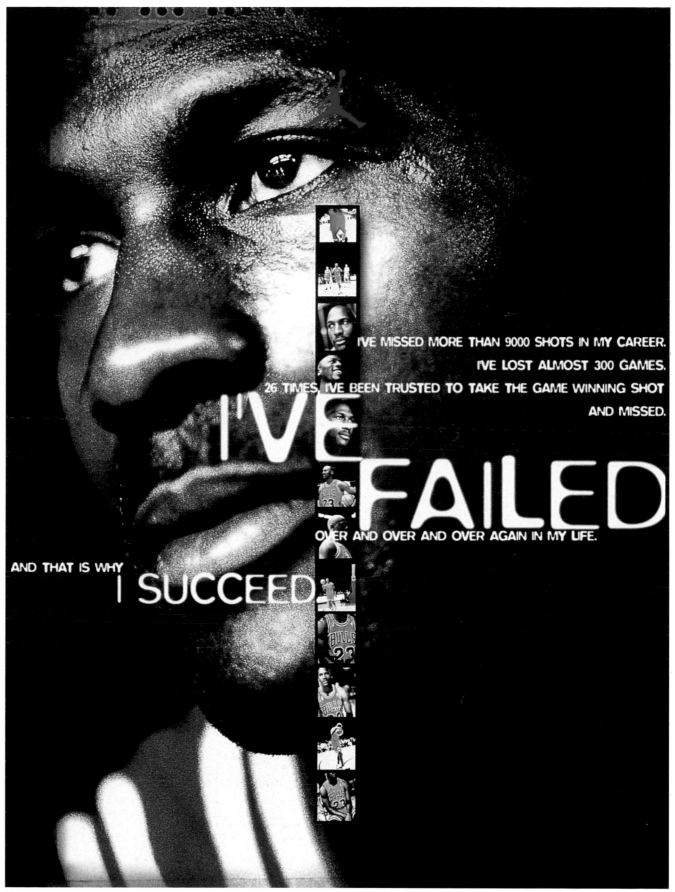

I'VE MISSED MORE THAN 9000 SHOTS IN MY CAREER.

I'VE LOST ALMOST 300 GAMES.

26 TIMES, I'VE BEEN TRUSTED TO TAKE THE GAME WINNING SHOT

AND MISSED.

I'VE FAILED

OVER AND OVER AND OVER AGAIN IN MY LIFE.

AND THAT IS WHY

I SUCCEED

Hello world.

I shot in the 70s when I was 8.

I shot in the 60s when I was 12.

Hello world.

I won the United States Junior Amateur when I was 15.

I played in the Nissan Los Angeles Open when I was 16.

I won the United States Amateur when I was 18.

Hello world.

I played in the Masters when I was 19.

I played in the United States Open when I was 19.

I played in the British Open when I was 19.

Hello world.

I am the only man to win three consecutive

United States Amateur titles.

Hello world.

There are still courses in the United States that I am

not allowed to play because of the color of my skin.

Hello world.

I've heard I'm not ready for you.

Are you ready for me?

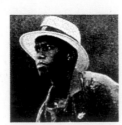

Just do it.

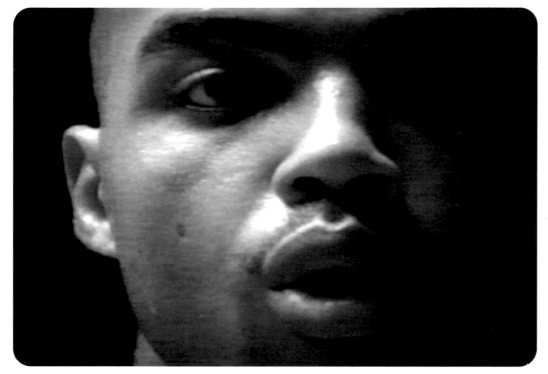

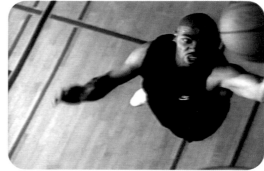

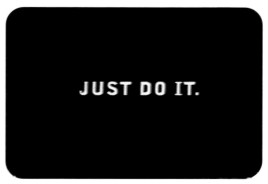

JUST DO IT.

24. **NIKE**
WIEDEN + KENNEDY,
PORTLAND, 1998
After Jordan, pro golfer Tiger
Woods became the new god of
advertising. Again, the ads told
the life story of the young man—
sometimes embellished for
dramatic effect.

25. **NIKE**
WIEDEN + KENNEDY,
PORTLAND, 1993
In the early 1990s, temperamental
basketball star Charles Barkley
played the role of advertising's
reluctant hero: "I am not a role
model," Barkley declared in this
famous TV commercial.

unburdened his soul in ads, most famously in a commercial in which he declared, "I am not a role model." (In the ad, Barkley goes on to say that parents, not ballplayers, should be role models for children.) Most recently, Nike has attempted—with very successful, though perhaps not quite Jordanesque, results—to turn the golfer Tiger Woods into the new god of advertising. When he was barely old enough to vote, Woods was unveiled to the ad public with a dramatic campaign entitled "Hello World." With that, the ad version of Tiger's tale began to unfold, in all its exaggerated glory and heartbreak ("There are still golf courses in America that I can't play on," the biracial Woods declared in one ad, which immediately led critics to question whether Woods, a prodigy who practically grew up on lush golf courses and in the spotlight, wasn't being a bit melodramatic with that line). Similar kinds of Nike legend-building have been going on around the world; the Amsterdam

office of Wieden + Kennedy has made larger-than-life figures of a number of European soccer stars in ads like the fiery one headlined "Sudden death: What any team faces without Eric." Who's Eric? For the record, his last name is Cantona and he plays for Manchester—but if you have to ask, you're not the targeted customer.

In recent years, there have been occasional backlashes against highly paid athlete endorsers; the sneaker company New Balance recently ran a campaign defiantly headlined, "Endorsed by no one." But for the most part, sports stars have continued to be a gold mine for advertisers—more effective, experts say, than actors, musicians, or any other type of performer. While all celebrities can, as research has shown, "transfer" positive feelings to the product, star athletes are a particularly rich source of transferable good feelings; when they appear in ads, one advertising creator told *USA Today*, viewers associate the products with the joy of watching

sports—hence, "what you're getting is the borrowed interest of the excitement."

Perhaps the only thing that can rival the athlete for sheer popularity as an endorser is the animal. Dog, cat, frog, chimpanzee: The particular species does not matter (well, perhaps it matters a little—the naked mole rat doesn't get too many endorsement opportunities, except in one ad for a New England zoo with the headline "The naked mole rat. As if being a rat weren't bad enough"). In American ads, talking animals have been the focal point of several of the most popular ad campaigns of the 1990s—including a Budweiser campaign that began with frogs croaking the name "Bud-wei-ser," and evolved into a subsequent series of ads in which lizards engaged in sarcastic banter with one another. But none of them could compete with the "spokesanimal" of the 1990s—the Taco Bell Chihuahua, one of the single most recognizable advertising characters created in recent years.

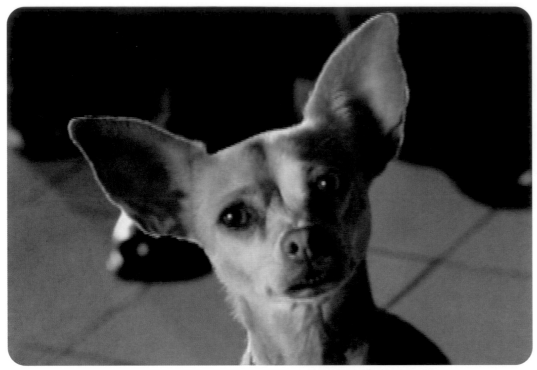

26

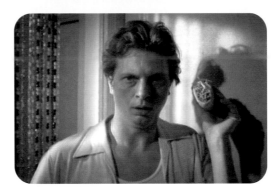

26. **TACO BELL**
TBWA/CHIAT/DAY,
LOS ANGELES, 1998
The Chihuahua's big piercing
eyes had a mesmerizing effect,
but the dog just didn't sell
enough tacos. The company
eventually said "*adios*" to the
corporate icon.

27. **BRITANNICA.COM**
DEUTSCH INC., NEW YORK,
1999
This ad for the on-line encyclope-
dia company delved inside the
mind of author Norman Mailer.

As is often the case with animal ads that strike gold, no one expected much from the Chihuahua—it was more or less a throwaway idea. The creators of the ads, TBWA/Chiat/Day's Chuck Bennett and Clay Williams, had been struggling to come up with ideas when, during an outdoor lunch break, they observed a passing Chihuahua "who looked like he was on a mission," said Bennett. They decided to try one ad about a little dog in search of a taco and thought that would be the end of it. But TV viewers loved it, and thus was born the tale of the Chihuahua on the endless quest for Mexican food. Does anybody really know why the Chihuahua struck a chord? Vada Hill, chief marketing officer of Taco Bell, theorized that it was because the Chihuahua was "a perfect personification of a quirky, iconoclastic, quasi-Mexican brand." More likely, it was the tiny dog's oversize, piercing eyes, which stared into the television camera with a mesmerizing effect

as she mouthed (via computer-generated effects) her lines. In the end, although the dog became a pop-culture phenomenon, it didn't sell enough tacos—and the company opted for a new canine-free ad approach.

The Chihuahua was just one in a parade of pitch-animals in recent years—including the Hofmeister bear and the PG Tips chimp in the UK, the koala bear for New Zealand's Qantas Airlines, Morris the Cat, or the whole menagerie that appeared in a series of ads for the Singapore SPCA—with each animal bearing a sign with a promise to behave well if adopted. Thompson believes that animals sell because, quite simply, they can be trusted: "They're the ultimate innocents," he said. Certainly they're the only performers in ads that haven't been paid off (except, perhaps, in peanuts). They're often adorable to begin with, and by the time advertising's special effects work their magic, piping in funny voices or enabling the creatures to dance,

the end result, Thompson noted, "is like a cruise missile to the heart."

In some ways, these technology-engineered talking animals of contemporary ads have filled a void left by the departed cartoon ad characters of old—creations like Charlie the Tuna and the Jolly Green Giant. However, Thompson asserts that the talking dogs and cats of today's ads—who, with rare exceptions, generally tend to come and go without leaving much of a lasting impression on the culture—are pale substitutes for the old-time ad characters, both animated and human. Those classic ad figures, from Mr. Whipple to Ronald McDonald, "contributed some of the most memorable, richest characters to the cultural pantheon," Thompson said.

And yet many of these characters were partially if not completely abandoned by brands and their ad agencies in the 1980s, as more contemporary, postmodern advertising approaches took hold, favoring elaborate style over simple

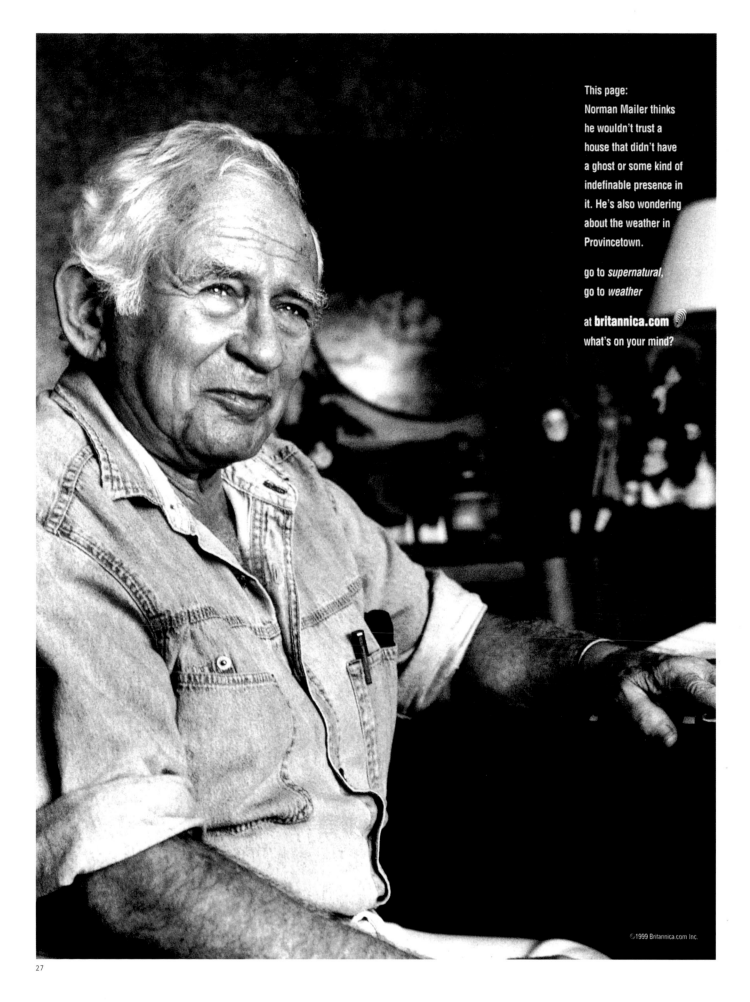

This page:
Norman Mailer thinks
he wouldn't trust a
house that didn't have
a ghost or some kind of
indefinable presence in
it. He's also wondering
about the weather in
Provincetown.

go to *supernatural*,
go to *weather*

at **britannica.com**
what's on your mind?

27

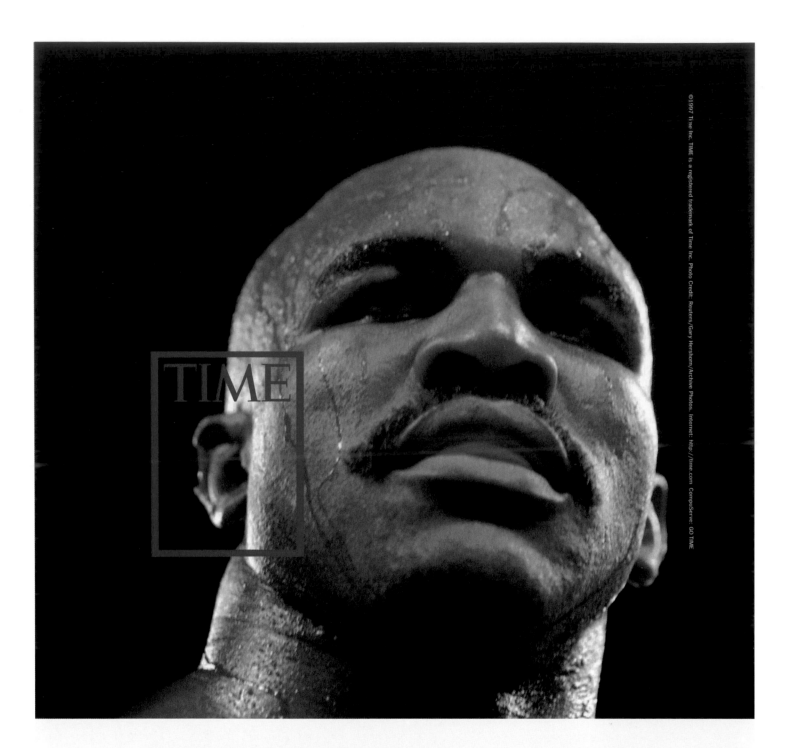

What kind of bandage can

boxing possibly put on this?

The world's most interesting magazine.

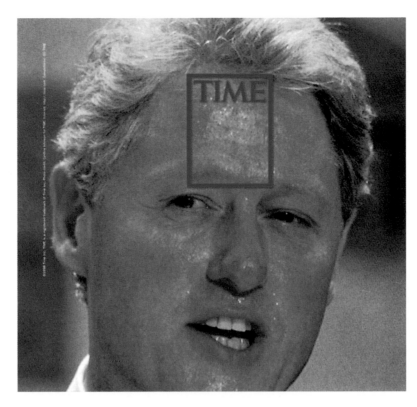

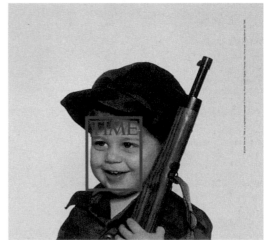

Make sense of anything.

Almost.

30

29

28, 29, AND 30.
TIME MAGAZINE
FALLON McELLIGOTT,
MINNEAPOLIS, MINNESOTA,
1997
Three faces of *Time* from the
long-running series of ads art-
directed by Bob Barrie. The red
box frames the significant details:
Boxer Evander Holyfield's chewed
ear, Bill Clinton's sweat, and the
angelic face of a child soldier.

THE FACES OF ADVERTISING.

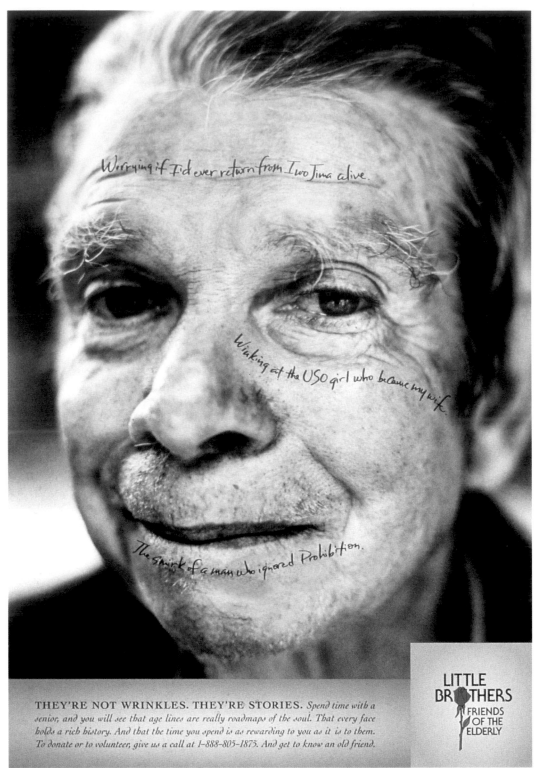

THEY'RE NOT WRINKLES. THEY'RE STORIES. *Spend time with a senior, and you will see that age lines are really roadmaps of the soul. That every face holds a rich history. And that the time you spend is as rewarding to you as it is to them. To donate or to volunteer, give us a call at 1-888-805-1875. And get to know an old friend.*

LITTLE BROTHERS FRIENDS OF THE ELDERLY

31

31. LITTLE BROTHERS
ODIORNE WILDE NARRAWAY +
PARTNERS, SAN FRANCISCO,
1998
Advertising has traditionally
shunned older faces, although
as this ad observes, there are
stories to be found in those
wrinkles.

**32. THE JOHN FITZGERALD
KENNEDY LIBRARY**
THE MARTIN AGENCY,
RICHMOND, VIRGINIA, 1997
Reliving history through adver-
tising: This series of ads explored
the complex relationship between
Jacqueline Bouvier Kennedy and
the man she married.

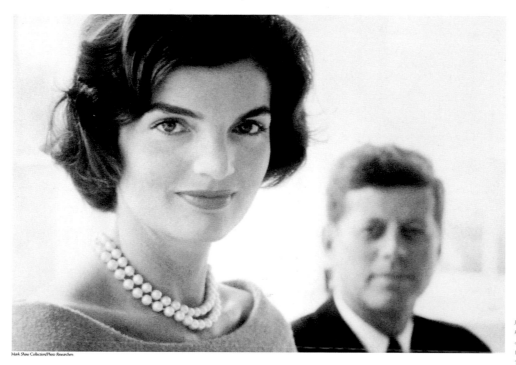

Mark Shaw Collection/Photo Researchers

Jacqueline Kennedy's historic restoration of the White House. Part of a new exhibit at **The John F. Kennedy Library & Museum.** *Boston, Massachusetts.*

32

characters. The assumption was that the new audience was far too cynical for the likes of the Jolly Green Giant. But it was also true that many creative people at ad agencies were eager to leave behind classic ad characters—which were considered both hokey and gimmicky. (Among advertising's creative cognoscenti, Mr. Whipple had become a kind of whipping boy, ridiculed along with old-fashioned jingles and earnest slogans. In the early 1990s, the award-winning American ad writer Luke Sullivan authored a book titled *Hey Whipple, Squeeze This!*—which opens with Sullivan joking about his longtime secret desires to gun down ad characters like Whipple and the Ty-D-Bol man.)

But it would take more than fantasy bullets to kill an icon like Whipple. To the surprise (and dismay) of many in advertising, the character resurfaced in Charmin's ad campaign in 1999, around the same time that a number of other classic ad characters—including the Jolly Green

Giant, KFC's Colonel Sanders, and Life Cereal's Mikey—were also being resurrected. Why? "These characters are part of the fabric of these companies, and there's an emotional attachment to them," said Ted Bell, chief creative officer at Young & Rubicam, the agency for KFC. Even after being on hiatus, Bell said, the classic characters remained known to consumers; "you see the Colonel, and it's instant recognition, with no explanation necessary," he said. What's more, Bell added, when the old characters reappeared, the new cynical audience actually seemed to like them. Younger consumers enjoyed them because they were corny and campy; for older viewers, they had nostalgic appeal. In some cases, the resurrected characters were modernized a bit—as with the KFC Colonel, who was brought back in animated form (originally, the character was played by a real person) and injected with a touch of hip-hop style.

It should come as no surprise that advertising would raid the coffins of its own characters;

death, it seems, is no impediment to being a successful advertising spokesperson. In recent years, special-effects technology has made it easier for advertisers to seamlessly insert old footage of deceased actors into new commercials, while also putting words in their mouths. Humphrey Bogart, James Cagney, and Louis Armstrong all showed up in Coca-Cola commercials in the 1990s, while Fred Astaire danced with a Dirt Devil vacuum cleaner. A recent South African ad for Dunlop tires featured the face of film icon James Dean, digitally retouched to make it appear as if Dean (who died at age 24 in a car accident) is an old man, alive and perched comfortably behind the wheel of his sports car. The point of the ad? To suggest that if only Dean had driven on Dunlop tires, he might be alive today. And if so, he could frolic with Judy Garland, who was resurrected in a commercial that ran during the January 2000 Super Bowl; using footage lifted from *The Wizard of Oz*, the

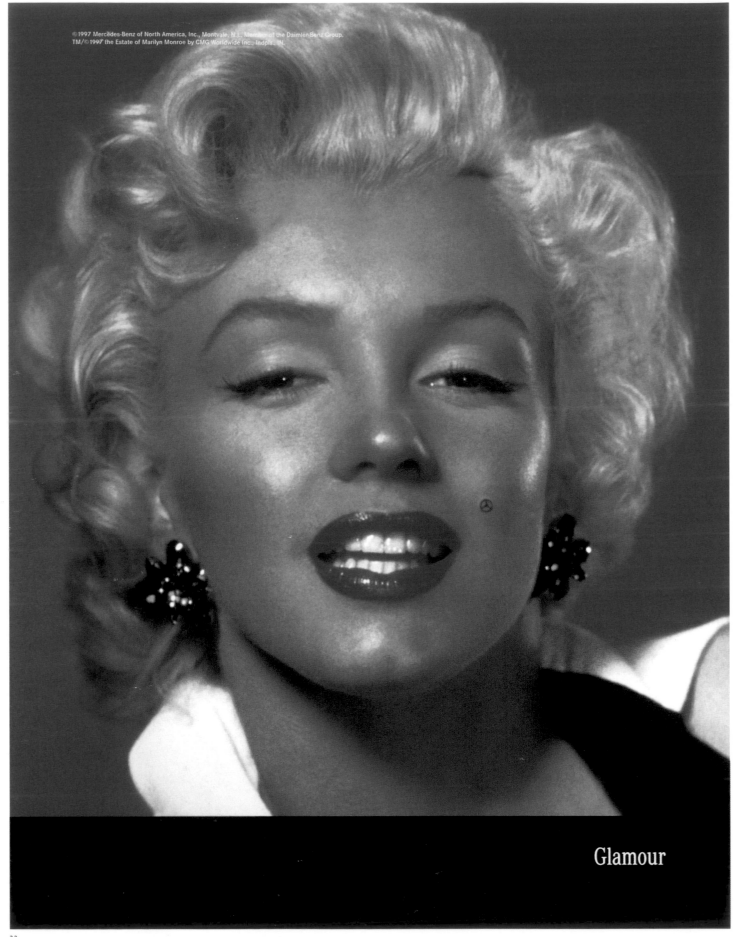

Glamour

33

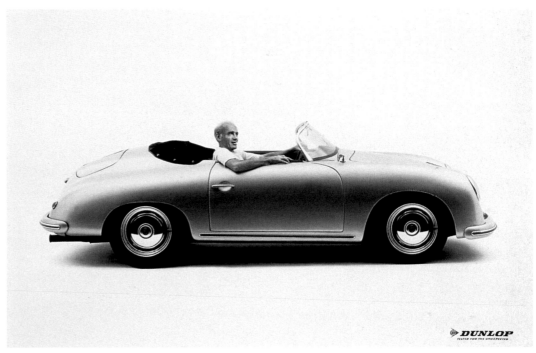

34

33. MERCEDES-BENZ
LOWE & PARTNERS/SMS,
NEW YORK, 1997
Marilyn Monroe continued to
land endorsement deals, three-
decades after her death. Here,
the advertiser has transformed
her beauty mark into a
corporate symbol.

34. DUNLOP TIRES
TBWA HUNT LASCARIS,
JOHANNESBURG, 2000
In this South African ad, an
image of film star James Dean
(killed in 1955 in a car crash) was
digitally aged to show what he
would look today. The implication:
Dean might still be with us if he
had driven on Dunlop tires.

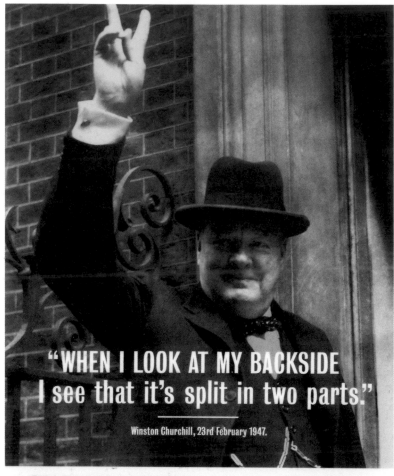

"WHEN I LOOK AT MY BACKSIDE
I see that it's split in two parts."

Winston Churchill, 23rd February 1947.

Quand je regarde mon derrière je vois qu'il est divisé en deux parties." OOH LA LA! What he really meant was when he looked at his past he could see it was split in two parts.

Maybe our wartime leader should have given us a call. At Wordbank, translation is handled by a national from the relevant country.

In fact, we have a network of over 3,000 translators living in their own country, which eliminates the risk of embarrassing mistakes.

If you want to make your foreign marketing and advertising make sense, call us on 0800 281 005. You can rest assured, our translators know their arse from their elbow.

WORDBANK
WORLD CLASS TRANSLATION

35

WHY DOES MAN EXIST?

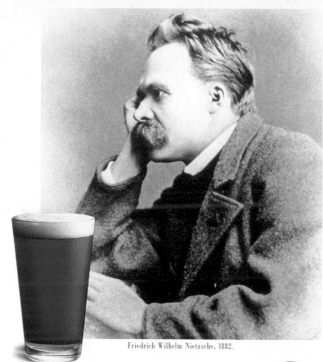

Friedrich Wilhelm Nietzsche, 1882.

**BASS HELPS YOU GET TO
THE BOTTOM OF IT ALL.**

36

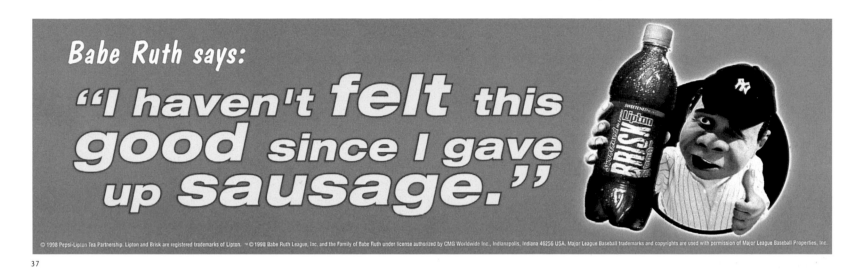

37

35. WORDBANK
LEO BURNETT, LONDON,
MID-1990s
Not everything Winston
Churchill said was inspirational:
this series of ads cites mis-
statements resulting from bad
translations. That a British
advertiser would dare to poke fun
at Churchill, however, is unusual.

36. BASS ALE
WEISS WHITTEN STAGLIANO,
NEW YORK, 1990
Friedrich Nietzsche probably
never contemplated a future
in advertising, but he is
used here to pitch beer to the
intellectual set.

37. LIPTON ICED TEA
J. WALTER THOMPSON,
NEW YORK, 1998
The legendary New York Yankees
baseball player, The Babe,
returns to pitching: Many dead
celebrities have more earning
potential now than when they
were alive.

ad plunked "Dorothy" down in the middle of a Federal Express commercial. (Also during that game's broadcast, the same computer-generation wizardry that raised Garland from the grave was used to lift the paralyzed American actor Christopher Reeve out of his wheelchair and make it appear as if he was walking—to some viewers, this was even creepier than watching the dead rise.)

While the use of deceased stars in ads has been widely criticized, ad agencies are free to use just about anyone in an ad if they can get the star's heirs and copyright holders of their films to agree to it, usually for a fee. The fact is, "many dead celebrities have more earning potential now than when they were alive," *The Chicago Sun-Times* observed recently. Consider the philosopher Friedrich Nietzsche, for example; shunned by advertisers during his lifetime (one can only assume they found him much too dour and seri-

ous), he's a perfect star for contemporary, slightly ironic Bass Ale ads positioning the beverage as the thinking man's beer. Gandhi, meanwhile, serves as a powerful symbol of "thinking differently" on behalf of Apple, as does the late Beatle John Lennon. The fact that some of these figures may have stood for anti-commercialism in their lifetimes doesn't trouble Apple. "The people that we're using in our ads are never used to sell the product," explained Allen Olivo, the company's former ad director. Instead, Olivo maintained, the ads "celebrate who they are, and we try to recognize them for their accomplishments." Perhaps Gandhi and Lennon would have welcomed that recognition—though it seems more likely they would have spurned offers or, at the very least, raised bothersome questions about what Apple does with its profits. No-questions-asked complicity is just one of the benefits of hiring dead pitchmen; they're also

cheaper—advertisers typically spend about only about $10,000 to use a deceased celebrity in a campaign—and far less likely to land in the midst of a scandal (though, given the "Bad is good" nature of some advertising today, that last point might actually be seen as a strike against them).

In the end, this much can be said about what it takes to qualify as a face of advertising in the modern commercial landscape: One doesn't necessarily have to be glamorous anymore. Or wholesome, or even law-abiding. Or well known. Or human. Or, for that matter, alive. In the age of the advertising anti-hero, what's required is only this: the attitude of a rebel, the authenticity of a "real" person, the pure dumb honesty of an animal, and the inner spirit of a legendary sports god. All of which, it turns out, can be bought as easily as the old point-and-smile pitchman of days gone by.

9. ADVE

AS AN A

SOCIAL

RTISING
GENT OF
CHANGE.

1. **FRIENDS OF PUBLIC EDUCATION**
FALLON McELLIGOTT, MINNEAPOLIS, MINNESOTA, 1995
Using a minimalist message to make that point that reading is fundamental.

When she was hired to pitch Lucky Strike cigarettes forty years ago, Janet Sackman seemed an ideal advertising spokes-model—fresh-faced and attractive, with a lilting voice that urged the public "to light up a Lucky." Sackman was so eager to do a good job that she took up smoking (following the suggestion of her employers, she said) so that she'd look more natural when holding a cigarette. That began a thirty-year smoking habit and, eventually, the onset of throat cancer. By the 1990s, Sackman no longer seemed like a likely candidate for a job as spokesperson—particularly since her voice box had been surgically removed as part of her cancer treatment. But then, in 1995, she returned to the advertising spotlight in a dramatic way.

Sackman was hired by the ad agency for the Massachusetts Department of Health, which was working on a series of anti-smoking ads. The agency and its client were looking for someone who could deliver a stirring indict-ment of the tobacco industry—and who better than Sackman? In an unsettling series of radio and television commercials, she apologized to the public—in a strained whisper of a voice—for having appeared in cigarette ads decades earlier. The ads won acclaim and awards throughout the industry, and were a centerpiece in a larger ad campaign that helped drive down smoking in Massachusetts by a remarkable 30 percent in the late 1990s.

Ads like Sackman's anti-smoking commercial represent, in effect, the conscience of advertising. In an industry that is often justifiably blamed for encouraging vanity, excessive spending, overeating, smoking, alcohol consumption, and any number of other bad habits, there is a growing category of ads that seeks to make amends for all of that. Commonly known as public-service advertising, it has billions of dollars and some of the ad industry's most creative minds behind it. And it is confronting virtually every critical social issue imaginable—including, in some cases, problems that were partly caused or at least exacerbated by advertising in the first place.

Increasingly, around the world, advertising is becoming a central part of the public discourse on matters of life, death, and much of what occurs in between. Some examples:

In the United States, more money than ever before is currently being spent on advertising to combat drug abuse, as part of a $2 billion initiative that began in 1998 and runs through 2003. In making such a huge commitment of resources, the U.S. Government has effectively pronounced that the best way to steer kids away from drugs is through advertising.

In the United Kingdom, an ongoing major ad campaign on the issue of child abuse has been so widely and thoroughly disseminated that it

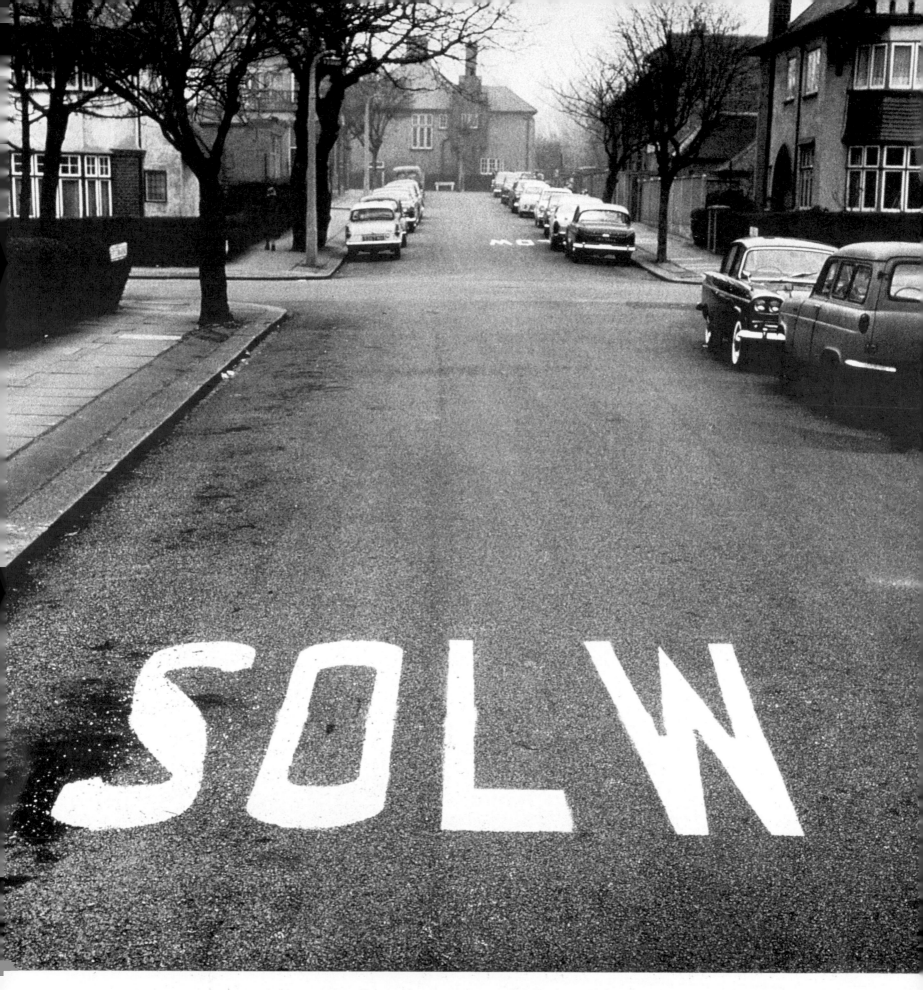

Stay in school.

Friends of Public Education · 1-800-353-4374

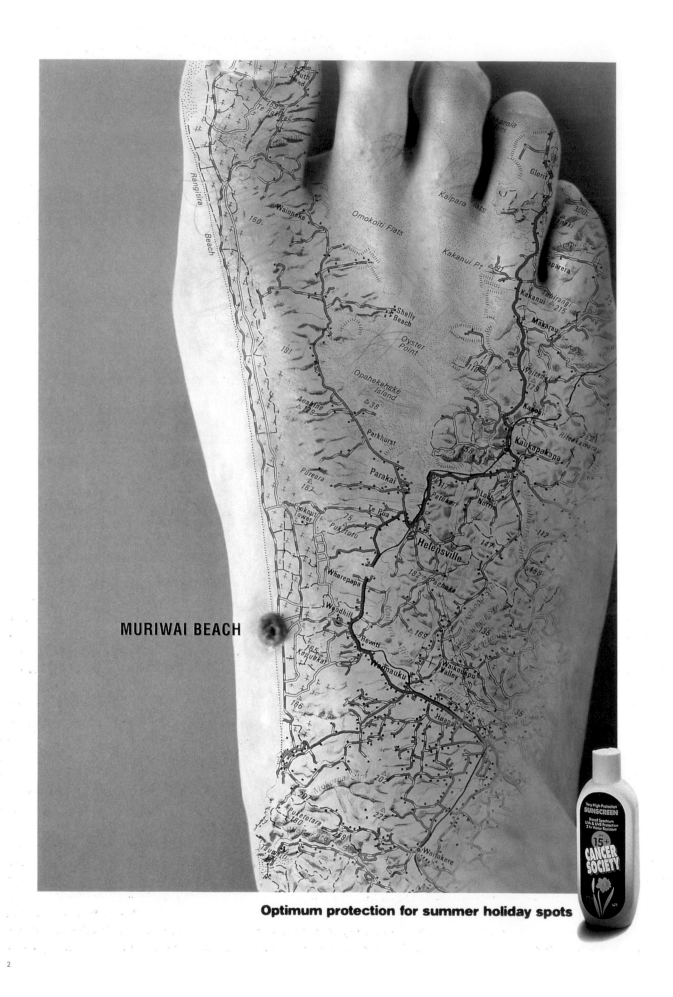

MURIWAI BEACH

Optimum protection for summer holiday spots

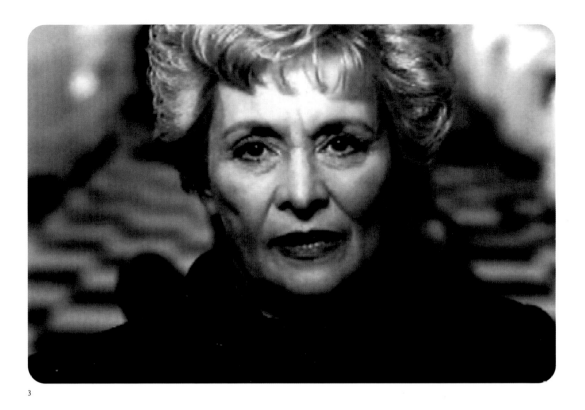

3

2. **CANCER SOCIETY
OF NEW ZEALAND**
WALKERS ADVERTISING,
AUCKLAND, 1997
In a part of the world where
the incidence of skin cancer is
particularly high, ads are
providing a road map to
prevention.

3. **MASSACHUSSETTS
DEPARTMENT OF HEALTH**
HOUSTON EFFLER HERSTEK
FAVAT, BOSTON, 1995
Janet Sackman, who lost her
voice box to cancer, became a
dramatic spokesperson in
anti-smoking ads.

has reached the attention of some 90 percent of the population. The campaign's ambitious goal: to actually wipe out child abuse.

In South Africa, advertising has taken on a central role in the sensitive and critical debate involving race and politics. In fact, many in the country believe that ads—by way of education or scare tactics, depending on one's viewpoint—were a driving force in mobilizing white support for apartheid reforms.

In Japan, recent public-service ads have attempted to change longstanding customs and behavior, including child-rearing participation among men. Addressing the problem of men neglecting their families to focus on work, one ad campaign showed well-known and respected Japanese men engaged in fathering, with the headline "You cannot call a man who doesn't care for his child a man." (The ads have stirred controversy among

some Japanese men, drawing complaints about meddling in private family affairs.)

Elsewhere around the world, public-service ads have addressed issues that are particularly critical in certain countries: educating on the need for birth control in India, or warning of the rise of xenophobic actions by neo-Nazi groups in Germany, or reminding people to stay out of the sun in New Zealand, whose population has one of the highest rates of skin cancer in the world. A look at a country's social-cause ads can be an eye-opener, bringing to light obscure issues that are unique to a given culture—as in the case of passionate, persuasive ads in Singapore urging citizens to refrain from eating tiger-penis soup (the popularity of this dish has threatened the tiger population).

But as advertising has become more concerned with social issues and causes, that has

in turn raised questions about the propriety and effectiveness of such ads. Skeptics reasonably wonder whether public education on complex social problems can, or should, be undertaken by the same people who peddle corn flakes (or, worse, liquor and cigarettes). And, too, there is the question of motive: If, as some suspect, advertisers address social issues primarily for self-serving reasons—i.e., to burnish their own image—does that diminish the value of the work they're doing in this area? Does it mean, perhaps, that advertising's public-service warnings and advice should be viewed with a wary eye?

It's fair to say that public-service advertising has been at least somewhat self-serving from the outset. In the U.S., such ads began to gain momentum in the early 1940s, after the industry leader James Webb Young, a consultant to the ad agency J. Walter Thompson, suggested that advertisers could offset mounting public criticism of their business by creating ads for good causes.

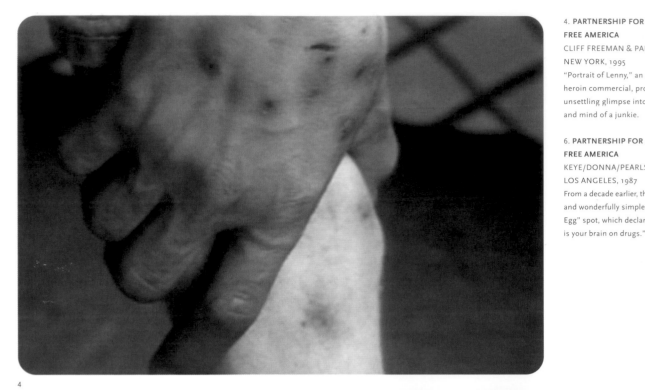

4

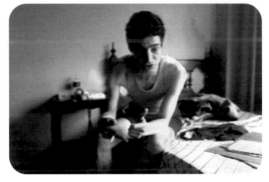

Young challenged his colleagues to use their persuasion skills "to confound the critics of advertising with the greatest demonstration of [advertising's] power they have ever seen." If ads could accomplish this, Young reasoned, the adversaries and critics of the business "will all be on our side."

The ad industry soon had an opportunity to put Young's plan into action. The onset of World War II led to the formation of an American group called the Advertising Council, which created ads serving the war effort by explaining food rationing, urging people to conserve, and so on. Some of the Council's more famous World War II ads became classics: "A slip of the lip can sink a ship" was one example of pithy Madison Avenue sloganeering brought to the cause, as was the emotional story told in "The Kid in Upper 4"— an ad that presented the thoughts of a fictional soldier on a train as he was heading off to war.

In creating wartime propaganda, these advertisers were not necessarily breaking new ground— similar work had been done previously in posters and short films not just in the U.S. but elsewhere, most infamously in Nazi Germany. But what was significant about America's wartime Ad Council was that it didn't disband when the war ended—instead, the group turned its attention and persuasive skills to peacetime domestic issues. In the late 1940s, the Ad Council brought to life one of advertising's most famous characters, Smokey the Bear, to educate the public on the dangers of forest fires. The success of Smokey suggested that advertisers could, in fact, use some of the same tools that sold cereal—lovable cartoon characters uttering catchy phrases—to tackle matters of grave importance.

Over the next three decades, advertising on behalf of various social causes developed into a multibillion industry in itself (in 1990, in America alone, roughly $2 billion worth of advertising time was devoted to public service announcements, or PSAs). Who paid for all of this benevolent advertising? To some extent, the public did, by way of donations to various charities, or through tax dollars that were subsequently allocated by government to address certain problems. However much of the tab for PSAs was picked up by ad agencies and the media; typically, ad professionals donated their time and creative ideas, while broadcasters and publishers donated airtime and pages to run the ads (the only part of the process that cost money was the actual production of the ads).

The creators of these ads realized that making dramatic commercials for important social causes also made them look good—and could help bring acclaim, awards, and new business to their agencies. Still, as PSAs began to proliferate in the 1960s, the spirit of the times was perhaps the primary motivator; as Doyle Dane Bernbach's Roy Grace noted, social activism and creative revolution were in the air. For the writers and art directors at top Madison

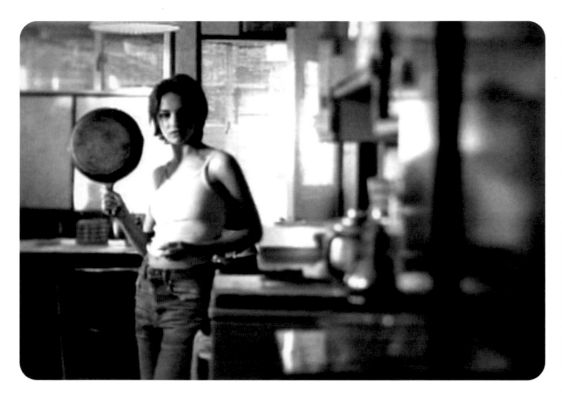

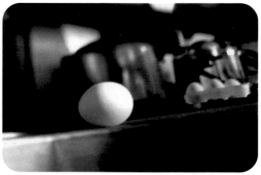

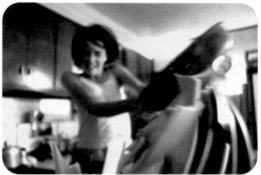

5

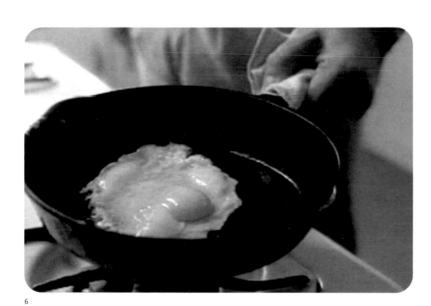

6

ADVERTISING AS AN AGENT OF SOCIAL CHANGE.

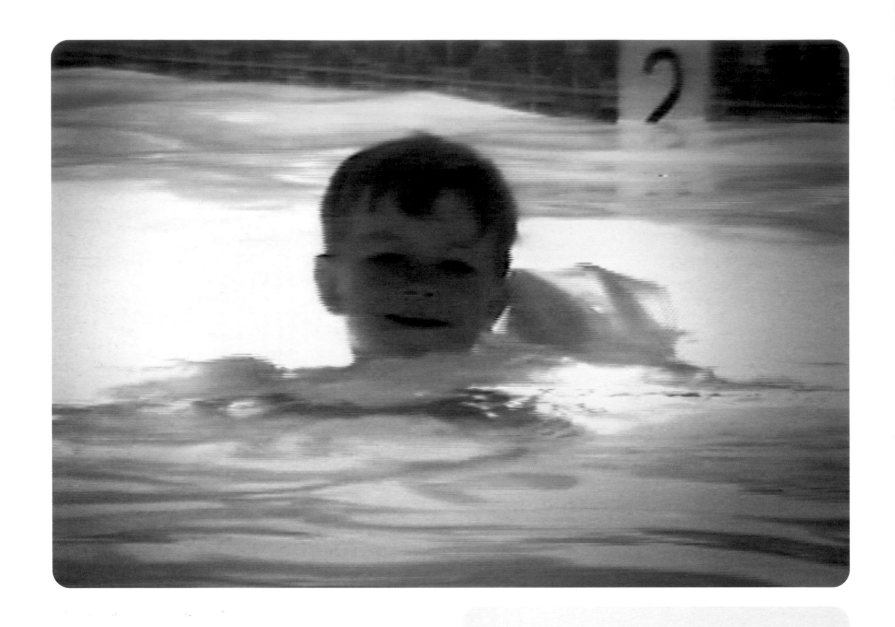

Alex Bishop.
Killed by a drunk driver
on November 8, 1992
on Kent-Kangley Road
in Kent, Washington.

7

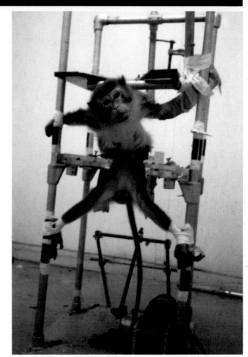

Imagine having your body left to science while you're still in it.

Three animals die every second in U.S. laboratories.

The monkey pictured here was surgically crippled and then forced to use his deadened arm.

Other animals, including rabbits, dogs, cats, pigs, rats, and primates, are routinely blinded, shocked, mutilated, decapitated, and force-fed poisons in tests that could easily be replaced with modern and more reliable methods.

These animal tests are being conducted by the government, universities, medical associations, and private corporations. And always behind closed, locked doors.

If you think these kinds of cruel experiments have no place in the 20th century, please join us: People for the Ethical Treatment of Animals.

PETA is America's leading animal rights organization. By working with medical and legal professionals, the media, members of Congress, and people like you, PETA has been able to stop some of the most horrifying animal experiments, including the one pictured here.

Please send me more information.
Name_____
Address_____
City_____State___Zip___
_Please send me a free copy of the book
Animal Liberation.
Please accept my tax-deductible contribution of:
_$20 _$35 _$50 _$100 _other $_____

PETA PETA, P.O. Box 42516
Washington, DC 20015

8

Avenue agencies like DDB, Young & Rubicam, and Marsteller, making a public-service message was the ad executive's equivalent to joining the Peace Corps or marching for equal rights. And all of those hot-button issues of the day—war overseas, growing urban poverty, civil rights, pollution, increased drug abuse—offered a wealth of dramatic subject material and inspired a golden era in public-service ads.

It was during this period that some of the most memorable, even haunting images of social advertising were produced. A commercial targeting litter and pollution featured a Native American named Iron Eyes Cody, who was shown paddling a canoe while observing the desecration of the American landscape; the character responded, wordlessly, by shedding a single tear, as the ad's tagline urged, "Keep America beautiful." Protecting the environment became a prevalent theme in ads; the San Francisco ad executive Howard Gossage—

who had long preached that advertising was too important to waste on commercial products— applied his logic and wit to championing the Sierra Club. Other public-service ads at the time took on sensitive issues such as racism and poverty, with heart-wrenching ads for the United Negro College Fund that featured the slogan "A mind is terrible thing to waste," as well as commercials for the Urban Coalition that rendered a stark portrayal of ghetto life. (One particularly unsettling ad trained the TV camera on a rat, while an off-camera child's voice beckoned, "Here, kitty, kitty.") Meanwhile, ads on road safety, urging the public to "buckle up" seat-belts and avoid driving after drinking alcohol, clearly began to alter behavior and shift public attitudes, thanks in part to dramatic imagery: One memorable "Don't drink and drive" commercial showed wineglasses being joined in a toast and shattering to bits. Outdoor ads for Mothers Against Drunk Driving installed parts of

wrecked cars upon the billboard, and topped that with the resounding headline "Sometimes it takes a family of four to stop a drunk driver."

Gradually, such advertising seemed to be developing its own style and tone, distinct from ads that sold products. Perhaps it was to be expected given the seriousness of the subjects, but in the 1970s public-service ads tended to be highly emotional and often harrowing. In a way, these socially conscious ads turned conventional advertising on its head—they dealt in brutal honesty, not upbeat fantasy. If anything, the ads became harsher in the 1980s, as advertising stepped up its own war on drugs with the formation of the Partnership for a Drug-Free America, which, unlike the Ad Council, focused on a single issue and attacked it fiercely. The group's early print ads targeting cocaine use showed close-ups of people pointing guns up their noses. And one of the Partnership's first TV commercials remains one of its most famous:

ADVERTISING AS AN AGENT OF SOCIAL CHANGE.

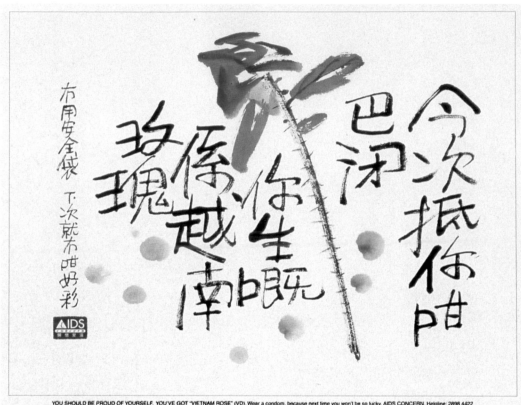

布用安全袋 下次就冇咁好彩

今次抵你啪
巴閉
你生既
係越南b
玫瑰

AIDS CONCERN

YOU SHOULD BE PROUD OF YOURSELF. YOU'VE GOT "VIETNAM ROSE" (VD). Wear a condom, because next time you won't be so lucky. AIDS CONCERN. Helpline: 2898 4422

9

9. **STD PREVENTION CAMPAIGN**
LEO BURNETT, HONG KONG, 1997
While American public service ads tended to shock, Asian ads were sometimes artfully designed; this one warned against the sexually transmitted disease known as "Vietnam Rose."

10. **PROMOTING CONDOM USE**
LEO BURNETT, MUMBAI, 1997
In India, this ad served as a highly visual reminder, avoiding the need to preach or persuade.

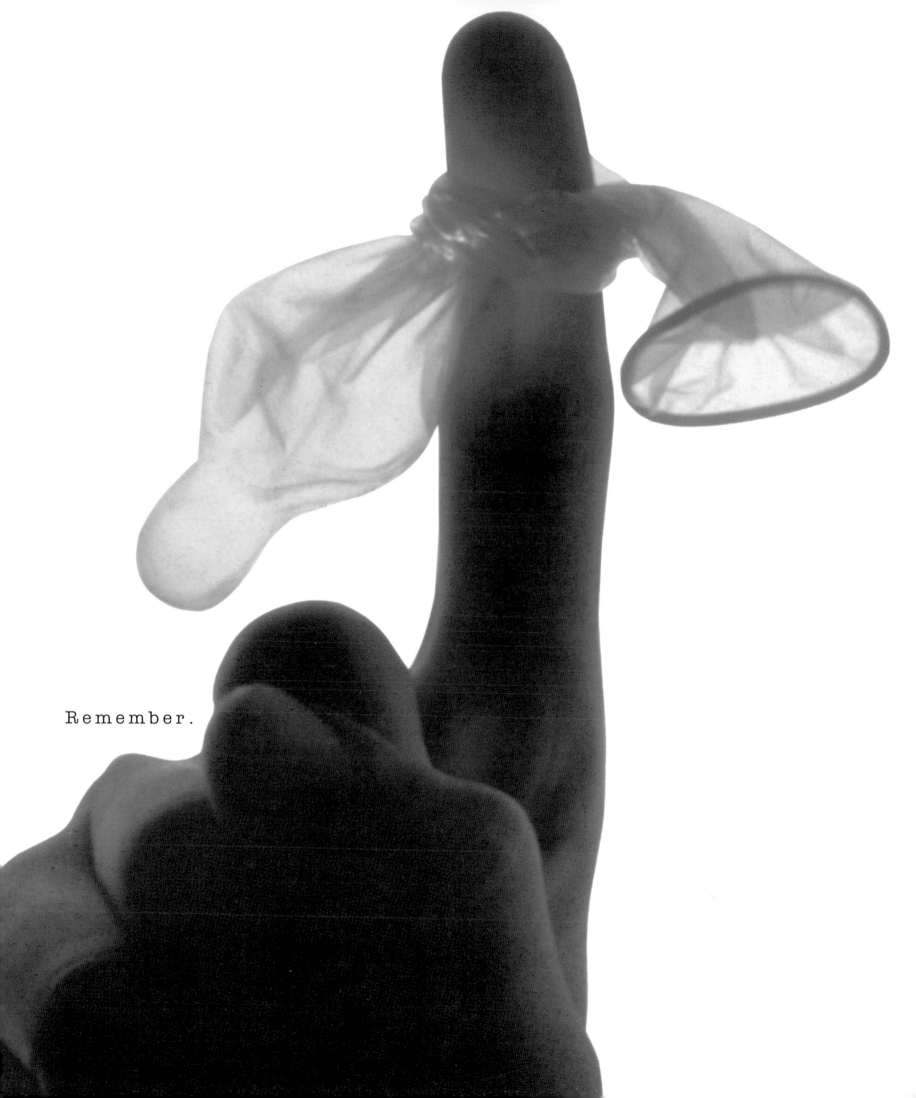

Remember.

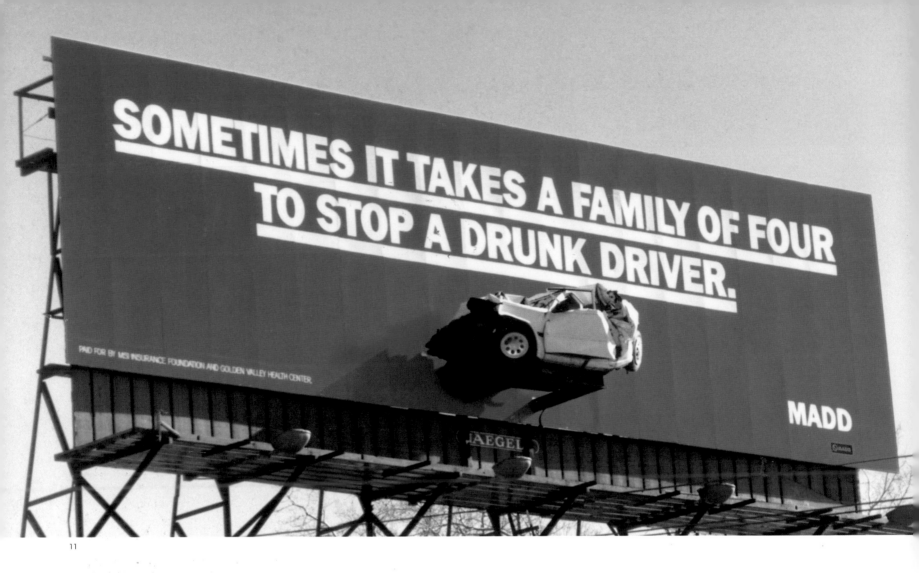

PAID FOR BY MSI INSURANCE FOUNDATION AND GOLDEN VALLEY HEALTH CENTER.

SOMETIMES IT TAKES A FAMILY OF FOUR TO STOP A DRUNK DRIVER.

MADD

11

"This is your brain," a voice-over declared as the camera focused on an egg; as the egg was broken and fried, the announcer added, "This is your brain on drugs. Any questions?"

The drug ads seemed tame compared with those produced on behalf of animal-rights activists such as the American group People for the Ethical Treatment of Animals (PETA). These ads included photographs taken inside animal-research laboratories; one showed a laboratory dog with its head in a viselike contraption, and the headline "There's a reason they cut the vocal cords first." Another featured a tortured monkey, as the accompanying headline, written by The Martin Agency's Luke Sullivan, asked the reader to "imagine having your body left to science while you're still in it."

Similar ads could be seen around the world by the 1980s—for example, European advertising for animal-cruelty prevention also featured images of tortured or dead animals. There are, not surprisingly, great differences in the levels

and kinds of public-service ads encountered from one culture to the next. No other country has come close to spending the billions of dollars that the U.S. pours into social ads, and in fact few have established large, powerful PSA organizations comparable to the Partnership or the Ad Council. Many countries take more of an ad hoc approach, turning to ads as a particular social problem is perceived to be worsening. Anti-drug advertising has been getting a lot of play in South America in recent years, but such ads are not nearly as prevalent, for example, in the Netherlands, which tends to have more relaxed attitudes about certain types of drug usage (on the other hand, the Dutch tend to use ads for social engineering—preaching tolerance for people of other races, those with disabilities, etc.). The different ways that ads in varying cultures address common problems, such as sexually transmitted diseases, can be interesting. Hong Kong ads warning against the STD known locally as "Vietnam Rose" featured artful design

and illustration; a campaign in India promoted safe sex by making a logical and sincere case for masturbation ("The best sexual partner you've ever had is someone you've known since you were born," declared one headline).

For the most part, though, the more successful social-issue ads around the world have had one thing in common—a reliance on disturbing imagery and blunt language. A British campaign created by Saatchi & Saatchi for the National Society for the Prevention of Cruelty to Children took the viewer inside a child's bedroom, as the camera showed teddy-bear wallpaper and pictures of the Spice Girls—while the soundtrack eavesdropped on rustling in the bed and a man's voice saying, "Not a word to anyone. It will be our little secret." The campaign brought scores of complaints from viewers across the UK who were upset by it—including victims of child abuse who said that it caused them to relive painful experiences. And one of the most

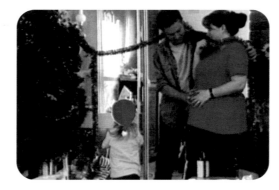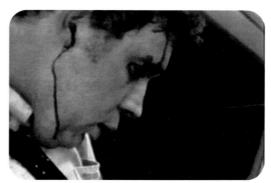

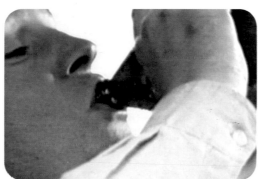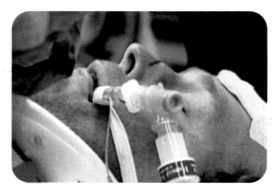

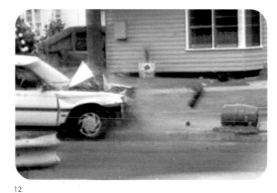

Should you
be driving home
tonight?

12

**11. MOTHERS AGAINST
DRUNK DRIVING (MADD)**
THE AD COUNCIL, NEW YORK,
1990
Not only is the headline powerful,
but it is accompanied by an
actual car crushed in a drunk
driving accident, which is
attached to the billboard.

12. AUSTRALIAN ROAD SAFETY
GREY ADVERTISING,
MELBOURNE, 1996
This campaign brought a new
level of realism to drunk driving
ads; crashes were simulated
on film with jarring force. The
commercials led to dramatically
lower local fatality rates.

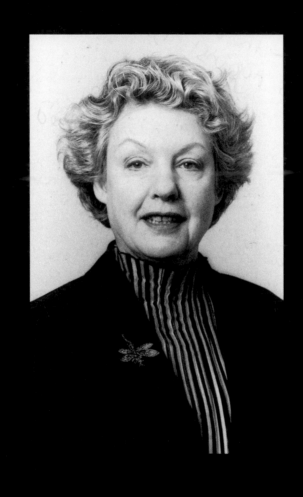

INTERVIEW: DORIA STEEDMAN

As the vice chairman of the Partnership for a Drug-Free America, Doria Steedman oversees a coalition of communications professionals who create most of the anti-drug advertisements produced in the United States—a huge and highly influential body of work, particularly since the Partnership received more than $3 billion worth of donated media exposure for its ads from 1987 to 1999. But the increased funding and visibility has also ratcheted up the pressure on the Partnership to produce quantifiable results and progress.

FIRST OF ALL, HOW DO ANTI-DRUG ADS GET MADE?
Sometimes ad agencies approach us, but it usually

proval. When awareness goes up in those two areas, drug use goes down.

IS ADVERTISING ABLE TO REACH AND AFFECT PEOPLE USING MORE ADDICTIVE DRUGS, LIKE HEROIN?
We have never tried to convince a heroin user to stop using it—because we have no evidence whatsoever that advertising can do that. We're trying to reach people before it gets to that point.

ANY SURPRISES YOU'VE FOUND IN TERMS OF WHAT WORKS AND WHAT DOESN'T?
When we launched an anti-heroin campaign, we learned that it would not be effective to tell young people they were going to die from this

6,000 kids and 800 parents across the country. There have been many other studies done showing the effectiveness of the ads. And drug use is down in this country, across the board.

THERE'S A FEELING OUT THERE THAT PEOPLE CREATE PUBLIC-SERVICE ADS FOR SELF-SERVING REASONS, TO GET ATTENTION AND WIN AWARDS. ANY VALIDITY TO THAT?
If that is true, I have never seen it. I am astounded by how involved agency creative people have gotten in the problem, sometimes going out and meeting kids and taking a personal interest in somebody. This drug problem is one that affects so many lives—so it's less likely someone's going to say, "This doesn't affect me; I'm just in

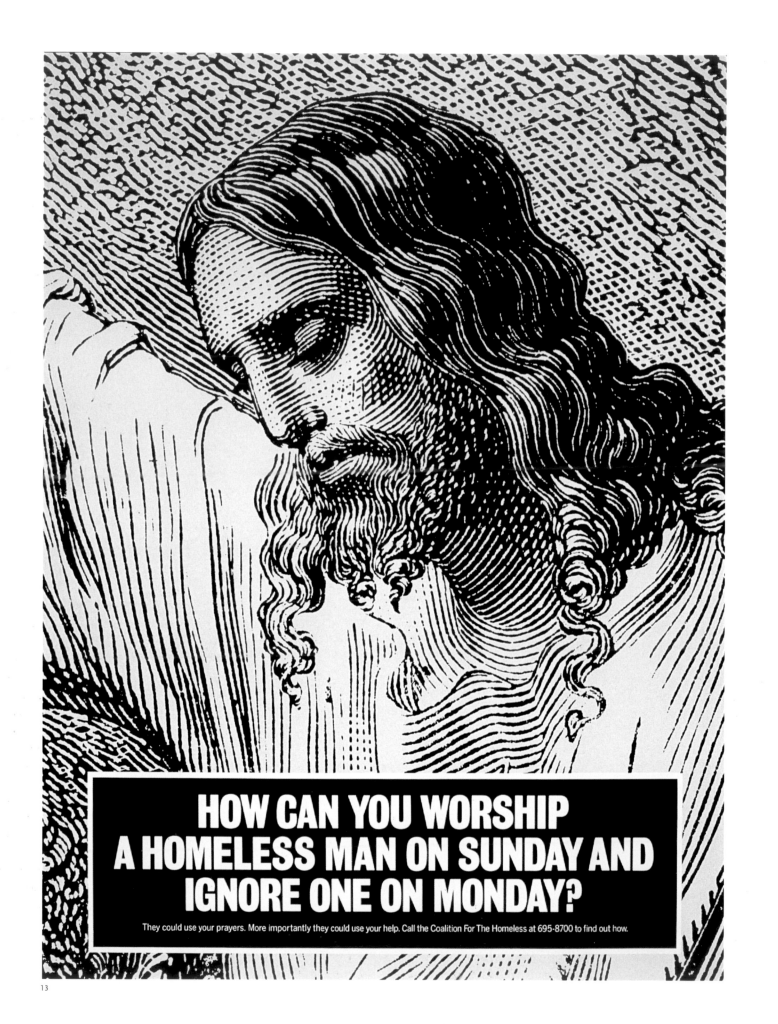

13

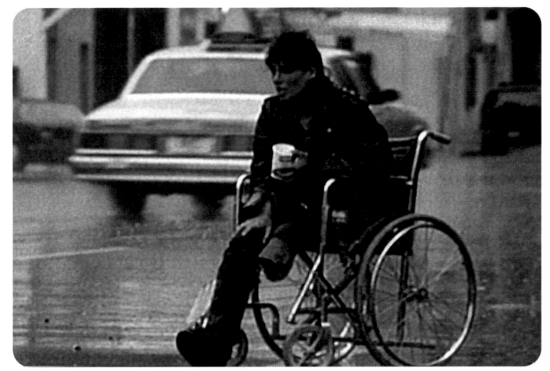

14

gripping ad campaigns in Australia in recent years has been a series of anti-drunk-driving commercials that show characters who've been drinking and then decide, against their better judgment and advice from others, to get behind the wheel. The ads then show the ensuing horrific car collisions—presented with jarring force and realism—as well as gory scenes taking the viewer into the emergency room post-crash. A mid-1990s American ad campaign on the same issue took a different, though no less compelling, tack: Rather than showing what happened to the drunk driver, "our attitude became 'Screw the drunks—let's focus on the real victims,'" said Steve Landsberg, one of the creators of the campaign from the agency Wells Rich Greene. So the ads featured children who had been killed in drunk-driving accidents, bringing them briefly to life for the TV viewer by showing scenes from old home videos obtained from the deceased children's families. One spot opened with footage of a boy learning to swim in the family pool as his mother cheered him on; gradually, the heart-warming scenes are intercut with onscreen text explaining when and how this child died.

Such advertising can be like a punch to the gut of the audience, and that is the intention. The American ad executive Sal DeVito, who created some of the aforementioned PETA work (including the "vocal cords" ad), said, "At first when I was working on that, I tried showing images that weren't as harsh—for example, showing one of these electrocution devices, without the animal in it. But I could see that it wasn't going to be as effective. With something like this, you need as much visual impact as possible. And then you have to balance it with a thoughtful headline, so it doesn't come across as just sensationalism." DeVito added, "I know people don't like seeing these pictures, but it's the reality."

But some question whether the barrage of shocking and disturbing images is the best way to address difficult social issues. Bob Garfield, a columnist for *Advertising Age*, recently wrote of PSAs, "Let's face it, the damn things are depressing. You're watching TV and at the commercial break, just when you think that you're going to see talking cars or adorable kittens or slow-motion images of women tossing their hair, on comes some gritty black-and-white film about spousal abuse." As the number of public-service ads have increased, the bombarded public can experience something akin to battle fatigue—particularly down in the trenches, in PSA-saturated places like subway trains, where ads about AIDS, child abuse, and rape are often placed side by side. One subway rider recently wrote to *The New York Times*, "Can't something be done to change the unrelentingly downbeat messages on display? Sure, people have problems, but one gets the impression that most of our fellow passengers are addicted, abused, diseased wretches living in roach-infested apartments."

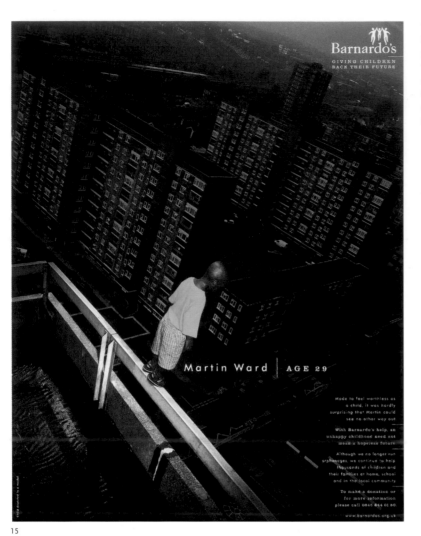

Barnardo's
GIVING CHILDREN
BACK THEIR FUTURE

Martin Ward | AGE 29

Made to feel worthless as
a child, it was hardly
surprising that Martin could
see no other way out

With Barnardo's help, an
unhappy childhood need not
mean a hopeless future

Although we no longer run
orphanages, we continue to help
thousands of children and
their families at home, school
and in the local community

To make a donation or
for more information
please call 0845 844 01 80.

www.barnardos.org.uk

15

15. **BARNARDO'S**
BARTLE BOGLE HEGARTY,
LONDON, 2000
The campaign for a children's
organization used dramatic
imagery to show that some
adults might not be here today if
they hadn't been helped as kids.

16. **SAN FRANCISCO
AIDS FOUNDATION**
J. WALTER THOMPSON,
SAN FRANCISCO, 1995
An attempt to encourage drug
users to participate in needle
exchange programs; the
placement of the words within
the picture turned the ad into
a puzzle.

The spread of such advertising is not limited to bargain-basement ad environments like the New York subway—increasingly the ads have begun to show up even in the priciest advertising slots (in January 2000, the first public-service ad appeared on the multimillion-dollar-a-minute Super Bowl). The Italian ad executive Marco Mignani, of Euro RSCG MCM, works on public-service ads himself but nevertheless recently observed, "On [TV] screens all over the world, anti-drug, anti-alcohol, anti-AIDS commercials follow one after the other; they raise social awareness, but they are powerless to offer an alternative." *Ad Age's* Garfield echoes that view, saying that such ads, for all of their noble intentions and attention-getting tactics, often leave the audience feeling overwhelmed by so many social problems and "powerless to help."

Of course, in many cases, the audience is not powerless; there are volunteer groups to join,

donations to be given, or individual behavioral habits—smoking, drinking, etc.—that can be reformed. The question is whether an ad is capable of providing enough motivation to spark that kind of action. There is evidence that ads can do this—sometimes. For example, since the American public was introduced to Vince and Larry—a couple of crash-test dummies that starred in a long-running "buckle up" ad campaign that debuted in the mid-1980s—American safety-belt usage tripled. Meanwhile, all of those horrifying Australian car-wreck commercials have been tied to measurable declines in drunk-driving accidents, year after year. And a number of local anti-smoking campaigns throughout the U.S. have been linked to declines in smoking rates.

But critics charge that these success stories are scattered, and that evidence of the effectiveness of social-issue ads is scant. Such ads are generally not held to the same rigorous standards as are ordinary soap and cereal ads; while the latter are

expected to produce immediate, measurable sales results in the marketplace, anti-drug ads, for example, are not expected to immediately reduce the number of drug users—only to "raise awareness" of the problem. Moreover, some believe that this type of advertising, for all of its high drama, is far less scientific and sophisticated than ads that sell products, in part because PSAs, with limited funds, typically are not subjected to the same kinds of research and testing as product ads. One study by the Harvard University School of Public Health found that melodramatic scenes in PSAs did not have a lasting impact on young people who viewed them; the study suggested that in order to truly effect behavioral changes, public-service ads needed to abandon shock-and-scare tactics and begin to incorporate some of the more sophisticated marketing approaches used in consumer ads—including product placements, sponsorships, more research and testing of ads, and manipulation of news programs to get the

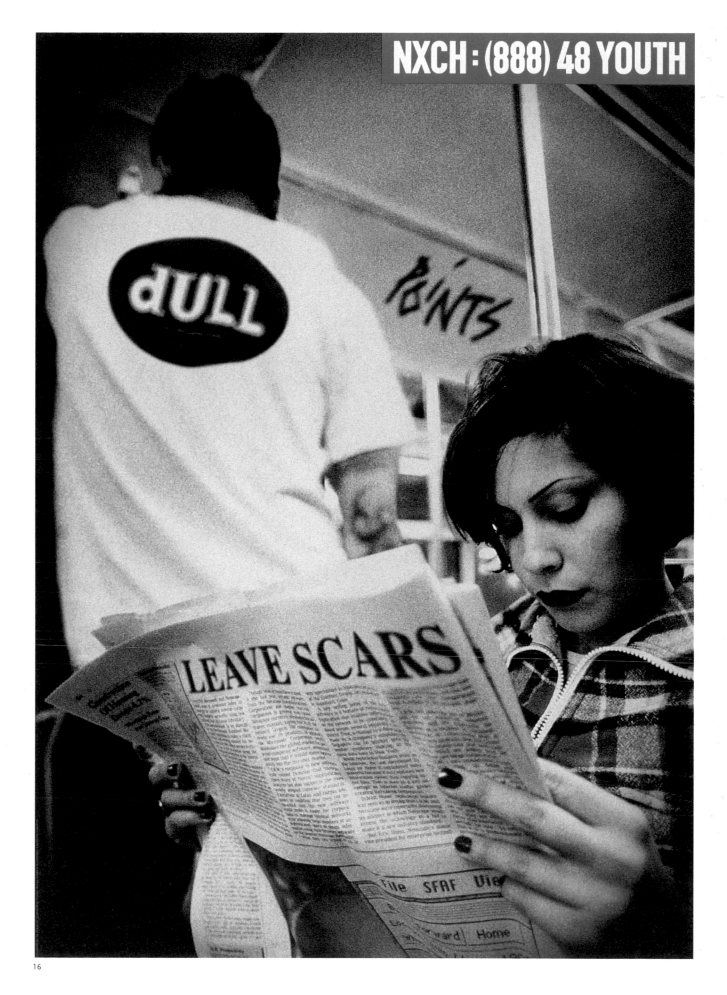

16

ADVERTISING AS AN AGENT OF SOCIAL CHANGE.

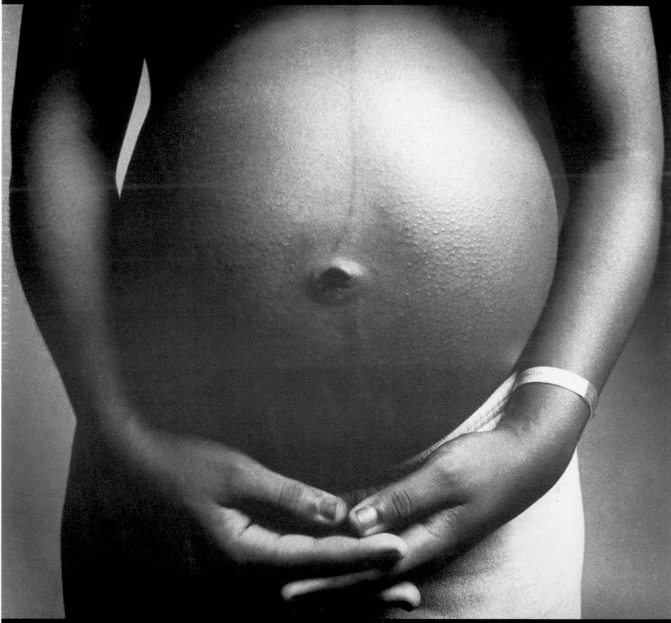

IF YOU'RE EMBARRASSED BY A PIMPLE TRY EXPLAINING THIS.

Being a teenager is tough enough. Why make things more difficult by becoming a mother too?

THE CHILDREN'S DEFENSE FUND

17

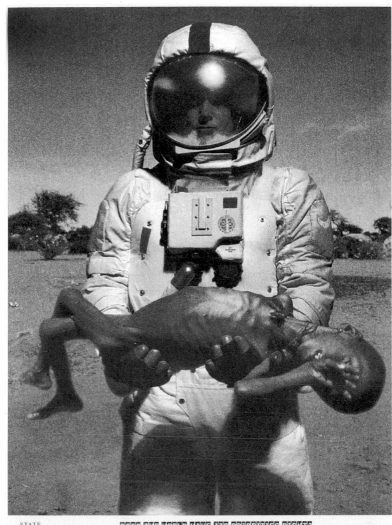

18

17. **THE CHILDREN'S
DEFENSE FUND**
FALLON McELLIGOTT,
MINNEAPOLIS, MINNESOTA,
1988
Part of a long-running series
of ads attempting to reach
disadvantaged youth.

18. **STATE OF THE
WORLD FORUM**
SAATCHI & SAATCHI
NEW ZEALAND, WELLINGTON,
1998
The photo may be melodramatic,
but it makes the point well; this
ad became a popular poster.

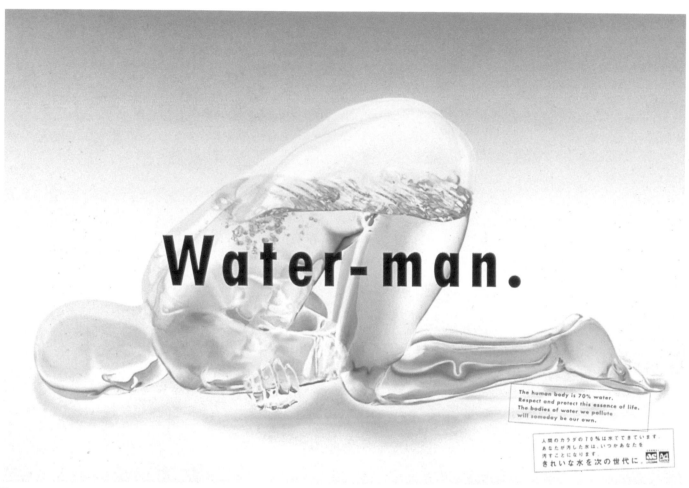

Water-man.

The human body is 70% water.
Respect and protect this essence of life.
The bodies of water we pollute
will someday be our own.

人間のカラダの70％は水でできています。
あなたが汚した水は、いつかあなたを
汚すことになります
きれいな水を次の世代に。

19

19. WATER CONSERVATION
DENTSU, TOKYO, MID-1990s
The campaign created a character,
"Water-man," to dramatize the
need to conserve.

20. KEEP AMERICA BEAUTIFUL
AD COUNCIL / MARSTELLER,
NEW YORK, 1971
In this classic campaign, a
Native American witnesses the
desecration of nature all around
him and sheds a single, memo-
rable tear.

**21. WORLD SOCIETY FOR THE
PROTECTION OF ANIMALS**
MULLEN, BOSTON,
EARLY 1990s
In the aftermath of the Exxon
Valdez oil tanker disaster
in 1989, this picture was
particularly poignant.

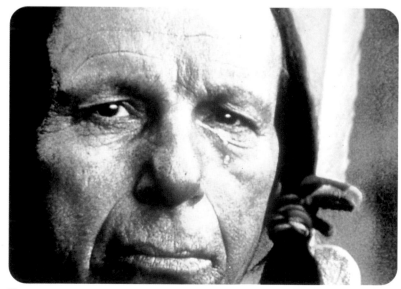

20

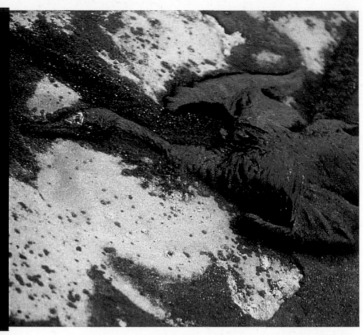

Could The Price Of Oil Be Any Higher?

If you think you pay a high price, consider what our beaches, coastlines and wildlife have to pay. Help us save the animals and clean up the spills. Donate what you can to WSPA, PO Box 190, Boston, MA 02130. Or call (617) 522-7000. We've been providing animal disaster relief for 30 years.

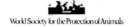

World Society for the Protection of Animals

21

messages across in a nonadvertising format. (It should be noted, however, that public-service messages can come under fire when they are delivered in such devious ways. When the U.S. government's Office of National Drug Control Policy recently began offering financial incentives and reviewing scripts in an effort to encourage producers of TV shows to weave anti-drug messages into their shows' story lines and dialogue, there was a public outcry—and a sense that the government was treading close to the dangerous areas of censorship and propaganda.)

In fairness, public-service ads shouldn't be expected to do the same job, in the same manner and with similar results, as product advertising; it is, after all, considerably easier to influence purchasing decisions than to change ingrained behavior among smokers, alcoholics, or abusive parents. The more realistic objective is that the ads become part of a public dialogue that gradually shifts public attitude, which in turn can lead to

changes in behavior. But it is a slow and multi-layered process, experts say. Dr. Gregory Connolly, who oversees the Massachusetts Department of Health anti-smoking campaign, acknowledges that the 30 percent decline in smoking achieved by the campaign was the result of a number of combined factors. "One thirty-second ad is not going to affect anybody's behavior," Connolly said. "But a series of ads, integrated with higher prices for cigarettes, clean indoor air [regulations] at the local level, and ready access to cessation services—all that together can result in hundreds of thousands of people quitting. We view advertising as the air cover for our ground troops. It frames the debate."

And that it seems to do well; when it comes to stirring discussion and placing a social issue on the radar of public consciousness, advertising has proved quite effective. When ads in America first targeted the issue of child abuse twenty-five years ago, the subject was still practically taboo. "People

didn't understand it and the media didn't want to get involved with it," according to Anne Cohn, who served as president of the National Committee for the Prevention of Child Abuse. The group started running a high-profile ad campaign headlined, "Child abuse hurts everybody" in 1976, and within five years, public attitudes on the issue had shifted dramatically—a 1982 Harris poll found that nine of ten people felt child abuse was a major social problem, compared with a previous study showing that only one in ten thought so.

Similarly, when the Partnership for a Drug-Free America began to saturate the American media with its messages in the late 1980s and early 1990s—producing a volume of ads second only to McDonald's at the time—the subject, as a result, was on everyone's mind: At one point, 92 percent of American teenagers reported that they had seen the "Fried Egg" spot (some drug users even took to joking, "Let's go fry an egg"). Did that growing awareness lead to

HERE'S A DEAD DOG. WHERE'S MY AWARD?

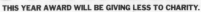

THIS YEAR AWARD WILL BE GIVING LESS TO CHARITY.

Community service and charity advertising has always been a special case when it comes to awards.

It has its own categories in every major advertising festival around the world. AWARD is no exception. However, we've spotted a problem.

Not only have community service and charity ads been able to enter their own categories, they've also been able to enter the general ones. A small space charity ad, for example, gets three bites at the guernsey; the Community Service and Charity section, the Small Space section and the Newspaper section.

Hardly fair on a packet soup ad that only gets one go. And often resulting in a book that looks more like a Charity Awards Annual.

So we've made a few changes for AWARD'91. Community Service and Charity ads will now only be judged in their own categories. Likewise, Small Space ads.

A minimum size for posters has been introduced to stop press ads being entered on the grounds they were pinned to the wall.

And Christmas cards, wedding invites, birth announcements, etc get their own category and are no longer a direct threat to direct mail for proper clients.

Details of changes are in the 13th AWARD Call for Entries booklet. If you still don't have a copy, call Mary or Sandra on (02) 267 6907 or (02) 267 6916.

But get a move on, the deadline for entries is June 7th. And if you've been pinning all your hopes on getting several gongs for one charity ad, all is not lost.

Just think of the money you'll save only having to enter it once.

1991 CALL FOR ENTRIES.

22

22. **AUSTRALIAN WRITERS & DIRECTORS ASSOCIATION**
BROWN MELHUISH FISHLOCK, SURRY HILLS, AUSTRALIA, 1991
A backlash against all the award-winning "help the animals" campaigns, this cynical ad suggested that it had become too easy for manipulative ads to win kudos.

23. **FRIENDS OF ANIMALS**
MAD DOGS & ENGLISHMEN, NEW YORK, 1997
Mad Dogs tried a postmodern approach to public service advertising, relying on irony instead of shock appeal.

changes in behavior and a decline in drug usage? That was a tough claim for the Partnership to prove; even in instances where some types of drug usage declined after the ads ran, as with cocaine in the early 1990s, there were various other factors aside from ads that could be credited. At the time, high-profile cocaine deaths among celebrities and other real-life horror stories in the news media may have had a larger impact than all of those make-believe ads. But various studies, such as one by the Johns Hopkins School of Medicine in 1991, indicated that teenagers exposed to anti-drug ads did seem to come away with a better understanding of the risks involved.

Such advertising can also have a kind of "ripple effect" that is difficult to measure, said Peter Cohen, one of the co-creators of a poignant, award-winning public-service commercial that ran in the early 1990s, featuring scenes of homeless people singing the lyrics to the song "New York, New York." Cohen says that that ad campaign, and others like it, succeeded in generating news-media attention, helped raise the visibility of the charitable organizations involved, attracted volunteers to the cause—and sometimes inspired individuals to take unexpected and spontaneous action. "I am constantly amazed," Cohen said, "by how many stories of goodwill and good deeds I still hear of that were generated by the 'New York, New York' ad we did years ago."

Of course, some of the people who are most affected by public-service ads are the people who create them. The most stark and striking ads tend to draw attention in the news media. And because such ads allow for more human drama than the usual recitations of product features and benefits, they are ideally suited for winning creative awards—which can help advance the careers of the award-winning creators. This not-so-hidden agenda has been the subject of much debate within the ad business (one

Australian creative team, frustrated at seeing shocking PSAs honored with prizes, ran a trade ad featuring a canine carcass and the headline "Here's a dead dog, where's my award?"). Dave Buonaguidi of the British agency St. Luke's believes that "probably less than 10 percent of the people who get involved in the production of [public service] ads give a damn about the end result." They do it, Buonaguidi suggested, because they see an opportunity to make high-profile ads that will, ultimately, boost their salaries.

Even if that's true, should anyone outside the business care? Certainly, the results of this advertising matter much more than the motives behind it—but it's also conceivable that the latter could influence the former. Skeptics in the ad industry believe melodramatic PSAs are sometimes designed for the press and award-show judges, rather than the target audience—which would raise questions about whether such ads may be neglecting their primary function and misusing

FUR WEARERS:

PLEASE REFRAIN FROM CLIMBING TRAFFIC LIGHTS, MARKING TERRITORY AND/OR SNIFFING OTHER PEDESTRIAN'S CROTCHES.

—BUREAU OF SANITATION

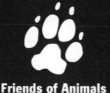

Friends of Animals

FUR IS A THING OF THE PAST. **EVOLVE.**

23

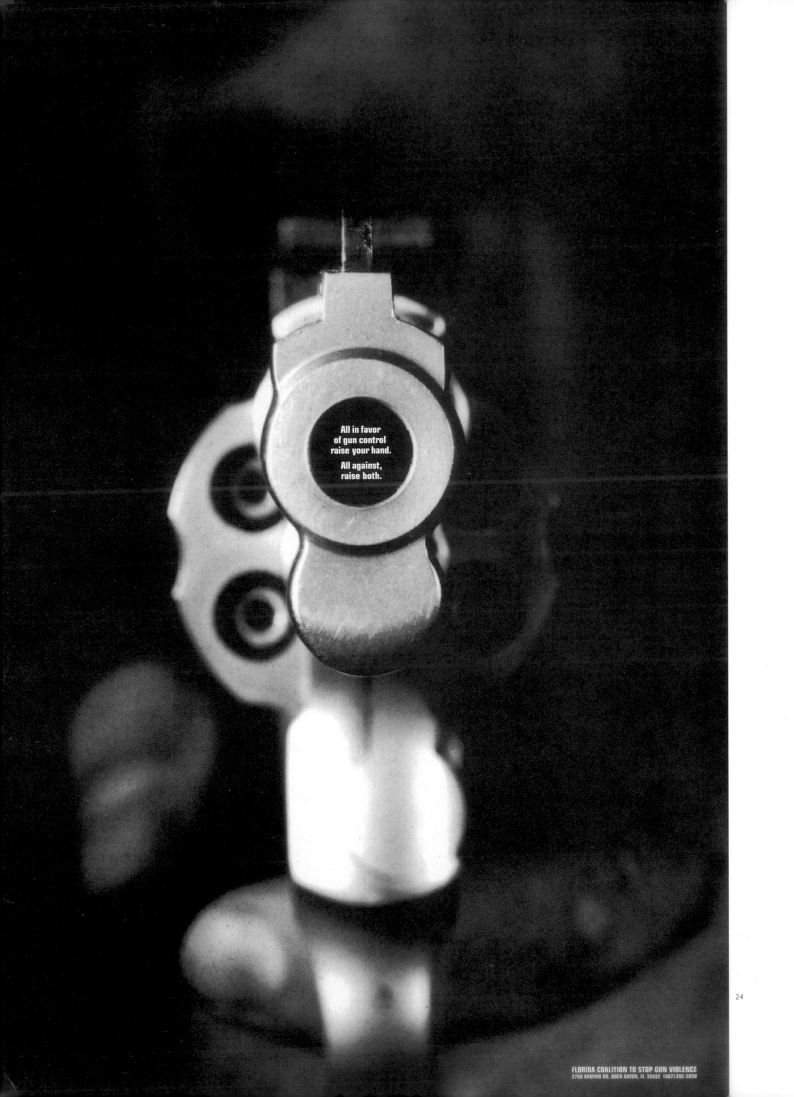

All in favor
of gun control
raise your hand.

All against,
raise both.

24

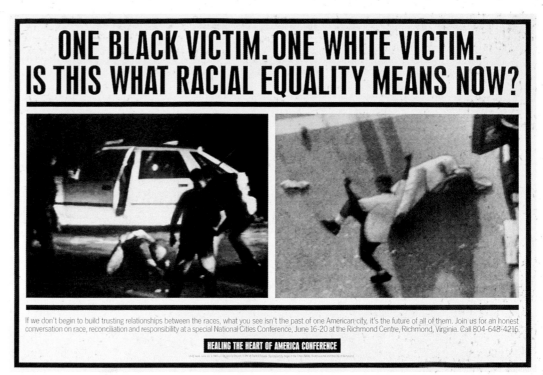

ONE BLACK VICTIM. ONE WHITE VICTIM. IS THIS WHAT RACIAL EQUALITY MEANS NOW?

If we don't begin to build trusting relationships between the races, what you see isn't the past of one American city, it's the future of all of them. Join us for an honest conversation on race, reconciliation and responsibility at a special National Cities Conference, June 16-20 at the Richmond Centre, Richmond, Virginia. Call 804-648-4216.

HEALING THE HEART OF AMERICA CONFERENCE

25

**24. FLORIDA COALITION
TO STOP GUN VIOLENCE**
CRISPIN PORTER +
BOGUSKY, MIAMI, 1995
Giving new meaning to the
phrase, "target marketing."

**25. HEALING THE HEART
OF AMERICA CONFERENCE**
THE MARTIN AGENCY,
RICHMOND, VIRGINIA, 1993
In the wake of the Los Angeles
race riots of 1992, this ad
appealed to all sides for calm.

donated funds and media time. But other ad experts insist that is a nonissue; what wins awards and what helps the cause is usually the same thing. John Hegarty of the London agency Bartle Bogle Hegarty noted that regardless of the personal motivations of people creating the ads, the point is that good talent prevails—and public-service advertising "gives worthy causes access to creative people they could not otherwise afford."

Meanwhile, for many agency creative people, the ads provide a rare chance to say something important and meaningful. As Stuart Elliott of *The New York Times* pointed out, in creating a PSA, "you can pour your heart out—in a way that you can't for dog food." Socially responsible ads have become a defining characteristic of some agencies, including the Amsterdam-based agency KesselsKramer. "We're interested not just in selling a product but in the social meaning of our work," said co-founder Johan Kramer. "People in

advertising should realize they have a big responsibility in creating social patterns." On an individual level, ad people often gravitate toward issues and causes that have special relevance to them. The American ad copywriter Richard Yelland, who has worked on anti-drug ads, said, "A couple of friends of mine had died because of heroin problems, and my partner and I felt desperate to do what we could to help."

Another concern about public-service ads is their tendency to inject some of the less desirable elements of advertising—the propensity to hype and oversell, to glamorize, to put a Madison Avenue spin on reality—into the public discourse on critical issues. One might assume that in the harsh world of PSAs there would be little room for glamorization, but advertising is still advertising. In one Partnership anti-drug ad—in which a young woman viciously wields a frying pan in a kitchen to make a point about the damage that

drugs can cause—the signals sent out by the ad were decidedly mixed. As noted by columnist Frank Rich of *The New York Times*, the woman in the ad doesn't look like an addict but more like "Winona Ryder; she's wearing a tight tank top; there are no visible track marks on her arms; and the kitchen representing her drug-induced hell is right out of the Pottery Barn, if not Williams-Sonoma." When not beautifying the image of problems such as drug addiction, ads can go the other way, creating an ersatz horror show; one recent campaign for battered women in New York showed disturbing images of women's bruised and swollen faces—however, the women in the ads were actresses, and their bruises had been created by a special-effects-makeup artist (the copy, too, could be considered less than authentic, considering that it was written by young male ad writers). Some feel that when ads take on serious, complex social problems in a superficial manner,

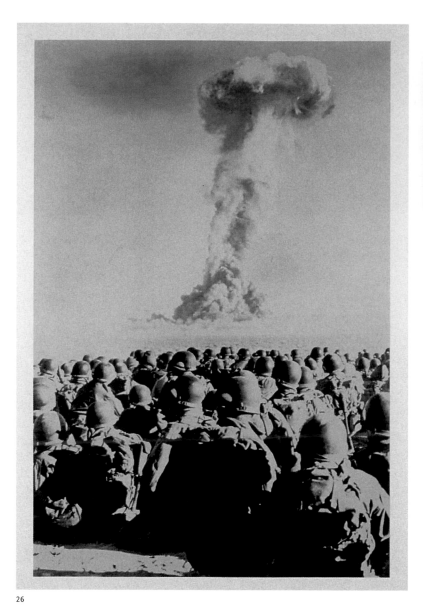

26

26. **NATIONAL ASSOCIATION OF ATOMIC VETERANS**
DOYLE ADVERTISING &
DESIGN, BOSTON, 1992
The campaign, from the early
1990s, gave voice to a group of
victims who had remained silent
for decades.

27. **NORTH KOREA FAMINE RELIEF**
SAATCHI & SAATCHI,
SINGAPORE, 1998
Using propaganda to counter
propaganda, the advertiser took
on those who tried to deny that
there was a crisis in North Korea.

28. **VIRGINIA HOLOCAUST MUSEUM**
THE MARTIN AGENCY,
RICHMOND, VIRGINIA, 2000
Each ad featured a bold
headline and told the story of
a concentration camp victim,
incorporating objects and
personal artifacts to provide
depth and detail.

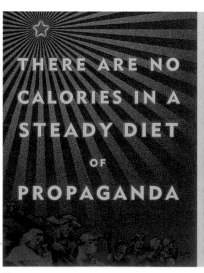

27

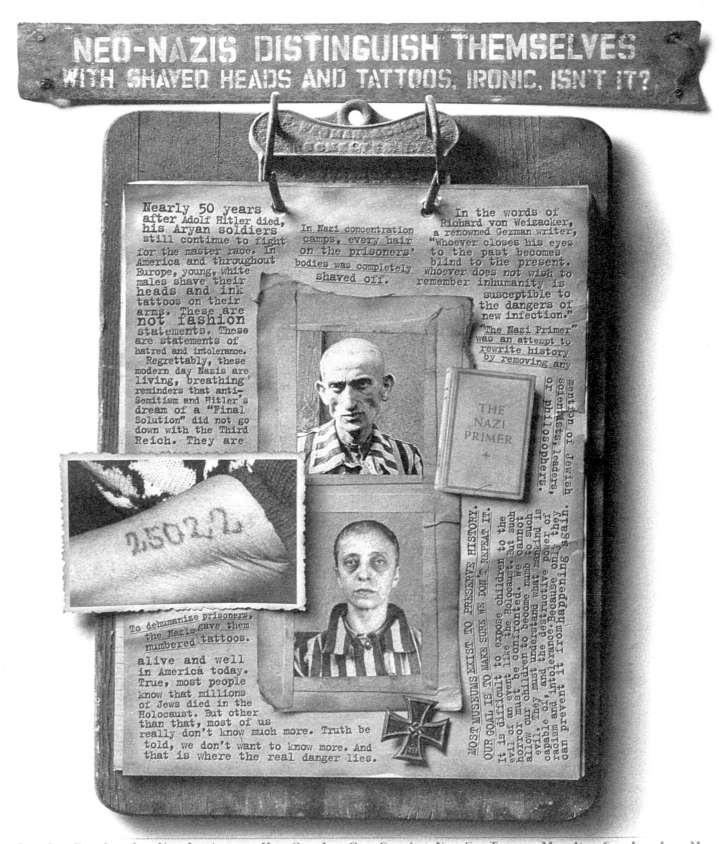

VIRGINIA HOLOCAUST MUSEUM

The Virginia Holocaust Museum was established in 1996. The museum is not intended to answer why the Holocaust happened. Rather, its sole mission is to teach tolerance through education. The startling exhibits trace the steps of the Ipson family from Lithuania's Kovno ghetto to a 9 x 12 x 4 foot underground hiding place where thirteen family members lived. Guided tours are available by calling 804-257-5400. The Virginia Holocaust Museum is located at 213 Roseneath Rd., Richmond, Virginia. Museum hours: Monday through Friday, 9 am-5 pm; Saturday, 2 pm-5 pm; and Sunday, 1 pm-5 pm. Admission is free.

28

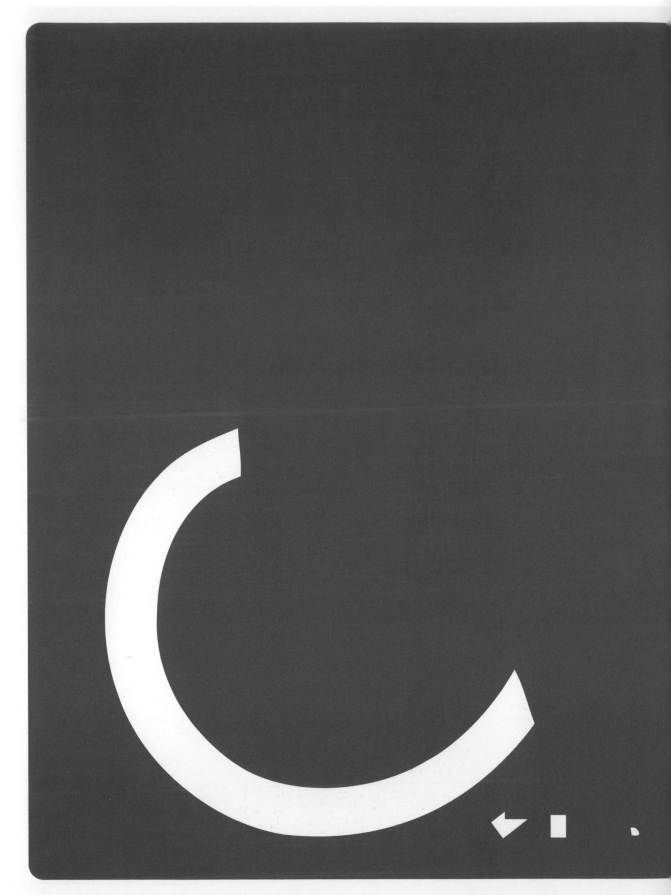

HELP CURE SPINAL CORD INJURIES. Send your donation to The Canadian Paraplegic As

, 520 Sutherland Drive, Toronto, ON M4G 3V9. (416) 422-5644. Or visit info@cpaont.org.

29. **THE CANADIAN PARAPLEGIC ASSOCIATION**
BUTLER SHINE & STERN,
SAUSALITO, CALIFORNIA, 1998
This ad altered a universal symbol
to convey an optimistic message.

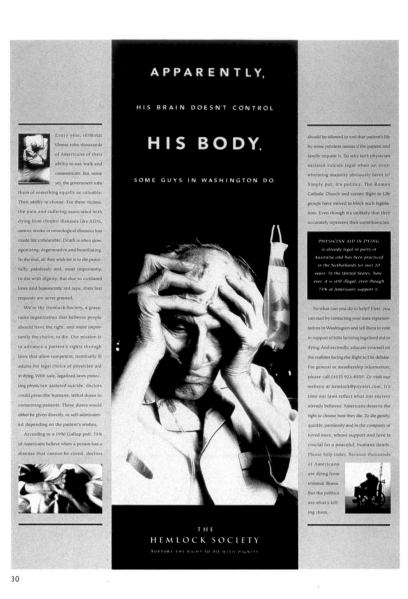

APPARENTLY,

HIS BRAIN DOESN'T CONTROL

HIS BODY.

SOME GUYS IN WASHINGTON DO.

THE
HEMLOCK SOCIETY
SUPPORT THE RIGHT TO DIE WITH DIGNITY

30

30. **THE HEMLOCK SOCIETY**
BUTLER SHINE & STERN,
SAUSALITO, CALIFORNIA, 1997
The creator of this campaign for
a pro-euthanasia organization,
Ryan Ebner, took a strong
personal interest in the subject
and decided to confront the
thorny issue with a series of ads.

31. **OREGON DONOR
PROGRAM**
BORDERS PERRIN NORRANDER,
PORTLAND, OREGON, 1991
Once again, using a familiar
icon to make a point.

they can do more harm than good. For example, a frequent criticism of some child-abuse ads has been that they tend to demonize and shame the abuser rather than reaching out to him or her (as child-abuse experts say the ads must do in order to have a positive effect). Shocking PSAs can occasionally further traumatize victims of abuse, as in the case of the aforementioned British child-abuse campaign. Or they can offend large segments of the population, as with recent South African rape-prevention ads, which alienated males who felt the ads seemed to be suggesting that all men are rapists.

Critics also worry about the blurring of the lines between bona fide public-service ads and hybrid ads that try to promote both a cause and a company at the same time. Increasingly, serious issues and causes are being adopted—or co-opted—by companies with a sales agenda. Nike has earned kudos for using its ads to promote more opportunities for women in sports,

as in the award-winning commercial "If You Let Me Play Sports. . . ." It's hard to take issue with that message, but it's also logical that as more girls and women "play," Nike will sell more sneakers to this demographic. At the same time, Anheuser-Busch increasingly uses ads to promote "responsible" drinking—which can seem like a mixed message from a company that so heavily promotes drinking. Recent commercials by Philip Morris, which owns numerous cigarette brands, have centered on the plight of battered women and the company's contributions to that cause; to a cynic, these ads might seem to be an attempt to divert attention from the public-health problems associated with this company's mainstay product. Perhaps the most obvious example of opportunism could be seen in a campaign from a British power company, which sent out promotional leaflets with the headline "Stop it, daddy, stop it"—yet another dramatic PSA, with the power company announcing its support for the national child-abuse fund.

But here was the catch: Money would be donated to the cause only if the recipient of the ad agreed to switch power companies.

Corporations aren't the only ones using ads to weigh in on social issues; so, too, are political-action groups, special-interest lobbies, private individuals and foundations, and academic think tanks, all of which have been fueling the growth of PSAs. The result, said issue-advertising specialist Victor Kamber, is that "TV has become a battleground of disparate voices, because groups realize the need to appeal to the public to effect change." And as this continues, the public will be exposed to more and more ads pushing something that can't be bought—a philosophy, a choice, a way of life.

Meanwhile, the ads themselves continue to evolve. Some have actually begun to move away from gloom and shock, opting for something more upbeat and contemporary. The Brazilian agency DM9 DDB recently unveiled an anti-gun

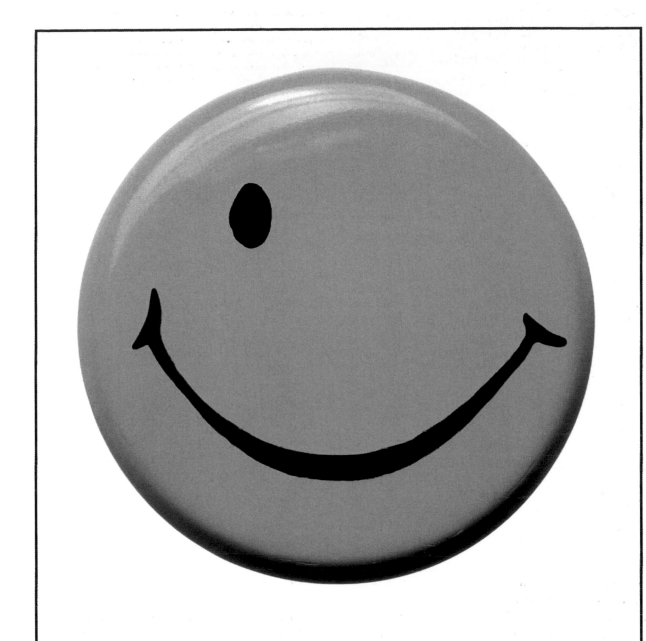

HAPPINESS IS BEING AN ORGAN DONOR.

OREGON DONOR PROGRAM

Feel good knowing you can help someone long after you're gone. Carry an organ donor card.

31

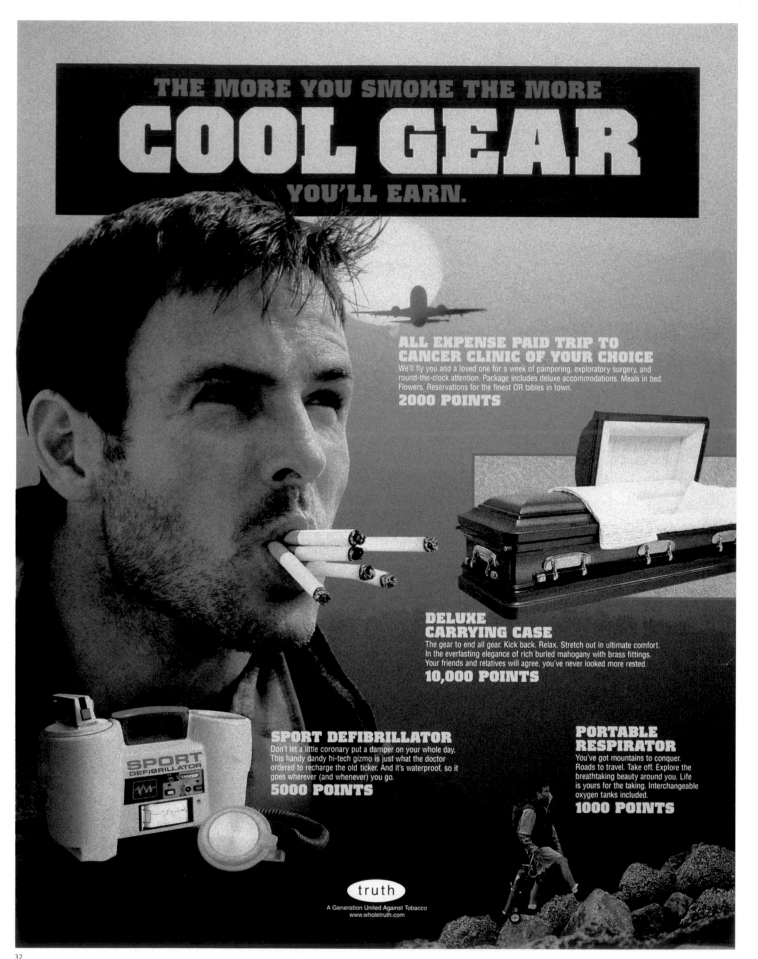

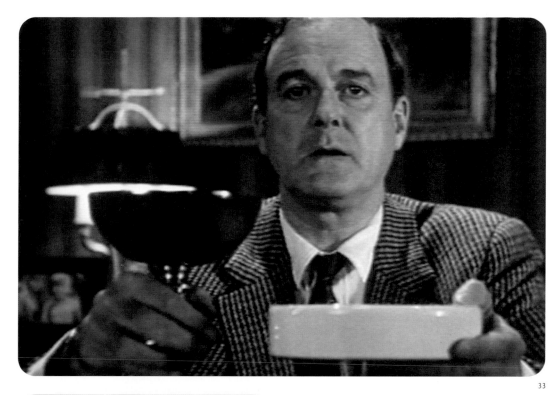

33

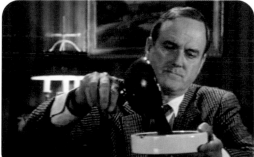

campaign, asking Brazilians to declare, *"Sou da paz,"* or "I am for peace," which borrowed the basic ingredients of product advertising—star endorsers, a slogan, a jingle (actually a peace song), and even a logo designed for the cause. And it seemed to be working, as more than 1,000 people in São Paulo turned in their guns in the first week of the campaign—far more guns than local police had been able to raise in three years of their own campaigns.

Some of the current ads have even begun to adopt an ironic attitude toward misery and death, using the kind of postmodern "anti-sell" approaches favored in hip commercials for sneakers and jeans. One ad titled "Everybody's Doing It," from the California agency Ground Zero, featured an upbeat jingle and copy promoting the virtues of heroin—while the screen showed images of a dirty, needle-scarred man convulsing on a bathroom floor. The sarcastic slogan: "Heroin, for the rest of your life." Another

ad, from the American Cancer Society, spoofed the typical TV sales offer; just buy enough cigarettes, the gushing announcer promised, and you'll be eligible for gifts including an oxygen mask, a chemotherapy discount . . . and even "a beautiful lung ventilator with matching tracheal tube!" (Some TV stations felt the ad's humor was in bad taste and refused to run it, but the cancer society stuck by it, believing it would appeal to teenagers because of the cutting-edge humor.) Still another popular anti-smoking campaign neatly turned cigarette advertising against itself: On billboards throughout California, the familiar Western-cowboy imagery of Marlboro advertising was recreated, but the ad agency, Asher & Partners, plugged in new headlines that were simultaneously disturbing and amusing. In one ad, a macho Marlboro Man was shown confiding to his fellow cowboy, "Bob, I've got emphysema."

As this more modern creative sensibility takes hold, public-service ads are also crossing

new media frontiers; recently the Ad Council brought Smokey the Bear into cyberspace, where the character has his own Web site. In some ways, the Internet may be the ideal environment for social-cause ads, and only partly because Web pages are inexpensive to produce. More important, this interactive medium allows PSAs to move beyond mere attention-grabbing to deliver more in-depth information on an issue or problem, while also helping to connect people with resources that can provide real help—rather than leaving viewers feeling helpless before an onslaught of grim images on their TV screens. That's not to suggest, however, that public-service ads won't continue to be at least somewhat unsettling, disturbing, and provocative, as the conscience of advertising faces up to its own demons and compels the rest of us to face ours. The adman DeVito noted that harsh problems demand harsh ads, and, he added, "If you can't stand looking at these pictures—well, that's the whole point, isn't it?"

10. TH
COMMA

E NEW
DMENTS.

The line wasn't terribly original. It wasn't particularly lyrical. It wasn't even grammatically correct. But when the Los Angeles ad agency TBWA/Chiat/Day coined the phrase "Think different" and placed it on a series of Apple Computer ads featuring the faces of well-known innovators and radicals, the campaign became a late-1990s cultural phenomenon. Interestingly, the line used by Apple echoed a similar "command" issued three decades earlier, when Volkswagen advertiser Doyle Dane Bernbach advised car buyers to "Think small." If those two campaigns represent a couple of the most well-known examples of advertisers telling us how to think, another famous series of ads, from the Nike agency Wieden + Kennedy, put forth a different kind of command, beginning in the late 1980s: Stop thinking about it, these ads barked, and "Just do it."

What connects all three of these slogans, aside from their immense popularity, is that each

seems to be urging us to do something much larger and more meaningful than purchasing a product. What these advertisers are really "selling" is a philosophy, a belief system, an attitude, a way of life. Increasingly, these are the kinds of loftier messages to be found in today's ads. These new commandments—sometimes clearly stated, sometimes slightly ambiguous ("Just do *what,*" exactly?)—constitute Madison Avenue's instruction book of rules to live by.

Why has so much advertising stopped telling us what to buy, opting instead to tell us how to live our lives? Like so many of the changes in advertising, this, too, can be at least partly attributed to the increase in product parity. As the award-winning ad writer Luke Sullivan pointed out, "It has become more difficult to find and promote a unique benefit to a particular product," and consequently, many advertisers have turned away from the product itself. As Sullivan observed, advertisers have elevated the

conversation from mundane product benefits to higher emotional benefits. Hence, an ad for a camera now is less likely to claim that the device takes better pictures, and more likely to urge you (or to gently order you) to get the most out of life by documenting and savoring experiences. And do it now, before it's too late.

Advertising's commandments are constantly changing to reflect cultural shifts and evolving public attitudes—because even as advertising seemingly orders us around, it is always careful to dispense only the kinds of orders that the current society is ready, willing, and, in fact, eager to obey. For example, in years past, ads were more apt to pressure the public to conform and to "keep up with the Joneses." And thus, advertising opened itself up to criticism for preying on insecurities: If you didn't use the right toothpaste or antiperspirant or a strong-enough floor polish, you risked potentially devastating embarrassment and ostracism, such ads suggested. "Ring around the collar," the

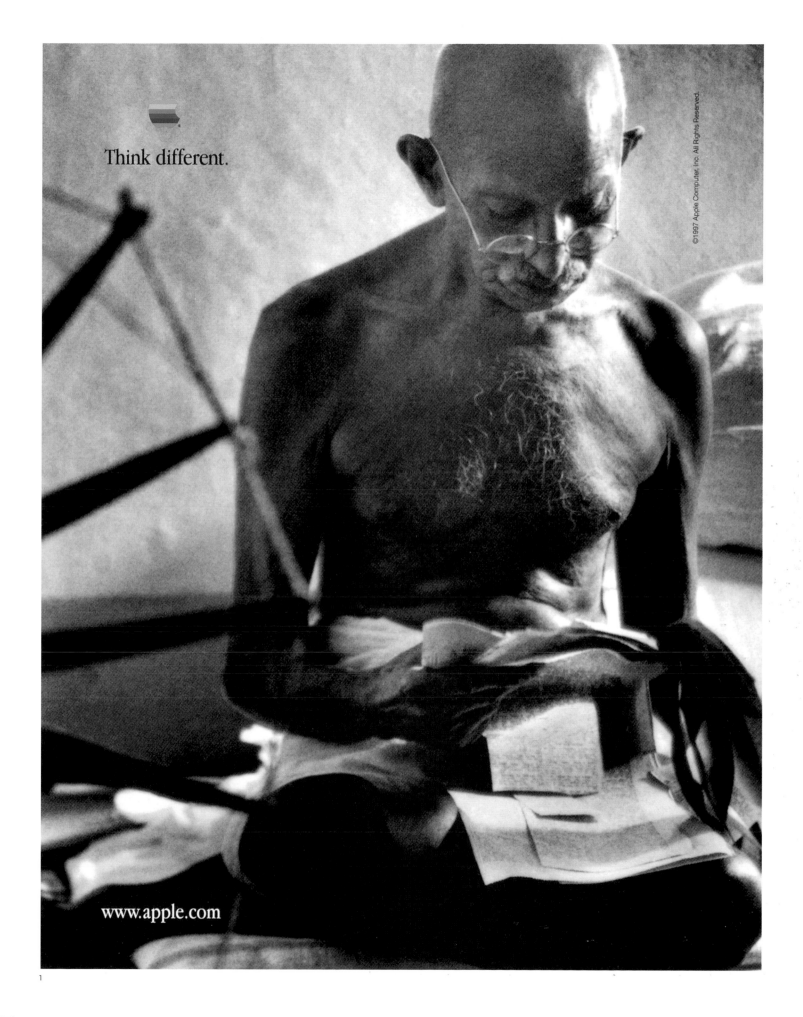

Think different.

www.apple.com

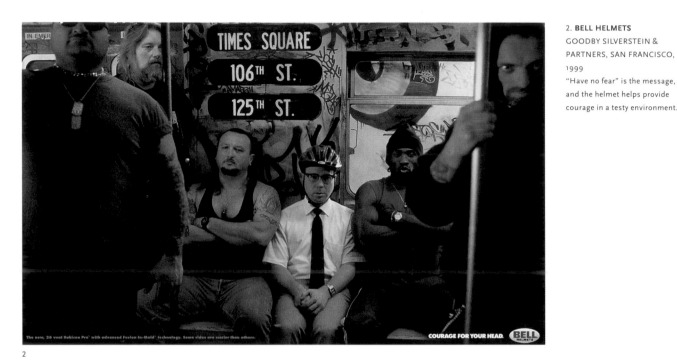

2

2. **BELL HELMETS**
GOODBY SILVERSTEIN &
PARTNERS, SAN FRANCISCO,
1999
"Have no fear" is the message,
and the helmet helps provide
courage in a testy environment.

3. **QWEST**
J. WALTER THOMPSON,
NEW YORK, 1999
In an era of sweeping change,
advertisers are fostering the
belief that everything can now
be recreated and improved.

line and image used in commercials by Wisk
detergent during the 1970s and early 1980s, was a
signal to the world—as visible and damning as a
scarlet letter—that one had failed at the most basic
kind of personal hygiene. During these times, ads
often issued one kind of warning or another, as in
the famous slogan for the credit-card company
American Express: "Don't leave home without it."

In more recent years, however, advertising has
tended to adopt a tone that is much more positive
and (to use a word that has been beaten nearly to
death in ad land) "empowering." According to the
research firm Iconoculture, which studies trends
and consumer attitudes, contemporary advertisers
in the 1980s and particularly in the 1990s gradually realized they were dealing with a much
more self-assured consumer, and "so it made
more sense to sell through positive empowerment, rather than through fear and insecurity,"
says Iconoculture's co-founder Larry Samuel. In
fact, if anyone had reason to feel insecure in the

new marketplace, it was the advertiser—because
increasingly, the customer was in control, with
endless options and brands to choose from. Mark
Waites, creative director at the British ad agency
Mother, observes, "In the 1980s, an ad might
have asked, 'Are you cool enough to drink our
beer?' Now if you say something like that, people
will tell you to screw off." If this newfound consumer confidence was true of the contemporary
male, it was even more true of the modern
woman—who, by the 1990s, was clearly rejecting
old-fashioned ad messages that in any way
suggested women could not be as outgoing,
adventurous, aggressive, or successful as men.

The new advertising was also tapping into a
lifestyle shift in America, Europe, and elsewhere.
Buoyed by economic prosperity and greater
political freedom around the world, the new-
millennium consumers—both male and
female—were no longer content with just fitting
in and getting by, according to Iconoculture and

other attitudinal researchers. The objective now
was to have adventures, to live well and fully, and
to make a mark as an individual. All of which has
made it a prosperous time to be an advertiser,
since this more adventurous lifestyle dovetails
well with the selling of everything from athletic
gear to sport-utility vehicles.

Responding to this new culture, ads in recent
years have done their best to reinforce the spirit of
rugged individualism, the desire for complete self-
fulfillment, and the hunger for experiences. And in
so doing, advertisers have taken on the combined
role of therapist and cheerleader—urging us to "go
farther" (Isuzu cars) and to "do more" (American
Express). Or, if you prefer, "the major brands have
become our new philosophers," says the American
ad executive Jeff Weiss. In so doing, they have
shifted some of the focus of ads away from themselves: Merrill Lynch used to describe itself as
"bullish on America," but now urges the rest of us
to "be bullish." The Prudential Insurance

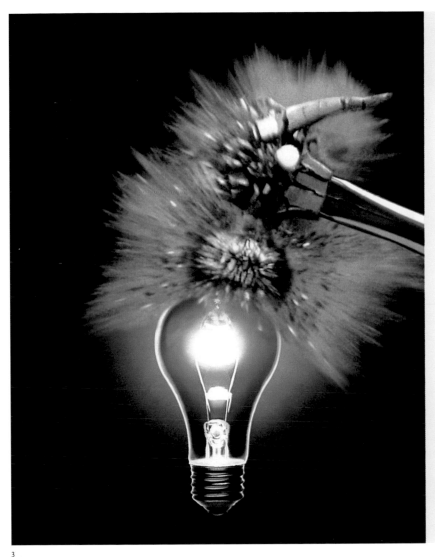

Change everything.

Finally, a network with the bandwidth that delivers the promise of the Internet.
It's called Qwest. And it can make all your expensive IT investments pay off. Because it's the network with the bandwidth to maximize multimedia applications, put e-business into overdrive, and make your kids start recognizing you again. Visit our Web site at **qwest.com** to find out about the bandwidth to change everything.

3

Unplug the phone. Mix plaids and stripes. Stop speaking to friends who begin every sentence with "I." Drink 6-8 glasses of water a day. When the oil light goes on in the car, add oil. Take deep breaths. Stay out of dark alleys. Listen when your boyfriend says he doesn't want a commitment. If it's collecting dust, throw it out. Stop feeling guilty. Don't surround yourself with off-white walls. Quit smoking. Don't lie to religious figures. Scratch the itch. Think of the thing you fear the most and do it. In the end, a spotless kitchen floor doesn't matter. Grow your own. Lower-watt light bulbs are more flattering. Move 3,000 miles away from your parents. Open a window. Smile when you say that. Kiss a baby. Go to church. Or a synagogue. Or a mosque. Or a mall. Play gin. Forgive somebody. Television isn't a role model. Laugh. And remember, sometimes all it takes is the right pillowcase. **Live better.** **IKEA**

It's a big country. Someone's got to furnish it.™

BALTIMORE • HOUSTON • LOS ANGELES • NEW YORK • PHILADELPHIA • PITTSBURGH • WASHINGTON DC

© Inter IKEA Systems. B.V. 1997.

4

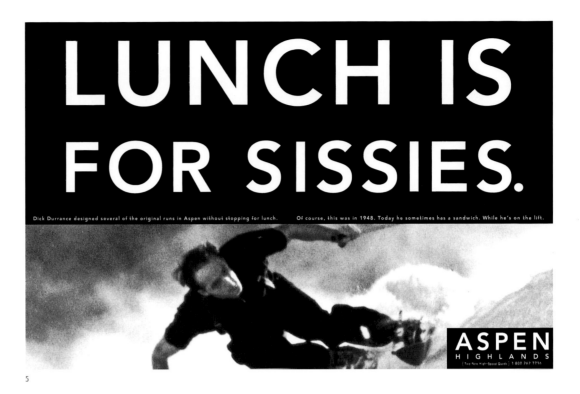

LUNCH IS FOR SISSIES.

Dick Durrance designed several of the original runs in Aspen without stopping for lunch. Of course, this was in 1948. Today he sometimes has a sandwich. While he's on the lift.

ASPEN
HIGHLANDS

5

4. **IKEA**
DEUTSCH INC., NEW YORK,
1997
Loading up on the commands,
the furniture company Ikea
sums it up last: Live better.

5. **ASPEN SKIING COMPANY**
COLE & WEBER, SEATTLE, 1994
The advertiser as bully: Mark
Fenske's no-nonsense campaign
for the Aspen, Colorado, ski
resorts chided the audience for
taking it easy. (Another headline
in the series: "April in Paris is
for wussies.")

Company of America's slogan evolved from "Own a piece of the rock" to "Be your own rock."

As advertising's new commandments increasingly reflected and fostered the confident "can do" spirit of the times, the messages have been largely aspirational—and in that regard, they can be viewed as a positive evolution from older ads that played on insecurities and fostered conformity. On the other hand, the new can-do ads are guilty of their own sins: appealing to vanity; encouraging a false sense of confidence bordering on arrogance; applauding behavior and attitudes that can be self-absorbed and antisocial. More than ever before, ad writers have resorted to flattery ("You are strong, you are special, you are one-of-a-kind" is the mantra of the sycophantic ad). And while they are no longer as apt to make false claims about the product being advertised, they've taken to proffering more grand illusions—often overpromising the opportunities and experiences available to today's "empowered" people. Having

death-defying adventures, becoming wealthy, enjoying great sex, answering to no one, having a rock-hard physique, attaining a deeper sense of fulfillment—it's all available to us if we get off the couch and "just do it."

Advertisers have promulgated countless new commandments in the past few years, but the ten that follow have been particularly prevalent. They may not last: Having been ushered in by various trends and economic developments, they could easily be swept away by more of the same. But for now, these commandments represent the dogma of advertising.

1. BREAK THE RULES.

It is perhaps the single most dominant message of contemporary advertising, running through ads for cars, computers, financial services, sneakers. No matter how generic and unoriginal their own products may be, advertisers are urging *us* to be different—to become rebels and nonconformists.

Of course, the other shoe drops with the suggestion, implied or stated outright, that the advertiser's products can somehow play a role in helping us to blaze our own trails.

This trend is ironic in that, for so many years, critics of advertising worried that Madison Avenue's overarching "Big Brother" agenda was to promote mindless conformity, with everyone buying into the same mass-marketed products and lifestyles. But now we find the modern advertiser's favorite message is "Reject the status quo. Be a rebel. Think different."

Advertising's rebel yell can be traced back to the 1960s. Led by Doyle Dane Bernbach's "Think small." campaign for Volkswagen, ads began to advance the proposition that a purchasing choice could be a bold statement of individuality and independent thinking, a chance to break from the pack. DDB had been prescient in identifying a burgeoning restlessness of spirit that would become much more apparent in the mid-to-late

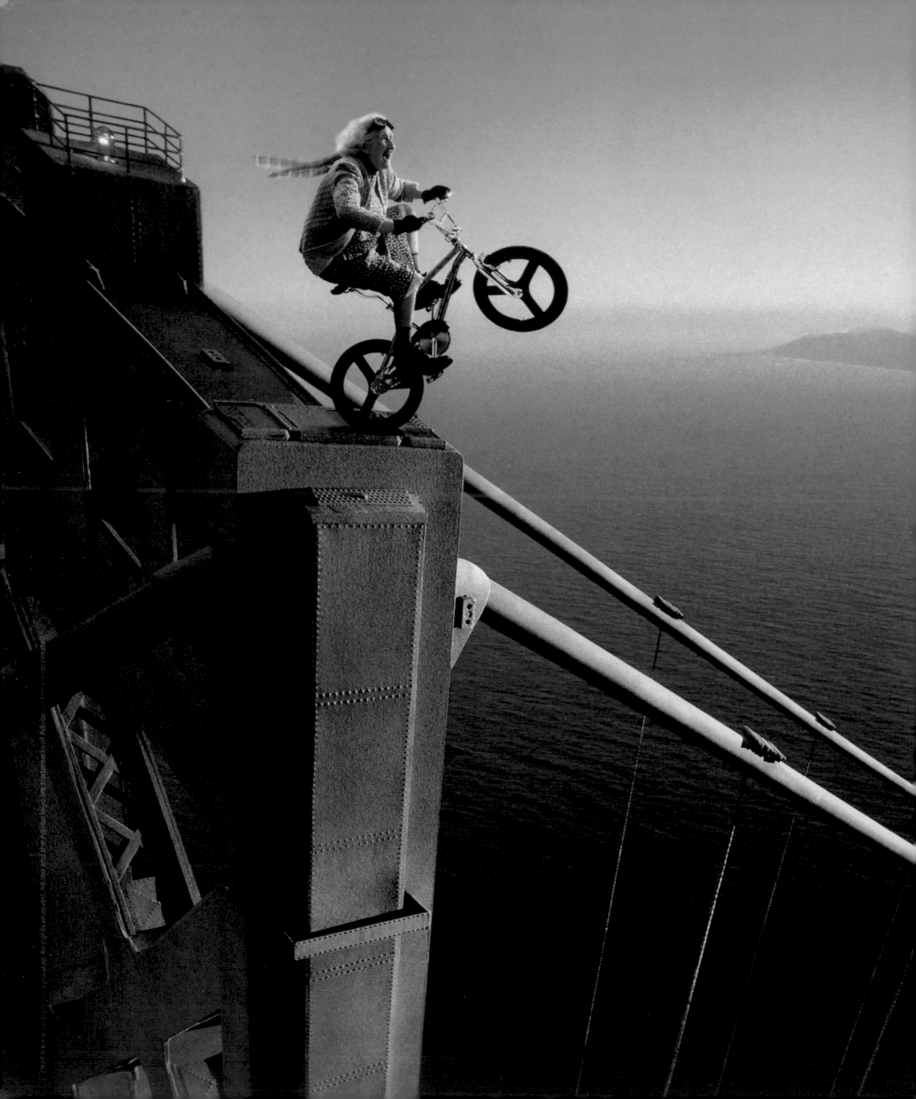

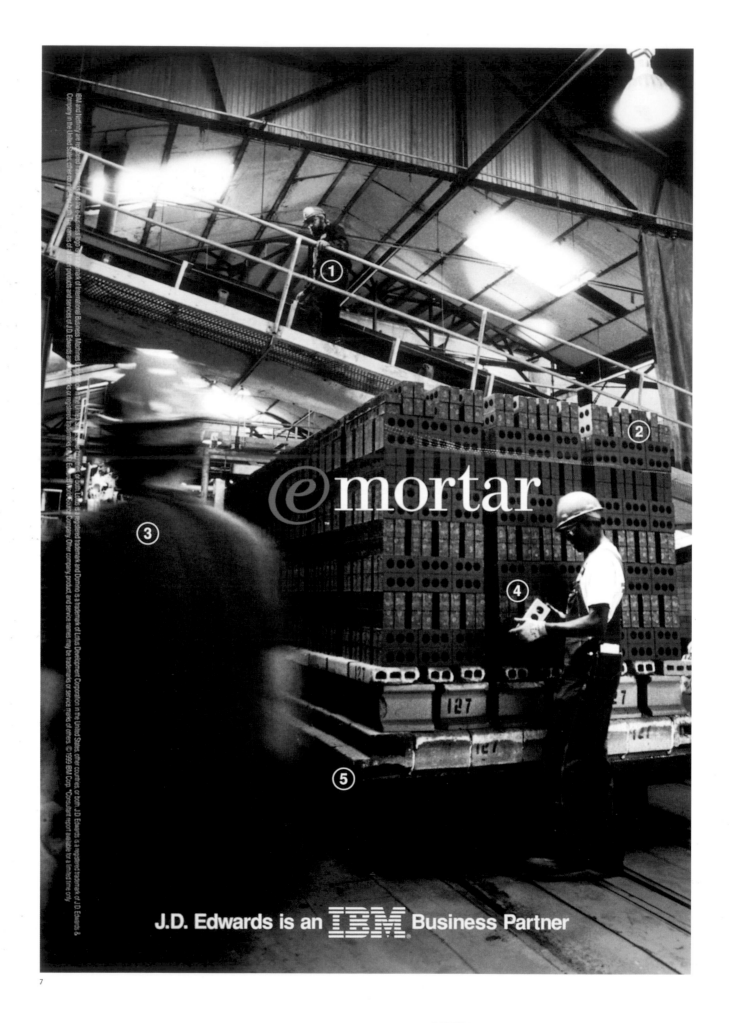

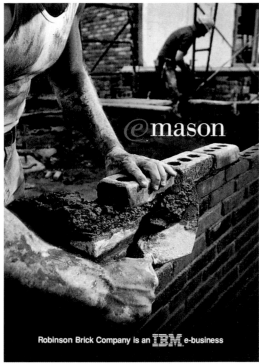

8

1960s—by which time many mainstream advertisers were encouraging consumers to "do your own thing" or "join a new generation," both in America and in Europe. While the 1960s strain of rebellious advertising quieted down somewhat in the more sober late 1970s and early 1980s, the "Break the rules" rallying cry returned in the mid-1980s, this time surging on the momentum of the computer revolution. The author Thomas Frank points to Apple's anti-establishment "1984" commercial as a leader in spreading the message that products could set us free and help us all to be the mavericks we really want to be. From that point forward, Frank believes, the nature of business theory itself was transformed: it became "about revolution, not status or hierarchy . . . about liberation, not order."

Nowhere has this philosophy held greater sway than in California's Silicon Valley, a culture rooted in the notion of breaking away from the established way of doing things, of leaving behind the safe company job to launch a dot-com business in a garage. The technology revolution in the 1990s certainly fueled the current wave of "Break the rules" advertising, and the message is delivered forcefully in the ads of Apple, Adobe, Qwest, and other high-tech companies.

But it isn't just the techies promoting revolution; even mundane, "old economy" businesses like fast-food chains have picked up the rallying cry (Burger King at one point was ending all its ads with the line "Sometimes you gotta break the rules," though the ads never made it clear who was breaking which rules and why). To some extent, the more traditional a company is, the more its advertising now screams about rule-breaking. In an age of too many look-alike products, advertisers are desperate to say, "We're not like everyone else. We're different. We break the rules. (How? By cooking the french fries longer!)."

It isn't just the advertisers who are "desperate to be different," however; it's the customer, too. The "Think different" entrepreneurial spirit "is all around us these days," says Tom Julian, a trend analyst with the agency Fallon Worldwide. "People now believe, 'I have to think out-of-the-box in order to be successful, and I must live my whole life that way.' " Cognizant that the voices in our heads are urging us to be bolder, advertisers are echoing back that command, again and again—sometimes verbally, sometimes through imagery of quirky, off-center behavior. Wearing a Mohawk hairstyle to the office, painting one's face blue, taking a bath in a public place (an image that appears in a Swedish ad for, of all things, Maxwell House coffee) becomes shorthand for "distinctive"—a quality that every brand, no matter how nondescript, must somehow claim for itself.

2. HAVE NO FEAR.

Of course, it's not enough just to decide to break the rules; you have to have the courage to act on your decision. And so "Have no fear" is a partner command to "Break the rules," though it also

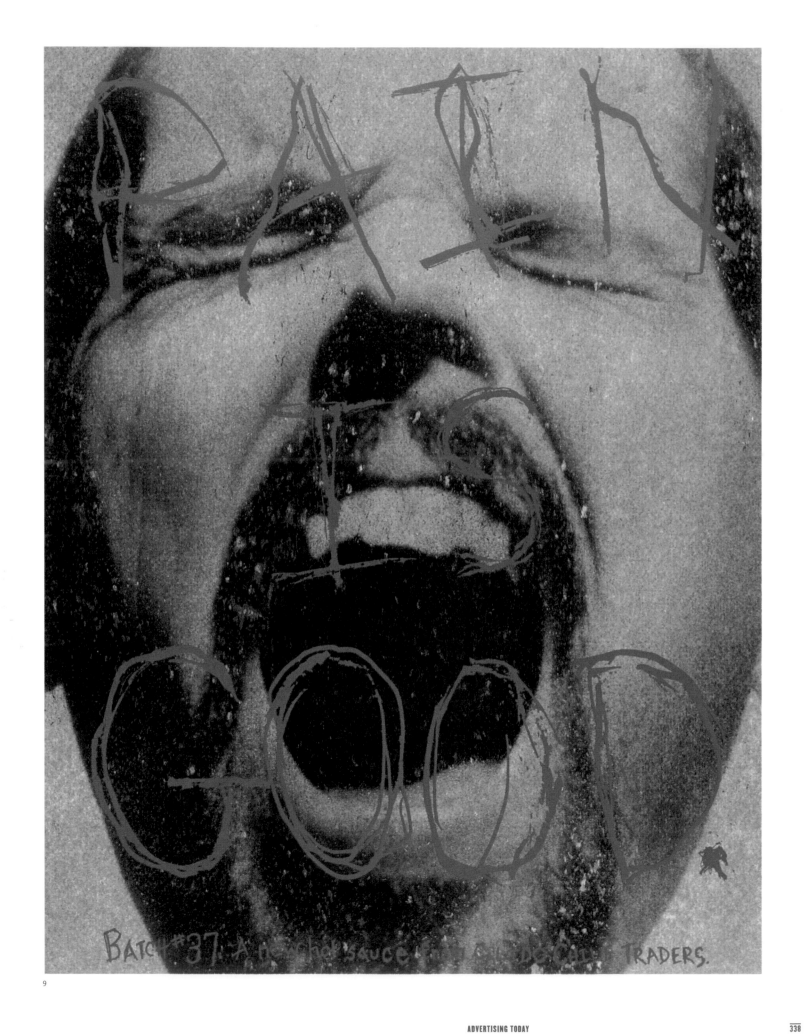

9

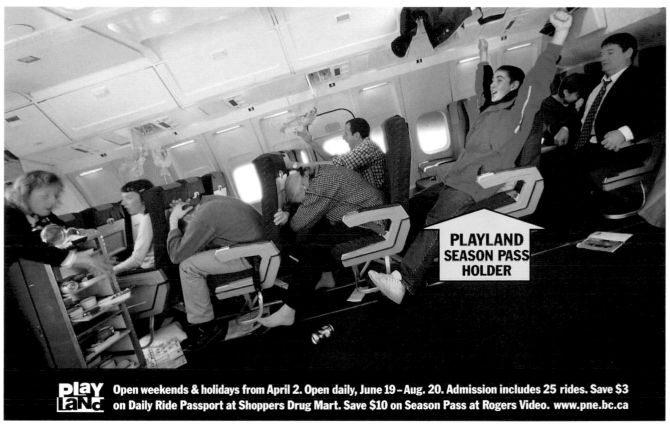

PLAYLAND SEASON PASS HOLDER

play land Open weekends & holidays from April 2. Open daily, June 19 – Aug. 20. Admission includes 25 rides. Save $3 on Daily Ride Passport at Shoppers Drug Mart. Save $10 on Season Pass at Rogers Video. www.pne.bc.ca

10

9. **CALIDO HOT SAUCE**
CORE, ST. LOUIS, MISSOURI,
1994
"Pain is good," this ad insisted;
when you feel your mouth on
fire, you know you're alive.

10. **PLAYLAND**
PALMER JARVIS DDB,
VANCOUVER, 1999
In "have no fear" advertising,
being a little crazy is encouraged;
it can help you enjoy life's twists
and turns.

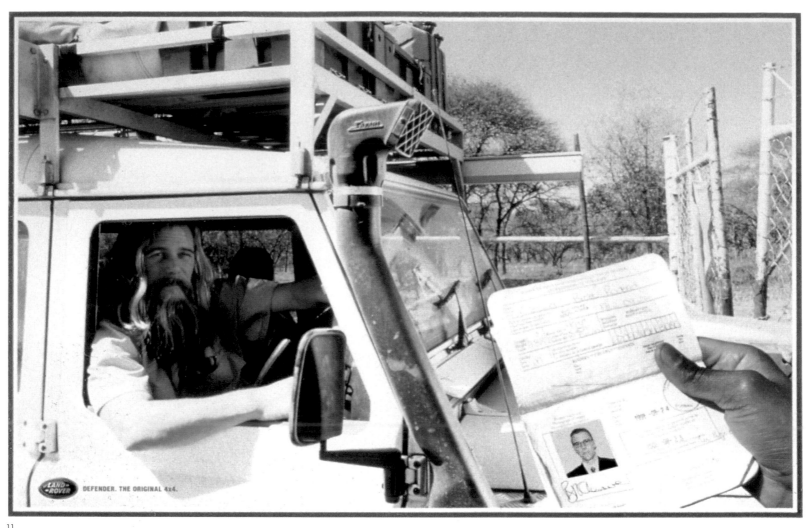

11

extends beyond taking entrepreneurial chances or dressing differently, and encompasses a whole lifestyle of risk-taking. Jumping off cliffs, braving storms, riding a jeep into untamed territories: These are the challenges that today's advertisers lay before us, like a dare. The big question: Do you have the guts? (After which comes the follow-up question: If you have the guts, do you have the right tires?)

This relatively new strain of kamikaze advertising is partly an outgrowth of the adventure-seeking culture that has evolved in recent years. Julian says today's thrill-seekers "want to experience something so pure that they're much more willing to take risks." And each adventure or experience they live through becomes a social "badge of accomplishment" that can be proudly shown off to others, Julian notes. Meanwhile, ads are offering the encouragement and the road map to adventure. New-millennium advertising has been filled with scenes of people skydiving or jumping off cliffs—

and the participants aren't just wild teenagers. A commercial for the Best Western hotel chain featured an older woman gleefully throwing herself from atop a waterfall because, the ad explained, "you always promised yourself you would." The promise of many of these ads is that "what doesn't kill us will make us stronger."

It's a philosophy that is being espoused by all sorts of product advertisers looking to jump on the "extreme" bandwagon, from a jeans company in Argentina (the brand, Nasa, takes this to a sadistic level with imagery of a bound woman and the headline "Face the pain, don't live in fear of it") to a hot-sauce-maker in the American heartland ("Pain is good," blared the headline of a condiment ad created by the St. Louis agency CORE). Not surprisingly, thrillseeker ads are particularly popular among advertisers peddling adventure-related products, including hiking boots, all-weather jackets, and of course, the sport-utility vehicle—presented in ads as the great

getaway machine, enabling us to break the boundaries of civilized life and explore the unknown. The former ad creator-turned-ad critic Jelly Helm has suggested that the fantasies spun in SUV ads border on recklessness by encouraging suburbanites to buy gas-guzzling trucks that end up being used to simply tool around the suburbs—at a higher cost to both the consumer and the environment. In such ads, "mountains and forests are playgrounds and racetracks for your cars," Helm says. "The entire world is an amusement park in which every natural object or creature exists in order to scratch whatever itch you want."

3. JUST BE YOURSELF.

In writing a Nike campaign of the early 1990s targeted at women, the Wieden + Kennedy copywriter Janet Champ began one ad with the line "You do not have to be your mother." If that sounded like something a psychiatrist might say to a patient on the couch, it was in some ways characteristic

It's what separates us from the animals.

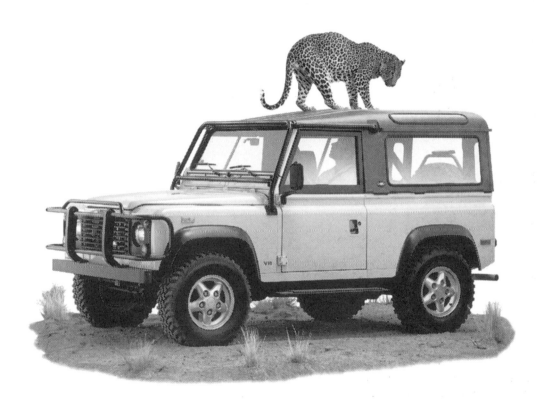

LAND ROVER **DEFENDER 90**

12

11. LAND ROVER
TBWA HUNT LASCARIS,
JOHANNESBURG, 2000
Reinvent yourself: This
adventurer crosses borders
and identities, thwarting a
customs official attempting
to read his passport.

12. LAND ROVER
GRACE & ROTHSCHILD,
NEW YORK, 1995
Not surprisingly, marketers of
sport-utility vehicles use ads
to encourage exploration and
adventure, even though the
typical SUV owner seems rarely
to venture beyond familiar suburban territory.

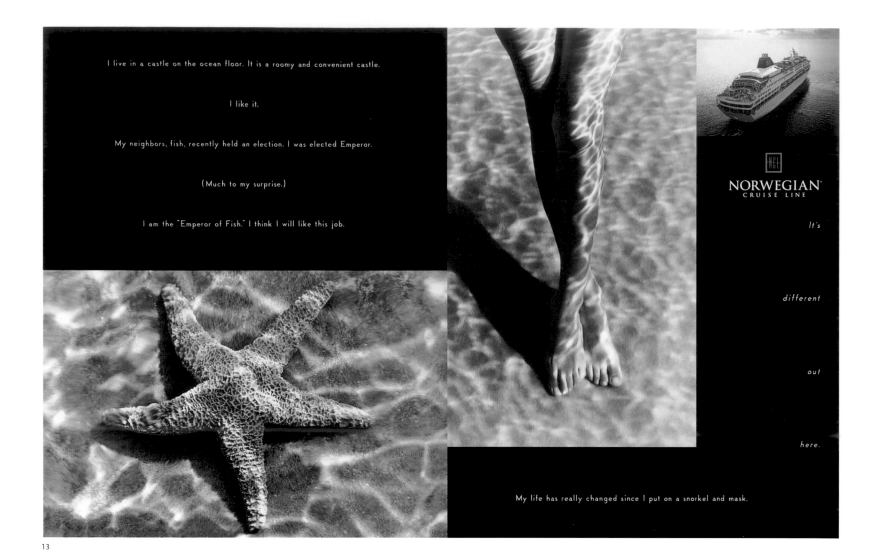

I live in a castle on the ocean floor. It is a roomy and convenient castle.

I like it.

My neighbors, fish, recently held an election. I was elected Emperor.

(Much to my surprise.)

I am the "Emperor of Fish." I think I will like this job.

NORWEGIAN
CRUISE LINE

It's

different

out

here.

My life has really changed since I put on a snorkel and mask.

13

13. NORWEGIAN CRUISE LINE
GOODBY SILVERSTEIN &
PARTNERS, SAN FRANCISCO,
1994
The sensuous ads suggested
that people could shed their
everyday inhibitions out on the
ocean, where the laws of the
land do not apply.

14. NIKE
WIEDEN + KENNEDY,
PORTLAND, 1991
You are not a goddess, and
you're not your mother. Nike's
early-1990s ads urged women to
forget about the expectations
of others.

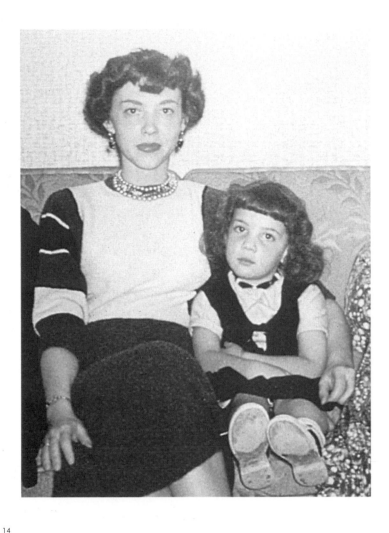

YOU DO NOT HAVE TO BE YOUR MOTHER UNLESS SHE IS WHO YOU WANT TO BE. YOU DO NOT HAVE TO BE YOUR MOTHER'S MOTHER, OR YOUR MOTHER'S MOTHER'S MOTHER, OR EVEN YOUR GRANDMOTHER'S MOTHER ON YOUR FATHER'S SIDE. YOU MAY INHERIT THEIR CHINS OR THEIR HIPS OR THEIR EYES, BUT YOU ARE NOT DESTINED TO BECOME THE WOMEN WHO CAME BEFORE YOU, YOU ARE NOT DESTINED TO LIVE THEIR LIVES. SO IF YOU INHERIT SOMETHING, INHERIT THEIR STRENGTH. IF YOU INHERIT SOMETHING, IN-HERIT THEIR RESILIENCE. BECAUSE THE ONLY PERSON YOU ARE DESTINED TO BECOME IS THE PERSON YOU DECIDE TO BE.

14

of a reassuring and therapeutic message that advertising in the 1990s began to disseminate, particularly in ads aimed at women. The essence: Don't try to live up to other people's expectations; stop worrying about what others think of you; live life on your own terms.

To propagate such a message (even if cynics suspected it of being as coldly calculating as any other ad message) was almost a kind of heresy in women's advertising, which had for so long fostered the notion that women *should* live up to other people's standards of beauty or accomplish-ment. Champ and her partner on the campaign, Charlotte Moore, sensed that women were ready for a new kind of individualistic, empowering advertising—and they were right. The Nike women's campaign was heralded as revolutionary within the ad industry, and was embraced by women across America; after it first appeared, Nike was swamped with 100,000 letters, the most ever received for any of its ads. The campaign also

triggered a wave of copycat empowering women's ads by other advertisers, all sharing a similar "Feel good about yourself" theme.

It wasn't the first time advertising had tried to modernize its message to women, but previous attempts at faux-feminist ads had been strident and sometimes woefully off-key. In the late 1970s and early 1980s, as advertisers projected unrealistic images of "Superwomen" who effortlessly balanced career and family life, looking sexy all the while, they only exacer-bated that old Madison Avenue problem of holding women to impossible and ridiculous standards. One of the more memorable misfires was a ludicrous 1980 commercial for Revlon's fragrance Enjoli, depicting a woman who could, according to the sultry theme song, "bring home the bacon . . . fry it up in the pan . . . and never let you forget you're a man." In contrast, the campaign from Champ and Moore took a distinct anti-Superwoman approach;

one ad, in fact, bore the headline "You are not a goddess."

In the years since the Nike campaign broke, many other advertisers have come up with their own versions of the "Be comfortable with yourself" message. Another athletic-shoe company, Avia, advised women, "The only competition is yourself." More recently, an ad for Sephora, a luxury-cosmetics-and-fragrances retailer, asked, "Have you ever wondered what other people see? Does it really matter?" And a striking Canadian ad campaign for Special K cereal urged women to be comfortable with their own bodies via a series of ads that ridiculed fashion designers and anorexic models. One ad showed a well-propor-tioned woman standing next to a pudgy man, with the headline "Ironically, she's the one who's worried about her weight." The ad went on to advise women to "Look good on your own terms." Of course, it also squeezed in a plug for Special K, which might, in the views of some,

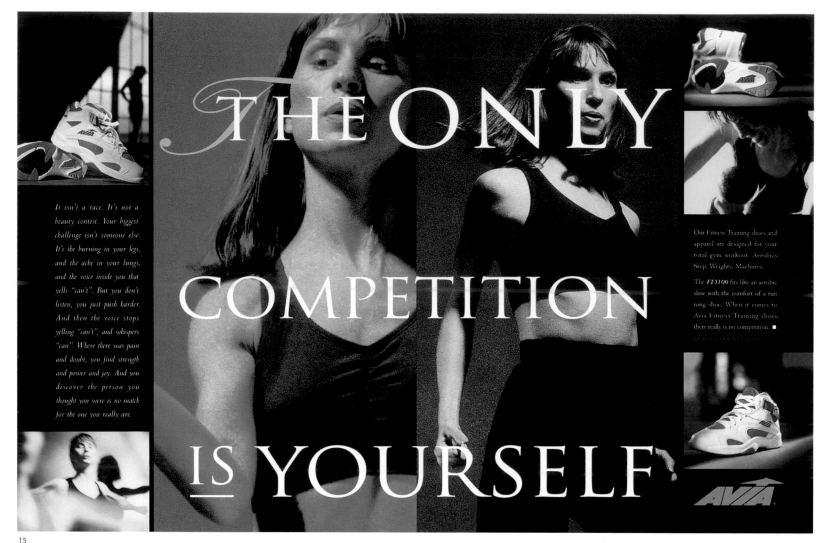

It isn't a race. It's not a beauty contest. Your biggest challenge isn't someone else. It's the burning in your legs, and the ache in your lungs, and the voice inside you that yells "can't". But you don't listen, you just push harder. And then the voice stops yelling "can't", and whispers "can". Where there was pain and doubt, you find strength and power and joy. And you discover the person you thought you were is no match for the one you really are.

THE ONLY COMPETITION IS YOURSELF

Our Fitness Training shoes and apparel are designed for your total gym workout. Aerobics. Step. Weights. Machines.

The *FT5100* fits like an aerobic shoe with the comfort of a running shoe. When it comes to Avia Fitness Training shoes, there really is no competition. ■

15

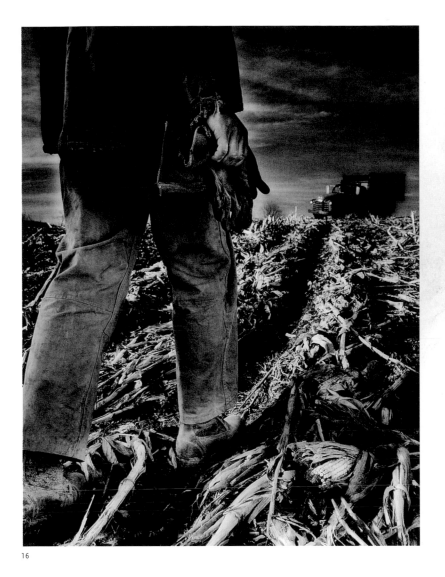

16

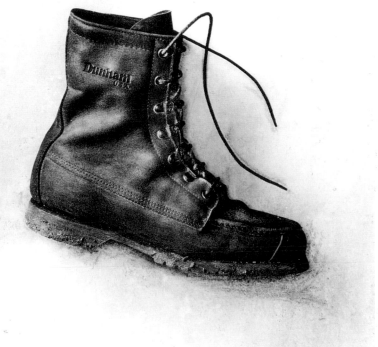

There are feet that have never seen a David Hockney. There are feet
that have never walked the streets of Cannes. There are feet unfamiliar with
beluga at midnight. Dunham. They get the job done.

15. AVIA
CITRON HALIGMAN
BEDECARRE, SAN FRANCISCO,
1993
Nike's empowerment theme
was picked up by many other
advertisers, particularly in the
athletic wear category.

16. DUNHAM BOOTS
DOYLE ADVERTISING &
DESIGN, BOSTON, 1990
While ads urged women to be
themselves, they called on men
to "get real," and to choose
authenticity over superficiality
or fads.

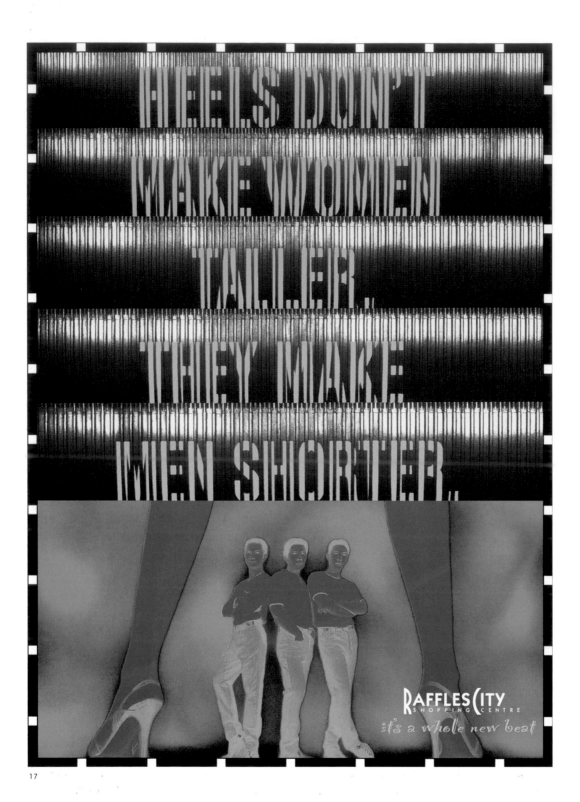

17

17. **RAFFLES CITY
SHOPPING CENTRE**
LEO BURNETT, SINGAPORE,
LATE 1990s
Ads that fostered group pride—
among women, men, or members
of ethnic groups—sometimes
took a good-humored "us-
against-them" tone.

18. **NORDSTROM**
FALLON McELLIGOTT,
MINNEAPOLIS, MINNESOTA,
2000
This campaign for an American
clothing store urged suburban
American "soccer moms" to
reinvent themselves via trendy
new shoes and garments.

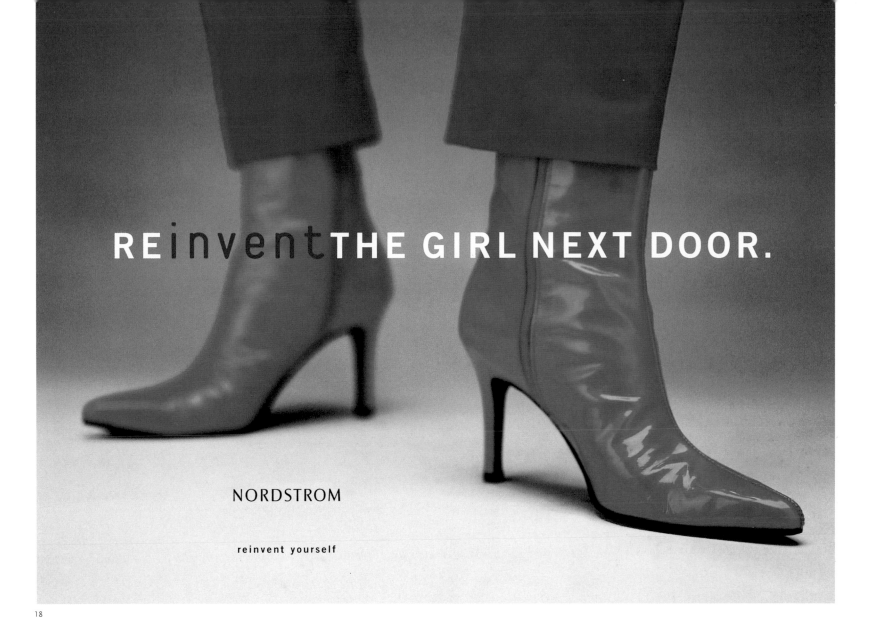

REinvent **THE GIRL NEXT DOOR.**

NORDSTROM

reinvent yourself

18

undercut the noble message slightly. Some critics have also suggested that empowering ads, for all their sensitivity and good intentions, can end up being condescending to women. Still, ads that encourage self-acceptance over the old self-loathing, and that replace the bacon-frying Superwoman with a realistic human being, must represent some kind of progress.

4. REINVENT YOURSELF.

This is, according to Syracuse University television professor Robert Thompson, "the first commandment of advertising, and always has been—the notion that you can change your life by way of a particular purchase." True, this message is not entirely new. But it may be more effective now than ever before—because many of today's consumers are predisposed to believe they can change their lives, and their identities, on an almost-daily basis. Fallon's Tom Julian points out that in today's culture of job-hopping, adventure-

seeking, Internet chat rooms, and diversified lifestyles, "people assume more identities than in the past." They're more flexible, more open to new experiences, and constantly eager to improve and enrich themselves, Julian noted. According to Iconoculture's research, many people today are refusing to be defined or limited by boundaries—whether physical, geographic, or age-related. "The popular thinking is that you can change your whole look with cosmetic surgery, or become a new person by taking kickboxing lessons," says Iconoculture's Larry Samuel. Advertising has helped to foster this new mind-set, consistently reassuring us that anyone can be anything. A "soccer mom" can reinvent herself as a hip woman of style, according to a Nordstrom campaign from Fallon; an aging baby boomer can feel like a kid with a rubber duck again, just by buying a Mercedes-Benz.

In some ads, reinvention of the self is linked to the notion of escape—the idea being that if you can just get away from your mundane surround-

ings, you'll discover another side of yourself. That was the essence of a brilliant Goodby Silverstein campaign for Norwegian Cruise Line. The lush, sensuous ads suggested that people could shed their everyday inhibitions—i.e., have more sex, for those not reading between the lines—by setting sail on the ocean, where the laws and restrictions and distractions of the land do not apply. Goodby's campaign was refreshingly candid in its acknowledgment that people tend to think of cruises as an opportunity to rekindle their sex lives; on the other hand, as ad executive Jack Supple of the Carmichael Lynch agency pointed out, the campaign may have been overpromising just a bit. "Will I really feel like being naked more on Norwegian Cruise Lines," Supple wondered, "or will I be fighting an old couple from Missouri for a deck chair?"

Ads also promise reinvention through the acquisition of instant wealth; the latter can come by way of savvy investment or just by playing the

WALK IN A DEMOCRAT.
WALK OUT A REPUBLICAN.

MYSTIC LAKE CASINO

19

19. MYSTIC LAKE CASINO
HUNT ADKINS,
MINNEAPOLIS, MINNESOTA,
1992
Nothing transforms a person
quite like instant wealth: this
wonderfully witty headline
is also a succinct lesson in
American politics.

20. BUDWEISER
DDB NEEDHAM, CHICAGO,
EARLY 1990s
In a popular series of commer-
cials from the early 1990s,
this character found himself
reinvented via mistaken identity.
Was he really rich and powerful?
"Yes I am!" he insisted.

lottery. In the classic commercial "Boardroom," created for the New York State Lottery by DDB Needham, we are introduced to Chuck, the mailroom clerk—who, after winning the lottery, turns the tables on his stodgy bosses and begins barking orders at them. Meanwhile, another advertisement, by the agency Hunt Adkins for Minnesota's Mystic Lake Casino, boiled the whole reinvention fantasy down to one extremely clever headline, which said simply, "Walk in a Democrat. Walk out a Republican."

If you're not lucky enough to win the jackpot, can't afford the sports car or the cruise or even the Nordstrom makeover, there is one other option—lie about yourself. That was the tack taken by a character in a series of humorous Bud Lite commercials from the mid-1990s. In a case of mistaken identity, the insignificant fellow was asked if he was a certain important and wealthy person, and he responded, with great conviction, "Yes, I am!" And off he rode in a

limousine, just another one of Madison Avenue's successful reinventions.

5. BE PROUD.

Faced with an increasingly multicultural society, advertisers have become adept at targeting consumers according to race, gender, age, ethnicity, and socioeconomic status. What has emerged is a new "tribal advertising"—which not only acknowledges diversity but celebrates it, urging consumers to identify with their own particular groups and take pride in them. As is often the case, advertisers putting forth this message are playing catch-up with social trends; group-identity politics has been gaining momentum on university campuses and in workplaces for years. "In society at large, the movement has been away from assimilation, and toward feeling proud of our own group's heritage and identity," says Iconoculture's Samuel. Still, for advertising to move in this direction took some

daring on the part of marketers—who were always more comfortable showing benign images of a homogenized society in which everyone played on the same team. The old approach was designed to appeal to the mainstream of society—the essence of mass marketing. The problem was, by the new millennium, there wasn't much of a "mass" to market to anymore, so advertisers had to begin to speak the language of each group.

Ads did this with some trepidation, because, as *New York Times* columnist Stuart Elliott noted, "sometimes members of minority groups appreciate it if an advertiser speaks to them in their own vernacular, but other times they may feel that it's pandering." McDonald's was among the first to use African-American slang in commercials whose characters referred to the restaurant as "Mickey D's"—a nickname that was first heard on the street, then incorporated into the ads. More recently, Budweiser achieved a cultural breakthrough with a humorous campaign

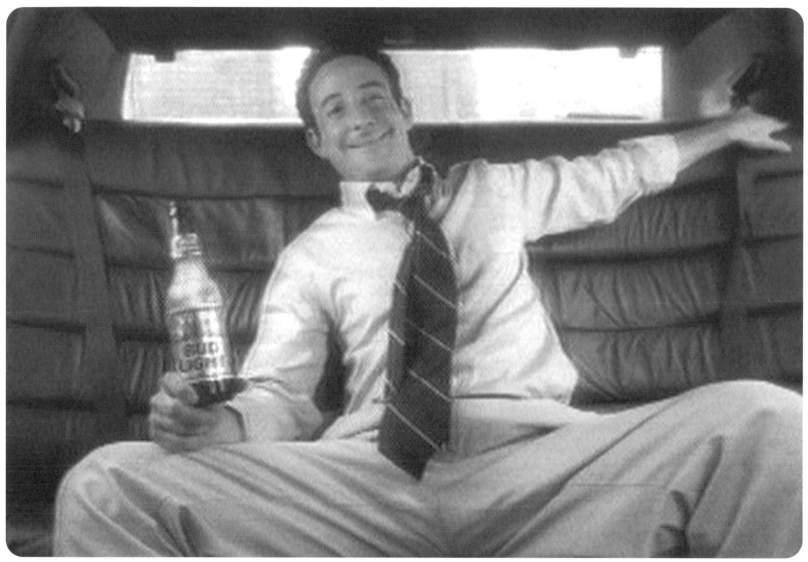

20

THE NEW COMMANDMENTS.

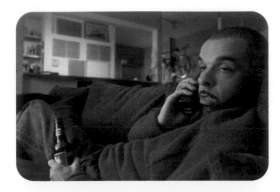

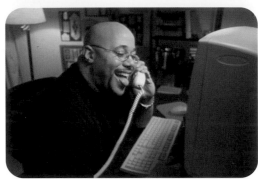

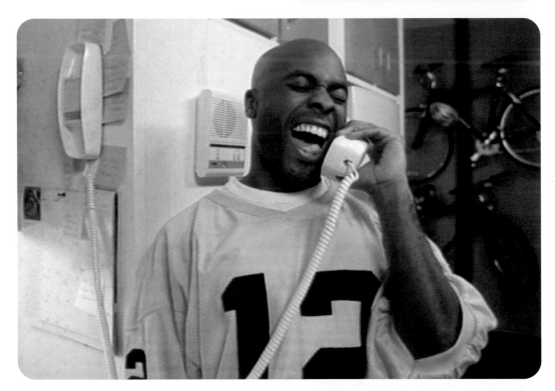

21

21. BUDWEISER
DDB WORLDWIDE, CHICAGO, 1999
Crossing the great divide in "group pride" advertising: The "Whassup?" campaign used an African-American expression, a question that was uttered again and again, with hilarious results. It achieved widespread mainstream popularity.

22. MILLER HIGH LIFE
WIEDEN + KENNEDY, PORTLAND, 1998
This campaign, artfully directed by Errol Morris, was a celebration of duct tape, greasy foods, and all things masculine.

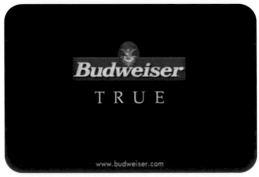

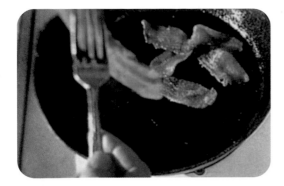

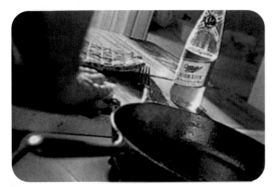

22

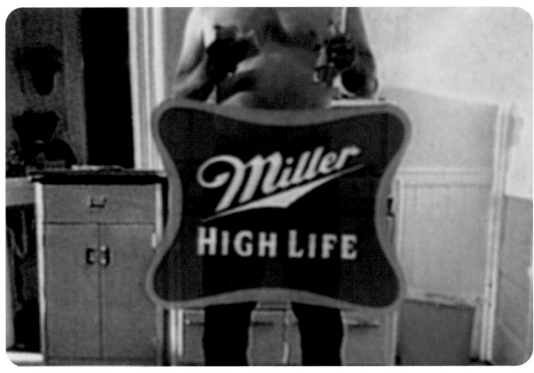

in which African-American characters use the expression "Whassup?" While the ads seemed to be targeted to a black audience, they played just as well with whites and other groups—eventually spawning fan clubs and Web sites. While the "Whassup?" commercials themselves are not deep (aside from the characters shouting the catchphrase to one another, not much happens in the ads), they may end up having a profound effect by demonstrating that ethnic advertising can have wide, across-the-board appeal. Similarly, advertisers have lately experimented with mainstream messages featuring apparently homosexual characters; a breakthrough spot was created by the agency Deutsch Inc., for the furniture retailer Ikea and showed two men shopping for furniture together. The commercial treated the subject with subtlety and humor, and proved to be one of the company's most popular ads.

While it's hard to find fault with advertising's long-overdue acknowledgment of the rich diversity in our midst, group-pride advertising can have its downside; at its worst, it can take on a divisive "us against them" tone. Recent ads targeted to blue-collar types have tended to sneer at yuppies; meanwhile, ads for the upper crust have been perhaps a little too candid in declaring that "greed is good." But the real battleground seems to be in gender-targeted advertising. The past few years have seen a spate of ads whose theme might be "It's good to be a guy." One campaign for Miller High Life, shot by the director Errol Morris, is a droll celebration of beer bellies, greasy hamburgers, duct tape, and other macho signifiers; the ads are stylish, self-aware, and funny, but still seem to have an edge of defensiveness. Other recent beer ads have shown men finding ways to trick women so they can avoid shopping or so they can watch football games without being nagged. Meanwhile, ads directed to women can be just as guilty of male-bashing; as Elliott noted, there has been a rash of them in

which women belittle men, and occasionally even whack them in the head. "It is becoming adversarial," Elliott noted. The newly aggressive "pride" message has even filtered down to little girls and Barbie, whose recent campaign declared, "Girls rule!"

6. GET REAL.

The quest for authenticity has become a near-obsession for marketers and their customers. The more that store shelves are packed with product knockoffs and look-alikes, the greater the appeal of those that can claim to be "the original" or "the real thing." Iconoculture's research has found that today's consumer is inclined to choose highly advertised products because they reinforce the feeling of being an individualist, the person who won't settle for generic products like everyone else. Of course, that's not entirely logical—choosing the original, best-known brand could actually be considered more conformist than experimenting with a no-name brand. But the "get real" ads make

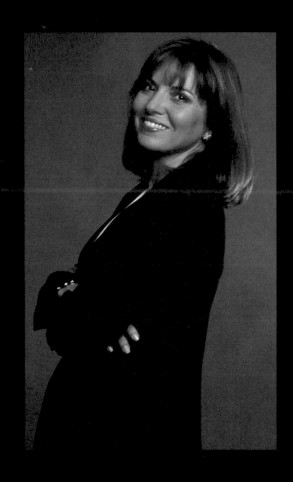

INTERVIEW: ANITA SANTIAGO

Anita Santiago's Los Angeles–based ad agency is one of the top specialists in the exploding field of ethnic advertising, which customizes and targets ads to various minority groups. In particular, Santiago helps advertisers tap into a Hispanic consumer market that spends an estimated $440 billion a year. She brings an interesting background (she started out writing TV soap operas in Venezuela), a keen understanding of Latin culture, and a master's degree in clinical psychology to her work for such clients as Wells Fargo Bank and the California Milk Board.

HOW HAS HISPANIC ADVERTISING EVOLVED?
I've been in the Hispanic ad market since the early 1980s, before it was really on the radar of major advertisers. Back then, it was a very minimal effort. It's now more sophisticated, with more strategic thought behind the message, and the production values are way up—because there's more money behind it now.

IN THIS CHAPTER, WE'RE LOOKING AT SOME OF THE PSYCHOLOGY DRIVING MODERN ADS, INCLUDING NEW COMMANDS LIKE "BREAK THE RULES." WHY DO YOU THINK THAT KIND OF MESSAGE IS RESONATING RIGHT NOW?
I think it's because such a huge portion of the American population—and the ones with so much of the real power right now—are baby boomers. And advertisers have analyzed the mind-set of the boomer and found someone who's accomplished, who's been at a job for a long time and maybe is tired of following the same routine. I do think the rich part of the U.S. population is going through midlife crises—and those crises are about who you are and who you want to be in society. That's why you see so much "Break the rules" and "Have no fear" and "Control your own destiny." It's because a lot of boomers are almost going through a second childhood right now.

DO THE SAME THEMES AND MESSAGES WORK IN THE HISPANIC MARKET?
No, not really. The mainstream American market is very individualistic. The average Anglo person in this country is out to make a name for him- or herself, and a career, and achieve his or her own goals. But in the Latin communities,

it's not so much about *me, me, me*—it's *us*. And people actually give up their own goals for the benefit of the larger community. Because of that, many of these themes, like "Break the rules," don't really work that well with this community. That rebel message represents too much of the me-oriented way of thinking. What connects much better with the Hispanic audience is something like "Show me how to better my lifestyle. Tell me what to do so I can work with this culture, your culture, so that I can improve my lifestyle — that's what I'm here for. And also, let me know that I'm welcome."

WE'RE ALSO SEEING A LOT OF ADS THAT URGE US TO "BE PROUD" OF OUR GROUP—WHETHER THE GROUP IS MEN, WOMEN, AFRICAN-AMERICANS, JOGGERS, YOU NAME IT. DOES THAT RESONATE WITH THE HISPANIC MARKET?
Well, there is a lot of pride in Hispanic heritage. But it's not really a matter of coming out and saying, "Hey, I'm proud to be Hispanic." It's more about taking pride in one's accomplishments. For example, you might see an ad with a father handing the car keys to a son—and that says a lot about how you've bettered your lifestyle and that you care for your family. Successful Hispanic advertising tends to be very aspirational and also emotional. You're less likely to see the kind of cool, sarcastic advertising you see for the Anglo audience now—that approach doesn't fly too well.

SHIFTING TO A DIFFERENT TARGET GROUP, WHAT DO YOU THINK ABOUT SOME OF THE CHANGES WE'VE SEEN IN ADVERTISING TO WOMEN IN RECENT YEARS—SPECIFICALLY, THE KIND OF "EMPOWERING" IMAGES AND MESSAGES PUT OUT THERE BY NIKE AND OTHERS?
I think it's been a great thing because it really did begin to focus ads on women's uniqueness. However, once again, the "women's empowerment" theme is a very Anglo message and doesn't really ring a bell in the Hispanic market. Hispanic women have a different mind-set— and, of course, I'm generalizing here. But if you tend to have more of an "us"-oriented way of thinking, then as a woman you don't want to separate yourself from family and talk about "doing my own thing." People in the Hispanic culture tend to set their own goals within the

landscape of family goals. The empowering message—"I am woman"—has an attitude that can be almost divisive. And that's not the attitude this audience responds to.

BY THE WAY, WHY DON'T WE SEE MORE FEMALE CREATIVE EXECUTIVES IN ADVERTISING?
I go back to my own experience starting as a copywriter, trying to rise up in this business. The battle was so intense to get your thoughts and concepts heard within a world of men. It is a very competitive, rough arena—and it's one in which you are exposed to ridicule. In advertising, anything you do creatively has to be put on the line, usually in front of a roomful of men, who will often shoot it down. And as a woman in these groups, you always run the risk of being perceived as a lightweight, so that adds to the pressure. I think all of this turns off some creative women—they might have great ideas and skills, but they don't want to deal with that part of the process.

ARE THERE ANY PRODUCTS YOU REFUSE TO ADVERTISE TO YOUR OWN ETHNIC COMMUNITY?
The beer companies are always waving offers under our noses, and we've turned down millions of dollars in business there—we just won't do it. Not because I don't drink beer and like beer, but I don't want to use my skills to do that, because I know I could sell a heck of a lot of it, and I'm aware of the problems it can cause. And the same with cigarettes; we won't do it—in fact, we did the first Hispanic anti-smoking ads in California. Turning down these products has probably slowed the agency's growth a little. But at least we sleep at night.

plane tickets to the town where she was born: $1,200

train to the house where she grew up: $63

pints at the pub where she met your dad: $8

finally understanding where your mother was coming from:

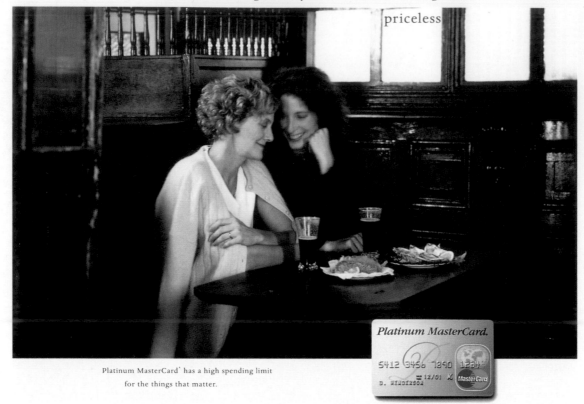

priceless

Platinum MasterCard® has a high spending limit
for the things that matter.

there are some things money can't buy.
for everything else there's MasterCard.™

23

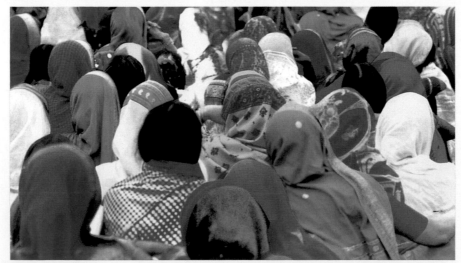

भारत तेरा रंग कैसा ?   पक्का. एरियल के वादे जैसा !

24

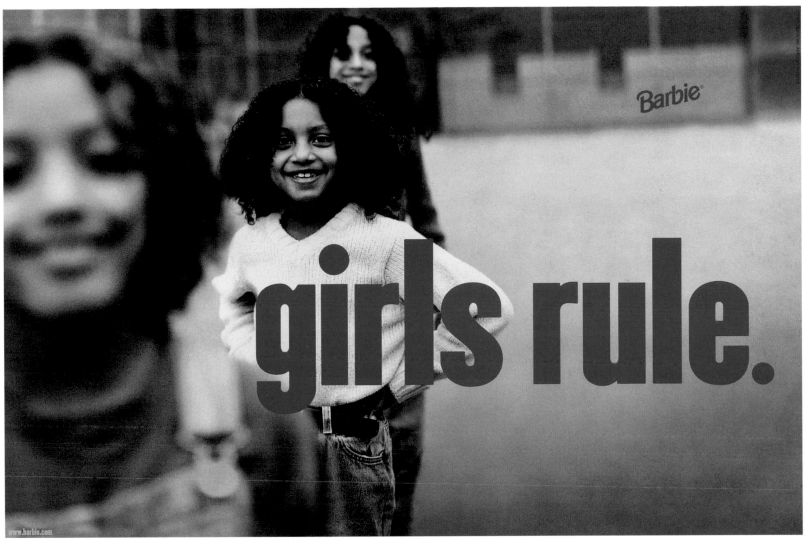

23. **MASTERCARD**
McCANN-ERICKSON,
NEW YORK, 1998
Prioritize your life: The "Priceless" campaign encouraged us to place a value on what is really important—even if it means using a credit card to do so.

24. **ARIEL**
LEO BURNETT, MUMBAI, 1997
The "break the rules" theme wasn't just a Western phenomenon; this ad from India for household detergent shows a woman standing out from the pack by slipping off her head-scarf.

25. **BARBIE**
OGILVY & MATHER,
NEW YORK, 1998
This ad declares that even little girls can be empowered, and that Barbie dolls (somehow) stand behind them.

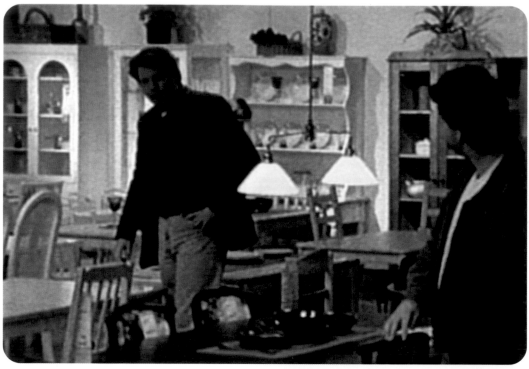

26

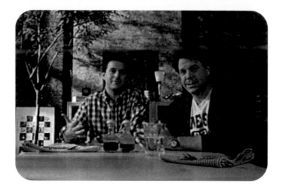

sure our thoughts don't stray down this path; they do their best to forge the associative link between "real" products and "real" people.

But how does a brand prove it's the real thing? One approach is to trot out the advertising-embellished history of the company, which may take the form of sepia-toned ads showing old bearded fellows from another era, perhaps cobbling shoes by hand; it's the most literal way to say "We're the original," but it's also, frankly, unoriginal. A more popular approach these days is to focus on the customer—not just any customer but a particular subset, the die-hard fanatic. Harley-Davidson sells its authenticity by populating its ads with Hell's Angel–type bikers, who wouldn't be caught dead on anything else; they may not be the most glamorous ad models, but they reek authenticity. Finally, some ads demonstrate the brand's authenticity by taking a down-and-dirty, we-don't-give-a-damn approach. Everlast got rid of the phony models in its ads and showed the

product in nonglamorous ways (such as showing a pair of Everlast shorts on a bird's legs). The unspoken message: We're too "legit" to pitch.

7. DON'T BELIEVE THE HYPE.

When the need to seem authentic collides with postmodernism, the result is this: advertising messages that urge us to disregard advertising messages. As described in Chapter 5, the past decade has seen the rise of a whole new genre of ironic, self-referential advertising that often mocks ad conventions; when done with a light touch, as in Wieden + Kennedy's early innovative work for Nike, the result can be engaging. But when "Don't believe the hype" is fairly screamed at the audience as a command, it tends to become, in effect, more hype. One of the leading proponents of this approach has been the soft drink Sprite, whose advertising campaign actually uses another command, "Obey your thirst," as its tag line. But the real point of the Sprite ads is to attack

advertising. The ads make fun of feel-good, overpromising commercials; they mock actors who affect street mannerisms, and they even ridicule one of advertising's most valuable tools, the athlete endorser (a commercial featuring the basketball star Grant Hill shows visions of dollar signs in his head as he does an advertising pitch). Rogier van Bakel, the editor of *Creativity* magazine, describes this approach as "advertising biting itself in the tail and chomping down hard. No one knows where it will end." As van Bakel points out, "this style of advertising plays on cynical, weary anti-advertising sentiments," but at the same time, "it only adds another layer of consumer cynicism. It confirms consumers' perception that advertisers are cunning salesmen who'll say just about anything—including anything 'self-deprecating'—to make a buck." Still, he adds, for the time being, "these messages seem to work quite nicely because they're paying consumers a compliment for being media-savvy 'individualists.'"

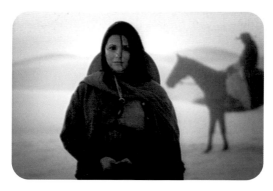

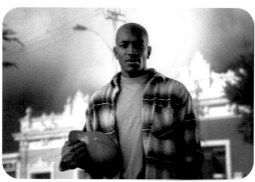

26. IKEA
DEUTSCH INC., NEW YORK,
1994
In rare instances, group pride
ads extended to gays. Deutsch
took a bold step forward when it
featured male living companions
in this mid-1990s commercial.

27. CISCO SYSTEMS
GOLDBERG MOSER O'NEIL,
SAN FRANCISCO, 1999
"Plug in," was the message
from the technology companies,
who promised that the Internet
would solve all of the world's
problems. This ad asked: "Are
you ready?"

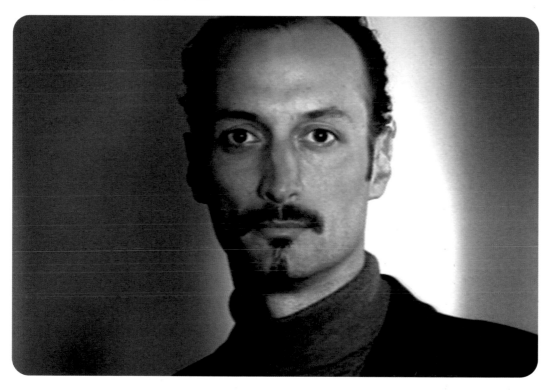

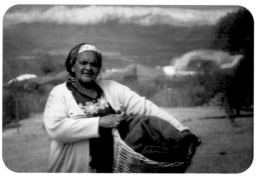

27

If your broker's so great, how come he still has to work?

It's time for 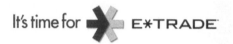 E✴TRADE

28

8. PLUG IN.

If there is any category of advertising that should come with a "Don't believe the hype" warning label, it is high technology. In this sector, advertising seems to be irony-free; on the contrary, ads for Internet-related technology have tended to be earnest and full of grand promises. Giant high-tech companies like Microsoft, Cisco Systems, and Nortel have used their ads to assure us that the Internet will soon solve all of the world's problems, provide equal education to everyone, and, in case that's not enough, enable us "to see every movie, ever made, any time of day or night" (a line from a popular commercial for Qwest broadband information networks). Sometimes this message is delivered by the industry's gods themselves: Microsoft chief Bill Gates recently appeared in his own ads promising "the best is yet to come," and that new technology will "anticipate your needs" and "help your children learn." For those who are just lonely and misunderstood, the Internet can

solve that problem, too; log on to Yahoo!, the company's ads show us, and you can search for kindred spirits who share your appreciation of punk rock and quilt-weaving.

Of course, to take advantage of all these wonders, you must "get wired"—hardware, software, high-speed modem, broadband Internet service connection (no one said admission to utopia would be cheap). And the unspoken warning from technology advertising is that if you're not quick about it, you'll fall hopelessly behind everyone else. "The message is 'Your life will be empty and meaningless unless you get on board the technology train,'" observes Helm, because "you are not only deprived of very cool stuff, but your relationships lack meaning, you are less fulfilled as a person, and you are not able to achieve all that you're capable of."

9. PRIORITIZE YOUR LIFE.

There's a problem with being so plugged-in,

empowered, and adventurous—you may become overwhelmed by your own life. Addressing this potential hazard is a series of ads that encourage us to always remember what's important: family, friends, helping the poor, relaxing with a cup of Maxwell House International Blend coffee. For those who have trouble sorting out what's really important and what isn't, a recent campaign for MasterCard, by the agency McCann-Erickson, helpfully offered a kind of valuation chart; in the ads, everyday activities like going to a ball game with the kids are deconstructed, with price tags flashed onscreen for each part of the experience (buying the tickets, the hot dog, etc.); the spots end by pointing that the most important part of the experience—seeing your son enjoy his first ball game—is, of course, "priceless."

One of the curious aspects of "Prioritize your life" ads is that they seem to be advocating a return to simplicity—but at the same time, they add to our collective stress overload by reminding

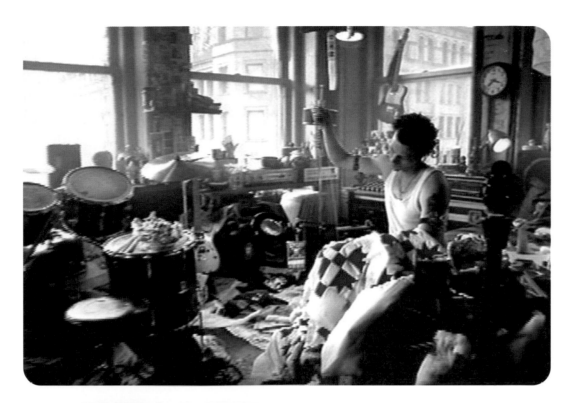

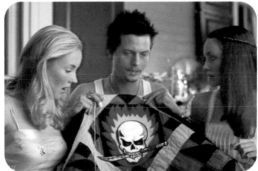

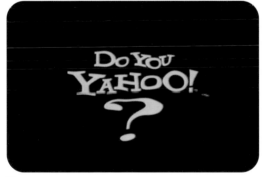

29

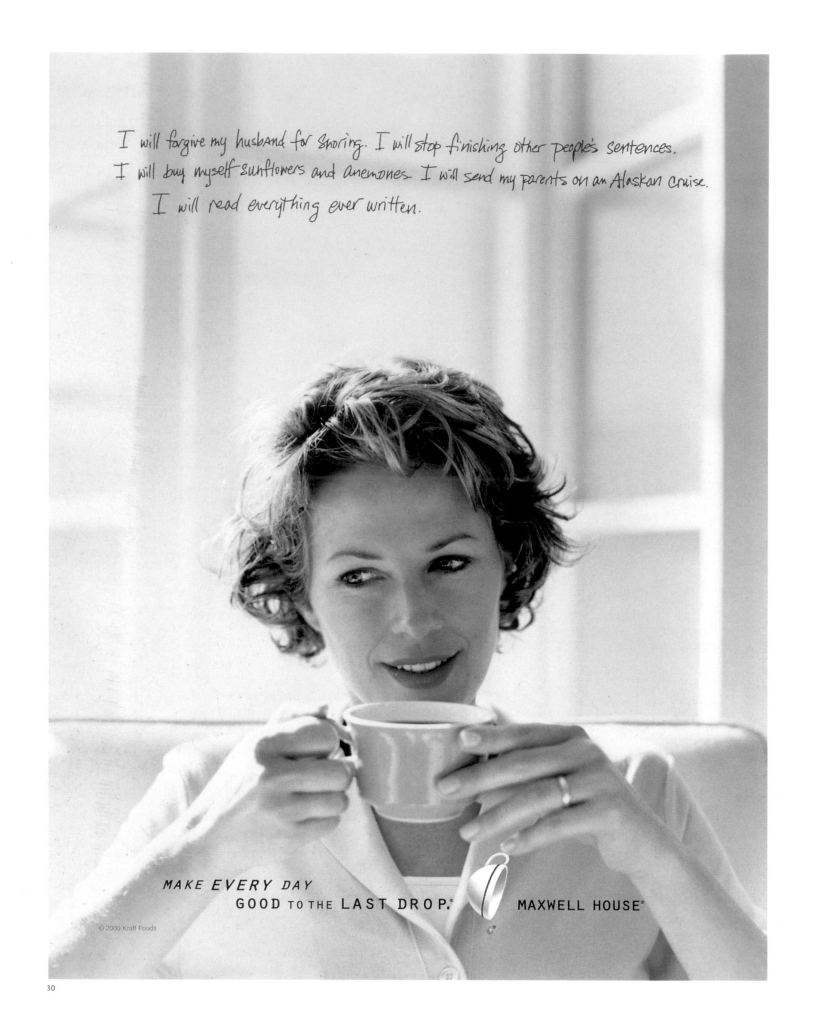

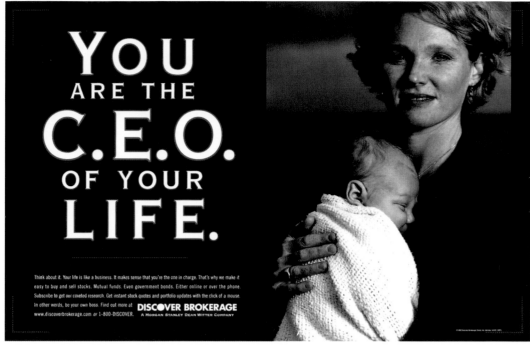

31

30. **MAXWELL HOUSE**
OGILVY & MATHER,
NEW YORK, 2000
Prioritizing your life can get
complicated; the woman in
this ad takes a coffee break to
mentally review her to-do list.

31. **DISCOVER BROKERAGE**
BLACK ROCKET,
SAN FRANCISCO, 1998
"Be your own boss," this ad
advises, appealing to the
corporate woman of the 1990s,
who balances career, home,
and family in affluent times.

us there are so many important things we should be doing. Some ads have even taken to printing "to do" lists for us. A recent Maxwell House ad features an Everywoman character who is shown thinking, "I will forgive my husband for snoring. I will stop finishing other people's sentences. . . . I will send my parents on an Alaskan cruise. I will read everything ever written." She'd better put down that coffee and get started.

10. CONTROL YOUR OWN DESTINY.

The last and most important thing advertisers would like us to realize is this: In today's every-man-for-himself world, you can't count on anyone or anything except yourself (and also the product being advertised). This is another variation of the "Go your own way" theme, but it specifically plays to growing concerns that we can no longer count on employers or government programs or hired financial experts to take care of us or guide us— we must do for ourselves. Iconoculture's Samuel

calls this the "free-agent mentality," and one of its preoccupations is the building of a nest egg that will provide for the individual when all else fails. How do you build the nest egg? If you are a free agent, "you're not going to do what some financial analyst might tell you—better to trust yourself and become your own day trader," noted Samuel. Cheering on the free agent is today's advertiser, with slogans like the Ameritrade line "Believe in yourself." Another on-line-trading company, E*Trade, created an ad campaign that told people to "fire your broker." (E*Trade's logic seemed pretty sound: "If your broker's so great," the ads wondered, "how come he still has to work?")

The ads for on-line trading certainly seem to be "empowering," but they've also come under fire for encouraging people to think of stock trading as a get-rich-quick option. E*Trade's agency, Goodby Silverstein, tried to counter some of this criticism recently by creating an ad in which a day trader sees his stock portfolio skyrocket and

promptly marches in to his boss to quit his job; by the time he gets back to his desk, his stocks have plummeted, forcing him to march back into the boss's office, full of apologies. But that message—suggesting that a real job with a real boss may actually be worth hanging on to—is an aberration in the ads of the free-agency world. More typical is the campaign for Discover Brokerage, which is headlined, "You are the C.E.O. of your life." The copy reads, "Your life is like a business. It makes sense that you're the one in charge." And it concludes with the words "Be your own boss." That was an appropriate message for the roaring late 1990s, but as the economy began to sputter early in the new century, one had to wonder: Where will the advertisers` who urged us to "go for it" be found as stocks crash and businesses fail? No doubt they are already crafting a fresh set of commandments for harder times, with a newly cautious tone: "Think safety." "Don't blow it." "Just watch it."

THE NEW COMMANDMENTS.

11. DREAMS

EAM.

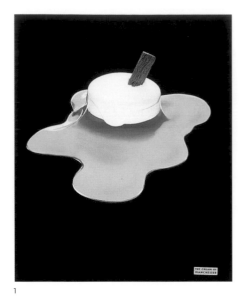

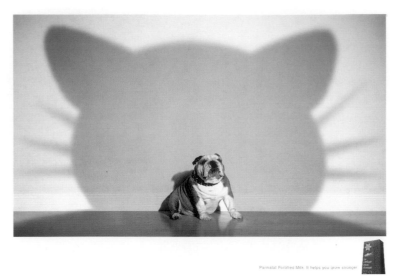

1. BODDINGTONS BEER
BARTLE BOGLE HEGARTY,
LONDON, 1997–98
To emphasize the creamy quality
of this beer, the basic beer glass
was transformed into various
images suggesting different
types of cream; UK readers
enjoyed playing along.

2. PARMALAT MILK
DM9 DDB PUBLICIDADE,
SÃO PAULO, 1999
Wordless ads playfully exaggera-
ted the power of milk; one series
featured dogs terrorized by cats
made enormous from drinking
Parmalat's high-nutrient blend.

3. CALIFORNIA MILK BOARD
GOODBY SILVERSTEIN &
PARTNERS, SAN FRANCISCO,
1995
This image became one of the
most popular in the campaign;
you can almost hear the cats
crying out for milk.

A great many advertisements come and go, unnoticed. A far smaller number of ads do slightly better than that, generating a brief blip on the cultural radar screen. And then there is that rarest of advertising miracles: the ad campaign that becomes a phenomenon, that permeates the culture down to the grassroots, lasts for years, and, even after it is gone, leaves a mark on the public consciousness. The creation of such ad campaigns is what brand marketers and ad creators lust after. But how does it come about?

To some extent, it is magic and dumb luck. But not entirely. Look closely at the making of any breakthrough ad campaign and you'll usually find there were critical ingredients and particular processes that had to be in place before the magic could occur. Often, it all begins with mind-reading: arcane, meticulous research that probes public attitudes, beliefs, and desires with regard to a particular product.

If the researchers are both good and fortunate, they may derive from this a key insight— a revelation of how people really feel about a product or an activity—that can help start the campaign on the right track. Then comes the hard part: A flash of inspiration is needed, a big idea that somehow speaks to these deep feelings of the audience but does so in a manner that is both original and intriguing. Even if the big flash occurs (and ad creators acknowledge that often, it never does), that's just another starting point; the idea must be sold to clients who are in need of original thinking yet at the same time tend to fear it. Then it must be executed in a way that brings the idea to life. And then it must be released upon the world in a manner that ensures it won't be simply ignored, like so much advertising. What happens after that is beyond the control of the ad creators or anyone else; it is at this point that the whims of the

zeitgeist take over. All the creators can do is wait and watch, to see if their idea is soon being discussed at water coolers and in pubs, joked about on the late-night talk shows, worn on T-shirts, lauded in the press, analyzed by academics, showered with awards. And even if all of that happens, it still won't mean a thing unless the campaign also causes the advertised product to sell like hotcakes.

During the past decade, not many ad campaigns have met all of these challenges. One that has is the California Milk Board series of ads from the San Francisco agency Goodby, Silverstein & Partners, which turned the simple question "Got Milk?" into one of advertising's most popular and powerful catchphrases. On the other side of the world, a separate and very different milk ad campaign created by the Brazilian ad agency DM9 DDB Publicidade, for the dairy company Parmalat, triggered a public

got milk?™

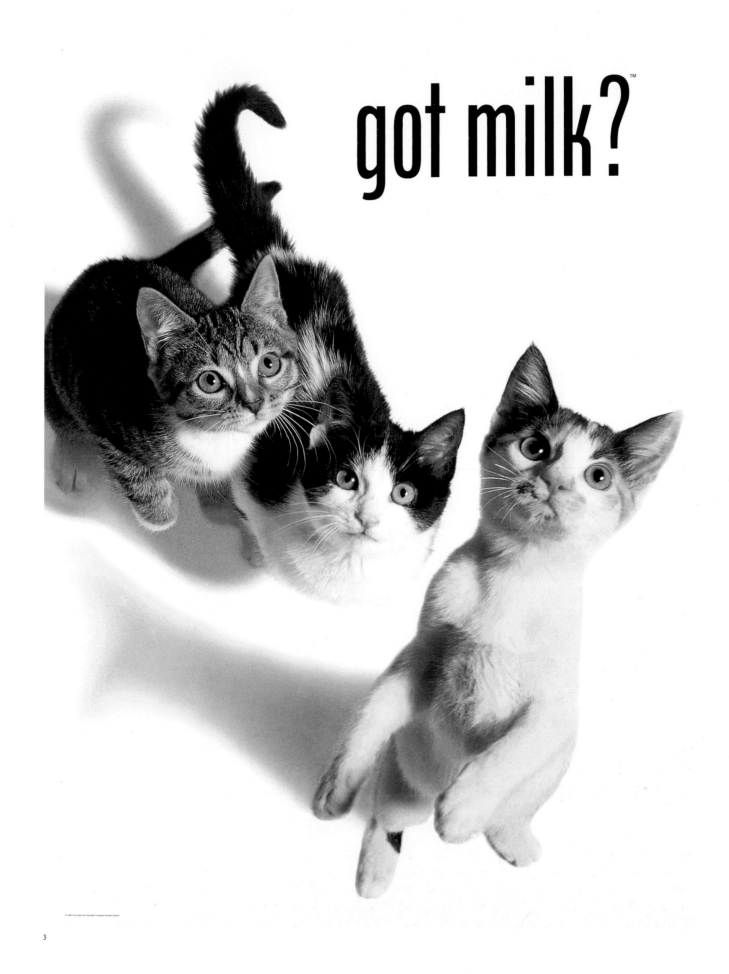

3

DREAMS OF CREAM.

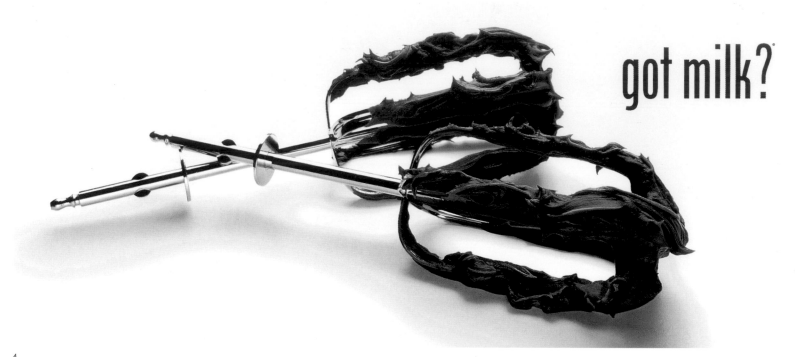

4

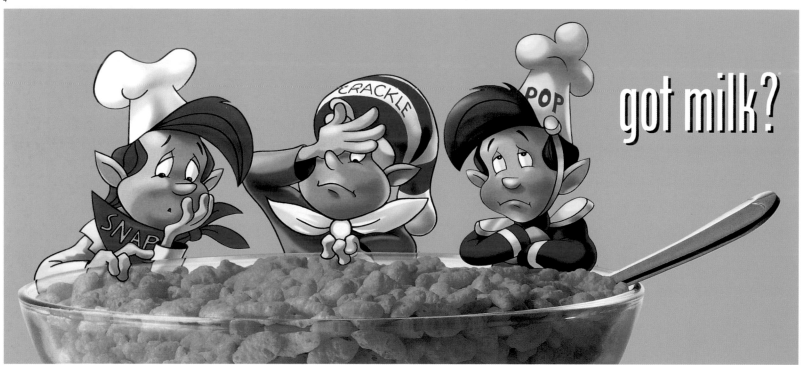

5

**4 AND 5. CALIFORNIA
MILK BOARD**
GOODBY SILVERSTEIN &
PARTNERS, SAN FRANCISCO,
1997
The billboard images featured
various foods that cry out for
milk, with chocolate topping
the list (top). The campaign
also borrowed freely from pop
culture: Snap, Crackle and Pop,
from the famous Kellogg's Rice
Crispies ads, were left high
and dry in the ad above.

6. CALIFORNIA MILK BOARD
GOODBY SILVERSTEIN &
PARTNERS, SAN FRANCISCO,
1995–96
The campaign's "deprivation
strategy" called for stories in
which characters run out of milk
at the worst times; here, the Trix
Rabbit realizes to his horror that
he (and his cereal) has run dry.

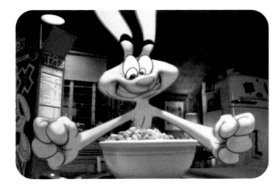

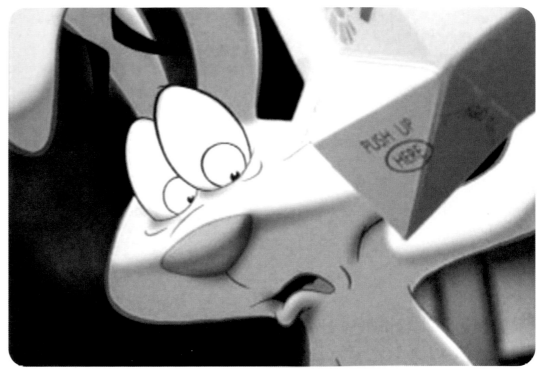

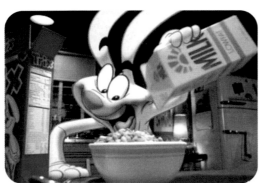

6

frenzy around milk, mammals, and stuffed toys. And in the United Kingdom—where, for some local denizens, beer quickly replaces milk as the source of life—a campaign for Boddingtons by the London agency Bartle Bogle Hegarty presented this beer as if it were a dairy product, and in doing so helped make both the brand and the ad agency legendary.

GOT MILK?

To some extent, milk is an advertising nightmare. The very things advertisers love to say about a product—"it's new, it's cool, it's different!"—do not apply to milk. It's generic, it's old-fashioned, it's bland. "What can you say about milk? It's white and comes in gallons," observed Jeffrey Manning, director of the California Milk Processors Board. Nevertheless, Manning's task, beginning in the early 1990s, was to try to encourage Californians to drink more milk, and he knew this would not be easy. The one thing

that had worked in milk's favor in the past was that it was thought to be healthful; hence, the old ad line that had been used for years by milk processors declared, "Milk does a body good." But in recent times, the public had become more concerned about fat and cholesterol, and milk is loaded with both. So the old health claims simply did not wash with the audience anymore, particularly in body-conscious California. Milk consumption in the state was plummeting, and had been for twenty years straight.

Manning needed something akin to an advertising miracle to turn this situation around. He called Jeff Goodby and Rich Silverstein. The two admen, who run the agency Goodby, Silverstein & Partners in an old waterfront warehouse in San Francisco, paid a visit to the milk board in the summer of 1993. Their agency was one of four that had been summoned by Manning to bid for the milk account. Goodby arrived with flowing, shoulder-length hair,

a self-effacing manner, and a razor-sharp wit, accompanied by partner Silverstein, a hyperactive exile from *Rolling Stone* magazine, known for riding a bicycle to work each day. The admen and their co-workers were so casual, Manning recalls, "I felt like we were having a cocktail party, not a meeting." Then Goodby slipped Manning a piece of paper with two words on it: "Got Milk?" That question—a minimalist slogan if ever there was one—summed up an entire strategy that Goodby had concocted before coming to the meeting.

In previous brainstorming sessions, the agency knew that it had to find some motivating principle, other than questionable health claims, that could rekindle people's interest in milk. As Goodby and his creative team discussed this, the beginnings of an idea started to surface: Someone made the observation that although milk is generally taken for granted, there is one time when it is fully appreciated—that desperate

DREAMS OF CREAM.

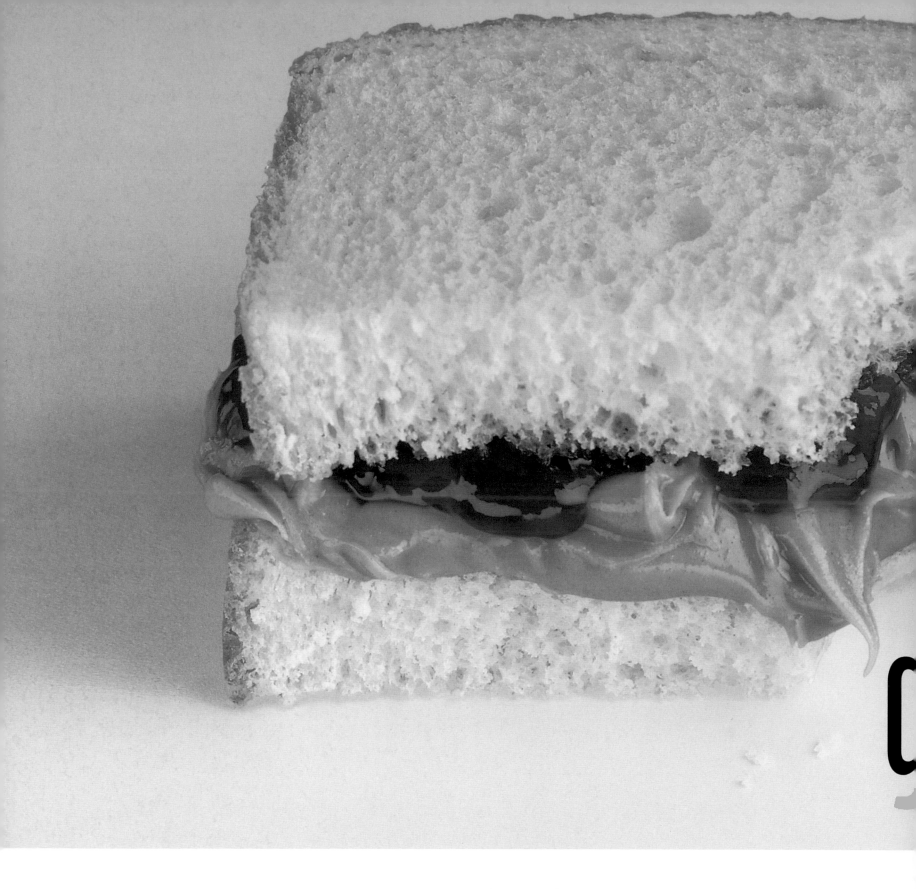

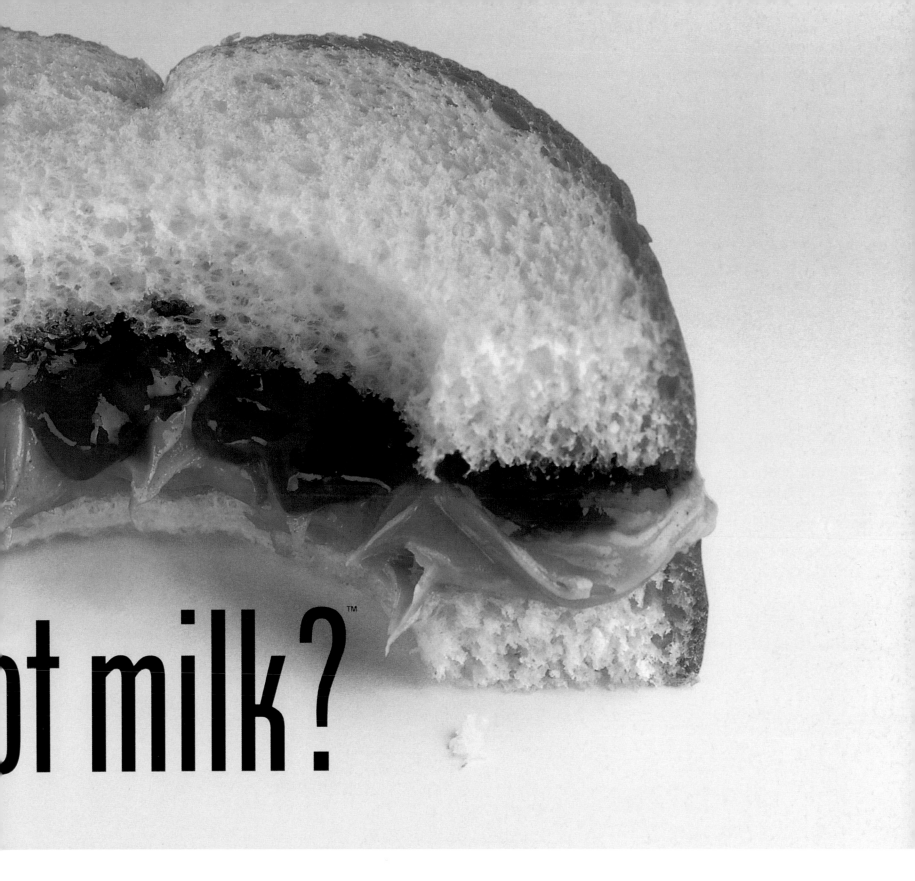

ot milk?™

7. **CALIFORNIA MILK BOARD**
GOODBY SILVERSTEIN &
PARTNERS, SAN FRANCISCO,
1994
Some photographs in the
campaign did a remarkable
job of pinpointing the moment
when milk is badly needed—
such as right after biting into
a peanut butter sandwich.

DREAMS OF CREAM.

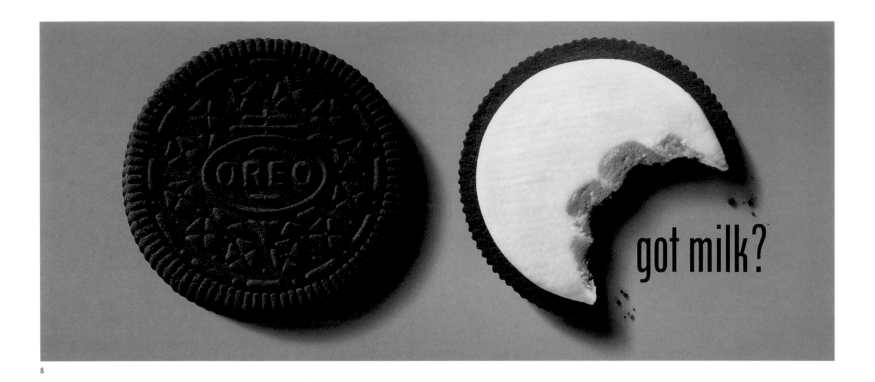

8

moment when you reach in the refrigerator and find that it is gone. Goodby and his cohorts immediately felt that this somewhat obvious observation actually represented a hidden truth; it was a feeling widely shared by people, but one that had not been articulated or expressed in advertising. The creative team began to toy with something Goodby would later call "the deprivation strategy"—which would, in effect, remove milk from all the ads and instead focus on its absence. Goodby reasoned that ads highlighting the horrors of being deprived of milk might not necessarily cause people to like milk more—but it just might scare them into buying an extra container just to avoid running out of the stuff.

Before proceeding too far with this somewhat heretical approach (removing the featured product from ads is always considered risky and is a tough sell to clients), the agency turned to its in-house planner, or consumer researcher,

Jon Steel, to find out if the idea was on the right track. In his research, Steel attempts to uncover inner, subconscious attitudes people have about products or brands, the kind of feelings that don't necessarily reveal themselves in standard surveys and interviews. "You have to dig deep for those feelings," Steel said. He conducted a number of unusual field tests involving milk. Steel spied on the ad agency's own employees by slyly planting a video camera in the back of the office refrigerator, to tape the distressed reactions of employees as they discovered there was no milk for their coffee. He also gathered members of the public into focus groups and asked them to deprive themselves of milk for a week and then report back to him. At the next session, "some pretty pissed-off people arrived," said Steel. "Somebody even said, 'When you're without milk, you want it so bad you'd steal it from the baby.'" (This statement would become one of Goodby's commercials, in which a

desperate man faces off against his own baby for the last of the milk, while the sound track plays the theme from the cowboy-showdown film *The Good, the Bad and the Ugly*.)

Armed with research, Goodby was able to sell the deprivation strategy to Manning, who realized the agency "was onto something big," and gave the green light to start making ads. Now came the fun part for Goodby, Silverstein— the creation of a series of ads that incorporated the deprivation theme into the most compelling, imaginative pictures and stories. The print ads were fairly easy: Just by showing food that cries out for milk—cupcakes, chocolate chip cookies, peanut butter sandwiches—they gave the two-word question that much more power. For the TV commercials, however, Goodby wanted to go further, creating a series of exaggerated thirty-second tales of protagonists for whom the missing milk is not just desired but desperately needed, like water in the desert.

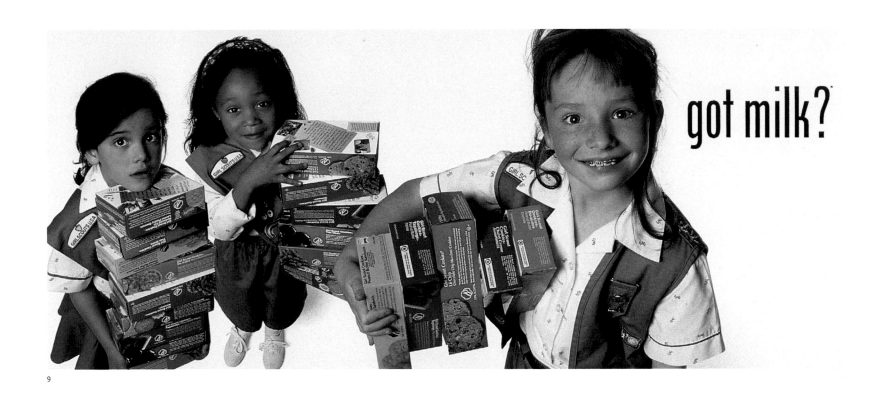

got milk?

9

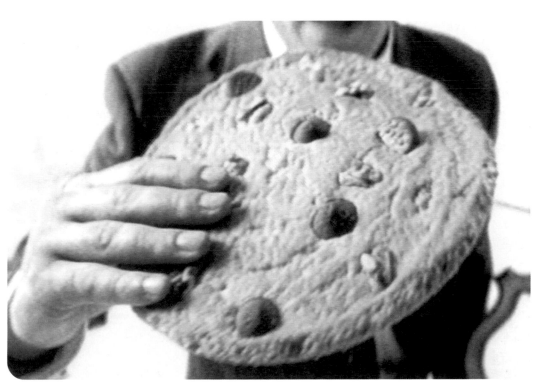

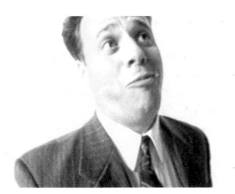

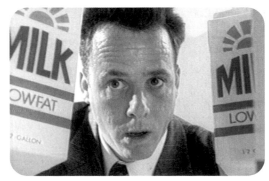

10

DREAMS OF CREAM.

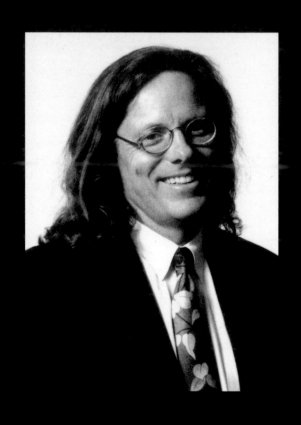

INTERVIEW: JEFF GOODBY

As co-founder and co–creative director of the San Francisco–based Goodby Silverstein & Partners, Jeff Goodby presides over what some regard as the best ad agency in the world. Goodby also helped produce one of the most memorable ad campaigns in recent years, promoting a certain dairy fluid with the minimalist slogan, "Got Milk?"

WHERE DID THE IDEA TO USE THOSE TWO WORDS, "GOT MILK?," COME FROM?
That line by itself never would have seemed like an interesting line. But when I thought of it, I was thinking of it being used in conjunction with all of these shaggy-dog stories, the kind of stories you'd watch and think, "Why am I watching this? What the hell is going on; what's the linchpin of this story?" Then the line at the end would be so tiny but so explanatory of the story that it would be kind of a humorous shock. That's the way I envisioned it.

THE "DEPRIVATION STRATEGY" YOU USED, WHICH BUILT THE WHOLE CAMPAIGN AROUND WHAT IT'S LIKE TO BE WITHOUT MILK—HOW DID YOU ARRIVE AT THAT?
That insight came somewhat from the research; someone in a focus group said something like "I never think about milk except when I run out of it." But the idea of the campaign was really having these incredibly elaborate stories about something as mundane, as tediously unimportant as milk. The deprivation strategy was important, but someone could have taken that same idea—that people think about milk only when they run out—and come up with something like "the magic milkman" who rushed in to give you milk as soon as you run out, or some stupid thing like that. I think that the planning community [researchers] gives you the impression that the commercials pretty much write themselves once you have the strategy. That's not the case.

WHEN DID YOU REALIZE THE ADS HAD BECOME A CULTURAL PHENOMENON?
When we had our Christmas party at a theater that wasn't in a particularly good part of town, and a few streets from the theater there was an X-rated bookstore. They had a sign out front that said, Got Porn. So I knew it was starting to take off.

SOME PEOPLE HAVE CITED "AARON BURR" AS ONE OF THE BEST COMMERCIALS EVER MADE, AND AN EXAMPLE OF HOW ADVERTISING CAN BE ART—BEAUTIFULLY CRAFTED, WITH ITS OWN HUMAN TRUTH TO IT, A STRONG CHARACTER, A REVELATION AT THE END. DO YOU LOOK AT THE COMMERCIAL THAT WAY?
I do. I think that's one of the best commercials we've ever done. And the reason is that it's based on something that is really true but is exaggerated in ways that are very pleasing. The obsession that character has is just esoteric enough to make it interesting. And the exaggeration made it work. I think that some of the things [director] Michael Bay did to it, particularly the wild set he created, with all the weird memorabilia, took the ad further than I thought it would go. The character lived in this crazy kind of apartment that happens to be in the middle of a warehouse—and you don't even wonder why, for some reason. It's a great piece of fantasy.

DO YOU FIND THAT A GREAT AD CAMPAIGN USUALLY STARTS WITH A MOMENT OF REVELATION AND THEN BUILDS FROM THERE?
Sometimes a great campaign starts with one really good commercial someone thinks of, and then you try to replicate it, or push it farther. Sometimes you can't do it. An example of that would be the Nissan commercial that Chiat/Day did with the dolls ["Toys"]. The rest of the campaign didn't live up to the promise of that commercial—they just couldn't replicate that feeling down the line. Making a good campaign is much harder than making a single piece of good advertising. You have to start out with a much deeper insight about the workings of a product and the way it really fits into people's lives. And the idea you come up with has to have a kind of depth and breadth that you'll be able to explore further down the line.

IS IT DIFFICULT TO KEEP A CAMPAIGN LIKE "GOT MILK?" FRESH AND INTERESTING OVER TIME? AND HOW DO YOU KNOW WHEN IT'S TIME TO MOVE AWAY FROM IT?
It's hard to keep the momentum going. You can change the people who are working on it—that's the easiest trick, and it usually gives you a new perspective on things. But actually, I find creative people and clients are sometimes too quick to give up on a campaign. Because all they've been

doing is thinking about this campaign, and they get sick of it. And the creative people get scared, like, "Maybe we won't be able to think of another round of ads." So the advertising people sometimes just want to start fresh, and they abandon a good campaign—even though the public might be just starting to get into it.

IN THE PAST, AD CAMPAIGNS OFTEN HAD ONGOING STORY LINES AND RECURRING CHARACTERS. WHY DON'T WE SEE THAT AS MUCH NOW?
I think some of it is fear on the part of creatives that they won't be able to come up with something else for Mr. Whipple to do, to keep him interesting. Also, I think the research that goes on now doesn't support that kind of campaign. You get research that says something like "Everyone remembers the Taco Bell dog, but they don't remember the burrito that was advertised. So the campaign's no good." So then, the creatives go back and try to come up with some way to integrate the burrito and the dog, with the dog asking for a burrito over and over—and the campaign starts getting bad because of that. Or maybe they start lessening the dog's role, thinking, The research shows that people remember the dog instead of the fajitas—so let's use the dog less. That's what you saw with that campaign. I think research really hurts that kind of campaign. If you took the classic Cracker Jack campaign now [starring the veteran actor Jack Gilford], the researchers would probably tell you, "Well, some consumers don't like to see old people." It's a mistake, because good characters and good stories can last a long time.

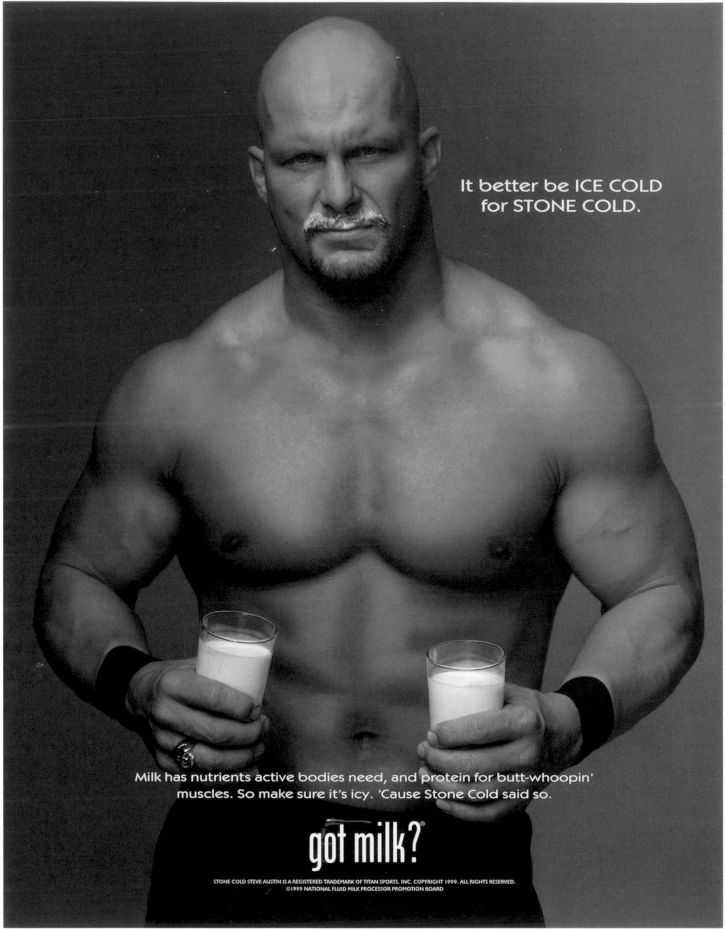

11. **NATIONAL MILK PROCESSOR PROMOTION BOARD**
BOZELL WORLDWIDE, NEW YORK, 1998
While the "Got Milk?" campaign ran in California, the national milk board's popular series of ads featured celebrities with milk moustaches (including the pro wrestler Steve Austin). The ads borrowed Goodby's headline, though it wasn't as appropriate in this context.

12. **CALIFORNIA MILK BOARD**
GOODBY SILVERSTEIN & PARTNERS, SAN FRANCISCO, 1993
The commercial "Aaron Burr" takes the viewer into the obsessive world of an American history fanatic who collects memorabilia from the famed 1804 duel between U.S. President Aaron Burr and Alexander Hamilton.

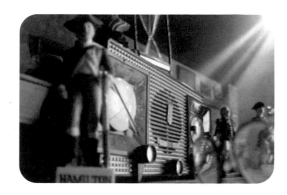

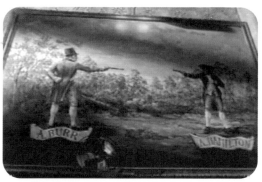

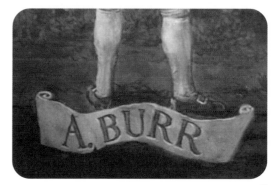

12

The first commercial, "Aaron Burr," featured a wild-haired history buff who is obsessed with the early American politician Alexander Hamilton, and who misses his opportunity of a lifetime—to answer the radio-contest question, "Who shot Alexander Hamilton?"—because he has no milk to wash down the peanut butter sandwich stuck in his mouth. ("Owum Buh!" he screams into the phone, to no avail.) Another early spot was the aforementioned father/baby showdown. A third featured the Trix Rabbit, star of a long-ago series of commercials in which the rabbit was always denied Trix cereal; in the new ad, Goodby created a clever scenario in which the rabbit finally gets the cereal—then is all the more heartbroken to discover there is no milk to pour on it.

The commercials worked on multiple levels, as entertainment and as a selling message. While almost every good ad agency tries to achieve that dual effect with its ads, "no one is

able to do it as well as Goodby, Silverstein," said the *Advertising Age* critic Bob Garfield. Garfield pointed out that the "Got Milk?" refrain serves not only as a punch line to the ads' jokes but also as a nagging question that follows consumers all the way to the supermarket. "The agency does all of this so smoothly it's almost sublime," Garfield said.

Perhaps the best ad in the bunch was the commercial titled "Heaven." In the opening scene, we meet a nasty yuppie executive snarling into his cellular phone. Stepping into the street, he's run over by a truck (one of the rare times a commercial has ever shown someone being killed), only to reappear in an ethereal world, where he's surrounded by chocolate chip cookies and containers of milk—Heaven, it would seem. Stuffing his mouth with cookies, he reaches for the milk and finds that each and every container is empty. This prompts him to pause and wonder, "Where am I?"—at which point a flaming "Got

Milk?" logo burns itself onto the screen.

Selling such a dark and complex commercial to a client is rarely easy, and "Heaven" was no exception. The idea originated with copywriter Harry Cocciolo. It hadn't tested particularly well in focus groups, but Cocciolo and his partner, Sean Ehringer, kept refining the script and presented it again to Goodby. According to Ehringer, "Goodby's reaction was warm but not overly positive. Kind of like when your kid proudly shows you his first poop in the toilet. I thought it was over, but Harry kept at Jeff [Goodby]. Day after day we would submit tiny changes." Goodby finally became convinced the spot could work. But the client didn't agree. "I didn't like it at first," Manning said. Goodby suspected that Manning was afraid of showing a man killed in a commercial, but Manning says, "I just thought the story was too complex to do in thirty seconds." Now it was Goodby's turn to nag. "Every meeting after that, I'd mention it,"

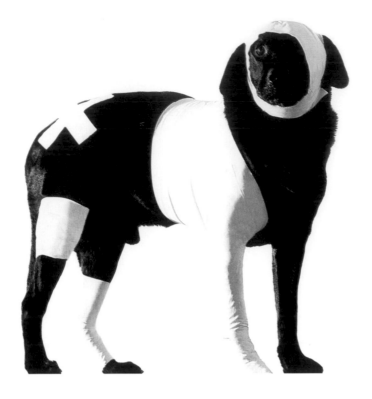

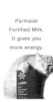

Parmalat
Fortified Milk.
It gives you
more energy.

13

13. AND 14. **PARMALAT MILK**
DM9 DDB PUBLICIDADE,
SÃO PAULO, 1999
One series of ads suggested an
uprising of milk-powered cats
against dogs, and the cats
were winning. A dog shows
the wounds of battle (above),
and a poodle is left a widow
(opposite).

says Goodby. "I'd say, 'Yeah, this new idea's pretty cool, but I keep thinking about that "Heaven" idea.' " He finally won Manning over by agreeing to direct the commercial himself. "I said, 'Fine, if you're going to put your rear end on the line, go do it,' " Manning said.

"Heaven," along with "Aaron Burr," became one of the most lauded commercials of the 1990s (Goodby even got a call from filmmaker Steven Spielberg, asking for a videotape of "Heaven"). *Time* magazine named "Got Milk?" the best advertising campaign of 1995. The Girl Scouts of America asked if they could be featured in the campaign, and Goodby obliged. Meanwhile, "the phrase 'Got Milk?' became part of the vernacular in California," says Manning.

But for the client Manning, the real news was in the sales figures: In 1994, the first full year the campaign was running, Californians drank 15 million gallons more milk than the previous year. It was the first time in two decades

that consumption increased. The California ads soon started running around the country and were successful everywhere. And eventually the question "Got Milk?" was licensed by a separate national milk-promotion group that had been running a series of ads featuring celebrities with milk mustaches. (While the milk-mustache campaign has been popular with the public for a number of years, it is generally not well regarded in advertising's creative community because of its easy reliance on celebrities; in fact, the grafting of the "Got Milk?" line onto this campaign displeased not only Goodby and Silverstein but others in the ad industry, such as TBWA/Chiat/Day creative director Lee Clow, who called it "a bastardization.")

Meanwhile, the original "Got Milk?" campaign was still running in the new millennium, as Goodby continued to spin tales of poor milk-deprived souls. And client Manning has continued to leverage the phenomenon in

every way possible, licensing the logo for T-shirts and putting the words on everything from pens to toy milk trucks. At this point, Manning said, "'Got Milk?' is more than an ad campaign. It has taken on a life of its own."

PARMALAT

While Goodby's challenge was to promote generic milk, the packaged-milk company Parmalat and its Brazilian agency, DM9 DDB Publicidade, had a more daunting task—they had to persuade Brazilians not only to drink more milk but specifically to choose Parmalat. Exacerbating this problem was the fact that, at the time, few people in Brazil knew or cared much about the brand.

Back in 1995, Parmalat's own research found that only 19 percent of Brazilian households were using the brand. Women, in particular, seemed to feel no connection to it, which was understandable—Parmalat's previous

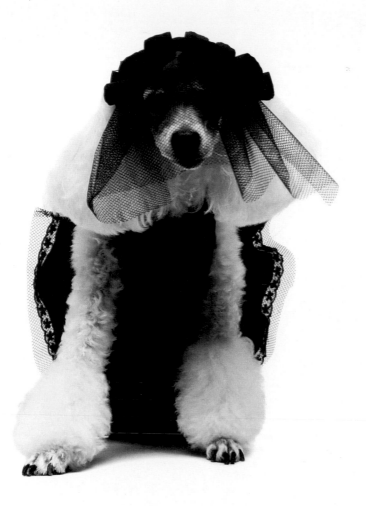

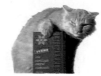

Parmalat
Fortified Milk.
It gives you
more energy.

promotional efforts had been aimed primarily at men. The brand's marketers had chosen to sponsor soccer matches, in an attempt to tie in with athleticism and good health. The problem was, men were not the ones making most household milk purchases—the real opportunity lay in appealing to mothers of growing families. And among this group, "we were still distant from our consumers," said Vania Machado, the brand's marketing manager. Moreover, as in many other places around the world, milk consumption in Brazil had declined in recent years. And those who were still drinking it tended to favor fresh pasteurized milk from local dairies; Parmalat, based in Italy, offered a packaged dairy product that was, in the minds of some, not as fresh.

When Machado presented her case to DM9, she understood what needed to be done but didn't know how to do it. Parmalat had to remind people that milk was an important and natural source of nutrition; at the same time, the ads had to transcend this informational message and somehow establish a special emotional bond with mothers and their children.

Erh Ray, a creative director at DM9, started out with a vague idea about tying in the notion of "mother's milk" with the ads. The point of that would be "to remind people that milk is the very first source of nutrition for all of us," he said. "This was not only about being fed but being taken care of, being loved, being near a gentle, caring mother—that whole universe of the moment when we first open our eyes to the world."

Ray was trying to come up with a scenario that might capture those sentiments when, on a visit to New York in 1996, he saw the work of the photographer Tom Arma, who specialized in photographs of young children in costume. "When I came back to Brazil I had this idea of using these kinds of photographs, with the kids dressed as animals," Ray said, but he still didn't have the idea fleshed out. He sketched some rough layouts of costumed children and showed them to his boss Nizan Guanaes. Guanaes looked at the pictures and immediately made the connection to a larger theme: The ads would feature kids portraying various mammals that are nursed on mother's milk. A slogan popped into Guanaes's head immediately: "Parmalat—because we are mammals."

The creative team decided that each ad would feature an Arma photo portrait of a different child in a different furry costume: a panda, a lion, a monkey, a sheep (and in each picture, the child/mammal would be shown clutching a package of Parmalat, of course). The agency knew the images of the cute kids, of varying ethnicities and races, would likely be irresistible to mothers, but they also reasoned that if the ads were crafted in the right way, children might be drawn to them, as well. So the creative team devised a theme song for the

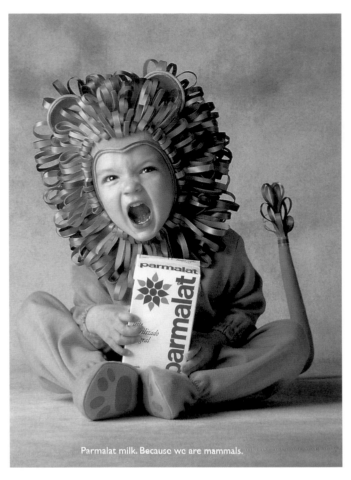

Parmalat milk. Because we are mammals.

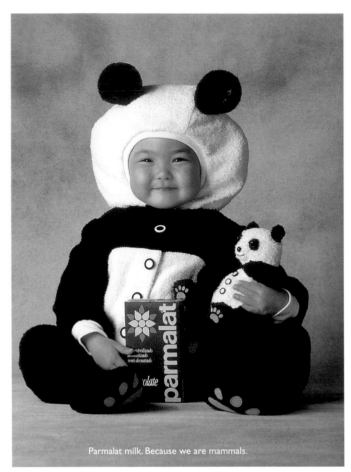

Parmalat milk. Because we are mammals.

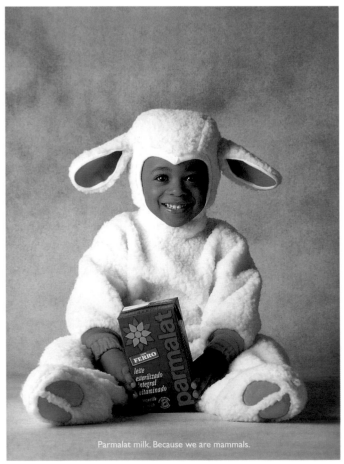

Parmalat milk. Because we are mammals.

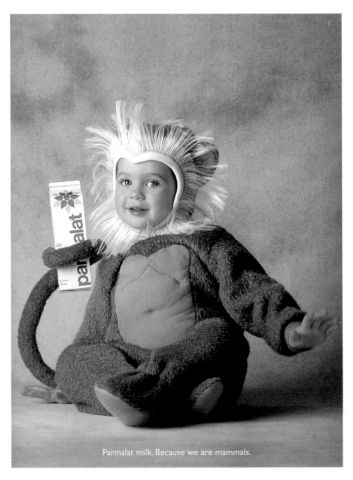

Parmalat milk. Because we are mammals.

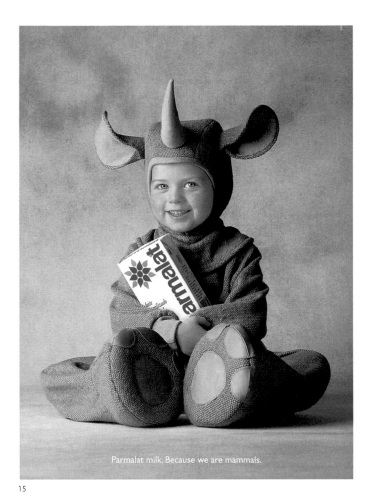

Parmalat milk. Because we are mammals.

15

15. **PARMALAT MILK**
DM9 DDB PUBLICIDADE,
SÃO PAULO, 1996–98
In portraits by photographer Tom
Arma, children were dressed up
in costumes of mammals that
drink milk. The campaign
became the talk of Brazil, and
soon created a feeding frenzy
for stuffed mammal dolls.

commercials that sounded like a lullaby. "The music was our 'secret-sauce recipe,'" said Ray. As soon as Machado saw the first versions of the ads, she knew that the idea was on target. "It was such a simple and obvious idea, and yet it managed to convey everything we wanted," Machado said, noting that the imagery tied up the various themes of nutrition, nature, family, caring, reliability, and more.

The campaign broke on Mother's Day. Ray wasn't sure what to expect but soon found that in his own neighborhood, a buzz was building. "Mothers were talking about the ads from day one," he said. And it just steamrolled from there. "People sang the mammals song, kids wanted to be mammals, at birthday parties the theme was . . . mammals! It was 'mammalsmania' everywhere," Ray said. "And not only here. It spread like a fever to all Latin America, and then all the way to China."

It's hard to figure why something as simple as children in furry suits can trigger a phenomenon. But when it happens, a smart advertiser seizes on the opportunity and leverages it. Parmalat and DM9 did that with one brilliant move: Once the mammal characters had been popularized through ads, the company began offering miniature stuffed dolls based on them—and soon a feeding frenzy was under way. Each day, some 60,000 Brazilians were lining up to exchange $7 plus twenty Parmalat bar codes for a mammal toy. Machado noted that people became fanatical collectors, wanting not just one or two but the entire collection of twenty-one animals. In subsequent ads, the agency started featuring the mammal toys being clutched (along with the milk) by the mammal-kids.

By now, the success of the campaign was being fueled by two separate but intertwined

forces: Parents had come to associate Parmalat with nurturing and nutrition; kids, meanwhile, were badgering parents to buy more Parmalat milk so they could collect more toys. Within a year, Parmalat's penetration into Brazilian households jumped by an astounding level— from 19 percent to 96 percent, virtually overnight. Meanwhile, the company was producing and redeeming mammal dolls as fast as it could, eventually selling more than 16 million of them.

As the company saw its milk-market share growing, it began to promote spin-off milk products, such as fortified milk and low-fat milk. But wisely, the ad agency didn't overplay its "mammals" hand. DM9 took a different tack with these products because the target groups were different. The low-fat milk, for example, was geared more to weight-conscious adults, so DM9 came up with a new twist on the animal

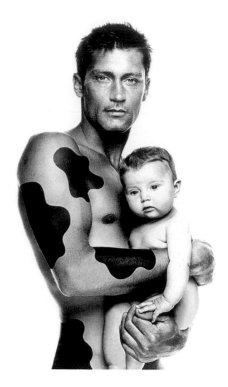

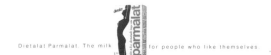

Dietalat Parmalat. The milk for people who like themselves.

16 AND 17. **PARMALAT MILK**
DM9 DDB PUBLICIDADE,
SÃO PAULO, 1997
For low-fat milk, the pitch was
aimed at body-conscious adults;
this time, instead of children in
cute costumes, slim adults
appeared with cow spots.

theme—this time, the ads featured adults whose bare skin was printed with cow spots. Unlike the cute and cuddly kids in the main campaign, the subjects of these ads were presented as being self-absorbed, reveling in their own bodies. The copy read, "The new light Parmalat. Milk for all those who are really into themselves."

Some of the most striking ads DM9 produced were for Parmalat's specially fortified milk. Here again, the agency wanted to connect with mothers and children, but because the milk was fortified the ads needed a much stronger emphasis on nutrition and physical growth. The agency again returned to the theme of animals, which had worked so well already. But this time, DM9 zeroed in on two particular species: dogs and cats. Obviously, the latter drinks milk, and the former doesn't. And so the creative team of Pedro Cappeletti and Jader Rossetto dreamed up a series of

exaggerated, humorous scenes showing what might happen if cats drank fortified milk—and suddenly grew larger and more powerful than their longtime canine nemeses.

In effect, the campaign presented images of a feline insurrection against dogs but did so without depicting any violence. Nor did the ads offer much in the way of explanation—the ideas were conveyed almost entirely through visual images (one of DM9's proven specialties is the ability to tell a story through still pictures). One ad shows a cat sitting majestically at the entrance to a doghouse; the name "Rex," above the doorway, has been scratched out, indicating that this particular battle has already been won. Another ad shows a dog, wide-eyed in terror; behind him on the wall, we can make out a giant cartoonish shadow of a cat's head. One of the most delightful ads is a DM9 picture-puzzle that is not immediately understandable unless you've

been following the campaign about the cat uprising; the ad simply shows a poodle dressed in widow's garb.

The overall campaign was such a resounding success that by the late 1990s, Parmalat had actually overtaken Coca-Cola and McDonald's as the most recognized and most popular brand among Brazilians. And don't expect its popularity to fade anytime soon. Perhaps the canniest aspect of this campaign is that it has begun to convert customers while they are still toddlers. Discussing the mammal-doll phenomenon with *Advertising Age* recently, Machado acknowledged, "Kids go to sleep cuddling your brand. That's the best branding you can have."

BODDINGTONS

People may have been drinking less milk in America and Brazil, but when it came to Brits and beer, declining consumption was never an

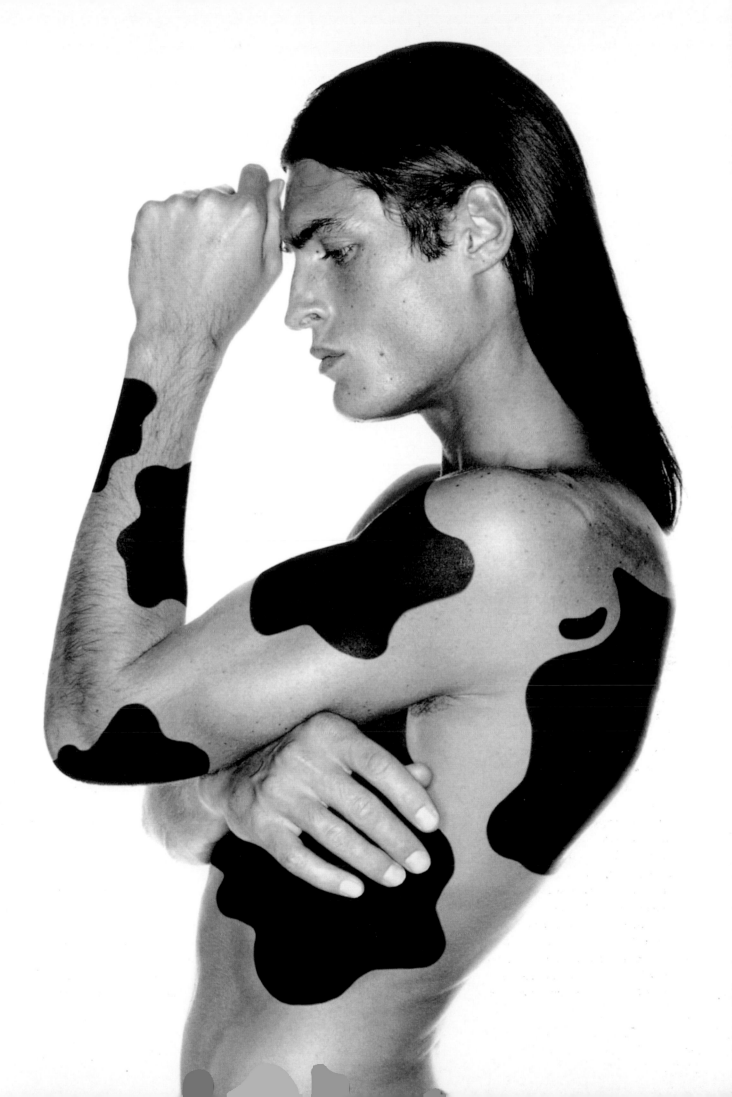

17

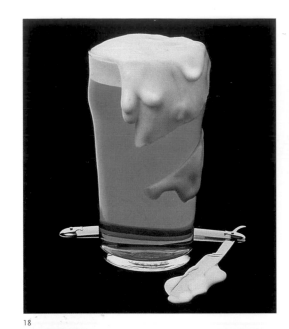

18

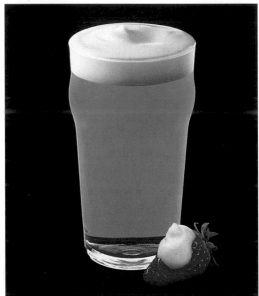

19

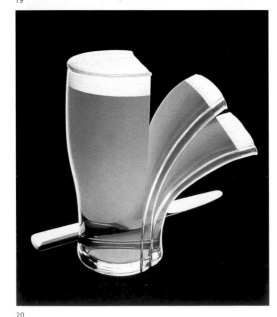

20

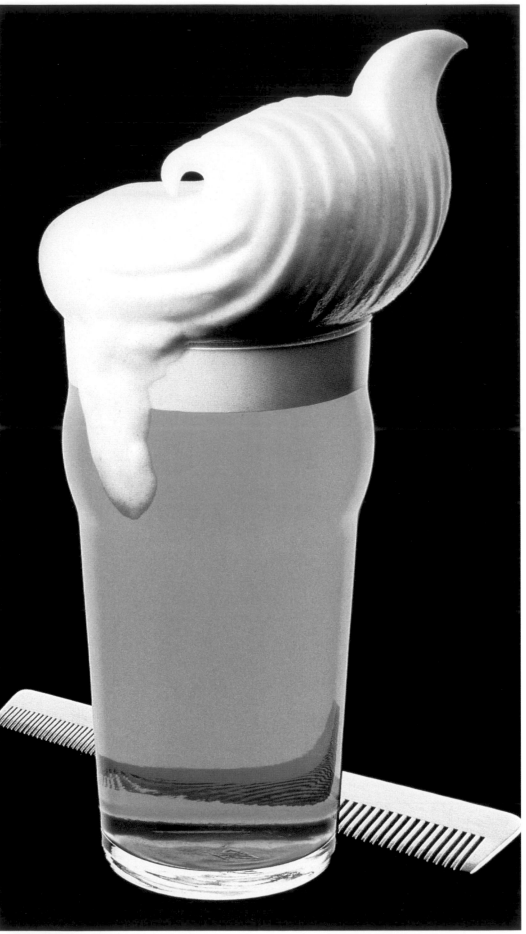

21

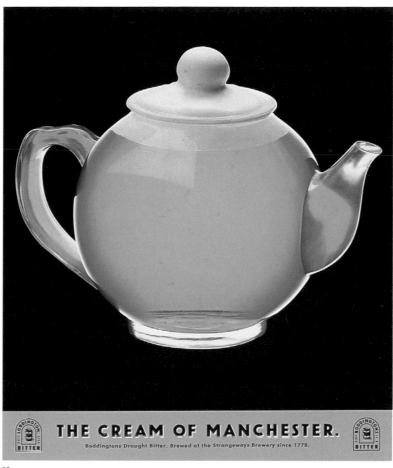

22

issue. However, there were plenty of other problems to be faced when Bartle Bogle Hegarty was called upon to advertise an obscure little brew known as Boddingtons.

Though the 200-year-old beer had a faithful following in its hometown of Manchester, that wasn't sufficient for its new owner, the large Whitbread Beer Company—which had acquired the Boddingtons brewery with an ambitious plan to take the beer national. It fell upon Bartle Bogle Hegarty, Whitbread's trusted agency and one of the hottest creative ad shops in England in the 1980s, to pull this off against several obstacles. For one thing, recent history had shown that when big beer companies took over little breweries, they usually ended up ruining the beer—something the public was aware of. "So we had to deal with the assumption that the takeover might ruin this local beer, too," said Martin Smith, the deputy chairman of the BBH agency. At the same time, Smith said, the agency

had to balance two conflicting agendas: "We had to maintain the heritage and authenticity of the beer and at the same time, go national with it— fast. Add to that the fact that half the country didn't care for this kind of beer [known as northern bitter] to start with, and you had a pretty difficult situation."

The first thing client and agency did was venture into the pubs of Manchester to find out what people liked about this particular old beer. What they learned was that the northern English treasure a beer with a thick, creamy head— unlike the thin-headed, weaker variations favored by southerners. The good news for BBH was that Whitbread had new technologies that would enable Boddingtons to maintain its distinctively northern creaminess, even after it was packed up in cans and shipped down south. That settled it for BBH: The advertising would have to focus on creaminess.

Of course, Boddingtons wasn't the only

creamy beer—far from it. Any number of competitors could have staked out this territory beforehand, noted BBH's Steve Kershaw. But they never did. According to Kershaw, the other brewers had "forgotten about the product," focusing their advertising on "male bonding, talking about sex or football." BBH decided to swoop in on this opening. By "owning creami-ness" (advertisers tend to believe they can "own" anything if they just get there first), BBH was able to link various wonderful qualities to the beer—not just richness and freshness and flavor but other connotations of the word cream, such as quality, premium, "cream of the crop." The agency, its executives freely admit, got lucky when it stepped in cream.

Still, just saying your beer is creamy isn't going to impress people much, BBH realized. They had to do something original and evoca-tive with the theme. Quickly, the creative team started playing with images of cream and just

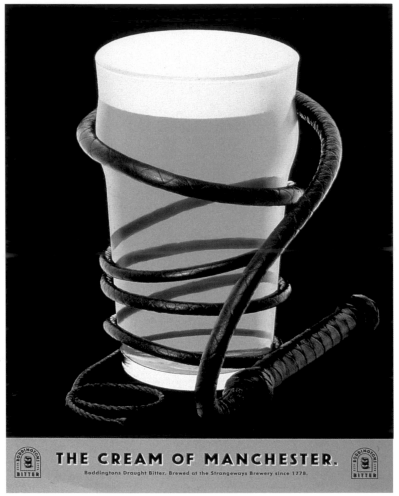

THE CREAM OF MANCHESTER.

Boddingtons Draught Bitter. Brewed at the Strangeways Brewery since 1778.

23

23 AND 24. **BODDINGTONS BEER**
BARTLE BOGLE HEGARTY, LONDON, 1996
Some of the "picture plays" in the campaign were trickier than others. "Whipping Cream" (above) took a bit of work, while "Hand Cream" (opposite) was easier to figure out.

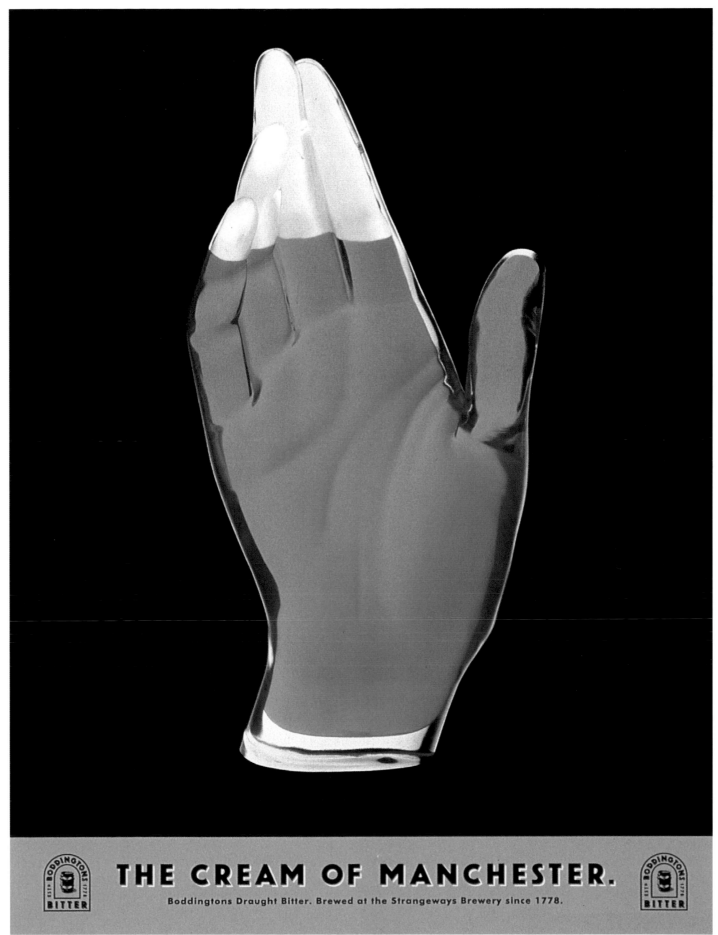

THE CREAM OF MANCHESTER.

Boddingtons Draught Bitter. Brewed at the Strangeways Brewery since 1778.

DREAMS OF CREAM.

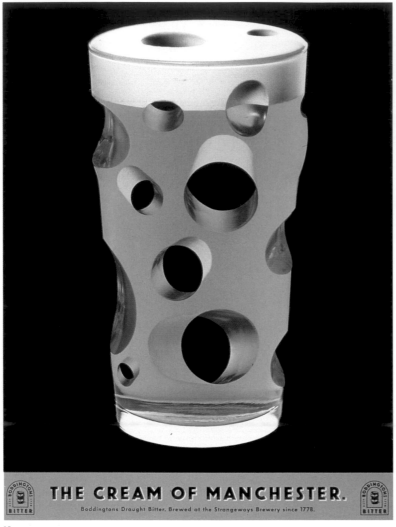

THE CREAM OF MANCHESTER.

Boddingtons Draught Bitter. Brewed at the Strangeways Brewery since 1778.

25

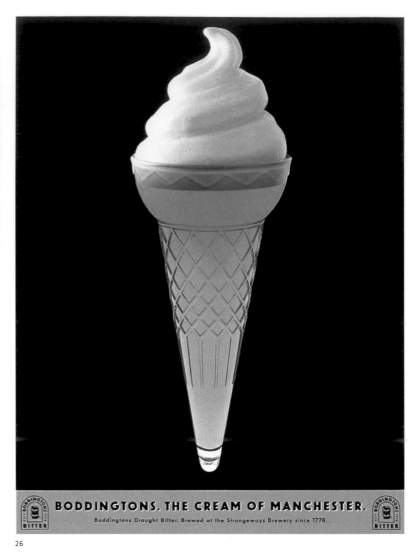

BODDINGTONS. THE CREAM OF MANCHESTER.

Boddingtons Draught Bitter. Brewed at the Strangeways Brewery since 1778.

26

one line of copy: "The cream of Manchester." (The agency didn't want people to forget where this beer came from.) That said, there wasn't much point in blathering on about creaminess—better to show than tell, BBH decided. What emerged from the drawing board was a series of playful images that substituted beer for cream: putting beer into an ice cream cone, pairing it with strawberries, turning it into shaving cream.

The picture riddles were undeniably clever, but within the agency, "there was dissension as to whether to present this to the client," said Smith. "It worked as a visual pun, but the taste expectations from some of these images were, frankly, a bit disgusting—who wants to eat a strawberry with a beer? And if you show a beer as shaving cream, does that mean it tastes like soap?" BBH creative director John Hegarty argued that the audience wouldn't draw those conclusions and would understand the game

being played in the ads. Still, just to be certain, the agency decided to get the opinion of real experts—which necessitated, of course, another run to the pub. "Our planner went in there and asked blokes what they thought of these pictures," said Smith (who admits the study "was ad hoc research—it wouldn't have stood up in a court of law"). Nevertheless, the reactions were exactly what BBH was hoping for: "They looked at it and said, 'Yeah, I get that,'" said Smith.

At this point, the BBH team began to feel they might be onto something big. "It was as if we'd created a whole new visual language," Smith said, "and suddenly every pun involving cream was open to us. The possibilities were endless." The agency explored them all, it seemed, from "cream tea" (beer poured in the shape of a teapot) to "cream cheese" (a glass of beer with Swiss-cheese holes in it). Part of what made the ads work was the richness and realism

of the images; rather than using illustrations or trick photography, BBH built lifelike models of the beer/cream objects, then photographed these creations against a dramatic black background. The result looked good enough to eat, or drink, though it was hard to tell which.

The finished work looked more like posters than magazine ads. But how to get those posters into the homes of millions? The agency purchased the back covers of Sunday newspaper magazines, and each week a different image appeared—then lay on kitchen tables or in cafés for days afterwards, inviting people to ponder the puzzle.

In 1992, within eighteen months of the campaign's debut, Boddingtons had become the number-one beer of its type in all of England. Meanwhile, the ads "became a kind of pop-culture art," said Smith, as well as a national pastime of sorts: Since the ads never actually explained the cream allusions being shown, it

 VANISHING CREAM.

Boddingtons. The cream of Manchester. Brewed at the Strangeways Brewery since 1778.

27

DREAMS OF CREAM.

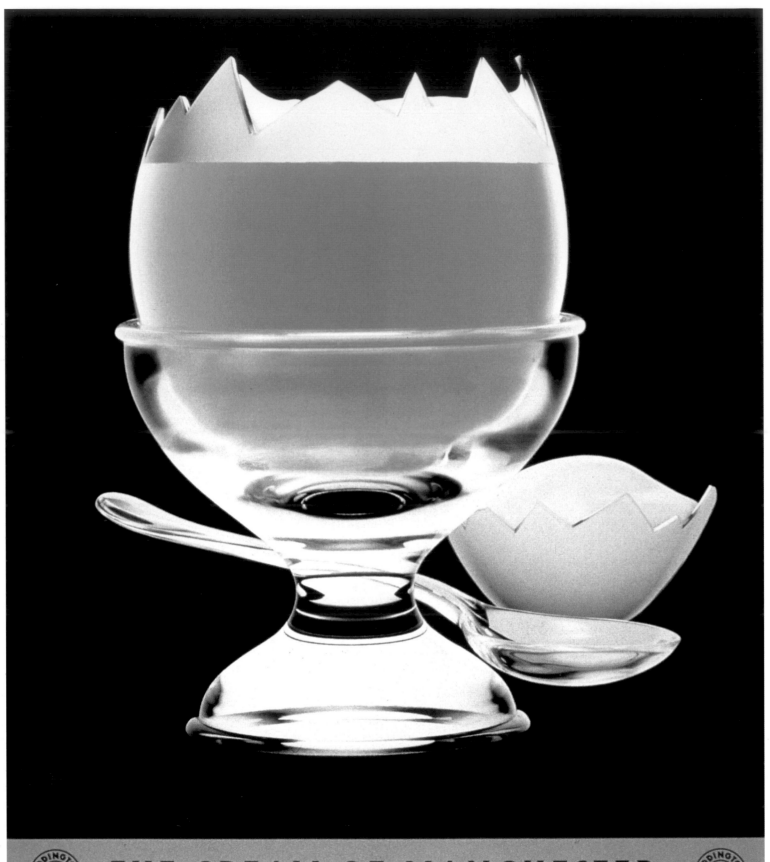

THE CREAM OF MANCHESTER.

Boddingtons Draught Bitter. Brewed at the Strangeways Brewery since 1778.

28

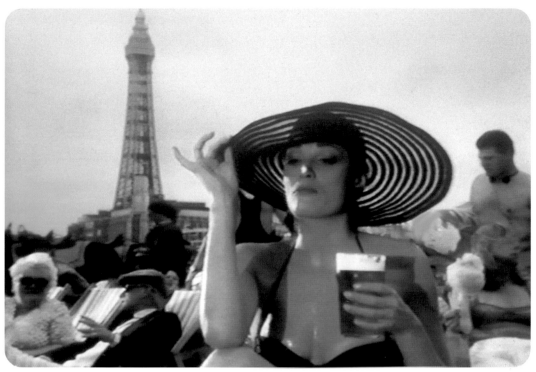

29

28. **BODDINGTONS BEER**
BARTLE BOGLE HEGARTY,
LONDON, 1996
In a more complex image,
"Cream Egg ," the beer glass is
transformed into an egg cup
holding the creamy contents.

29. **BODDINGTONS BEER**
BARTLE BOGLE HEGARTY,
LONDON, 1994
In the commercial "Sun Cream,"
sunbathers are shown rubbing
the beer into their bodies;
another TV spot showed a
glamorous woman using it
as a face cream.

was left for the audience to figure out each one—and BBH kept making them a little harder to solve. "People liked it that way," said Smith. "They wanted to be challenged." One slightly kinky ad wrapped the beer glass with a cat-o'-nine-tails (whipped cream). Another had an all-black page, with no beer at all (vanishing cream, of course).

Gradually, the brewer, ecstatic with the success of the print campaign, wanted to bring it to life on television. The first commercial appeared in 1993, picking up on the print advertising's cream theme, but taking it in a quirky new direction. The spot starts out looking like a glamorous cosmetics commercial: A beautiful woman in an elegant setting is massaging her face with what appears to be face cream. Gradually we see that she's actually dipping her hand into a glass of Boddingtons, skimming off the creamy head, then rubbing it into her face. The commercial ends with her distinguished

tuxedo-clad paramour arriving, embracing her, and then declaring—in a completely incongruous broad cockney accent—"By 'eck, you smell gorgeous!" Subsequent spots pulled off equally effective spoofs of advertising for suntan cream and ice cream. The commercials were hip and postmodern enough to appeal to the most sophisticated viewers, but they were particularly well loved in the working-class pubs, where, Smith says, "You'd hear guys at the bar joking to each other, 'By 'eck, you smell gorgeous tonight!'" One more thing that made the commercials stand out: They featured women, something that just wasn't done in British beer ads (traditionally, beer advertising in the UK has almost always featured three men in a pub because, as the British adman Trevor Beattie once observed, "Four or more was a potential riot . . . two could only be a gay couple . . . and one was just sad!").

By the late 1990s, the Boddingtons

campaign was industry legend. In England, it was so recognizable that 84 percent of consumers could identify a Boddingtons ad without any name or logo. In the final stages of the campaign (Boddingtons finally stopped running it after nearly a decade, having finally exhausted the seemingly endless supply of cream puns), the advertiser was so confident of recognition that it did, in fact, pull its name off the ads, leaving just the picture and the "Cream of Manchester" line. "Everyone knew from the look that they were Bodd's ads," said Kershaw, so removing the brand name was one more way to "make the ads work harder and re-engage with the audience." It meant everyone now had to figure out not just the riddle but the identity of the advertiser. Most of them could do this easily, but it still made them feel quite clever, said Kershaw. "But of course, if you asked them they would say it was the ads that were clever. Funny how psychology works in cases like this."

12. TH
GLOBAL H

E NEW
OT SPOTS.

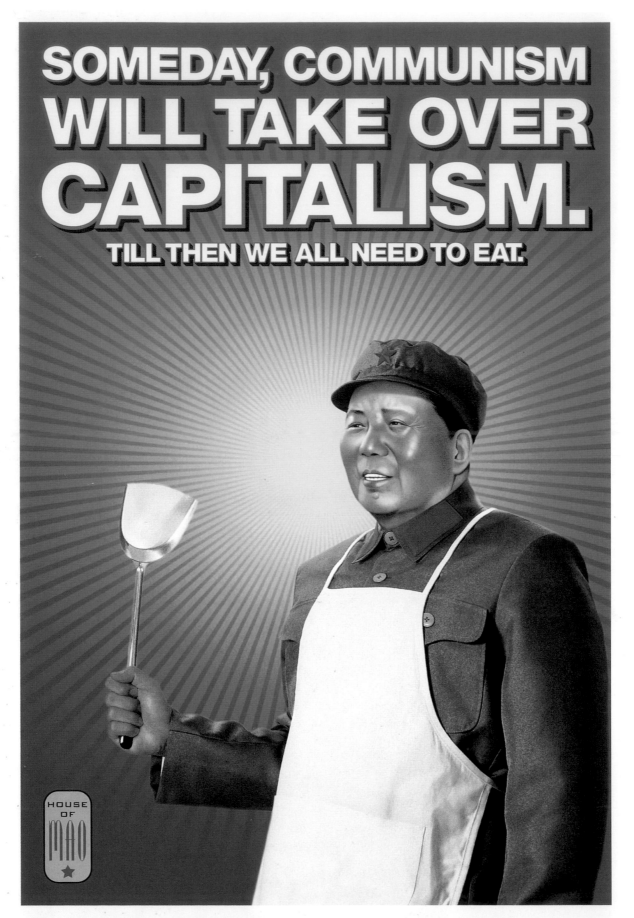

A REVOLUTIONARY RESTAURANT, NOODLE BAR AND CAFE AT CHINA SQUARE FOOD CENTRE. TEL: 5330660.

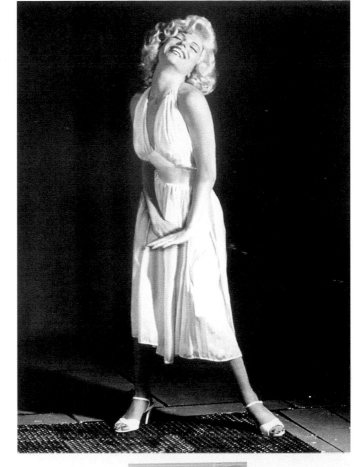

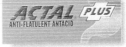

NO WIND.

2

It was, perhaps, to be expected that the ad revolution based in New York in the 1960s would quickly spread to London and throughout Europe; after all, the heavy interaction between American and European cultural and business communities almost guaranteed that the fever would be transmitted. But how did this particular bug—whose symptoms included an unshakable urge to apply conceptual thinking, clever language, and stylistic design to the selling of products—find its way to places like Singapore or São Paulo?

In recent years, sophisticated advertising has been bursting forth from somewhat unexpected places, in locales far removed from the advertising epicenters of New York and London. No one has been more surprised by all of this than American and European ad creators, who had every right to assume that creative advertising was a form they alone had mastered. In the past, when advertising's creative cognoscenti gathered

annually on the French Riviera to select the world's best ads at the International Advertising Festival, the only real mystery each year was "Would the most-honored ad agency be American or British this time around?"

But by the mid-1990s, the party in Cannes was being stormed by outsiders. They arrived from Asia, South America, and Africa, unveiling their elegantly simple and striking posters and their thirty-second TV gems of humor and pathos—all rooted in ideas and concepts that needed no translation to connect with an audience of any nationality. Increasingly in recent award festivals, the outsiders won over advertising's most discerning judges and ended up taking many of the top creative trophies home with them. More important, their work was refreshingly different; it was rewriting some of the rules of advertising communication and demonstrating that ads from the other side of the planet could, in fact, be bolder, more styl-

ized, and more innovative than what was being produced by the most experienced practitioners of the craft.

On one level, of course, this should have come as no surprise; good ideas know no boundaries and are apt to emerge anywhere and everywhere. But at the same time, modern creative advertising was a uniquely Western creation. It had to be carried to far-off cultures and then nurtured. The major agencies based in America and Europe were, in many cases, the ones that initially foisted the advertising culture on countries with developing commercial business markets. However, as these big ad-agency networks put down roots in Asia, South America, and elsewhere, they tended to export a bland version of "global advertising" in the 1970s and 1980s. "International advertising was a creative graveyard," said John Hegarty of the British agency Bartle Bogle Hegarty. "Nobody wanted to work on it, and most of the advertising

THE NEW GLOBAL HOT SPOTS.

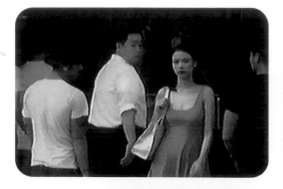

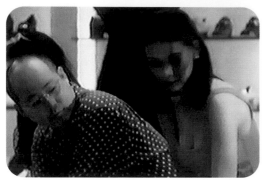

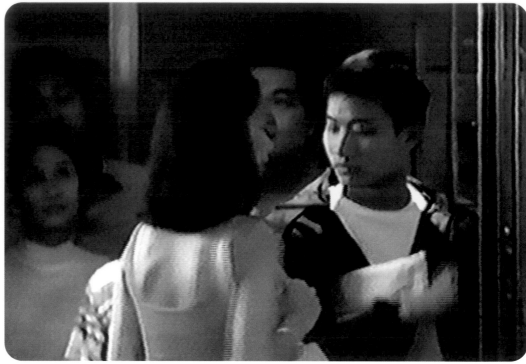

3

produced was dull and creatively dead." Hegarty says that such ads "tended to overemphasize cultural differences," while missing the point that a good idea expressed a certain way can often transcend cultural differences.

There were exceptions, however. In a few scattered markets throughout Asia, South America, and Australia, a handful of creative "missionaries" were spreading the gospel of Bill Bernbach and David Ogilvy and the UK's Collett Dickenson Pearce—in effect, putting forth the notion that ads could be more compelling if they were stylish, unpredictable, and relatively candid with the public. In some regions, that philosophy was quickly seized upon by local writers and artists who, for the first time, began to see advertising as a place to express ideas.

Meanwhile, the regional barriers that had at first impeded the spread of the Creative Revolution began to dissolve as a new global culture emerged. The "McDonald's effect," as some called it, was more accurately "the MTV effect"—dominated not so much by big business as by American youth culture. By the mid-1990s, British ad executive Tim Delaney of Leagas Delaney had observed, "one culture is sweeping across the entire planet. It is the only game in town. Whether you go to India, Australia, or South America, agencies with a global perspective are selling American culture. It's going to be the only 'kids culture' in the future."

Delaney noted that the emergence of this common global youth culture played to the strengths of creative advertisers. "It has helped us to find shared interests among people around the world, and connect with them. The big ideas are beginning to work in a way that crosses borders. All of those old rules that made global advertising so dreadful—'Humor doesn't travel,' and so forth—make no sense when you're dealing with a world that is totally media-literate and plugged into one culture. More and more, if you

write great, simple, and true ads, the audience, no matter where they are, will reach for them and embrace them."

This one-world approach has been labeled "global consumer culture positioning" by the *Journal of Marketing*, and is based on the idea of "associating a brand with a widely understood and recognized set of symbols." Put simply, it explains why images of Michael Jordan and Marilyn Monroe show up not just in American ads but in Asian and South American ones, too. As the new advertising popping up in regional "hot spots" around the world has become increasingly multicultural, it is often relying more on visual images than language—enabling the ads to move easily from one country to another. In these markets, "advertisers are realizing they have to live beyond their own borders," said BBH's Hegarty. "Agencies in these places find themselves with a client saying, 'Listen, our ads are going to have to run in eight

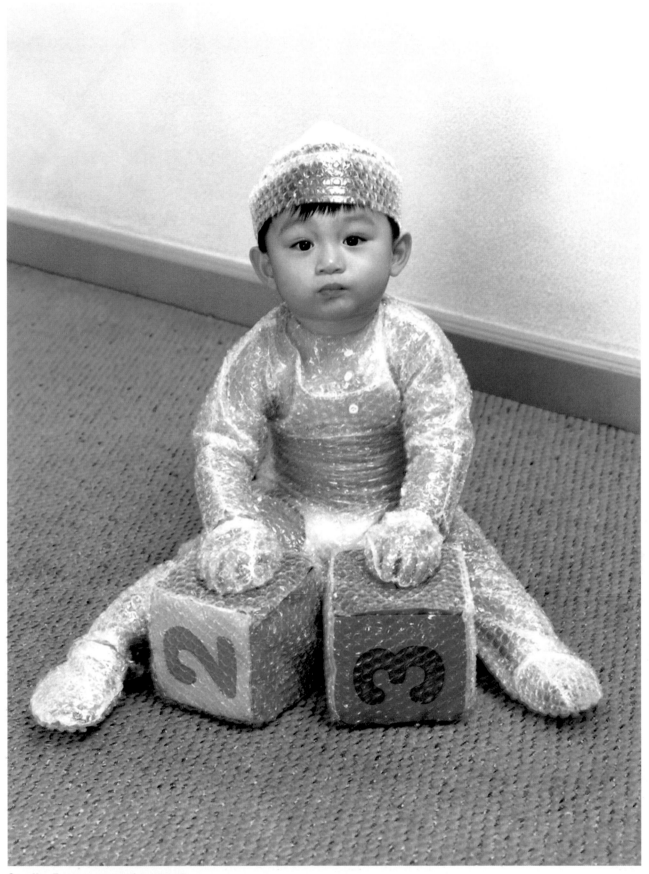

Corolla. For overprotective parents.

Dual airbags, self-tensioning seat belts, collapsible steering column, energy-absorbing reinforcements in the roof-side rails and pillars, side impact protection beams, rigid passenger safety cell, ABS and shatter-resistant glass. ⊕ **TOYOTA**

4

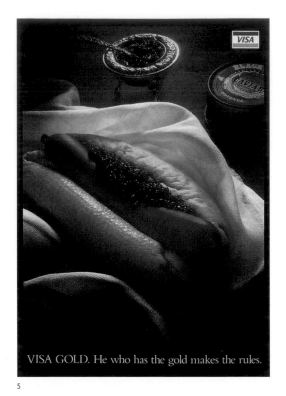

VISA GOLD. He who has the gold makes the rules.

5

6

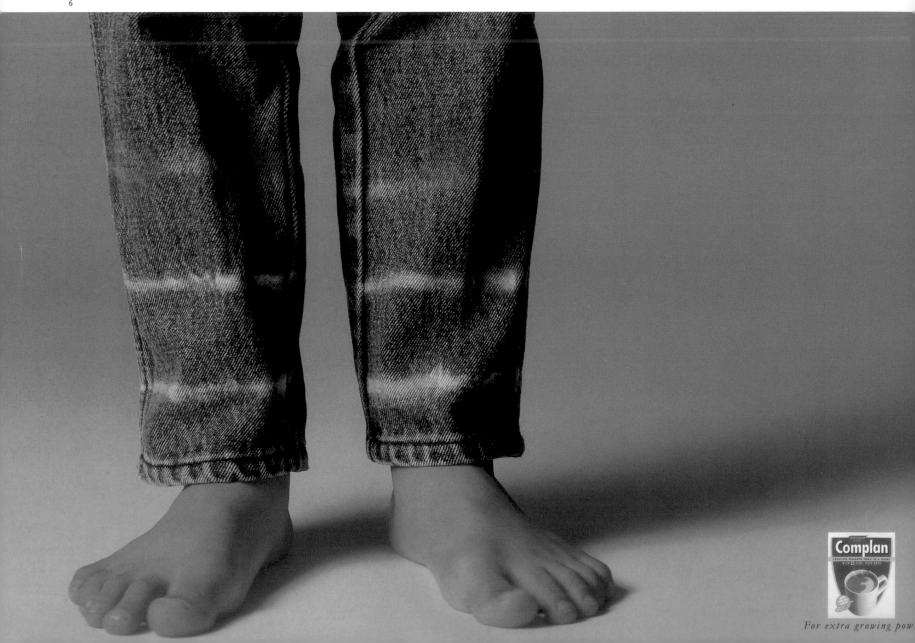

Complan

For extra growing pow

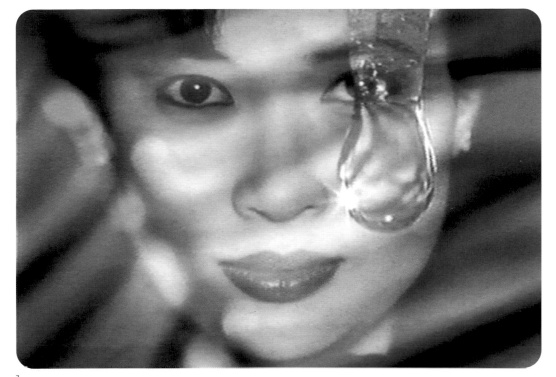

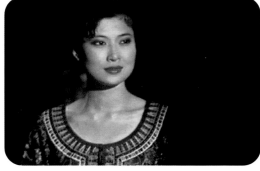

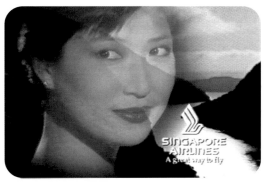

7

5. **VISA GOLD**
BATEY ADS, SINGAPORE, 1996
With the widespread availability
of credit cards in Asia, new
attitudes came to the fore. This
mid-1990s campaign promoted
self-indulgence.

6. **COMPLAN**
CHAITRA LEO BURNETT,
MUMBAI, 1998
Ads in India have tended to be
highly visual; this one makes
its point without a word of
body copy.

7. **SINGAPORE AIRLINES**
BATEY ADS, SINGAPORE, 1994
The "Singapore Girl" campaign
promoting the airline's hostesses
has portrayed women in a
traditional subservient role,
though recent ads have taken
a more modern approach.

different markets, and they all speak different languages.' You have to find a way of reaching all those people, while still creating advertising that communicates to a very advertising-literate young audience." As a growing number of international ad agencies have risen to this challenge, a handful of countries in particular have emerged as new creative hot spots on the continents of Asia, South America, Australia, and Africa.

ASIA

Asian advertising, which is still relatively young and growing up fast, can confound one's expectations at every turn. In a part of the world often associated with traditionalism and conformity, it's not uncommon to find an ad in Hong Kong or Bangkok that challenges convention, attacks stereotypes, advocates individuality—and flashes some skin, too. (Although in mainland China, some restrictions remain; recent ads have been censored for mentioning politics or showing women in miniskirts.) But for the most part, ads in Asia increasingly celebrate—indeed, revel in—the consumer culture of spending, status symbols, and self-indulgence. Such ads can seem strangely disconnected from traditional Asian values, as well as from the codes of conduct associated with some Asian countries' Communist history. But in many parts of Asia, including China, attitudes began to change as the public got its first taste of real consumerism in the early 1990s: Branded consumer products flooded in from the West, credit cards became available, the Asian media expanded—all of which helped fuel a burgeoning Asian consumer class.

Naturally, advertising is pouring as much fuel on this fire as it possibly can. But the best Asian advertising does so with a light touch and an awareness of local culture and history. As one restaurant ad from O&M Singapore recently declared, "Someday Communism will take over Capitalism. Till then, we all need to eat."

Singapore has been at the forefront of creative advertising in Asia. Because the former British colony has had a heavy Western influence and a substantial English-speaking population for some time, it was a natural entry point, along with Hong Kong, for Western advertisers trying to penetrate the Asian marketplace. As a number of agencies put down roots in the early 1970s, Ogilvy & Mather, and in particular the O&M creative director Neil French, seemed to have the most formative effect. "The map in Singapore was changed by Neil French," observed the Asian ad writer Kash Sree. Prior to French's arrival, the local advertising "was all about not making waves," said Sree. "But French brought an irreverent English sensibility." In a very proper society, French's ads spoke candidly about human behavior ranging from sex to flatulence.

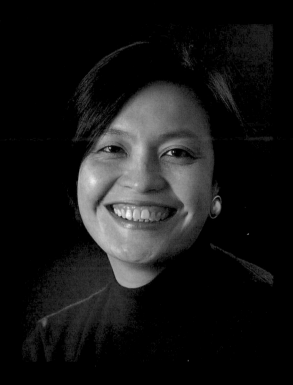

INTERVIEW: KITTY LUN

As the former creative director of Euro RSCG's renowned Hong Kong agency, Kitty Lun was one of the most respected creative leaders in Asian advertising and one of the highest-ranking female executives in the region. With a flair for design and a willingness to take on controversial themes (her ads for Chinese modern art shocked some in the Hong Kong ad community), Lun represents a new generation of Asian ad creators who are helping to modernize advertising throughout the continent.

WOULD YOU SAY ASIAN ADVERTISING HAS HAD A CREATIVE REVOLUTION OF ITS OWN IN RECENT YEARS?
Yes, in different places and at different times. Thailand was one of the first Asian markets to awaken to the need for its own creative style. In the 1980s, a unique brand of Thai advertising emerged with emphasis on local culture and Thai humor. During that time, Hong Kong and Singapore were supposed to be the most sophisticated ad markets, but the style in those two countries was very much influenced by the West. Global clients ruled. Even ads developed locally took on the globally accepted formulas. I am not saying there was no great creative work—but it lacked a unique local culture. Most creative directors in Hong Kong and Singapore were expatriates. So Thailand's revolution came as a breath of fresh air. After Thailand came Taiwan. A new style emerged there—very unique, highly art-directed and MTV-ish, with messages always focused on social issues. Western rational approach was not emphasized. The revolutions I'm referring to are a departure from conventional Western wisdom of what an ad, or an idea, should look like. They represent a completely different-thinking path, a kind of Oriental way of thinking. Usually not linear and not rational, hence very lateral and amazing. The next market to watch would be China.

A LOT OF ADVERTISING AROUND THE WORLD, ESPECIALLY PRINT, HAS BECOME VERY SIMPLE AND VISUAL—OFTEN USING ONE STRIKING IMAGE WITH FEW WORDS. HAS THIS CAUGHT ON IN ASIAN ADVERTISING?
Yes, especially in Singapore and Hong Kong. Singapore consumers are very sophisticated and can understand the simplicity and can draw their own conclusion with minimum clues given. Also,

Singapore was groomed by a group of very sophisticated admen from the West who favored this kind of approach. And when done cleverly, these ads win awards easily—hence attracting younger creatives to do more of the same.

AMERICAN ADVERTISING HAS COME TO FEATURE MORE WILD SCENARIOS, BIZARRE CHARACTERS, OFFBEAT MESSAGES—"ODDVERTISING." DOES THIS KIND OF APPROACH WORK IN THE ASIAN MARKETS? THE COMMON PERCEPTION IS THAT THE AUDIENCE THERE MIGHT BE MORE CONSERVATIVE.
Japan was probably one of the first to use Oddvertising. Years ago, Japanese advertising started to catch the eye of the world, with award-winning Cup Noodles commercials—not much of a strategy, very left-field, very unusual. And Thailand and Taiwan are very used to this kind of offbeat approach—even more so than the West. Many people have a perception that China is a conservative market. However, time and again, the consumers surprise us. After all, a piece of communication is more than just science. It is art that appeals to the emotion, the soul, the aesthetics. Chinese consumers react mostly the same ways as consumers around the world. They react with their hearts. They may not be as worldly, because the country was not exposed to the outside world in the last century. But being such a virgin market, they are even more open to unusual ideas.

IS IT UNUSUAL FOR A WOMAN TO BE A TOP AD EXECUTIVE IN ASIA?
Actually, I find the opportunities are good. The best person gets the job, period. In fact, we find a higher proportion of women in top creative and management positions in Hong Kong, Taiwan, and China than in the U.S. and in Europe. With advertising being seen as a "soft" business, it is a female-dominated industry over here.

WHAT ABOUT PORTRAYALS OF WOMEN IN CHINESE ADS—WOULD YOU SAY THEY ARE PROGRESSIVE OR MORE OLD-FASHIONED AND TRADITIONAL?
The answer is both. The portrayal of business-women is pretty progressive, and comparable to anywhere in the world. However, there is still a large number of ads portraying women as the "plaything." It was particularly true a few years

back when cognac and beer were big players in the industry. Also, in traditional household products like cooking oil, rice, and detergent, women are still confined to the standard good-housewife image. For cosmetics, shampoo, and other beauty products, women are still portrayed as trying to look their best for their men. Apart from being a social and sexist issue, it is also a creative issue—it's about finding new ways to represent the users of these products.

OBVIOUSLY, MANY AMERICAN ADS ARE BASED ON THE IDEA OF PEOPLE TREATING THEMSELVES WELL AND INDULGING DESIRES FOR EXPENSIVE THINGS. DO CHINESE ADS TEND TO HAVE CERTAIN ATTITUDES ABOUT SHOWING WEALTH AND SELF-INDULGENCE— MIGHT THAT BE CONSIDERED INAPPROPRIATE IN SOME ASIAN CULTURES?
No, it is extremely appropriate. This is the market for conspicuous spending and indulgence. The higher the price tag, the bigger the "face." It is always glorified as "aspiration"—and the ad agencies are often forced to present products in a light much superior to what they really are. Categories that do this include real estate, selling dreams rather than homes; luxury goods— watches, jewelry, designer labels like the rest of the world; self-indulgent products like chocolates, airlines, and hotels. Advertising people often struggle to present things in a more earthy, back to basics light. But it is very seldom that clients have the insight to portray the true value of the products. However, that situation is improving now.

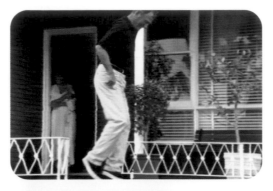

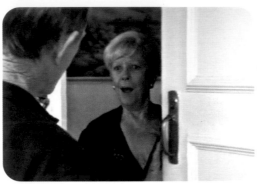

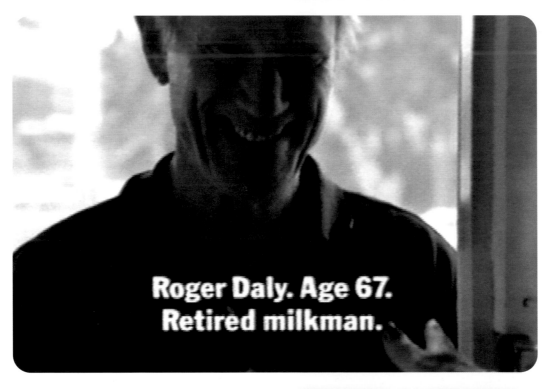

Roger Daly. Age 67. Retired milkman.

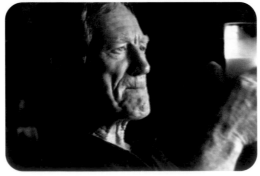

10

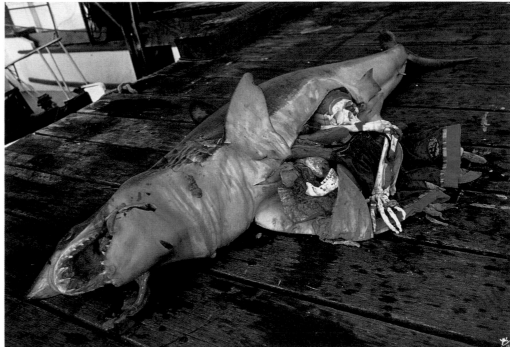

11

**10. AUSTRALIAN MILK
ASSOCIATION**
CLEMENGER, MELBOURNE,
1998
This risqué Australian campaign
used sex to sell milk, portraying
the milkman as a door-to-door
Romeo. The milk is what keeps
his juices flowing.

11. KADU CLOTHING
ANDROMEDA, SYDNEY, 1994
Shocking imagery has been
part of Australian advertising
for years; this ad showed a
disemboweled shark, whose
contents included a human
skeleton.

ad for picture frames, showing a wall filled
with photographs, in a variety of frames, all
containing the same scowling woman's face; it
was headlined, "There's more than one way to
hang your mother-in-law."

A couple of places in Asia where humor is
more welcome and usually wilder are Thailand
and Japan. In the past few years, Thailand has
earned a reputation for quirky outrageousness in
its commercials, which have been known to
feature spontaneous kung fu brawls, slapstick
humor, and even silver-painted transvestites
(known as the Lead Devils, these characters
created by the Bangkok office of Leo Burnett
invade cars filled with the wrong type of
gasoline, and can be dispatched only by fueling
up with the right kind of gasoline). According to
Rutaiwan Wongsirasawad, creative director at
JWT in Bangkok, "You can make fun of the
product, of yourself—nothing is out of bounds."
Even the country's military leaders aren't shielded

from the barbs of advertisers; in one popular
commercial from Bangkok's Results agency,
an army general tries to talk a kidnapper into
giving up his hostage—and ends up getting a
hole blown in his stomach. Then, a working-
class hero named "tractor man" comes to the
rescue in his Mitsubishi tractor, which plows
right into the kidnappers' hideaway. Bhanu
Inkawat, regarded as one of the creative leaders
of Thai advertising, says the wild humor in ads
"is based on the comic-book and slapstick-come-
dy style we grew up with. You can see this kind
of entertainment everywhere, in the coffee shops
across the country, on the TV game shows."

The advertising of Thailand has been compared to that of Japan, which is known for
bursts of wild humor and outrageous antics—
though Japanese advertising can also be subtle
and stylish. In either case, Japanese ads have
long tended to favor emotional appeals, fantasies, and soft sell, rather than straightforward

sales pitches. Having embraced industrializa-
tion and capitalism relatively early, Japan was
well ahead of other countries in Asia when it
came to mastering the craft of advertising; in
fact, it had its own ad creative revolution back
in the mid-1960s, just a few years after the
American one. Subsequently, Japanese ads
became very image-oriented—they tended to
promote the company, not the product itself,
and gently tried to forge bonds of goodwill.
Critics from abroad often said that Japanese
ads didn't sell at all, but Jun Yoshitake, a top
executive at the Dentsu agency, explains that
for Japanese consumers, who have a strong
tendency toward brand loyalty, the soft sell was
often preferable. Hard-sell pitches could be
seen as a form of bragging.

In recent years, Japanese ads have lost some
of their stylishness, and have come to rely more
on celebrities and on quick sales pitches packed
into the now-popular fifteen-second commercial

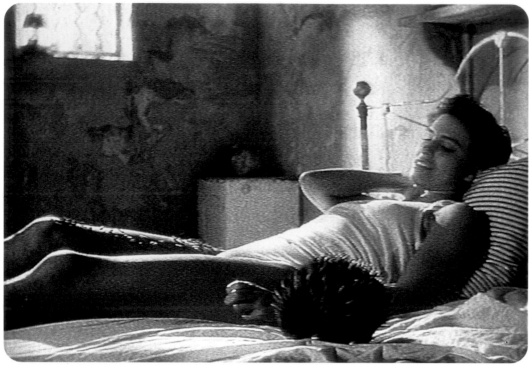

12

format. Yoshitake attributes this to the economic downturn in Japan, which pressured advertisers to gravitate toward hard sell. But there are still bright spots and surprises, as in the slapstick humor of a long-running campaign that always ends with the bizarrely enthusiastic exclamation "Hungry? PotNoodles!" And a recent Dentsu commercial for a cable movie channel shows there's still room for lively storytelling. The commercial opens with a dinner scene in which a Japanese expatriate in America informs his blonde girlfriend that he must return to Japan immediately. In an overly dramatic manner, he slowly journeys back to his homeland, while we hear his girlfriend screaming over and over, "Why? Why?" In the end, the truth is revealed: He's gone back because he misses the Wowow TV channel.

If Japan is slumping creatively these days, other Asian countries are picking up the slack. India, for example, produces lively commercials

that borrow heavily from the country's thriving "Bollywood" film industry and tend to feature "lots of music, chaos, and beautiful women," Aitchison observes. Kash Sree adds, "Whereas jingles have lost their power in the West, you can sell almost anything with a song in India." India has also served as a rich source of English-language copywriters for Asia. The country that gave us Salman Rushdie (a onetime advertising writer himself, before he gave the craft up for novels) has also produced a host of other copywriting stars, who "have beaten a path to Hong Kong and Singapore," Aitchison notes, because they can earn much more money there than back in India.

Many believe the next stage in the evolution of Asian advertising will be a rediscovery of local culture. After a decade of trying to copy and learn from Western advertising, says Inkawat, the Asian ad community is now feeling more confident and secure in its own identity. He

thinks that will be reflected more and more in the Asian ads created in days ahead. "I believe every country is now looking inward for its inspiration, for insights and stories from its own culture, rather than looking toward the U.S. or England like before," said Inkawat. "It's a good sign of progress."

AUSTRALIA

Down Under, they're still talking about the dancing penis. An Australian commercial featuring a singing, dancing penis (promoting a gay radio station in Sydney) not only attracted attention locally but ended up stealing the show at a recent gathering of the International Advertising Festival in Cannes. It wasn't the first time that those randy and mischievous Australians had shocked the international ad community.

Each year, it seems, Australian advertising pushes the boundaries of good taste a little farther, which recently prompted one Australian

WHAT THE BITCH WHO'S ABOUT TO STEAL YOUR MAN WEARS.

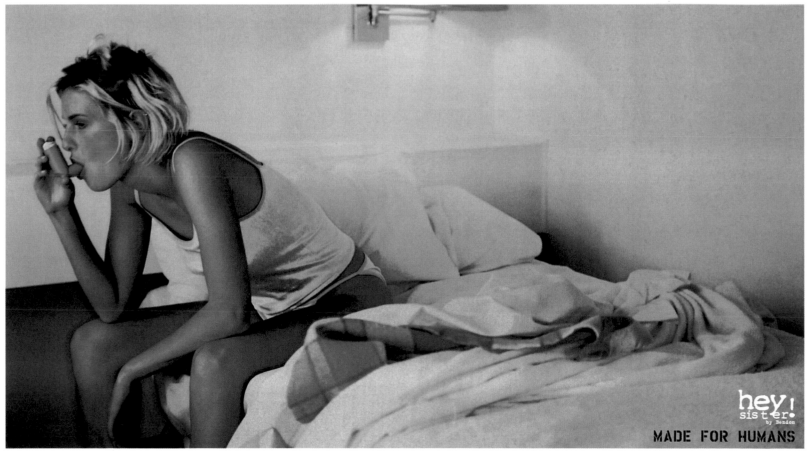

13

14

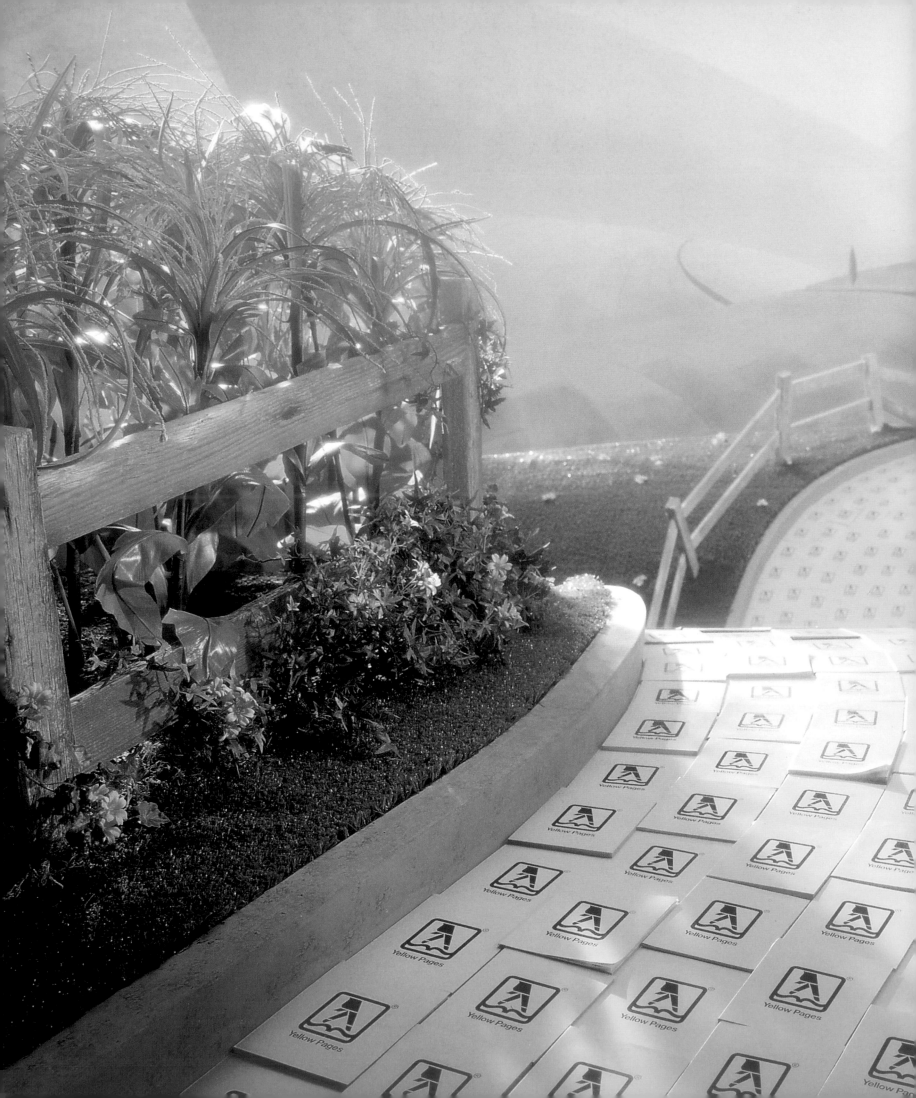

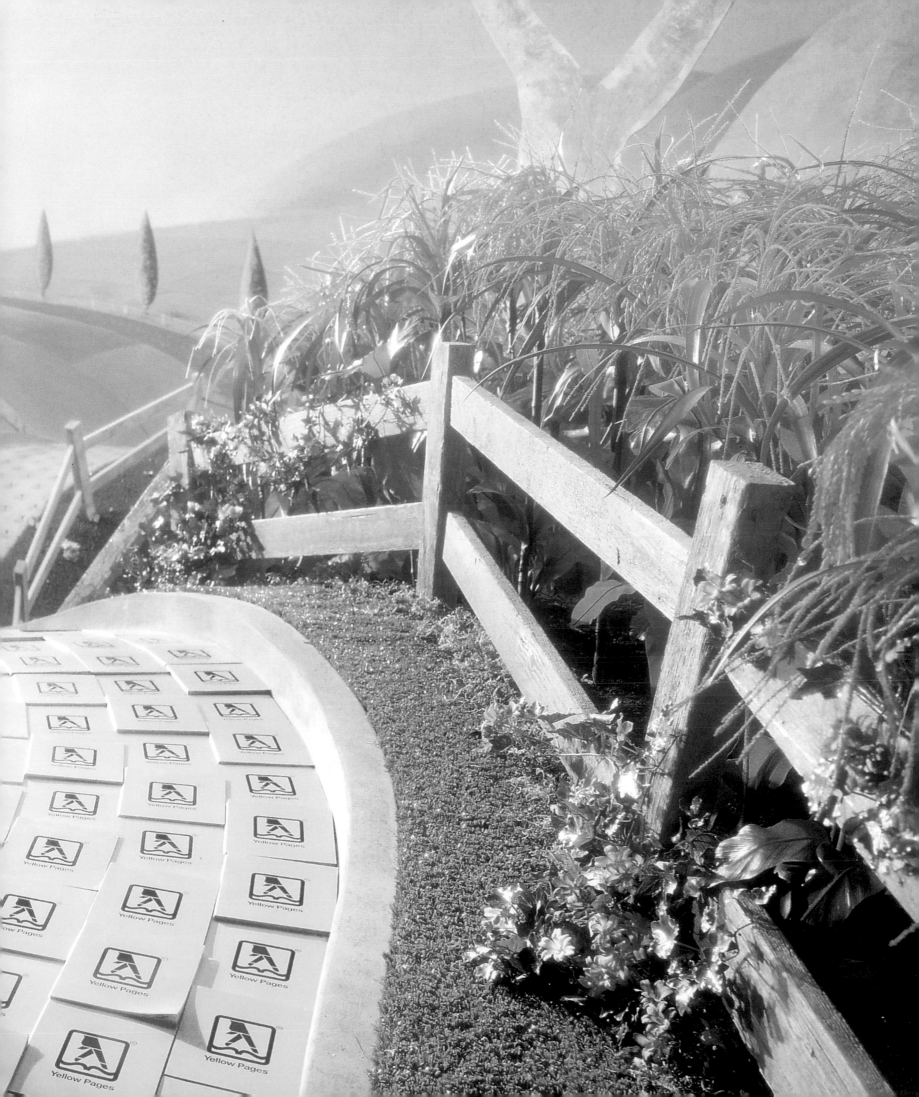

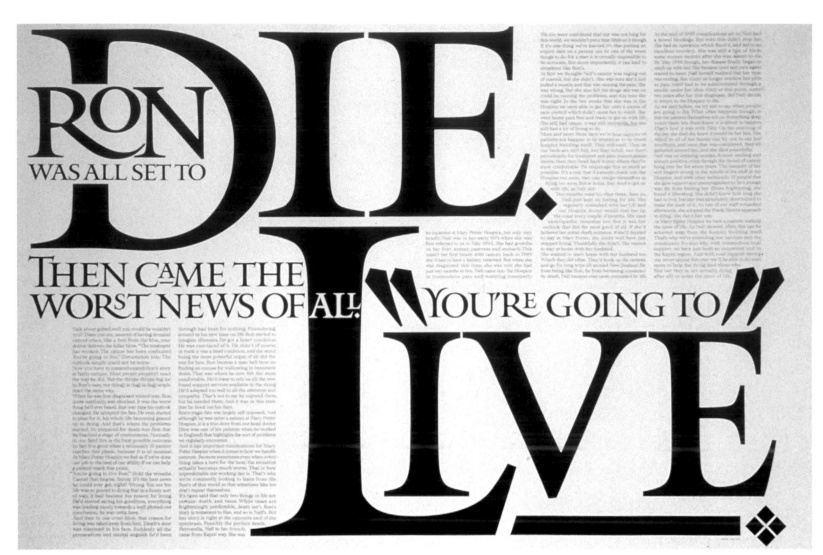

16

15. (PREVIOUS SPREAD)
YELLOW PAGES
CLEMENGER, MELBOURNE,
1996
Building a yellow brick road out
of Yellow Pages books, this ad
promised the world without
saying a word.

16. **MARY POTTER HOSPICE**
SAATCHI & SAATCHI NEW
ZEALAND, WELLINGTON, 1996
New Zealand has emerged as an
advertising hotbed, and leading
the way has been Saatchi's local
office; here, experimental use of
type produces dramatic results.

17. **COALITION FOR GUN
CONTROL**
SAATCHI & SAATCHI,
SYDNEY, 1999
More brashness from Down
Under: This time, the ad shows
both sides of a bullet wound.

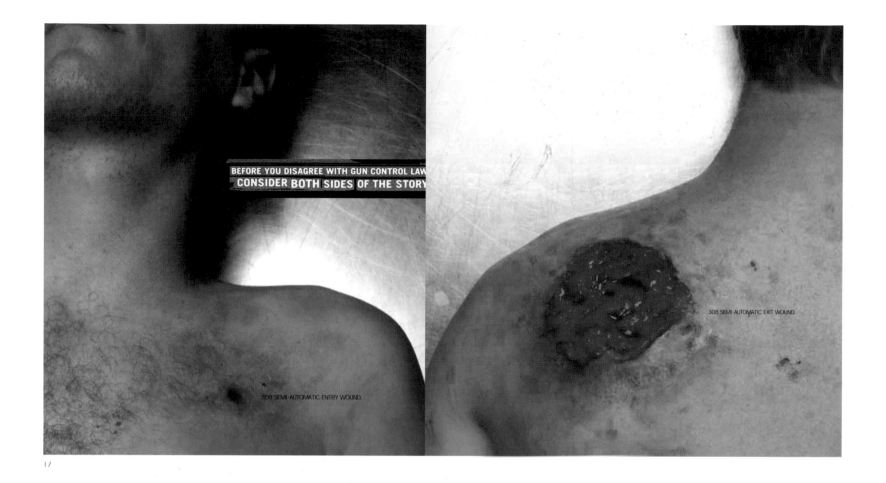

BEFORE YOU DISAGREE WITH GUN CONTROL LAW
CONSIDER BOTH SIDES OF THE STORY

.308 SEMI-AUTOMATIC ENTRY WOUND.

.308 SEMI-AUTOMATIC EXIT WOUND.

17

expatriate, Paul Bernasconi, to wonder aloud in an *Advertising Age* editorial, "Why is Australian advertising so hilariously obnoxious? How do they get away with it?"

The examples abound, as Bernasconi pointed out. An infamous commercial from Campaign Palace featured a semi-naked girl who rids her underwear of ants with the help of an aggressive anteater. Another showed a transvestite cleaning a public toilet, then declaring it "fit for a queen." One of Bernasconi's favorites: "a beer commercial showing a man in a confessional box tricking a priest into revealing the names of wayward women."

Even the most wholesome of products, milk, is promoted with a healthy dose of sexual innuendo in Australia. A hugely popular ad campaign from the Clemenger Melbourne agency features a spry 67-year-old retired milkman who continues to make his rounds— but it's not milk he's delivering to the house-

wives at each stop. Another ad in the series acknowledges the cliché of the milkman as door-to-door Romeo, and points out, "It was never the postman, always the milkman." The only explanation for this, the ads suggest, is the power of milk.

When not using outrageous or risqué humor, Australian ads have been known to feature shockingly gritty scenes: An award-winning print ad for Kadu clothing company showed a photograph of a disemboweled shark, with the ingredients of its stomach (including a human skeleton) spilling out on the ground. And a long-running series of commercials promoting traffic safety, from Grey Advertising in Melbourne, presents some of the most devastatingly realistic simulations of car accidents ever seen on television—showing not only the bone-jarring collisions but also the ensuing bloodshed and tears in the hospital emergency room.

It's not entirely clear why Australian

advertising has tended to be so bold and occasionally shocking. Bernasconi theorized, "Australia is an island, physically and culturally. And as such, within a very short time, Australians have developed into a breed apart. We have our own sense of humor. . . . We brandish our crudeness like a sword, repelling the creeping sameness, the choking homogeneity of the rest of the English-speaking world. We wear vulgarity and brashness like a badge, declaring to the world that we will not be Canadianized. And as America and Britain continue to dominate the global conversation, we make our voice heard by behaving like the spoiled bastard child that we are. . . . We misbehave."

Whether the contributing factors are geography, genetics, or something else, Australian ads have been attention-grabbers since the local ad creative community first started to take shape, back in the early 1970s, under the guidance of Lionel Hunt, who came

THE NEW GLOBAL HOT SPOTS.

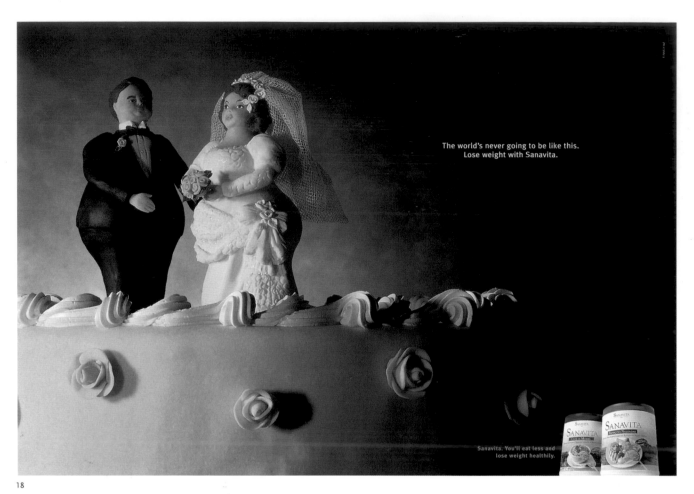

The world's never going to be like this.
Lose weight with Sanavita.

Sanavita. You'll eat less and
lose weight healthily.

18

from the UK and helped set up the pioneering creative agency Campaign Palace. From the outset, the advertising was—and to some extent remains—derivative of the English irreverent style. As Rob Dow of Grey Melbourne said, "Australians tend to follow the UK style with subtle wit rather than the belly laugh." At the same time, Australian advertising was also heavily influenced by America, which may have contributed to its brassy, in-your-face sensibility.

The frankness of Australian ads extends beyond sex or blood and guts. Ads to women have tended to be refreshingly candid. One award-winning fashion ad from a few years back bore the provocative headline "What the bitch who's about to steal your man wears." Another, for the body-pillow mattress, engaged in a bit of playful male-bashing by describing the product as "the perfect male substitute. Warm, cuddly, and totally brainless." And advertisers in the region have been willing to challenge the beauty

myth: the New Zealand underwear marketer Bendon created a campaign featuring young models who bore the scars of real life, including a woman with her arm in a plaster cast and using an asthma inhaler. The advertiser said that local teens "do not necessarily relate to the cover girl and supermodel look. . . . The images they find most powerful are those closer to their own individual reality."

A surprising level of candor about race can be seen in some Australian commercials. In pitching suntan lotion, Young & Rubicam in Sydney featured black characters who are amused by the fact that Caucasians get burned in the sun and need sunscreen "to get the protection the black man has naturally." After one character concludes, only half-jokingly, that "Mother Nature must be black," the commercial closes with the ironic tag line "For whites who want equality."

Though the public seems to enjoy provocative ads, there is the occasional backlash.

For example, a Johnson & Johnson TV campaign for Meds tampons seemed innocuous enough; the ads posed the question "What tampon does your lady use?" and showed men reacting in various ways—some grimace at the query; some laugh; some actually answer the question ("Meds. If she's busy, I buy them for her," said one very progressive fellow). Yet the campaign was pulled from the air after a barrage of complaints—mostly from women. And the Australian Standards Council called the ads "a bit gauche."

Australian advertising's brashness is tempered by a sense of style; the region is known for its elegant design, particularly in New Zealand—which is heavily influenced by the Australian culture but at the same time exhibits its own flair. The agency Saatchi & Saatchi in Wellington has specialized in arresting imagery that seems to scream out its messages. Its work includes an eye-opening type treatment for a

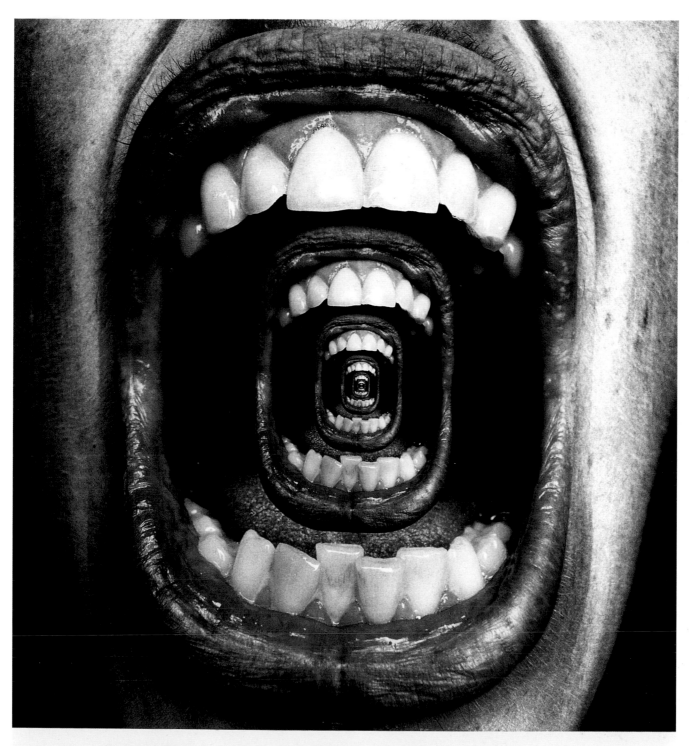

THE ABUSE YOU YELL AT YOUR KIDS STAYS IN THE FAMILY FOR GENERATIONS

You're useless. You're dumb. I wish you'd never been born. Shout verbal abuse like this at your kids and you don't just hurt them, you teach them to be abusive parents too. Break the cycle. Call 0800 222 999 for a free parenting booklet that will help.

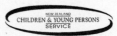

NEW ZEALAND
CHILDREN & YOUNG PERSONS
SERVICE

19

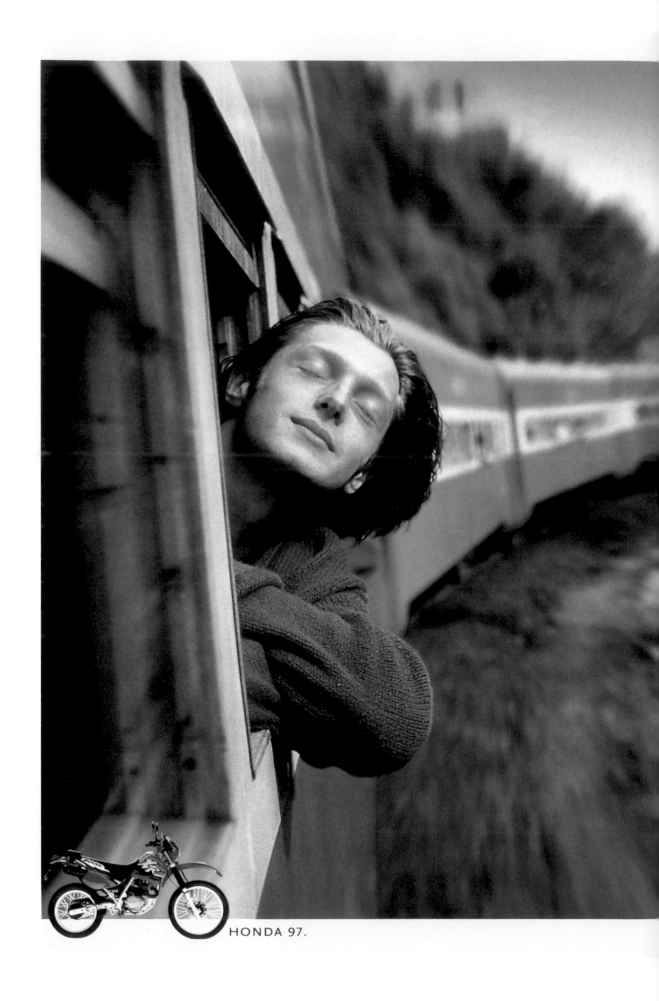

HONDA 97.

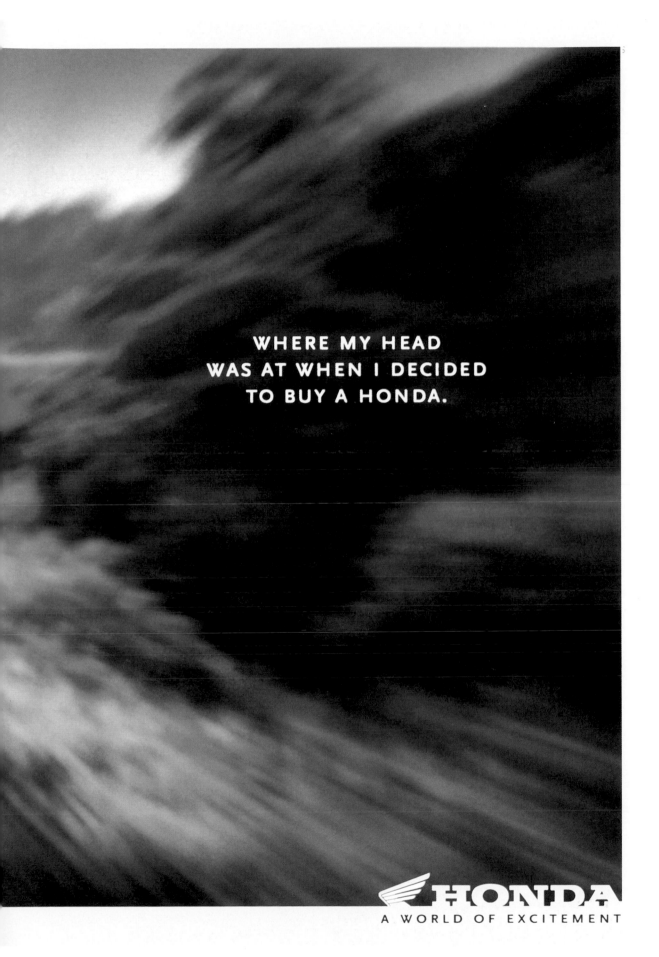

WHERE MY HEAD
WAS AT WHEN I DECIDED
TO BUY A HONDA.

HONDA
A WORLD OF EXCITEMENT

20. **HONDA**
DM9 DDB PUBLICIDADE,
SÃO PAULO, 1997
Selling a motorcycle by showing
a train: DM9 focuses not on the
product itself but the feelings
associated with it.

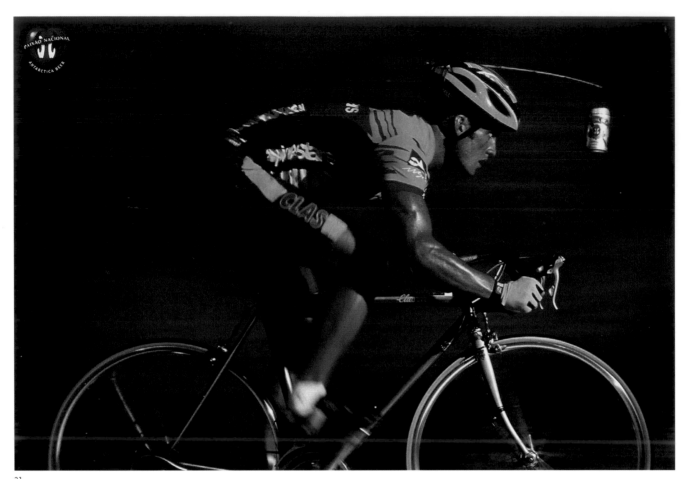

21

21. **ANTARCTICA BEER**
DM9 DDB PUBLICIDADE,
SÃO PAULO, 1997
A funny image, and a lesson in
motivational strategies: Here,
the beer can becomes the carrot
that we're all chasing.

22. **DIET GUARANÁ**
DM9 DDB PUBLICIDADE,
SÃO PAULO, 1999
This Brazilian agency
specializes in using a simple
picture to tell a story and sell
the product; showing a tight
squeeze reminds us why we
should opt for a diet drink.

local hospice, as well as a child-abuse ad that features a screaming mouth within a screaming mouth within a screaming mouth, and the headline "The abuse you yell at your kids stays in the family for generations." Even more than Australia, New Zealand is a cost-conscious ad market, and there's little opportunity for elaborate Hollywood-style production and special effects. Given those limitations, says Saatchi New Zealand art director John Fisher, "a strong idea becomes even more important here, because it can get the job done even if the production values aren't quite where you'd want them to be in an ideal world."

SOUTH AMERICA

In the 1990s, South America, and particularly Brazil, fell madly in love with advertising. Suddenly, commercials were being passionately discussed in bars. Students who formerly might have opted for a career in medicine or

engineering now wanted to make ads. And award-winning admen became local celebrities, "granted the status of pop stars," observed the veteran Brazilian adman Washington Olivetto.

The love affair has, over the past few years, produced a body of creative advertising that has been sweeping international award shows and introducing a new language in the ad world. As befits the region it springs from, South American advertising tends to be bold, colorful, emotional, and playful. But what is perhaps most striking about it is the economy with which it communicates big ideas. The advertising produced by São Paulo's DM9 DDB Publicidade, the preeminent agency in the region over the past few years, often conveys emotion through one simple image: A picture of ketchup coming out of a bottle is all that's needed, in one ad, to suggest that this particular condiment will set your mouth ablaze. And the agency used nothing more than a picture of a

man trying to squeeze out of a car door in a tight parking space to make its case for a diet soft drink.

When asked why his ads invariably tried to say so much by saying so little, DM9's longtime creative director Nizan Guanaes blamed it on Brazil. "I live in a simple country," Guanaes said, noting that Brazilians have no desire to wade through tedious explanation and no tolerance for ads that take themselves too seriously. "No one here wants to spend a lot of time reading an ad," Guanaes said. "They want to know immediately what it is about."

That may explain the prevalence of visual riddles and puns in South American advertising, running the gamut from subtle and emotional (a car key being passed from one hand to another in a Volkswagen ad headlined "Forever") to obvious and a bit tacky (a Colgate mouthwash ad that turns a human mouth into a toilet seat). There is another explanation for all of these ads:

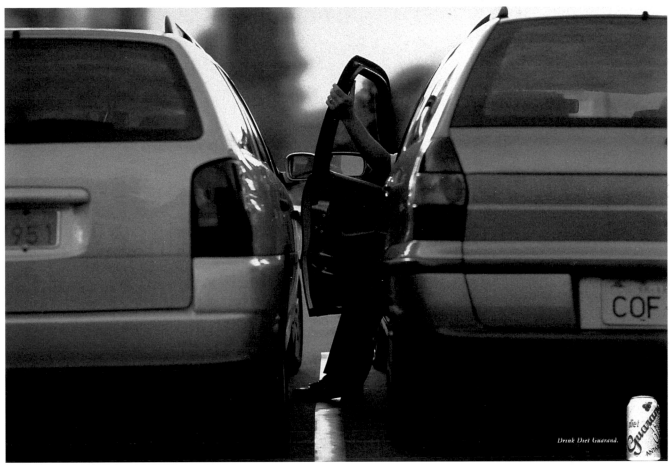

Drink Diet Guaraná.

22

They tend to fare well at international award shows and have reaped top prizes for the agencies that created them. "In the 1990s some professionals, eager to be well renowned, started producing advertising for festivals only," said Olivetto, who runs the Brazilian agency W/Brasil. The hallmark of such ads, he noted, is their tendency to be "preeminently visual, easily understandable in any language, but inappropriate to the Brazilian reality. I myself consider this to be extremely bad and unreal, so much so that I have labeled this 'ghost advertising.' "

Olivetto's opinion on such matters cannot be discounted, considering that he is regarded as South America's creative ad pioneer, the Bill Bernbach of Brazil. He served as creative director at the agency DPZ, which first began draw attention in the late 1970s and early 1980s with advertising that blended humor, emotion, and sensuousness—traits that are "typical of the Brazilian people," Olivetto said. While Olivetto

and his peers were developing their own approach, they also drew on the influences of Doyle Dane Bernbach as well as British advertising. The blending of these all of these styles, Olivetto said, "gave birth to a type of advertising that aims at selling but is also conscious that entertainment is necessary."

Olivetto, after moving on to form W/Brasil, also helped to train a new generation of South American creative leaders, including the young copywriter Guanaes. During the 1980s, Guanaes was already experimenting with a postmodern style of advertising that seemed light-years ahead of the kinds of ads previously seen in South America. One of his ad campaigns for a local bank parodied other hyperbolic commercials by using the character of a bank spokesman who made boastful claims about the bank; as it became clear he was exaggerating, the character desperately tried to cover up and make excuses. Guanaes was practicing "anti-advertising"

before most of his peers had even grasped straightforward advertising.

Guanaes was just one of a handful of talented young creative leaders who were poised to take the mantle from Olivetto in the 1990s. As both creative fervor and entrepreneurial fever began to rage in Brazil, a third factor fueled the 1990s ad revolution—the Brazilian economy, which had suffered through years of hyperinflation, kicked into gear in the mid-1990s and created a thriving consumer market. Brazil emerged as one of the top-selling markets in the world for a vast array of consumer products, from beer to detergent to TV sets. By the mid-1990s, *Advertising Age* noted, "global marketers rushed in to win the hearts and wallets of Brazilian consumers."

These big agency outsiders from America and Europe—including the Saatchis, BBDO, and the DDB network—realized the way to do that was to align themselves with Brazil's most talented admen. That led to the formation of

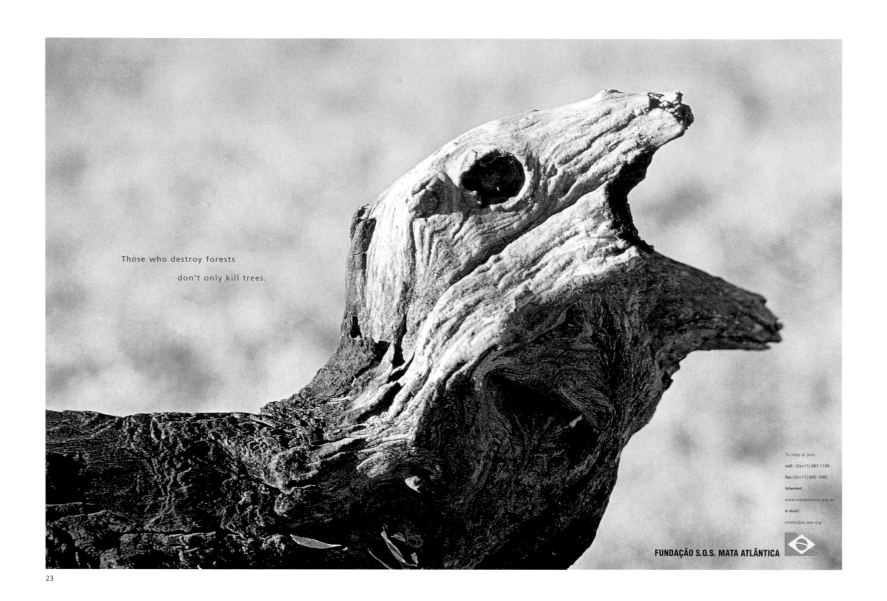

Those who destroy forests
don't only kill trees.

FUNDAÇÃO S.O.S. MATA ATLÂNTICA

23

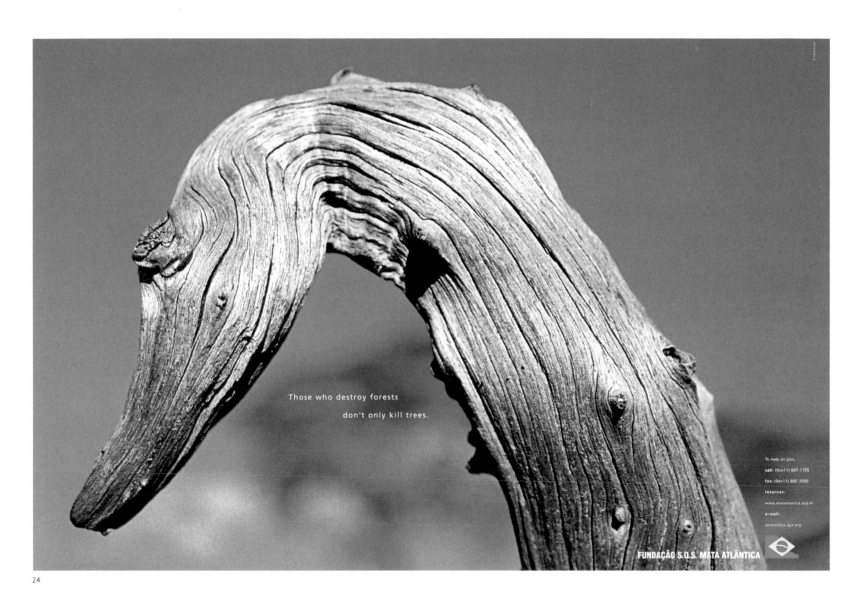

Those who destroy forests
don't only kill trees.

To help or join,
call: (0xx11) 887-1195
fax: (0xx11) 885-1680
Internet:
www.mataatlantica.org.br
e-mail:
smata@ax.apc.org

FUNDAÇÃO S.O.S. MATA ATLÂNTICA

24

23 AND 24. **SAVE THE**
FOREST CAMPAIGN
F/NAZCA SAATCHI & SAATCHI,
SÃO PAULO, 1998
The campaign could have shown
trees, or it could have shown
endangered animals; by showing
animals carved from trees, the
image is far more striking
and effective.

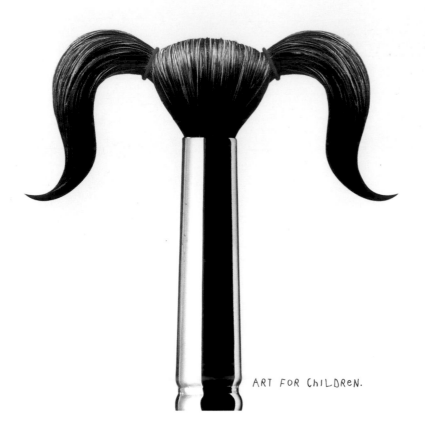

ART FOR CHILDREN.

MASP

25

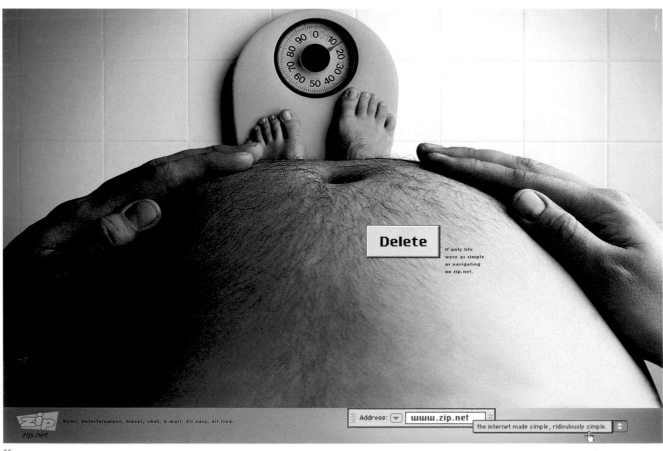

26

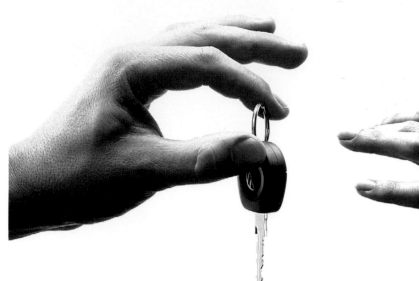
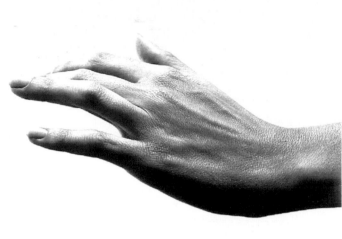

Forever

27

25. **SÃO PAULO MUSEUM OF ART**
W/BRASIL, SÃO PAULO, MID-1990s
South American ads are designed to travel across cultural and language barriers. Here, the paintbrush with ponytails becomes the headline.

26. **ZIP.NET**
F/NAZCA SAATCHI & SAATCHI, SÃO PAULO, 1999
As in North America, dot-com ads below the equator tend to suggest that technology can solve even the most intractable problems; this campaign made fun of that notion.

27. **VOLKSWAGEN**
ALMAP BBDO, SÃO PAULO, LATE 1990s
Instead of using text to discuss tradition, family values, and a sound automobile, the agency decided to let the picture do the talking.

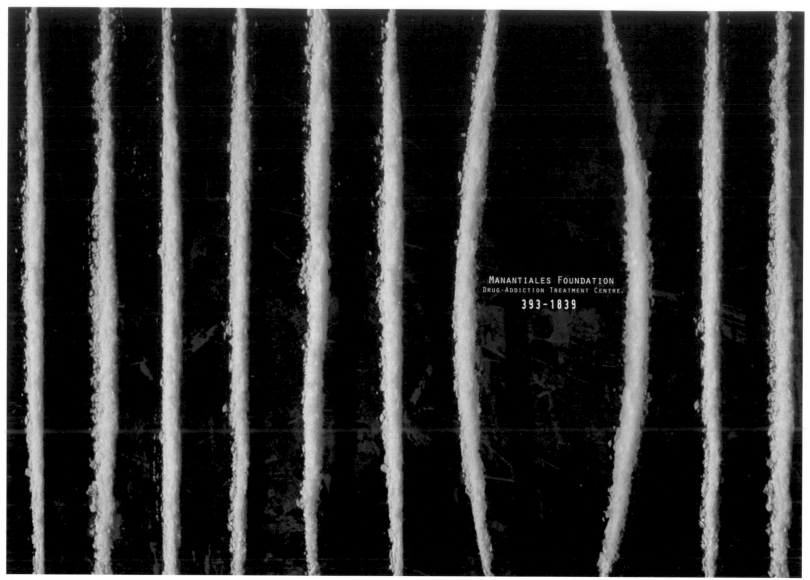

MANANTIALES FOUNDATION
DRUG-ADDICTION TREATMENT CENTRE.
393-1839

28

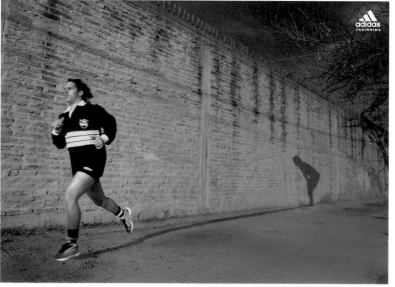

29

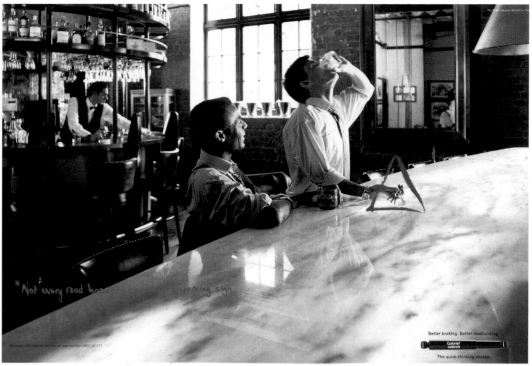

30

agencies such as DM9 DDB, Almap/BBDO, and F/Nazca Saatchi & Saatchi—all well funded by the international networks but still operating under the autonomous creative leadership of local ad stars like Guanaes, Marcello Serpa, and Fabio Fernandes. With resources and creative freedom, the revolution was under way—and it wasn't limited to Brazil. Argentina also emerged as a red-hot creative market, producing ads that were often just as visually striking as the work from Brazil.

Not all South American advertising has achieved the level of sophistication found in Brazil and Buenos Aires. That was made painfully evident recently in Peru, where a late-1990s controversy erupted over an overtly racist commercial that showed Africans preparing to eat white tourists—then opting for Nabisco pudding instead. In fact, several well-known brands had to deal with fallout when a news report uncovered a number of ads featuring

caricatures or stereotypes of blacks (in a Goodyear ad made in Peru, a pitchman compared the thickness of tires to the lips of his black partner). Even in Brazil, it sometimes seems that the attitudes expressed in the ads are not as advanced as the style; a recent commercial that sensuously compared a glass of beer to various parts of a woman's body, including hips and legs, was elegantly and stylishly art directed, but the idea itself was outdated. If the region can over-come such lapses—and resist the temptation to overindulge in the occasional gimmickry of some visual-pun ads designed for award shows— South America may be central to the future of global advertising.

SOUTH AFRICA

When the apartheid system came tumbling down in South Africa, it had an unexpectedly liberating effect on the country's advertising community. Previously, explains the Johannesburg adman

John Hunt, "we lived in a very strict Calvinist society, and we knew all about barriers and how to confine things, how to split things into black and white." Hunt believes that those confining attitudes—not to mention the old regime's tendency to stifle dangerous ideas—kept advertising from being as freethinking and creative as it could be. "Then came 1994 and the celebration of freedom of the new South Africa, and advertising was ready to blossom," Hunt said. "With the liberalization of South Africa, there was also a liberalization of advertising norms and trends. The old censorship—'Don't show certain things, or talk about certain things'—gave way to a new freedom. There was a whole lightness of attitude that emerged." Today, South African ads are known worldwide for their stylishness and their sense of humor. "We've learned to laugh at ourselves," says Hunt. "Before, we were so busy having our wrists slapped, we weren't too hot on humor."

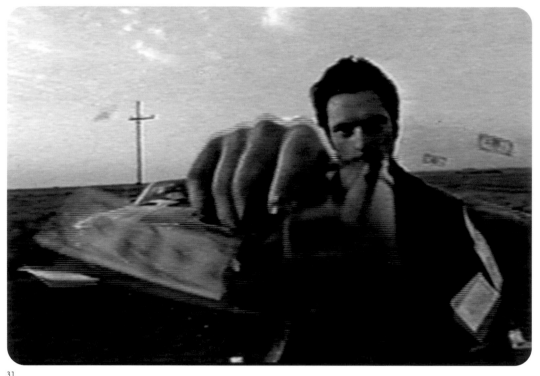

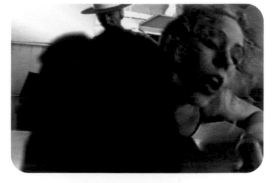

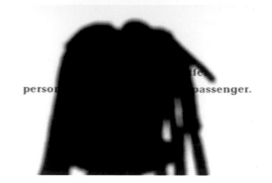

31

Hunt's agency, TBWA Hunt Lascaris, has been one of the driving creative forces behind the rise of South African advertising in the past decade. But he's had plenty of company. Agencies like Ogilvy & Mather Rightford Searle-Tripp & Makin, the Jupiter Drawing Room, and Net#work have also joined in, forming a vibrant creative community.

Like Brazilian advertising, ads in South Africa tend to be visually bold and direct—the ideas are conveyed with minimal explanation. "That might have something to do with the fact that we have eleven official languages in South Africa," said Hunt. "We also have extreme wealth to extreme poverty—a little like Brazil, I guess— so when you're selling something, you've often got to catch all those different people. You tend to be simple, be visual, make the point, and then get the hell out."

Examples of this can be seen in Hunt's own advertising for clients like Nando's chicken restaurants. To inform the public that this purveyor of spicy food was now serving kosher food as well, the agency simply showed a picture of a red pepper—with the tip sliced off. To convey the driving power of one of its clients' four-wheel-drive trucks, Hunt Lascaris showed the vehicle being driven off by newlyweds— but instead of dragging the customary tin cans, the speeding truck has huge kegs tied to its rear bumper.

But South African advertising is interesting these days not just because of its cleverness. Many of the ads are providing a mirror— surprisingly faithful to reality, at times—of a society adjusting to sweeping changes. Advertising has, in fact, been in the midst of the country's social upheaval. In the election leading up to government reform, ad agencies played a role in assuring the public that there was no reason to fear change. As it became clear that apartheid was ending, Schweppes used in its

advertising the line "Everything you wanted to know about mixing in the new South Africa." And finally, after Nelson Mandela came to power (partly on the strength of Hunt Lascaris's advertising), advertising helped white-owned companies overcome some of the ill will felt by black consumers. For example, one government-owned oil company that had been linked to the apartheid regime was advised by Hunt Lascaris to start addressing blacks in its ads; the resulting commercials showed a black child dreaming of being a soccer star, and it proved popular with both whites and blacks.

By the mid-1990s, it was normal for advertisements to show racial mixing—which had been practically taboo in the old days (as one local ad executive explained in the press, ads used to cut from showing blacks to showing whites, but "now we can show a more extended interaction," he said). Of course, portraying inte-gration in ads wasn't simply an act of goodwill by

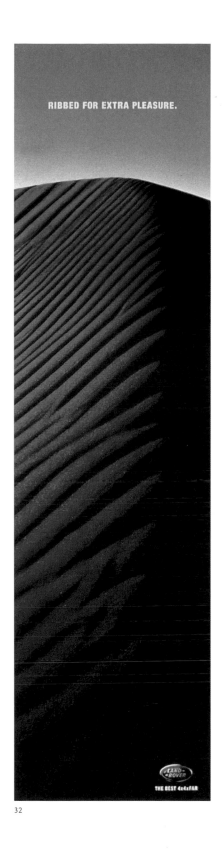

RIBBED FOR EXTRA PLEASURE.

THE BEST 4x4xFAR

32

Circulation up 94%.

An explosion you can categorically blame on the Blacks.

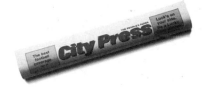

From 134 389 (ABC July-Dec 1991) to 261 057 (ABC July-Dec 1995). It makes us the biggest Black newspaper in the country. And it makes sense to buy a page in it, don't you think? Call City Press for the damage.

33

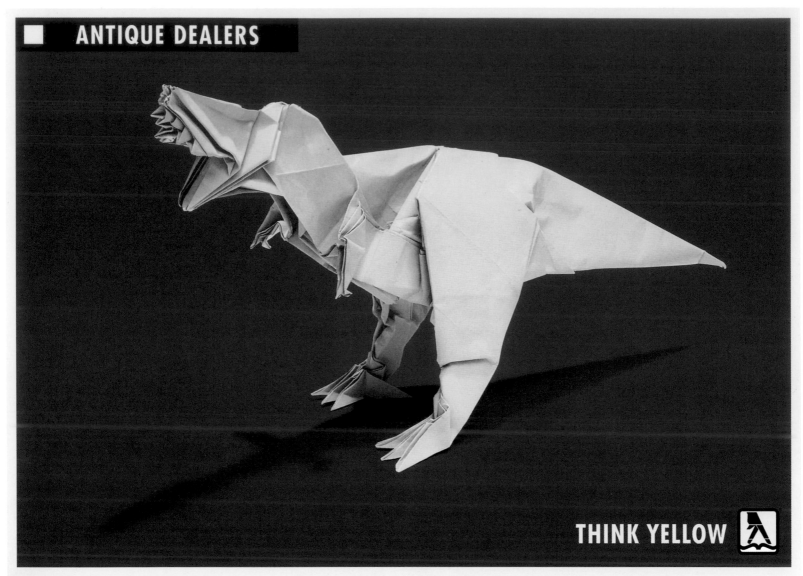

ANTIQUE DEALERS

THINK YELLOW

34

34 AND 36. **YELLOW PAGES**
JUPITER DRAWING ROOM,
JOHANNESBURG, 1996–97
In one Yellow Pages campaign,
the agency constructed familiar
shapes from paper; in a separate
series of ads, type was used to
create the images (in the ad on
the opposite page, the names
of businesses form the shape
of a key).

35. **NANDO'S RESTAURANT**
TBWA HUNT LASCARIS,
JOHANNESBURG, 1998
The agency used this picture
to announce that Nando's
restaurant was now serving
kosher food.

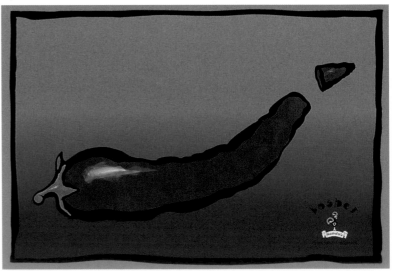

35

13. GUERRILLA ADVERTISING IT TO THE

RRILLA

NG: TAKING

STREETS.

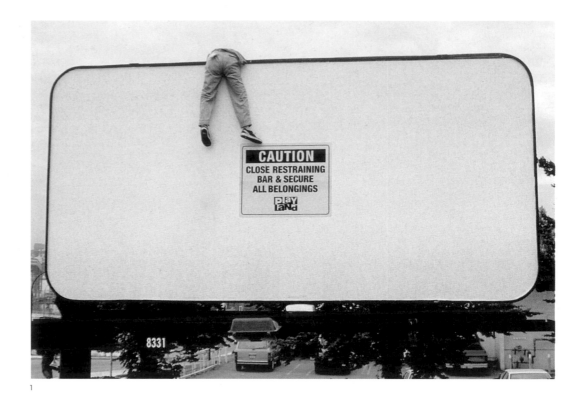

1

If you happened to visit a certain dark and trendy nightclub in New York City on a given evening several years ago, you might have noticed a handsome couple at the bar engaged in a spirited conversation about a new cocktail. Gradually, others surrounding them might have joined in the conversation about this so-called Hennessy martini. Meanwhile, as you inched toward the bartender to place your order, you might have found yourself drawn into the discussion and asked for your views: Had you heard of this hot new drink everyone was talking about? Eventually, the attractive couple perhaps would have decided to settle this whole matter once and for all, telling the bartender: "Let me try one of these Hennessy martinis—and while you're at it, how about a round for my friends here at the bar." As you walked away, sipping your strange new drink and trying to decide if you liked it, it still might not have occurred to you that you had just participated in a living advertisement.

The Hennessy martini stunt was a classic bit of "guerrilla advertising" staged in the mid-1990s by the New York ad agency Kirshenbaum Bond & Partners, which was, at the time, trying to stir up interest in Hennessy cognac among young people who don't usually drink cognac. The first thing agency chief Richard Kirshenbaum did was to concoct a cocktail and name it; thus was born the Hennessy martini. Next, the agency wanted to create a "buzz" around town, so attractive actors and models were hired and planted in fashionable bars, with orders to initiate fake conversations about this "popular" drink that no one had ever heard of. According to Kirshenbaum, the tactic worked quite well; the Hennessy martini actually did become somewhat popular and helped boost sales of the cognac. Would ordinary advertising have worked as well? Kirshenbaum doesn't think so; he believes that increasingly, advertisers must sneak "under the radar" of consumers who are adept at tuning out conventional sales messages.

And the best way to do that, Kirshenbaum and many other advertisers believe, is via some form of unconventional guerrilla-style advertising— which lurks all around, hits us where we live, and invariably takes us by surprise.

Increasingly, around the world, ads are breaking the boundaries that once kept them contained on the printed page or in thirty-second slots on broadcast media. They are now materializing on sidewalks, in bathroom stalls, on the covers of schoolbooks, at the bottom of a drinking glass, on pieces of fruit—or, as with Hennessy, in the midst of a conversation. It is a trend that has already triggered alarms among those who see this as a form of environmental pollution that shows no sign of letting up until every surface—and perhaps the atmosphere, too—has been claimed. Writing in *Time* magazine in 1998, the journalist Jeffrey Kluger lamented the spread of ads everywhere, noting, "In the past few years, it seems, the endgame, the D-day, the final storming of the last

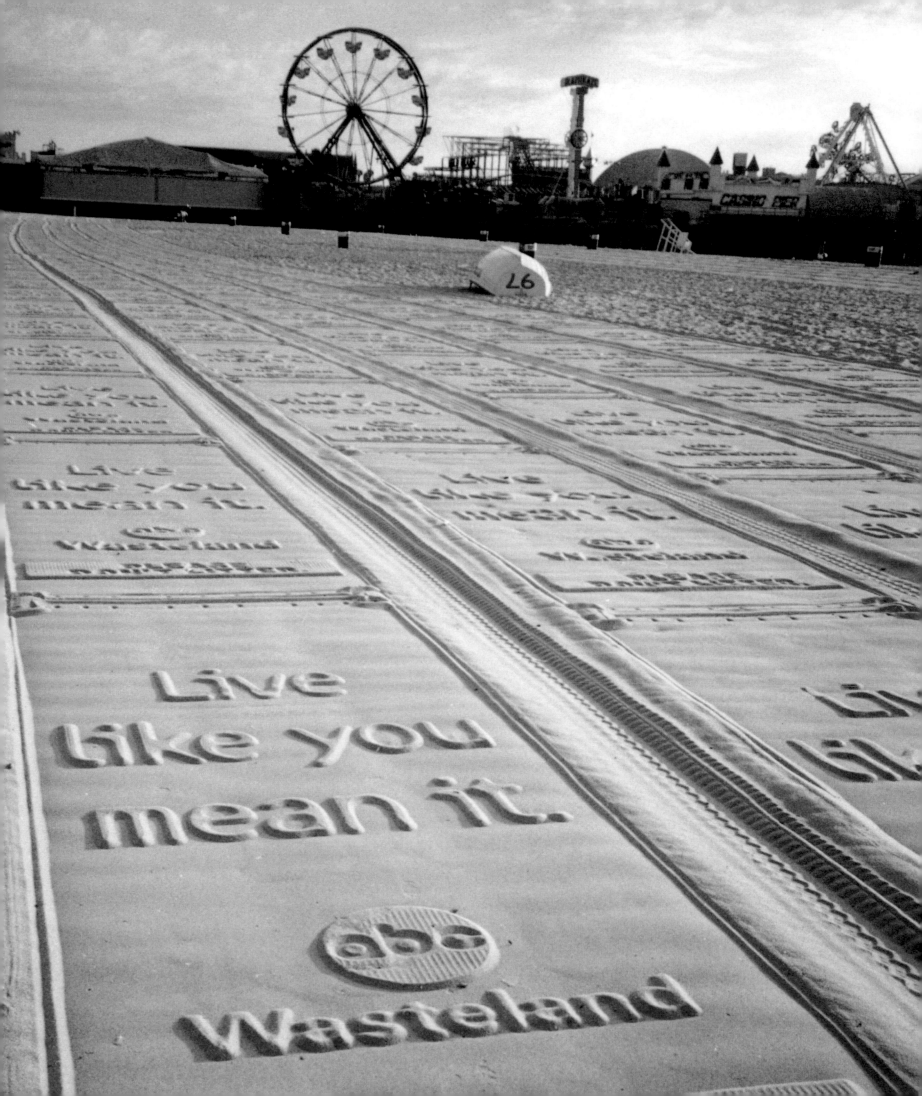

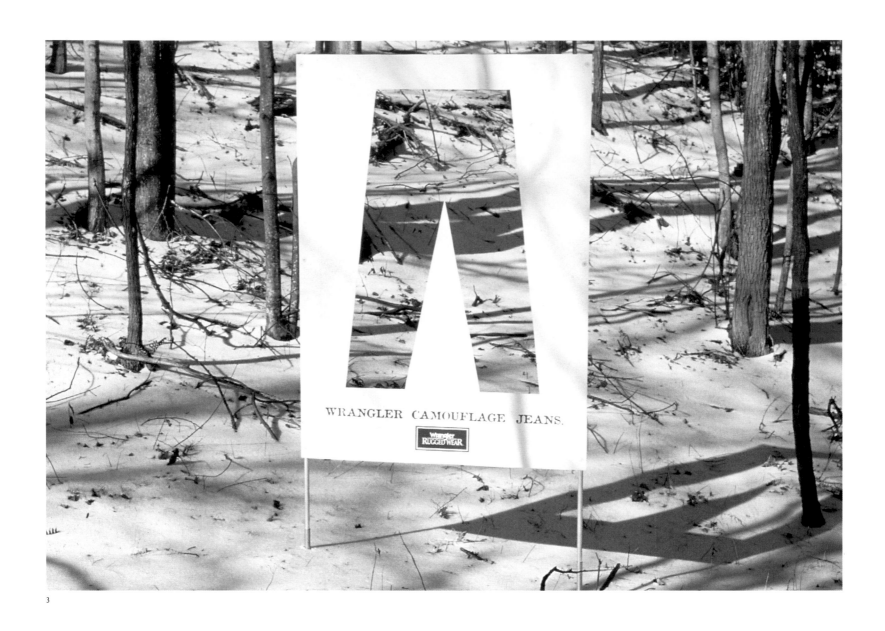

3

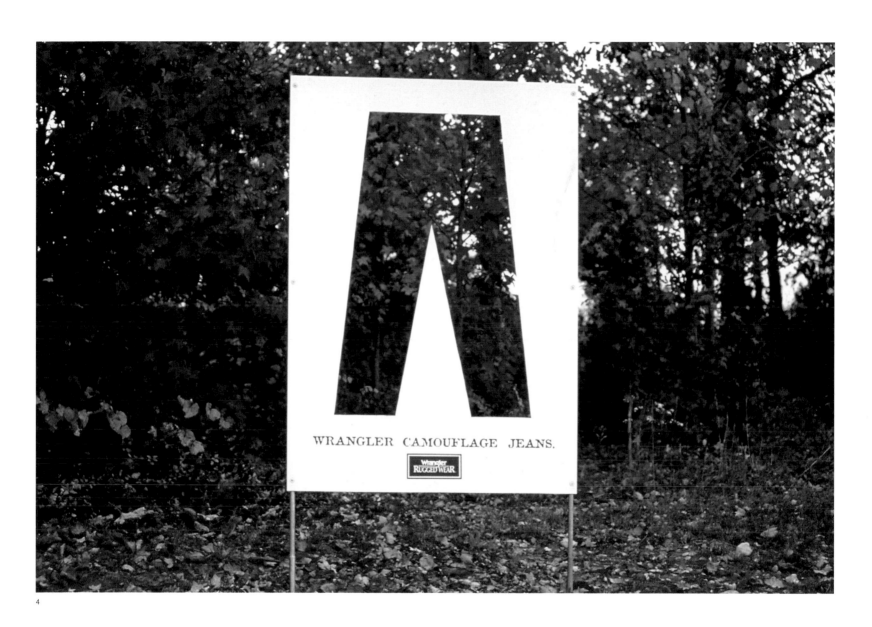

4

3 AND 4. **WRANGLER JEANS**
THE MARTIN AGENCY,
CHARLOTTE, NORTH
CAROLINA, 1998
A transparent salespitch: The
advertiser used cut-out billboards
to promote camouflage jeans.

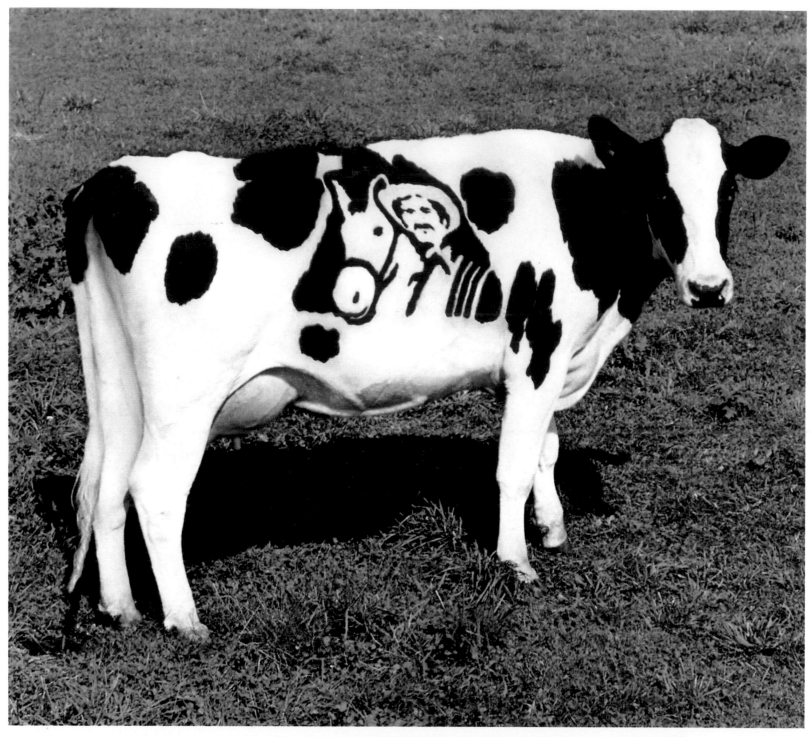

Cream good enough for Colombian Coffee isn't exactly easy to find.

100% Colombian Coffee

The richest coffee in the world.™

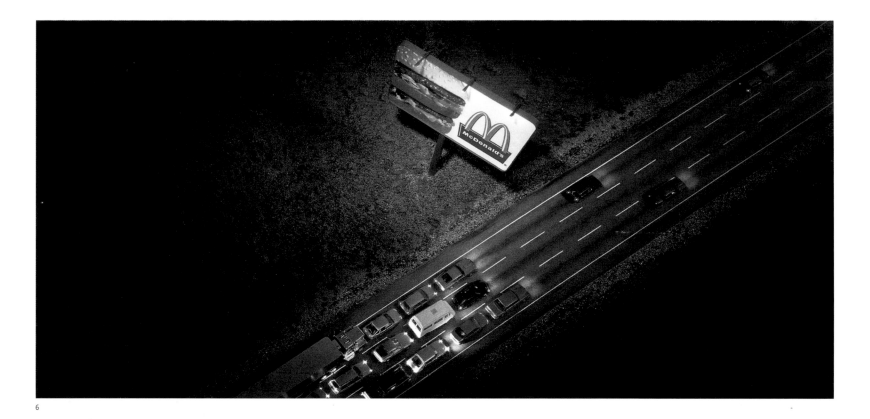

6

untrademarked beaches has begun." (What Kluger perhaps didn't know at the time was that the beaches had already been taken: On the shores of New Jersey, Skippy Peanut Butter and an entrepreneur with a customized tractor were imprinting the Skippy logo in the sand.)

In Kluger's military analogy, advertisers are cast as the ruthless invaders, continuing to advance upon new borders until the entire free world has been commercialized. But from the perspective of advertisers, the guerrilla movement is not so much an advance as a reaction—to a changing media landscape and an increasingly elusive consumer. "It used to be that with the three basic media of TV, radio, and print, you had enough reach to get your message out to just about everybody," said Rick Boyko, the creative chief of Ogilvy & Mather in New York. "But that's not true anymore. Everything has become so fragmented in terms of the way people use media today—they're no longer all watching the same

TV programs and reading the same publications." In addition, Boyko noted, lifestyles have become more varied and more mobile. "So you have to try to find all kinds of new points of contact with people," he said. Mary Warlick, director of The One Club for Art & Copy, a New York–based ad-industry group that promotes creativity, predicts, "Guerrilla advertising will continue to grow. It can be extremely effective because it is unexpected."

This new world of ubiquitous ads is not necessarily a utopia for advertisers. In fact, their lives were simpler (and it was more profitable for ad agencies) when all that was required was a handful of commercials that could be run and rerun and rerun on three major broadcast networks. The new guerrilla landscape requires advertisers to be more innovative not only in crafting the message but also in choosing—if not actually creating—the medium for that message. Or, to return to the military analogy, marketers who once plowed straight ahead with that

Sherman tank of advertising known as the TV commercial now must engage in small-arms sharpshooting from up on the rooftops and down in the toilet stalls.

Interestingly, as advertisers have tried to chase after the newly elusive consumer, it has become clear that one of the more effective tools also happens to be one of the oldest forms of advertising: the outdoor billboard. The big boards had become almost passé as TV commercials grew in popularity; they were reduced to carrying the ads that TV wouldn't accept, for liquor and tobacco. Many top ad creators thought billboard work was beneath them; in fact, one of the industry's foremost executives, Howard Gossage, suggested in the 1960s that billboards be abolished altogether on grounds that they were unsightly and intruded on the natural landscape. But by the mid-1990s, billboards were suddenly back in vogue as ad sales in this medium grew sharply. Times Square and its electronic billboards

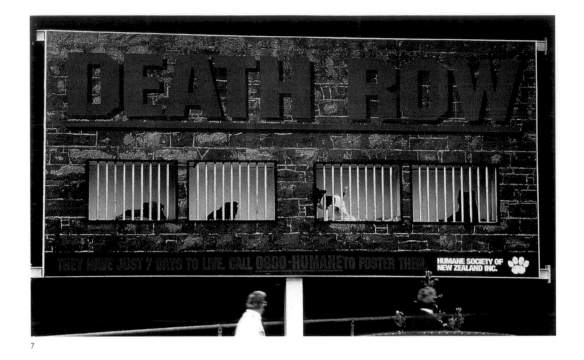

7

once again became an epicenter of the ad world. And on the other side of America, in Silicon Valley, billboards became a medium of choice for the new dot-com entrepreneurs.

The reason for the revival was that billboards addressed some of the critical issues in an increasingly fragmented media marketplace. With TV viewers armed with remote controls enabling them to surf through a sea of channels, it had become easier than ever to dodge TV spots. A billboard, on the other hand, was immovable, "unzappable," and therefore unavoidable. It was also an ideal medium for reaching particular demographic groups that advertisers were lusting after: busy two-income couples, travelers, weekend outdoorsmen, young party animals—the kind of active people who tend to watch less TV. In the case of dot-com advertisers, billboards in strategic locations were sometimes targeted to small groups of venture capitalists in an effort to raise investment money. Whoever the target

groups might be, and however little media they consumed, they all had to travel a certain route to work or play—and advertisers could use billboards to stalk them on that path.

It also helped that billboard technology took several leaps forward in recent years. The use of computer graphics and digital printing on new surfaces, such as vinyl, yielded images that were not only sharper but more dynamic; they could move and change. The old flashing neon of Times Square was augmented by huge video screens, electronic strips, and vinyl ads that transformed themselves every few seconds. And throughout New York and other major cities, huge "wallscapes" began to appear, digitally printed on vinyl and draped over the entire sides of buildings hundreds of feet tall; the images just grew larger and larger. Advertisers also began to take advantage of the three-dimensionality of billboards, sometimes incorporating lifelike objects into the ad, with startling effects. For

example, the Canadian agency Palmer Jarvis DDB created a billboard promoting a roller-coaster ride that featured what looked like a man's body draped over the top of the board. And in Auckland, New Zealand, billboards for the Humane Society actually had built-in cages with live dogs in them, beneath headlines like "Every dog has its day. His is Monday." (The board included a number to call in order to adopt the dog before it was euthanized.)

But even as advertisers were embracing improved billboards, they were also looking beyond these roadside signs toward other, newer forms of street-level communication. They began to, in effect, hijack trains and buses (which had always carried small, assorted promotional messages) and turn them into singularly focused moving ads; it's now common in New York to find oneself aboard a "brand train" in which all the ads are bought by one advertiser, enveloping the rider in a wall-to-wall sales pitch. Even

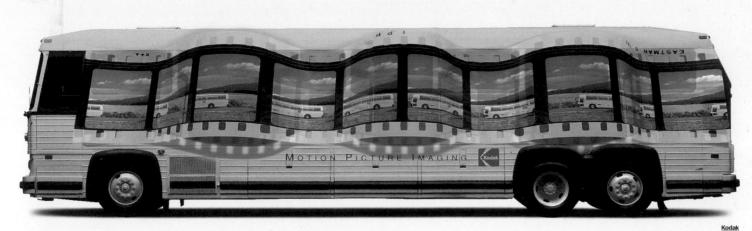

KODAK MOTION PICTURE IMAGING

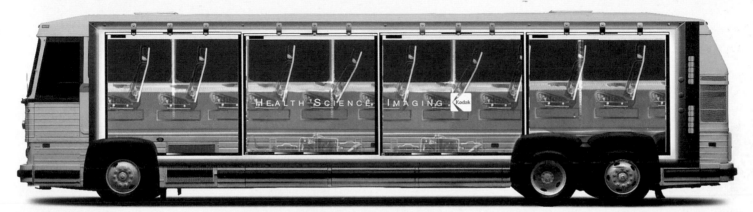

KODAK HEALTH SCIENCE IMAGING

8

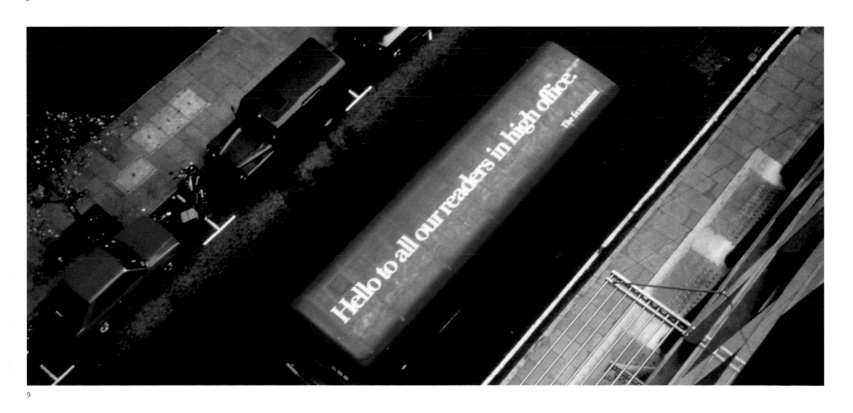

9

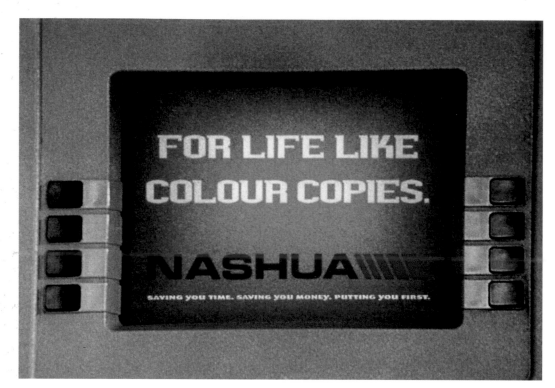
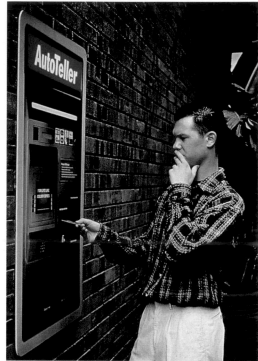

10

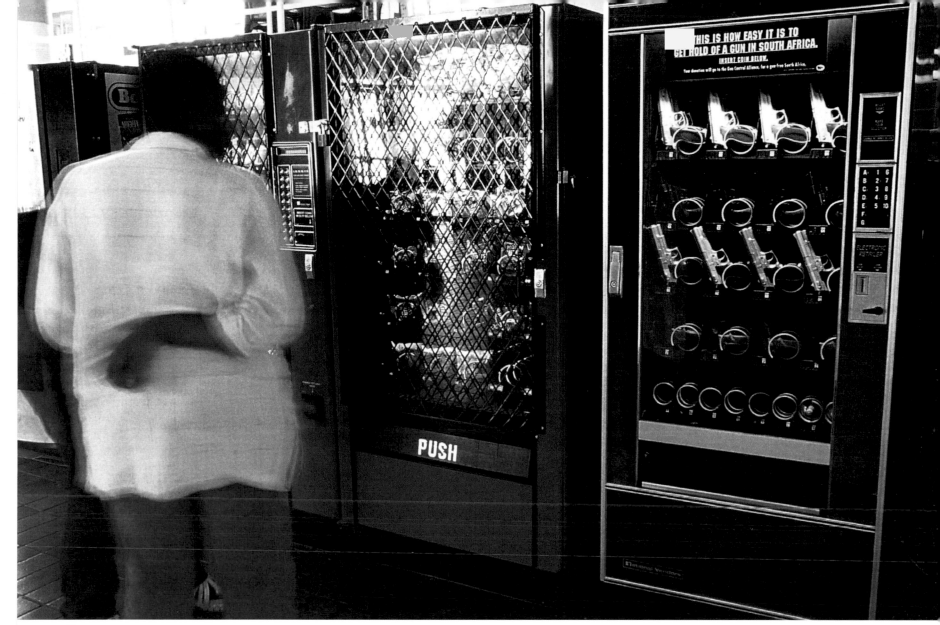

11

10. **NASHUA COPIERS**
TBWA HUNT LASCARIS,
JOHANNESBURG, 1999
South Africa has been a big
market for guerrilla-style ads.
This one touted the lifelike
reproduction capabilities of
Nashua photocopiers by creating
fake ATM machines.

11. **SOUTH AFRICAN
GUN CONTROL/ KFM
BROADCASTING**
JUPITER DRAWING ROOM,
JOHANNESBURG, 1998
Another South African ad, for
gun control, was designed to
look like a vending machine
filled with pistols.

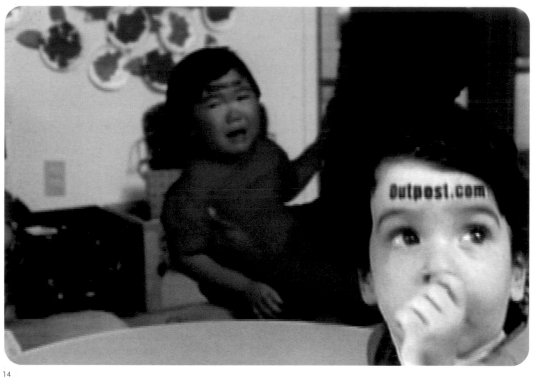

14

machines (who better to advertise to than someone with a fresh fistful of cash?) and gasoline pumps; in both venues, ads have been flashing messages for some time but are now becoming more advanced to include talking sales pitches. In South Africa, airports have become a testing ground for all kinds of unusual guerrilla tactics. For example, in Johannesburg, Virgin Atlantic airlines placed cartons of eggs on the baggage-claim carousel; as the eggs went round and round, so did the accompanying message to passengers that Virgin treats baggage with care. At the same airport, the agency TBWA Hunt Lascaris came up with a unique way to promote a chicken restaurant—on the runway, as planes were guided in, the guider's batons were replaced with chicken drumsticks. (Guerrilla advertising is widely practiced in South Africa, where many companies have limited ad budgets. "We use it because it's inexpensive, and it works big-time," says local ad executive John Hunt.)

The bathroom used to be a place of refuge, but no longer—it has become a favorite advertising venue because it is not only a captive environment but also gender-specific, making it ideal for targeted ads. Messages have been showing up directly above urinals (where it's almost impossible not to look), inside toilet stalls, on walls opposite the mirror (printed backwards of course). Ads are even being printed on toilet paper. Who would advertise on toilet paper? A company as reputable as SmithKline Beecham, for one. Or the young ad student who recently tried to get a job at the agency Kirshenbaum Bond & Partners by going into the agency bathroom and hand-printing a self-promotional message on the toilet paper, announcing, "I'm willing to start at the bottom." (The agency liked his cheeky approach, and hired him.)

One might suppose advertising couldn't get any lower than the toilet, but there's always the floor—of shopping malls, supermarkets, stores of

all kinds, as well as outside on the sidewalk. The guerrilla masters at Kirshenbaum Bond were stenciling messages on the sidewalks of New York as far back as the early 1990s. One of the agency's more infamous sidewalk ads was for a lingerie company, and the message to pedestrians was "From here, it looks like you could use some new underwear." Not all sidewalk ads are played for laughs, however: In Australia, Young & Rubicam placed small round stickers on the ground that adhered to the shoes of people who stepped on them; when you tried to peel the ad off your foot and noticed the copy, it explained that, assuming the sticker were a land mine, "there's a 50% chance you will die within minutes." (The ad was asking for support to ban land mines around the world.) Meanwhile, in Amsterdam, pedestrians had to be particularly careful about stepping on ads for the Hans Brinker Budget Hotel. The hotel's agency, KesselsKramer, had placed tiny flags in dog

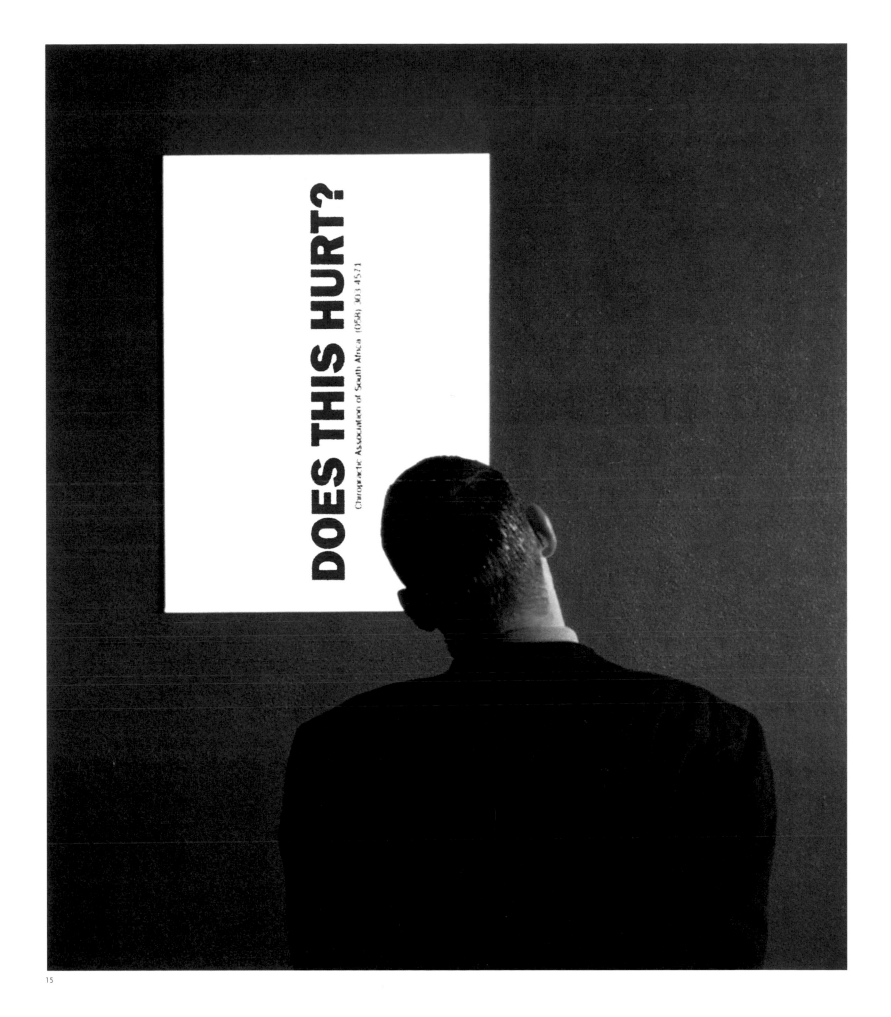

DOES THIS HURT?

Chiropractic Association of South Africa (0548) 903 4571

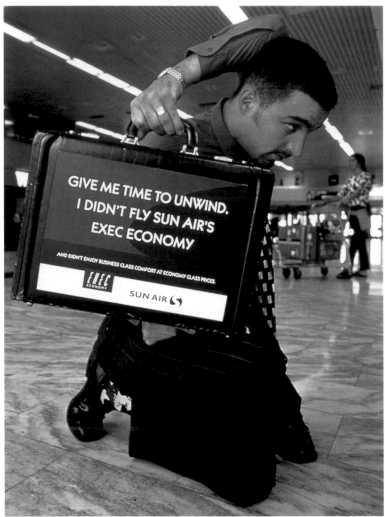

19

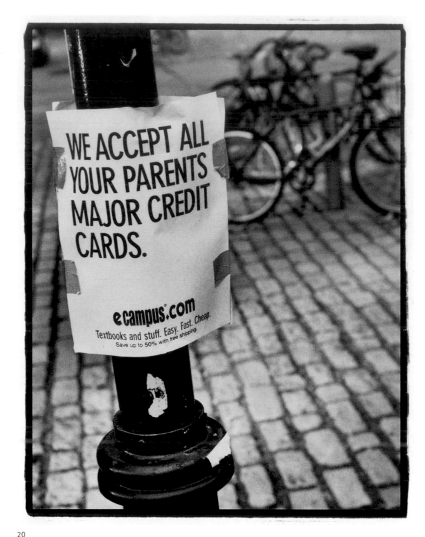

20

then interact with the company's advertising when it appeared on the screen (the woman would rise from her seat and shout at the characters on-screen; in turn, their lines had been scripted so that it seemed as if they were responding to what she was saying).

It's interesting to note that some kinds of guerrilla invasions irritate the public much more than others do. For example, turning people into ads doesn't seem to have bothered anyone, but stickers on fruit has. "I didn't want my apple defiled with advertisements," a Dallas woman complained to *The New York Times*, after noticing that the fruit in her supermarket was being used to promote a new movie. Invading the home is also risky: In the summer of 2000, the American Broadcasting Company was criticized for a plan to insert prerecorded messages on home telephone-answering machines; the messages were in the voices of TV stars, asking viewers to watch their new shows (ABC backed

off the plan, but this new technology, voice-mail broadcasting, is drawing interest among many marketers who believe that ads left on answering machines may be more effective than "live" sales pitches from telemarketers).

One of the most volatile areas has been advertising's ongoing attempts to infiltrate schools and schoolbooks. The textbook publisher McGraw-Hill was criticized for publishing a sixth-grade math book peppered with references to Nike, Gatorade, and other brands. The book publisher insisted that no sponsors had paid their way into the book; the writers had simply decided the math problems would seem more relevant if they involved products the kids used. (A typical entry: "Will is saving his allowance to buy a pair of Nike shoes that cost \$68.25. If Will earns \$3.25 per week, how many weeks will Will need to save?") Nike is not only inside the books but covering them, too—the company has distributed logo-drenched book covers free at

schools. Some schools, faced with budgetary pressures, have also begun to accept corporate sponsorships that can turn the school building itself into an ad. In Colorado Springs, for example, school hallways are plastered with billboards for soft drinks and other products (and to get to school, the kids ride in schoolbuses covered in corporate logos).

While ads in schools have sparked much debate, in most other instances, the advancement of guerrilla ads has been largely accepted by the public, which seems to be of two minds about it. There is certainly a keen awareness and some concern that ads are taking over more and more public spaces, but many people have also grown accustomed to this proliferation; in particular, younger people tend to be least likely to object to the trend because "their life is completely subsumed in commercial advertising," the advertising professor James Twitchell has observed. Trend analyst Tom Julian of the ad

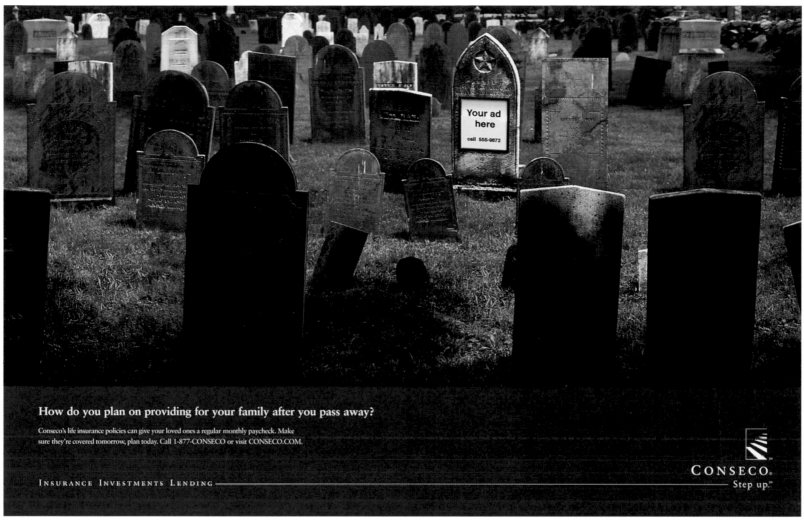

How do you plan on providing for your family after you pass away?

Conseco's life insurance policies can give your loved ones a regular monthly paycheck. Make sure they're covered tomorrow, plan today. Call 1-877-CONSECO or visit CONSECO.COM.

INSURANCE INVESTMENTS LENDING

CONSECO.
Step up.℠

21

19. **SUN AIR**
FCB BOSMAN JOHNSON, JOHANNESBURG, 1998
The use of people as "living ads" is becoming more popular; this advertiser hired a contortionist and stationed him at the airport.

20. **ECAMPUS.COM**
DEVITO VERDI, NEW YORK, 1999
In street advertising, the idea is to not look too professional; homemade-looking fliers and posters can be effective. (This ad appeared, as photographed, in magazines.)

21. **CONSECO INSURANCE**
FALLON WORLDWIDE, MINNEAPOLIS, MINNESOTA, 2000
This ad addresses one of the driving forces behind the spread of guerrilla marketing: Every space is for sale these days, including those once considered off-limits.

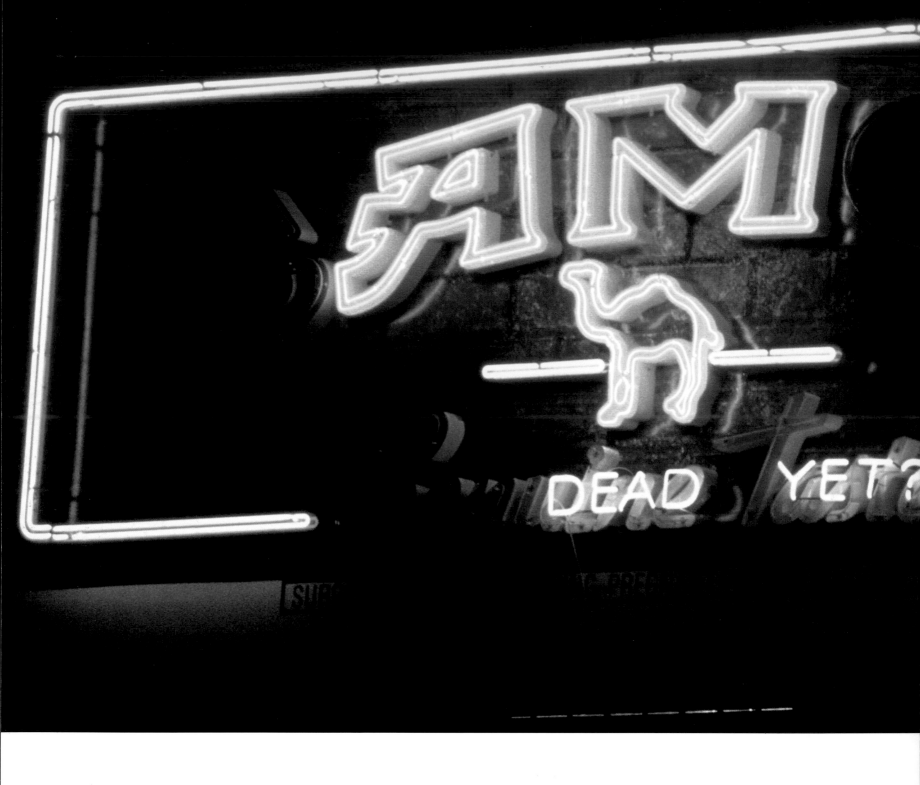

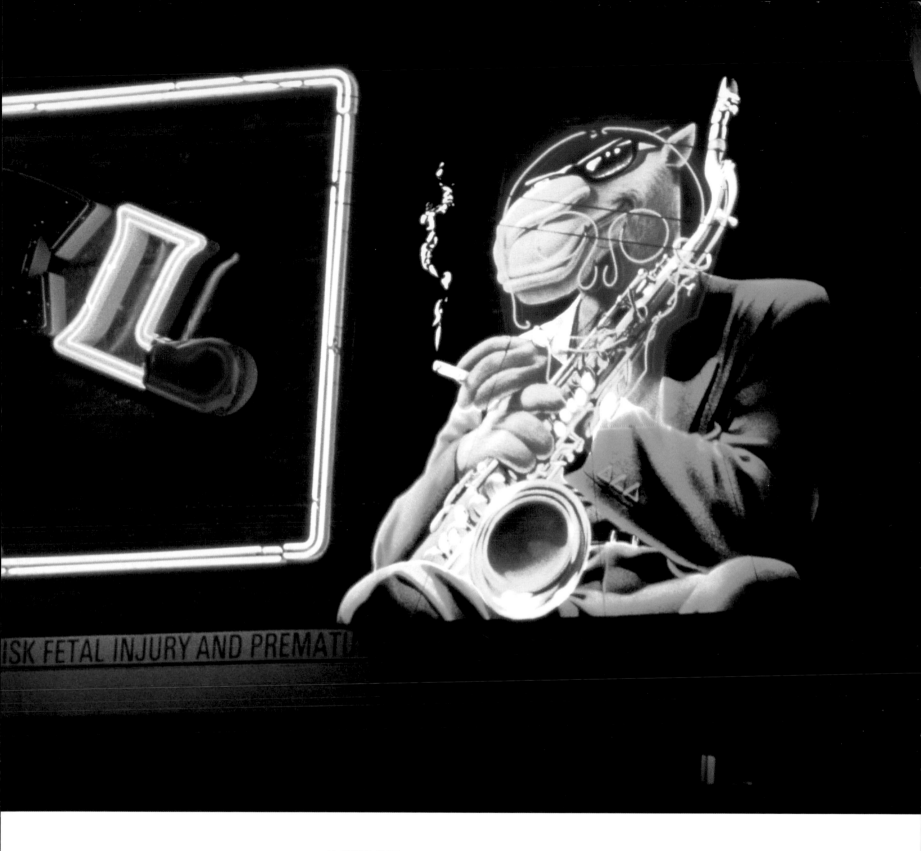

22. **ALTERED CAMEL**
BILLBOARD
BILLBOARD LIBERATION
FRONT, SAN FRANCISCO, 1995
The "culture jammers" have
been waging a counteroffensive
against the spread of ads. This
San Francisco anti-advertising
group rewired an electronic
Camel billboard to read "Am
I dead yet? "

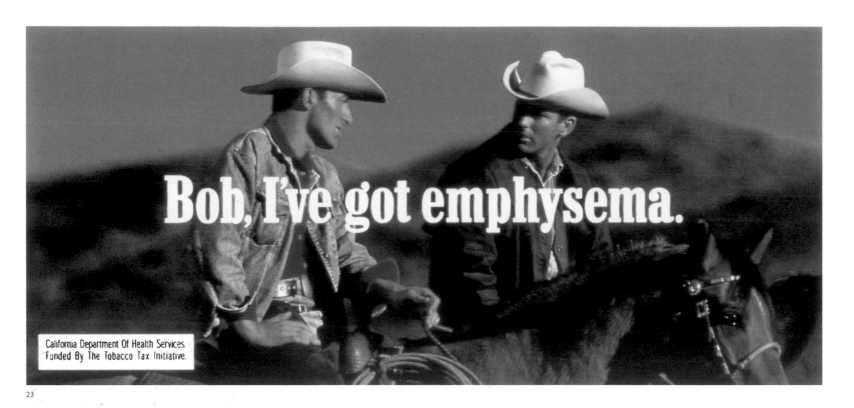

Bob, I've got emphysema.

California Department Of Health Services.
Funded By The Tobacco Tax Initiative.

23

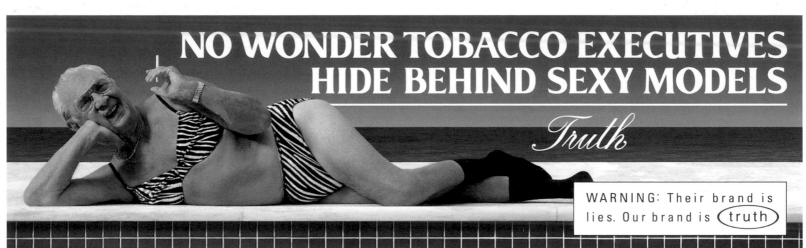

NO WONDER TOBACCO EXECUTIVES
HIDE BEHIND SEXY MODELS

Truth

WARNING: Their brand is
lies. Our brand is truth

24

**23. CALIFORNIA
DEPARTMENT OF HEALTH**
ASHER & PARTNERS,
LOS ANGELES, 1997
In recent years, ad agencies have
mimicked the style of culture
jammers. An anti-smoking
campaign put a new headline
on a classic Marlboro image.

**24. FLORIDA ANTI-SMOKING
CAMPAIGN**
CRISPIN PORTER + BOGUSKY,
MIAMI, 1999
Here again, an anti-smoking
campaign created a billboard
that looked like a defaced
cigarette company billboard.

**25. FAKE MCDONALD'S
BILLBOARD**
RON ENGLISH, NEW JERSEY,
1990
Some artists have begun to use
billboards both to display their
work and to make anti-commercial
statements; here, Ron English
takes on McDonald's.

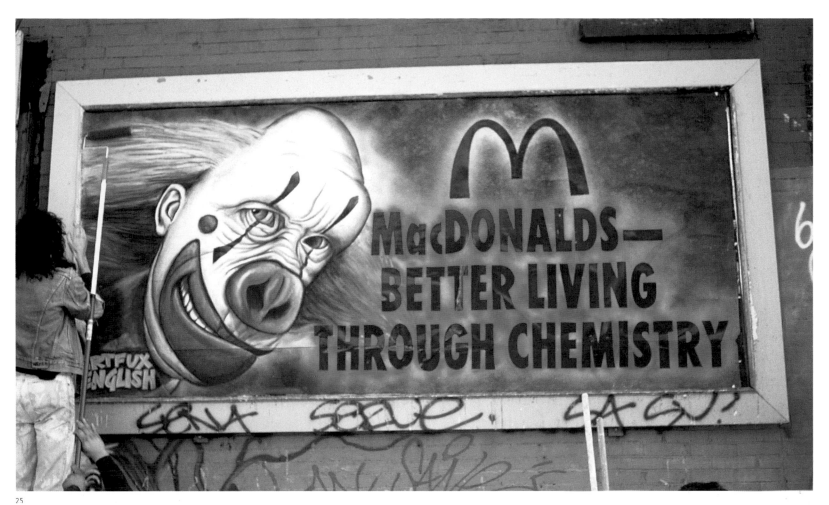

25

agency Fallon McElligott says that while today's consumers sometimes feel that ads in the surrounding environment are invasive, they also tend to appreciate the uniqueness and the appropriate placement of such ads. And many don't particularly mind being ambushed by guerrilla ads if they are done with a certain level of wit and style.

However, there is also a growing minority faction that has taken an active role in resisting the creeping commercialism in the environment; in a sense, these are the authentic "guerrillas" in the battle to control street-level mass communication. Sometimes calling themselves "culture jammers," they can be found around the world, waging war against advertising by creating their own strain of communication—which often consists of altering and subverting existing ads. Culture jamming burst on the scene in the U.S., Europe, and Australia in the 1980s, when underground groups with names like Guerilla [sic]

Girls and Negativland began altering and ridiculing messages from advertisers via pirate TV and radio broadcasting, public posters, elaborate media hoaxes, and various other stunts. But most often, culture jammers target what they consider the most intrusive form of advertising— the billboard. The often colorful and clever alterations on billboards have evolved into an engaging form of protest art.

A pioneer in this underground movement was San Francisco's Billboard Liberation Front (BLF), which first began altering billboards back in 1977. Members of the group were known for scaling billboards by rope and ladder in the dead of night and pasting "new and improved" headlines over the old ones. On a Camel cigarettes electronic billboard, the BLF rewired the neon lettering in 1995, so that the glowing message became "Am I Dead Yet?" In the late 1990s, the BLF targeted some of the most prevalent new outdoor campaigns, including

Apple's "Think different" boards. The headline of a "Think different" billboard featuring mogul Ted Turner was changed to "Think dividends." For the tragic aviator Amelia Earhart, the headline became "Think doomed."

Culture jamming became so popular by the early 1990s that the movement had its own ad-spoofing magazine, *AdBusters* (which is still published from its base in Canada). American magazines like the *Utne Reader* and *Wired* portrayed the BLF and other groups as "media heroes," while academic scholars wrote weighty theses on culture jamming, with some likening it to the Russian samizdat movement that defied government censorship by printing and circulating defiant messages among the public.

But advertising gradually became very aware of the enemy in its midst, and soon began to do what it has done to the pop and street culture for the past two decades—copy, co-opt, and absorb. By the late-1990s, the rough-hewn look and

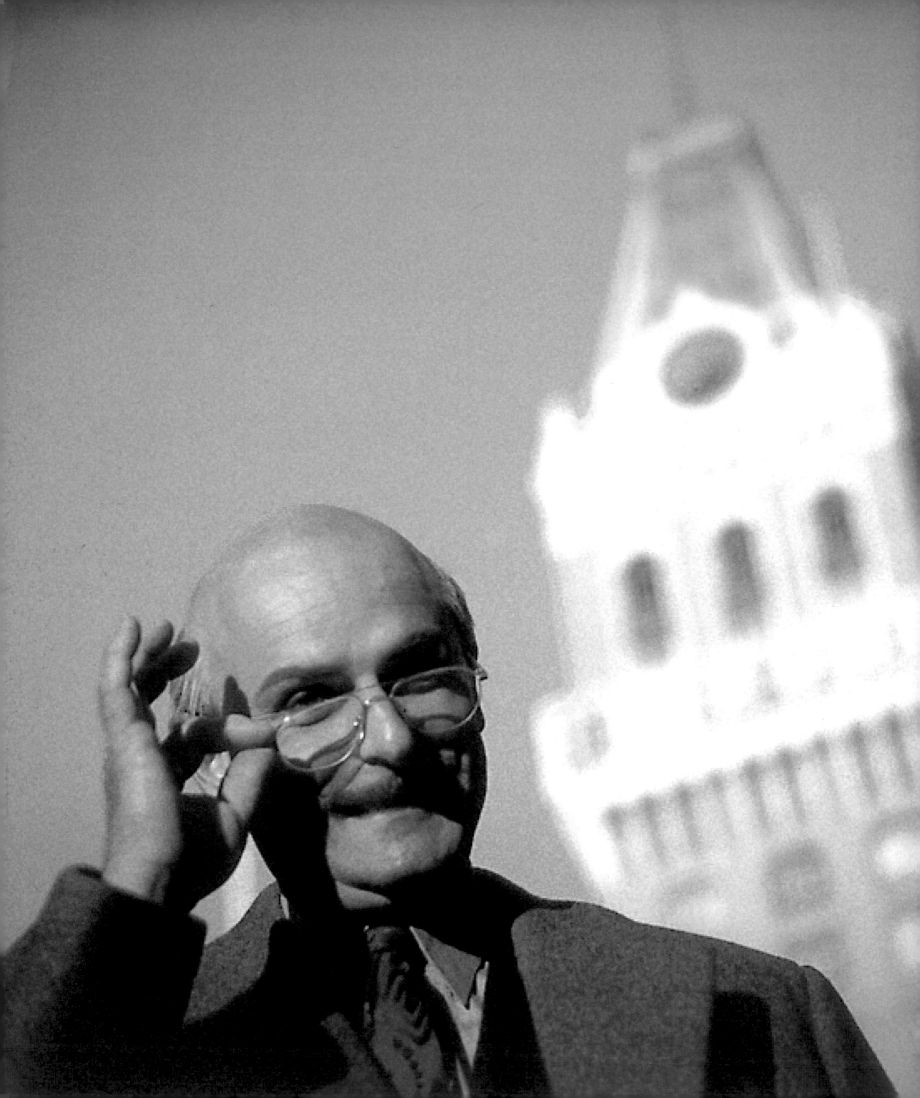

INTERVIEW: "JACK NAPIER"

For the past 25 years, the San Francisco–based Billboard Liberation Front has pioneered the art of "culture jamming." The group, which has remained underground through the years, specializes in altering billboards in creative ways, subverting the ad message in order to make a statement (whether political or just humorous). The BLF has been called "the Monkey Wrench Gang of outdoor advertising" by *Wired* magazine, and was named "one of the top 10 media heroes" by the *Utne Reader*. One of the founders and the current spokesman of the group goes by the nom de guerre of "Jack Napier" (pictured opposite in cosmetic disguise).

AT THE TIME THE BLF WAS GETTING STARTED IN THE LATE 1970S, WAS ANYONE ELSE DOING THIS KIND OF THING?
Apparently, there was a group in Michigan in the late 1960s, and an Australian group, called Bugger Up, in the late 1970s. In our own San Francisco area, another group started in 1979 called Truth in Advertising. But it goes way back—if you go back as far as World War II, there were advertisements and political posters being jammed.

WHAT'S YOUR PHILOSOPHY ABOUT ADVERTISING?
I have nothing against advertising, per se. I actually like a lot of ads, anything that's clever. But I have to admit I'm pretty irate that a handful of [outdoor advertising] corporations control all the public spaces. I find that to be completely undemocratic. I think all of us should be able to have a say in what appears on these billboards in public spaces. Whenever I see a billboard, I find myself thinking, Wouldn't it be funnier if it said this? So I change it.

WHAT SEPARATES GOOD BILLBOARD ALTERATION FROM ORDINARY GRAFFITI?
The first thing is coming up with a good idea. Something that works as a concept and something that'll work graphically. I think that if the messages are blatantly and stodgily political, that's just not going to get through to anyone except those who already agree. My favorite billboards are ones that are enigmatic, that people might have a hard time figuring out at first—but that stick in their minds.

WHAT ABOUT THE TECHNICAL ASPECTS OF ALTERING A BILLBOARD?
Well, the idea is to make it look as though the message came from the billboard company. If you're going to add an image, you want it to look like it's part of the background image. You've got to take your measurements. We often do layouts and sketches in advance to see what it looks like. We use computer-aided design, PhotoShop, and laser-cut vinyl for paste-overs. And we go to great pains to make sure everything we add to the billboard is removable.

WHY IS THAT IMPORTANT?
Because we're not anti-property, and we don't want to damage private property. We look at what we're doing as just borrowing the space. So all someone has to do is go up on a ladder to remove our work in order to restore the original billboard—sometimes we even leave a six-pack of beer up there for the guy who has to do that. We're also protecting ourselves. If there are no damages to the billboard, it's harder for us to be prosecuted.

IT SEEMS THAT SOME PEOPLE WHO ALTER BILLBOARDS HAVE A POLITICAL AGENDA, WHILE OTHERS ARE MORE INTERESTED IN CREATING ARTWORK, RIGHT?
Yes, you have someone like Ron English, who was just a good painter who couldn't get a gallery show, and he wanted people to see his work. So he went out and started putting up these giant paintings on billboards. He got a lot of attention for it, and it helped him establish his art career. The Cicada group on the East Coast would be an example of a more political group, going after cigarette billboards—but they do it with a sense of humor. I don't mind being hit with a blatant political message as long as it's funny.

WHAT KINDS OF REACTIONS DO YOU GET FROM ADVERTISERS AFTER THEIR BILLBOARDS HAVE BEEN HIT?
The billboard companies have responded in the press several times to our activities, and a number of times they've acknowledged that we don't damage the billboards. There was a controversy over our Apple [alterations]. An internal E-mail barrage went on at the company for some time; they were definitely aware of what we were doing. Some people thought it was funny; others didn't get it. Some even thought we were shills for Microsoft.

WHAT ARE YOUR THOUGHTS ON THE WAY THAT ADVERTISERS HAVE CO-OPTED THE LOOK OF THE ANTI-ADVERTISING MOVEMENT?
It was inevitable. I knew it was going to happen years ago. I was a little surprised and angry when I first saw ads crossing out their own headlines and writing in something self-mocking—my first reaction was "They should be paying residuals to the BLF!" But after the initial shock wore off, it made perfect sense. That's what I would do if I were one of those guys. They're continually mining what's hip. It seems like now you can't have any kind of subculture pop up that has originality or meaning to kids without it being co-opted immediately. They won't leave these poor kids alone to have their own culture. I have thought about this question of whether it's even possible anymore to question or ridicule advertising, given that it has become so accepted as the language of the culture. All I can say is, you have to at least try. If there isn't some kind of insurgent spirit popping up between the cracks, you might as well give it up as a society. We're not at that point yet—not even close.

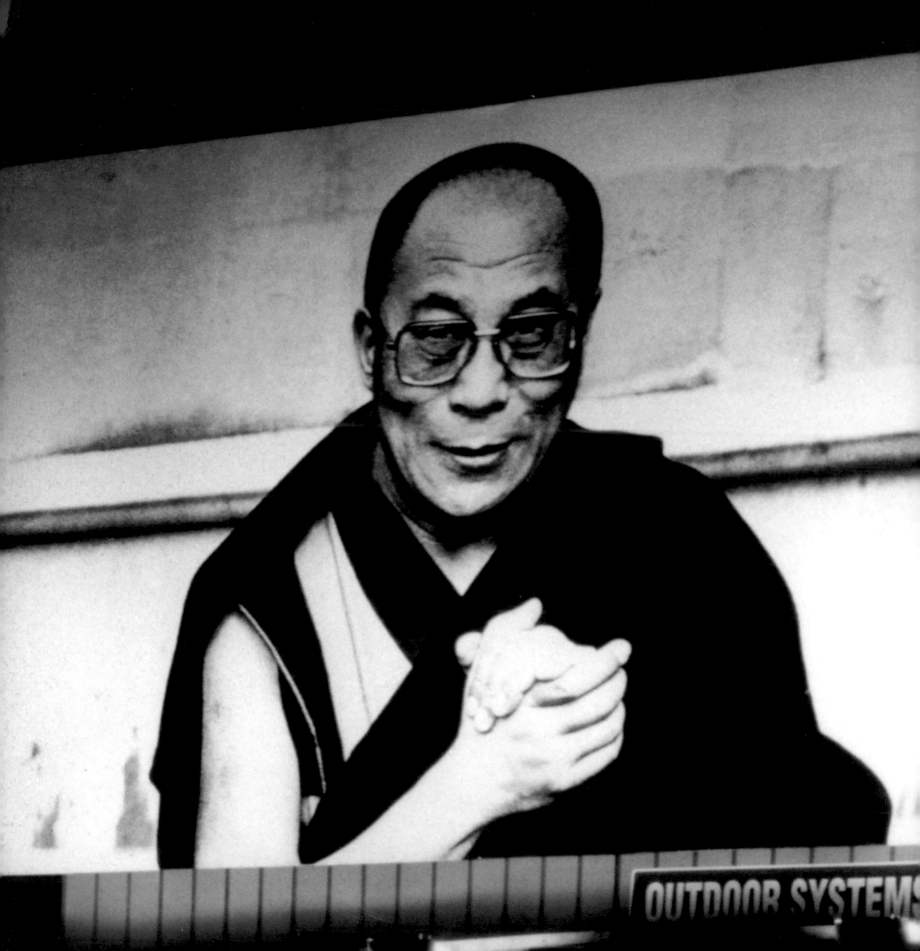

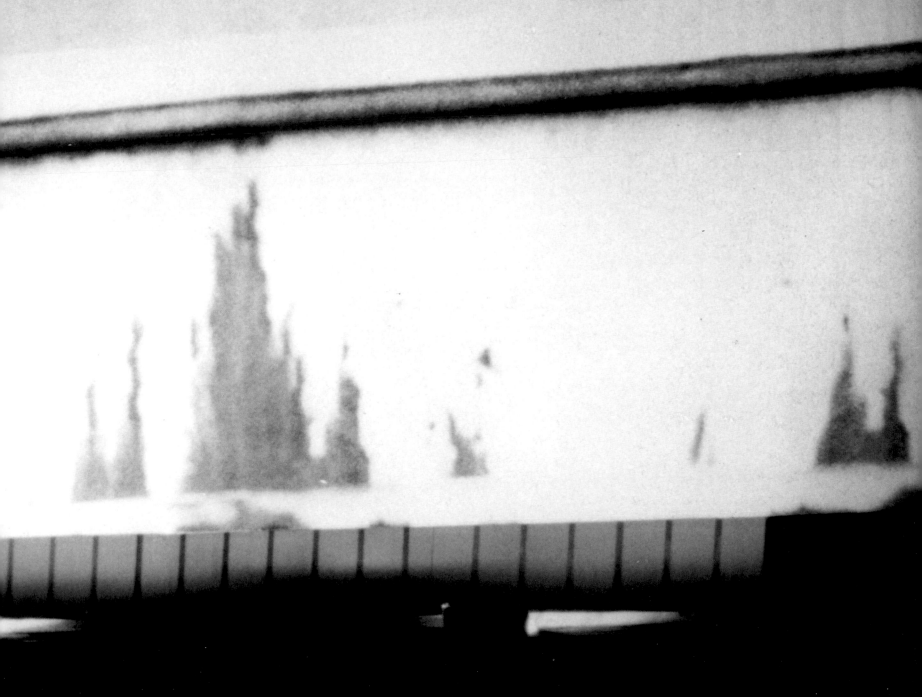

STOP
The MADNESS!!!
Potato on pizza is
unnatural, subversive
AND
WRONG!

ATTENTION! ATTENTION! ATTENTION!
LET THE SHOCKING TRUTH BE KNOWN: A RADICAL GROUP
OF NONCONFORMISTS COMMONLY KNOWN AS CPK
(CALIFORNIA PIZZA KITCHEN) IS RIGHT NOW SERVING POTATO ON
PIZZA IN THIS COMMUNITY! THIS GOES AGAINST EVERYTHING OUR
FOREFATHERS INTENDED PIZZA TO BE! Whatever happened to
COMMON DECENCY?? Who died and gave CPK the RIGHT to CROSS
THE INVISIBLE LINE between the *Four Food Groups*?? Potatoes should
NOT be integrated with Rosemary Chicken,
let alone PIZZA! If people start
adopting a permissive attitude
towards potato on pizza. Next thing
you know, it's the COLLAPSE OF
CIVILIZATION IN THE FREE WORLD!!!
Right now, MILLIONS OF CPK PIZZA-
CRAZED "ZOMBIES" walk our streets!
And the scourge is spreading!

Rosemary Chicken-Potato Pizza =
Radical propaganda thinly veiled in a
thin, flaky crust. Don't be fooled by its
pizza-like appearance. IT IS THE ENEMY.

WE MUST TAKE ACTION NOW!!
Consider the cold, hard, irrefutable FACTS!
Fact: "Savory" Rosemary Chicken-Potato Pizza is cooked with fire.
Fact: Fire is a destructive element.
Conclusion: "Savory" Rosemary Chicken-Potato Pizza is destructive!!!

We must STAND UP to protect pizza from being transformed
into a tool of "COUNTERCULTURE" factions. Let's go back to
a simpler time when pizza was a place for
pepperoni. Not Tandoori Chicken, Shrimp
Pesto, Peking Duck, Goat Cheese
(Blasphemy!) or Rosemary Chicken-Potato.
If we were intended to taste two different
"exotic" foods at the same time, we would
have been BORN WITH TWO TONGUES!!
WAKE UP AND SMELL THE GARLIC!!! Every
one of CPK's 27 highly addictive, unholy
combinations must be ELIMINATED. TOGETHER, we can
stop the crispy, wood-fired menace! A return to traditional
pizza MORALS is OUR BEST SECURITY FOR OUR FUTURE!!!

BOYCOTT
ANTI-ESTABLISHMENT
PIZZAMONGERS!
Whatever you do, don't go to
any of these CPK locations:
- 437 S. Highway 101,
Solana Beach, (619) 793-0999.
- 3363 Nobel Dr., La Jolla,
(619) 457-4222.
- 11602 Carmel Mountain Rd,
San Diego, (619) 675-4424,
And, by all means, don't call
for take-out orders.

Support our grassroots action group, C.R.U.S.T.
(Crusaders Resisting Unnatural Subversive Toppings).

Potatoes Belong on a PLATE!!
Not a PIZZA!!!

guess.com

26. (PREVIOUS SPREAD)
ALTERED APPLE BILLBOARD
BILLBOARD LIBERATION
FRONT, SAN FRANCISCO, 1998
The BLF targeted the popular
Apple "Think different"
billboards, changing one
word in the headline each
time. (For mogul Ted Turner,
the headline was changed to
"Think dividends"; for Amelia
Earhart, "Think doomed.")

27. **CALIFORNIA PIZZA
KITCHEN**
RUBIN POSTAER &
ASSOCIATES, LOS ANGELES,
1996
Another advertiser imitating
a culture jammer: this ad for
a pizza chain was designed
to look like a rant from an
underground radical.

28. **ALTERED GUESS JEANS AD**
KAWS, NEW YORK, 1999
The graffiti artist known as
"Kaws" uses outdoor ads as his
canvas, typically painting a new
head or one of his signature characters on the model in the ad.

29. **FAKE CALVIN KLEIN AD**
ADBUSTERS MAGAZINE,
VANCOUVER, 1995
The Canadian magazine
AdBusters emerged as the
journal of the culture jamming
movement. The magazine
created its own fake ads, like
this one for Calvin Klein.

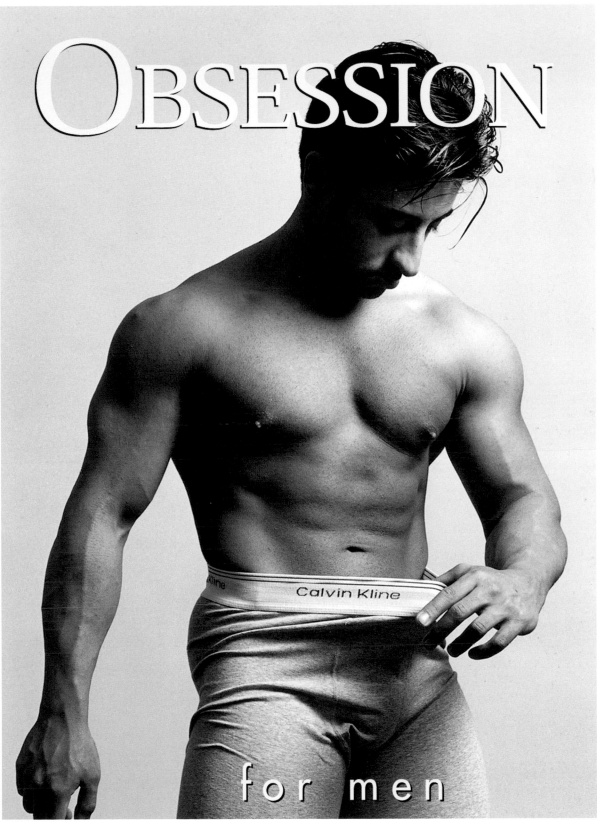

29

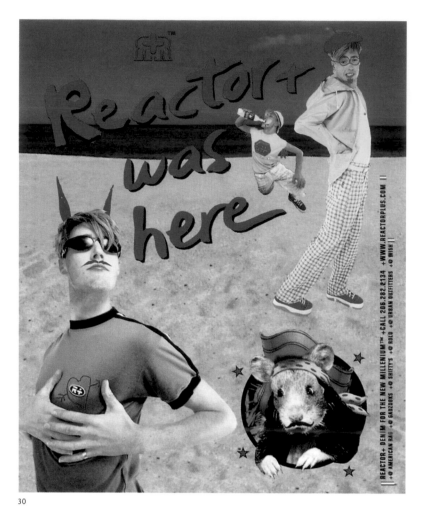

30

subversive attitude of altered billboards and street posters was being imitated in ads for jeans and beer. Some advertisers, such as the Captain Morgan rum brand, even took to "jamming" or altering their own billboards, by crossing out headlines or putting fake graffiti on the ads. Why would advertisers deface their own ads? To strike an anti-establishment pose, thereby making the brand seem more irreverent, hip, and self-aware. One of the more extreme examples was seen in a billboard campaign featuring ad copy that seemed to have been written by an anarchist urging the public to avoid Amstel Lite "at all costs," and warning of "impending doom"—the posters were, of course, created by Amstel Lite.

The look and language of anti-advertising has even found its way into million-dollar TV commercials—which have increasingly adopted a rough cinema-verité style and a self-mocking tone. As Sprite commercials began to point out that ad slogans were bogus and spokespersons

were bought and paid for, the advertiser was, in effect, doing the culture jammers' job for them.

It wasn't hard for advertising's creative Young Turks to adopt the style of culture jammers, considering how much the two groups have in common: the same irreverent attitude, absurd sense of humor, and compulsion to put one's cleverness on public display. Annie Finnegan, an ad executive who has taught a guerrilla-advertising course at the ad school Creative Circus in Atlanta, pointed out that the culture jammers and some of today's cutting-edge ad creators "both are products of the same culture, with the same sensibilities—they just went in opposite directions." Consider, for example, the Philadelphia ad executive Steve Grasse, founder of the hot agency Gyro: A specialist in targeting disaffected young audiences, Grasse claims to hate conventional advertising, and enjoys playfully defacing ad imagery in much the same way that culture

jammers do. But Grasse does it for mercenary purposes: His self-mocking, intentionally amateurish-looking ads are financed by huge client companies that sell liquor and cigarettes to the "twentysomething" market.

While it can be increasingly difficult to distinguish between real protest communications and advertising's ersatz version, culture jamming is continuing to survive and even flourish—not only in altered headlines on billboards but also in other forms that include painted outdoor signs and wall murals that reinterpret advertising images. The American culture jammer Ron English is known for impressionistic anti-advertising art on billboards around the East Coast of the U.S. Another American artist, Dick Detzner, creates Renaissance-style frescoes—but in place of religious figures are ad characters like Snuggles the Fabric Softener Bear. In a few instances, anti-advertising artists have jumped to the other side; one team of New York

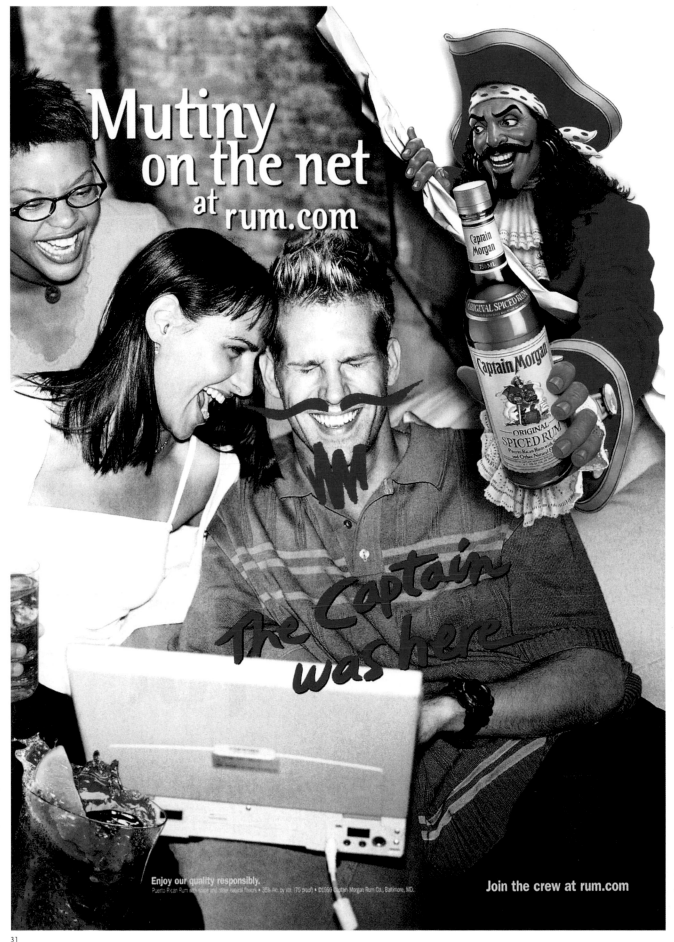

31

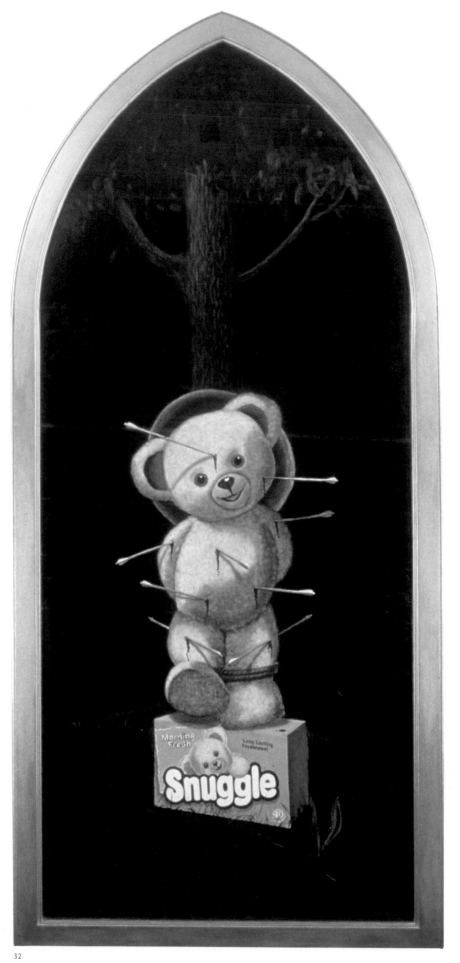

32

32. *ST. SNUGGLEBEAR*
DICK DETZNER, ARTIST, 1998
Anti-advertising artists like
Detzner, in the U.S., use ad
characters (including Snuggles
the Fabric Softener Bear) as
the subjects of their work.

33. **BUZZ MAGAZINE**
DEUTSCH INC., LOS ANGELES,
1995
The ad as prank: These fake
billboards prompted people in
Los Angeles to call for more
information; on the other end
of the line was the real advertiser,
Buzz magazine.

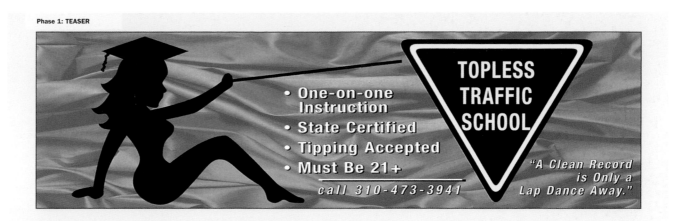

BUZZ OUTDOOR

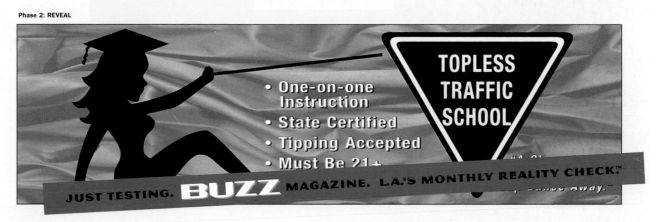

33

graffiti artists signed on to produce street murals for Coca-Cola and others. Even those jammers who steadfastly refuse to "sell out" are well aware that they have no chance of winning the street-level communication war against the ever-growing, co-opting ad machine. But they persist anyway: The longtime leader of the BLF, who goes by the nom de guerre of Jack Napier, said that even though ads have copied the style and language of culture jammers, the movement still provides an alternative viewpoint on the street.

Meanwhile, ad agencies continue to expand their own arsenal of tricks, pranks, and stunts. One Swedish agency produced an ad for travel insurance that was placed in a wallet and glued to the sidewalk of a busy street—this was one advertiser who knew how to get people's attention. The Los Angeles office of the agency Deutsch Inc. recently fooled large numbers of people in Los Angeles with a series of fake billboards for "topless traffic school" and other

nonexistent businesses; when curious people called the number they were connected to the advertiser that sponsored the campaign. One of the more recent forms of ad pranksterism has targeted the much-sought-after venture-capitalist investors in Silicon Valley. The adman Michael Dweck has made an art of stalking and tricking these financiers on behalf of his dot-com clients, who will try anything to draw the attention (and money) of investors. Dweck has infiltrated delicatessens in order to slip client advertising messages into some of the lunch delivery bags bound for bankers' offices. Staking out bars frequented by the venture capitalists, he has planted actors there and instructed them to pretend to talk on cell phones and to repeatedly mention the name of the company that Dweck was slyly promoting. Knowing the investors tended to take certain taxi routes, Dweck left printed messages, touting his clients, in the backseats of cabs. And just in case these

subtleties were missed, he also turned loose a bunch of trained chimps, wearing promotional T-shirts, in the offices of one investor.

The trend of advertisers resorting to pranksterism to draw attention is perhaps the most extreme form of guerrilla marketing, and although it can be amusing and creative, it can also backfire. "Sometimes people become angry when they discover they've been tricked by an advertiser," Finnegan points out. But those who are troubled by the kind of "stalker advertising" practiced by the likes of Dweck had better brace themselves, because advertising that snoops on us and invades our space will very likely be part of the next wave. In fact, new technology will enable advertisers to know exactly where you are at any given time . . . what you're doing . . . and maybe even what you're thinking. So say goodbye to your privacy, and hello to the advertising of the future.

14. THE N

EXT WAVE.

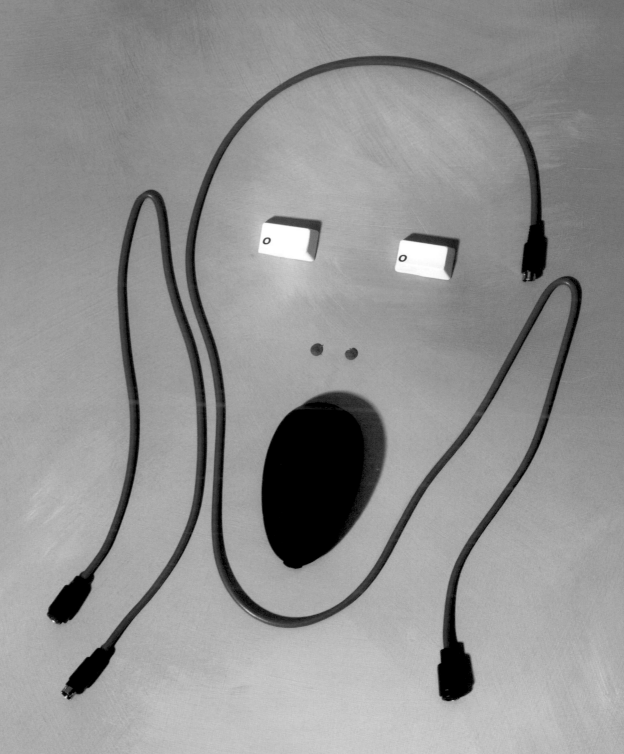

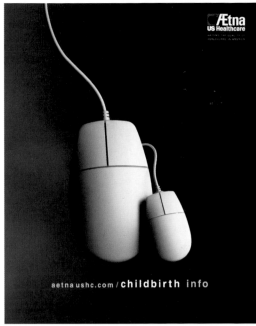

2

1. **SELF-PROMOTIONAL AD**
PETER McARTHUR STUDIO,
LOS ANGELES, 2000
Edvard Munch's famous painting,
The Scream, gets wired. Art and
technology are beginning to
come together, albeit slowly,
in some of the ads produced
at the beginning of the twenty-
first century.

2. **AETNA**
McKINNEY & SILVER,
RALEIGH, NORTH CAROLINA,
1999
The technology revolution has
given birth to a new generation
of ads, recognizable by their
computer and electronic
imagery and ever-present
Web site addresses.

To the question "Where does advertising go from here?" the answer would seem to be obvious: everywhere. As noted in the preceding chapter, ads have already permeated the environment to such a degree that sanctuary can be found (for the moment at least) only in houses of worship. And if the major advertising agencies have their way—as they usually have before—the ad cocooning effect should continue. Consider that the agency Ogilvy & Mather, for example, has rooted much of its future in a strategy called "360-degree branding," whose primary purpose is to ensure that ads shadow us wherever we go.

Technology will continue to make it easier to do that. Dave Westreich, a futurist at Ogilvy & Mather, points out that through the use of satellite technology, it will be possible to track someone's movement and send him messages through devices he wears or carries—advanced Palm Pilots, for example, or "augmented reality"

eyeglasses. (Unlike the more familiar "virtual reality" helmets that envelop you in an artificial world, augmented reality might use translucent eyewear that would allow you to continue to see the real world around you—but with an overlay of images and messages.) "This means you would be able to stream advertising content to people based on where they're standing," says Westreich. "If I happen to be a few steps away from the delicatessen, today's menu might pop up in my eyewear." This kind of "stalking advertising" might follow you anywhere. For example, Westreich envisions the beach towel of the future as having a built-in receiver that will play the kind of music you happen to like—while also trying to sell you concert tickets for your favorite musicians.

While it may become increasingly difficult to get away from ads, we will have more control over their content, experts believe. Watts Wacker, whose firm FirstMatter helps companies plan

for the future, predicts: "Ads will be stratified, based on your needs at a given time. So if you're looking to buy a washing machine, you'll turn on 'the advertising channel' on your TV and it will show you continuous ads for washing machines—until you indicate that you want something else."

Even the faces we see in those ads may be customized for each of us. The high-tech guru Jaron Lanier (who coined the phrase "virtual reality") envisions next-generation advertising that will make us all stars of our own commercials. Internet test labs are already hooking up digital cameras to computers and refining the process of photographing the computer user's face, then recreating that image and inserting it into the midst of Web content—such as online movies or commercials. In effect, your face would replace that of an actor in a commercial, and you would even speak his or her lines. So, instead of seeing the rock star

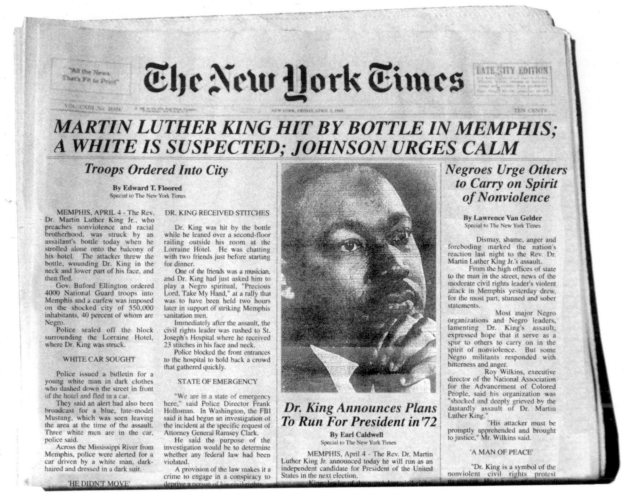

We can live without guns.

3

Sting behind the wheel in a Jaguar ad, you'll see yourself. And that could prove to be a very compelling sales presentation because, as Lanier notes, "we may find that vanity trumps celebrity."

Such changes are still to come, but to some extent the future has already arrived in the form of interactive marketing on the Internet—which is allowing companies to track customers on the Web, engage in a dialogue with them, and, in effect, "read their minds" better than conventional advertisers ever could. In the past, advertising was mostly a one-way street, with all the messages going from the advertiser to the audience. But the Internet, and eventually interactive TV, is transforming it into a two-way thoroughfare, with information constantly flowing back and forth between the advertiser and the customer.

In some ways, this represents "the end of advertising as we know it" (a phrase that is constantly on the lips of new-media executives these days). Even within some of Madison

Avenue's oldest ad agencies, many are bracing for a world without thirty-second commercials. Bob Jeffrey, the president of J. Walter Thompson's flagship New York office, has already declared the conventional TV commercial to be obsolete. Jeffrey and many others believe that the convergence of television and computer will form a multifaceted, interactive medium wherein old-fashioned sales pitches simply won't work. The viewer will be in control, dictating what appears onscreen—and who in his right mind will request commercials? Instead, viewers may use digital personal video recorders, known as PVRs, to fetch, assemble, and present the kind of shows they want to watch, with commercials edited out; or they may simply download programming right off the Internet.

This scenario doesn't mean that companies will stop pitching to us—only that the pitching will take a very different form. In the new model, marketers will still be disseminating

information about their products, but they will need to be much craftier about it: weaving product plugs into programs, or creating "infotainment" that somehow promotes a brand, or offering us incentives to click a button on the TV screen that transports us to the company Web site—whereupon they will attempt to lavish us with information, advice, and coupons as they "build relationships" with us.

To some degree, all of this should be welcome news to anyone who has ever lamented that "the ads never tell me what I need to know before I buy." In the new advertising environment, detailed information about products will be readily available and tailored to the customer's questions and needs. The advertising of the future, says Clement Mok of the high-tech design and consulting company Sapient, will "no longer rely on clever sound bites" that try to "blast out a sales pitch to people." Rather, Mok says, it will provide detailed editorial-style information, will

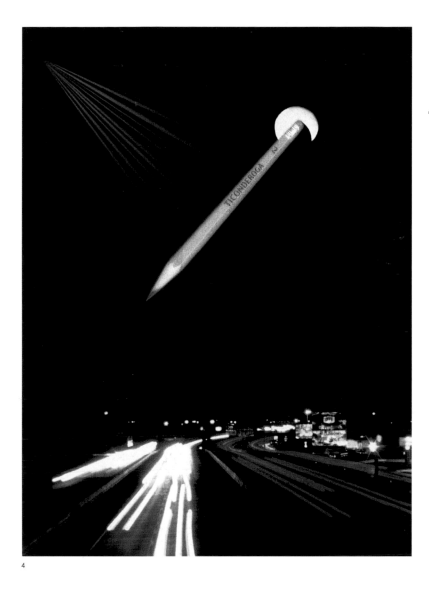

4

respond to questions, and will tend to reward you for your interest by offering something of substance and value (a coupon, say, or free expert advice, or a piece of entertainment). Bob Herbold, a top executive at Microsoft, concurs that "you're going to see more brands do good things for people in terms of providing a service, as opposed to running a traditional message that pounds the attributes of a brand." The public, armed with the power to point-and-click not just on its computers but on its TV screens, will have more control over when and how ad messages are received; the marketers, meanwhile, will benefit by being able to communicate more directly with us, finding out what we really want and need from them. It certainly sounds like an "Everybody wins" scenario.

Of course, marketers *would* tend to make it sound that way. The reality of the new advertising environment will have its downside, and it may be a big one. The most explosive issue will be—

and in fact, already is—privacy. As advertisers use technology to get closer and closer to their customers, trying to discern details about our tastes and habits and peccadilloes that we might not be anxious to share, backlashes are inevitable. Already, a few opening shots have been fired across the Internet. One of the first skirmishes involved DoubleClick, America's biggest on-line advertising company, which has been amassing detailed information on consumers—including tracking people as they surf the Internet. Whenever a Web surfer visits any one of hundreds of sites in the DoubleClick network and clicks on certain ads, a bug, or "cookie," is immediately planted on that person's hard drive, without his knowledge. The cookies contain an identifying number that enables DoubleClick to watch where you surf and what you do on the Web long after you leave its site. DoubleClick is just one of many companies planting cookies on unsuspecting Web surfers'

computers, but in early 2000, the company tried to go a step further; it announced plans to combine the tracking information gathered from cookies with other personal data collected separately—to assemble complete "on-line profiles," which would then be shared with various advertisers (conceivably, this could have included revealing to advertisers everything from one's taste in ice cream to one's predilection for kinky Web sites). A storm of protest followed, causing DoubleClick to back off the plan. And in the summer of 2000, the U.S. Federal Trade Commission reached a voluntary agreement with advertisers promising that in the future, Web surfers would be informed of on-line advertisers attempts to "profile" them.

But it was clear that the DoubleClick controversy was just the tip of the iceberg. To think that marketers will exhibit self-restraint when it comes to gathering and disseminating information about customers is naive; the very

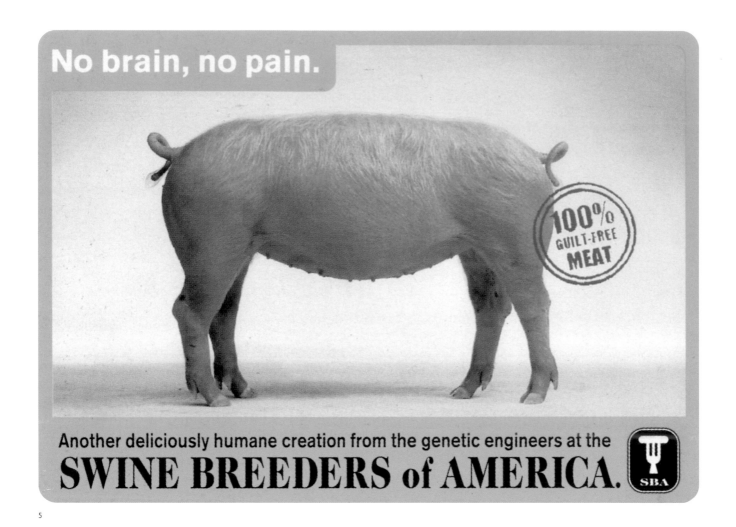

No brain, no pain.

100% GUILT-FREE MEAT

Another deliciously humane creation from the genetic engineers at the
SWINE BREEDERS of AMERICA.

SBA

5

5. **"SWINE BREEDERS OF AMERICA"**
TBWA/CHIAT/DAY,
LOS ANGELES, 1999
This mock ad, created for
Advertising Age's "Next Century"
issue, promotes genetic engineering. In the future, advertising
will probably be called upon to
make radical technology seem
less scary.

6. **AMERICAN STANDARD**
CARMICHAEL LYNCH,
MINNEAPOLIS, MINNESOTA,
1999
In the Internet age, even old
products must be given a new
spin; here, a toilet becomes
"interactive sculpture."

7. **TOASTMASTERS**
TBWA HUNT LASCARIS,
JOHANNESBURG, 1998
The less said, the better: The
new global advertising will
have little use for words.

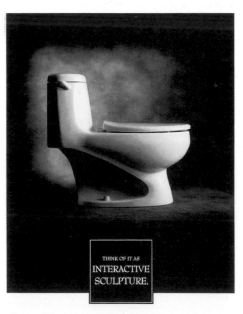

THINK OF IT AS
INTERACTIVE SCULPTURE.

Behold the *Savona* toilet, the product of a unique artistic collaboration. We asked people what their ideal toilet would look like. Then we sculpted this. Call 1-800-524-9797 ext. 484 for a guidebook full of similarly inspired creations. *American Standard*

6

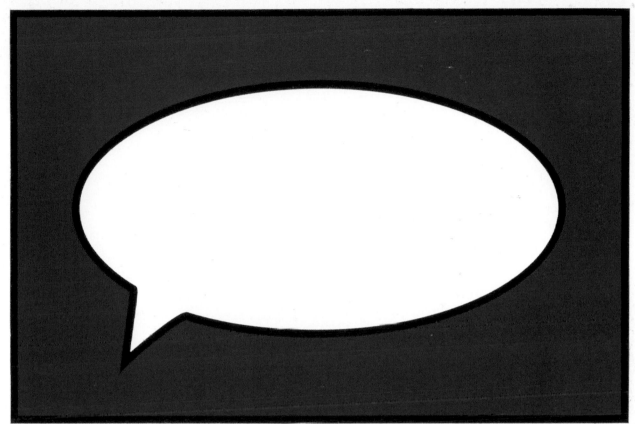

TOASTMASTERS: (011) 646 9451

7

reason they are rushing to the Internet is to be "closer" to customers—by talking to us on-line, building databases on us, tracking our on-line movements and purchases, and getting inside our heads in a way that the old focus-group research never could. And, of course, this is not limited to adults; already marketers have been using the Internet to build marketing profiles on children, offering kids rewards for giving up personal information. Herbold of Microsoft is right that marketers "will be doing more things for people" on the Web—but what they'll want in return is more and more access to our thoughts, habits, and lives.

Whether the convenience of being provided with more customized information and more free "perks" from marketers will outweigh the attendant loss of privacy is a question that can't be answered here. But what can be examined is the impact of the current changes on the style and the craft of advertising. Because as technology

promises (or threatens, depending on one's view) to usher in "the end of advertising as we know it," the questions arise: What form of communication will be offered in its place? Will the new incarnations of advertising be more aesthetically pleasing and emotionally satisfying, or less? Will there still be room for creative expression by writers and designers, or will engineers and technologists rule the day?

For those who value creativity in ads, the early stages of the revolution have not been particularly encouraging. The beauty of interactivity is that it makes advertising more measurable, more controllable—on the Web, advertisers can immediately see how you respond to every offer, every image, every word. Naturally, this tilts the balance that advertising has maintained between art and science much more in the direction of science. And it begins to shift the power from the ad creators to the researchers and technicians.

This is seen as good news to many advertisers who never truly bought into the value of creativity, because they couldn't properly measure it. True, an ad might be highly pleasing to the audience, it might be recognized and honored for its style and creativity, but to what extent was it actually moving product off the shelf? That's always been a difficult question to answer with precision—until now. As Grey Advertising's Norman Lehoullier told *The New York Times*, the precise measurement provided by interactive advertising is a kind of "Holy Grail" for advertisers, allowing them to "figure out what works and what doesn't" as they track the responses and actions of someone interacting with ads on a Web site. In this new environment, Lehoullier said, "increasingly money will be spent not on lore or art—but on science."

But the problem for the audience on the receiving end of the communication is that science has rarely produced interesting or

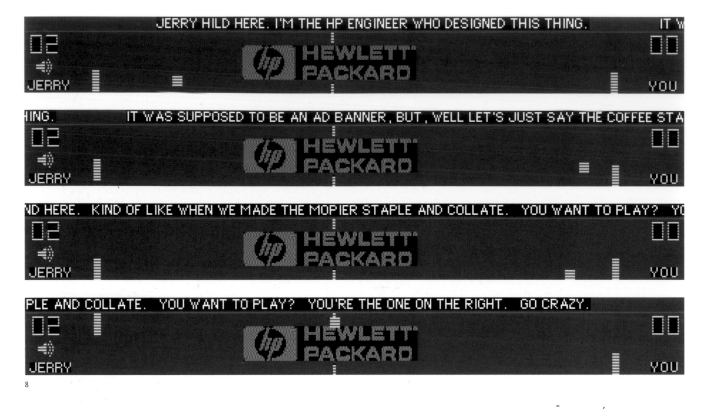

JERRY HILD HERE. I'M THE HP ENGINEER WHO DESIGNED THIS THING. IT W

ING. IT WAS SUPPOSED TO BE AN AD BANNER, BUT, WELL LET'S JUST SAY THE COFFEE STA

ND HERE. KIND OF LIKE WHEN WE MADE THE MOPIER STAPLE AND COLLATE. YOU WANT TO PLAY? YO

PLE AND COLLATE. YOU WANT TO PLAY? YOU'RE THE ONE ON THE RIGHT. GO CRAZY.

8

8. HEWLETT PACKARD
GOODBY SILVERSTEIN &
PARTNERS, SAN FRANCISCO,
LATE 1990s
This banner ad introduced a
fictional HP employee named
Jerry, who challenged the public
to play him at the computer
game Pong, right there in the ad.

9. IBM
OGILVY & MATHER,
NEW YORK, 1999
Advertising, and in particular
the IBM campaign, is creating
a new language, wherein every
word begins with "e".

creative advertising. As the top creators of ads frequently attest, there is practically an inverse relationship between research and creativity in the ad world; generally speaking, the more that an advertising idea is tested, prodded, and manipulated on the basis of customer research, the more watered down it becomes. It is the reason larger, more bureaucratic, and research-driven companies have invariably produced more bland ads than small, entrepreneurial, risk-taking companies. As Tim Delaney of the agency Leagas Delaney noted, the best advertising more often results from intuition and leaps into the creative unknown—not from parroting back what the customer wants to hear. Of course, this truism extends beyond advertising to other creative fields such as filmmaking, where it's widely accepted that formulaic approaches often result in the worst movies. However, this is something of an alien concept so far in the Internet-marketing realm—which, as the

journalist Randall Rothenberg has pointed out, tends to follow the philosophies and principles of "direct" marketing, a field that slavishly adheres to research and formula. The producers of direct-mail promotions generally have no interest in winning style points or generating good feelings about a brand; rather, they strive to elicit an immediate response from consumers, by any means necessary—including resorting to empty promises on envelopes ("You may already be a winner!"). In its early stages, Internet advertising bears a much closer resemblance to the direct-mail business and is quite different from the commercials and print advertising that often attempt to build positive feelings about a brand through soft-sell emotional storytelling. According to *The Economist,* "on the Internet, brand-building is out and straight selling is in," because, as the magazine noted, "the combination of interactivity and precision makes the Internet ideally suited to the hard sell."

That may explain why, so far, advertising on the Internet has failed to stoke the imagination of the public. There's certainly no shortage of it out there: In 1999, advertisers spent more than $4 billion on Internet ads, and that figure is expected to climb to $30 billion by 2004, according to Forrester Research, a high-tech consultancy. All of those on-line pop-up windows, banners, and buttons are trying to do the same job that TV commercials try to do—but they don't seem to be doing it nearly as well. "We have abominable creative [advertising] on-line, the worst of the worst," a leading Internet advertising-industry spokesman, Rich LeFurgy, acknowledged. Another industry executive complained of "cheesy banners that obnoxiously scream out a free offer." Most Web banner ads are like old-fashioned billboards, and not very good ones at that; they seem to lack the capacity for charm or wit, and many simply flash a teaser message, often with the word *free* in it.

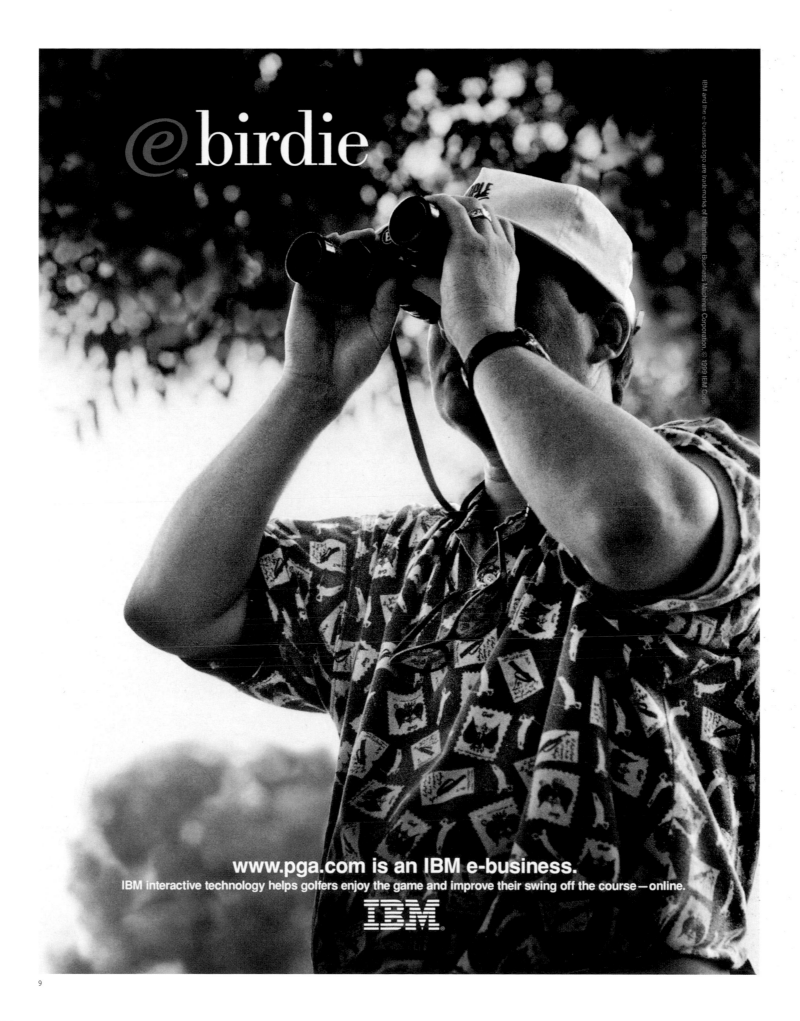

@birdie

www.pga.com is an IBM e-business.
IBM interactive technology helps golfers enjoy the game and improve their swing off the course—online.

IBM

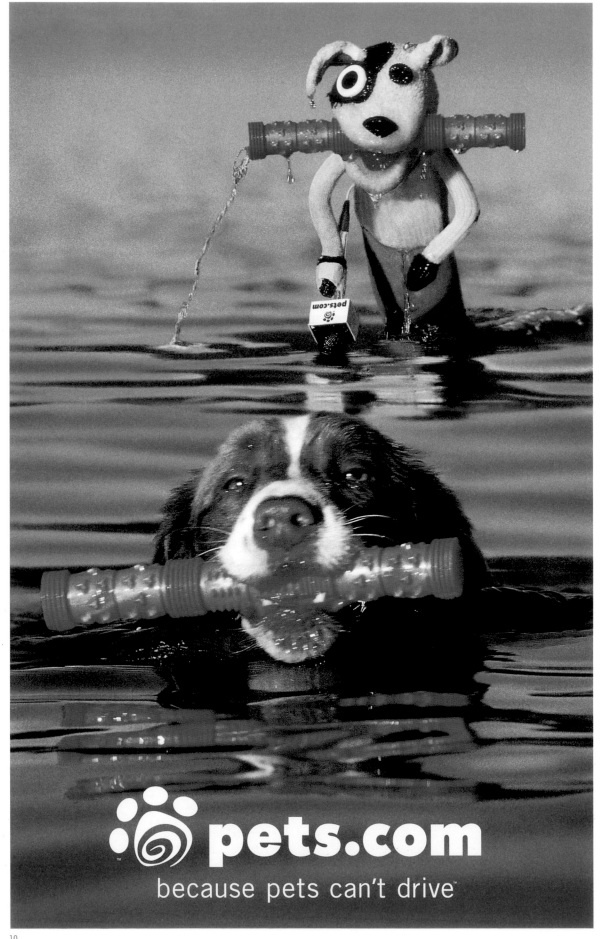

10

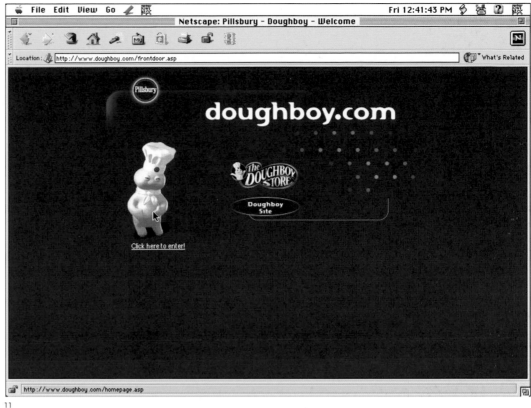

11

Not surprisingly, travelers on the information highway have been speeding past them and not bothering to click; most banners are experiencing minuscule click-through rates of less than half of one percent.

Banner ads have tried various means of engaging the audience, often by utilizing the ace in the hole of interactivity. Some have used the available technology to incorporate game-playing, which can be effective and amusing. Among the first to draw attention with this approach was a series of banner ads for Hewlett-Packard that introduced a fictional HP employee named Jerry, who challenged the public to play him in a game of Pong (played right there on the banner). Similarly, an IBM banner promoting its E-business partnership with the Professional Golf Association turned the banner into a tiny putting green, with the user's cursor serving as the putter. While some have played games, others have resorted to trickery—designing banners

that, for example, resembled a computer-error warning prompt on the user's screen (if you tried to respond to the warning by clicking an "OK" button, you were immediately hijacked to the advertiser's Web site). Even more bothersome than trick banners are "interstitials"—ad screens that pop up to interrupt Web surfing, and which must be removed from the screen before you can proceed. Some Internet advertisers argue that this form of advertising is no more intrusive than a TV commercial or roadside billboard, but in truth, the interstitial is like a roadside billboard that has been dragged to the middle of the road and left there, forcing drivers to stop and maneuver around it.

In fairness, the relatively poor quality of on-line ads is partly a function of the newness of the medium. The banner ads appearing now are only the first-generation versions of Internet marketing, and will rapidly evolve and improve. Andy Berlin of the agency Berlin Cameron &

Partners draws comparisons to the early days of television advertising, which tended to yield clumsy efforts. Part of the problem, Berlin notes, is that "technical revolutions tend to be led by the people that understand the technology and the people that finance it. And that's the sensibility early on. And then eventually they recognize that artistic people have to get involved or they won't get the full benefit of it." So far, the art crowd of the ad world—the award-winning creators of the best advertising in recent years— have been largely detached from advertising's Internet revolution, often by their own choice. According to Bob Schmetterer, who heads the Euro RSCG international advertising-agency network, a schism has developed in the ad business in which the Internet advertising arena is perceived to be a kind of ghetto, shunned by top creative stars who prefer to work in TV and print. "There is a very big and very prevalent belief that the Internet is the province of

THE NEXT WAVE.

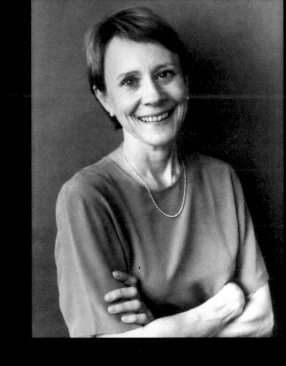

INTERVIEW: ESTHER DYSON

Esther Dyson has emerged as one of the preeminent thinkers and leaders of the new digital culture. Dyson's highly influential newsletter, "Release 1.0," and her book, *Release 2.1: A Design for Living in the Digital Age*, have provided a road map to what's unfolding and what is yet to come as the high-tech revolution reshapes the world. Today Dyson serves as chairman of the New York–based company EDventure Holdings, Inc., while also advising the WPP Group advertising conglomerate. She also oversees the governmental body dealing with registration of Internet domain names.

IS THE THIRTY-SECOND COMMERCIAL GOING TO BE EXTINCT SOON?
Like everything else, the changes being brought about by the Internet are cumulative, rather than things being suddenly replaced. I don't think mass-market commercials will go away. But I think people are using the Net wrong by putting mass-market commercials onto it. The Net is for one-to-one communication and customer support. It's not a place for making promises about the brand—it's the place to deliver on those promises.

SO FAR, A LOT OF MARKETERS HAVE TRIED TO USE BANNER ADS, AND THEY HAVEN'T BEEN THAT EFFECTIVE.
Yes, because it's not interactive. So it's sort of like going to a store where you expect to talk to a salesperson—and all you see is billboards surrounding you.

WHAT WILL ADVERTISERS HAVE TO DO TO BRING MORE INTERACTIVITY TO THEIR COMMUNICATION ON THE WEB?
You do it by paying attention to the consumer, rather than just clamoring for his attention. You can use the Net to listen to people and to help them talk to one another. And in that sense, maybe what we're talking about is not really advertising at all. It may be more a matter of providing information—maybe about someone's air-miles account or about using the product or creating a sense of community among users. There are lots of good things you can do, but simply saying, "Wow, I'm great" isn't one of them.

IT SOUNDS LIKE YOU'RE SAYING THERE'S NO PLACE ON THE INTERNET FOR MAKING CLAIMS ABOUT A PRODUCT OR USING SOUND BITES TO GET ATTENTION.
No, the Internet will still be a medium for delivering that. But that kind of message won't be considered native to the Internet format. What will be native is interactive communication. That can include storytelling ads, though they might be presented in a different way—probably more like serials or continuing cartoons. Or letting viewers vote on what they see. Right now, advertisers try to guess what the consumer wants to see. But why not just let consumers select from a list of what kinds of ads they want to see? Presumably they'll pay more attention to ads they've chosen, and they'll change the list when they change their mood. Seems like a very sensible idea—and it's something that interactivity allows you to do.

AS ADVERTISING INCREASINGLY DRIVES PEOPLE TO WEB SITES, WHAT DO THE WEB SITES HAVE TO DO TO ENGAGE PEOPLE ONCE THEY ARRIVE?
When you walk into a restaurant, usually you can tell whether it's the kind of fast-food place where you have to stand in line with a tray, or a fancier restaurant where you sit down and get waited on. But sometimes you walk into a restaurant and you can't tell—and that's annoying. With a Web site, people should know what to do and what to expect when they get there. Fundamentally, a Web site is not a window that people look through; it's a door, and when people walk through it they expect to interact with what they find inside.

AS ADVERTISING BECOMES MORE OF A TWO-WAY DIALOGUE INSTEAD OF THE OLD ONE-WAY SALES PITCH, IS THIS A POSITIVE DEVELOPMENT FOR EVERYONE INVOLVED?
Well, I think it's positive for consumers. But it's tough for marketers, because it's very expensive, people-intensive, and it's hard to do well. You can't simply produce a message at headquarters and slap it out to millions of people. And what's also disconcerting in this new communication is that people are uppity—they talk back. And they don't necessarily believe what you tell them. So I think it will be good for the world, but it's kind of tough for traditional advertising agencies.

DO YOU THINK THOSE TRADITIONAL AD AGENCIES—THE MADISON AVENUE ESTABLISHMENT—WILL CONTINUE TO CONTROL ADVERTISING AND MARKETING AS IT SHIFTS MORE TOWARD THE WEB?
Some agencies will and some won't. It's a matter of who understands how to use the new medium, and who is smart and open-minded. It's not a matter of big or small. In fact, being small usually correlates to being open-minded because you have less to protect. So that favors the newer companies.

IN TERMS OF THE TWO-WAY DIALOGUE BETWEEN ADVERTISER AND CONSUMER, ONE AREA OF CONCERN IS PRIVACY AND THE SENSE THAT WE SHOULD BE WORRIED ABOUT HOW THE INFORMATION WE GIVE TO MARKETERS ENDS UP BEING USED. WILL THIS BE A PROBLEM IN INTERNET MARKETING FOR A LONG TIME TO COME?
Not if people handle it right. I don't see it as a plague; I see it as a misunderstanding right now. When I give my money to a bank, it's still my money—and the same is true with the data I give to companies. But I think companies don't understand that; they think it's their data. What people can do about this is to make a contract with marketers about how they can and can't use those personal data. Companies need to begin to understand this, and consumers need to understand it. A lot of consumers are very happy to share the information if it means they'll get better offers in return—but you've got to ask them first. And people should be able to make different choices; we don't have to find one way that suits everyone. It's like choosing a credit card that has an expensive rate: People choose those for a reason, because it gives them credit they couldn't get otherwise. The challenge marketers will face is managing their data effectively and tagging them for what they can and can't do with them, based on the choices consumers have made. But the consumer should set the guidelines about which information can be used and where. In that regard, the balance of power is changing, and most companies don't get that yet.

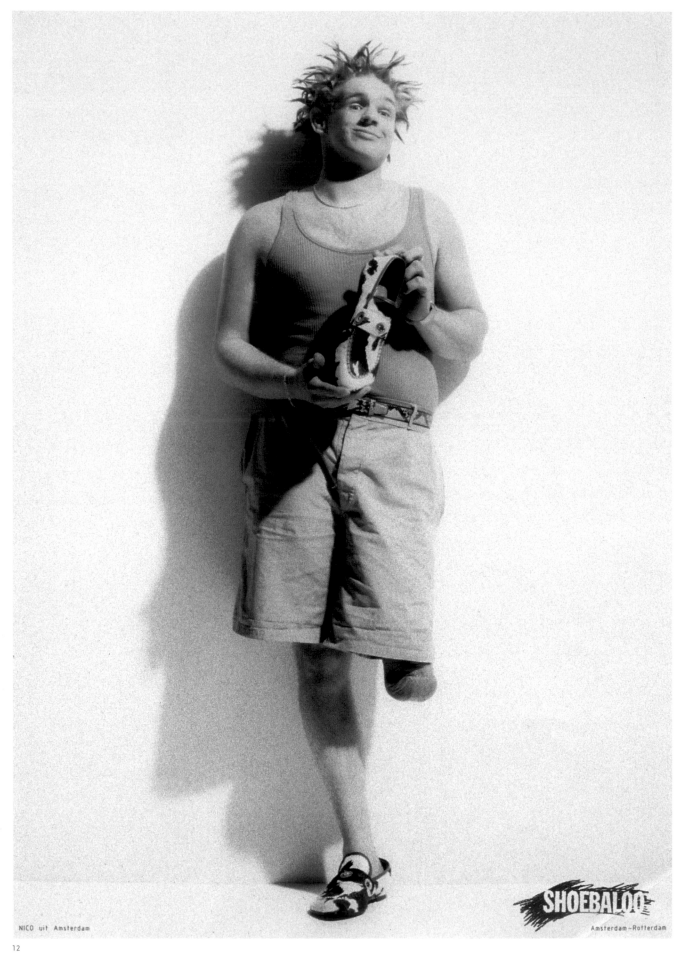

NICO uit Amsterdam

SHOEBALOO

Amsterdam-Rotterdam

12

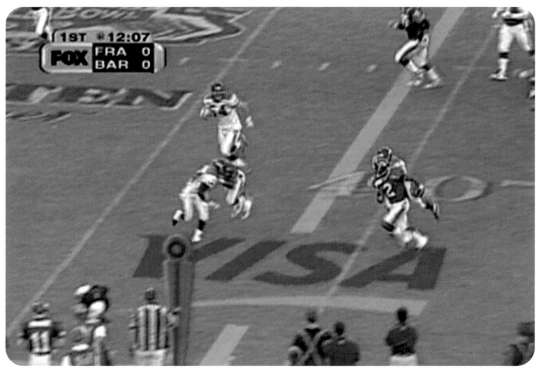

13

12. **SHOEBALOO**
KESSELSKRAMER, AMSTER-
DAM, 1996
KesselsKramer holds that
advertising must become more
socially conscious to succeed
in the twenty-first century; the
Dutch agency features disabled
people in ads.

13. **VISA**
PRINCETON VIDEO IMAGING,
PRINCETON, NEW JERSEY,
1999
"Virtual ads" can now be digitally
planted into the television
picture. It may look like that
logo is painted on the football
field, but it exists only in the
eye of the viewer.

technocrats," Schmetterer wrote recently, "while TV, print, and other traditional media remain the province of *real* creative people. This is a huge problem for our industry."

One reason advertising's best storytellers and creators have ignored new media is that so far it's still difficult to bring emotion and story to life on the Internet, partly because of technical limitations. But as Internet access and data transmission improve via the growth of broadband information-delivery systems, advertisers on the Web will be able to make better use of "rich media," combining high-grade graphics with audio and interactive capabilities. They will, in effect, be able to bring video storytelling qualities to more and more on-line ads (some advertisers already use rich media, but it's costly and can't be viewed by computer users with inadequate equipment).

While there's little doubt that technology will gradually provide the capability to bring more

emotional advertising to the Internet, some Internet experts maintain that emotional appeals have no real place in cyberspace—a world where speed and functionality are the top priorities. "Today, brands on the Web are all about how quick and easy it is for a consumer to find what he's looking for," according to Web analyst Jim Nail of Forrester Research. Nail argues that emotional appeals are needed by only those marketers who must draw people to a store with a promise; "but on-line, the delivery of that promise is one click away," he says. Sapient's Mok believes that in place of emotional sales pitches, Internet marketers will "craft and create real content and editorial," perhaps taking a form more similar to on-line magazines. But other advertisers still see a critical role for emotional appeals, storytelling, and entertainment. In fact, some believe that in the new media environment, emotional advertising will blend and blur with entertainment programming offered on the Web

and on TV—to the extent that it may be difficult to tell where the programming ends and the ad starts.

Ad agencies are already gearing up for this new form of "stealth advertising." A number of them have been creating in-house entertainment divisions or forging alliances with television and film producers; for example, in January 2000, J. Walter Thompson formed a creative alliance with Hollywood's Basic Entertainment, producers of the hit HBO television series "The Sopranos." The plan is for the ad agency to become more involved in the development of TV programs. This could go well beyond the kind of standard product placement that has been a part of moviemaking for years—it may involve coming up with concepts for shows in which the client's product is an integral part of the entertainment. J. Walter Thompson's Marina Hahn, who is overseeing the alliance, offers the following example: Listerine, a JWT client, might sponsor a comedy show in which some of the jokes and

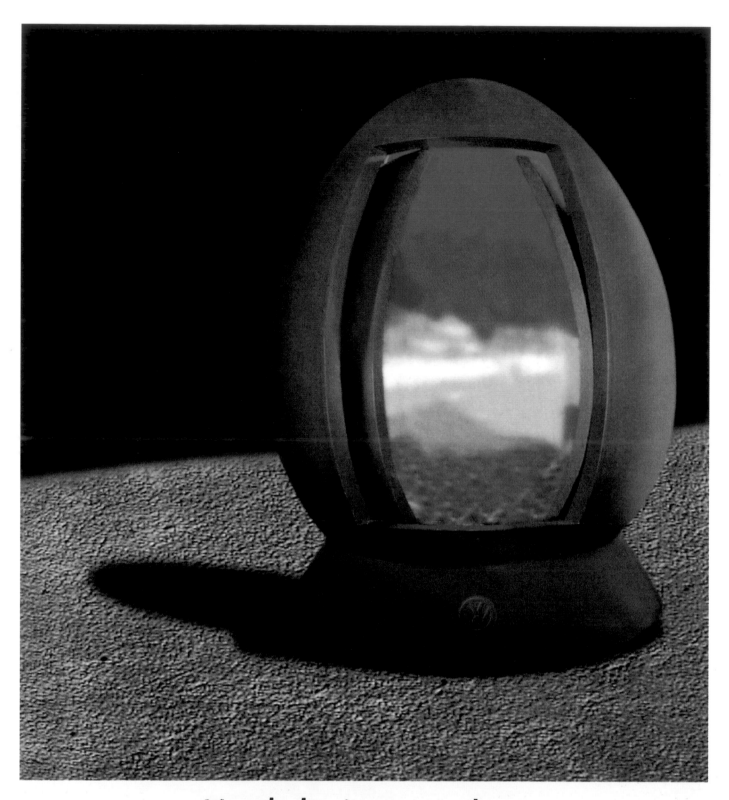

It's ugly, but it gets you there.

The new Volkswagen Time Machine.

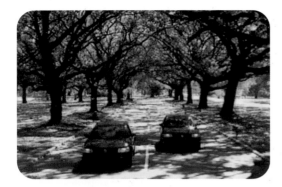

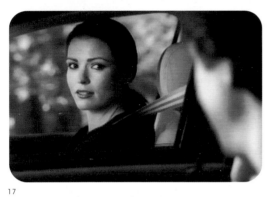

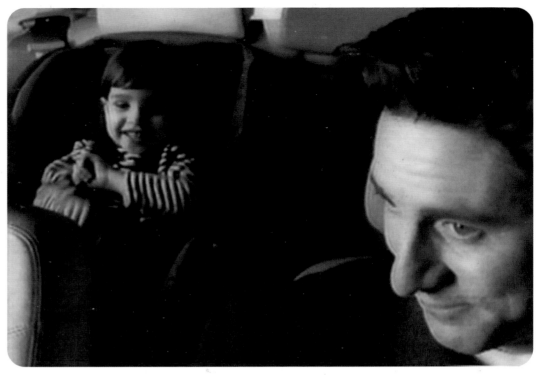

17

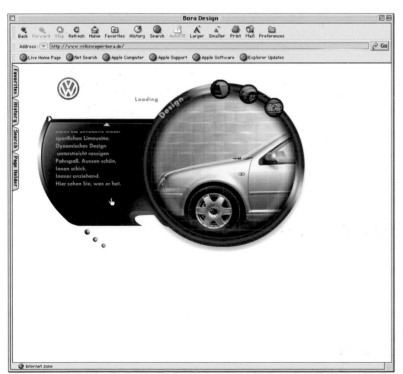

18

16. **VOLKSWAGEN "TIME MACHINE"**
DM9 DDB PUBLICIDADE,
SÃO PAULO, 1999
This mock ad was originally
created for *Advertising Age's*
"Next Century" issue in Fall
1999. This time, DM9 took a
crack at promoting a VW time
machine.

17. **VOLKSWAGEN**
ARNOLD COMMUNICATIONS,
BOSTON, 1999
VW's current TV commercials
have begun to feature more
"visual narratives," like this
wordless tale of a flirtatious
encounter between two parents
driving a VW Passat.

18. **VOLKSWAGEN WEB SITE (GERMANY)**
BBDO INTERACTIVE GMBH,
DUSSELDORF, 2000
The new, uncluttered ads are
now designed to drive consumers
to the Web site—which then
uses detailed information to
close the sale.

19. FORD FOCUS
J. WALTER THOMPSON,
DETROIT, 2000
Ford Motors and its agency
used interactivity to allow TV
viewers to assemble their own
commercial. The result was a
messy Frankenstein's monster
of an ad.

20. PHILIPS ON-LINE CATALOG
EURO RSCG INTERACTION,
AMSTERDAM, 1999
So far, the on-line sales pitch
has been more direct and
less artful. To some extent,
on-line marketing is more like
direct-mail promotion than
advertising.

21. BMW WEB SITE
DUFFY DESIGN/FALLON,
MINNEAPOLIS, MINNESOTA,
1999
The BMW Web site allows
viewers to get an inside look
at the vehicles. According to
technology consultant Esther
Dyson, a Web site is "a door,
and when people walk through
it they expect to interact with
what they find inside."

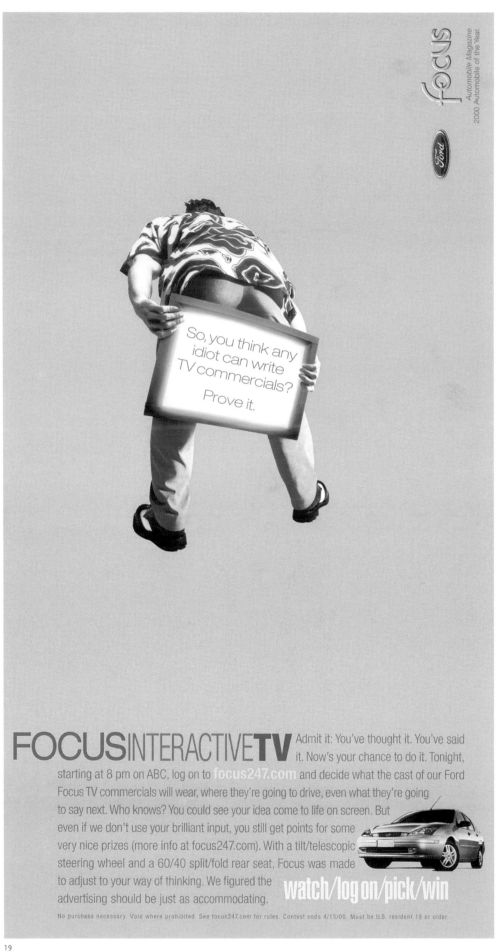

19

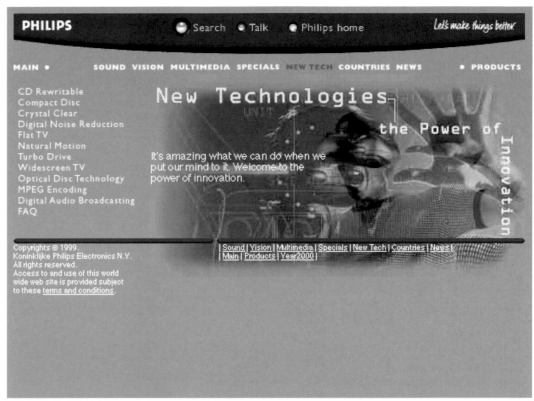

20

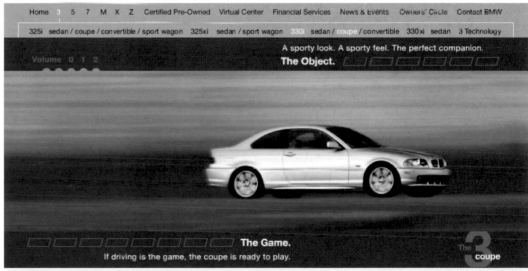

21

THE NEXT WAVE.

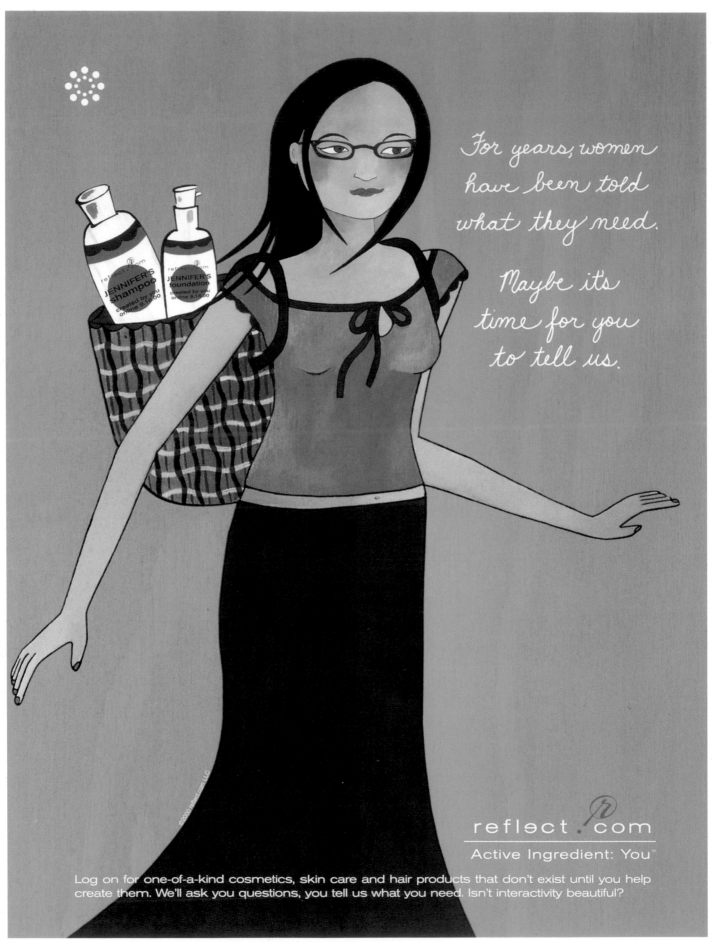

22

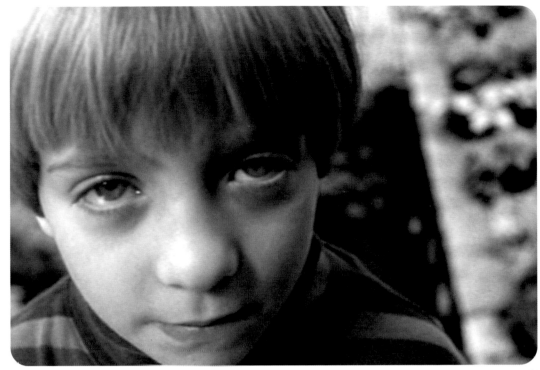

23

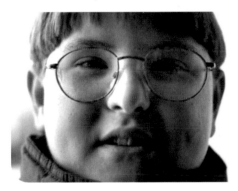

true, Boyko insists. "People had the means to zap commercials a long time ago," he points out, referring to remote controls, mute buttons, and VCRs. "The fact that they haven't done it suggests that commercials have become a part of our life that we've accepted and sometimes enjoy. Look at the Super Bowl, and the way some people pay more attention to the ads than to the game itself."

Moreover, even as customized Web marketing becomes more prevalent, there will still be a need for something to drive people to the Web site—a task for which today's entertainment-heavy, info-light commercials are actually well suited. Already, most commercials list Web-site addresses, though some recent ads have tried to create a more compelling link to the Internet. One series of Nike commercials featured scenes in which a character is being chased; in mid-chase, the commercial stops and directs viewers to visit a Web site in order to find out how the story ends (once there, the viewer

could see several different endings to the com-mercial). It was a clever idea, but might have been ahead of its time; in the pre-convergence world, this required someone to actually get up and move from TV to computer, which is a lot to ask of the average couch potato. (There was another problem with the ads: A couple of TV networks declined to run them, fearing they might end up pulling viewers away from the TV and the show they were watching.)

Similarly, Ford and its agency J. Walter Thompson produced a series of live commercials in the spring of 2000 that tried to entice viewers to the Web site by offering to turn over creative control of the advertising to the audience. Once at the Web site, viewers could actually dictate the content of the next commercial in the series—by voting on which characters would appear, what they would wear and say, etc. Not surprisingly, the Frankenstein's monster of a commercial that resulted from this experiment was a bit awkward;

the lesson there may be that even in the brave new "viewer controlled" media world, perhaps we'd best leave admaking to the professionals.

Evidence suggests that even without resorting to such gimmickry, commercials can do a good job of funneling people to Web sites. During the 1999 Super Bowl, a new employment Web site named Monster.com gambled a large portion of its start-up funds on a striking commercial that featured children fantasizing about dreary, dead-end careers ("I want to work my way up to middle management!" dreamed one boy). In the twenty-four hours after the commercial ran, traffic to the Web site jumped from 600,000 searches a day to over 2 million—and it spiked particularly high in the moments right after the ad ran, indicating that people had actually risen from the couch, turned away from the game, and gone to their computers. Monster.com's enormous success prompted a host of other dot-com companies to snap up ad time (at a

THE NEXT WAVE.

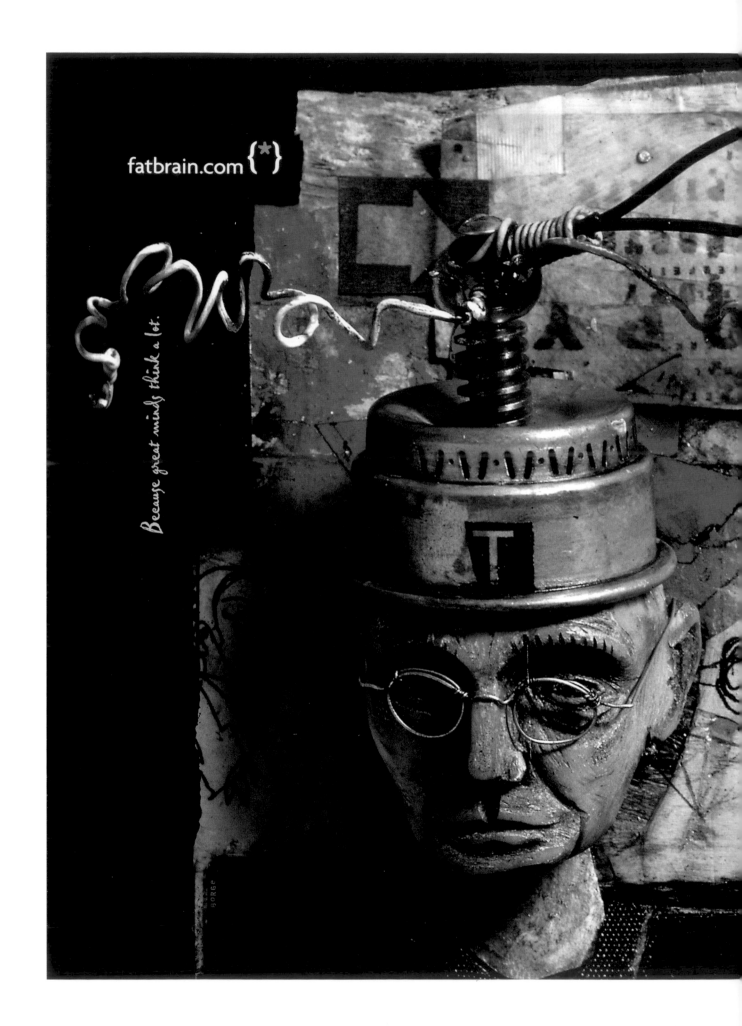

fatbrain.com {*}

Because great minds think a lot.

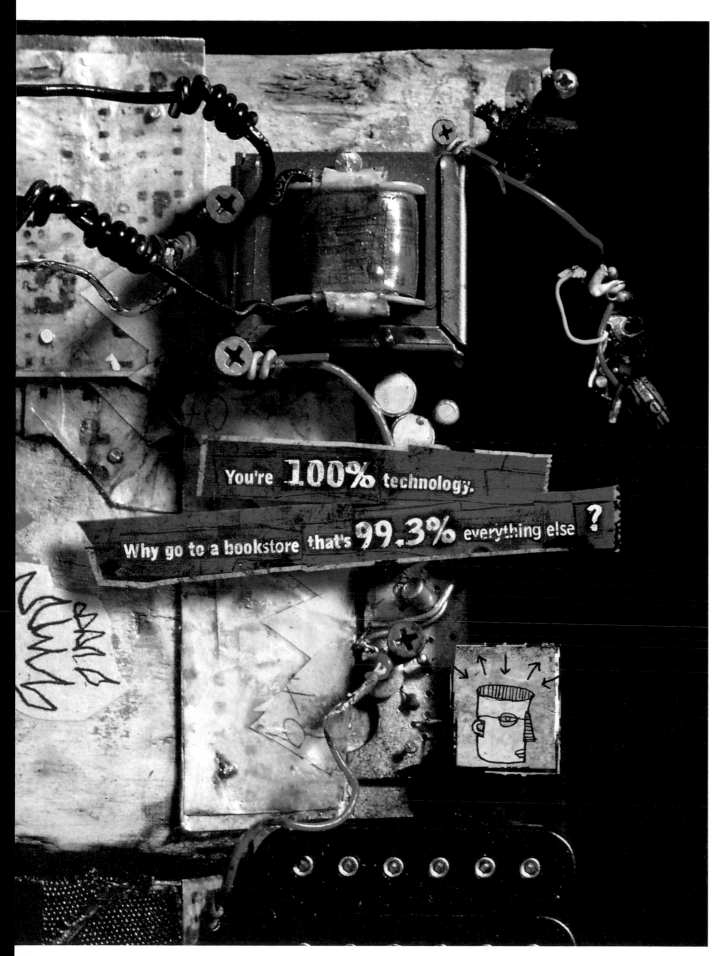

You're **100%** technology.

Why go to a bookstore that's **99.3%** everything else **?**

27. FATBRAIN.COM
GOLDBERG MOSER O'NEILL,
SAN FRANCISCO, 1999
Traditional print advertising
was a huge beneficiary of the
technology boom. Magazines
such as *Wired* overflowed with
wild ads like this one for a Web-
based business information
manager.

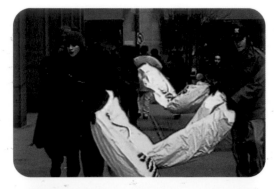

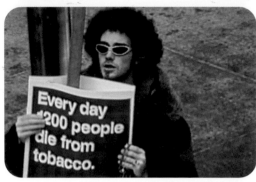

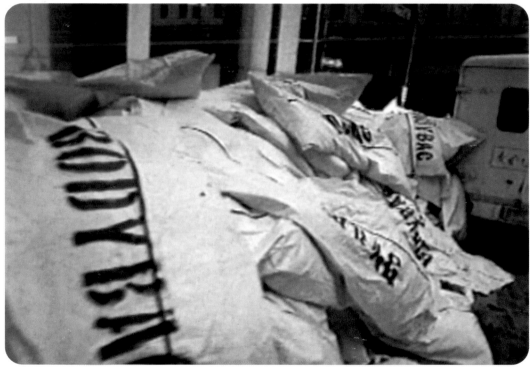

28. AMERICAN LEGACY FOUNDATION
ALLIANCE (CRISPIN PORTER + BOGUSKY, MIAMI / ARNOLD COMMUNICATIONS, BOSTON), 2000
The "Truth" anti-smoking ads are like short documentary films, following rebellious teenagers who challenge tobacco marketers. In this commercial, "Body Bags," kids piled body bags outside the offices of a cigarette company.

29. BRODERBUND SOFTWARE
SAATCHI & SAATCHI, SAN FRANCISCO, 1997
This series of ads promoting the Riven CD-ROM turned the print ad itself into a kind of game (can you find the Web site address in this picture?)

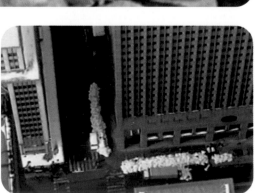

28

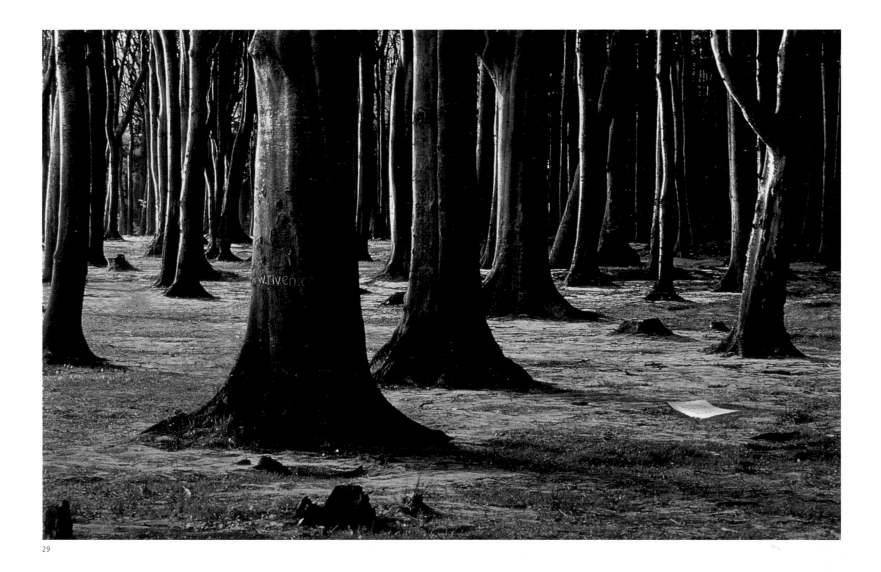

29

know what they're selling; I don't know what the benefits are to them." Many dot-coms, including Outpost.com and its flying gerbils, failed at this. In the new millennium, some forty years after DDB's Bill Bernbach laid down the law that advertising had to balance art and commerce, and that it needed to entertain yet never lose sight of the product and the message, the problem was still the same—many advertisers just couldn't seem to figure out how to achieve that very delicate balance.

The balancing act won't get easier in days ahead, and may in fact become more difficult. Among the new challenges facing ads in the future: The need to connect with an audience that is, itself, divided into many distinct and very separate groups. According to the futurist Jim Taylor, coauthor of the book *The 500-Year Delta*, the coming years will bring "the deconstruction of the concept of collective, so-called mass society. We will see the growth of small, highly

ethnocentric 'tribal' societies." Reaching a more culturally diverse society of consumers, new ads will travel by way of a more fragmented and splintered delivery system. How splintered? One major marketer recently experimented with an advertising delivery system that would send customized versions of its commercials to different rooms within the same house—so that children upstairs might see one version of the commercial, while one parent in the den would see another version, and the other parent, in the kitchen, would see yet another version of that ad. O&M's Westreich foresees the possibility of software that could take a single ad and "create two-hundred versions of it automatically," so that the ad is seen differently by each ethnic or demographic group; the perception and interpretation of such advertising will truly be in the eye of the beholder. Meanwhile, the targeting of ads is expected to zero in on ever-narrower and quirkier audience segments. (Already, one

pet-food advertiser has created and run a TV commercial targeted to cats; it features a montage of scenes involving a fish swimming, a ball of yarn, and a mouse, with a sound track of actual catcalls.)

But for advertisers to be able to connect with the various tribes in an increasingly global and multicultural world, the business itself must diversify. As the new millennium began, advertising in America and Europe was still a predominantly white male bastion, particularly in creative departments of top agencies. Executives throughout the ad industry are attuned to the problem, but many seem at a loss as to how to resolve it. Training programs and scholarships have been tried, but the cycle has been difficult to break; for members of minority groups, there are "no heroes to emulate in advertising," says Ron Seichrist of the Miami Ad School. And while advertising must learn to speak the language of ethnic groups, it must avoid the

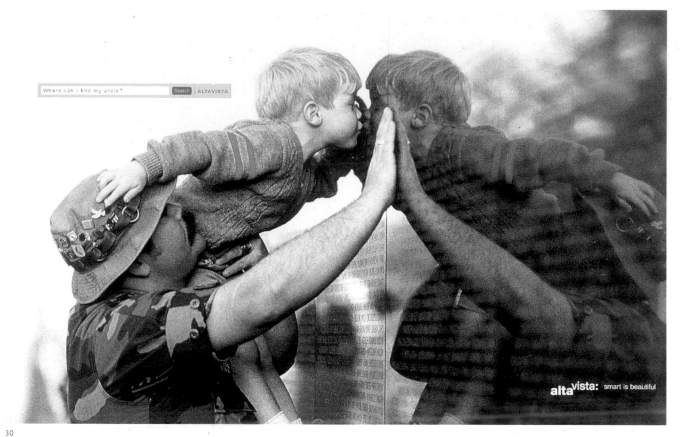

30

30. ALTA VISTA
WIEDEN + KENNEDY,
PORTLAND, 1999
This ad for the Web search
engine Alta Vista used a touching
image of visitors at the Vietnam
Veterans Memorial in Washington, D.C. The successful ad must
strike a balance between art and
commerce, emotion and logic.

31. PROJECT MILLENNIUM
McCONNAGHY STEIN
SCHMIDT & BROWN,
CHICAGO, 1999
Some within the industry
believe it is now time for
advertising to take on its
toughest challenge: to become
more socially responsible.

kind of pandering that has, so far, caused ads targeted to minority groups to be among the least creative of all advertising. "An idea whose primary purpose is to convey ethnicity is likely to be weak," noted Jo Muse, who runs the agency Muse Cordero Chen, a specialist in ads to the African-American, Asian, and Hispanic communities. "The fact is, a compelling idea has no color; it has its own truth and texture."

As advertising of the future struggles to become more diverse and to do a better job of reflecting a changing world, it may also increasingly have to confront matters of ethics. While some may think of "ethics in advertising" as an oxymoron, younger practitioners of advertising seem to be more socially conscious now than in years past. In the U.S., Jelly Helm, a former creative star at Wieden + Kennedy, has become the leader of a homegrown movement advocating ethical advertising—wherein advertisers question the kinds of products they

promote, whether it's proper to advertise to children, and so forth. Helm says that just as advertising has in recent years weeded out most of the old sexist and racist imagery, it must now go to the next level—"applying the same standards to work that advocates reckless and irresponsible consumption." Helm's views have sparked lively debate in the industry and have particularly drawn interest at ad schools around the U.S. A similar attitude can be found in Europe, where agencies like St. Luke's in London and KesselsKramer in Amsterdam have adopted socially responsible stances. "We think that just as the engine of twentieth-century economic growth has been marketing, the engine of the twenty-first century economic future will be ethics," said Johan Kramer, co-founder of KesselsKramer. "We try to work for clients and products that benefit human and social development. And we try to make ads that avoid promoting reckless consumption." For advertis-

ing's own ethical watchdogs, the challenges ahead will involve not just certain products but also questionable practices—such as high-tech trickery that alters images and engages in sly product placement, or the use of psychological profiling information gathered on the Internet.

With all of these swirling issues and turbulent changes in the air, advertising in the early part of the twenty-first century could be said to be in the midst of a revolution more jarring and profound than the one led by Bernbach forty years ago. That particular insurrection brought forth advertising that was more sophisticated and stylish than what had come before; indeed, it established that advertising could be, at least in the view of some, a vital and interesting form of communication and might even, on rare occasions, aspire to the level of art. If the current revolution advances that cause and yields similar progress, it will be worth watching. For now all that can be said is, stay tuned.

SOMETHING TO KEEP
IN MIND AS WE CONTINUE
—TO SCREW UP—
THE EARTH'S ENVIRONMENT:
THE SPACE SHUTTLE ONLY SEATS FIVE.

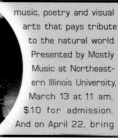

The last 200 years of human activity have left our planet with a wicked hangover. So what will the next 200 bring? Will we balance the demands of civilization and nature? Or turn the earth into a giant polluted strip mall? During March and April, Project Millennium invites you to ask these questions by presenting 100 events focusing on the Environment. Check out *Our Letter to the World*, a multimedia performance of music, poetry and visual arts that pays tribute to the natural world. Presented by Mostly Music at Northeastern Illinois University, March 13 at 11 am, $10 for admission. And on April 22, bring your family to *Earth Day* at the Lincoln Park Zoo, a free event running from 10 am to 1 pm. Enjoy fun activities while learning about endangered species and what you can do to make a difference for wildlife and the environment.

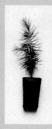

SAY "THANK YOU" TO A TREE FOR PROVIDING SHADE AND OXYGEN. WE SUGGEST DOING IT WHEN NO ONE'S LOOKING.

Make a tree happy by visiting the Morton Arboretum for their *Arbor Day Celebration*, April 30–May 1. Program includes tree plantings, nature art activities, tours and more. Admission $7 per vehicle. Free on Arbor Day, April 30, 10 am–4 pm. Asian Longhorn Beetles are not welcome. Or take a *Treekeepers Class* to learn basic tree care skills, including insect and disease recognition, planting, pruning techniques and tree identification. Presented by Openlands Project at the North Park Village Administration Bldg., call 312.427.4256 to register; course fee $65. Classes are held on seven consecutive Saturday mornings, March 14–April 25, 9:30 am–12:30 pm.

When you consider that water covers three-fourths of the earth, maybe our appreciation of the sea should extend beyond a Long John Silver's Value Platter. Marine biologist and deep sea explorer Dr. Sylvia Earle would agree, having spent 6,000 hours of her life diving underwater. A 1998 recipient of the United Nations Environment Prize, she has helped bring attention to

how pollution and overfishing threaten our oceans and, ultimately, our own existence. In the second installment of *Future Perfect: Conversations for the New Millennium*, Earle and author/naturalist Diane Ackerman discuss

Throughout 1999, more than 190 organizations will present nearly 1,000 exhibits, performances, film series, tours, lectures and kid's events. To learn more, visit **www.ProjectMillennium.org** or contact us at 312.322.8889.

AN EXHIBITION OF WORMS, BEETLES AND EARWIGS. NO WONDER BUSINESS AT THE MUSEUM CAFÉ IS SLOW.

Get a "bug's-eye" view of the soil beneath your feet at The Field Museum's newest permanent exhibit, *Underground Adventure*. This 15,000-square-foot total immersion environment lets you walk through a soil ecosystem recreated at 100 times life-size and visit a mud room chock full of live dirt-dwelling creatures. Opening on March 27, special admission fee. Those of you seeking a different kind of beauty should visit the Terra Museum of American Art for *From Forests to Farms*, a lecture/tour on 19th-century American landscape paintings that illustrates how farming and development have changed the physical appearance of our country. March 16 at 6 pm, free, reservations required.

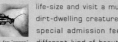

Earwig, Latin for "gross"

WILL THE MOST DANGEROUS THING IN OUR OCEANS SOON BE THE WATER?

how we can begin to reconcile the effects of human enterprise with the natural world. Ackerman's works include "The Rarest of the Rare," about the plight of endangered animals and the best-selling "A Natural History of the Senses." Moderated by Bill Kurtis, *Conversations for the New Millennium* takes place March 3 from 7–8 pm and will be broadcast live on Channel 11, WTTW. And be sure to visit the Shedd Aquarium for a behind-the-scenes look at their amazing *Coral Construction* program. March 9, 6:30 pm, admission is $20. Just call 312.692.3324 to register.

SEE WHAT HAPPENS WHEN A TOXIC WASTE SITE CHECKS INTO REHAB.

Sometimes, a polluted piece of land gets a second chance. Like the Wisconsin Steel Works, the subject of *Cleaning Up 101*, a free lecture by EnvironCom Inc. that describes the environmental cleanup at the site of an old steel mill. March 24, 6:30 pm at the Chicago Public Library, Vodak/East Side Branch, call 312.747.5500 for info. The theme of transformation is also explored in *Footprints on the Land* at the Spring Valley Nature Sanctuary in Schaumburg. This workshop uses a new trail to show changes that have taken place in both human and natural landscapes. April 18, 1–4 pm, free admission.

31

NOTES

Excerpts are listed in italics, by page number, followed by their source or attribution.

CHAPTER 1

p. 10: More than $400 billion a year is spent on advertising worldwide.
Projections from universal McCann forecasting director Robert J. Coen, announced Dec. 4, 2000.

p. 10: A recent survey by the Starch Roper research firm found people today actually like watching commercials more than ever before, no doubt because ads have evolved to become far more watchable in recent years.
Survey published in **AMERICAN DEMOGRAPHICS**, Nov. 1997. Other studies conducted by **ADVERTISING AGE** for its special issue "The Next Century," Fall 1999, found that people are more likely to "view advertising as an entertainment medium in its own right."

p. 10: "Art is something that reinterprets for people the life they're leading, it allows you to experience what you know about life," Fenske says. "And because advertising deals with the minutiae of everyday life, any art that comes out of it is going to be particularly relevant and powerful."
Fenske's comments originally appeared in **ONE. A MAGAZINE**, Vol. 1, Issue 2, 1997.

p. 16: (In the U.S. last year, companies spent more than $100 million researching and testing their own ads).
THE NEW YORK TIMES, April 13, 2000.

p. 16: "They have a talent they're born with, and they happen to wander into advertising, where that particular talent begins to grow and flower," says the celebrated British advertising writer Tim Delaney.
From my interview with Delaney for the newsletter **ONE-TO-ONE**, Nov./Dec. 1994.

p. 16: George Lois . . . believes Pablo Picasso's observation that "art is the lie that tells the truth" can be applied to great advertising. "Almost all products are comparable in quality," Lois has noted, "but when advertising is great advertising—when it's inventive, irreverent, audacious and loaded with chutzpah—it literally becomes a benefit for the product, and Picasso's 'lie' becomes the truth."
From **WHAT'S THE BIG IDEA?** by George Lois, 1991.

p. 17: "There used to be a lot of pride taken in the creation of very utilitarian things," observes Dan Wieden of Wieden + Kennedy. "In fact we dig them up all over the world now, we look at vases and bowls and forks and spoons from different eras and cultures. At the time, they were basically commodities—but the person making them cared enough about them to put something special into them, and that made them art."
From my interview with Wieden, originally published in **ONE. A MAGAZINE**, Vol. 2, Issue 3, 1999.

pp. 17–18: "Advertising has become so entrenched in the Brazilian culture that it is one of the preferred topics of conversation in bars, along with soccer and politics," says Sergio Caruso of the Brazilian agency Carillo Pastore Euro RSCG. Caruso adds that "the names of some of Brazil's advertising people have become part of the layman's repertoire," and "more Brazilians now want to become advertising people than doctors, engineers, or journalists."
STAR MAGAZINE, published by Euro RSCG, Spring 1999.

p. 20: As one industry pundit commented recently, "the creatives have taken over the asylum."
Rance Crain, **ADVERTISING AGE**, special issue, "The Advertising Century," Spring 1999.

p. 28: The author Marshall McLuhan called advertisements "the richest and most faithful daily reflections that any society ever made of its entire range of activities."
Marshall McLuhan, **UNDERSTANDING MEDIA: THE EXTENSIONS OF MAN**, 1964.

p. 39: The Sulk Institute . . . once said of him, "He could explain us to ourselves."
From **BILL BERNBACH'S BOOK,** by Bob Levenson, 1967.

CHAPTER 2

p. 46: The idea was to identify a compelling reason people should buy a product—Reeves called this the "Unique Selling Proposition"—and then harp on that point, over and over. Reeves's mission, and that of advertising as a whole, was simply to "get a message into the heads of as many people as possible at the lowest possible cost."
Rosser Reeves introduced and explained the USP theory in his book **REALITY IN ADVERTISING**, 1961.

p. 46: The impact of an ad, [Bernbach] reasoned, "is a direct result of how fresh and original it is, because you react strongly to something you've never seen or heard before."
Interview between Richard Coyne and Bill Bernback, 1971. Republished in **COMMUNICATION ARTS**, March/April 1999.

pp. 46–49: Bernbach felt that "if two good people get together, an art director and a copywriter, sometimes you don't know who's writing the copy and who's doing the art because you get excited about the thought—which is the important thing."
Ibid.

p. 49: "Listen to the ideas percolating up from your unconscious," Bernbach advised his creative troops.
From **THE MIRROR MAKERS**, by Stephen Fox, 1984.

p. 50: [The Levy's ads] "helped people feel comfortable with America's ethnic diversity in a way that any number of human relations commissions could not," wrote the journalist Michael Kinsley.
HARPER'S, Jan. 1983.

p. 50: "Bernbach took the exclamation point out of advertising," Krone would later remark, "and I put in the period."
From my interview with Marty Cooke, biographer of Helmut Krone.

p. 59: "You would have to look to Toulouse Lautrec's posters to find another artist with as wide an influence on the printed advertising message," she says.
Phyllis Robinson tribute to Bob Gage, in **ONE. A MAGAZINE**, Vol. 4, Issue 1, 2000.

p. 59: At the time, says Roy Grace, "A funeral was the worst thing you could have in a commercial—and that's why it was so right."
ENTERTAINMENT WEEKLY, special issue, "Fab 400 TV," 1999.

p. 67: "My attitude," he later explained to a journalist, "was that I could wait for Ford."
From Craig Reiss's profile of Ed McCabe in **SMART** magazine, Oct. 1990.

p. 73: The author Thomas Frank has noted that the writers and artists driving the Creative Revolution were truly part of the 1960s spirit of the counterculture; they may have worked within the "establishment" of Madison Avenue, but they were also trying their best to overthrow that old bureaucracy and its conservative ways.
From **THE CONQUEST OF COOL**, by Thomas Frank, 1997.

p. 73: According to McCabe, "We wanted to be able to tell our family and friends that we were in advertising, and when we told them [which ads] we were doing, watch the disdain on their faces melt into something almost like admiration."
ONE. A MAGAZINE, Vol. 1, Issue 2, 1997.

p. 73: "The cocktail circuit buzz found television commercials, for the first time, more compelling than the programs," observed one publication, and advertising's creative stars "were favored guests of talk show hosts . . . and their entrances at the rococo photographer's parties of the 1960s set off a stir the way hot young fashion designers do in trendy nightclubs today."
Ron Gales, "Where have the ad giants gone?," **ACROSS THE BOARD**, June 1993.

p. 81: Harper's magazine was one of the few to observe this at the time, noting that Bernbach "probably had a greater impact on American culture than any of the distinguished writers and artists who have appeared in the pages of Harper's during the past 133 years."
HARPER'S, Jan. 1983.

CHAPTER 3

p. 87: As TBWA/Chiat/Day executive Bob Kuperman noted, "With more product parity, the differences and unique benefits became increasingly slight, and more easily copied by competitors that didn't have one of their own."
ONE. A MAGAZINE, Vol. 1, Issue 3, 1998.

p. 93: The co-creator Geoff Hayes came up with the idea at home one evening, while watching an episode of the television show The Honeymooners.
ADWEEK, "20th Anniversary Issue," Nov. 9, 1998.

p. 115: Hegarty says the language-driven advertising that has been popular in the UK "obviously becomes a problem if you're going to talk to lots of people in different countries. Consequently, we now have to think of advertising as being more driven by the image. This doesn't mean you can't use words—only that you have to think about the words you're using in a different way."
ONE. A MAGAZINE, Vol. 3, Issue 2, 1999.

CHAPTER 4

p. 124: "Most of my stuff wouldn't be funny on the page," Sedelmaier acknowledged.
BACK STAGE, Sept. 15, 1989.

p. 125: "There is no time to build character in a commercial," the director told Adweek, "so you have to find characters."
ADWEEK, "20th Anniversary Issue," Nov. 9, 1998.

p. 125: (Esquire magazine dubbed Steve Horn "The Thirty Second David Lean").
ESQUIRE, August 1983.

p. 132: ("I use fear and intimidation," said Pytka of his approach to dealing with clients. "It works for the Catholic Church, and it works for me.")
ONE. A MAGAZINE, Vol. 3, Issue 1, 1999.

p. 132: Dektor would ask actors to improvise, and, as Adweek magazine noted, he relied on non-intrusive film techniques, such as long-lensed cameras.
ADWEEK, Nov. 9, 1998.

p. 132: "I watch them and I feel like I'm in a nuthouse or something," Sedelmaier commented. "It's like the guy running the camera is on something."
THE LOS ANGELES TIMES, Dec. 20, 1987.